Textbook of
Running Medicine

Textbook of Running Medicine

Francis G. O'Connor, MD FACSM
Assistant Professor of Family Medicine
Director of Primary Care Sports Medicine Fellowship
Uniformed Services University of the Health Sciences
F. Edward Herbert School of Medicine
Bethesda, MD

Robert P. Wilder, MD FACSM
Assistant Professor of Physical Medicine and Rehabilitation
Director Division of spine and Sports Care
Medical Director, The Runner's Clinic at UVa
University of Virginia
Charlottesville, VA

Surgical Section Editor:

Robert Nirschl, MD, MS
Director, Orthopedic Sports Medicine Fellowship
Nirschl Orthopedic Clinic/Arlington Hospital Arlington Virginia
Clinical Professor Orthopedic Surgery Georgetown U. Medical Center
Washington, DC

McGraw-Hill
Medical Publishing Division

New York Chicago San Francisco Lisbon London Madrid Mexico City
Milan New Delhi San Juan Seoul Singapore Sydney Toronto

McGraw-Hill

*A Division of The **McGraw·Hill** Companies*

Textbook of Running Medicine

1234567890 CCICCI 09876543210

ISBN 0-07-135997-X

This book was set in Palatino by TechBooks.
The editors were Darlene Cooke, Susan Noujaim and Regina Brown.
The production supervisor was Catherine H. Saggese.
The cover designer was Mary McKeon.
The index was prepared by Jerry Ralya.
Courier Kendallville was the printer and binder.

This book is printed on acid-free paper.

Catalog-in-Publication Data is on file for this title at the Library of Congress.

This book is dedicated to our families;
our wives, Janet and Susan, and our children, Ryan, Sean
Brendan, Lauren, Stephen, Ryan and Caroline
for their support and patience through this
"ultramarathon" effort

Contents

Preface

Since the running boom of the 1970's, track and field and distance running has enjoyed an ever increasing participation. This has created the necessity for sports clinicians who understand the specific demands of the sport and the injuries and medical conditions commonly associated with running. This need has also resulted in the development of specific running injury and sportsmedicine clinics such as the ones we have at The University of Virginia and DeWitt Army Community Hospital. Physicians treating runners realize that running injuries can be challenging conditions to evaluate and treat. Most often related to overuse, running injuries are often associated with a host of intrinsic and extrinsic factors which must be addressed in addition to the presenting injury itself. Runners also present with certain common medical problems which require specific management and clear guidelines for participation. The satisfaction of assisting a runner back to activity, be it to a recreational level or elite competition, is very rewarding.

As physicians with a special, personal interest in running, we desired to compile a source that would serve as a definitive reference for all clinicians—physicians, podiatrists, chiropractors, therapists, trainers, and nutritionists who treat runners. Our first goal was to recruit a list of internationally known authors with special interest and expertise in various areas of running medicine. The response was overwhelmingly favorable.

The text is divided into seven major sections. Section I, General Considerations, reviews epidemiology, biomechanics, principles of training, and histopathology of overuse tendinosis. Section II reviews available clinical and ancillary methods for evaluating injuries and medical conditions in runners. Section III details etiology, presentation, and management of common running injuries. Section IV discusses the diagnosis and management of medical problems. Section V reviews special considerations of unique running populations inlcuding pediatric, geriatric, female, and disabled runners and ultramarathon runners as well as nutrition and the organization of a race medical team. Section VI details the principles of rehabilitation. Section VII details specific indications and techniques for surgical intervention of selected running injuries.

We thank all the contributors for assisting in compiling this text.

Acknowledgements

We wish to acknowledge our mentors, both in running and in medicine, who have encouraged and inspired us to this project: David Brennan, Marion Dell, MD, Richard Edlich, MD, Bill Guerrant, Thom Lacie, Mark Lorenzoni, Tom McNichol, Pat Miller, Robert Nirschl, MD, Ralph Oriscello, MD, Steve Price, and Barry Smith, MD.

Special thanks is extended to Susan Noujaim of McGraw-Hill for her tireless work as a publisher, and to Robert P. Nirschl MD, who as our fellowship director and as our mentor continues to encourage us in word and in example.

Contributors

William B. Adams, MD
Primary Care Sports Medicine
Naval Medical Clinic Annapolis
United States Naval Academy
Annapolis, MD

Venu Akuthota, MD
Clinical Instructor
Department of Physical Medicine
and Rehabilitation
Northwestern University Medical School
Chicago, IL

Keith S. Albertson, MD, LTC, MC, USA
Chief, Orthopaedic Surgery Service
DeWitt Army Community Hospital
Fort Belvoir, VA

Thomas Allen, MD
Assistant Chief of Nuclear Medicine
Department of Radiology
Walter Reed Army Medical Center
Washington, DC

Eduardo Amy, MD
Co-Director, Sports Injuries Unit
Center for Sports Health and Exercise Sciences
Puerto Rico Olympic Training Center
San Juan, PR

Michael Andary, MD
Associate Professor
Michigan State University
College of Osteopathic Medicine
Department of Physical Medicine and Rehabilitation
East Lansing, MI

William J. Barrish, MD
Clinical Instructor, Physical Medicine
& Rehabilitation
Fellow, Spine & Sports Care
University of Virginia
Charlottesville, VA

Jeffrey R. Basford, MD, PhD
Associate Professor
Department of Physical Medicine
& Rehabilitation
Mayo Clinic and Mayo Foundation
Rochester, MN

LTC Kenneth B. Batts
Department of Primary Care
Womack Army Medical Center
Fort Bragg, NC

Kim L. Bennell, B App Sci, PhD
School of Physiotherapy, Faculty of Medicine, Dentistry,
and Health Sciences
University of Melbourne
Melbourne, Australia

Richard B. Birrer, MD, FAAP, FACSM
Professor of Family Medicine
SUNY Health Science Center Brooklyn
Professor of Medicine
Cornell University
Senior Vice President and CMO
St. Joseph's Hospital Medical Center
Patterson, New Jersey

Barry P. Boden, MD
Adjunct Assistant Professor
Uniformed Services University of the Healthy
Sciences
The Orthopaedic Center
Rockville, MD

David K. Brennan, MS
President, Houston International Running Center
Houston, TX

Fred H. Brennan, DO, FAOSM, FAAP
Head Team Physician, Methodist College
Director, Primary Care Sports Medicine
Womack Army Medical Center
Fort Bragg, North Carolina

Fred H. Brennan, Jr., DO, FAOASM, FAAFP
Primary Care Sports Medicine Director
Dewitt Army Community Hospital
Fort Belvoir, VA

Peter D. Brukner, MBBS, FACSP, FACSM
Olympic Park Sports Medicine Center
Melbourne, Australia

David Brown, MD
Clinical Assistant Professor of Family Medicine
Uniformed Services University
Staff Family Physician
Dewitt Army Community Hospital Residency
Fort Belvoir, VA

Cary Bucko, PT
Director, The Spine Center
Overlake Hospital Medical Center
Bellevue, WA

Janus D. Butcher, MD
Associate Clinical Professor of Family Practice
University of Minnesota-Duluth School of Medicine
Staff Physician, Sports Medicine
Duluth, MN

Steven Buzermanis, DPM
Chief Resident, Podiatric Surgery
Catholic Medical Centers of Brooklyn and Queens
Jamaica, NY

Larry H. Chou, MD
Assistant Professor
Department of Rehabilitation Medicine
University of Pennsylvania
School of Medicine
Philadelphia, PA

MAJ Eric M. Chumbley, MD
59th Aerospace Medicine Squadron
Flight Medicine Clinic
Lackland AFB, TX

John C. Cianca, MD
Assistant Professor of Physical Medicine & Rehabilitation
Baylor College of Medicine
Medical Director, TIRR Human Performance Center
Medical Director, Compaq Houston Marathon
Houston, TX

C. Randall Clinch, MD
Assistant Professor of Family Medicine
Director, Division of Predoctoral Programs
Department of Family Medicine
Uniformed Services University
Bethesda, MD

Andrew J. Cole, MD, FACSM
Northwest Spine and Sports Physicians, PC
Bellevue, WA
Clinical Assistant Professor

Dept of Rehabilitation Medicine
University of Washington
Seattle, WA

Diane L. Dahm, MD
Assistant Professor
Mayo Clinic Medical School
Rochester, MN

Gregory G. Dammann, MD
CPT, MC, USA
Chief Resident in Family Medicine
DeWitt Army Family Medicine Program
Fort Belvoir, VA

W. Scott Deitche
Family Physician
Guthrie Ambulatory Health Care Clinic
Fort Drum, NY

Michael DellaCorte, DPM, FACFAS
Director of Podiatry
Mary Immaculate Hospital Division
Jamaica, NY

Patricia A. Deuster, PhD, MPH
Professor and Director of Human Performance
    Laboratory
Department of Military and Emergency Medicine
Uniformed Services University of the
    Health Sciences
Bethesda, MD

Nancy M. DiMarco, PhD RD
Department of Nutrition and Food Sciences
Texas Women's University
Denton, TX

Ted Epperly, MD
Deputy Commander for Clinical Services
Eisenhower Army Medical Center
Fort Gordon, GA

Gregory P. Ernst, PhD, PT, SCS, ATC
CDR. Assistant Professor
US Army-Baylor University Graduate Physical
    Therapy Program
Fort Sam Houston, TX

Karl B. Fields, MD
Director of the Family Practice Residency and Sports
    Medicine Fellowship
Moses Cone Hospital/Greensboro AHEC
Greensboro, NC

Catherine M. Fieseler, MD
Staff Physician Depts of Orthopaedic Surgery
    and Family Medicine
Cleveland Clinic Foundation
Cleveland, OH
Primary Care Physician for WNBA
    Cleveland Rockers

Scott D. Flinn, MD
CDR, Medical Corps. US Navy
Branch Medical Clinic Parris Island, Bldg. 669
Parris Island, SC

Michael Fredericson, MD
Assistant Professor of PM&R
Stanford University School of Medicine
Team Physician, Stanford Cross-Country & Track Teams
Department of Functional Restoration
Division of Physical Medicine & Rehabilitation
Stanford University Medical Center
Stanford, CA

George F. Fuller, MD
White House Physician
Clinical Assistant Professor of Family Medicine
Uniformed Services University of the Health Sciences
Bethesda, MD

Patrick J. Grisalfi, DPM, FACFAS
Chairman, Dept. of Podiatry
St. Vincent's Catholic Medical Center
New York, NY

John E. Glorioso, Jr., MD
Director, Primary Care Sports Medicine
Department of Family Practice and Emergency
    Medical Services
Tripler Army Medical Center, Hawaii
Honolulu, HI

Jonathan S. Halperin, MD
Department of Orthopaedics and Rehabilitation
UC San Diego School of Medicine
Sharp Rees Stealy Medical Group
La Mesa, CA

Brian Hoke, PT, SCS
Atlantic Physical Therapy
Virgina Beach, VA

Debra Horn, MS
Houston, Texas

Thomas M. Howard, MD
COL, MC, USA
Chief, Family Practice and Assistant Fellowship
    Director, Primary Care Sports Medicine
DeWitt Army Community Hospital Fort Belvoir,
    Virginia
Assistant Professor of Family Medicine
Uniformed Services University of the Health Sciences
    School of Medicine
Bethesda, Maryland

Inku Hwang, MD
Nuclear Medicine Staff
Department of Radiology
Walter Reed Army Medical Center
Washington, DC

Arlon H. Jahnke Jr., MD
Augusta Orthopaedic Specialists
Sports Medicine
Augusta, GA

Carlos E. Jiménez, MD
Deputy Commander, Rodriguez
Army Health Clinic
Ft. Buchanan, PR

John A. Johnson, MD
Department of Family Practice
Womack Army Medical Center
Fort Bragg, NC

MAJ Michael W. Johnson
Director, Primary Care Sports Medicine
Department of Family Practice
Madigan Army Medical Center
Tacoma, WA

Karim Khan, MD, PhD
School of Human Kinetics
University of British Columbia
Vancouver, Canada

Joseph Kosinski, MD
Family Physician
Fort Campbell, KY

Barry S. Kraushaar, MD
President Advanced Orthopedics and Sports Medicine
Spring Valley, New York

John P. Kugler, MD
Uniformed Services University of the
    Health Sciences
Fredricksburg, VA

Wade A. Lillegard, MD
Clinical Assistant Professor, University of
    Minnesota-Duluth
Co-Director, Sports Medicine
Department of Orthopedics
St. Mary's/Duluth Clinic
Duluth, Minnesota

Frederick G. Lippert III, MD
Professor of Surgery
Uniformed Services University of the Health Sciences
Department of Orthopaedics
National Naval Medical Center
Bethesda, MD

Bryant R. Martin, MS
Department of Military and Emergency Medicine
USUHS, School of Medicine
Bethesda, MD

Mark T. Messenger, DPM
Thompson Podiatry
Thompson, GA

John P. Metz, MD
Primary Care Sports Medicine Fellow
DeWitt Army Community Hospital
Fort Belvoir, Virginia

William Micheo, MD
Chairman, Department of Physical Medicine,
    Rehabilitation, and Sports Medicine
University of Puerto Rico
Co-Director, Sports Injuries Unit
Center for Sports Health and Exercise Sciences
Puerto Rico Olympic Training Center
San Juan, PR

Josef H. Moore, PhD, PT, ATC, SCS
LTC Director, Sports Medicine-Physical
    Therapy Residency
Chief, Physical Therapy
Keller Army Community Hospital
United States Military Academy
West Point, NY

Bradley J. Nelson, MD
Chief, Sports Medicine
Orthopaedic Surgery Service
Dwight D. Eisenhower Army Medical Center
Fort Gordon, GA

Robert P. Nirschl, MD, MS
Director, Orthopedic Sports Medicine Fellowship
Nirschl Orthopedic Clinic/Arlington Hospital
    Arlington Virginia
Clinical Professor Orthopedic Surgery Georgetown
    U. Medical Center
Washington, DC

Koji D. Nishimura, MD
Director, Sports Medicine Clinic
Department of Family Medicine
DeWitt Army Community Hospital
Fort Belvoir, VA

Francis G. O'Connor, MD FACSM
Assistant Professor of Family Medicine
Director of Primary Care Sports Medicine Fellowship
Uniformed Services University of the Health Sciences
F. Edward Herbert School of Medicine
Bethesda, MD

Ralph G. Oriscello, MD
Associate Prof Medicine
Selvn Hall University
Prof Grad Medical School
Director, Critical Care Medicine
Trinitus Hospital
Elizabeth, NJ

Paul F. Pasquina, MD
Assistant Professor of Neurology
Program Director Uniformed
    Services University

Department of Physical Medicine & Rehabilitation
Walter Reed Army Medical Center
Washington, DC

Joel Press, MD FACSM
Associate Professor
Department of Physical Medicine
    & Rehabilitation
Northwestern University Medical Center
Director, Center for Spine, Sports, and
    Occupational Rehabilitation
Rehabilitation Institute of Chicago
Chicago, IL

Carlos Rivera-Tavares, MD
Physical Medicine and Rehabilitation
University of Puerto Rico
San Juan, PR

William O. Roberts, MD, MS, FACSM
Clinical Associate Professor of Family Medicine
Department of Family Practice and
    Community Health
University of Minnesotta Medical School
Medical Director, Twin Cities Marathon
Minn Health Family Physicians
White Bear Lake, MN

Christopher S. Robinson, PhD
Department of Family Medicine
Uniformed Services University of the
    Health Sciences

Carolyn M. Ruan
Northwest Spine and Sports Physicians, PC
Bellevue, WA

Matthew Samuels, MS, RD
Corinth, Texas

Marcy Schlinger, DO
Assistant Professor
Michigan State University
College of Osteopathic Medicine
Department of Physical Medicine
    and Rehabilitation
East Lansing, MI

Steve Simons, MD
Sports Medicine Institute
St. Joseph's Regional Medical Center
South Bend, IN

Jay Smith, MD
Assistant Professor
Mayo Clinic Medical School
Rochester, MN

David A. Soto-Quijano, MD
Physical Medicine and Rehabilitation
University of Puerto Rico
San Juan, PR

Seth John Stankus, DO
Chief, Neurology
Eisenhoner Army Medical Center
Augusta, GA

Steven I. Subotnick, DPM, ND, DC
Family Health Center Building
San Leandro, CA
Diplomate, American Board of Pediatric Surgery
Fellow, American College of Foot Surgery

LTC Dean C. Taylor, MD
Orthopaedic Surgery Service
Keller Army Hospital
West Point, NY 10996

Andrew W. Torrance, MD
Director of Primary Care Sports Medicine
Family Practice Residency
Dwight D. Eisenhower Army Medical Center
Ft. Gordon, GA

Robert H. Vaughan, PhD
Chairman of Training Theory
Division of Coaching Education for USA
    Track & Field
Baylor/Tom Landry Sports Medicine
    Research Center
Dallas, TX

Joseph A. Volpe
Texas Sports Medicine
Austin, TX

Russel D. White, MD
Associate Director, Family Medicine Residency
Director, Sports Medicine Fellowship
Bayfront Medical Center
St. Petersburg, Florida
Clinical Associate Professor
Department of Family Medicine
University of South Florida College of Medicine
Tampa, FL

John H. Wilckens, MD
Orthopaedic Sports Medicine and Team Physician
United States Naval Academy
Annapolis, MD

Robert P. Wilder, MD, FACSM
Assistant Professor, Physical Medicine & Rehabilitation
Director, Division of Spine & Sports Care
Medical Director, The Runner's Clinic at UVa
University of Virginia
Charlottesville, VA

MAJ Mark S. Williams
Director, Primary Care Sports Medicine
Department of Family Practice and Community Medicine
Martin Army Community Hospital
Fort Benning, GA

Stuart E. Willick, MD
Assistant Professor
Department of Physical Medicine and rehabilitation
University of Utah
Salt Lake City, UT

A Tribute to Dr. George Sheehan

George Sheehan always traveled as a runner. We were scheduled to appear on the David Susskind Show, a nationally televised discussion program, to debate the value of exercise with the author of "The Exercise Myth", Dr. Norman Solomon. George arrived in blue jeans, running shoes and a turtleneck sweater. In his gym bag were rolled-up khakis, a rolled-up blue button-down shirt and a rolled-up blue blazer. After "dressing", George asked if anyone had an extra tie. He appeared without a tie.

George was a cardiologist in the era before coronary angiography, bypass grafting, angioplasty, ablative therapy, cardiac transplantation, cardiac ultrasound, and nuclear scanning. He was trained in taking a history, doing a physical exam, interpreting an electrocardiogram, reading a chest X-ray, and evaluating barium swallows for atrial size in those with rheumatic heart disease and mitral stenosis. He recognized his limitations.

I am convinced that if I had not beaten him in a race more than 20 years ago, we would never have become friends. It was at the end of a 10K race in Cranford, N.J., the Fall Classic. In front of me was a grunting, moaning, shirtless, gray-haired man 20 years my senior nearing the finish line in less than 41 minutes. I thought he would cross the line and die. I crossed the line about 50 meters in front, turning in anticipation of catching a collapsing man in my arms. He brushed past me paying me no mind. I asked if he needed help, explaining I was a cardiologist. He said he needed none, this was how he always finished a race (later confirmed by many who ran with him), and he, too, was a cardiologist—still with no name. In the cool down after the race he approached me, extending his hand for the first time, introducing himself. It was the beginning of one of the most rewarding personal and professional relationships of my career.

"The marathon, you see, is my benchmark. It is the status symbol in my community, the running community. It is my credibility factor, not only for others but for myself as well. My marathon time is in fact my most valued possession. By it, I can establish my value as a runner, and each year I raise or lower that value according to what I do in the Boston Marathon".[1] This was written shortly after the 1979 Boston Marathon, a race he completed in 3:15. He felt it was the best race he could run that day.

He was asked by a spectator after the race: "Who are you?" "Just a runner," he replied.

He was in reality at least two people, the racing person to the public and a more humble realist to his friends. He believed that a marathon was stress enough and that extraneous conditions did not have to be added. There was strength. Then there was sanity.

Before I knew of his sanity, I knew of his strength. I saw George at the beginning of the 1981 Jersey Shore Marathon on a horrific weather day, the wind-chill factor along the Atlantic Ocean being in the low teens-high single digit numbers. The wind was so severe that at the 20 mile mark it lifted the leader in the air, smashed him against a car, broke his wrist, causing him to withdraw.

At the end of the race I could not find George. I was embarrassed, feeling my time was so poor that he had finished, cooled down and left. I wrote to him telling him I was about to fold at 20 miles but prayed to God for strength similar to what he had given George in the past. Several days later I received his response:

"My prayers were answered at 20 miles. The Lord heard me and sent help. Not strength, but sanity. I quit right then and there.

Nevertheless, congratulations. A fine effort on a terrible day. It was a heartless combination of elements that destroyed abler runners than either of us. I think the marathon is a once or twice a year venture and then only when all conditions are favorable. The 26.2 miles is test enough. No need to add any additional stress."

Christopher Columbus, Neil Armstrong, Jonas Salk, and others are considered pioneers. George Sheehan was a pioneer in motivating and mobilizing people, of great and of limited athletic ability, to run in order to improve their perception of life. He was instrumental

---

[1] Sheehan, George. *This Running Life.* Simon and Schuster. 1980.

in fostering good habits to improve health, both physical and mental. He knew that the gain in life expectancy might be small but the improvement in the quality of life would be so great as to be immeasurable.

This book is designed to treat and prevent problems that tend to limit people's running. It is designed to keep us physically and mentally fit for our own personal pleasure and for keeping us desirable company for those burdened by being members of our families. The less agony and the more ecstasy running produces the more pleasure we give ourselves and others.

Ralph G. Oriscello, M.D., F.A.C.C., F.A.C.P.

Foreword

Timothy Noakes

It is appropriate that the cover of this important book should feature the late Dr George Sheehan, the Red Bank, New Jersey physician who pioneered the modern, post-1970's understanding of the runner's medical problems. For it was Sheehan who, shortly after the 1968 Olympic Games, began to write a weekly column on the running life. His weekly columns became the diaries of his life and the source of the 7 books he authored. At first his interest was in the orthopaedic and medical problems he encountered both in himself and in those pioneering runners who consulted him. Later he turned to the philosophical and begat a literary legacy that may never be matched.

Sheehan's first book, The Encyclopaedia of Athletic Medicine (Runners World Publication, Mountain View, CA), was published in 1972. It ran to a modest 96 pages and included sections on the causes and prevention of running injuries, a description of the common running injuries, medical problems and care, and environmental issues. For many of us, it was our first textbook of running medicine. How quaint and outdated that book now seems. Yet its opening sentence captured Sheehan's greatest legacy and his eternal message: "The athlete has brought a new dimension to medicine Health."

How Sheehan would have loved to read The Complete Book of Running Medicine, published 29 years after his more grandly titled Encyclopaedia, and 9 years after his own untimely death. How he would have marvelled at the growth of knowledge in the discipline that he, in so many ways, pioneered. Mostly he would have been struck by the passion that exudes from its pages—the passion of the true experts. So those who are passionately interested in the runners' problems, often because they have themselves experienced the same conditions and all the frustrations that injury or a medical condition means to a runner.

For just as Sheehan's books arose from his desire to bring novel medical ideas directly to the runners, so too the origins of this book stem from the concerns of its authors that now is the time also for all the runner's caregivers to have access to the best information, necessary to provide an optimum care.

So the authors conclude that many of the books that are currently available were written for the entire running community, not for the more specialized needs of those professional caregivers who daily minister to the growing tribe of runners. In addition, those books usually focus either on injuries or medical problems, but seldom on both in appropriate detail. Normally they take the self-help approach to care whereas health professionals need to know all the possible treatment options. The need for a new book is even more urgent given that the knowledge and wisdom in this discipline have increased exponentially in the last decade. Thus the authors conceived the opportunity to create THE text that the clinician can consult for almost any problem with which a runner of whatever ability might present.

In selecting their authors, the editors have chosen those clinicians who see many patients including many runners in busy clinics and who have had to find the practical answers to both the simple and the complex problems with which their runners present. Their choice of topic has been equally meticulous and the 7 sections cover the runner's medical problems in quite remarkable detail. The writing of these experts is concise and practically relevant.

So the editors have succeeded admirably in their goal. They have produced a book of the highest quality, covering the discipline in the appropriate practical detail. Here indeed is the one-stop textbook that the care provider can access in order to elucidate the runner's problems, their causes and their cures.

I am sure that George Sheehan would agree. It is time for even his most ardent fans to retire their oldest classic—the Encyclopaedia of Athletic Medicine. May its most worthy successor—Textbook of Running Medicine—prove to be equally as successful, educational and inspirational.

Part I

GENERAL CONSIDERATIONS

Chapter 1

EPIDEMIOLOGY OF RUNNING INJURIES

Ted Epperly and Karl B. Fields

INTRODUCTION

Running is rapidly becoming one of the most popular leisure sports in America. It is estimated that there are over 30 million runners of which more than 10 million run on more than 100 days per year, and about 1 million enter competitive races per year.[1-3] Part of the growing popularity of running is its easy accessibility and health benefits. All that is needed is a good pair of running shoes, a relatively safe training surface, and the strength of will and discipline to make running part of one's behavior. The benefits of running include improved health, pleasure, relaxation, competition, fitness, stress reduction, and pride of personal performance. Reductions in cardiovascular morbidity and mortality as well as coronary artery disease have been documented with the expenditure of 1400 kcal to 2200 kcal/week.[4]

Running injuries can be defined in a number of ways and their treatment suffers from the lack of a single consistent set of defining parameters. The literature variously defines a running injury to have occurred when it is severe enough to reduce the number of miles run and causes the runner to take a medication or see a health care professional.[5] Others define a running injury as "any injury that markedly hampers training or competition for at least 1 week."[6] With this degree of variability in case definition, the incidence of injuries secondary to running is difficult to quantify exactly. When the literature is examined to determine the incidence of running injuries, in studies of 500 or more participants the yearly incidence rate ranges from 37% to 56%.[1,5] To better understand this incidence rate in relationship to exposure in days or hours, the calculation of injury incidence is expressed in terms of injuries per 1000 hours of running, and this injury rate ranges from 2.5 to 5.8 injuries per 1000 hours of running.[1,6] The lower rate of 2.5 per 1000 hours is seen in long-distance and marathon runners. Sprinters have the highest rate of 5.8 per 1000 hours, and middle-distance runners are between the two at 5.6 per 1000 hours.[6] Despite the relatively high incidence rate of running injuries per runner per year, this incidence rate is still 2 to 6 times lower than in all other sports.[1]

Runners will reduce or cease their training in about 30% to 90% of all injuries, will seek medical care in about 20% to 70% of all injuries, and will miss work in about 0% to 5% of running-related injuries.[1] With nearly 70% of runners seeking medical care or advice on their injuries, it behooves family physicians and all others that engage in primary care sports medicine to have a good understanding of risk factors, common injury sites, common injury types, and appropriate treatment and prevention strategies.

TABLE 1–1. TOP 14 RUNNING INJURIES

Diagnosis	n	Percent
Patellofemoral pain syndrome	568	32.2
Tibial stress syndrome "shin splints"	306	17.3
Achilles tendinitis	128	7.2
Stress fractures	127	7.2
Plantar fasciitis	119	6.7
Iliotibial band syndrome	111	6.3
Patellar tendinitis	100	5.7
Metatarsal stress syndrome	58	3.3
Adductor strain	52	3.0
Hamstring strain	45	2.6
Posterior tibial tendinitis	45	2.6
Ankle sprain	42	2.4
Peroneus tendinitis	34	1.9
Iliac apophysitis	29	1.6
Total	1764	100

Source: Adapted from Van Mechelen[1] and Ballas.[2]

COMMON INJURY SITES

Most running injuries are musculoskeletal overuse syndromes related to cumulative overload of the lower extremity. Of all running injuries, 70% to 80% occur from the knee down. Table 1–1 lists the 14 most commonly seen and treated running injuries. Of note, the knee is the most common site of injury and accounts for approximately 25% to 33% of all running-related problems. Figure 1–1 reveals the locations of the various running injuries.

The pattern of injury varies among different types of runners. Although there are no age- or gender-related differences, there are differences in injury pattern between sprinters, middle-distance runners, and long-distance runners. Hamstring strains and tendinitis are more commonly seen in sprinters, backache and hip problems are more commonly seen in middle-distance runners, and foot problems are more common among long-distance and marathon runners.[6]

Common minor injuries such as blisters, skin chafing, and muscle soreness are not considered here because they usually do not interfere with training, decrease number of miles run, or usually result in seeking treatment from a health care professional. Fortunately, running injuries are rarely associated with major medical problems such as trauma (ankle sprains, fractures), animal bites, environmental injuries (from cold or heat), or cardiovascular conditions (myocardial infarction, cerebrovascular accident, dehydration).

Thus, although all studies that review individuals coming to a particular clinic have an inherent selection bias based on its patient population, a fairly consistent

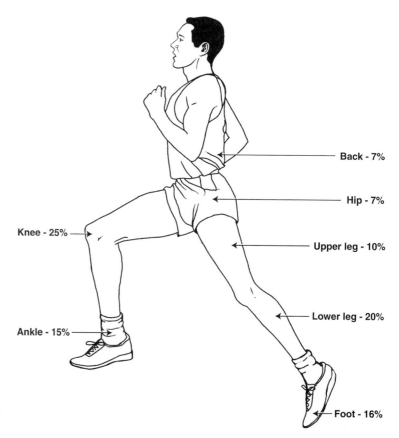

Figure 1–1. Sites of common running injuries.

distribution and occurrence rate of running injuries has been reported in the major studies published since 1974.

RISK FACTORS FOR RUNNING INJURIES

Multiple studies have analyzed the potential risk factors that contribute to running injuries.[1,3,5,6–12] These risk factors can be broadly separated into extrinsic factors (training errors, improper running surface, worn shoes, etc.) and intrinsic factors (flexibility, prior injury, malalignment, etc.). The two most important predictors for the overall risk of running injuries are training miles per week and a history of a previous running injury.[5,13] Increased risk starts at 19 miles per week and the relative risk for running injuries in runners averaging 40 miles or more per week is 2.88.[8,13] Both increased duration and increased frequency of running produces more injuries. Previous injury (in the preceding 12 months) carries a relative risk of injury of 1.51.[8]

There are several other factors that have been shown to put runners at some increased risk. Inexperienced runners (those that have been running less than 3 years) are at greater risk for injury. Errors in training such as running too often, too fast, and too long can increase injury rates. Highly motivated runners also are more predisposed to injuries. This is probably multifactorial and relates to more competitive training with harder and longer workouts, and the fact that more motivated runners tend to ignore the early symptoms of injuries, thus allowing the injury to worsen.[1]

There are several risk factors that have been studied and found to have equivocal, contradictory, or unclear evidence supporting a direct link with running injuries. These include flexibility (both hyperflexibility and hypoflexibility), malalignment problems, warm-up and stretching exercises before or after runs, running shoes, shoe orthotics, running on roadsides, height of runners, intensity of running type or speed (interval training or hill training), and time of day or season of run.[1,3,4]

Several studies clearly show no risk of running injuries in association with genu varum, genu valgus, high Q-angle, femoral neck anteversion, pelvic obliquity, knee and patella alignment, rear foot valgus, and leg length discrepancy.[1,8,9] A study done on male Army infantry trainees, however, found that the rate of overuse injury was higher with genu valgus (RR = 1.9), and that Q-angles more than 15° were significantly associated with stress fractures (RR = 5.4).[10] Warm-up and stretching exercises have not been shown to reduce the incidence of running injuries. In fact, there

TABLE 1–2. RISK FACTORS FOR RUNNING INJURIES

Important Risk Factors
Training miles per week
Previous running injury
Inexperienced runner
Training intensity
Equivocal Risk Factors
Hyper- or hypoflexibility
Stretching exercises
Running shoes
Shoe orthotics
Roadside running
Malalignment problems
Unrelated Risk Factors
Age
Gender
Body morphology
Running surface
Cross training
Time of day
Warm-up or cool-down periods

may be an increase in running injuries in runners that "sometimes, usually, or always stretch" compared with those that "never stretch."[1] Further studies are needed to sort out this conundrum. Running shoes have mixed data on their association with injury rates. Similarly, rear foot strikers versus mid-foot and forefoot strikers have no increased risk. Several observations, however, are worthy of consideration regarding running shoes. Running shoes that are wet lose their shock-absorbing ability and all shoes will lose about 30% to 50% of their shock-absorbing characteristics after 400 km of running.[1] Although there is no clear seasonal predilection to running injuries, one would expect that the spring and summer will see more injuries as dormant runners and increased competitive running occurs in many locales in these seasons.[5]

Risk factors that have *not* been associated with an increase in running-related injuries include age, gender, body mass index, running on hard surfaces, cross training in other sports, time of day, and cool-down procedures.[1,4] Table 1–2 summarizes risk factors that are important, equivocal, and unrelated to risk of running injuries.

COMMON INJURIES OF RUNNERS

Patellofemoral Stress Syndrome

The knee is generally the most common anatomic site of injury in runners, and they most often experience anterior knee pain. Pain originating around the patella typically results in a diagnosis of patellofemoral stress syndrome (PFSS). This entity encompasses a range of possible causes including inflammation of the tendons, joint capsule, plica, and bursae, or retropatellar cartilage. Most individuals do not demonstrate chondromalacia with pathologic changes in the cartilage. In skeletally immature athletes, osteochondroses such as Osgood-Schlatter or Sinding-Larsen-Johannson may be the cause of the symptoms.

Studies of running injuries include different types and age groups of runners, which influences injury distribution. Frequency of patellofemoral injury in some of the larger running studies follow:

Clement et al.[15]	25.8%
Brubaker and James[14]	14.7%
Lysholm and Wiklander[6]	~15%
Marti, et al.[16]	27.9%*
Ontario Cohort Study[5]	~27%*

(*Marti and co-workers and the Ontario cohort study merged all knee injuries into one category.)

PFSS frequency ranked higher in the study by Clement and colleagues and knee injuries in general were common in the Ontario Cohort and Marti studies. The Marti and Ontario studies looked at runners of all age groups and both genders participating in road races. Clement looked at all patients coming to a primary care sports medicine practice. In contrast, the studies by Brubaker and Lysholm looked at young competitive track racers. While PFSS still commonly occurred, the overall injury pattern differed between studies of young competitive runners and those examining a more general population.

Iliotibial Band Syndrome

Lateral knee pain typically arises near the lateral femoral condyle where the iliotibial band (ITB) may impinge while the knee is flexed from 28 to 32 degrees during weight bearing. This injury occurs at different running paces and causes sharp and sometimes incapacitating pain. In most studies the frequency of ITB problems is approximately half that of PFSS. The incidence of ITB injury in runners ranges from 1.6% to 12% in various reports.[17] In general, PFSS accounts for approximately 50% of runners' knee overuse problems, while ITB injury leads to 10% to 25%. The remaining knee injuries fall into a wide variety of categories. The frequency of ITB would be expected to vary between elite versus recreational runners. This is primarily because of the differing degree of knee flexion required for speed running and interval training as opposed to that of long, slow distance training. In the study by Clement et al., ITB caused only 4.3% of all injuries, because many of the patients were recreational athletes.[15] A few of the patients with ITB symptoms had a lateral meniscus injury or popliteal tendinitis.

Medial Tibial Stress Syndrome and Tibial Stress Fracture

A routine complaint of young runners is that of shin pain. Often labeled as "shin splints," most shin pain occurs medially and arises from a variety of causes. In the inexperienced runner the pain often results from tendinitis or inflammation of the posterior tibialis, flexor hallucis, flexor digitorum, or soleus muscle medially or the anterior tibialis and peroneal muscle groups in other areas of the shin. In the more experienced runner, medial tibial pain arises after overtraining and often represents a continuum, ranging from periosteal irritation to tibial stress fracture. Limited information exists about the frequency of this injury in high school athletes, but running studies give a general idea of the occurrence. James et al. reported "shin splints" in 13% of track runners visiting their office.[18] Brubaker and James found stress fractures in 15.6% of the runners in their study with 41.2% of these occurring in the tibia.[14] In a group of competitive runners, tibial stress syndrome accounted for 13.2% of injuries with confirmed tibial stress fracture in an additional 2.6%.[15] Similar numbers were seen in the Ontario Cohort Study.[5] Some of these runners probably have compartment syndromes, but the actual frequency of this entity remains difficult to assess without more common use of compartment pressure measurement.

Achilles Tendinitis

Analysis of a variety of studies of runners reveals that Achilles tendinitis occurs more often than any other tendon pathology, accounting for approximately 10% of all running injuries. The Achilles functions with the calf complex to provide the power in the push-off phase of the gait cycle. Most injury to the tendon occurs with eccentric contraction and the Achilles routinely undergoes forceful eccentric stress that is exaggerated by uphill running or sprinting. Aging is another factor that appears to play a major role in Achilles and calf pathology. The study by Marti et al.[16] best demonstrated this, in that Achilles and calf problems were the most common overuse injuries, with Achilles tendon injuries in 11.6% and calf injuries in 8.9% of their subjects. In runners over age 40, Achilles tendon and calf injuries ranked ahead of those of the knee or any other anatomic area.[16] Achilles tendinitis accounted for a major portion of the 11.6% of tendinitis patients seen by Brubaker and James[14] and for 14.9% of those seen by Clement et al.[15] Classically, Achilles tendinitis leads to inflammation of the tendon at the insertion to the calcaneus or several centimeters proximal to it. However, broad tendinous attachments higher in the calf may break down leading to rupture of the medial head of the gastrocnemius muscle.

Plantaris muscle rupture or strain of the soleus also cause calf pain.

Plantar Fasciitis

Heel pain troubles numerous runners. While the absolute frequency of the injury is unknown, reports suggest a range of 5% to 10% of all running injuries[19] (e.g., Clement et al.[15] noted it in 4.7% and James[18] in 7% of office visits). The long duration of symptoms means that prevalence is high; resolution of plantar fasciitis may require 12 months or longer in many athletes. Even therapy such as injections, night splints, or orthotics rarely results in relief of symptoms in less than 12 to 16 weeks. In rare situations calcaneal stress fracture, plantar nerve entrapment, or systemic disease may mimic plantar fasciitis.

The five conditions listed above (six for those who separate patellar tendinitis from PFSS) rank among the most common injuries, according to published studies of runners. Although the injuries that follow typically occur less frequently, factors such as use of spiked racing shoes, differing surfaces and training regimens, and overall mileage can influence the occurrence of particular problems.

Stress Fractures

Recent studies indicate that factors such as bone architecture may play a role in stress fracture equal to that of decreased bone mineral density. High mileage, hard training surfaces, excessive pronation, and poor shoe support are other contributors to higher injury frequency. In most studies, stress fractures cause in the range of 10% of the total number of injuries, and this rate is somewhat increased in highly competitive groups (15.6% were found in the Brubaker and James study[14]). Tibial stress fractures predominate, followed by those of the metatarsal, fibular, and tarsal bones. Navicular stress fractures account for 5% to 6% of stress fractures and can lead to nonunion and more serious injury. Less common stress fractures occur in the shaft of the femur, femoral neck, pubic rami, sacrum, sesamoid bones, and tibial plateau.

Groin Pain

Osteitis pubis causes pain in the groin, adductor compartment, and/or directly over the symphysis. Symptoms may persist for 12 months or longer.[20] Groin pain should trigger a differential diagnosis that includes osteoarthritis of the hip, avascular necrosis of the hip, femoral neck stress fracture, or tendinitis of the iliopsoas or other hip flexors. In pediatric athletes, considerations include Legg-Calvé-Perthes disease, slipped capital femoral epiphysis, and snapping hip syndrome. Rarely, malignancy or infection may mimic injury.

Metatarsalgia

Pain in the forefoot, usually proximal to the second metatarsal head, arises from strain or collapse of the transverse arch. Inflammation and bruising can cause severe pain even in the absence of a stress fracture. Freiberg's infarction or avascular necrosis of the second metatarsal head remains a concern, particularly in adolescents. Morton's neuroma also causes forefoot pain, but more often at the third metatarsal interspace.

Piriformis Syndrome

Pain in the buttocks often associated with sciatica typically arises from injury to the piriformis muscle or one of the other hip rotators. Spasm or scarring leads to a compression neuropathy of the sciatic nerve. The differential always requires consideration of lumbar disk disease, particularly since many older runners have a prior history of low back pain or disk injury. In the Ontario Cohort Study, 11% of runners reported back pain (5% as a new injury).[5]

Knee Pain With Swelling

While PFSS may occasionally cause a knee effusion, other differential diagnostic concerns include degenerative injury of the meniscus, degenerative joint disease, and rarely, intraarticular stress fracture. In young patients, osteochondritis dissecans is also a rare cause.

Hamstring Strain

For runners who participate in sprints, hurdles, or speed workouts, hamstring injury poses a substantial risk. The hamstring acts to check the forward translation of the knee of the lead leg during late swing phase and at foot strike of running gait.[21] Overstriding or a foot that slips can accentuate an already stressful eccentric contraction and cause a strain or a tear. Hamstring flexibility of runners is often poor and this may contribute to injury. The true incidence of this injury remains difficult to assess since the risk varies greatly with the type of training or competition, but hamstring injury accounted for 32.4% of all strains in one study[14] and 60% of upper leg strains in another.[15]

Traumatic Injury

Ankle sprains occur frequently in all running and jumping sports. Uneven surfaces such as those found in cross-country racing or trail running may contribute to increased risk. Estimates of 15% to 30% of running injuries appear high because of extrapolation from databases that include contact sports.[20] Nevertheless, this injury ranks as the most frequent traumatic occurrence in runners. In addition, a number of upper extremity fractures from falls and a variety of injuries including head trauma are reported in all large series of runners.

Tarsal Tunnel Syndrome

Excessive pronation may cause impingement of the tibial nerve in the tarsal tunnel. This condition has been recognized as a cause of plantar surface foot pain. However, running injuries can also affect a number of other nerve branches and the peroneal nerve.

UNCOMMON RUNNING INJURIES AND PROBLEMS

Sudden Cardiac Death

Sudden cardiac death occurs in approximately 1 in 250,000 young athletes (below the age of 30), but very few of these have been runners. In athletes over 30 years of age the risk appears closely related to the prevalence of coronary artery disease, with a small percentage relating to congenital heart problems. Estimates suggest approximately 1 death annually for each 7620 joggers (1 per every 396,000 hours of participation). This number falls to 1 per 15,240 runners if those with known coronary artery disease are excluded.[22,23]

The Physicians Health Study, a prospective case study, found that the absolute risk of sudden death during or immediately following vigorous exertion was 1 sudden death per 1.51 million episodes of exertion. Additionally, habitual vigorous exercise diminishes the risk of sudden death even further.[24]

Environmental Injury

Hot, humid conditions, extreme cold, and high air pollution levels all pose specific risks for outdoor running. Researchers observing the Peachtree Road Races, held the July 4th weekend in Atlanta, Georgia, found that during three of the hotter years, severe heat injury occurred in approximately 1 of every 1000 to 1500 competitors. Heat stroke guidelines released by The American College of Sports Medicine were developed in part because of the high number of heat injuries occurring at races held in periods of unacceptably high wet bulb temperature readings (in excess of 82°F or 28°C).[25]

Similarly, conditions that promote hypothermia raise the risk of serious injury. Winter sports obviously occur in temperature ranges that increase risk, but athletes in water sports and endurance events may also experience hypothermia in conditions that would generally be considered lower risk. Exhaustion with depletion of glycogen stores limits the ability of internal thermogenesis to balance heat loss. Chronic illness, older age, medication use, poor nutrition, and particularly alcohol use all may elevate risk.

Air pollution levels more often lead to asthma attacks, but also have led to postrace increased susceptibility to respiratory infections.

Rhabdomyolysis and Acute Renal Failure

Muscle breakdown from extreme exertion occurs more commonly in situations where runners are dehydrated or overheated.[26] Other factors such as recent infection, use of certain medications, and other systemic illnesses may contribute. Individuals with sickle cell trait appear to be at greater risk.[27] Severe cases can result in acute renal failure.

Exercise-Induced Anaphylaxis

The etiology of this condition remains elusive. However, atopic individuals perhaps with other cofactors such as ingestion of certain foods (e.g., seafood) may develop true anaphylaxis during exercise. The exact role of the running remains to be defined.

Hematuria

Numerous reports document the occurrence of hematuria following running. Incidence ranges from 17% to 69% in long-distance running, with the highest risk occurring in ultramarathons. Bladder contusion and aggravation of preexisting vascular malformations of the bladder wall are two suggested mechanisms. Adequate hydration appears to be protective.[26]

Gastrointestinal Bleeding

Positive occult blood stool tests occur in many runners after strenuous exertion. Irritation throughout the GI tract can be causal. Postrace endoscopic evaluation of marathon runners demonstrated gastric mucosal lesions consistent with local ischemia. The frequency of postrace bleeding has been reduced by the prophylactic use of cimetidine. NSAID use also may play a role in GI irritation in runners. While "cecal slap" or other traumatic irritation may cause microscopic bleeding, frank lower GI bleeding suggests the likelihood of an arteriovenous malformation of the colon or some other pathologic lesion that bleeds secondary to regional ischemia or trauma.[28]

Cardiac Arrhythmia

Irregular heartbeat occurs frequently in well-trained athletes. Some conditions such as atrial fibrillation have clinical significance, and for runners with structural heart disease arrhythmia might indicate worsening disease. Pantano and Oriel[22] studied well-trained runners and found premature ventricular contractions in 27% on treadmill testing but in 60% on monitored training runs. Higher-grade arrhythmias occurred on free running, with up to 25% having grade 2 or higher ventricular arrhythmia. They concluded that arrhythmias in runners do not necessarily imply pathologic conditions. Similar studies demonstrating marked bradycardia due to excessive vagal tone also suggest cautious interpretation of data before any finding of pathologic heart disease is made.

CONCLUSION

Running injuries severe enough to reduce or stop all training or cause the runner to seek medical care occur in approximately 37% to 56% of runners each year. These injuries are almost exclusively musculoskeletal overuse injuries, with 70% to 80% affecting the body from the knee down. The knee is the most commonly injured site, accounting for about 25% of all injuries.

Injury patterns and types have remained fairly constant over the last 25 years despite better education, training, and shoe design. The two most important risk factors for running injuries are the number of miles run per week and a history of a previous running injury. It is important for all physicians who deal with primary care sports medicine to understand the most common injury sites, types, and modifiable risk factors, in order to maximize and maintain your running patients' health.

REFERENCES

1. Van Mechelen W: Running injuries, A review of the epidemiological literature. *Sports Med* 1992:14, 320.
2. Ballas M, Tytko J, Cookson D: Common overuse running injuries: Diagnosis and management. *Am Fam Physician* 1997:55, 2473.
3. Jacobs S, Berson B: Injuries to runners: A study of entrants to a 10,000 meter race. *Am J Sports Med* 1986:14, 151.
4. Hambrecht R, Niebauer J, Marburger C: Various intensities of leisure time physical activity in patients with coronary artery disease: Effects on cardiorespiratory fitness and progression of coronary atherosclerotic lesions. *J Am Coll Cardiol* 1993:22, 468.
5. Walter S, Hart L, McIntosh J, Sutton J: The Ontario Cohort Study of running-related injuries. *Arch Intern Med* 1989:149, 2561.
6. Lysholm J, Wilkander J: Injuries in runners. *Am J Sports Med* 1987:15, 168.
7. Jones B, Cowan D, Tomlinson J, et al.: Epidemiology of injuries associated with physical training among young men in the army. *Am Coll Sports Med* 1993:25, 197.
8. Macera C, Pate R, Powell K, et al.: Predicting lower-extremity injuries among habitual runners. *Arch Intern Med* 1989:149, 2565.
9. Wen D, Puffer J, Schmalzried T: Lower extremity alignment and risk of overuse injuries in runners. *Am Coll Sports Med* 1997:29, 1291.
10. Wen, Puffer J, Schmalzried T: Injuries in runners: A prospective study of alignment. *Clin J Sport Med* 1998: 8, 187.
11. Cowan D, Jones B, Frykman P, et al.: Lower limb morphology and risk of overuse injury among male infantry trainees. *Am Coll Sports Med* 1996:28, 945.
12. Cowan D, Jones B, Robinson J: Foot morphologic characteristics and risk of exercise-related injury. *Arch Fam Med* 1993:2, 773.
13. Fredericson M: Common injuries in runners. Diagnosis, rehabilitation, and prevention. *Sports Med* 1996:21, 50.
14. Brubaker CE, James SL: Injuries to runners. *Sports Med* 1974:2, 189.
15. Clement DB Taunton JE, Smart GW, et al.: A survey of overuse running injuries. *Physician Sportsmed* 1981:9, 47.
16. Marti B, Vader JP, Minder CE, et al.: On the epidemiology of running injuries: The 1984 Bern Grand-Prix Study. *Am J Sports Med* 1988:16, 285.
17. Messier SP, Edwards DG, Martin DF, et al.: Etiology of iliotibial band friction syndrome in distance runners. *Med Sci Sports Exerc* 1995:27, 951.
18. James SL, Bates BT, Osternig LR: Injuries to runners. *Am J Sports Med* 1978:6, 40.
19. Kibler WB, Goldberg C, Chandler TJ: Functional biomechanical deficits in running athletes with plantar fasciitis. *Am J Sports Med* 1991:19, 66.
20. Fricker PA, Taunton JE, Ammon W: Osteitis pubis in athletes: Infection, inflammation or injury? *Sports Med* 1991:12, 266.
21. Stanton P, Purdam C: Hamstring injuries in sprinting—the role of eccentric exercise. *J Orthop Sports Phys Ther* 1989:March, 343.
22. Pantano JA, Oriel RJ: Prevalence and nature of cardiac arrhythmias in apparently normal well-trained runners. *Am Heart J* 1982:104, 762.
23. Rich BS: Sudden death screening. *Med Clin North Am* 1994:78, 267.
24. Albert CM, Mittleman MA, Chae CU, et al.: Triggering of Sudden Death from Cardiac Causes by Vigorous Exertion. *N Engl J Med* 2000:343, 1355.
25. Gambrell RC: Hyperthermia and heat-related illness, in Fields KB, Fricker PA (eds.), *Medical Problems in Athletes*, Blackwell, Malden, Mass, 1997:279.
26. Batt ME: Nephrology in sport, in Fields KB, Fricker PA (eds.), *Medical Problems in Athletes*, Blackwell, Malden, Mass, 1997:209.
27. Kark JA, Ward FT: Exercise and hemoglobin. *S Semin Hematol* 1994:31, 181.
28. Hughes, D: Gastroenterology and sport, in Fields KB, Fricker PA (eds.), *Medical Problems in Athletes*, Blackwell, Malden, Mass, 1997:151.

Chapter 2

BIOMECHANICS OF RUNNING

Richard B. Birrer, Steven Buzermanis,
Michael P. DellaCorte,
and Patrick J. Grisalfi

INTRODUCTION

Over the past few decades, much emphasis has been placed on physical fitness. This heightened awareness has led to an increase in walking, power walking, jogging, and running as a means of achieving fitness goals. Running has become an important aspect of exercise routines whether for aerobic training or recreational sport. This has also led to an increase in the number of acute traumatic injuries and chronic injuries caused by overuse or improper training. It has been estimated that between one fourth and one half of all runners sustain an injury that is severe enough to cause a change in practice or performance.[1] A better understanding of the intricate mechanisms of the lower extremity as the body propels itself forward is essential to understanding how to treat the pathologies that often arise.

The walking gait cycle can be likened to controlled falling. One limb is pushed ahead of the other as the body tries to catch up to itself. The major action is accomplished by the stance limb. During running, most of the forward force is provided by the swinging arm and leg rather than by the stance limb.[2] Much has been written about the biomechanics of human ambulation and the normal walking gait cycle. This chapter focuses on the biomechanics of running and its impact on the athlete.

THE WALKING GAIT CYCLE

The gait cycle is defined as the period from initial contact of one foot until initial contact of that same foot. It is divided into a stance phase and a swing phase. The stance phase begins with initial contact of the foot with the ground. The swing phase begins at toe-off (TO) of the limb that has just completed the stance phase.

During walking the stance phase occupies approximately 60% of the gait cycle. It is further divided into four periods, or subphases. The first subphase is loading response (LR). This begins after initial contact (IC) of the leg with the ground. It is the first time during the cycle that both feet are on the ground at the same time, known as double support. Double support occurs during the first and last segments of the stance phase. The next period is midstance (MS), which occurs when the foot makes full contact with the ground and is adapting to the external environment. This is also the beginning of single support. Single support of the stance limb is equal to the duration of the swing phase of the contralateral limb. Terminal stance (TST), which is the time when the foot is preparing to lift off, follows. The last subphase is preswing (PSW), which is the second instance during the walking gait cycle in which there is a period of double support.

The remaining 40% of the walking gait cycle is occupied by swing phase. The swing phase begins with the instantaneous event of TO and ends with IC.[3] The swing phase is further divided into three subphases. The first is initial swing (ISW), followed by midswing (MSW), and then completed with terminal swing (TSW).

THE RUNNING GAIT CYCLE

During running, the gait cycle is quite different. There is an approximate temporal reversal between the stance and swing phases. In running, the stance phase occupies only about 40% of the gait cycle. It is divided into two subphases, the first being absorption and the second propulsion. These are separated by MS. The swing phase now occupies most of the gait cycle for the remaining 60%. It is divided into ISW and TSW. ISW occupies the first 75% and TSW the last 25%. The point at which ISW becomes TSW is termed MSW.

Walking differs from running in that walking has two double support periods in stance, whereas running has two periods of double float in swing. Double float is the time during the gait cycle when neither limb is in contact with the floor. This occurs at the beginning and end of each running swing phase.

Some other terms that are useful in describing gait are stride length, step length, and cadence. Stride length is the distance from IC of one foot until IC of the contralateral foot. Step length is the distance from IC of one foot until IC of that same foot, or one complete gait cycle. Cadence is the number of steps in a given period of time. Winter[4] determined that average natural cadence ranged from 101 to 122 steps/min. In general, women have a natural cadence of between six and nine steps a minute higher than that of men.

As velocity increases, there is an initial increase in step lengths followed by increased cadence. Stride length is limited by an individual's limb length and height, as well as by individual ability. Increased stride length is associated with an increase in velocity.[5] Once optimum stride length is attained, further increases in velocity can occur only with increases in cadence.

As previously reported by Mann,[2] during the stance phase of walking the duration of the LR is equal to 15%, MS is equal to 15%, TST is equal to 15%, and PSW is equal to 15% of the gait cycle. ISW and TSW are equal to approximately 20% each. Changes in duration of the stance phase are therefore decreased as velocity increases. According to Mann and Hagy,[6] the stance phase is decreased from 62% in walking to 31% in running and 22% in sprinting.

KINEMATICS

Kinematics is a description of motion of joints or body segments that occurs independent of forces that cause that motion to occur. According to Oonpuu,[3] kinematics refers to the variables that describe the spatial movement between segments such as joint angular motion measured in degrees. The kinematics of walking differs greatly from that of running. Generally there is an increase in joint range of motion as velocity increases. However, there are no major differences between walking and running kinematics in the coronal and transverse planes. Most kinematic differences occur in the sagittal plane.[6] The body lowers its center of gravity (COG) with increased speed by increasing flexion at the hips and knees and by increased dorsiflexion at the ankle.[7]

The Hip

The hip demonstrates an overall increase in range of motion (ROM) as velocity increases. The most significant motion occurs in the sagittal plane. Most of this increase occurs in flexion, and the amount of extension actually decreases slightly. In a study by Oonpuu,[3] overall ROM was determined to be 43 degrees with maximum flexion and extension, measuring 37 and 6 degrees, respectively, for normal walking. In running, however, overall range of motion was increased to 46 degrees with the hip flexing and never quite returning past neutral into extension. Maximum hip extension occurs at TO and maximum flexion in TSW.[4] Coronal plane ROM in walking was determined to be 13 degrees, with maximum adduction and abduction measuring 6 degrees and 7 degrees, respectively. This increased slightly to 14 total degrees during running, with the extra degree coming from abduction. The pelvis begins the gait cycle with 8 degrees of external rotation at IC. Hip range of motion carries through to 8 degrees of internal rotation at TO.[6]

The Knee

As in the hip, the most significant motion occurs in the sagittal plane. The knee joint demonstrates increased flexion as velocity increases, but extension is, as in the hip, decreased. The knee flexes during the absorption phase of stance in running. This helps absorb the force of impact, accommodating the increased ground reactive forces placed on the limb. After IC, there is approximately 10 degrees of knee flexion during walking and 35 degrees during running, after which extension occurs.[7] At MS of running, the knee begins to reverse motion for the propulsive phase. In general, the average knee range of motion is 60 degrees during walking and 63 degrees during running. It must be understood that neutral (0 degrees of flexion or extension) never occurs. Maximum flexion in walking reaches 64 degrees, and extension is −8 degrees (8 degrees of flexion). In running, maximum flexion reaches 79 degrees, and extension is −16 degrees (16 degrees of flexion).

The Ankle and Foot

The ankle acts primarily as a dorsiflexor and plantarflexor, whereas most of the foot joints exhibit biplanar or triplanar motion. The major triplanar motions are termed pronation and supination. Pronation is a combination of dorsiflexion with abduction and eversion. Supination is a combination of plantarflexion with adduction and inversion. The subtalar, oblique midtarsal, longitudinal midtarsal, and fifth ray produce pronation and supination. The first ray is triplanar but not pronatory/supinatory. Motion about the first ray is dorsiflexion with adduction and inversion, and plantarflexion with abduction and eversion. The metetarsophalangeal joints are biplanar, with mostly dorsiflexion and plantar flexion and approximately 10 degrees of abduction and adduction. The interphalangeal joints are similar to the metatarsalphalangeal joints but with even less abduction and adduction.

During walking, the ankle plantarflexes after IC and during LR. This is followed by dorsiflexion once the foot has made complete contact with the floor. Oonpuu[3] determined overall ROM at the ankle during walking to be 30 degrees, with maximum plantarflexion of 18 degrees and maximum dorsiflexion of 12 degrees. This is in accordance with Winter,[4] who reported maximum plantarflexion of 19.8 degrees and maximum dorsiflexion of 9.6 degrees during normal walking. Running produces a greater overall ankle ROM of 50 degrees due to increased hip and knee flexion during running.

During running, motion about the ankle is quite different. At IC, although the heel makes contact with the ground first in most runners, due to the increased hip and knee flexion the ankle undergoes rapid dorsiflexion during the absorption phase. In running, because the ankle never quite reaches the amount of plantarflexion that it undergoes while walking, the amount of supination in the subtalar joint is limited but the degree of pronation is increased. It has been suggested that this is the cause of the vast number of running injuries. It has been shown that running barefoot results in an even greater amount of pronation.[8] This is cause for arguing that shoe gear limits pronation and reduces the time for supination.

Subtalar motion is determined by muscular activity as well as response to ground reactive forces. Midtarsal joint motion, however, is determined by subtalar position. The relationship between the rearfoot position and midtarsal axes can be seen in Fig. 2–1. When the calcaneus and talus are neutral, an individually determined amount of motion is available at the midtarsal joints.

When the calcaneus and talus are supinated, the axis is such that an increased obliquity is produced across the oblique and longitudinal midtarsal joints. This serves to lock the midtarsal joint functionally, thereby resulting in a decrease in available motion and allowing the foot to become a "rigid lever." This occurs during late TST and PSW.

When the calcaneus and talus are pronated, the axis is such that an increased parallelism exists between the oblique and longitudinal midtarsal joints. This results in an increased available motion in these joints, serving to unlock the midtarsal joint and allowing an increased ROM for adaptation to the ground surface as well as absorbing the ground reactive forces, which lets the foot become a "mobile adapter." This occurs during MS.

As the foot makes contact with the floor, the pelvis, femur, and tibia begin the process of internal rotation (Fig. 2–2). This internal rotation lasts through loading

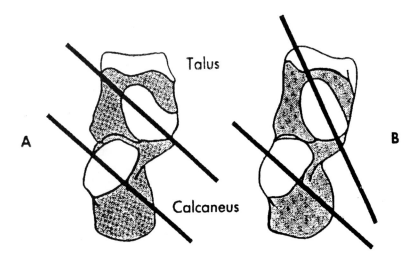

Figure 2–1. Axes of transverse tarsal joint. (*A*) When calcaneus is in eversion, conjoint axes between talonavicular and calcaneocuboid joints are parallel to one another so that increased motion occurs in the transverse tarsal joint. (*B*) When calcaneus is in inversion, axes are no longer parallel, and decreased motion and increased stability of the transverse tarsal joint are found. (*Source: From Mann.[2]*)

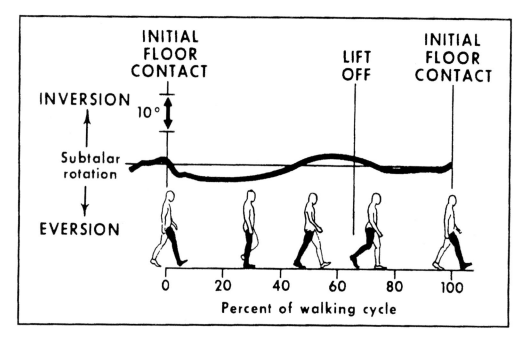

Figure 2–2. Motion in subtalar joint during normal walking cycle. At initial floor contact, rapid eversion is followed by progressive inversion until lift-off, after which eversion recurs. (*Source: From Mann,[17] as adapted by Wright et al.[18]*)

response and into MS, resulting in eversion and unlocking of the subtalar joint. This results in subtalar pronation, which allows unlocking of the oblique and longitudinal midtarsal joints, resulting in further pronation.

The pelvis, femur, and tibia then begin to rotate externally, which causes inversion and locking of the subtalar joint (Fig. 2–3). This, as stated previously, results in increased obliquity of the oblique and

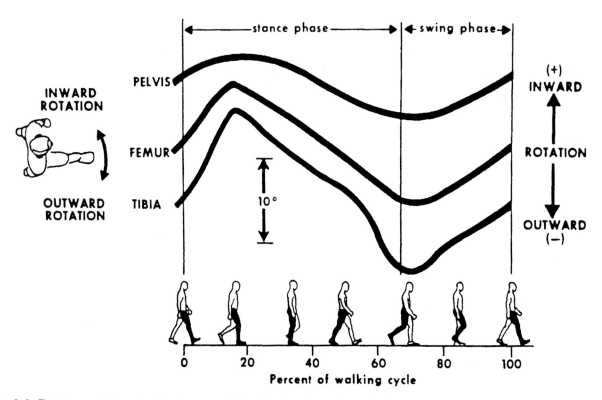

Figure 2–3. Transverse rotation of pelvis, femur, and tibia. Maximum internal rotation is achieved by approximately 15% of the walking cycle, and maximum external rotation occurs at time of TO. (*Source: From Mann.[17]*)

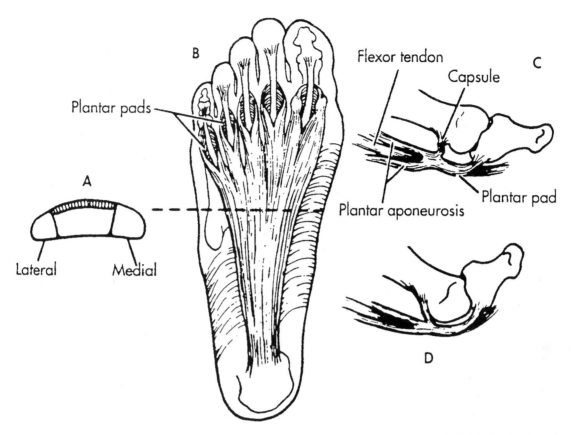

Figure 2–4. Plantar aponeurosis. (*A*) Cross section. (*B*) Plantar aponeurosis divides as it proceeds distally to allow flexor tendons to pass through. (*C*) Plantar aponeurosis combines with joint capsule to form plantar pad of metarsalphalangeal joint. (*D*) Dorsiflexion of toes forces metatarsal head into plantarflexion and brings plantar pad over head of metatarsal. (*Source: From Mann.*[17])

longitudinal midtararsal joints, causing supination of the forefoot and allowing the foot to become a "rigid lever."

Aside from the joint motions and alignments, several other factors are important in allowing the foot to proceed through its course. The plantar fascia originates from the plantar calcaneal tubercle and extends distally to the toes (Fig. 2–4). This structure helps to stabilize the foot by increasing the medial longitudinal arch and inverting the heel, as the toes are dorsiflexed during propulsion.

Another factor important in aiding normal kinematic motions during gait is the metatarsal break (Fig. 2–5). This is an axis represented by an oblique line across the metatarsal heads. As the toes are forced into dorsiflexion, this oblique axis helps promote hindfoot inversion during TO, which facilitates external rotation of the stance leg.

The joints of the lower extremity all move together in a well-orchestrated concert to provide us with locomotion. The joints are dependent on muscular action and inertia for their movement. They are also dependent on each other to allow certain degrees of freedom of motion from

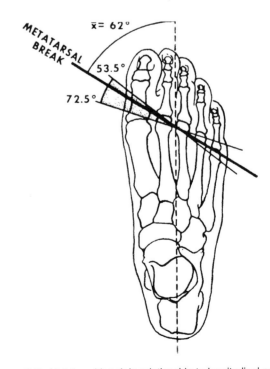

Figure 2–5. Metatarsal break in relationship to longitudinal axes of foot. (*Source: From Mann.*[17])

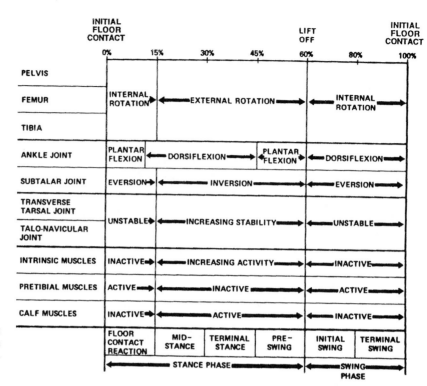

	INITIAL FLOOR CONTACT 0%	15%	30%	45%	LIFT OFF 60%	80%	INITIAL FLOOR CONTACT 100%
PELVIS							
FEMUR	INTERNAL ROTATION	←————EXTERNAL ROTATION————→				INTERNAL ROTATION	
TIBIA							
ANKLE JOINT	PLANTAR FLEXION	←——DORSIFLEXION——→		PLANTAR FLEXION	←——DORSIFLEXION——→		
SUBTALAR JOINT	EVERSION→	←————INVERSION————→			←——EVERSION——→		
TRANSVERSE TARSAL JOINT	UNSTABLE→	←——INCREASING STABILITY——→			←—UNSTABLE—→		
TALO-NAVICULAR JOINT							
INTRINSIC MUSCLES	INACTIVE→	←——INCREASING ACTIVITY——→			←—INACTIVE—→		
PRETIBIAL MUSCLES	ACTIVE→	←————INACTIVE————→			←—ACTIVE—→		
CALF MUSCLES	INACTIVE→	←————ACTIVE————→			←—INACTIVE—→		
	FLOOR CONTACT REACTION	MID-STANCE	TERMINAL STANCE	PRE-SWING	INITIAL SWING	TERMINAL SWING	
	←————STANCE PHASE————→				←——SWING PHASE——→		

Figure 2–6. Schema of complete walking cycle, showing rotations in various segments and joints and activity in foot and leg musculature. (*Source: From Mann.*[17])

one joint to the next down the line, of limb. A summary of the events of the gait cycle is depicted in Fig. 2–6.

KINETICS

Kinetics is defined as the study of forces that cause movement, both internally and externally. Internal forces are related to muscle forces, and external forces are related to ground reactive forces. Muscle activity is most easily determined by electromyography (EMG). Muscle activity increases during running in all muscles, as does the duration of muscle activity. Ground reactive forces are the forces exerted on the foot during foot contact. The data are collected with a force plate. This is in accordance with Newton's third law, which states that for every action there is an equal and opposite reaction.

Ground reactive forces involve three component forces: fore-aft, medial-lateral, and vertical. The greatest and most significant component is the vertical one. Walking produces vertical ground reactive forces equal to 1.3 to 1.5 times body weight.[3] These peaks occur during LR and PSW, giving a "double bump" appearance (Fig. 2–7). During running, the vertical ground reactive force begins with a small impact force peak in the first 20% of stance followed by a more gradual and larger peak in the remainder of stance.[3] These ground reactive forces equal three to four times that of normal body weight.[9]

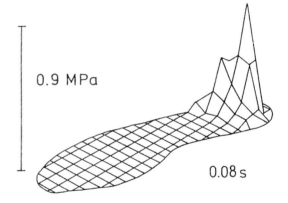

0.9 MPa

0.08 s

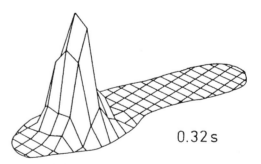

0.32 s

Figure 2–7. Pressure between the shoe and the ground at two instances of the stance phase of normal slow walking. (*Source: adapted from Cavanagh et al.*[11])

The fore-aft ground reactive force represents braking and propulsion in the first and last halves of stance phase, respectively. The peak amplitude only accounts for about 30% of body weight.

The medial-lateral ground reactive force is a very small component and accounts for only about 10% of body weight, according to a study performed by Oonpuu. These results were similar to those of Roy, who measured medial-lateral ground reactive forces and found that they ranged from 10% to 20% of body weight.

In walking, the heel contacts the ground first, followed by foot flat. Most runners (80%) make IC with the posterolateral border of the foot. These are referred to as rearfoot or heel strikers. The remainder of runners, known as midfoot strikers, usually make contact with the midlateral border of the foot (Fig. 2–8). In sprinting, IC is usually made with the toes.[10] The ground reactive force pattern also depends on the type of running style. Heel strikers have a center of pressure (COP) path beginning along the outer border of the rear foot and progressing along the lateral border for approximately two thirds of the stance phase. The center of pressure then progresses across the forefoot in a medial direction toward the first and second metatarsal heads. Midfoot strikers have a COP path that begins on the lateral midfoot and progresses

posteriorly. This corresponds to the heel contacting the floor. The COP then rapidly moves to the medial forefoot, as in heel strikers.[11]

Generally speaking, the percentage of muscle activity increases throughout stance phase during running. It is rare to see a muscle group active for than 50% of the stance phase during walking, but in running, activity is noted for 70% to 80% of the stance phase.[12]

During walking, the gluteus maximus is active from the end of the swing phase until the foot is flat on the floor. This serves to decelerate the limb and stabilize the hip joint for initial contact. During running, however, it is active from TSW through 40% of the stance phase. This helps to produce hip extension.

The hip abductors function during TSW and throughout 50% of the stance phase during walking and running. This serves to stabilize the stance leg pelvis at IC, which prevents excessive sagging of the swing leg.[13] The hip adductors are active during the last one third of the stance phase during walking. During running, they are active during the entire stance and swing phases, but data are difficult to obtain, and the results are quite variable.[12] The hip extensors provide the main source of power during late swing and early stance (Fig. 2–9). The hip flexors provide the main source of power during push-off and early swing.[14]

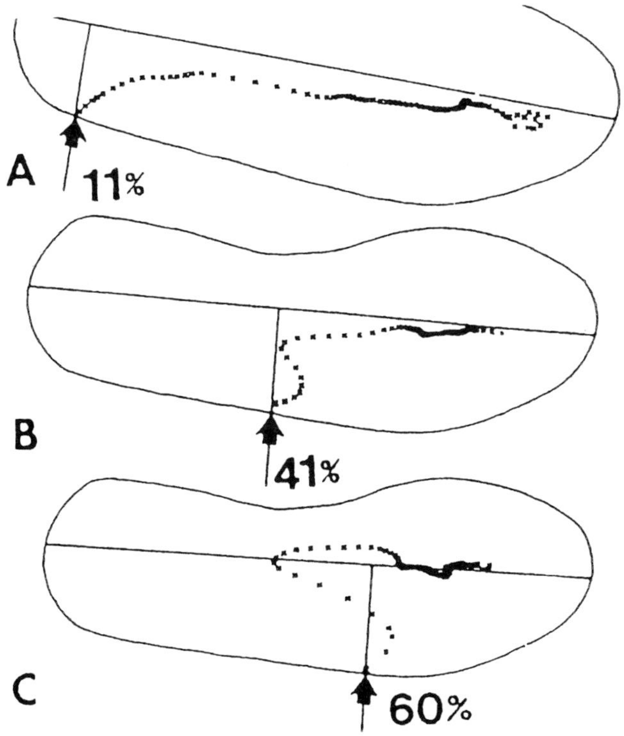

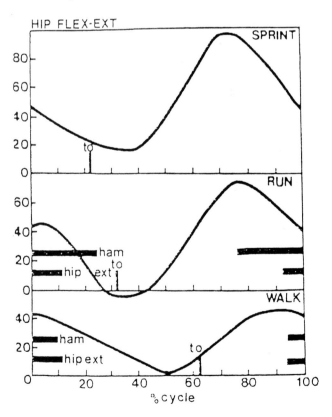

Figure 2–8. Center of pressure patterns of three subjects all running at the same speed. Note great differences among subjects despite matched running speeds. (*A*) Rearfoot striker. (*B*) Midfoot striker. (*C*) Forefoot striker. (*Source: From Cavanagh et al.[11]*)

Figure 2–9. Electromyographic activity of the hip ROM during sprinting, running, and walking. (*Source: From Mann et al.[7]*)

The quadriceps are composed of four separate muscles acting together. One of the component muscles, the rectus femoris, is a two-joint muscle that crosses both the hip and knee joints. This allows for different functions at either joint at any given point during the gait cycle. The quadriceps are active at the end of the swing phase to bring about terminal knee extension and to aid in hip flexion, through a concentric contraction. They also help stabilize the knee joint at initial contact, through an eccentric contraction. In running, they are highly active during the absorption phase of stance to deal with the greater requirements of weight acceptance. They are continually active throughout knee flexion eccentrically to limit the rate at which knee flexion occurs. They are active for 50% to 60% of the running stance phase and for only 25% of the walking stance phase (Fig. 2–10).

The hamstrings constitute another two-joint muscle complex that crosses both the hip and knee joints. During walking, the hamstrings are active at the end of swing phase and into stance phase until the foot is in full contact with the ground. This occurs at about 10% of the walking gait cycle. During running, they are active during the last third of the swing phase during hip and knee extension. Here they are acting concentrically across the hip joint but eccentrically across the knee joint. This action initiates hip extension and resists knee extension simultaneously.

During walking, the anterior tibial muscle group is active from late stance phase through the swing phase and then for the first 10% to 15% of the next stance phase. This produces dorsiflexion of the ankle during the swing phase through concentric contraction. It also helps to control plantarflexion by IC through eccentric contraction, thereby preventing foot slap. During running, they are active from late stance phase, through the swing phase and for the first 50% to 60% of the next stance phase (Fig. 2–11). For their duration of activity they are undergoing concentric contraction. During walking, they decelerate foot plantarflexion at IC; however, during running they appear to accelerate movement of the leg over the fixed foot.

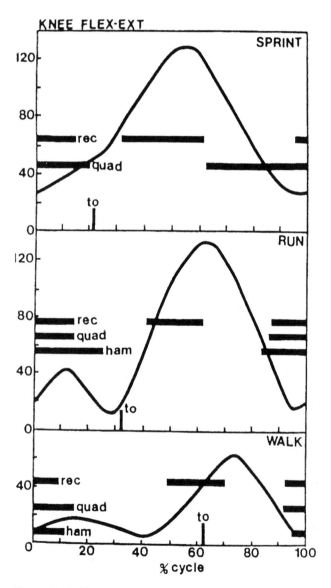

Figure 2–10. Electromyographic activity in the knee ROM during sprinting, running, and walking. (*Source: From Mann et al.*[7])

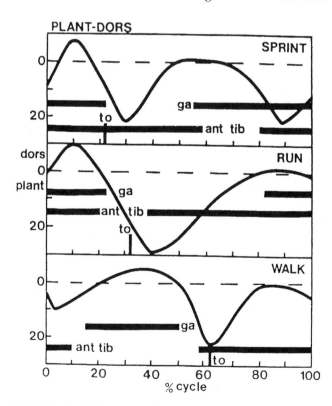

Figure 2–11. Electromyographic activity in the ankle ROM during sprinting, running, and walking. (*Source: From Mann et al.*[7])

In heel strikers, a greater degree of activity is found in the anterior tibial muscle group than in midfoot strikers.

Activity of the posterior leg musculature begins during TSW of gait. During walking, these muscles act to resist forward movement of the tibia over the fixed foot during the stance phase. They are active from 25% to 50% of the stance phase through mostly eccentric contraction. During their last 25% of activity, they undergo concentric contraction to initiate active plantarflexion. During running gait, IC is a period of rapid dorsiflexion. Here the triceps undergo eccentric contraction, again to resist this motion. They are active for approximately 60% of the stance phase. Initially they serve to stabilize the ankle joint at IC, and then to provide for propulsion.

CONCLUSIONS

Running adds complexity to the normal gait cycle. This complexity varies from athlete to athlete, making evaluation and management of running disorders and injuries difficult. Understanding the biomechanical differences between walking and running arms the physician with increased knowledge to diagnose running injuries more accurately. Once the appropriate diagnosis is made, the physician may then develop a focused treatment and rehabilitation plan.

(For further discussion of the biomechanics of running, see Vaughn[15] and Novacheck.[16])

REFERENCES

1. Hoeberigs JH: Factors related to the incidence of running injuries. A review. *Sports Med* 1992:11, 771.
2. Mann RA: Biomechanics of running, in Mack RP (ed.), *AAOS Symposium on the Foot and Leg in Running Sports,* St. Louis, Mosby, 1982:1.
3. Oonpuu S: The biomechanics of walking and running. *Clin Sports Med* 13, 843.
4. Winter DA: *The Biomechanics and Motor Control of Human Gait,* Waterloo, Ontario, Canada, University of Waterloo Press, 1987.
5. Fenn WO: Work against gravity and work due to velocity changes in running: Movements of the center of gravity within the body and foot pressures on the ground. *Am J Physiol* 93, 433.
6. Oonpuu S: The biomechanics of running: A kinematic and kinetic analysis. *Instru Course Lect* 1990, 305.
7. Mann RA, Hagy J: Biomechanics of walking, running and sprinting. *Am J Sports Med* 8, 345.
8. Chan CW, Rudins A: Foot biomechanics during walking and running. *Mayo Clin Proc* 1994:69, 448.
9. Rodgers MM: Dynamic Biomechanics of the normal foot and ankle during walking and running. *Phys Ther* 68, 1822.
10. Thordarson DB: Running biomechanics. *Clin Sports Med* 1997:16, 239.
11. Cavanagh PR, Lafortune MA: Ground reaction forces in distance running. *J Biomech* 1980:13, 397.
12. Mann RA: Biomechanics of running. *Spine Lower Extremity Sports* 335.
13. Inman VT: Functional aspects of the abductor muscles of the hip. *J Bone Joint Surg* 1947:29, 607.
14. Novacheck TF: Running injuries: A biomechanical approach. *J Bone Joint Surg Am* 80-A, 1220.
15. Vaughan CL: Biomechanics of running gait. *CRC Crit Rev Biomed Eng* 1986:12, 1.
16. Novacheck TF: Walking, running, and sprinting: A three-dimensional analysis of kinematics and kinetics. *Instru Course Lect* 1995:44, 497.
17. Mann RA: Biomechanics of the foot, in *Atlas of Orthotics: Biomechanical Principles and Application*, St. Louis, Mosby, 1975:257.
18. Wright DG, Desai SM, Henderson WH: *J Bone Joint Surg Am* 1965:46, 361.

Chapter 3

PRINCIPLES OF TRAINING

Robert H. Vaughan

INTRODUCTION

Since the turn of the 20th century coaches and athletes have trained for the previous Olympic Games just as generals traditionally prepared for and fought the last war. Success by an athlete or coach in the Olympic Games bred a confusing assortment of training theories, based on belief and practical experience. Theory has begun to be replaced by scientific principles as science has gradually has become more important in the training of elite athletes. First, we shall attempt to define and explain six essential principles. Second, we shall describe the physiology of fatigue for each of the three energy systems and attempt to make a connection with the six principles. Finally, we shall describe several of the current training concepts.

Training may be random or planned. While it is possible to achieve improved performance without systematic planning, it is certainly more difficult. The more impact failure has, such as the loss by a microsecond of a berth on an Olympic team, the more careful planning becomes essential. Failure could cost a prospective Olympic champion millions of dollars as well as years spent in preparation. The six principles that appear most frequently in the numerous publications focused on training theory are adaptation, individualization, overload, restoration, reversibility, and specificity.[1-3] Each is related to the others and, as you will see, no single principle stands alone.

TRAINING PRINCIPLES

Adaptation

An adjustment in function or dimension of an organism, which results from the demands placed upon it, is known as adaptation. Hypertrophy, for instance, is an adaptation to the metabolic cost and amount of resistance applied during strength training.[4] However, adaptation to either endurance or strength-related stress is not only specific to the type of stress, but also fiber type and genetics.[5-7]

One of the first adaptations to endurance training is increased plasma volume. This is in response to a reduction in central blood volume following a bout of exercise. Reduced blood volume is a consequence of pooling of blood in the peripheral vessels and dehydration that occur during a training session.[8] The reduction in central blood volume temporarily lowers venous return and right atrial pressure. The body adjusts to reduced atrial pressure and dehydration by increasing sodium and fluid retention, which eventually results in increased plasma volume, increased venous return to the heart, and increased end-diastolic volume.[8-10] Increased cardiac volume allows a larger stroke volume which produces a reduced heart rate at rest and during submaximal work. Consistent endurance training is a chronic stimulus to plasma volume expansion and, therefore, training bradycardia.[8]

Individualization

The principle of individualization states that there is a need to tailor training programs to the physiological and psychological responses of each athlete. No two persons, not even identical twins, respond in the same way to a training program or training session.[6,11,12] Genetic factors may be identical, but social, environmental, and physiological interactions vary even among individuals who are raised together. Training age, chronological age, gender, emotional maturity, motivation, and fitness are but a few of the differences among athletes that require an individual approach in the construction of a training schedule.[13–16]

The capability to meet the energy demands of an event also varies from individual to individual. An 800-meter runner with an oxygen uptake of 75 ml/kg and a personal best of 47.7 seconds for 400 meters would approach training for the 800 differently than would an 800 runner with an oxygen uptake of 55 ml/kg and a 400-meter personal best of 45.5 seconds. An athlete with a well-developed aerobic-energy system might not respond, or have the capacity to respond, to a training program that concentrates on improving anaerobic energy delivery. Nor would an athlete with a preponderance of type II fibers thrive on a training program weighted toward development of the aerobic energy system.

Overload

In order to initiate the adaptation process, a training stimulus must be of sufficient strength to disturb homeostasis. The use of increased volume, duration, or intensity to produce change is known as overloading. Examples of overloading are

1. Loads at near peak levels in weight training sessions, which result in larger strength and power gains than do lower loads.[17]
2. Long-term aerobic exercise that depletes glycogen stores, and stimulates the storage of glycogen in excess of previous levels.[18]
3. Improvement in the lactate threshold which results from training at or just above the current threshold.[19]

Loads that produce change early in a training cycle will fail to elicit similar improvements when applied during the latter stages of that cycle. The workload must be increased as the training process continues to elicit a response. If the load is well within the individual's current exercise capacity, no change will occur. However, if the load is too great, exhaustion or injury may be the result (Figure 3–1).[2,20]

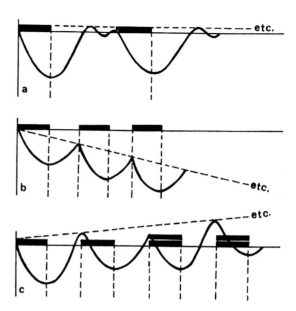

Figure 3–1. Effective overloading. Training that is too infrequent to improve performance: a. Training that is too intense or too frequent causes a decrease in fitness: b. A gradual increase in intensity and volume produces an optimal increase in fitness: c. (Reproduced with permission from G Schmolinsky, Basic Elements of Track and Field Training. In: Track and Field: Text-Book for Coaches and Sports Teachers. 1983 p. 57, Sports Books Publisher, Toronto. Ont.).

Restoration

Restoration is a principle too often ignored among highly motivated athletes. Restoration refers to the period of time following a training stimulus when the work capacity returns to prestimulus levels. If recovery time is optimal, supercompensation results.[21] If the recovery period is too short, fatigue and overtraining follow.[22–24] When there is too much time between training bouts the response is attenuated.[1,2] In addition to rest, restoration may include massage, antioxidant supplementation, hydration, and various mental diversions that allow for emotional restoration.[25–27] The time necessary for full restoration of exercise capacity may be several minutes after a single repetition, or 24 to 48 or even 72 hours following a vigorous training session. The emotional and physical drain of an especially taxing competition such as the Olympic trials may require several weeks or months for recovery.[28,29]

Reversibility

Adaptations may be lost through imposed or selected inactivity. This process is known as reversibility. The loss of fitness is known as detraining. The effects of detraining are directly related to the length of the training interruption. Aerobic endurance declines rapidly, but $\dot{V}o_2$max decays only after several weeks of inactivity.[30,31] Also, athletes who have trained over a number of years lose those adaptations more slowly than do

TABLE 3–1. THE RELATIONSHIP OF WORLD RECORD TIMES, IN METERS PER SECOND, OF RUNNING EVENTS RANGING FROM 100 METERS TO THE MARATHON

Men				Women			
Distance	Time	MPS	% Difference	Distance	Time	MPS	% Difference
100	9.79	10.21		100	10.49	9.53	
200	19.32	10.35	1.01	200	21.34	9.37	0.98
400	43.18	9.26	0.89	400	47.60	8.40	0.90
800	101.11	7.91	0.85	800	113.28	7.06	0.84
1500	206.00	7.28	0.92	1500	230.46	6.51	0.92
1609	223.13	7.21	0.99	1609	252.56	6.37	0.98
5000	759.36	6.58	0.91	5000	868.09	5.76	0.90
10000	1582.75	6.32	0.96	10000	1771.78	5.64	0.98
42199	7542.00	5.60	0.89	42199	8443.00	5.00	0.89

Note the close relationship of the 100–200 and the 5,000–10,000.

those who more recently began endurance training.[32] In addition, detraining results in a loss of capillary density, mitochondrial number and volume, a decrease in both glycolytic and oxidative enzymes, and eventually a decline in fitness to the untrained state.[32,33] Reduced fitness that stems from overtraining may be caused by factors such as an increased incidence of upper respiratory infections or muscle catabolism resulting from a decreased testosterone to cortisol ratio.[29]

Specificity

Training should mimic the physiological and biomechanical demands of competition. Each running event has a unique set of physiological demands that necessitate a specific training approach.[34] Training should produce improvements in the specific energy delivery systems critical for success to obtain optimal results.[35] One reason for specificity in training is to use time most efficiently. Time spent engaged in medium-intensity aerobic training, such as that often used in preparation for middle-distance events, will increase general endurance, but will have limited effects on high-intensity endurance, such as anaerobic capacity.[36] Not every training session must contain high-intensity work, but during the specific preparation and competition phases, event-specific activities should be included every 48 to 72 hours.

When a coach or athlete applies the principles of training he or she must consider the energy demands of the activity and the energy delivery capability of the athlete. Each event has its own unique demands so that a person proficient in one, such as the 100 meters, will not necessarily excel at the 200 meters, although many of the energy demands are the same. Occasionally an athlete will succeed at the international level in two somewhat dissimilar events, such as Tatyana Kazankina and Peter Snell in the 800 and 1500 meters, Jarmila Kratochvilova and Alberto Juantorena in the 400 and 800 meters, and Marie-Jose Perec and Michael Johnson in the 200 and 400 meters. There is a close relationship in terms of speed in meters per second (mps) between the 100 and 200 meters and the 5000 and 10,000 meters, where success as measured by double gold medals and world records is more common (Table 3–1). Very rarely, however, will there be a Haile Gabriselassie, who in 1998 was ranked second in the world indoors at 1500 and who set indoor world records in the 2000 and 3000 meters, and outdoor marks for the 5000 and 10,000 meters.

FATIGUE AND THE ENERGY SYSTEMS

Training is designed to postpone the onset of fatigue. Fatigue differs in relation to the intensity and duration of the exercise that determines the relative contribution of the alactic (high-energy phosphate), the anaerobic, and the aerobic energy systems. The high-energy phosphate system provides the majority of energy during the first 15 to 20 seconds of intense exercise. The anaerobic system produces the majority of necessary energy for the next 90 seconds, and from 2 minutes on the aerobic energy system is dominant (Figure 3–2).[37]

Alactic

During intense work, such as sprinting 100 meters, utilization of available adenosine triphosphate (ATP) in cells produces the first 2 to 3 seconds of the necessary energy. As exercise continues, phosphate (P) is donated from creatine phosphate (CP) to the adenosine diphosphate (ADP) resulting from ATP utilization. There is sufficient CP in the cell to allow approximately 4 to 6 additional seconds of work at that same intense rate.[3] As CP is depleted, the exercise rate falls. Even elite 100-meter runners slow after 70 to 80 meters due to a rapid reduction of available ATP and CP. There is a linear

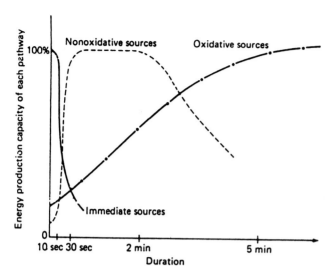

Figure 3–2. The time frame and relative contribution of each of the energy systems to intense exercise. (Reproduced with permission from Dee W. Edington and V. Reggie Edgerton, Classifications and Definitions. In: The Biology of Physical Activity. 1976 p. 8, Houghton Mifflin Co., Boston, MA).

relationship between exercise intensity and depletion of CP. As the distance run increases from 100 to 200 and 400 meters, the reduction of CP takes somewhat longer.[32,38–40] The consumption of ATP within the cell is never complete, however. In fact, fatigue, or the slowing of energy production, serves to protect remaining ATP stores.[41] The engagement of the high-energy phosphate system produces a stimulus for both the anaerobic and aerobic energy systems and thus serves to further protect ATP.[41] In addition, the time delay of 15 to 20 seconds from the onset of exercise provided by the high-energy phosphate system allows time for the anaerobic system to become fully functional.[42]

Anaerobic

Fatigue resulting from high-intensity anaerobic work has both metabolic and nonmetabolic origins.[41] Metabolic fatigue may be caused by a buildup of hydrogen ions, heat, or both, within the working muscle.[43,44] Nonmetabolic fatigue follows disruption in the structure of the cell that leads to muscle weakness lasting up to several weeks.[41]

Anaerobic energy production provides the majority of energy for exercise after 15 to 20 seconds, following reduction of available ATP and CP in the cell, when there is a greater demand for oxygen than the aerobic energy system can supply. The anaerobic production of energy is very inefficient, in that only 2 percent of energy contained in a mole of glucose is utilized in the formation of ATP.[45]

In the anaerobic production of energy, the excess hydrogen ions produced are donated to pyruvic acid in the

cytoplasm of the cell to form lactic acid. Lactic acid is a small, easily diffusible molecule. As long as egress from the cell is maintained, so that the internal pH does not fall below critical levels, muscle function continues.[45] When the pH within the cell falls below 6.5, all cellular function slows dramatically.[32] The slowdown is caused by inhibition of the glycolytic enzymes, phosphofructokinase and actomyosin ATPase. Diminished enzyme action inhibits ATP, and therefore energy production.

Anaerobic fatigue is not caused by the buildup of lactic acid.[45] Lactate is used for fuel by the heart and nonworking muscle tissue. Most of the excess lactate created during intense work is completely removed from the cell and reconverted, first to pyruvic acid, and then glucose, within the liver. Within 3 to 5 hours of the exercise bout, all traces of lactic acid have been removed from the cell and converted.

Aerobic

During aerobic exercise metabolic fatigue is directly related to depletion of muscle and/or liver glycogen, or the buildup of heat. Carbohydrates, muscle and liver glycogen, and blood glucose are the primary, but not exclusive, fuels utilized in the mitochondria to produce ATP during intense aerobic exercise above 65% of maximal oxygen consumption (Figure 3–3).[46] Below approximately 60% to 65% of maximal oxygen consumption, fatty acids are the primary energy source. Aerobic energy production occurs within the mitochondria. As long as exercise intensity, and therefore carbohydrate flux, is low, fatty acids enter the

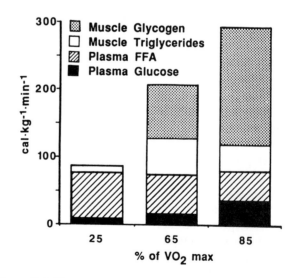

Figure 3–3. The contribution of glucose and FFA to energy production at 25%, 65%, and 85% $\dot{V}O_2$max. (Reproduced with permission from JA, Romjin, EF, Coyle, LS, Sidossis, Regulation of endogenous fat and carbohydrate metabolism is relation to exercise intensity and duration. In: American Journal of Physiology. Vol. 41, American Physiological Society, Bethesda, MD).

mitochondria to be used as fuel. However, as exercise intensity increases, carbohydrate flux interferes with fatty acid entry into the mitochondria and the depletion of glycogen progresses rapidly.[46,47] Under ordinary conditions there is sufficient glycogen stored in the muscle and liver of an elite athlete for approximately 1.5 to 2 hours of intense activity.[48] Beyond that point, as the level of blood glucose is reduced, the work rate slows dramatically. As a result of the quantity of glycogen normally found in muscle and the liver, only the marathon and longer events require exogenous glucose supplementation. However, reduced glycogen stores are found in dieters and individuals on rigorous training programs without sufficient rest.[49,50] Glycogen depletion could have a negative impact on 5000- and 10,000-meter performance in those individuals.

Recovery from an aerobic training session parallels muscle glycogen repletion.[51] Nonmetabolic post-exercise fatigue evidenced by muscle weakness may have several causes, which include an increase in proteolytic enzymes, free radical release, and hydrolysis of lysosomal acid.[41] Recovery from nonmetabolic fatigue may be prolonged and intense exercise should not be attempted as long as muscle weakness and soreness persist.

TRAINING THEORY

Elements of Training

The basic elements of training are speed, strength, endurance, recovery, and flexibility. These elements are the main ingredients of a training program and continuous, fartlek, interval, repetition, and resistance training are the typical methods used to improve the elements. There may be some variation in the meaning or definition of the various methods among coaches, but the elements are the same the world over. The ultimate result of training—enhanced performance—derives from how well the principles are applied to the methods to improve the elements of training.

Speed

The first element, speed, is defined as "the ability to move the body, or parts of the body, through a given range of motion in the least time."[52] Speed is a primary requirement for success in the 100, 200, and 400 meters. Even though the events 800 meters through 10,000 meters place increasing emphasis on endurance, speed is also vital in those events. Speed may be divided into acceleration, maximal speed, speed-reserve, and speed-endurance. Meckel et al. report reaction time is not critical to sprint performance.[53]

Acceleration is a measure of the rate of increase in speed. The ability to generate great force in the

TABLE 3–2. 10-METER SPLITS FOR THE FIRST- AND SECOND-PLACE FINISHERS AT THE ATHENS WORLD CHAMPIONSHIPS

	Men		Women	
	Greene	*Bailey*	*Jones*	*Pintusevich*
0–10	1.71	1.77	1.81	1.86
10–20	1.04	1.03	1.11	1.11
20–30	0.92	0.91	1.02	1.01
30–40	0.88	0.87	0.97	0.97
40–50	0.87	0.85	0.95	0.94
50–60	0.85	0.85	0.94	0.94
60–70	0.85	0.85	0.95	0.94
70–80	0.86	0.86	0.95	0.96
80–90	0.87	0.87	0.97	0.98
90–100	0.88	0.9	0.99	1
Finish	9.86	9.91	10.83	10.85

The splits clearly follow the model that suggests an early peak velocity results in a rapid loss of velocity. (Reproduced with permission from UG, Kersting, Biomechanical Analysis of the Sprinting Events. In: Biomechanical Research Project Athens 1997. 1999 pp. 19,33, Meyer & Meyer Sport, Germany).

starting blocks and during acceleration is an important aspect of successful performance in the sprint events.[54] The model for optimal performance in sprint events is a long acceleration phase, maintenance of maximal speed, followed by a relatively short deceleration phase. Athletes competing in the 100 meters follow this model, with an acceleration phase lasting 50 to 60 meters, maintenance of peak speed for 20 to 30 meters, and finally a loss of velocity over the last 20 to 30 meters (Table 3–2).[55]

Maximal speed is the peak velocity achieved by an athlete during the course of an event, usually measured in 10-meter increments. Peak velocity, in the 100-meter dash, is usually attained near the 60-meter mark for men and the 50-meter mark for women. That peak may be maintained, as we have seen, for approximately 20 meters. Results from the 1997 I.A.A.F. World Championships in athletics confirm the validity of the theory (Table 3–2).[55] The winning time for the 100 meters was 9.86 seconds for the men's champion Maurice Greene, and 10.83 seconds for Marion Jones, the women's winner. The fastest 10-meter segments run by Greene were between 50 and 60 meters and 60 and 70 meters, both timed at .85 second, or 11.76 mps. The actual top speed attained by Greene was 11.87 mps at the 58.1 meter mark in the race. Jones' fastest 10-meter segment occurred between 50 and 60 meters, which she ran in .94 second, or 10.64 mps. Jones' actual top speed, 10.68 mps, was recorded at 58.8 meters. Greene covered the last 10 meters of the race in .88 second, a deceleration of .03 second from his fastest 10-meter segment. Jones ran the last 10 meters in .99 second, a loss of .05 second.

The capacity to attain maximal speed is facilitated by the rapid excitation, contraction, and relaxation, of opposing muscle groups.[2] Fatigue causes a prolonged relaxation phase, which could lead to fused summation of action potentials, cramping, and performance decrements.[56] Training to improve neuromuscular coordination is essential to increase maximal speed.

Stride length and stride rate also play important roles in absolute speed. The stride length must be optimal so that the foot strikes the ground as close to the center of gravity (COG) as possible. The foot strike of elite sprinters is about 8 inches in front of the COG, which causes a slight braking action. Lower body movement just prior to and following foot strike is important to reduce the braking action and maximize propulsive force.[54] The stride rate must be such that optimal force will be applied to the ground during each foot strike in the least amount of time.[57] A comparison of Carl Lewis and Ben Johnson during the 1987 I.A.A.F. World Championships and the 1988 Seoul Olympic Games confirms the importance of stride rate (Table 3–3).[55] Johnson's stride was shorter and his turnover faster than Lewis' on both occasions. Johnson's explosive acceleration was the result of an increased ability, developed over the previous years, to apply force. What portion of that improved acceleration was a purely training response and what portion was due to exogenous testosterone usage plus training is a point in question.

Ground contact time increases as the distance of the event lengthens. The following times were reported by Mann at the Elite Sprint-Hurdle Olympic Development Clinic held in Orlando, Florida, on December 12 to 17, 1996[58]: Total amount of time spent with the foot in contact with the ground during each stride is approximately .089 second in the peak speed phase for elite 100-meter sprinters. The ground contact time for each step in the 200 meters is nearly identical for the first 100 meters of the race, but increases to around .095 second in the fatigued state, within 20 meters of the finish. Ground contact time in the 400 meters for elite male sprinters in the nonfatigued state is around .10 to .105 second, which increases to .110 to .120 second in the fatigued state at 380 meters.

Speed reserve is the result obtained when an athlete's best speed over 100 or 200 meters is subtracted from the average speed over a 100- or 200-meter segment of the competition event. In theory, the greater the speed reserve, the greater the potential to perform at competition speeds, assuming endurance is equal. Michael Johnson's sprint performance makes a case for this concept. Johnson's best time for 100 meters is 10.1 seconds. When he ran 43.18 seconds for a world record in the 400 meters, his average time per 100-meter segment was 10.8 seconds. That gave him a speed reserve of 0.7 second. Another 400-meter competitor might have a best of 10.5 seconds for 100 meters. In an attempt to run 43.18 seconds, this hypothetical individual would have a speed reserve of only .3 second. He would have difficulty maintaining a 10.8-second pace, because the work necessary to perform at or near peak speeds increases dramatically as one nears his or her capacity.

Strength

Strength is defined as the ability to apply force. Strength, as are speed and endurance, may be divided into several distinct parts: absolute strength, power, and strength endurance. When we discuss absolute, or maximal, strength, we mean the ability to apply force during a single muscle contraction. In running events, absolute strength is correlated with maximal speed.[58] Power, the ability to produce force over time, is associated with improved acceleration.[59] Strength endurance means the ability to maintain force production over time. Speed endurance, mentioned above, and strength endurance are complementary, if not precisely identical concepts. An athlete who maintains pace during the last 50 meters of a 200-meter dash, with minimal slowing, demonstrates excellent strength and speed endurance.

Endurance

While vital to success in running events, speed is of little consequence without the capability to sustain it. Endurance is the ability to maintain speed or intensity for a specified time or distance. There are numerous

TABLE 3–3. A COMPARISON OF STRIDE LENGTH AND STRIDE RATE BETWEEN BEN JOHNSON AND CARL LEWIS*

	Johnson		Lewis	
Distance	Rate	Length	Rate	Length
1987				
0–30	4.5	1.79	4.12	1.94
30–60	4.96	2.34	4.71	2.46
60–100	4.73	2.45	4.49	2.6
0–100	4.72	2.22	4.4	2.36
Time	9.83		9.93	
1988				
0–30	4.26	1.8	4.15	1.93
30–60	5.02	2.36	4.73	2.46
60–100	4.74	2.44	4.42	2.6
0–100	4.76	2.22	4.4	2.36
Time	9.79		9.92	

*From the 1987 I.A.A.F. World Championships and the 1988 Seoul Olympic Games. Ben Johnson's faster turnover and shorter stride prevailed over Lewis' longer stride and slower cadence. (Reproduced with permission from UG, Kersting, Biomechanical Analysis of the Sprinting Events. In: Biomechanical Research Project Athens 1997. 1999 p. 26, Meyer & Meyer Sport, Germany).

categories of endurance, such as aerobic, alactic, and anaerobic endurance, as well as long-term and short-term endurance. Here we will divide endurance into two major categories: basic and specific.

Basic endurance may be defined as the capacity to resist general (central nervous system [CNS], neuromuscular, and cardiorespiratory) fatigue over an extended period of time. Basic endurance is closely related to aerobic fitness.[1,2] Training used to improve basic aerobic endurance, which may include continuous runs and extensive intervals, causes an expansion of blood volume, a larger cardiac volume, higher capillary density, increased number and volume of mitochondria, and improved arterial-venous oxygen dif-ference.[60,61] The net result of these changes is an improved ability to run at high speeds with reduced lactate production and increased lactate removal (Figure 3–4).[62] Basic endurance training reduces glucose uptake for a given load, reduces muscle glycogen degradation, and increases glycogen storage.[63–65] Along with reducing the utilization of glucose, endurance training increases the contribution of fatty acids as fuel during submaximal work.[66] Although fatty acids may be used as an energy source, they utilize more oxygen than do glucose or glycogen for the same work rate.

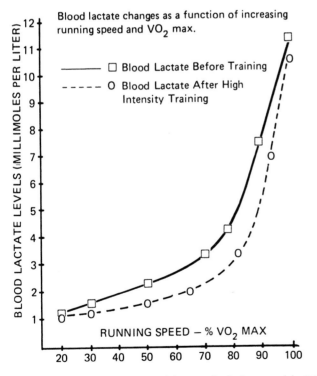

Figure 3–4. Intense aerobic training results in increased lactate clearance and decreased lactate production at the same absolute speeds. (Reproduced with permission from S Powers and RE Steben: Shifting the Anaerobic Threshold in Runners. In: Track Technique Annual '83. 1982 p. 108.

Athletes who wish to successfully compete in cross-country, track, or road racing, must develop endurance specific to the physiological requirements of that event. Depending on the event, that endurance may involve one or all of the energy systems. The following section, speed endurance, further explains the need for specificity in the construction of a training program.

Speed Endurance

Specific endurance is often synonymous with speed endurance in the training literature. The capacity to maintain pace over the course of a race, or a portion of the race distance in training, is known as speed endurance.[2] Each event, from 100 meters to the marathon, necessitates a measure of speed endurance specific to that event. Speed endurance in the 100 meters is a product of efficient use of the high-energy phosphate system combined with excellent neuromuscular coordination that results in the least amount of deceleration over the last 20 to 30 meters.

The ability to sustain near maximal velocity in the presence of increasing fatigue is a prerequisite for success in the 200 meters. The resistance to or postponement of fatigue in the 200-meter dash is due to development of neuromuscular coordination, the alactic energy system, and the anaerobic energy system. 400 meter runners, with well-developed anaerobic energy systems, have often demonstrated the value of anaerobic endurance in the last 30 to 40 meters of the 200 meters.

The 400 meters and 400-meter hurdles are events that produce overwhelming fatigue over the last 40 to 60 meters. Training for the 400 meter and 400-meter hurdles necessitates full development of the anaerobic energy system. Training must mimic the intensity of those events to improve specific anaerobic performance. Because high-intensity training may have negative consequences, such as injury or illness, careful design of training is necessary.[67] The anaerobic fatigue that develops during a 400-meter dash is peripheral rather than central. Therefore, the training for and adaptation to anaerobic training must have a local, rather than systemic, focus.[68]

Anaerobic energy production is best accomplished by type IIb (fast twitch glycolytic) muscle fibers. Although type II fibers are able to produce rapid and forceful muscle contractions, the onset of fatigue is also rapid. Not only does fatigue develop rapidly in type II fibers, in addition, the lack of mitochondria and reduced capillary supply of oxygen to these fibers cause a slow recovery from fatigue. Adequate time for restoration is important in the design of training programs, to allow recovery from both metabolic and nonmetabolic fatigue. In addition, a careful warm-up has been shown to improve anaerobic performance and may prevent some of the nonmetabolic causes of fatigue.[69]

Middle-distance events such as 800 and 1500 meters demand a high level of speed endurance in order to maintain a velocity that, while not near maximal, exceeds the body's ability to utilize oxygen. The 800 and 1500 meters are thought of as combination events and success in either or both events requires thorough development of the anaerobic and aerobic energy systems.[70]

The 3000 steeple and 5000- and 10,000-meter runs are performed, for the majority of the race, at or near $\dot{V}O_2$max. However, success in the longer middle distances is related to improvements in the lactate threshold rather than maximal oxygen uptake.[19] As a result, events from 3000 to 10,000 meters necessitate training programs designed to improve the lactate threshold.

Recovery

Restoration of full work capacity following exercise depends on which energy systems (alactic, anaerobic and/or aerobic) were stressed and to what degree. Recovery of the high-energy phosphate system following dynamic exercise, such as a 30-meter sprint, should be 95% to 100% complete within 3 minutes.[71] Thirty-meter sprints could, theoretically, be repeated indefinitely at three-minute intervals barring dehydration and the buildup of heat. An anaerobic repetition of 300 meters might require 20 to 30 minutes for near-complete recovery, or 7 to 10 minutes for an incomplete but worthwhile break. Aerobic intervals run at near $\dot{V}O_2$max would require very short recovery bouts of $1/2$ to 2 times the time of the repetition to maintain the worthwhile break. Jogging rather than passive rest speeds recovery from steady state and interval running.[72,73]

Recovery between strength training sessions that stress the high-energy phosphate system should provide time for restoration of the neural activation pathways of the CNS, which are especially stressed with heavy-resistance training.[74,75] High intensity sessions that fatigue the anaerobic energy system must allow time for healing of the myofibrils and for repletion of glycogen stores in type II fibers.[41] Continuous and intermittent aerobic endurance training cause depletion of glycogen in both the type II and type I fibers as well as dehydration.[76] Complete restoration of performance capacity normally takes 48 to 72 hours, but that time will increase if intense training sessions are too frequent or prolonged (Figure 3–5).[77]

Flexibility

The importance of flexibility in high-performance athletics has been debated for years. Two of the purposes of flexibility training are to increase range of motion and to prevent injury. Numerous articles have stated

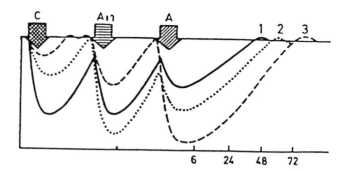

Figure 3–5. Training loads that are too frequent or too intense cause delayed recovery. C = speed; An = anaerobic; A = aerobic. (Reproduced with permission from A Viru[77])

that increased flexibility reduces the incidence of injury.[78–80] Others have claimed that muscle and tendon injuries resulted from improved flexibility.[81] Still others have found no relationship between flexibility and injury.[82–84] Acute injury may result more from an imbalance of strength or flexibility than a lack of flexibility.[85] It is possible that an overzealous approach to improving flexibility may predispose an athlete to injury and may lead to decreased running economy.[86,87]

Although stretching cannot be shown conclusively to prevent acute muscle or tendon injury, flexibility training improves range of motion during injury rehabilitation.[88] Also, a program designed to equalize flexibility following injury has been demonstrated to prevent reinjury.[89] And, as opposed to acute injury, prevention and treatment of chronic or overuse injuries may benefit from a stretching program.[78]

Methods of Training

Steady State

Submaximal, steady state exercise may be defined as a continuous run, during which oxygen consumption equals oxygen demand.[32] After an initial rapid increase at the onset of exercise, oxygen consumption, diastolic blood pressure, ventilation, and lactate levels remain relatively constant.[90] Heart rate also increases initially, and continues a minimal rise throughout the duration of the run. The length of such a session may vary from 20 minutes to several hours. A 20-minute steady state, also known as a tempo run, might be performed just below the lactate threshold. In this intense form of steady state training, the chief adaptation is a shift to the right of the lactate threshold. The lactate threshold is the pace at which lactate production exceeds lactate removal. The shift in the lactate threshold results in part from increased buffer capacity and improved oxidative phosphorylation.[41] In addition to a shift in the lactate threshold, at the typical training pace, running economy has been shown to improve.[91] Running economy is measured by the oxygen cost of the exercise. The more oxygen consumed at a training or racing pace, the lower the running economy.

A long-distance runner performs a 3-hour steady-state run well below the lactate threshold and at a much lower ventilation and heart rate. Long runs improve basic aerobic fitness by increasing aerobic enzyme activity, capillary density, the size and number of the mitochondria, and by decreasing glycogen dependency.[41] These adaptations have the effect of allowing the athlete to run nearer his or her $\dot{V}O_2$max with a lower accumulation of metabolic by-products and a reduced glycogen consumption.

Fartlek

Imagine the play of a child. It is without restraint, free. Substitute athletes for children and fartlek, a Swedish term meaning "speed play," is the result. When Swedish coach Gosta Holmer created fartlek, he envisioned unstructured periods of intense running, followed by recovery breaks composed of easy running, or walking.[92] Holmer believed fartlek should be performed in the forest, over undulating terrain. The feeling of release, from running on forest trails, was thought to reduce the perception of fatigue.[3] Even though fartlek is free and unstructured, it can be very rigorous. Fartlek's uninhibited character is diametrically opposed to interval training where the pace, distance run, and the period of recovery are precisely stated. When a fartlek workout contains prescribed distances, pace, and recovery times, it ceases to be fartlek.

Intervals

Designated periods of work followed by rest bouts of a predetermined length describe interval training.[3] The theory behind it holds that a greater volume and intensity of work may be accomplished with less fatigue using interval training, rather than continuous running.[93] Additionally, as opposed to continuous running or fartlek, the precise nature of interval training increases the coach's ability to monitor the volume and intensity of an athlete's program, and therefore to more accurately assess the athlete's progress.

The break between exercise bouts is the focus of interval training, thus the name. Research in Germany during the 1930s by coach and physiologist Waldemar Gerschler and cardiologist Hans Reindell supported their belief that endurance performance was dependent on the size of the heart. Gerschler and Reindell demonstrated that venous return to the heart was found to peak in the first few seconds of recovery immediately following a short bout of exercise, and proposed interval training as a means to increase cardiac volume.[94]

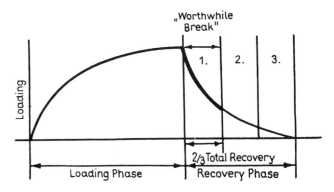

Figure 3–6. Gerschler and Reindell's model for interval training. The next repetition should begin at the end of the worthwhile break. (Reproduced with permission from G Schmolinsky, Basic Elements of Track and Field Training. In: Track and Field: Text-Book for Coaches and Sports Teachers. 1983 p. 57, Sports Books Publisher, Toronto, Ont.).

Gerschler and Reindell also observed 70% of a full recovery took place in the first third of the time necessary for full recovery (Figure 3–6).[2] The first third of a full recovery became known as a worthwhile break. If another exercise bout began immediately after the worthwhile break, the designated exercise rate could be maintained for a considerable period. There would be increasing fatigue with each repetition, but not so much that it required termination of the training session before completion of at least $1\frac{1}{2}$ to 2 times the racing distance. Gerschler and Reindell concluded that the volume and intensity of a workout could be increased without overstressing the athlete if bouts of work were interspersed with rest intervals.[95] Therefore, one of the advantages of interval training is to provide a strong stimulus for adaptation that does not result in complete exhaustion.

An interval training session designed to stress either the aerobic, anaerobic, or combination of the two energy systems may be classified as extensive or intensive. Extensive intervals are by definition high in number and low in intensity, with short rest intervals. Extensive intervals stress the aerobic energy system, with some low-level involvement of anaerobic metabolism, and are especially suited for development of 5000 and 10,000-meter runners. Lactate levels remain low during extensive intervals, though they tend to rise during the course of a training session. Volume rather than intensity is responsible for the fatigue of extensive interval training. The improvement of basic aerobic fitness would be the primary purpose of including extensive intervals in a training program. Early adherents of interval training, such as Vladimir Kuts and Emil Ztopek, were reported to have run up to 90 × 400 meters in a single training session.[96]

Intensive intervals are performed at a higher percentage of work capacity than are extensive intervals. The break between repetitions is directly related to the strenuousness of the exercise. Also, as the speed of the repetitions increases, the volume or quantity must be reduced. Lactate levels are higher following each repetition and at the end of the session than during extensive intervals. Fatigue in intensive interval work is the result of the buildup of hydrogen ions within the muscle, rather than the depletion of muscle and liver glycogen. Intensive interval training improves speed endurance by enhancing the production of anaerobic enzymes, inducing muscle hypertrophy, and increasing buffering capacity. Roger Bannister, as a medical student with limited time to train, used a workout of 10 × 400 meters on a weekly basis prior to his successful attempt to break the 4-minute mile.[97]

Repetitions

Repetitions differ from intervals in terms of density, intensity, and volume. Because the ability to perform repeated, high-intensity work is limited, the time period between each repetition approaches a full recovery of 20 to 30 minutes. Repetitions are performed at speeds equal to or exceeding that of the competition distance. Normally, two to four repetitions constitute a training session. The length of each repetition varies from $^1/_8$ to $^3/_4$ of the competition distance.

Time Trials

Fartlek, interval, and repetition training sessions target specific aerobic and/or anaerobic adaptations. Time trials, on the other hand, simulate the general physiological responses of actual competition. Time trials are most often run at some fraction of the main competition distance, although they are occasionally run at or above the full distance. Time trials allow the athlete to experience the fatigue of the actual event, as well as practice techniques under near-race conditions. They may also be useful in predicting performance and in enhancing the athlete's ability to determine the correct pace. One and rarely two time trials are run during a training session, to duplicate the physiological response to competition.

Strength Training

The principles of strength training will be covered in detail in Chapter 48, so we shall only briefly discuss them here. The function of resistance training is to improve strength and/or anaerobic power.[98] Although resistance training causes hypertrophy, especially in the type II fibers, the greatest strength gains are the result of increased activation and modulation of motor units and improved neuromuscular coordination.[99,100]

Traditional training programs have utilized three workouts per week, with three sets per exercise to increase strength.[32,101] Maintenance of strength gains has been documented using one or two training sessions per week.[102] However, there are some data to indicate the advisability of a nontraditional approach. Hakkinen and Kallinen suggest that reducing the volume of a single strength training session by dividing it into two daily sessions will produce a more powerful training effect.[103] Also, recent research indicates that there is no benefit to the use of three sets over one set in regard to strength gains or muscle hypertrophy.[104] We have previously mentioned the importance of strength training in the sprint events, but there is no consensus as to whether strength training should be used in conjunction with endurance training. Kraemer and colleagues state that a combination of strength and endurance training may result in attenuated strength gains.[105] However, Tanaka and Swensen demonstrated a beneficial effect of strength training on short- and long-term endurance.[98]

Load Characteristics

Training must be of sufficient intensity, duration, volume, or density to interrupt homeostasis and stimulate adaptive changes.[1,2] In order to explain the terms listed above we will use them in a practical example: a training session that includes 10 repetitions of 400 meters, in 65 seconds each, with a 2-minute jogging interval. Stimulus duration refers to the time of each 400-meter repetition, or the total time for all 10. The single stimulus duration is 65 seconds, or 650 seconds for the stimulus duration of the entire training session. A 2-hour run has a stimulus duration of 2 hours. Density is the time relationship between the training stimulus and the recovery period. In our example, the suggested interval between each 400-meter repetition is 2 minutes. The density is approximately 1:2, or for every minute of work, there are 2 minutes of recovery. Stimulus intensity is the percentage of maximal effort elicited by the stimulus. If an athlete is capable of running 400 meters in 50 seconds and has been requested to run each 400 in 65 seconds, the intensity would be 69%. For a 60-second 400 meter runner it would be 92%. Stimulus volume is the total time or distance of all repetitions, or the total time or distance of a continuous effort, in this case 10 × 400 meters or 4000 meters. The 4000-meter total does not include warm-up or warm-down distance or the distance covered during the 2-minute recovery jog between each repetition. If all the additional distance were to be included, the total volume of the training session could exceed 14,000 meters.

Periodization of Training

Periodization is a term used to describe the organization of a comprehensive training plan, one that emphasizes gradual adaptation and the compartmentalization of the various aspects of the training process. The use of periodization in conditioning programs has been highly praised as a means to maximize performance, and to reduce chances for overtraining and injury.[106–108] Verhoshansky argues that periodization is outdated, impractical, and arbitrary.[109] However the principles, if not the name periodization, have been used with great success by Nurmi, Lydiard, Coe, and others over the past 80 years.

Periodization gained prominence as a tool for improving athletic performance after the concept was introduced by Matvyev, who in 1962 divided a training cycle into its various component parts.[3] Those divisions are the training session, microcycle, mesocycle, phase, macrocycle, and annual plan. The following definitions are a compilation of the writings concerning periodization of Schmolinsky,[2] Bompa,[1] and the coaching education division of USA Track and Field.[110]

Training Session

A training session is typically made up of three parts, called the preparatory, main, and concluding portions. The preparatory portion of a training session may include instructions, warm-up, flexibility, and drills. The main portion, or body, of the workout might be composed of a steady-state run, intervals, repetitions, or a time trial, as designated by the coach to accomplish that day's training task. Warm-down including flexibility is the concluding portion. A training session may be made up of several distinct sections, such as the workouts mentioned above, or a single section, as a long run. Each session should be designed to accomplish specific objectives from the training plan.

Microcycle

A microcycle consists of several primary training sessions separated by recovery days. Typically it spans 1 to 2 weeks. Two to three intense sessions may be performed during a week-long microcycle. One to two recovery sessions are scheduled after each intense workout. A well-designed microcycle results in the proper relationship between training and restoration, which ensures accomplishment of the goals set out in the annual plan.

Mesocycle

The next division of the annual plan, a mesocycle, is made up of two or more microcycles and normally lasts between 3 and 6 weeks. The mesocycle allows enough time for training to produce physiological changes, but the relatively short 3- to 6-week period decreases boredom that might result from too much time spent on one activity.[111] A mesocycle is designed to emphasize one aspect of training, such as endurance, speed, or speed endurance. This is not to say that all other components are ignored during the mesocycle, but only that one aspect is stressed.

Phase

A number of mesocycles, arranged to produce specific physiological adaptation, are known as a phase. There are traditionally three phases: preparatory, competition, and transition (Figure 3–7).[1] The preparatory phase may then be subdivided into the general and specific preparatory phase, and the competition phase into the pre- and main competition phase.

Improvement of overall physical fitness is emphasized during the general preparation phase. Development of aerobic endurance, anaerobic endurance, and basic strength take precedence when designing the preparatory phase of the annual plan. One reason to emphasize aerobic endurance in the preparatory phase is that a base of aerobic fitness improves recovery between anaerobic exercise bouts.[112] Normally the preparation phase is the longest of all the phases in the annual plan.[1] The precise length of the preparatory phase depends on the amount of time available before the competition phase and the amount of time necessary to achieve basic fitness. Current research indicates that positive changes in aerobic enzymes, capillary density, and volume and number of mitochondria begin to occur within the first 3 weeks after beginning an endurance training program.[41]

The specific preparatory phase serves as a bridge to connect the general preparatory phase to the competition phase. During the specific preparation phase volume is gradually reduced and intensity gradually increases. There is a greater emphasis on event-specific training, although general fitness is maintained. Even though competition may be weeks away, the improvement of high-quality performance during the specific preparatory phase is stressed.

The precompetitive phase further refines the gains made during the specific preparatory phase. Time trials and off-distance races are often used to predict the athlete's performance capacity and to identify weaknesses that were not apparent in the preparatory phase. The precompetition phase could be used to improve specific fitness or rehearse racing tactics prior to the main competition phase. Races during the precompetition phase test the race readiness of the athlete, but training is still of greater importance during this period and is not reduced to produce peak performance.

The main competition phase emphasizes reduced training volume, maintenance of intensity, and numerous

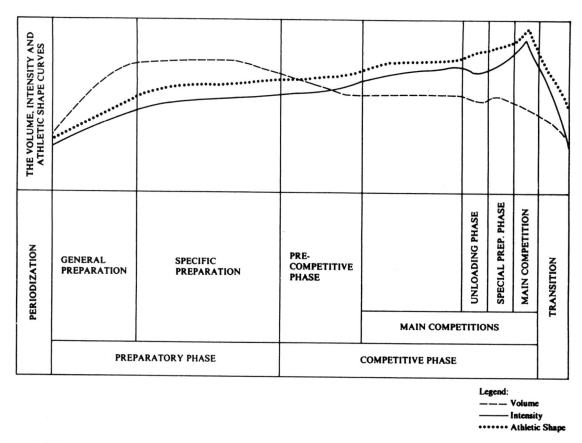

Figure 3–7. The division of the annual plan into preparatory, competition, and transition phases, with volume, intensity, and athletic condition curves. Form of credit: From *Theory and Methodology of Training: The Key to Athletic Performance*, Third Edition by Tudor O. Bompa. Copyright © 1994 by Kendall/Hunt Publishing Company. Used with permission.

competitions. The focus of the main competition phase is a peak performance in the ultimate competition for that season. The races preceding the main competition serve as stepping-stones or means to the end of peak performance. The primary competition may be a state meet, the NCAA championships, the Olympic Trials, the World Championships, or the Olympic Games. The last 2 to 3 weeks before the primary competition may include a reduction in volume, known as a taper, designed to reduce fatigue and allow the physical and mental capabilities of the athlete to be fully energized.

A transition phase follows each main competition phase. The length of time devoted to transition, recovery, or restoration following completion of a macrocycle (see below) varies depending on factors such as health of the athlete, stresses associated with the main competition phase, and amount of time available before the next preparatory phase must begin. The stress of competition is not solely physical, but psychological as well.[113,114] In fact, the negative effects of psychological stress may be more long lasting than physical training stress. There has been a great deal of

research documenting the harmful effects of psychological stress on training and competition.[115,116] The transition phase should be of sufficient length to allow a significant reduction or elimination of those harmful effects.

Macrocycle

Three to four phases make up a macrocycle. A macrocycle includes the buildup to and completion of a competition season, such as the cross-country or outdoor season. Each macrocycle contains at minimum a preparatory phase, a competition phase, and a transition phase. There may be one, two, or three macrocycles per year, each with a main competition phase.

Annual Plan

Planning should include long-term goals such as the 4 years of an Olympiad or the 4 years of college eligibility. The annual plan is designed to complete a portion of the 4-year program. The annual plan for a collegiate middle-distance runner, who may compete in cross-country, indoor track, and outdoor track would contain three full macrocycles. An elite

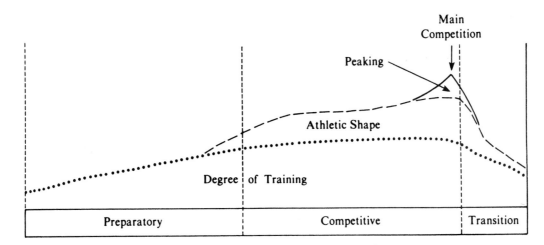

Figure 3–8. An illustration of peaking resulting from increased athletic fitness at the end of the competitive phase. Form of credit: From *Theory and Methodology of Training: The Key to Athletic Performance*, Third Edition by Tudor O. Bompa. Copyright © 1994 by Kendall/Hunt Publishing Company. Used with permission.

middle-distance runner preparing for an international competition such as the World Championships or Olympic Games might have but one complete macrocycle per year. A macrocycle with one main competition phase is known as a monocycle, or single periodization model. An annual plan with two main competition phases is known as a bi-cycle, or double periodization model, and the aforementioned three-competition phase model is a tricycle, or triple periodization model.

Peaking

The purpose of training is to provide the basis for improved performance in competition. Physiological and psychological training designed to produce optimal results on a given day, such as an Olympic final, is known as peaking. A peak occurs when fatigue is low, combined with a high level of physical fitness and emotional arousal (Figure 3–8).[1] Peaking is not solely a reduction in training volume for the few days prior to competition, but is a culmination of physiological and psychological forces, based on fitness, self-confidence, motivation, and an ability to tolerate frustration.[1] Peaking for a major competition actually begins when an athlete first identifies his or her goal. Peaking culminates with a performance at the highest level of the athlete's mental and physical powers.

Tapering, one of the last aspects of a peaking program, is a gradual reduction in training volume leading to an important competition. In a traditional taper, unloading, or a gradual reduction in training volume, begins 2 to 3 weeks prior to the main competition. Intensity remains high throughout the unloading period. The gradual reduction in the volume of work allows fitness to remain at peak levels.[117–119]

CONCLUSION

Adherence to a specific training theory by coaches and athletes is not unlike the allegiance of dieters to the most recent weight-loss fad. Although theories based on magnets, pyramids, and aromatherapy may influence athletes and coaches for a few months or years, sound physiological principles are timeless. If an athlete organizes his or her training around those principles, focuses on long-term goals, and understands how the body responds to training, the likelihood of a successful outcome to training increases dramatically. Adaptation over a period of years to gradually increasing levels of stress is the message to athletes and coaches from theoretical and applied scientists, as well as experienced practitioners of the sport. A lack of knowledge of the adaptation processes, or the desire to find the "secret" for instant success leads to illness, injury, and unfulfilled promise. A need to produce immediate results fosters a mindset that accepts all suggestions and pursues every means for improvement. Those means often include banned substances. When the athlete becomes convinced that "everyone's doing it," or "I have to because I am not as gifted as my competitors," perception becomes reality. This chapter is dedicated to everyone who tried, and is trying, to train and perform within the rules.

REFERENCES

1. Bompa TO: *Theory and Methodology of Training: The Key to Athletic Performance*, 2nd ed., Dubuque, Iowa, Kendall/Hunt, 1990.

2. Schmolinsky G (ed.): *Track and Field: Text-Book for Coaches and Sports Teachers,* 2nd ed., Berlin, Sportverlag, 1983.

3. Doherty K: *Track and Field Omnibook,* 4th ed., Los Altos, Calif, Tafnew Press, 1985.

4. Smith RC, Rutherford OM: The role of metabolites in strength training. I. A comparison of eccentric and concentric contractions. *Eur J Appl Physiol Occup Physiol* 1995:71, 332.

5. Pette D: Training effects on the contractile apparatus. *Acta Physiolo Scand* 1998:162, 367.

6. Karjalainen J, Kujala JM, Stolt A, et al.: Angiotensinogen gene M235T polymorphism predicts left ventricular hypertrophy in endurance athletes. *J Am Coll Cardiol* 1999:34, 494.

7. Thomis MA, Beunen GP, Maes HH, et al.: Strength training: Importance of genetic factors. *Med Sci Sports Exerc* 1998:30, 724.

8. Boushell R, Snell P, Saltin B: Cardiovascular regulation with endurance training, in Saltin B, Boushel R, Secher W, Mitchell J (eds.), *Exercise and Circulation in Health and Disease,* Champaign, Ill, Human Kinetics, 1999:225.

9. Giada F, Bertaglia E, De Piccoli B, et al.: Cardiovascular adaptations to endurance training and detraining in young and older athletes. *Int J Cardiol* 1998:65, 149.

10. Fagard FH: Impact of different sports and training on cardiac structure and function. *Cardiol Clin* 1997:15, 397.

11. Uusitalo AL, Huttunen P, Hanin Y, et al.: Hormonal responses to endurance training and overtraining in female athletes. *Clin J Sport Med* 1998:8, 178.

12. Rodas GF, Calvo M, Estruch A, et al.: Heritability of running economy: A study made on twin brothers. *Eur J Appl Physiol* 1998:77, 511.

13. Malina RM, Beunen G, Wellens R, et al.: Skeletal maturity and body size of teenage Belgian track and field athletes. *Ann Hum Biol* 1986:13, 331.

14. Brown RT, McIntosh SM, Seabolt VR, et al.: Iron status of adolescent female athletes. *J Adolesc Health Care* 1985:6, 349.

15. Hall EG, Davies S: Gender differences in perceived intensity and affect of pain between athletes and nonathletes. *Percept Motor Skills* 1991:73, 779.

16. Kircaldy BD: Performance and circadian rhythms. *Eur J Appl Physiol Occup Physiol* 1984: 52, 375.

17. Moss BM, Refsnes PE, Abildgaard A, et al.: Effects of maximal effort strength training with different loads on dynamic strength, cross-sectional area, load power and load-velocity relationships. *Eur J Appl Physiol Occup Physiol* 1997:75, 193.

18. Griewe JS, Hickner RC, Hansen PA, et al.: Effects of endurance exercise training on muscle glycogen accumulation in humans. *J Appl Physiol* 1999:87, 222.

19. Jones AM: A five year physiological case study of an Olympic runner. *Br J Sports Med* 1998:32, 39.

20. Lehmann M, Foster C, Dickhuth HH, et al.: Anatomical imbalance hypothesis and overtraining syndrome. *Med Sci Sports Exerc* 1998:30, 1140.

21. Princivero DM, Lephart SM, Karunakara RG: Effects of rest interval on isokinetic strength and functional performance after short-term high intensity training. *Br J Sports Med* 1997:31, 229.

22. Kentta G, Hassmen P: Overtraining and recovery. A conceptual model. *Sports Med* 1998:26, 1.

23. McKenzie DC: Markers of excessive exercise. *Can J Appl Physiol* 1999:24, 66.

24. Steenland K, Deddens JA: Effect of travel and rest on performance of professional basketball players. *Sleep* 1997:20, 366.

25. Tiidus PM: Massage and ultrasound as therapeutic modalities in exercise-induced muscle damage. *Can J Appl Physiol* 1999:24, 267.

26. Vasankari T, Kujala U, Sarna S, et al.: Effects of ascorbic acid and carbohydrate ingestion on exercise induced oxidative stress. *J Sports Med Phys Fitness* 1998:38, 281.

27. Mack GW: Recovery after exercise in the heat—factors influencing fluid intake. *Int J Sports Med* 1998:19, S139.

28. Newsholme EA, Blomstrand E, McAndrew N, et al.: Biochemical causes of fatigue and overtraining, in Shephard RJ, Astrand P-O (eds.), *Endurance in Sport.* Boston, Blackwell Scientific, 1992:351.

29. Shepard RJ: Medical surveillance of endurance sport, in Shephard RJ, Astrand P-O (eds.), *Endurance in Sport.* Boston, Blackwell Scientific, 1992:409.

30. Linossier MT, Dormois D, Perier C, et al.: Enzyme adaptations of human skeletal muscle during bicycle short-sprint training and detraining. *Acta Physiol Scand* 1997:161, 439.

31. Madsen K, Pedersen PK, Djurbuus MS, et al.: Effects of detraining on endurance capacity and metabolic changes during prolonged exhaustive exercise. *J Appl Physiol* 1993:75, 1444.

32. Aastrand P-O, Rodahl K: *Textbook of Work Physiology: Physiological Bases of Exercise,* 3rd ed, New York, McGraw-Hill, 1986.

33. Henriksson J: Cellular metabolism and endurance, in Shepard RJ, Astraand P-O (eds.), *Endurance in Sport,* Boston, Blackwell Scientific, 1992:46.

34. Nummela A, Rusko H, Mero A: EMG activities and ground reaction forces during fatigued and nonfatigued sprinting. *Med Sci Sports Exerc* 1994:26, 605.

35. Abernethy PJ, Thayer R, Taylor AW: Acute and chronic response of skeletal muscle to endurance and sprint exercise. *Sports Med* 1990:10, 365.

36. Tabata I, Nishimura K, Kouzaki M, et al.: Effects of moderate-intensity endurance and high-intensity intermittent training on anaerobic capacity and $\dot{V}O_2$max. *Med Sci Sports Exerc* 1996:28, 1327.

37. Edington DW, Edgerton VR: *The Biology of Physical Activity.* Boston, Houghton Mifflin, 1976:8.

38. Hirvonen J, Rehunen S, Rusko H, et al.: Breakdown of high-energy phosphate compounds and lactate accumulation during short supramaximal exercise. *Eur J Appl Physiol Occup Physiol* 1987:56, 253.

39. Bogdanis GC, Nevill ME, Lakomy HK, et al.: Power output and muscle metabolism during and following recovery from 10 and 20 s of maximal sprint exercise in humans. *Acta Physiol Scand* 1998:163, 261.

40. Brooks GA, Fahey TD (eds.): *Exercise Physiology: Human Bioenergetics and Its Applications,* New York, John Wiley & Sons, 1984.

41. Green HJ: Mechanisms of muscle fatigue in intense exercise. *J Sports Sci* 1996:15, 247.

42. Newsholme EA: Application of principles of metabolic control to the problem of metabolic limitations in sprinting, middle distance, and marathon running. *Int J Sports Med* 1986:7, 66.

43. Layzer RB: Muscle metabolism during fatigue and work. *Baillieres Clin Endocrinol Metab* 1990:4, 441.

44. Miller RG, Boska MD, Moussavi RS, et al.: 31P nuclear magnetic resonance studies of high energy phosphates and pH in human muscle fatigue. Comparison of aerobic and anaerobic exercise. *J Clin Invest* 1988:81, 1190.

45. Guyton A: *Textbook of Medical Physiology,* 9th ed., Philadelphia, Saunders, 1995.

46. Romjin JA, Coyle EF, Sidossis LS, et al.: Regulation of endogenous fat and carbohydrate metabolism in relation to exercise intensity and duration. *Am J Physiol* 1993:265, E380.

47. Sidossis LS, Wolfe RR, Coggan AR: Regulation of fatty acid oxidation in untrained vs. trained men during exercise. *Am J Physiol* 1998:274, E510.

48. Essen B: Intramuscular substrate utilization during prolonged exercise, in Milvy P (ed.), *The Marathon: Physiological, Medical, Epidemiological, and Psychological Studies.* New York, *Ann NY Acad Sci* 1977:30, 301.

49. Snyder AC: Overtraining and glycogen depletion hypothesis. *Med Sci Sports Exerc* 1998:30, 1146.

50. Grandjean AC, Ruud JS: Nutrition for cyclists. *Clin Sports Med* 1994:13, 235.

51. Friedman JE, Neufer PD, Dohm GL: Regulation of glycogen synthesis following exercise. Dietary considerations. *Sports Med* 1991:11, 232.

52. Winckler G, O'Donnell K, Seagrave L, et al.: Sprints, hurdles, relays. USATF Level II Coaching Education Program, 1992.

53. Meckel Y, Atterbom H, Grodjinovosky A, et al.: Physiological characteristics of female 100 meter sprinters of different performance levels. *J Sports Med Phys Fitness* 1995:35, 169.

54. Mero A, Komi PV, Gregor RJ: Biomechanics of sprint running. A review. *Sports Med* 1992:13, 376.

55. Kersting UG: Biomechanical analysis of the sprinting events, in Bruggemann G-P, Koszewski D, Muller H (eds.), *Biomechanical Research Project Athens 1997.* Oxford, Meyer & Meyer Sport, 1999:13.

56. Bentley S: Exercise-induced muscle cramp. Proposed mechanisms and management. *Sports Med* 1996:21, 409.

57. Young W, McLean B, Ardagna J: Relationships between strength qualities and sprinting performance. *J Sports Med Phys Fitness* 1995:35, 13.

58. Mann R: Elite Sprint-Hurdle Olympic Development Clinic, Orlando, Fla, December 12–17, 1996.

59. Delecluse C, Van Coppenolle H, Willems E, et al.: Influence of high-resistance and high-velocity training on sprint performance. *Med Sci Sports Exerc* 1995:27, 1203.

60. El-Sayed MS: Effects of exercise and training on blood rheology. *Sports Med* 1998:26, 281.

61. Li K, Lu S: Study on adaptive changes of myocardial ultrastructure after endurance training at different intensities in rats. *Chung-Kuo Ying Yung Sheng Li Hsueh Tsa Chih* 1997:13, 193.

62. Powers S, Steben RE: Shifting the anaerobic threshold in distance runners, in Gambetta, V (ed.), *Track Technique Annual '83,* Los Altos, Calif, Tafnews Press, 1982.

63. Richter EA, Kristiansen S, Wojtaszewski J, et al.: Training effects on muscle glucose transport during exercise. *Adv Exper Med Biol* 1998:441, 107.

64. Azevedo JL Jr, Lindeman JK, Lehman SL, et al.: Training decreases muscle glycogen turnover during exercise. *Eur J Appl Physiol Occup Physiol* 1998:78, 479.

65. Holloszy JO, Kohrt WM, Hansen PA: The regulation of carbohydrate and fat metabolism during and after exercise. *Frontiers Biosci* 1998:3, D1011.

66. Kiens B: Training and fatty acid metabolism. *Adv Exp Med Biol* 1998:441, 229.

67. Billat V, Renoux JC, Pinoteau J, et al.: Times to exhaustion at 90, 100 and 105% of velocity at $\dot{V}o_2max$ (maximal aerobic speed) and critical speed in elite long-distance runners. *Arch Physiol Biochem* 1995:103, 129.

68. Cahill BR, Misner JE, Boileau RA: The clinical importance of the anaerobic energy system and its assessment in human performance. *Am J Sports Med* 1997:25, 863.

69. Stewart IB, Sleivert GG: The effect of warm-up intensity on range of motion and anaerobic performance. *J Orthopaed Sports Phys Therapy* 1998:27, 154.

70. Bhattacharya AK, Panda BK, Das Gupta PK: Pattern of venous lactate and pyruvate after submaximal exercise in athletes training in different disciplines. *Int J Sports Med* 1983:4, 252.

71. Harris RC, Edwards RHT, Hultman L-O, et al.: The time course of phosphorylcreatine resynthesis during recovery of the quadriceps muscle in man. *Pflugers Archiv: Eur J Physiol* 1976:367, 137.

72. Takahashi T, Miyamoto Y: Influence of light physical activity on cardiac responses during recovery from exercise in humans. *Eur J Appl Physiol Occup Physiol* 1998:77, 305.

73. Faye J, Cisse F, Manga M: An attempt to analyse the recovery mode effects on heart rate and performance in a series of 400 meter flat race. *Dakar Med* 1993:38, 11.

74. Stojnik V, Komi PV: Neuromuscular fatigue after maximal stretch-shortening cycle exercise. *J Appl Physiol* 1998:84, 344.

75. Hakkinen K, Kallinen M: Distribution of strength training volume into one or two daily sessions and neuromuscular adaptations in female athletes. *Electromyog Clin Neurophysiol* 1994:34, 117.

76. Gisolfi CV, Duchman SM: Guidelines for optimal replacement beverages for different athletic events. *Med Sci Sports Exerc* 1992:24, 679.

77. Viru A: Some facts about the construction of microcycles in training, in Jarver J (ed.), *Middle Distances: Contemporary Theory, Technique and Training,* Los Altos, Calif, Tafnews Press, 1991:15.

78. Krivickas LS, Feinburg JH: Lower extremity injuries in college athletes: Relation between ligamentous laxity and lower extremity muscle tightness. *Arch Phys Med Rehabil* 1996:77, 1139.

79. Garrett WE Jr: Muscle strain injuries. *Am J Sports Med* 1996:24, S2.

80. Jones BH, Cowan DN, Knapik JJ: Exercise training and injuries. *Sports Med* 1994:18, 202.

81. Bennell KL, Crossley K: Musculoskeletal injuries in track and field: Incidence, distribution and risk factors. *Aust J Sci Med Sport* 1996:28, 69.

82. Gleim GW, McHugh MP: Flexibility and its effects on sports injury and performance. *Sports Med* 1997:24, 289.

83. Orchard J, Marsden J, Lord S: Preseason hamstring muscle weakness associated with hamstring muscle injury in Australian footballers. *Am J Sports Med* 1997: 25, 81.

84. Twellaar M, Verstappen FT, Huson A, et al.: Physical characteristics as risk factors for sports injuries: A four year prospective study. *Int J Sports Med* 1997:18, 66.

85. Fredericson M: Common injuries in runners: Diagnosis, rehabilitation and prevention. *Sports Med* 1996:21, 49.

86. Hebbelinck M: Flexibility, in Dirix H, Knuttgen G, Tittel K (eds.), *The Olympic Book of Sports Medicine,* London, Blackwell Scientific, 1988:212.

87. Craib MW, Mitchell VA, Fields KB, et al.: The association between flexibility and running economy in sub-elite male distance runners. *Med Sci Sports Exerc* 1996:28, 737.

88. Noonan TJ, Garrett WF Jr: Muscle strain injury: Diagnosis and treatment. *J Am Acad Orthop Surg* 1999:7, 262.

89. Clanton TO, Coupe KJ: Hamstring strains in athletes: Diagnosis and treatment. *J Am Acad Orthop Surg* 1998:6, 237.

90. Rostrup M, Westheim A, Refsum HE, et al.: Arterial and venous plasma catecholamines during submaximal steady-state exercise. *Clin Physiol* 1998:18, 109.

91. Svedenhag J: Endurance conditioning, in Shephard RJ, Astrand PO (eds.), *Endurance in Sport,* Boston, Blackwell Scientific, 1992:290.

92. Down MG: Interval training: An appraisal of work-rest cycle applications to training for endurance running. Masters thesis, Loughborough University, 1966.

93. Fisher AG, Jensen CR: *Scientific Basis of Athletic Conditioning,* 3rd ed., Philadelphia, Lea & Febiger, 1990.

94. Nett T: Examination of interval training, in Wilt F (ed.), *Run Run Run,* Los Altos, Calif, 1964:197.

95. Sprecher P: Visit with Dr. Woldemar Gerschler, in Wilt F (ed.), *Run Run Run,* Los Altos, Calif, 1964:150.

96. Nelson C: *Track & Field: The Great Ones,* London, Michael Joseph Ltd., 1970.

97. Bannister R: *The Four-Minute Mile,* New York, Lyons & Burford, 1989.

98. Tanaka H, Swensen T: Impact of resistance training on endurance performance. A new form of cross-training. *Sports Med* 1998:25, 191.

99. Henriksson J, Tesch P: Current knowledge on muscle training: Endurance and strength yield complementary effects. *Lakartidningen* 1999:96, 56.

100. Ozmun JC, Mikesky AE, Surburg PR: Neuromuscular adaptations following prepubescent strength training. *Med Sci Sports Exerc* 1994:26, 510.

101. Klausen K: Strength and weight-training, in Reilly T, Secher N, Snell P, Williams C (eds.), *Physiology of Sports,* New York, E & FN Spoon, 1990:41.

102. Bell GJ, Syrotuik DG, Attwood K, et al.: Maintenance of strength gains while performing endurance training in oarswomen. *Can J Appl Physiol* 1993:18, 104.

103. Hakkinen K, Kallinen M: Distribution of strength training volume into one or two daily sessions and neuromuscular adaptations in female athletes. *Electromyog Clin Neurophysiol* 1994:34, 117.

104. Carpinelli RN, Otto RM: Strength training. Single versus multiple sets. *Sports Med* 1998:26, 73.

105. Kraemer WJ, Patton JF, Gordon SE, et al.: Compatibility of high-intensity strength and endurance training on hormonal and skeletal muscle adaptations. *J Appl Physiol* 1995:78, 976.

106. Stone MH: Muscle conditioning and muscle injuries. *Med Sci Sports Exerc* 1990:22, 457.

107. Kibler WB, Chandler, TJ: Sports specific conditioning. *Am J Sports Med* 1994:22, 424.

108. Stone WJ, Steingard PM: Year-round conditioning for basketball. *Clin Sports Med* 1993:12, 173.

109. Verhoshansky Y: The end of periodization in high performance sport. *Track Coach* 1999:148, 4737.

110. Freeman W, Vaughan R, Gambetta V: USATF Level II Training Theory, 1999.

111. Dawson B, Fitzsimmons M, Green S, et al.: Changes in performance, muscle metabolites, enzymes and fiber types after short sprint training. *Eur J Appl Physiol Occup Physiol* 1998:78, 163.

112. McMahon S, Wenger HA: The relationship between aerobic fitness and both power output and subsequent recovery during maximal intermittent exercise. *J Sci Med Sport* 1998:1, 219.

113. Kentta G, Hassmen P: Overtraining and recovery. A conceptual model. *Sports Med* 1998:26, 1.

114. Kuipers H: Training and overtraining: An introduction. *Med Sci Sports Exerc* 1998:30, 1137.

115. McKenzie DC: Markers of excessive exercise. *Can J Appl Physiol* 1999:24, 66.

116. Shepard RJ, Shek PN: Acute and chronic over-exertion: Do depressed immune responses provide useful markers? *Int J Sports Med* 1998:19, 159.

117. Mujika I: The influence of training characteristics and tapering on the adaptation of highly trained individuals: A review. *Int J Sports Med* 1998:19, 439.

118. Houmard JA, Kirwan JP, Flynn MG, et al.: Effects of reduced training on submaximal and maximal running responses. *Int J Sports Med* 1989:10, 30.

119. Morgan WP, Brown DR, Raglin JS, et al.: Psychological monitoring of overtraining and staleness. *Br J Sports Med* 1987:21, 107.

Chapter 4

TENDINOSIS AND TENDON INJURY

Barry S. Kraushaar and Robert Nirschl

INTRODUCTION

The treatment of athletic tendon injuries depends upon an understanding of the structure and normal behavior of tendon tissue. When tendon is injured, various events occur to determine the ultimate outcome, which is self-resolution, rehabilitative resolution, or failure to heal. Failed tendon healing may best be avoided when the treating physician understands the nature of the injury and then applies the appropriate treatment plan based upon sound rehabilitative principles. Specifically, it is important to remember that not all tendon pain is "tendinitis," and in fact many tendon injuries are actually best called *tendinosis*.[4,8] This chapter discusses the properties of normal and abnormal tendon tissue and the factors that relate to the healing process.

NORMAL TENDON

Anatomy

Tendons form the strong fibrous linkage between fleshy muscle tissue and rigid bone. This brilliant white material is capable of bending with minimal elongation and no contractility. The structural components of tendon are well documented. Tendon is composed primarily of Type I collagen organized into fibrils surrounded by parietal paratenon, which make up fibers surrounded by endotenon, which become bundles that make up the overall tendon contained in a sheath or epitenon-type covering.[10]

Tendons derive their blood supply from capillaries that penetrate the sheath that surrounds the individual fascicles (epitenon and endotenon, but not the parietal paratenon). The individual fascicles normally do not contain vascular structures or nerve endings.

Microscopy

Tendons are composed of collagen, matrix (proteoglycans, glycosaminoglycans, water), and fibroblast cells. In summary, the basic composition of normal tendon fascicles are fibers organized into long parallel strands, matrix that acts as a ground substance, and sparsely distributed inactive fibroblast cells that are capable of monitoring local tendon health. The fibroblast cell is capable of producing and repairing collagen and matrix, affording a form of regional maintenance to the tendon (Figure 4–1).

TENDON INJURY

Vulnerable Tendon Types

There is an increased chance of injury in tendons that belong to a muscle-tendon unit crossing two or more joints. For example, the quadriceps originates on the pelvis, crosses the hip, and crosses the knee before inserting on the tibia. Tendons that pass over a convex

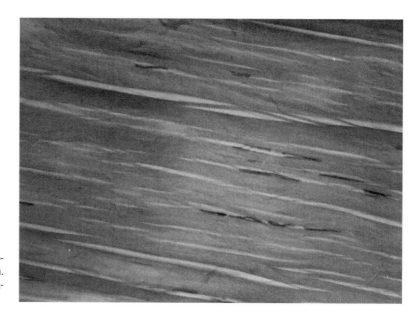

Figure 4–1. Normal tendon. Inactive fibroblasts between parallel bundles of collagen. No blood vessels are present within the matrix (hematoxylin and eosin, ×100).

surface are also at higher risk, as is seen with the rotator cuff that is draped over the head of the humerus near its insertion. When these tendons are exposed to the high straining forces of eccentric contractions, internal structural damage may occur. Tendons involved in locomotion and ballistic performance (throwing) are susceptible to injury[5,6,10] (Table 4–1).

The Achilles' tendon is particularly vulnerable to injury because it is a tendon of locomotion, belongs to a muscle-tendon group that crosses two joints (the gastrocnemius originates on the distal femur and inserts onto the calcaneus), and is exposed to repetitive eccentric contractions. There is a watershed area of poor blood supply in the Achilles' tendon just proximal to its insertion on the calcaneus.

Mechanism of Injury

Tendon injury can be divided conceptually into three categories: acute trauma, chronic overuse injury, and trauma superimposed upon repetitive overuse.

Acute trauma is an event that suddenly causes serious damage to previously normal tendon. An example is laceration of any tendon by a sharp object, transecting the tendon and its surrounding tissues. This causes obvious bleeding and mechanical disruption of tendon and peritendinous structures. As a result, the body's wound healing response pathway is activated. A well-documented series of events divided into four stages follows: clotting, inflammation, proliferation, and remodeling. These stages are described below (see section on Tendon Healing).

TABLE 4–1. TENDONS VULNERABLE TO INJURY

	Crosses 2 Joints	Convex Surface	Ballistic/ locomotion
Wrist extensors	Elbow, wrist	Radial head	Ballistic
Wrist flexors	Elbow, wrist		Ballistic
Rotator cuff		Humeral head	Ballistic
Scapular muscles			Ballistic
Lumbosacral muscles			Locomotion
Quadriceps origin	Hip, knee		Locomotion
Iliotibial band	Hip, knee	Hip greater trochanter	Locomotion
Hip adductors			Locomotion
Hamstrings	Hip, knee	Medial tibia	Locomotion
Patellar tendon		Patella	Locomotion
Achilles' tendon	Knee, ankle	Calcaneus	Locomotion
Plantar fascia	Multiple foot		Locomotion
Posterior tibial tendon	Ankle, subtalar, tarsometatarsal	Medial malleolus	Locomotion
Peroneal tendons	Ankle, subtalar, tarsometatarsal	Lateral malleolus	Locomotion

Chronic overuse injury refers to repetitive events that result in cumulative damage to the tendon. Forces that overcome the ability of tendon to withstand tension cause internal microtears of the collagen matrix. Even lower-intensity forces can cause damage when they are repeated without rest long enough to generate heat damage within the tendon. Overuse injury does not result in mechanical failure of the tendon, but internally the tendon loses some efficiency in force load transmission. Overuse injuries may not result in internal tendon bleeding because blood vessels are not disrupted. Examples are tennis elbow and Achilles' tendinosis.

Trauma superimposed upon repetitive overuse occurs when previous overuse has created internal damage to the integrity of collagen fibers, and then a sudden overload event occurs which results in traumatic disruption of the tendon. This causes regional bleeding and often separation of tendon fibers. An example is rupture of the Achilles' tendon, which has been shown to usually contain evidence of preexistent tendinosis at the time of sudden rupture.[4-6,8]

Degrees of Disruption

Structurally, tendons may be thought of as a form of bundled rope enclosed in a sheath. *Microscopic* tendon damage is analogous to fraying of the rope within the tendon sheath. Unlike rope, human tendon is capable of a healing response, and if the fraying of collagen is mild, a local response by fibroblast cells already present within the tendon is often enough for self-healing. The fibroblasts are capable of producing all the materials necessary for minor repairs, and the same cells direct the remodeling and cross-linking of minimally injured tendon.

Full thickness tearing of a tendon involves the entire rope and sheath. Disruption of the tendon sheath causes bleeding which incites the body to activate a complete inflammatory healing response. Unfortunately, full tendon rupture usually results in retraction of the torn ends and a gap that may be impossible to bridge without surgical reattachment.

Partial thickness tendon tears are ruptures of some but not all of the bundles of tendon. The tendon sheath may be torn as well, but it may also remain intact. If the tendon sheath is torn local bleeding occurs, and in this case the tendon ends do not retract very far because the remaining intact bundles prevent separation. The tendon may heal through the cascade of events described below. However, if the tendon sheath is not torn and a partial thickness tendon tear occurs, the only source of scar tissue is from fibroblasts residing in the torn tendon. These fibroblast cells are able to manufacture collagen but are unable to remodel the

material produced over large gaps. Instead of good quality tendon, an unhealthy scar is produced. This material is called *tendinosis* and represents a failed healing process.

TENDON HEALING

Extrinsic Healing

When a tendon is lacerated or surgically divided, the tendon sheath is injured, and bleeding accompanies damage to the collagen bundles. The series of events that follow such trauma are well documented.[1,5,6,10] There are four phases of normal tendon healing:

1. *Clot formation:* Local bleeding forms a blood clot. The clot becomes firm and rubbery, providing a scaffold for further healing and a structure that retains needed healing elements in the injured area. Importantly, the clot contains strong chemical attractants for the body's immune system to activate a true inflammatory response.
2. *Inflammation:* The immune system mediates the increased cellular activity in the region. Removal of debris and recruitment of mesenchymal cells to the region is well coordinated. Local warmth, erythema, and swelling are a reflection of the increased local metabolic activity in the inflammatory stage. During this stage there are numerous lymphocytes, neutrophils, and macrophages present.
3. *Proliferation:* Eventually fibroblast cells from the clot matrix and inflammatory recruitment begin to predominate. These cells produce collagen and ground substance in order to establish a fundamental structure that is capable of withstanding some tensile load.
4. *Remodeling:* This stage is controlled by the fibroblasts present in the repairing tissue, rather than by the immune system. Collagen crosslinking and the proper geometric orientation of collagen are optimized. Tensile forces in the tendon are sensed by mechanoreceptors in the fibroblasts which arrange collagen longitudinally in order to resist tension, giving greater structural and mechanical integrity to the tissue.

Intrinsic Healing

When a tendon is minimally damaged internally, the tendon sheath may not rupture and there may be no associated bleeding. Internal tendon damage results in the disruption of collagen fibrils and their cross-links with other fibrils. Cleavage planes between parallel bundles have been observed microscopically. The tenocytes (inactive fibroblasts) within the tendon at the site of microscopic damage have long cytoplasmic projections within the tendon. These cells and their stellate projections are able to monitor tendon disruption, and to respond with a collagen proliferation response. Microscopic damage and self-healing by local fibroblast response is probably the most common reason for self-limited tendon pain which is known an *tendinitis*. Tenocytes are capable of becoming active fibroblasts that secrete collagen, coordinate the remodeling process, and then become quiescent cells again after the healing process is complete (Figure 4–2).

Remodeling of microscopic tendon injury is dependent upon the same factors as remodeling of traumatic tendon lacerations. Avoidance of reinjury during the healing process is important. This means protection not only from sudden, intense forces, but also from repetitive low-demand motions. It is also important to avoid complete immobilization of tendon in the remodeling phase because tendon cross-linking is oriented to optimally resist tensile forces. The well-known Wolff's Law of Bone (increased strength in response to increased demand) applies to tendons, as long as the demands do not overcome the tensile strength of the tendon (Wolff's Law of Tendon).[1]

Failed Healing: Tendinosis

It is unnecessary for a health care practitioner to intervene in tendon injuries that resolve quickly by themselves. On the other hand most complete tendon ruptures and lacerations will require the help of someone capable of managing the repair process. Between

TABLE 4–2. REPORTED HISTOPATHOLOGIC FEATURES OF TENDINOSIS*
Hemorrhage
Histiocytes ± lipid
Fibrinoid degeneration
Hyaline degeneration
Vascular proliferation
Fibroblastic proliferation
Granulation tissue in subtendinous space
Necrosis of tendon fascicles
Calcific debris
Crystalline debris
Cellular infiltrate
Polymorphonuclear leukocytes
Lymphocytes

Source: Regan et al. 1992

these two extremes lies a population of athletes with tendon injuries that take unbearably long to resolve, and may never heal normally. The practitioner needs to understand the underlying pathology of failed tendon healing, known as tendinosis.[7]

When a tendon suffers a partial thickness tear that does not disrupt the outer sheath, the internally torn structure is required to heal by a local response. The proliferation of local tendon cells in a damaged region of tendon is densely populated with metabolically active mesenchymal cells including activated fibroblasts, vascular endothelial cells, fat cells, and the products of these cells (Table 4–2). It is speculated that tenocytes residing quiescently in normal tendon are capable of dedifferentiating into other types of mesenchymal cells.

Nirschl termed the abnormal finding of primitive vascular structures and dense fibroblast populations

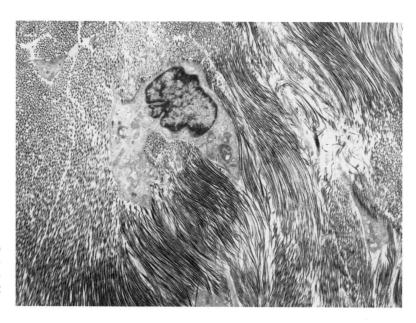

Figure 4–2. Normal fibroblast. Stellate shape, condensed nucleus, quiescent cytoplasm, and an organized surrounding collagen matrix characterize the tendon fibroblast (electron microscope, ×5130).

angiofibroblastic hyperplasia, more commonly known as tendinosis.[7] Notably absent from tendinosis are cells derived from hematopoietic cell lines, such as lymphocytes, neutrophils, macrophages, plasma cells, basophils, eosinophils, mast cells, megakaryocytes, and monocytes. Without a true inflammatory response, a torn tendon must either bridge a torn region and remodel the material internally or it is destined to fail the healing process. The result of failed healing is a poor quality scar that contains debris, tendinosis, unremodeled ground substance, disorganized collagen fragments, and chemical remnants.[4–6]

Macroscopically, tendinosis material appears dull and gray in comparison to normal tendon, which is bright white. The abnormal scar tissue appears edematous and amorphous, lacking the typical striped pattern of healthy tendon. Microscopically, tendinosis appears as patches of cellular density with swirls of fibroblasts and vessel lumens (Figure 4–3). Under the electron microscope, tendinosis appears as a field of debris containing unconnected collagen strands and fragments of material without a pattern of tendon structure.

The same tendinosis appearance is seen in tennis elbow, Achilles' tendinosis, partial thickness rotator cuff tears, and all of the aforementioned areas that are vulnerable to tendon injury. The common themes are repetitive reinjury, vulnerable anatomy, a poor environment for self-repair, and possibly iatrogenic harm by injudicious use of cortisone injections. Cortisone damages tendons by disrupting the beneficial inflammatory healing process, pressurizing fluid into the tendon, and possibly directly harming remaining tendon quality. Nirschl described the predisposition that some

patients have for acquiring multiple areas of tendinosis as *mesenchymal syndrome*.[3,4,6,7]

CONSEQUENCES OF FAILED TENDON HEALING

Internal Tendon Dysfunction

If a tendon is torn and retracted, or if it is torn and has developed tendinosis in the injured region, the function of the tendon is altered. The role of a tendon is to transmit forces between bone and muscle. This function requires a highly organized cross-linkage system between collagen strands, and the tendon continually repairs and remodels itself to maintain its mechanical strength and force-directing ability. Injured tendon tissue does not resist tension well. This causes the tensile forces to be magnified in the remaining uninjured portion of tendon. Eventually uninjured tendon may be damaged by exposure to increased demands. At some point the demands on the remaining tendon result in catastrophic failure and tendon rupture. This concept is supported by reports that approximately two-thirds of acute ruptures of the Achilles' tendon are associated with histologic evidence of chronic pathologic changes within the tendon.[2,3]

Even if tendon with internal tendinosis damage does not progress to rupture, force transmission is compromised by painful inhibition of its corresponding muscle. It is not clear why tendinosis is painful. Histologic analysis does not reveal any increase in pain receptors in the tissue. It is possible that the chemicals in tendinosis tissue that are as yet unknown

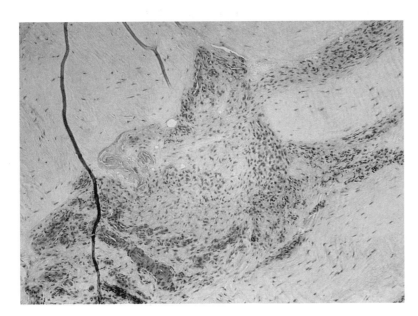

Figure 4–3. Tendinosis contains rudimentary vascular structures, nests of fibroblast hyperplasia, and a disorganized collagen matrix (elastin, ×40).

are irritating. Although tendinosis contains angiomatous hyperplasia, these channels are not proven to be true vascular channels, and tendinosis is functionally avascular. Local anoxia might explain the pain of tendinosis, which Nirschl has called the "heart attack of tendon."[4,6]

Disruption of the Kinetic Chain

Pain inhibition of a muscle-tendon unit will result in the interruption of function of a segment of the kinetic chain. This translates into disruption of normal movement patterns and can result in an abnormal gait, change in posture, altered arm swing, and other forms of unconscious avoidance of pain. With time, regional weakness may occur, and secondary injuries appear. If a tendon is chronically painful, the athlete may eventually decrease his running mileage and eventually lose global strength, endurance, and aerobic capacity. If chronic tendon pain causes cessation of tendon use, the tendon will be unable to remodel properly and a cycle of tendon failure continues.

TRUE INFLAMMATION

This chapter emphasizes tendinosis because this term best represents the usual pathology found in microscopic studies of injured tendons. A region of true inflammation may occur without tendinosis or it may accompany tendinosis. In the period immediately following a tendon injury the initial physiologic response may in fact be a true inflammation of the region. The paratenon that surrounds tendon is richly vascularized, and can develop paratenonitis. When tendon courses around a bony prominence, bursitis (i.e., retrocalcaneal, prepatellar, hip trochanteric, and subacromial bursitis) may arise, even in the absence of tendinosis. When pain occurs close to a joint, various forms of arthritis are to be suspected. Pain that develops in muscle mass may represent injury or pathology of that muscle that is unrelated to tendon injury. Tendinosis is usually swollen and tender, but generally lacks the increased warmth and erythema associated with true inflammation. An MRI may be useful when intratendinous and peritendinous pathology are hard to separate.

TREATMENT PRINCIPLES

The main goals of the treatment of tendinosis are the control of pain; preservation of motion, flexibility, and strength; and the development of endurance over time.[4,6,7]

Pain Control

Oral medications such as nonsteroidal anti-inflammatory drugs or COX-2 inhibitors are used for their analgesic properties and to treat the component of injury that may be true inflammation. Cortisone injections into tendon are not recommended but specific sites of bursitis and paratenonitis sometimes require injection. Ice, topical analgesics, electrical stimulation, ultrasound, and cortisone modalities (ionto- and phonophoresis) are various examples of pain-control interventions.

Rehabilitative Exercise

The actual reversal of tendinosis damage requires the development of strength, flexibility, and endurance. These properties are the result of resistive exercise, stretching, and gradually increasing aerobic activities. Rehabilitation is aimed at realigning the collagen of tendinosis during the remodeling phase of healing. The exercise program should not exceed the tendon's capacity to resist force, but light resistive exercise is more beneficial to tendon remodeling than complete rest.

Rehabilitation works to restore functional control of the injured muscle-tendon unit. Ultimately, the injured functional segment is reincorporated into the series of muscle firings that constitute the kinetic chain. For example, the treatment of patellar tendinosis ultimately involves restoring the appropriate release/contraction cycle that the quadriceps shares with the hamstrings. These two muscle groups must participate properly in the whole series of events that make up the gait cycle.

Avoidance of Reinjury

If tendinosis is the result of sudden or accumulated tendon overuse, then avoidance of reinjury is achieved by correcting the original problems of technique, intensity, and frequency of activities. Bracing or orthotics are used to help protect reinjury. An athlete's goal should be well-balanced strength and flexibility. It is generally accepted that painful warning signs should be heeded rather than ignored.

Surgery

When noninvasive measures fail to resolve the unhealthy, abnormal scar tissue of tendinosis, surgical inspection and resection may be the only remaining option. The decision to operate is usually the last resort after the physician and patient have shared a full historical review of the problem and a thorough physical examination. Studies such as x-rays and MRI are commonly part of the evaluation process. When a course of quality rehabilitation (not just palliative measures) is unsuccessful, surgery is indicated with the specific purpose of removing damaged tissue, assessing the quality of remaining tissues, and repairing them if they require reconstruction or augmentation.

REFERENCES

1. Amadio PC: Tendon and ligament, in *Wound Healing: Biomechanical and Clinical Aspects,* Cohen IK, Diegelman RF, Lindblad WJ (eds.), Philadelphia, Saunders, 1992:384.
2. Jozsa LG, Kannus P (eds.): Overuse injuries in tendons, in *Human Tendons: Anatomy, Physiology, and Pathology,* Champaign, Ill, Human Kinetics, 1997:253.
3. Kannus P, Jozsa L: Histopathological changes preceding spontaneous rupture of a tendon. A controlled study of 891 patients. *J Bone Joint Surg* 1991:73-A, 1507.
4. Kraushaar BS, Nirschl RP: Tendinosis of the elbow (tennis elbow). *J Bone Joint Surg* 1999:81A, 259.
5. Leadbetter, WB: Cell-matrix response in tendon injury. *Clin Sports Med* 1992:11, 533.
6. Nirschl RP: Patterns of failed tendon healing in tendon injury, in *Sports-Induced Inflammation: Clinical and Basic Science Concepts,* Leadbetter WB, Buckwalter JA, Gordon SL (eds.), Park Ridge, Ill, American Academy of Orthopedic Surgeons, 1990:609.
7. Nirschl RP, Pettrone FA: Tennis elbow. The surgical treatment of lateral epicondylitis. *J Bone Joint Surg* 1979:61-A, 832.
8. Puddu G, Ippolito E, Postacchini F: A classification of Achilles tendon disease. *Am J Sports Med* 1976:145, 150.
9. Regan W, Wold LE, Coonrad R, Morrey BF: Microscopic histopathology of chronic refractory lateral epicondylitis. *Am J Sports Med* 1992:20, 746.
10. Woo S L-Y, An K-N, Arnoczky SP, et al.: Anatomy, biology, and biomechanics of tendon, ligament, and meniscus, in *Orthopedic Basic Science,* Simon SR (ed.), Rosemont, Ill, American Academy of Orthopedic Surgeons, 1994:45.

Part II

EVALUATION OF THE RUNNER

Chapter 5

EVALUATION OF THE INJURED RUNNER

Robert P. Wilder and
Francis G. O'Connor

INTRODUCTION

Evaluation of the injured runner emphasizes the identification of intrinsic and extrinsic risk factors, in addition to establishing an injury-specific diagnosis. The history attempts to identify changes in the training regimen or technique that might have contributed to injury. The physical examination includes a biomechanical screening to identify related imbalances in posture, alignment, strength, and/or flexibility. Additionally, each runner is observed walking and running, as running is a dynamic activity. Subtle abnormalities not evident on static or open-chain examination may become evident on dynamic evaluation. This comprehensive, running-specific approach to diagnosis will assist the clinician in developing optimum rehabilitation programs.

ETIOLOGY OF RUNNING INJURIES

Most running-related injuries are caused by overuse. Overuse injuries result from repetitive microtrauma that leads to inflammation and/or local tissue damage in the form of cellular and extracellular degeneration. This tissue damage is cumulative, resulting in tendinitis and/or tendinosis, stress fracture, joint synovitis, ligamentous strains, and/or muscle myositis. Running overuse injuries are multifactorial in origin, with numerous contributing risk factors. Predisposing risk factors have intrinsic or extrinsic causes (Table 5–1).[1]

Intrinsic risk factors represent biomechanical abnormalities unique to the individual athlete. Running necessitates a single-leg support phase that accentuates biomechanical abnormalities. In addition, it has been estimated that running places three to eight times the weight of the body on the lower extremity.[2] Subtle abnormalities or variations in normal anatomy, which may have no clinical significance during walking, may lead to abnormal stress concentrations, with subsequent injury during running. Accordingly, functional asymmetries, muscular imbalance and inflexibility patterns, malalignment, and poor foot mechanics can all potentially lead to injury.[3]

Extrinsic risk factors represent the most common cause of running injuries. Commonly cited areas of concern include improper equipment, poor technique, inadequate running surfaces, and a hostile training environment. Running shoes assist in preventing injuries by providing the athlete with good rear foot stability and shock absorption. Running surfaces vary in their pitch and shock-absorbing capacity, uniquely contributing to running injuries. Training errors,

TABLE 5–1. RISK FACTORS THAT CONTRIBUTE TO OVERUSE INJURIES

Intrinsic	Extrinsic
Malalignment	Training errors
Muscle imbalance	Equipment
Inflexibility	Environment
Muscle weakness	Technique
Instability	Sports-imposed deficiencies

however, are consistently identified as the most important predisposing element to injury.[1,4–6]

Training errors include a number of factors such as inadequate warm-up, lack of stretching before and after running, and/or repetitively running on a banked surface. Doing too much, too soon, and too fast is what frequently predisposes runners to overuse injuries. Excessive mileage, precipitous changes in workouts, excessive hill running, and/or inadequate rest can all overwhelm the body's ability to accommodate, with resultant overuse injury. Individual athlete vulnerability to extrinsic overload varies with intrinsic characteristics. Brody[6] observed few intrinsic abnormalities in accomplished long-distance runners and subsequently postulated that they would not have achieved their level of performance if there were significant biomechanical problems.

EXAMINATION OF THE RUNNER

The history and physical examination are of paramount importance in establishing a diagnosis for the injured runner. In orthopedic sports medicine, the history frequently establishes the diagnosis, and then the physical examination is used for confirmation. In evaluating runners, a detailed history can consistently help to illuminate a diagnosis; however, a complementary biomechanical examination is required to identify asymptomatic contributors to the injury. The entire examination can be performed rapidly, particularly if specialized runner examination forms are used; these are often utilized in runners' clinics (Fig. 5–1). The history and physical examination thus attempt to explore the chief complaint and also to analyze and identify contributing risk factors.

In the identification of risk factors, we have found two guiding principles to be of great assistance. Leadbetter's[7] "principle of transition" seeks to identify extrinsic risk factors through a careful review of systems. This principle states simply that injury is most likely to occur when the athlete experiences a change in the mode or the use of the involved part. If the transition is so rapid that the tissue is unable to accommodate for ongoing demands, injury results. Most running injuries occur when the athlete has a specific change in training, i.e., in running volume, equipment, and/or running surfaces. Accordingly, the history carefully searches to identify the change or transition.

The second principle is applied to the physical examination of the runner. The "victim and culprits" principle of Macintyre and Lloyd-Smith[8] underscores the importance of the biomechanical examination. The presenting injury represents "the victim," and it occurs as a result of an inability to compensate for a primary dysfunction at another site, "the culprit." Accordingly, the entire kinetic chain must be examined to rule out asymptomatic injury or dysfunction. It is well known, for example, that the "malicious malalignment syndrome" (femoral anteversion, knee valgus with increased Q angle, external tibial torsion, heel valgus, and pronation) can, with faulty training techniques, contribute to injury.[9] Such injuries may include lateral hip pain (glutei overload syndrome), patellofemoral syndrome, shin splints, and plantar fasciitis. Varus alignment has been associated with iliotibial band syndrome, plantar fasciitis, and Achilles' tendonopathy, and plantar fasciitis has been associated with gastrocsoleus, hamstring, and/or gluteal inflexibility.

History

A thorough history includes the past medical and surgical history, medications, and a detailed review of systems. Review of the past medical history should detail all ongoing medical problems, with particular emphasis on musculoskeletal, rheumatologic, cardiac, and respiratory conditions. The surgical history should likewise be inclusive, with an emphasis on prior orthopedic operations. Medications and allergies are reviewed, since overuse injuries are frequently treated with nonsteroidal anti-inflammatory drugs (NSAIDs). In addition, prior injuries should be noted, as well as their treatment and ongoing disability.

The review of systems begins with an assessment of the runner's premorbid running history. It is important for the examiner to query the athlete concerning weekly mileage, pace, number of pairs of running shoes worn, frequency of hill work and interval training, and running surfaces. Of utmost importance is a detailed review of flexibility and warm-up exercises.

The history of the current injury must be extremely detailed. Because overuse injuries are often asymptomatic in their origin, the history must include the period well before symptoms first appeared. Were

The Runner's Clinic at UVa
Robert P. Wilder, MD, FACSM, Director

Name: _____ Date: _____ Birthdate: _____ Age: _____

Date of Injury: _____

Briefly Describe Symptoms and How They Occurred: _____

_____

_____

_____

Previous Treatments for This Injury: _____

Past Injuries (List): _____

_____

Medical Problems (List): _____

_____

_____

Past Surgeries: _____

Medications (List): _____

Allergies: _____ Job: _____

Last Menses: _____ Pregnant: Y/N

Time Between Injury and This Visit: _____ Number Years/Months Running: _____

Levels of Competition (Circle):   1. Elite/Sponsored
                                    2. Competitive Club Level
                                    3. NCAA Division I
                                    4. NCAA Division II, III, College
                                    5. High School
                                    6. Recreational Competitive
                                    7. Recreation only

Current Running Club: _____

Current Weekly Mileage: _____ Current Long Run (Miles or Minutes): _____

No. Track Workouts/Week: _____ No. Hill Workouts/Week: _____

Running Surface: (Road, Track, Trail, Other): _____

Brand Training Shoes: _____ Age: _____

Brand Racing Shoes: _____ Age: _____

Orthotics: Y/N   Bracing: Y/N (Explain): _____

Races Run in Last 6 Months (Dates & Mileage): _____

_____

Goals: Short-term (≤ 3 mos.): _____

        Long-term (> 3 mos.): _____

Cross-Training Methods and Frequency: _____

Stretching (Circle):   Daily   Frequently   Sometimes   Never

Figure 5–1. Record forms for the Runner's Clinic at UVa. *(a)* History. *(b)* Physical examination. *(Courtesy of Robert P. Wilder, MD, Director.)*

there antecedent changes in training routines, running shoes, or surfaces? What has been the transition or change? When during running does the pain occur (Table 5–2)? Does the pain only occur with hills, after a certain distance, or when only running on a particular surface? Does the pain occur during and after running? Is there any initial improvement with periods of warm-up? In addition, the examiner should question the athlete about self-treatment or prior medical treatment. All previous diagnostic tests should be reviewed. Finally, the health care provider should always ask the runner what he or she believes the problem to be.

The Runner's Clinic at UVa
Robert P. Wilder, MD, FACSM, Director

STANDING:

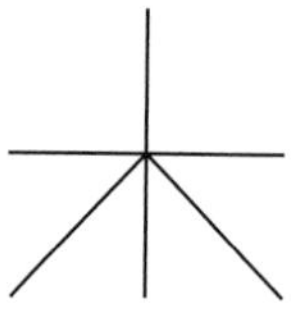

Posture
Pelvis
Sacroiliac
Genu varus/valgus
Foot type
Tibia vara
Rear foot alignment
Subtalar motion
Navicular drop
Stand on toes test
Gastrocsoleus
Gluteal strength

SITTING: Pelvis
Patella position
Tubercle sulcus angle
Knee crepitus
Patella tracking
Straight leg raise
Hamstring flexibility

Strength   hip flexor
quadricep
hamstring

Neurovascular screen
Interdigital palpation

SUPINE: Leg length
Femoral torsion
Tibial torsion
Q angle
Patella tilt
Patella glide
Thomas test
Hip internal rotation
Hip external rotation
Hamstring flexibility

SIDELYING: Ober test
Abductor strength

PRONE   Quad flexibility
Dorsiflexion
Soles
Subtalar   inversion
eversion

Midtarsal mobility
Neutral   leg – rearfoot
rearfoot – forefoot
1st ray mobility
Hamstring strength

SITE SPECIFIC:

DYNAMIC   PLAN   Ice   Reevalution
Walk   NSAID
Run   PT
Video   X-ray
MRI
Bone scan
CT
EMG

SHOE

DIAGNOSIS

Figure 5–1. *(continued)*

TABLE 5–2. FUNCTIONAL CLASSIFICATION OF PAIN

Type	Characteristics
1	Pain after activity only
2	Pain during activity, not restricting performance
3	Pain during activity, restricting performance
4	Chronic, unremitting pain

Examination

Examination of the injured runner includes a sequential biomechanical screening, site-specific examination, gait analysis, shoewear assessment, and appropriate ancillary tests.[6,9–11]

Biomechanical Assessment

STANDING. The examination of the runner begins in the standing position on a noncarpeted surface. The athlete should be in running shorts, without shirt, shoes, or socks on. The female athlete should be in an appropriate sports bra or gown. The examiner should have adequate space to step back for assessment of posture. Posture is assessed by having the athlete face the examiner, face sideways, and stand with his or her back to the examiner. The physician should start by observing the general contour of the spine, noting abnormal curvature, shoulder or pelvic tilt, flank creases, or prominent scapula, which may suggest scoliosis. The athlete is observed bending forward and sideways, while any spinal deformities or segmental dysfunction are noted. Having the athlete bend forward also allows the examiner the opportunity to assess lumbopelvic rhythm. The normal lumbar lordosis should reverse with forward flexion.

The examiner then screens for leg length discrepancies. The examiner palpates the iliac crests as well as the anterior and posterior superior iliac spines and notes any asymmetries. Asymmetries can represent functional or anatomical leg length discrepancies. Functional leg length discrepancies imply that the actual leg lengths are equal. Functional differences are not uncommonly secondary to varying degrees of foot pronation or sacroiliac, pelvic, or hip dysfunction. Anatomical leg length discrepancies imply that one leg is actually shorter than the other.

In the standing position, sacroiliac (SI) joint function can be quickly assessed by the SI fixation or flexion tests.[12] With the SI fixation test, the inferior slope of the posterior superior iliac spine and the medial spinous process of S2 are identified with the thumbs bilaterally. The patient is then asked to flex the hip. With the SI flexion test, the patient bends forward with the examiner's thumbs on the posterior superior iliac spines bilaterally. A negative test occurs when the examiner's thumb swings downward and lateral. A positive test (indicative of SI dysfunction) occurs when the examiner's thumb swings upward or does not move relative to the other side.

Alignment of the lower leg is assessed by sequentially observing the knees, lower legs, and feet. The knees are observed for genu valgum and varum, which is measured with a goniometer. Genu varum is not uncommon in men, with 5 degrees representing the upper limit of normal. Genu valgum is not uncommon in women, with 5 degrees again representing the upper limit of normal. Genu recurvation is also noted, as well as patellar position. Normally, in the standing position the patellae face directly forward; "squinting" or excessively laterally displaced patella should be noted.

From the standing position the examiner can quickly make an assessment about foot type. Most feet can be identified as either cavus, neutral, or pronated. The cavus foot is highly arched and rigid, with calcaneal inversion. The pronated foot is flexible, with little to no arch. The neutral foot represents the middle ground between the cavus and pronated foot. Although overpronation has commonly been linked with numerous overuse injuries, a recent review that assessed the role of high, neutral, and low arches in musculoskeletal overuse injuries found that high arches had an odds ratio of nearly 6:1 compared with low arches for overuse running injuries.[13] In this study a radiographic bone arch index was utilized to clarify foot types.

The lower extremity is also examined in the subtalar neutral position. In the standing position, the foot is placed in neutral position by placing the talonavicular joint in a position of congruency. Talonavicular congruency is obtained by having the examiner place the thumb just distal to the medial malleolus at the talonavicular joint, with the middle finger just distal to the tibiofibular syndesmosis. The foot is then moved into pronation, where the thumb will appreciate a bulge from the talus. When the foot is supinated, the middle finger will appreciate a bulge from the talus. Talonavicular congruency, or subtalar neutral position, is appreciated when the talus is felt equally by both the thumb and the middle finger. From this position the examiner can determine the neutral tibial stance by bisecting the posterior lower one-third of the tibia, and measuring this angle with the sagittal perpendicular. Normal individuals in neutral stance will have 0 to 4 degrees of tibial varus. The navicular drop can then be measured by having the runner relax the feet from

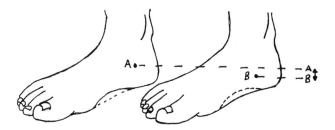

Figure 5–2. Navicular drop test. *(A)* The navicular is marked with the foot in the subtalar neutral position . *(B)* The foot is then relaxed and the subsequent navicular position noted. The distance from A to B is the navicular drop.

the neutral position. The amount of movement of the navicular toward the floor is termed the navicular drop. Up to 1 cm is considered normal. A drop of greater than 1.5 cm is abnormal and may indicate a heightened need for motion control, either via shoes or corrective orthoses (Fig. 5–2).

Before beginning the sitting examination, a quick dynamic assessment of lower extremity flexibility and strength can be performed. The examiner first asks the patient to place the feet shoulder-width apart and face away from the examiner. The athlete is then asked to stand up on his or her toes, allowing assessment of plantarflexor strength and rearfoot motion. Normally the calcaneus swings into inversion, demonstrating normal posterior tibialis function, and adequate subtalar motion. From the lateral position, the examiner observes the patient flex at the knees without lifting the heels from the floor, for assessment of functional gastrocsoleus flexibility. The normal running gait requires 10 to 15 degrees of ankle dorsiflexion. The strength of the gluteal muscles (medius + minimus), important pelvic stabilizers, is tested by asking the runner to stand on one leg. Any dip in the pelvis may indicate weakness in the gluteals of the weightbearing limb. Gluteal strength can be further assessed by having the runner perform a single-legged squat. When squatting, the runner should be able to maintain the center of the patella in line with the second toe and should be able to maintain the patella posterior to the toes. If the knee projects beyond the toes, gluteal weakness may be present. In all cases in which either static or dynamic motion is assessed, symmetry and range of motion are carefully noted.

SITTING. The athlete is then asked to sit on the end of the examination table with the knees hanging over the table in 90 degrees of flexion. The sitting position allows the examiner to reassess pelvic position and leg length and to initiate an examination of the knee, including the patellofemoral joint.

Functional leg length discrepancies that are detected on the standing examination are further evaluated in the sitting position. Abnormalities or obliquities detected by palpating the iliac crests and/or posterior superior iliac spines are rechecked in the sitting position. If the aforementioned become level in the sitting position, a discrepancy in the leg should be suspected. If the asymmetry persists, hip, sacroiliac joint, and/or spinal dysfunction should be suspected.

Patellar position and tracking are conveniently assessed in the sitting position. In the normal individual, the patella should face directly forward when the knees are flexed 90 degrees. Patella alta may exist if the patellae are oriented obliquely toward the ceiling. In this static position the examiner may also measure the tubercle-sulcus angle. This angle is calculated by first constructing an imaginary line through the medial and lateral epicondyles of the femur. Then a perpendicular to this line is drawn through the center of the patella. The sulcus angle is then determined by measuring the angle between this vertical line and a line drawn from the center of the patella to the center of the tibial tubercle. Normal is less than 8 degrees in females and 5 degrees in males.

By then actively and passively flexing and extending the knee, the examiner can appreciate patellar tracking. The examiner first observes active patellar tracking. With normal active extension the patella tracks straight superior or lateral to superior in a 1:1 ratio. An abnormal lateral pull will move more lateral than superior. The examiner than places a hand over the patella and palpates for crepitus, noting the severity as well as the point of occurrence during knee flexion. Passive extension of the seated patient's legs also allows the examiner a quick assessment of hamstring tightness and neural irritation. Stress testing of the knee and ankle is performed to assess ligamentous stability. Any laxity or asymmetry is noted. The sitting position allows for screening of hip flexor, quadriceps, hamstring, and foot and ankle strength. A neurovascular screen including motor strength, sensation, reflexes, pulse palpation, and measurement of capillary refill is made. Finally, palpation of the interdigital spaces, especially between digits 3 and 4, may reveal the presence of a neuroma.

SUPINE. The supine examination permits a more detailed examination of leg lengths, lower extremity alignment, patellar tracking, and flexibility. The leg lengths are assessed by measuring the distance between the anterior superior iliac spines and the medial malleoli. Discrepancies of even 0.5 to 1.0 cm may be significant in a runner and may require correction.

Assessment of the lower extremity alignment includes determination of the degree of femoral and tibial torsion. Femoral torsion is assessed by first palpating the greater trochanter of the leg to be examined. By internally and externally rotating the leg at the medial and lateral femoral condyles, the other hand positions the greater trochanter in its most lateral position. From this point the relationship between the plane of the femoral condyles to that of the examining table is determined, allowing the examiner to determine the degree of anteversion or retroversion. Eight to 15 degrees of anteversion is considered normal in the adult.

To assess tibial torsion, the medial and lateral femoral condyles are placed in the frontal plane. The examiner then palpates the medial and lateral malleoli. An imaginary axis between the medial and the lateral malleoli is measured against the plane of the examining table. Normal individuals have 15 to 25 degrees of external tibial rotation.

The next angular rotation to be assessed in the supine position is the Q angle. By convention, measurement is performed with the knee extended and the quadriceps contracted. The Q angle is formed by the intersection of a line from the anterior superior iliac spine through the midpatella and a secondary imaginary line from the midpatella to the tibial tubercle. A normal Q angle is up to 10 degrees in males and 15 degrees in females. Angles greater than normal may predispose to lateral tracking and patellofemoral pain.

The supine position next permits examination of the patella by assessing passive patellar tilt as well as medial and lateral patellar glide.[14] Passive patellar tilt is assessed by having the examiner place the thumb on the medial edge of the patella and the index finger on the lateral edge. The examiner then tries to elevate the lateral facet from the lateral condyle. The plane of the patella is compared with the axis of the medial and lateral condyles. The tilt is recorded as positive when the lateral edge of the patella rises above the transcondylar axis. The tilt is negative when the edge is below this line. Males normally have a tilt of (+)5 degrees and females (+)10 degrees. Lesser degrees of tilt may be associated with a tight lateral retinaculum and thus a predisposition to patella tracking problems.

Medial and lateral patella glides are assessed with the knee resting in 30 degrees of flexion with passive support provided by a pillow or towel. The patella is longitudinally divided into imaginary quadrants. The patella is then pushed with the thumb medially and laterally. If the medial glide is less than two quadrants, a tight lateral restraint is said to be present. A lateral glide of one quadrant suggests a competent medial restraint. On the other hand, a lateral glide of greater than three quadrants suggests an incompetent medial restraint. Patellar apprehension should be noted.

Further assessment of knee range of motion and stability is performed including anterior and posterior drawer testing and varus/valgus stress testing.

The last aspect of the supine biomechanical examination involves testing for adequate lower extremity flexibility. Normal hip flexibility is as follows: flexion is 110 to 120 degrees; extension is 10 to 30 degrees; abduction is 30 to 50 degrees; adduction is 20 to 30 degrees; internal rotation is 30 to 40 degrees; and external rotation is 40 to 60 degrees.[15] From the supine position, the examiner can quickly perform a Thomas test, which can identify a hip flexion contracture.[12] The patient flexes the contralateral hip and knee against the abdomen, with the lumbar spine flat against the table. If the other thigh elevates from the table, a hip flexion contraction is present. Furthermore, in this position the knee should remain flexed to 90 degrees. If the knee passively extends, a tight rectus femoris may be present. Hip internal and external rotation is conveniently assessed with the hip and knee in 90 degree of flexion.

Hamstring flexibility is also assessed with the hip flexed to 90 degrees. The athlete places both hands in the popliteal space, maintaining this position. The knee is then passively extended as far as possible. In the runner, the long axis of the femur and the fibula should have an angle of 0 degrees. Any popliteal angle greater than 0 degrees is consistent with hamstring tightness.

SIDELYING. The sidelying position allows open-chain testing of abductor strength (gluteus medius and minimus). The runner should be able to offer resistance during abduction, maintaining the hip in neutral flexion and slight external rotation and thus isolating the gluteals. If the athlete flexes or internally rotates the hip during abduction, a substitution pattern exists.

Flexibility of the tensor fascia lata is measured by the Ober test.[16] The patient is asked to turn on the side, facing away from the examiner. The examiner then stabilizes the pelvis and maintains the hip in neutral position. The upper leg is then abducted 30 to 45 degrees, extended at the hip, flexed at the knee, and allowed to adduct passively behind the lower leg. Twenty degrees of cross adduction is considered normal. Less motion is noted in runners with a tight tensor fascia lata or (to a lesser degree) tight gluteals.

PRONE. The final segment of the biomechanical examination is in the prone position, allowing further assessment of flexibility and the soles of the feet, as well as a detailed subtalar neutral examination. To measure quadriceps flexibility, the examiner fully flexes the athlete's knee; adequate flexibility is demonstrated if the heel can touch the buttocks. Ankle dorsiflexion is

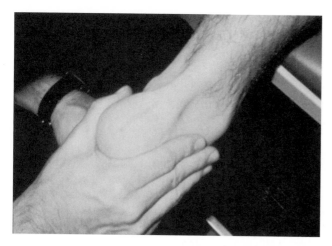

Figure 5–3. Assessment of subtalar motion by evaluating calcaneal inversion and eversion.

passively assessed with the foot in slight eversion and should be at least 10 degrees.

The examiner then observes the soles of the feet. Excessive wear and abnormal shear forces can be implied by the callus pattern. Subtalar range of motion is then assessed with the examiner grasping the calcaneus with the palm of one hand, while stabilizing the tibia with the other. By then passively inverting and everting the foot, subtalar mobility is measured (Fig. 5–3). The normal ratio of inversion to eversion is 3:1, with inversion around 30 degrees, and eversion 10 degrees. Midtarsal joint motion is assessed by stabilizing the calcaneus with one hand, while inverting and everting the forefoot, comparing for symmetry with the other foot.

The foot is then placed in the subtalar neutral position (Fig. 5–4), with the examiner at the patient's feet; with the thumb and index finger, the examiner grasps

the fourth and fifth metatarsal heads. The other hand's thumb and index fingers are then used to palpate the talar head. When examining the right foot, the right hand grasps the metatarsal heads, and the left hand appreciates talonavicular congruency. When examining the left foot, the left hand grasps the metatarsal heads, and the right hand finds the subtalar neutral position.

The talus is most easily found by placing the thumb just distal to the medial malleolus at the talonavicular joint, with the middle finger distal to the tibiofibular syndesmosis. The foot is then moved through pronation and supination, with the examiner's thumb appreciating a bulge during pronation, and the index finger feeling a bulge during supination. The neutral position is identified when the bulge is felt equally on both sides. The neutral position, therefore, is that position where there is talonavicular congruency.

Once subtalar joint neutral is identified, it is then possible to establish the relationship of the lower leg to the rearfoot (Fig. 5–5) and the rearfoot to the forefoot (Fig. 5–6). To determine the former, the examiner creates imaginary (or water-soluble) lines that bisect the calcaneus and the lower one-third of the lower leg. The relationship is measured with a goniometer. Up to 4 degrees of varus alignment is considered normal.

The second angular relationship measured is that of the rearfoot to the forefoot. The examiner first ensures that the subtalar joint is in neutral, and the midtarsal joint is locked by loading the forefoot. This is accomplished by passively dorsiflexing the ankle by exerting a forward pressure on the fourth and fifth metatarsal heads until resistance is felt. The examiner then measures the angle between the bisected calcaneus and an imaginary line drawn through the heads

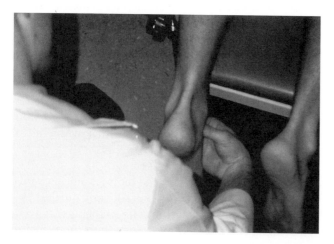

Figure 5–4. The subtalar neutral position is defined as that point where the talus is felt equally by the thumb and middle finger. *(Source: From O'Connor et al.[18])*

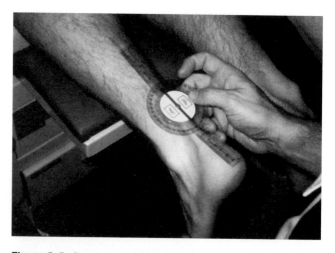

Figure 5–5. Assessment of leg-rearfoot alignment. *(Source: From O'Connor et al.[18])*

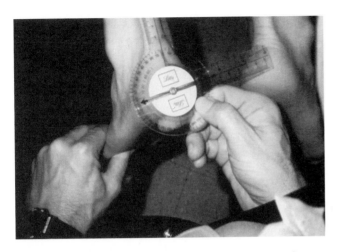

Figure 5–6. Assessment of rearfoot-forefoot alignment. *(Source: From O'Connor et al.[18])*

of the first through fifth metatarsals. The forefoot is neutral if the relationship is perpendicular. If, however, the first metatarsal head lies on a higher plane than the fifth metatarsal head, the forefoot is in a position of varus. If the first metatarsal head is on a lower plane in relationship to the fifth metatarsal head, then there is forefoot valgus. These measurements can be estimated or determined with a swivel goniometer. The forefoot normally is in a slight varus position of 2 to 3 degrees.

In addition to determining rearfoot and forefoot relationships, it is important to assess first-ray (first metatarsal) mobility (Fig. 5–7). The range of motion is determined by grasping the heads of the first and the second metatarsals.[6] The first metatarsal is then moved up and down in relationship to the second. The first ray can be rigid, have normal movement, or be

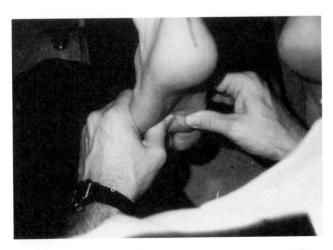

Figure 5–7. First ray mobility. *(Source: From O'Connor et al.[18])*

hypermobile. A first ray with normal motion can be moved just above and below the second metatarsal. A hypermobile first ray should be aligned with the second through fifth metatarsal heads when assessing the forefoot-rearfoot relationship; otherwise, the degree of forefoot pronation may be misinterpreted. The prone position also allows for assessment of hamstring strength by resisting knee flexion, as well as further examination of the sacroiliac joints and spine with palpation, spring testing, and the femoral stretch test.

Site-Specific Examination

After a thorough biomechanical examination has been performed, the examiner moves on to a site-specific examination. The systematic examination includes the following: inspection; bone palpation; soft tissue palpation; range of motion; neurologic examination; specialized testing; and examination of related areas. The examiner again is reminded to search for functional and structural asymmetries throughout the kinetic chain.

Dynamic Evaluation

Subtle abnormalities absent on static examination may become evident with dynamic assessment. Each runner should, therefore, be examined both walking and running. Spinal posture, joint motions, and arm and leg swing are assessed. Balance is noted at the shoulder, pelvis, hips, knees, feet, and ankles, recognizing the relationship throughout the kinetic chain. Any asymmetries are recorded and assessed for contributing factors. Antalgia is always significant.

Video gate analysis is generally reserved for recalcitrant cases and can be useful in identifying subtle imbalances in alignment, flexibility, strength, and mobility (see Chapter 6). Athletes should be familiar and comfortable with treadmill running. Video analysis should include whole-body assessment in multiple planes to examine the entire kinetic chain in addition to foot and ankle mechanics.

Shoe Evaluation

The runner is encouraged to bring in for examination all previous running shoes. The shoes should be examined for specific wear patterns. Most runners heel strike on the lateral aspect of the heel, so wear in the posterolateral heel is not uncommon. Excessive lateral heel wear, however, can lead to excessive varus load with subsequent lateral knee pain. Determinations about the runner's degree of pronation and supination, however, are best made by examining the forefoot.

Excessive pronation causes excessive wear along the medial forefoot. Wear in the midsection of the forefoot indicates a probably normal toe-off. Wear on the lateral side is indicative of a runner with supinated gait. Excessive pronation is additionally identified by a medially tilted heel counter, whereas a supinated gait causes the heel counter to tilt laterally.

The shoes are additionally assessed for the type of last and construction. Unique combinations of last and construction offer varying degrees of motion control and shock absorbency. Quality control is also inspected for by examining areas of the shoe that require gluing or stitching. A more detailed assessment of shoes and orthoses is given in Chapters 46 and 47.

Ancillary Testing

As with musculoskeletal injury, ancillary testing is useful in identifying injury and grading severity.

Radiologic Testing

Plain films should be ordered whenever fractures or joint instabilities are suspected. Plain films may also be useful in identifying alignment abnormalities such as when measuring the congruency angle in the patient with patellofemoral pain. Technetium bone scanning is more sensitive than plain films for identifying stress fractures and should be ordered if fracture is suspected in spite of normal plain films. Bone scanning is also useful in differentiating medial tibial stress syndrome from tibial stress fracture. Magnetic resonance imaging (MRI) is most useful in assessing soft tissue (muscle, tendon, ligament, cartilage) injury. MRI may also be used to detect stress fractures and has been useful in some cases of exertional compartment syndrome. Computed tomography scanning is useful in assessment of bone and intra-articular injury (see Chapter 7).

Electrodiagnostic Testing

Electrodiagnostic testing is requested when nerve injury is suspected. In runners, electrodiagnostic testing is most useful in evaluating for lumbosacral radiculopathy, tarsal tunnel syndrome (tibial/plantar), or peroneal nerve injury. Studies may be performed both statically and after running (see Chapters 8 and 20).

Pressure Monitoring

Compartment pressure monitoring is performed when exertional compartment syndromes of the leg are suspected.[17] Testing should be performed at rest as well as after exercise in all four compartments (anterior, lateral, superficial posterior, deep posterior) as symptometically indicated. Normal resting compartment pressure measures 0 to 8 mmHg. During exercise in normal subjects, pressure will rise to more than 50 mmHg. After exercise, pressure will decrease below 30 mmHg immediately and should be at preexercise levels by 5 minutes. In patients with exertional compartment syndromes, pressures rise to greater than 75 mmHg after exercise, remaining greater than 20 mmHg for 5 minutes or longer, and may be associated pain and paresthesias (see Chapter 9).

CONCLUSIONS

The injured runner is one of the most challenging athletes the sports medicine physician will encounter. A comprehensive history and biomechanical examination can assist the practitioner in diagnosing and managing running injuries successfully. The extra time and effort given to the initial evaluation provides the runner with the best opportunity to return to running and remain injury-free.

REFERENCES

1. O'Connor FG, Sobel JR, Nirschl RP: Five-step treatment for overuse injuries. *Physician Sportsmed* 1992:20, 128.
2. Miller DI: Ground reaction forces in distance running, in Cavanaugh PR (ed.), *Biomechanics of Distance Running*, Champaign, IL, Human Kinetics Books, 1990:203.
3. James SL, Jones DL: Biomechanic aspects of distance running injuries, in Cavanaugh PR (ed.), *Biomechanics of Distance Running*, Champaign, IL, Human Kinetics Books, 1990:249.
4. Brody DM: *Running Injuries*, Summit, NJ, Ciba Clinical Symposium, 1980.
5. Clancy WG: Running, in Reider B (ed.), *Sports Medicine: The School Age Athlete*, Philadelphia, WB Saunders, 1991:632.
6. Brody DM: *Running Injuries: Prevention and Management*, Summit, NJ, Ciba Clinical Symposium, 1987.
7. Leadbetter WB: Cell-matrix response in tendon injury. *Clin Sports Med* 1992:11, 533.
8. Macintyre JG, Lloyd-Smith DR: Overuse running injuries, in Renstrom PA (ed.), *Sports Injury–Basic Principles of Prevention and Care*, Boston, Blackwell Scientific Publications, 1993:139.
9. Brody DM: Evaluation of the injured runner. *Tech Orthop* 1990:5, 15.
10. When the feet hit the ground everything changes. Toledo, OH, Basic Course, American Physical Rehabilitation Network, 1986.
11. Drez D. Examination of the lower extremity in runners, in D'Ambrosia RD, Drez D (eds.), *Prevention and Treatment of Running Injuries*, Thorofare, NJ, Slack, 1989:36.
12. Magee DJ: *Orthopedic Physical Assessment*, Philadelphia, WB Saunders, 1992:319.

13. Cowan DN, Jones BH, Robinson JR: Foot morphologic characteristics and risk of exercise-related injury. *Arch Fam Med* 1993:2, 773.

14. Paulos LE, Kolowich PA: Patellar instability and pain, in Reider B (ed.), *Sports Medicine: The School Age Athlete,* Philadelphia, WB Saunders, 1991:332.

15. Hoppenfeld S: *Physical Examination of the Spine and Extremities,* East Norwalk, CT, Appleton-Century-Crofts, 1976.

16. Ober FB: The role of the iliotibial and fascia lata as a factor in the causation of low-back disabilities and sciatica. *J Bone Joint Surg* 1936:18, 105.

17. Mubarak SJ: Exertional compartment syndromes, in D'Ambrosia RD, Drez D (eds.), *Prevention and Treatment of Running Injuries,* Thorofare, NJ, Slack, 1989:133.

18. O'Connor F, Wilder R: Evaluation of the injured runner. *J Back Musculoskel Rehab* 1995:5, 281.

Chapter 6

VIDEO GAIT ANALYSIS

Francis G. O'Connor, Brian Hoke,
and Andrew Torrance

INTRODUCTION

Human gait analysis has been in practice since at least the late nineteenth century.[1] Various methods of analysis are available, from the very simplistic with no technical support, to those performed with complex and expensive equipment. These methods may include observation, videotaping, electromyography, kinematics, kinetics, and energetics.[2] They are frequently utilized at the elite level in attempts to make minor adjustments in order to maximize running efficiency.

With advances in technology and computers it is now possible to rapidly perform much more sophisticated gait analysis with essentially instantaneous feedback.

Advances in bioengineering technology have allowed for precise measurements of specific gait characteristics including joint angles, forces, and power; angular velocities and accelerations; ground reaction forces; and electromyographic data.[3] However most of these advances have occurred in the laboratory and their application to daily clinical practice has remained impractical, expensive, and difficult to implement. Review of the current literature on gait analysis finds most articles appearing in the bioengineering and/or rehabilitation journals. They pertain primarily to the sophisticated analysis of gait in the laboratory, or the application of gait analysis in the evaluation of individuals with pathologic gait difficulties (e.g., patients with cerebral palsy, cerebrovascular accidents, muscular dystrophy, amputees). The intent of this chapter will be to provide a brief overview of the latest technological advances in gait analysis, but our primary focus will be a discussion of the practical application of gait analysis within our everyday clinics, without the benefit (or expense) of sophisticated laboratory instruments.

VIDEOTAPED OBSERVATIONAL GAIT ANALYSIS

Gait analysis can be broadly classified as either kinetic or kinematic. Kinematic analysis describes movement patterns without regard to the forces resulting in movement or the resultant forces from the movement.[4] Kinetic analysis evaluates the forces which are involved in gait: joint forces and powers, and ground reaction forces. Observational gait analysis is frequently utilized in clinical practice, but it provides little quantitative data. In previously published reports, the intrarater and interrater reliability of videotaped observational gait analysis (VOGA) has been shown only to be slightly to moderately reliable.[5,6] However, both studies utilized patients with grossly abnormal gaits in their assessments. One utilized 15 children with lower limb disabilities requiring utilization of corrective bracing.[5]

The most recent report involved 54 licensed physical therapists observing three patients with abnormal gait secondary to rheumatoid arthritis.[6] One analysis of preliminary results demonstrated a similar correlation between intra- and interrater reliability using VOGA in a healthy active duty military population.[7]

Observational gait analysis can be a useful clinical tool. Because it requires no equipment, it is the most common form of gait analysis performed in clinical practice. Patients are frequently observed while ambulating the length of clinic hallways. Useful information can be obtained from this simple application of gait analysis. However, it provides no quantitative data, and the results are often fraught with error, as it is impossible to observe multiple body segments and events simultaneously. VOGA is capable of improving the accuracy of gait analysis by allowing slow motion single-frame review, thus allowing the observer to review in detail the kinematics of each body segment individually. It has been shown that reviewing videotapes in slow motion provides more consistent results than observing repetitive walking cycles.[5] James and Jones[8] concluded in their review of kinematics that while current methods of applying foot and leg biomechanics are still somewhat inexact, from a practical standpoint in an office environment they nevertheless are often very effective in diagnosis and treatment.

Equipment

Paramount in the performance of VOGA is the proper equipment, including an adequate video camera and accompanying tripod, a videocassette recorder with accompanying color monitor or television, adequate lighting, and a treadmill.

The video camera is the most important element of the procedure. The camera should have slow motion, single-frame review capability, and ideally a zoom lens (4× or greater) with automatic focus capabilities, as well as the capability to provide high quality video in low light situations (a low lux capacity of 2 or less). The camera should have high shutter speeds of $^1/_{500}$ per second or greater. Many inexpensive commercially available video cameras fulfill these requirements. The more recent digital 8 mm technology is felt to provide a better picture for reviewing in slow motion.

A camera tripod is also required for gait analysis. A standard, commercial, readily available tripod will suffice; however, the tripod should be sturdy and allow the camera to be mounted 18 inches from the ground.

A television monitor and videocassette recorder (VCR) for playback/review are required. The monitor is for use by the examiner during his evaluation and by the examinee for educational instruction. The VCR remote control should have pause, slow motion, and frame-by-frame capability. A video printer is also a useful addition as it can provide a hard copy of the monitor screen display, which is useful to include with a report.

A lighting source may be needed. If required, lights should be added in pairs to avoid shadows. In our experience, however, lighting other than normal room light is only rarely required.

The final element required is a treadmill. Any commercial treadmill capable of multiple speed adjustments should be suitable. Various speeds have been utilized during VOGA, but the runner should determine his or her most comfortable pace. During the videotaped session, the treadmill should be set to provide little or no incline (grade). The treadmill should have the capability for unobstructed posterior and lateral viewing as well as speeds of 10 to 12 miles per hour. The treadmill should also be able to accommodate a grade of 10% to 20% in case the need arises to create a grade to re-create a particular clinical situation. There is no preference of AC or DC motor drive; most important is to obtain it from a reputable manufacturer with good warranty coverage.

Data Collection

Data collection is accomplished through the use of angular measurements and observations during the testing. These data are logged on a kinematic gait analysis form (Fig. 6–1). Angular measurements are made using the pause feature on the VCR and measuring on the video screen. These measurements are facilitated through the use of carefully placed retroreflective markers (Table 6–1 and Fig. 6–2). We suggest the use of Scotchlite™ retroreflective tape (silver/white and red/orange) in selected locations. These markers have the advantage of providing easier visualization of segmental movement. When the markers are coupled with sophisticated systems, computerized collection of data points can be achieved. Disadvantages of using reflective markers, however, are that there may be difficulty in locating anatomic landmarks, which can result in large changes in joint angle measurements leading to misinterpretation of data. In addition, joint axes are not always constant with some varying with joint angle. The adhesive on the markers may cause minor skin irritation. Also, they may not reflect bony structure movement.

Planning the Taping Session

The actual videotaping is a systematic process that evaluates the entire kinetic chain during running. The patient should be examined statically prior to the VOGA. A complete evaluation of the runner is detailed in Chapter 5. However, a brief evaluation should precede testing to screen for obvious static alignment abnormalities.

Evaluation of gait should begin as soon as the patient enters the examination room. The examiner should observe the patient's posture, noting any obvious limp or deformity. Most runners being evaluated with VOGA will present without obvious pathology on normal ambulation. Ideally, the gait should be observed from the anterior, posterior, and lateral aspects, with the examiner in each instance observing from proximal to distal in an organized, systematic manner. The examiner should initially screen for leg length discrepancy by palpating the posterior superior iliac spines and iliac crests. Any asymmetry may be caused by either a functional or true anatomic leg length discrepancy. Any apparent asymmetry or

pelvic obliquity should be delineated further. Functional leg length discrepancies are often due to pelvic malrotation or sacroiliac dysfunction. Particular attention is also paid to the patient's head, upper extremities, trunk, back, hips, knees, ankles, and feet. The patient should be examined in bare feet first, followed by evaluation in their current running shoes. Static abnormalities should be noted and recorded.

Assessment of gait should be performed in all three planes of movement: sagittal, coronal, and transverse. In the sagittal plane, pelvic tilt, hip and knee flexion and extension, and ankle dorsiflexion and plantarflexion are noted. In the coronal plane, attention is paid to the amount of pelvic obliquity, hip abduction/adduction, knee valgus/varus position, and foot inversion or eversion. In the transverse plane, one can appreciate pelvic, femoral, tibial, and foot rotation.[3]

Kinematic Gait Analysis Form

Name: _____ Tape Number: _____

Referring Physician: _____ Index Number: _____

Footwear (Describe): _____

_____

Orthotic Devices (Describe): _____

_____

Treadmill Speed: _____ m.p.h.   Treadmill Incline (Grade): ___ %

	Posterior		Lateral	
	R	L	R	L
HEAD				
Position	—	—	—	—
Vertical Displacement	—	—	—	—
SHOULDER				
Max. Extension			—	—
Max. Flexion			—	—
ELBOW				
Max. Extension			—	—
Max. Flexion			—	—
TRUNK				
Rotation	—	—		
Lateral Lean	—	—		
Forward Backward Lean			—	—
PELVIS				
Pelvic Drop	—	—		
Anterior Rotation			—	—
Transverse Rotation	—	—		
HIP				
Rotation	—	—		
Max. Flexion			—	—
Max. Extension			—	—
KNEE				
Position at Foot Strike			—	—
Cushioning Flexion			—	—
Propulsive Extension			—	—
Max. Swing Flexion			—	—
Valgus Varus	—	—		

A

Figure 6–1. Kinematic gait analysis form. (Source: *Reproduced with permission from Hoke et al.*[9]).

Kinematic Gait Analysis
Page 2

Name: _____

	Posterior		Lateral	
	R	L	R	L
LOWER LEG				
Tibial Attitude (Valgus Varus)	—	—	—	—
ANKLE				
Position at Foot Strike	—	—	—	—
Max. Stance DF	—	—	—	—
Max. Propulsive PF	—	—	—	—
Swing Phase DF	—	—	—	—
SUBTALAR (Calcaneal Angle)				
At Foot Strike	—	—		
At Max. Pronation	—	—		
At Heel Lift	—	—		
At Toe-Off	—	—		
FOOT				
Stride Length				
Cadence			—	—
Foot Strike (RF, FF, Total)			—	—
Angle of Gait			—	—
Base of Gait	—	—		
Arch Height	—	—		
Swing				
Early Stance			—	—
Late Stance			—	—
Swing Phase Foot Position	—	—	—	—

SUMMARY OF FINDINGS

_____

_____

_____

Figure 6–1. *(Continued)*   **B** _____

The VOGA should be performed with the participant running on a standard treadmill, ideally with zero degrees of inclination, at a self-determined, comfortable pace for each individual runner. VOGA is first done with the runner in bare feet, followed by identical VOGA with the runner in current running shoes. The VOGA is recorded on standard videotape, and is immediately available for review by both the runner

TABLE 6–1. RETROREFLECTIVE TAPE BONY LANDMARKS

Lateral	Posterior	Anterior (optional)
Head: zygomatic arch	Lower back: PSIS	Hip: ASIS
Shoulder: acromion	Knee: popliteal fossa	Patella: midpoint
Elbow: lateral epicondyle	Lower leg: bisection of distal	Lower leg: tibial tuberosity
Wrist: ulnar styloid	third of tibia and fibula	Foot: midline of second metatarsal
Hip: greater trochanter	Foot: calcaneal bisection	
Knee: central femoral condyle		
Ankle: fibular malleolus		
Foot: lateral border parallel to floor		

PSIS = posterior sacroiliac spine; ASIS = anterior superior iliac spine.
Source: Reproduced with permission from Hoke PT et al.[9]

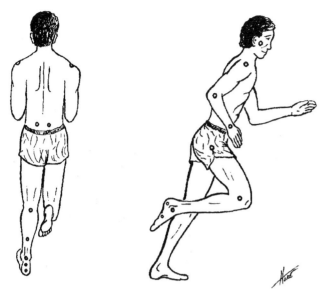

Figure 6–2. Location of bony landmarks for placement of reflective markers.

Source: Reproduced with permission from Hoke et al.[9]

TABLE 6–2. TAPING SESSION PROTOCOL

Static posture: head to feet
Anterior (10 sec)
Lateral (10 sec)
Posterior (10 sec)

Posterior view:
Head to feet (30 sec)
Hips to feet (30 sec)
Lower leg and rear foot
  Shoes on (30 sec)
  Shoes off—walking (30 sec)
  Shoes off—running (30 sec)

Lateral view:
Head to feet (30 sec)
Hips to feet (30 sec)

Anterior view (optional):
Head to feet (30 sec)
Hips to feet (30 sec)
Lower leg and feet (30 sec)

and the examiner. The taping session should proceed in a logical and predetermined fashion; we employ the protocol developed by Hoke (See Table 6–2).[9]

Data Analysis[9–14]

Key to the data analysis is knowledge of the biomechanics of the normal running gait and typical range of motion parameters during running (see Chapter 2). While each runner is unique and there are wide variations, there are some recognized normal values (Table 6–3). As we discuss the data analysis working from head to toe, we will comment on normal biomechanics, as well as commonly observed variations from normal and their clinical implications.

Beginning cephalad and working caudally, identify the position of the head and the amount of vertical

TABLE 6–3. TYPICAL RANGE-OF-MOTION VALUES FOR THE LOWER EXTREMITIES DURING RUNNING

Running Phase	Joint	Motion
Foot strike[a] to midsupport[b]	Hip	45–20 degrees flexion at midsupport
	Knee	20–40 degrees flexion by midsupport
	Ankle	5 degrees plantar flexion to 10 degrees dorsiflexion
Midsupport to takeoff[c]	Hip	20 degrees flexion to 5 degrees extension
	Knee	40–15 degrees flexion
	Ankle	10–20 degrees dorsiflexion
Follow-through[d]	Hip	5–20 degrees hyperextension
	Knee	15–5 degrees flexion
	Ankle	20–30 degrees plantar flexion
Forward swing[e]	Hip	20–65 degrees flexion
	Knee	5–130 degrees flexion
	Ankle	30 degrees plantar flexion to 0
Foot descent[f]	Hip	65–40 degrees flexion
	Knee	130–20 degrees flexion
	Ankle	0–5 degrees dorsiflexion to 5 degrees plantar flexion

[a]Foot strike begins when the foot first touches the ground and continues until the foot is firmly fixed.
[b]Midsupport starts when the foot is fixed and continues until the heel leaves the ground.
[c]Take-off begins when the heel starts to rise and continues until the toes leave the ground.
[d]Follow-through begins as the trailing foot leaves the ground and continues until the foot ceases rearward motion. It concludes the airborne period.
[e]Forward swing starts with forward motion of the foot and stops when the foot reaches its most forward position.
[f]Foot descent starts after the recovering foot has reached its most forward position, reverses direction, and then terminates with foot strike.
Source: Reproduced with permission from McPoil et al.[10]

displacement. The head normally sits straight on the shoulders with the earlobe in line with the tip of the shoulder. The examiner should notice lateral, anterior, or posterior positioning. An altered head position may be the result of a torticollis, prior trauma, or muscular weakness. During dynamic assessment the head should not have any rotational or anterior/posterior displacement. In addition there should not be any vertical displacement of more than 4 cm. A bouncy gait, resulting from a leg length discrepancy or early heel lift, will result in excessive vertical displacement. Early heel lift may be secondary to an equinus deformity of the foot or a tight gastrocsoleus mechanism.

Next observe the upper extremities noting presence of any asymmetry of arm swing. The shoulders should move symmetrically in a relaxed fashion. An asymmetrically depressed or decreased shoulder range of motion is frequently compensation for a contralateral lower extremity dysfunction.

Ideally the elbow should be carried at 80 to 110 degrees of flexion in the recreational runner; angles greater than 100 to 110 degrees are thought to result in wasted energy. The arm swing should be parallel to the direction of movement and should not cross the mid-line because the amount of pelvic rotation and strain will become exacerbated. In addition, arms that swing across the body are inefficient and impair forward progression.

When examining the trunk, note the amount of rotation, presence of any lateral lean, and the amount of forward or backward lean. There should be no forward or backward lean; lateral lean should be no greater than 4 cm in each direction. A forward leaning posture may be the result of weak back extensors or tight hip flexors. Excessive lateral lean may be the result of either a leg length discrepancy compensation or hip abductor weakness. If the hip abductors are weak, the stabilizing effect of these muscles is lost, and the patient exhibits an excessive lateral list in which the thorax is thrust laterally to keep the center of gravity over the stance foot. A positive Trendelenburg sign is also demonstrated as the contralateral hip droops because the ipsilateral hip stabilizers fail to stabilize the pelvis. If the runner has excessively tight hip flexors, he or she may not be able to acquire adequate extension through toe-off for propulsion and require excessive external hip/pelvis rotation. Internal hip rotators are overstretched while external rotators are overworked (e.g., piriformis syndrome).

Hip rotation and pelvic symmetry should be noted, as well as the degree of maximum hip flexion and extension. Hip excursion is dependent on the running speed. The pelvis should not drop more than 4 degrees, with both anterior and transverse rotation limits being approximately 7 degrees.

The hip at contact is approximately 45 degrees flexed at heel strike, then extends to 20 degrees of flexion. During midstance the hip continues to extend from a 20 degree flexed position to slight extension. During propulsion, the hip extends to peak (5 degrees) then begins to flex reaching a peak of 65 degrees in the final third of swing phase. Hip rotation should be no more than 8 degrees. Hip rotation is inferred because direct measurements would require an overhead camera angle. The clinician should once again observe for weak hip abductors as this may result in a secondary iliotibial band lesion on the affected side. In addition, tight hip flexors may impair extension, leading to excessive hip rotation to accommodate toe-off and propulsion.

The knee on first contact (heel strike) is initially flexed at about 15 to 20 degrees and then flexes to 40 degrees. At midstance and entering propulsion, the knee extends to about 15 degrees anatomic flexion. During propulsion the knee further extends to 5 degrees anatomic flexion. During swing flexion the knee continues peaking in the first 50 percent of swing phase to a maximum flexion angle of 120 degrees and then extends until heel strike. The cushioning flexion range is calculated by measuring the difference between the position of the knee at foot strike and at maximum stance flexion. Values less than 20 to 25 degrees reflect quadriceps weakness, and are indicative of a need for quadriceps eccentric rehabilitative exercise, particularly plyometric exercise.

Propulsive phase extension of the knee should be around 5 degrees; values lower than this may demonstrate a muscular contracture. Limited swing phase knee flexion (less than 115 to 120 degrees) may be significant for hamstring weakness. An arthrogenic or stiff knee may be demonstrated by several findings, including exaggerated plantar flexion of the opposite ankle to clear the knee, a circumducted gait, and a smaller stride length on the affected side.

The ankle at heel strike is slightly plantarflexed and then progresses to 10 to 15 degrees of dorsiflexion as the knee flexes through the stance phase. During midstance the ankle reaches peak dorsiflexion at heel lift and begins plantarflexing to approximately 20 degrees. During propulsion the ankle plantarflexion increases to about 30 degrees at toe-off. If at heel strike there is marked plantarflexion, there may be anterior tibialis weakness or evidence of a chronic exertional compartment syndrome with a steppage or drop foot gait. The more common pathologic condition involving the ankle, however, is limited dorsiflexion as a result of anterior tibial impingement or gastrocsoleus inflexibility. As the knee is generally flexed during stance, most of the flexibility deficit is secondary to the soleus mechanism. Early heel-off without adequate dorsiflexion results in overload of forefoot structures that have not had an opportunity to resupinate. Resulting clinical conditions include plantar fasciitis, metatarsalgia, and hallux limitus.

The final event to observe during VOGA is foot function, with particular attention paid to the subtalar joint. During the contact phase the subtalar joint is slightly supinated at heel strike, pronating to a maximum of 6 to 8 degrees at the end of contact. At midstance the subtalar joint resupinates from a maximally pronated position to a slightly supinated position. During propulsion, supination continues peaking just prior to toe-off. During the swing phase the subtalar joint pronates initially from the supinated position, then hovers near subtalar neutral for the remainder of the swing phase.

Foot biomechanics also involve the midtarsal joint. At contact the midtarsal joint is supinated around the longitudinal axis and pronated around the oblique axis. At midstance the joint remains pronated around the oblique axis, but progressively pronates around the longitudinal axis. At heel lift both axes are fully pronated. At propulsion, the midtarsal joint is fully pronated around the longitudinal axis, but progressively supinates around the oblique axis to peak at toe-off. Finally, during the swing phase the midtarsal joint pronates around the oblique axis early in swing, and supinates in later swing around the longitudinal axis.

Subtalar angular motion is measured through the calcaneal angle. The calcaneal angle is measured by placing a mark in the middle of the proximal calcaneus at the insertional site of the Achilles tendon, followed by another mark also bisecting the calcaneus, several centimeters distal to the first. A line is then drawn connecting these two marks. Two similarly placed marks along the calf are also connected and serve as the longitudinal axis of the tibia. The angle created by the intersection of these two lines is considered the calcaneal angle. Normal parameters for the calcaneal angle include 6 degrees inversion at foot strike; 6 to 8 degrees eversion at maximal pronation; 0 degrees or slight inversion at heel lift; and 6 to 8 degrees inversion at toe-off. If the calcaneus is still everted at heel-off, this is most consistent with excessive pronation, probably compensating for a forefoot varus.

In addition to the calcaneal angle, the posterior view allows assessment of the angle of gait and the base of gait. The foot should demonstrate no more than 7 degrees of an external rotation angle with the line of forward progression. Angles greater than this may be indicative of alignment torsional abnormalities, a weak posterior tibialis, or an equinus deformity limiting ankle dorsiflexion. The base of the gait should be between 0 and 1.5 inches. Excessively wide gaits may be the result of tight iliotibial bands or large thigh muscle mass. Narrow crossover gaits, on the other hand, may induce iliotibial band overload. Heel-off and swing phase assessment also allows for the detection of calcaneal whips and circumduction. A heel whip occurs after heel rise and is an exaggerated rotatory twist. A medial calcaneal whip is a compensation for late pronation, while a lateral calcaneal whip is a compensation for late supination. Circumduction occurs with an accompanying lifting of the affected extremity with a rotational element. Circumduction may be the result of weakness in the anterior tibialis, joint restriction (arthrogenic joint or postsurgical), or weak hip flexors.

Force Plate Analysis

When patients fail to respond to interventions that have been suggested by the VOGA, such as footwear changes or rehabilitative exercise programs, the provider may want to consider more advanced testing. In our setting, we have observed that orthotics often are beneficial, particularly in those runners identified as demonstrating excessive pronation. While there are a number of means by which to prescribe orthotics (see Chapter 47), one of the authors (F.O.) has found force plate biomechanical analysis to be helpful. A commercially available system from Footmaxx™ provides a dynamic, weightbearing biomechanical patient assessment and enables digital data to be transmitted for the purpose of generating a gait and pressure analysis report, as well as the prescription for custom foot orthotics (Fig. 6–3). The author's (F.O.) anecdotal experience with this system of biomechanical analysis and orthotic fabrication has been favorable.

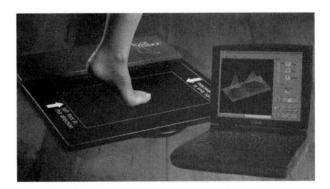

Figure 6–3. Footmaxx force plate for biomechanical assessment. Footmaxx digital readout assessment of biomechanical gait assessment. (Reproduced with permission from Footmaxx.)

CONCLUSION

VOGA is an office assessment tool that offers the clinician an opportunity for dynamic assessment of the runner. While many of these observations outside of the laboratory setting are somewhat subjective and have limitations of reliability, dynamic assessment affords a unique opportunity to witness mechanism of injury. While still in its clinical infancy, this evaluation tool has tremendous potential. In the hands of a skilled provider, VOGA can assist in the understanding of biomechanical abnormalities that contribute to injury that we cannot ascertain during static assessments.

REFERENCES

1. Marey EJ: *Movement*, New York, Arno, 1895.
2. Kopf A: Clinical gait analysis—methods, limitations and possible applications. *Acta Med Austriaca* 1998:25:27.
3. Harris GF, Wertsch JJ: Procedures for gait analysis. *Arch Phys Med Rehabil* 1994:75, 216.
4. Norkin CC: Gait analysis, in O'Sullivan SB, Schmitz TJ, (eds.), *Physical Rehabilitation: Assessment and Treatment*, 3rd ed., Philadelphia, Davis FA, 1994:168.
5. Krebs DE, Edelstein JE, Fishman S: Reliability of observational kinematic gait analysis. *Phys Ther* 1985:65, 1027.
6. Eastlack ME, et al.: Interrater reliability of videotaped observational gait-analysis assessments. *Phys Ther* 1991: 71:465.
7. Brannen SJ, Torrance AW, Robinson CS: Interrater and intrarater reliability of videotaped observational gait-analysis assessments. (Preliminary results, unpublished data).
8. James SL, Jones DC: Biomechanical aspects of distance running injuries, in Cavanagh PR (ed.), *Biomechanics of Distance Running*, Champaign, Ill, Human Kinetics, 1990:249.
9. Hoke BR, Lefever-Button SL: *When the Feet Hit the Ground, Everything Changes, Level Two: Take the Next Step*, American Physical Rehabilitation Network, Toledo, Ohio, 1994.
10. McPoil TG, Cornwall MW: Applied sports biomechanics in rehabilitation: Running, in Zachazewski JE, MaGee DJ, Quillen WS, (eds.), *Athletic Injuries and Rehabilitation*, Philadelphia, W.B. Saunders, 1996:356.
11. Novacheck TF: The biomechanics of running and sprinting, in Guten GN (ed.), *Running Injuries*, Philadelphia, Saunders, 1997:4.
12. Milliron MJ, Cavanaugh PR: Sagittal plane kinematics of the lower extremity during distance running, in Cavanagh PR (ed.), *Biomechanics of Distance Running*, Champaign, Ill, Human Kinetics, 1990:65.
13. Hinrichs RN: Upper extremity function in distance running, in Cavanagh PR (ed.), *Biomechanics of Distance Running*, Champaign, Ill, Human Kinetics, 1990: 107.
14. Edington CJ, Frederick EC, Cavanagh PR: Rear foot motion in distance running, in Cavanagh PR (ed.), *Biomechanics of Distance Running*, Champaign, Ill, Human Kinetics, 1990:135.

Chapter 7

DIAGNOSTIC IMAGING OF RUNNING INJURIES

Carlos E. Jiménez, Thomas Allen, and Inku Hwang

With our society's enthusiasm for exercise, running-related injuries are becoming increasingly common. Epidemiological studies indicate that most running injuries occur in the lower body with the knee being the most frequent site of involvement.[1] The mechanism of most running injuries is overuse, predominantly the patellofemoral stress syndrome, tibial periostitis, iliotibial band syndrome, plantar fasciitis, stress fractures, and various heel and foot syndromes.[2,3] Other less common running injuries, such as femoral neck and navicular stress fractures, are important because, if left untreated, they may result in long-term disability.[4]

Although many running injuries may be diagnosed with a thorough history and physical examination, imaging evaluation may be necessary when the clinical examination is equivocal and the clinician wants to exclude a serious injury. Moreover, when an injured runner fails to respond to suitable conservative therapy, exploration of alternative diagnoses with diagnostic imaging is appropriate. When injured, runners are often reluctant to tolerate inactivity or delay in diagnosis, imposing a greater pressure on physicians to expedite diagnosis and treatment. Since the risk of serious reinjury exists if the runner inappropriately returns to his or her training routine, clinicians are often inclined to secure their clinical diagnoses with correlative imaging studies.

Radiology is a rapidly evolving specialty in which constant innovations in imaging techniques are occurring. Because of the ever-increasing variety of imaging studies available to the practitioner, good communication and cooperation between the referring physician and the radiologist are essential in order to properly select and apply imaging studies. This chapter provides the primary care and sports medicine physician a basis from which to select appropriate musculoskeletal imaging studies in order to properly manage the injured runner. The first portion of this chapter briefly reviews the most common radiological studies applicable to the injured runner, and the second portion discusses the appropriate imaging modalities for various running injuries by anatomical location.

IMAGING STUDIES

Despite the recent technological advances in diagnostic imaging, the plain film radiograph remains the mainstay in the initial evaluation of running injuries. Inexpensive and readily available, radiographs are the most specific means to diagnose musculoskeletal injuries as well as other processes, such as neoplasia and arthritis, that may clinically mimic overuse or post-traumatic injury and therefore may be confused with musculoskeletal injuries. In other instances, plain films are also helpful to correlate osseous abnormalities detected on other more-sensitive but less-specific imaging modalities such as the bone scan and magnetic resonance imaging (MRI).

An adequate plain film radiograph consists of at least two perpendicular views of the injured area. In cases of suspected long-bone injury, it is important to radiograph the joints above and below the site of symptomatology, because occasionally referred pain from an unsuspected joint injury may occur. Sometimes oblique projections and special views are required in complex regions such as the joints, particularly if the initial film fails to identify any abnormality. For example, when evaluating anterior knee pain in a runner, a merchant view may demonstrate an osteochondral fracture or any loose material from the undersurface of the patella. These special views will be discussed in the next section.

One of the limitations of plain films is that early stress fractures and many nondisplaced fractures may not be detected on the initial radiographs. When the clinical suspicion for a fracture is high and initial radiographs are negative, a follow-up plain film examination in 10 to 14 days may identify an occult fracture by the presence of callus formation along the fracture margin.[5] In some cases, nondisplaced fractures are not detected during sequential follow-up radiographs due to hyperemia, inflammation, and new bone formation at the fracture site that may obscure the lucent fracture line. Another shortcoming of plain films is that they provide a very limited evaluation of the soft tissues, usually restricted to the presence of abnormal calcifications, significant soft-tissue swelling, distortion and obscuration of normal soft-tissue planes, and the presence of gas and metallic foreign bodies.

Fluoroscopy is another fundamental diagnostic imaging modality that, like plain film radiography, uses an x-ray beam to create an image. However, unlike plain radiographs where the x-ray beam strikes a piece of film, in fluoroscopy the x-rays strike a fluorescent screen. The light emitted from the fluorescent screen is amplified for a very sensitive electronic image intensifier and the real-time image is displayed on a video screen. Fluoroscopy permits continuous, dynamic imaging that can be used to monitor invasive procedures and permits visualization of moving anatomic structures. For example, fluoroscopy is used to assess bones and joints during motion for subluxation and instability. Fluoroscopy should be performed by an experienced radiologist whose responsibility is to perform an adequate study while minimizing radiation exposure to the patient and staff.

Although the exposure from one fluoroscopic study is minimal, the cumulative dose from many studies may be significant. Therefore, using adequate shielding and modern fluoroscopic equipment, and minimizing the actual time the x-ray beam is turned on are important radiation protective measures for the patient and staff.[6]

Plain radiography in conjunction with intraarticular instillation of iodinated contrast material, referred to as arthrography, has been used in the past to visualize joint volumes, articular cartilage defects, and periarticular ligament tears. However, recently MRI imaging has mostly replaced arthrography in the evaluation of intraarticular soft-tissue injuries.[5]

Computed tomography (CT) is a technology that uses a computer to reconstruct cross-sectional images of the body based on differences in x-ray transmission through a thin section of the body. Since its introduction in the early 1970s, CT has been used in musculoskeletal imaging because of its excellent spatial resolution and depiction of cortical bony detail. Specifically, CT is most often used to detect and delineate occult nondisplaced fractures when the plain film is unremarkable or equivocal, and there is a high clinical suspicion of a fracture. For traumatic injuries involving the hip, acetabular injuries are poorly visualized on plain radiographs and are best assessed with CT.[7] Furthermore, CT provides superior information about the position of intraarticular loose joint fracture fragments as compared with plain radiographs and MRI.[8] The most recent generation of CT scanners, referred as helical CT scanners, acquires data continuously as the patient is translated through the gantry. This allows the acquisition of larger volumes of CT data and an increased number of tomographic sections in shorter periods of time as compared with conventional CT scanners. In musculoskeletal imaging, helical CT is very useful when motion may compromise the study and when evaluating small anatomic regions such as the foot, where small slice thickness (1 to 2 mm) reconstruction images can be obtained.[9]

CT scanning with intravenous contrast is sometimes performed to differentiate distinct soft-tissue processes; however, this technique offers inferior soft-tissue contrast resolution as compared with that produced by MRI. The CT arthrogram, intraarticular injection of contrast material within a joint followed with CT scanning, is performed to better visualize the soft tissues within a joint. This technique detects tendon and ligamentous tears with improved accuracy.[10]

MRI, the most complex and expensive of imaging modalities, is the result of over 6 decades of research in physics and chemistry. MRI uses magnetic fields and radiofrequency waves to create tomographic images of the body. Because of its inherent ability to analyze multiple soft-tissue parameters including hydrogen or proton density, intrinsic tissue T_1 and T_2 relaxation times, and the presence of flowing blood within tissue, MRI produces images with exquisite contrast resolution and respectable spatial resolution. This is a distinct advantage over CT scanning, which analyzes a single soft tissue parameter, x-ray attenuation. Because of this, MRI is the test of choice for evaluating multiple soft-tissue appendicular injuries, including meniscal, ligamentous, and tendinous injuries.[5,11] Because of its ability to produce noninvasive high-resolution images of the ligaments, MRI has largely supplanted arthrography for diagnosing ligamentous injuries. MRI possesses comparable sensitivity to radionuclide bone imaging for the detection of osseous abnormalities with the added advantage of demonstrating soft-tissue pathology in superb anatomic detail.

In MRI imaging, the patient is placed within a large magnet with a strong magnetic field that causes a small percentage of the mobile hydrogen protons in various tissues to align themselves with the external magnetic field. These protons are then perturbed through the periodic application of radiofrequency waves called pulse sequences. Based on the ability of these protons to absorb and release applied radiofrequency energy, a signal is generated and detected by a receiver coil, and the signal is then processed by a computer to create an image. The rate of absorption and release of applied radiofrequency energy is unique for each tissue, and this forms the basis for MRI's excellent soft-tissue contrast resolution.

MRI images can be reconstructed in any anatomic plane, but are typically displayed in multiple orthogonal planes consisting of coronal, sagittal, and transverse views. The MR operator controls image contrast by selecting specific pulse sequences. The two major components of pulse sequences are the TR, the time between administered radiofrequency pulses, and the TE, the time allowed for absorbed radiofrequency pulses to be emitted and detected. The MR technologist selects these times to emphasize a particular soft-tissue parameter such as proton density, T_1 or T_2 relaxation time, and blood flow.

A discussion of MRI physics is beyond the scope of this chapter but understanding the appearance of both normal and abnormal tissues using these parameters is clinically useful. T_1-weighted MR images offer the best anatomic detail and are helpful for identifying fat and subacute hemorrhage. T_2-weighted images most sensitively depict pathologic lesions. Proton-density images minimize T_1 and T_2 effects and display the differences in proton concentration among various tissues.

On MR imaging, cortical bone normally has low signal intensity on all pulse sequences because it contains no mobile protons; therefore, cortical bone is visualized primarily because of contrasting increased signal within the surrounding tissues. Similarly, tendons, ligaments, and cartilage are primarily composed of hard fibrous tissue containing few mobile protons, and likewise these structures normally appear dark in all pulse sequences. Muscle has detectable mobile protons and displays low to medium signal intensity on T_1- and T_2-weighted images. Subcutaneous fat and marrow fat appear bright on T_1-weighted images, moderately bright on proton-density and T_2 images, and dark on short TI inversion recovery (STIR) images. Free water in normal or abnormal areas has lower signal intensity than muscle on T_1-weighted images and higher signal intensity than fat on T_2-weighted images.[6]

Most pathology of tendons, ligaments, and cartilage is seen as alterations in size or continuity of these structures and regions of associated increased signal within the affected structure on T_2-weighted and STIR images. Some pulse sequences will visualize abnormalities better than others. For instance, ligament tears are best seen on T_2-weighted pulse sequences and meniscal tears are generally best observed on proton-density images.[12,13] Abnormalities within the marrow fat due to fractures or osteonecrosis typically will appear darker than the surrounding marrow fat on T_1-weighted images and brighter than the surrounding marrow fat on T_2-weighted images. Gadolinium-based contrast agents are sometimes used in MRI to shorten the T_1 relaxation time of tissues with increased perfusion and/or capillary leakage. This results in signal enhancement of these tissues on subsequent T_1-weighted images.

MRI is generally safe and well tolerated; however, it is not recommended during pregnancy or after recent surgery. Among the limitations of MRI is the time required for image acquisition. The MR signal is weak and often requires acquisition times of up to 10 to 20 minutes to obtain a single set of optimal spin-echo images. The lengthy time required for MR image formation may require a patient to remain motionless for intervals of up to 10 minutes. Recently, more rapid imaging sequences such as gradient refocused echo (GRE) and fast spin echo (FSE) have been developed to shorten acquisition time somewhat. Another limitation of MRI is that the imaging chamber is a very cramped tubular space. Some patients experience claustrophobia within the MRI unit and may require sedation, and others are simply unable to tolerate the confined environment of a MRI scanner. Newer, less-confining MRI scanners called open magnetic resonance units are being developed to address the issue of claustrophobia and to increase patient comfort. Because of the strong magnetic field, MRI is unsafe and is contraindicated in patients with cardiac pacemakers, implantable drug infusion pumps, cochlear implants, and bone-growth stimulators. Ferromagnetic aneurysm clips and vascular clips are at risk of movement in the MRI scanner and are therefore a contraindication to MRI scanning. Bullets, shrapnel, and other penetrating metallic objects, particularly in the orbit, may become mobile in the strong magnetic field and cause further injury. These patients should be carefully evaluated with plain radiographs prior to any planned MRI examination. Most orthopedic hardware including screws, plates, and joint prostheses as well as nonferromagnetic vascular clips do not prohibit MRI imaging, although they may produce artifacts which significantly degrade image quality.

Currently ultrasonography is not commonly used in the United States to evaluate the musculoskeletal system. This is mainly due to the inability of the high frequency sound waves to penetrate bony or joint structures, and to the fact that its accuracy is much more operator-dependent than are the other imaging modalities. In Europe and in only a few centers in the United States, ultrasonography is effectively used to detect bursitis, joint effusions, hematomas, muscle ruptures, tendinitis, and tendon tears and ruptures. With continued experience, research, and technical advances, the role of this modality in future musculoskeletal imaging may significantly impact clinical diagnosis and therapy.[5,14]

Even with the advent of high-resolution anatomic studies, such as MRI and CT, the radionuclide bone scan remains a highly effective tool for evaluating patients presenting with intractable skeletal pain, particularly when the physical examination and radiograph are inconclusive. Its strengths are its ability to provide early physiologic information on osseous abnormalities, often preceding their detection on anatomic imaging studies, as well as its ability to evaluate the entire skeleton in a single short and relatively inexpensive examination. For instance, bone scans are commonly used to detect occult fractures, particularly in the frequently injured carpal scaphoid bone. Scintigraphy can become positive as early as 7 to 24 hours following a scaphoid fracture, and within 2 days its sensitivity approaches 100%.[15] A negative bone scan reliably excludes an acute fracture in clinically questionable cases.

It is not unusual for patients to have symptoms in a particular anatomic location with an inconclusive or negative radiograph, MRI, or CT study. Because it is a physiologic study, the bone scan can differentiate between those abnormalities that are metabolically active and possibly responsible for symptoms and those which are inactive or just normal variants.

Another key advantage of the radionuclide bone scan over anatomic radiologic studies is that bone scans can effectively distinguish referred pain from the true source of pain. Referred pain is frequently a problem in spinal and pelvic injuries where athletes may have pain in one area but the causative lesion is in another location. With the newer multiheaded gamma cameras, a whole body bone scan can rapidly distinguish between sites of referred pain and the actual site where the pain originates. In addition, the bone scan frequently reveals additional unsuspected abnormalities.[16]

The development of single photon emission computed tomography (SPECT) has enhanced the contrast resolution of bone scans by eliminating the effect of overlying soft tissues. This has resulted in improved detection and localization of small abnormalities, especially in the spine, pelvis, and knees. In some cases increased metabolic activity not seen or only vaguely detected on the planar views can be easily seen with SPECT imaging. SPECT bone scan images can also be reprojected and displayed in a dynamic rotating format on computer monitors to create a three-dimensional effect. These rotating or cine SPECT images facilitate the detection and demonstration of lesions to referring physicians. Bone scans, although extremely sensitive, have been criticized for being notoriously nonspecific. However, over time nuclear medicine physicians have increased the diagnostic specificity of the bone scan by developing more accurate imaging techniques and by learning the classic scintigraphic patterns of several musculoskeletal disorders, such as stress fractures, periostitis, plantar fasciitis, sesamoiditis, piriformis muscle syndrome, pathologic accessory navicular bone, iliotibial band syndrome, rhabdomyolysis, and reflex sympathetic dystrophy.[17-23]

Although many traditional pharmaceuticals and radiologic contrast agents are known to cause toxicity and certain adverse reactions, toxicity from the use of nuclear medicine isotopic tracers is essentially nonexistent. Moreover, patient radiation exposure during diagnostic nuclear medicine procedures is very low and has never been associated with cancer induction or development of genetic abnormalities. In addition to being very safe, a bone scan typically costs about one third to one half as much as a CT or MRI study.[24]

IMAGING EVALUATION OF PAIN SYNDROMES IN RUNNERS FROM PELVIS TO FEET

Physical examination of the pelvis and hips can be difficult because these areas contain large amounts of soft tissue overlying the bony structures. When a runner presents with hip or groin pain, the differential diagnosis includes injuries to bones, tendons, ligaments, and muscles that result from a variety of pathologic processes, including stress and complete fractures, avulsion injuries, sprains, strains, bursitis, traumatic arthritis, and myositis. Imaging plays an important diagnostic role in the pelvis when the clinical picture is unclear or when injury confirmation is imperative. The initial radiographic evaluation begins with plain film radiographs, which offer excellent depiction of the bony structures. If these are normal and a pelvic fracture is suspected, a radionuclide bone scan can be diagnostic. One pelvic fracture that is common in joggers and long-distance runners is the inferior pubic ramus stress fracture.[25] This fracture is usually nondisplaced, occurs primarily in women, and produces pain in the groin, buttock, or thigh. Unlike other stress fractures, pubic stress fractures do not usually occur when initiating a new running regime or when changing track surfaces, but instead occur during or following a marathon race or with intensification of a running regime. This injury is caused by the extensive cyclic muscular contractions of the strong muscles that insert into the inferior border of the lateral pubis.[26] Radiographic findings of a pubic ramus stress fracture, if present, are often subtle and consist of a radiolucent fracture line with surrounding callus formation. Since radiographs are often negative for the first few weeks after the onset of symptoms, a bone scan or MRI may be helpful follow-up examinations to confirm a suspected pubic ramus stress fracture. In pubic ramus stress fractures, the bone scan shows increased focal uptake in the inferior pubic ramus (Fig. 7–1), helping to differentiate it from other causes of groin pain in runners, such as pubic symphysis injuries and referred pain from femoral neck stress fractures. MRI is equal in sensitivity to the bone scan for the detection of pubic ramus stress fractures. On T_1-weighted MRI pulse sequences stress fractures appear as areas of relatively low signal intensity in comparison with the contrasting brighter signal within adjacent bone marrow. Sometimes observed within this area of relatively low signal intensity is a line of very dark signal representing the actual fracture line. On T_2-weighted or STIR MRI pulse sequences, stress fractures appear as regions of high signal intensity, representing edema within bone marrow.[27]

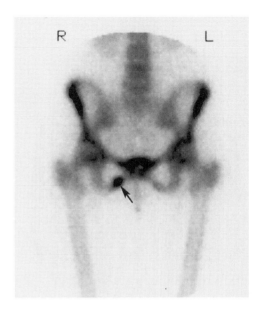

Figure 7–1. Anterior pelvis bone scintigraphy of a runner demonstrating increased focal uptake in the right inferior ramus (arrow) consistent with a stress fracture.

Running injuries to the pubic symphysis are clinically and radiographically referred to by many names, including osteitis pubis, pubic symphysitis, osteochondritis of the symphysis pubis, adductor avulsion injuries, and the gracilis syndrome. Avulsion injuries of the large and powerful adductor and gracilis muscles are suspected to be the major etiologic factors.[25] Similarly to pubic stress fractures, these patients present with a history of groin pain that may radiate to either the peroneal region or thigh and is exacerbated during running and jumping. Physical examination is often unremarkable, but may demonstrate tenderness to palpation over the pubic symphysis and pain with resisted adduction of the thigh. Radiologic evaluation for pubic symphysitis begins with plain film anteroposterior pelvic radiographs; positive findings include loss of cortex and sclerosis or irregularities along the articular surface of the symphysis pubis, as well as widening of the symphysis pubis. Since the radiographic findings may not be present early in the course of the disease, a bone scan should be obtained if the diagnosis is in doubt or to exclude a stress fracture. Findings on bone scan include bilateral or unilateral increased focal uptake in the region of the symphysis pubis[28] (Fig. 7–2). Although it is more expensive, MRI is also very sensitive for detecting pubic symphysitis.[27,29]

Other important pelvic avulsion injuries occur as a result of sprinting and jumping. These are due to sudden and forceful muscle contractions that pull the involved muscle from its point of origin. The peak

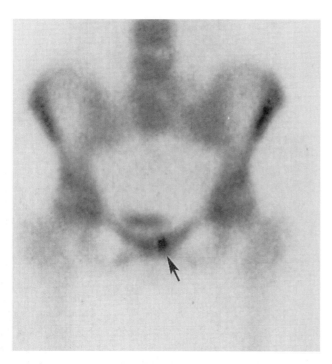

Figure 7–2. Anterior pelvis bone scintigraphy of a runner demonstrating increased focal uptake in the left pubic symphysis (arrow) consistent with pubic symphysitis.

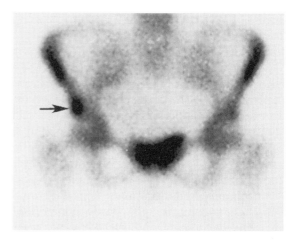

Figure 7–3. Anterior pelvis bone scintigraphy of a runner demonstrating increased focal uptake in the right anterior-inferior iliac spine (arrow) consistent with rectus femoris avulsion fracture.

incidence of these pelvic avulsion injuries is during the second and third decades, when the hip apophyses are closing and are relatively weak. One of the most common pelvic avulsion injuries occurs at the ischial tuberosity, the attachment site of the strong hamstring muscles. Other pelvic avulsion sites include the lesser trochanter (iliopsoas), anterior-inferior iliac spine (rectus femoris), anterior-superior iliac spine (sartorius), greater trochanter (gluteus medius and minimus), and the iliac crest (external oblique). Clinically, avulsion injuries are categorized as incomplete and complete.[30] An incomplete avulsion injury is nondisplaced and generally causes chronic local pain with mild limitation of activity. When the avulsion injury is complete, displacement of the avulsed fragment can cause sudden significant pain and loss of function. Plain film radiographs are the radiologic procedure of choice when an avulsion injury is suspected. Typically, an avulsion injury appears as a small displaced osseous fragment near a muscular or ligamentous attachment site. If there is high clinical suspicion of an incomplete or minimally displaced avulsion injury which is not visualized radiographically, osseous scintigraphy can identify such a lesion with high sensitivity. On bone scans, avulsion injuries appear as a well-defined focus of increased tracer activity at a musculotendinous attachment site (Fig. 7–3).[31]

Stress fractures must be considered in any runner with hip or leg pain, because if undetected they can progress to completion and potentially to displacement. Runners may develop stress fractures within the femoral neck and along the entire femoral diaphysis. Femoral neck stress fractures are among the most significant lesions encountered in sports medicine due to their potential for causing long-term disability. This is a relatively rare injury that most commonly occurs in distance runners or in runners who suddenly increase their training load.[32] Femoral neck stress fractures are biomechanically classified as two types: tensile and compression.[33] Tensile stress fractures occur in the superior cortex of the femoral neck and are more common in older patients. These fractures are generally considered unstable and should be stabilized internally to prevent fracture completion and displacement. Compression stress fractures, on the other hand, involve the cancellous bone along the inferomedial femoral neck without disruption of cortical bone (Figs. 7–4, 7–5, and 7–6). Displacement of femoral neck compression stress fractures is extremely rare. Consequently these fractures are considered stable and are usually treated nonoperatively with protected weight-bearing and frequent radiographic follow-up.

Patients with femoral neck stress fractures typically present with groin, anterior thigh, or knee pain that is exacerbated by activity and is relieved with rest. On physical examination, bony tenderness may be difficult to elicit due to overlying soft tissue. The diagnosis of femoral stress fracture is frequently delayed because its nonspecific presentation is often mistaken for more common injuries such as muscle strains, bursitis, and degenerative joint changes. The radiographic appearance of stress fractures is dependent on the time

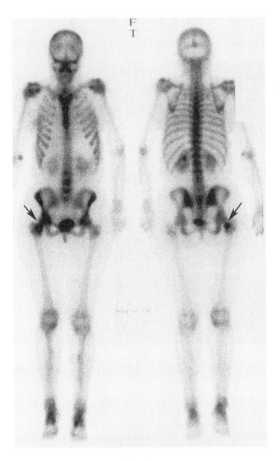

Figure 7–4. Whole body bone scan of a runner showing increased focal uptake in the right inferior femoral neck (arrow) consistent with a right femoral neck compression fracture.

interval between symptom onset and radiographic examination. Initially, plain film radiographs may be negative for 2 to 6 weeks following the onset of symptoms. Later, during the remodeling phase of the stress fracture, endosteal and periosteal thickening develops, and occasionally a radiolucent fracture line may be visible. Patients with suspected femoral stress fractures whose plain film radiographs are negative should have osseous scintigraphy or MRI performed urgently because early diagnosis is associated with the most favorable prognosis.[34] The bone scan is very sensitive and typically demonstrates an increased focus of abnormal activity within the femoral neck (Figs. 7–7 and 7–8). On MR T_1-weighted images, a femoral neck stress fracture appears as a line of very low signal intensity surrounded by a poorly-defined zone of somewhat brighter but low signal intensity. On T_2-weighted or STIR MR images of the femoral neck, a line of low signal intensity surrounded by a wider area of high signal intensity is consistent with a stress fracture (Fig. 7–9).

Runners and joggers can commonly develop stress fractures at other sites in the lower extremities, such as the tibia, fibula, and metatarsals. Abrupt increases in the duration, intensity, or frequency of physical activity without an adequate period of rest are predisposing factors for developing stress fractures. Other factors, such as nutritional deficiencies, hormonal imbalances, hard surfaces, and poor footwear may also contribute to their development.[35] These stress

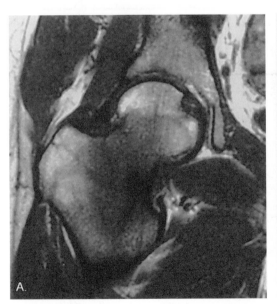

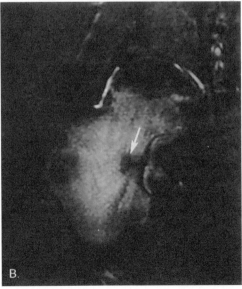

Figure 7–5. MRI of the patient shown in Fig. 7–4 demonstrating the right femoral neck stress fracture. Focal low signal intensity line in the inferior femoral neck (arrow) represents the sclerotic fracture site. Associated bone marrow extension edema appears as diffuse surrounding low signal on T_1-weighted coronal image *(A)* and as diffuse surrounding high signal on T_2-weighted coronal image *(B)*.

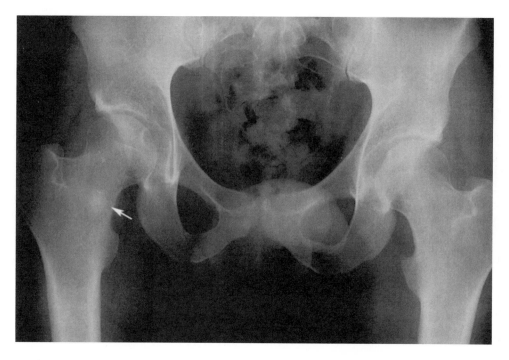

Figure 7–6. Plain radiograph of the same patient as in Fig. 7–5 showing sclerotic stress fracture involving cancellous bone of right inferior femoral neck (arrow).

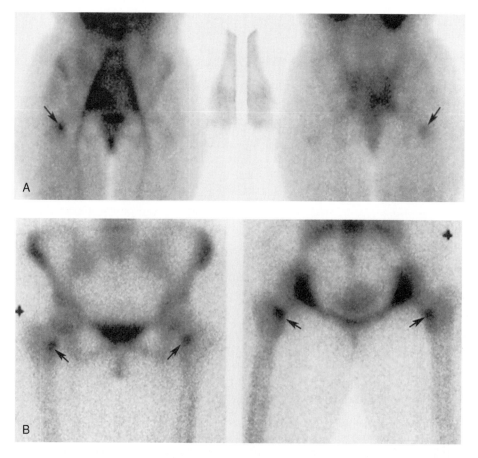

Figure 7–7. Runner with bilateral compressive femoral neck stress fractures. Blood pool *(A)* and delayed *(B)* bone scan images show focal uptake along the inferomedial aspect of both femoral necks.

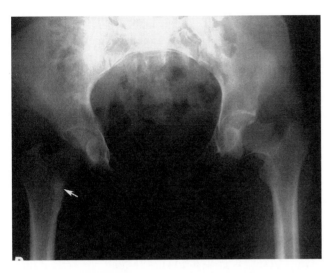

Figure 7–8. Plain radiograph. Rare instance of a complete and displaced left femoral neck compressive stress fracture in a runner (same patient as in Fig. 7–7) who continued training despite femoral neck stress fractures. Sclerotic region in the inferomedial aspect of right femoral neck (arrow) is a stress fracture.

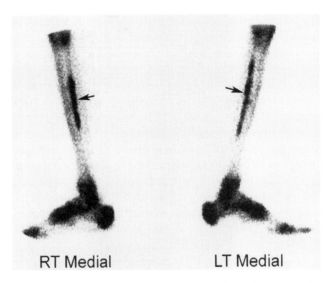

Figure 7–10. Bone scintigraphic lateral tibial views of a runner with medial tibial stress syndrome (MTSS). There is bilateral linear tracer uptake along the posteromedial tibial periosteum (arrows).

fractures can be broadly categorized as either high-risk or low-risk. High-risk stress fractures are lesions with potential to cause long-term disability and which may require surgical intervention. Critical anatomic sites for high-risk stress fractures include the tarsal navicular, femoral neck, anterior tibial cortex, medial malleolus, and stress fractures in long bones with intraarticular extension.[34,36,37] The treatment of lower extremity high-risk stress fractures in runners should be individualized, but many are managed with an aggressive nonsurgical protocol consisting of nonweightbearing cast immobilization. Others with complete and displaced fractures or chronic radiographic changes may benefit from surgical intervention.

Low-risk stress fractures are normally uncomplicated and can usually be effectively treated with rest followed by a gradual return to activity. Among runners, a stress fracture in the posteromedial tibial diaphysis is the most common low-risk stress fracture. The importance of this injury is that it can be confused with medial tibial stress syndrome (MTSS). MTSS refers to the tearing of Sharpey's fibers that connect muscle to bone along the posteromedial and anterolateral aspects of the tibiae, corresponding to the origins of the soleus and/or posterior tibialis muscle(s) (posteromedial) and the anterior tibialis muscle (anterolateral). Radionuclide bone scanning can readily distinguish between MTSS and stress fractures. Characteristic vertical linear increased activity along the tibial periosteum is seen in MTSS, which differs from the more focal fusiform increased radiotracer uptake exhibited by stress fractures (Fig. 7–10).[16,17,38]

Although most stress fractures are suspected by the history and physical examination, several imaging studies may aid in confirming and grading stress

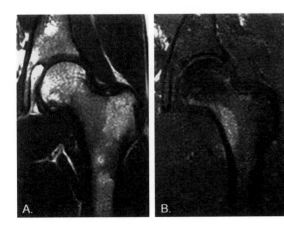

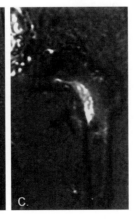

Figure 7–9. Coronal MRI of left femoral neck stress fracture. Free water (due to marrow edema) appears as a focus of low signal intensity on T_1-weighted image *(A)*, increased signal intensity on proton density image *(B)*, and hyperintense signal on T_2-weighted image *(C)*.

fractures. Anteroposterior and lateral radiographs of the involved area may be normal during the first 2 to 4 weeks following symptom onset. Later in the course of the injury, radiographs may demonstrate periosteal and endosteal changes, sometimes associated with a lucency. In the long bones of the lower extremities such as the tibia, a horizontal or oblique line of sclerosis traversing the bone shaft is considered diagnostic of a stress fracture. However, only about 50% of stress fractures are visible on radiographs.[34] The three-phase radionuclide bone scan is the diagnostic gold standard for the detection of stress fractures. It is extremely sensitive for stress fractures and may become positive as early as 48 hours following the onset of symptoms. The characteristic scintigraphic appearance of a stress fracture is an area of focally increased radionuclide uptake with an oval or fusiform shape involving the bone cortex (Fig. 7–11).

Stress fractures may be graded by their morphology on bone scans. There is an established scintigraphic grading system for long-bone stress fractures

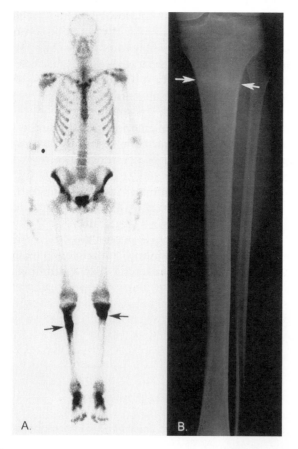

Figure 7–11. (A) Whole body bone scan images in an army recruit demonstrating bilateral Grade IV proximal tibial stress fractures (arrows). (B) A follow-up left tibial radiograph of the same patient demonstrates the proximal tibial transcortical stress fracture.

that consists of four categories[39,40] and requires the analysis of at least two orthogonal views of the involved bone. A Grade I fracture demonstrates a small, mildly active lesion confined to the bone cortex. A Grade II fracture is a larger lesion with moderate activity but is still confined to the cortical area. A Grade III fracture extends from the cortical shaft into the medullary region and shows markedly intense activity. Finally, a Grade IV fracture occupies the full bone shaft width and appears as a transcorticomedullary complete fracture with markedly intense uptake. Treatment during the early stages of a stress fracture (Grades I and II) will stop the progression of the fracture and return the patient sooner to his or her normal level of activity. Identifying a Grade IV stress fracture is important because if it is not treated correctly it may progress to complete fracture and/or nonunion.

The three-phase bone scan, consisting of blood flow, blood pool, and 3-hour delayed images, is particularly useful in determining the acuity of stress fractures. A positive study on all three phases is consistent with an acute injury of approximately 0 to 4 weeks duration. A scan showing an abnormality on blood pool and on delayed images suggests a subacute injury of 4 to 12 weeks' duration. A scan demonstrating an abnormality only on delayed images implies a chronic injury of greater than 12 weeks' duration. Furthermore, an area of focal increased uptake on the blood flow and pool images, with normal uptake on the corresponding delayed bony images, suggests a soft-tissue inflammatory process and rules out skeletal pathology. The delayed osseous uptake seen in a healing stress fracture usually persists for about 3 months and gradually diminishes during the next 3 to 8 months. Occasionally some degree of abnormal uptake can be present for up to 12 months.

MRI is also a very valuable imaging tool for diagnosing stress fractures. It has sensitivity comparable to that of bone scanning but also provides information regarding soft-tissue injury unavailable with osseous scintigraphy. The major disadvantage of MRI at this time is the cost. In clinical practice at certain centers MRI is mostly being utilized to diagnose or further characterize high-risk stress fractures that occur in the pelvis and feet, such as femoral and navicular stress fractures. However, for common low-risk potential stress fractures of the tibia and fibula, MRI images do not provide additional information that may change the clinical management. Therefore, in these cases MRI is not routinely recommended over plain radiographs or radionuclide scintigraphy.

Knee injuries associated with running activities are very common. Most are secondary to overuse

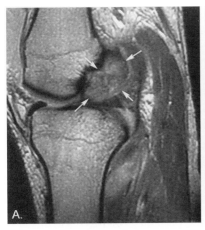 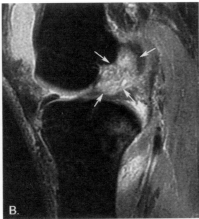

Figure 7–12. Complete proximal rupture of the anterior cruciate ligament (ACL). *(A)* Sagittal proton density image shows complete rupture of the ACL from its normal insertion site on the medial aspect of the lateral femoral condyle. The ACL is displaced by abnormal signal (arrows) running along the normal ligament course. *(B)* Fast spin echo T_2-weighted image with fat suppression shows diffuse abnormal hyperintense signal (arrows) along the normal course of the ACL. Other associated injuries also identified are a hyperintense bone bruise to the posterior lateral tibial plateau, a hyperintense strain injury of the popliteus muscle, and a large knee effusion.

syndromes, such as patellofemoral syndrome, stress fractures, and osteoarthritis.[1,3] Other running-related knee injuries, like ligamentous tears, meniscal disruptions, and chondral defects, may occur after an acute event involving sudden "cutting" (i.e., tibial rotation while bearing in a partially flexed position) and deceleration or from traumatic contact. The history and physical examination in patients complaining of knee pain may help to ascertain the specific lesion. On other occasions, a patient's knee pain will not allow enough relaxation to perform a proper knee examination, making it difficult to arrive at a diagnosis. There are clinical guidelines for efficient use of radiography in acute knee injuries. One set of guidelines recommends radiographic evaluation when the patient age is 55 years or older, tenderness is present at the head of the fibula or if there is isolated patellar tenderness, inability to flex to 90 degrees, and inability to bear weight (four steps) both immediately after injury and in the emergency department.[41,42] When supplemental imaging is required, plain film radiographs, including anteroposterior, lateral, oblique, tunnel, and merchant views, should first be obtained to exclude bony injuries or degenerative changes. The merchant view can be helpful in determining whether there is predisposition for patellar subluxation or dislocation. A tunnel view is useful in evaluating the patellofemoral articulation and the femoral condyles. The lateral knee radiograph can detect joint effusions, one of the best indicators of intraarticular pathology.[43]

If plain radiographs are negative and the patient continues to show signs and symptoms of suspected intraarticular knee injury, MRI is the imaging modality of choice because it can superbly demonstrate abnormalities of the menisci, cruciate ligaments, extensor mechanism, collateral ligaments, and periarticular soft tissues. It can also demonstrate stress fractures,

osteoarthritis, chondromalacia, patellar fracture or dislocation, osteonecrosis, iliotibial band syndrome, avulsion fractures, and infiltrative marrow disorders.[11–13] Bone scanning with SPECT can also be valuable in diagnosing some causes of chronic knee pain, including occult or stress fractures, infrapatellar tendinitis, osteochondritis, Osgood-Schlatter disease, painful bipartite patella, and osteoarthritis; however, bone scanning cannot compete with MRI for diagnosing meniscal and ligamentous injuries because it lacks the ability to show the required anatomical soft-tissue detail (Fig. 7–12).

Myositis ossificans is a form of heterotopic bone formation which is a common sequela to muscle contusion occurring most commonly in adolescents and young adults. The thighs, elbows, gluteal muscles, legs, and shoulders are the most frequent sites of myositis ossificans. Trauma is the most frequent inciting factor for myositis ossificans; however, the antecedent trauma is often imperceptible, and in one series only 60% of patients with myositis ossificans reported a history of trauma.[44] Forcible stretching of muscles during aerobic exercise such as running may cause a subtle muscular injury that may progress to ossification.[45,46] Clinically, myositis ossificans presents as a warm and painful soft-tissue mass within the first 2 weeks after injury.

On plain radiographs, myositis ossificans initially presents as a soft-tissue mass and periosteal reaction. After 4 to 6 weeks, ill-defined floccular calcifications develop within the mass. Following 2 to 3 months maturation, the mass develops a characteristic well-defined peripheral zone of dense calcification with a lucent center, as well as a radiolucent cleft separating the mass from adjacent bone (Fig. 7–13 A & B). These features help distinguish traumatic myositis ossificans from malignant parosteal osteogenic sarcoma, which

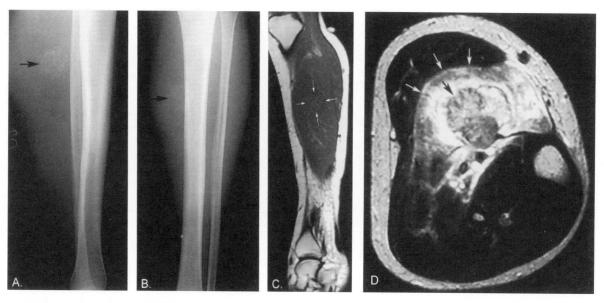

Figure 7–13. *(A)* Lateral and *(B)* anteroposterior radiographs of the left leg reveal a peripherally calcified soft-tissue lesion lying in the posterior aspect of the proximal left leg. *(C)* Sagittal T_1-weighted MRI of the left leg demonstrates a soleus muscle mass that is nearly isointense to the muscle and causes some displacement of the surrounding fascial planes. Thin rim of dark signal around the periphery of the mass represents calcification. *(D)* Axial T_2-weighted MRI of the proximal left leg shows extensive heterogeneous high signal within the soleus muscle that is less intense centrally. These findings, in conjunction with those in Fig. 7–12, are consistent with myositis of the soleus muscle with a central focus of myositis ossificans.

may mimic myositis ossificans both histologically and radiographically.

MR imaging, because of its excellent soft-tissue contrast, is well suited for detecting a wide spectrum of muscle injuries, including strain-related injuries, delayed onset muscle soreness, chronic overuse injuries, rhabdomyolysis, and myositis ossificans.[47] On STIR and T_2-weighted images of muscle injuries, increased signal within the muscle represents muscle edema (Fig. 7–14). In myositis ossificans, focal regions of low signal intensity representing heterotopic bone formation are seen within larger areas of muscle edema (Fig. 7–13 C & D).

Surgical resection of myositis ossificans is only undertaken after maturation of the process; excision of an active lesion can lead to further bone production and a high rate of recurrence. Serial skeletal scintigraphy has been shown to be useful for determining the state of maturity of myositis ossificans.[48,49]

Injuries to the ankle and foot are quite common among runners, and these conditions range from acute problems such as sprains, fractures, and dislocations to chronic overuse syndromes such as stress fractures and enthesopathy. Most ankle sprains are mild to moderate and usually recover fully with conservative therapy. The majority of ankle sprains do not require radiography, but some patients may present with significant injuries that may benefit from imaging. According to the Ottawa ankle rules,[50,51] films are rec-

ommended if the patient is unable to bear weight (four steps) initially after injury and later when examined. Also if bony tenderness is reproduced at the posterior edge of the medial or lateral malleolus or the proximal

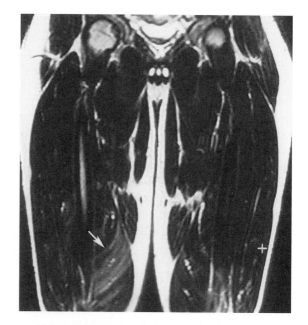

Figure 7–14. Rhabdomyolysis. Coronal T_2-weighted spin echo image of the thighs. Strands of increased signal within the distal thighs, most prominent in the right vastus medialis muscle (arrow), represent interstitial muscle edema.

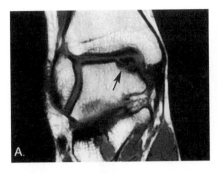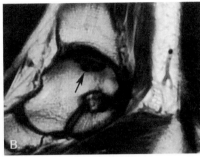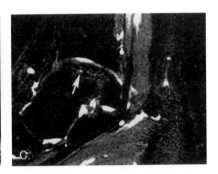

Figure 7–15. Osteochondral lesion of the talus. T_1-weighted spin echo coronal *(A)* and sagittal *(B)* images demonstrate a complete, nondisplaced osteochondral fracture of the medial right talar dome (arrows). The osteochondral fragment shows low signal intensity sclerosis. STIR sagittal *(C)* image reveals a small amount of fluid with high signal intensity beneath the osteochondral fragment.

fifth metatarsal, radiographs are recommended. Standard radiographic evaluation of an acute ankle sprain consists of anteroposterior, lateral, and mortise views of the ankle joint. Significant findings that would alter treatment include distal fibular fracture, osteochondral injury, syndesmosis widening, or tarsal fracture. When ankle radiographs are normal, yet the patient continues to complain of ankle pain after an adequate course of conservative therapy, supplemental evaluation with a CT scan or an MRI should be done to evaluate for an occult osseous injury, such as talar or calcaneal fractures (Fig. 7–15).

A runner's tendons may be injured either through direct trauma or overuse. MRI imaging, because of its exquisite soft-tissue contrast, is ideally suited for depicting the spectrum of tendinous injuries of the ankle and foot. Intact tendons and ligaments have low signal intensity on all MRI pulse sequences. Tenosynovitis, an inflammation within the sheath surrounding a tendon, manifests on MRI as fluid within the tendon sheath surrounding a normal low signal intensity tendon (Figs. 7–16 and 7–17). Tendinitis, a partial-thickness tendon tear, is seen on MRI as focal tendon swelling with associated increased signal within the tendon on T_2-weighted pulse sequences. In advanced cases of tendinitis, thinning of the tendon may herald an impending tendon rupture. Complete tendon rupture, the most severe of ankle tendon injuries, usually occurs in middle-aged males and in athletes. On MRI, complete tendon rupture manifests as the absence of a normal low-signal tendon in its usual location on one or more transaxial images (Fig. 7–18). MRI helps the sports medicine physician to differentiate tendinitis from complete tendon rupture because the clinical findings are not always obvious. This is an important distinction since the former entity is always treated conservatively while the latter entity is sometimes treated surgically.[52]

Plantar fasciitis, an inflammation of the plantar fascia at its calcaneal attachment, is a common cause of chronic heel pain among runners. This condition is characterized by an insidious onset of heel pain that is worse after rising in the morning or after a brief period of inactivity. In most patients, the diagnosis of plantar fasciitis can be established clinically, without the need for imaging studies. However an MRI or a three-phase bone scan can be useful in patients not responding to conservative therapy and for evaluating other causes of heel pain, such as calcaneal stress fractures (Fig. 7–19) and avulsion injuries. MRI findings of plantar fasciitis include thickening and increased signal within the plantar aponeurosis on STIR and T_2- weighted images.[52] On bone scan, plantar fasciitis demonstrates linear increased radiotracer uptake along the fascia in the blood pool phase, and focal increased radiotracer uptake at the plantar fascial insertion site on delayed imaging (Fig. 7–20).[18]

Chronic medial plantar forefoot pain in a runner may be related to hallux sesamoiditis. This disorder results from repetitive stress or direct trauma to the first metatarsal phalangeal region, causing inflammation of the sesamoid and surrounding structures. Physical examination will demonstrate localized tenderness over the medial or lateral sesamoid and pain on passive dorsiflexion of the great toe. The initial radiographic examination should include weightbearing anteroposterior, lateral, oblique, and axial views of the first metatarsophalangeal joint. If the plain radiographs are unremarkable, a bone scan may be diagnostic, showing increased uptake in the affected sesamoid bone (Fig. 7–21). Another cause of forefoot pain among runners is the metatarsal stress fracture, particularly involving the second and third metatarsals, because they are the least mobile of the five metatarsals.[53] Metatarsal stress fractures are especially common in long-distance runners and walkers, and in middle-aged runners who suddenly increase or alter their running regimen.

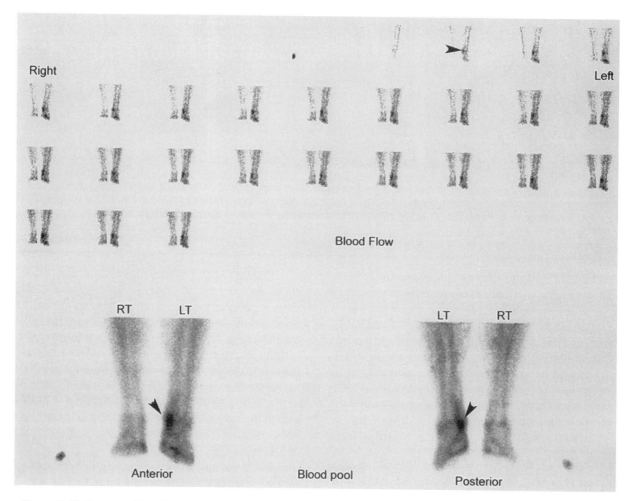

Figure 7–16. Tenosynovitis of flexor hallucis longus tendon. Flow and blood pool phase images from a bone scan of the ankles and feet demonstrate increased flow and blood pool activity around the medial left ankle (arrows). Delayed images of the ankles (not shown) were normal; therefore the flow and blood pool abnormalities represent nonspecific soft-tissue inflammation.

Radiographic examination of a suspected metatarsal stress fracture generally includes anteroposterior, lateral, and oblique views of the foot in question; however, most metatarsal stress fractures are not initially visible on radiographs. A three-phase bone scan is highly sensitive for the detection of metatarsal stress fractures and should be performed if the initial radiographs are negative (Fig. 7–22). Another foot stress

Figure 7–17. Flexor hallucis tenosynovitis MRI (same patient as in Fig. 7–16) with hyperintense fluid within the tendon sheath surrounding the flexor hallucis longus (FHL) tendon (arrows) on STIR *(A)* sagittal and fat-suppressed T$_2$-weighted fast spin echo axial MR images of the left ankle *(B).*

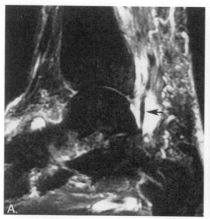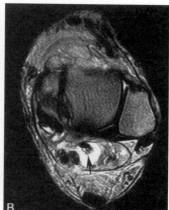

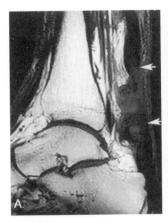
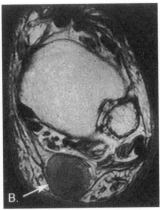
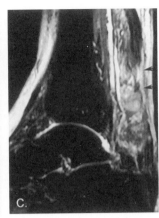

Figure 7–18. Complete Achilles tendon rupture. *(A)* Sagittal T_1-weighted image of the ankle shows a large intermediate signal intensity gap between the dark signal intensity proximal and distal portions of the Achilles tendon. *(B)* T_1-weighted axial image shows absence of the normal dark signal Achilles tendon in the posterior ankle. *(C)* STIR sagittal image shows associated hemorrhage and edema in the peritendinous soft-tissue structures.

fracture that deserves particular attention because of its potential for long-term disability is fracture of the tarsal navicular bone. A tarsal navicular stress fracture should be considered when a patient complains of dorsal medial midfoot pain combined with a history of overuse.[54] Radiographs are rarely positive. A bone scan will help to make the diagnosis (Fig. 7–23).

A number of accessory ossicles with associated pain syndromes have been described in the foot. Among these, two types of accessory navicular bones exist: type I is a separate ossicle in the posterior tibialis tendon, and type II appears as an accessory ossification center in the tubercle of the navicular bone.

Though considered a normal variant, injury to the synchondrosis between the accessory ossicle and the adjacent navicular bone may produce pain. Another accessory foot ossicle that may become injured is the os peroneum. A painful os peroneum refers to an injury of the peroneus longus tendon associated with a fracture of the os peroneum, an intratendinous sesamoid bone similar to the type I accessory navicular.[55]

The os trigonum is an accessory bone in the lateral tubercle of the posterior talus found in approximately 10% of the population. The os trigonum can become symptomatic from physical activities that result in

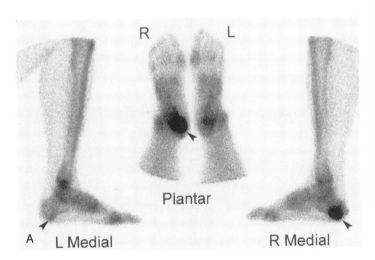
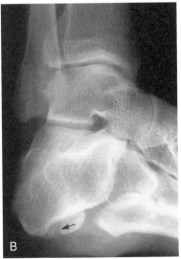

Figure 7–19. *(A)* Delayed bone scan of a runner showing increased focal uptake in the inferoposterior aspect of both calcaneal bones (arrows), but much more prominently on the right side. Blood flow and pool images (not shown here) demonstrated a similar pattern suggestive of a stress fracture. *(B)* Follow-up right foot radiograph subsequently demonstrated the calcaneal stress fracture (arrow).

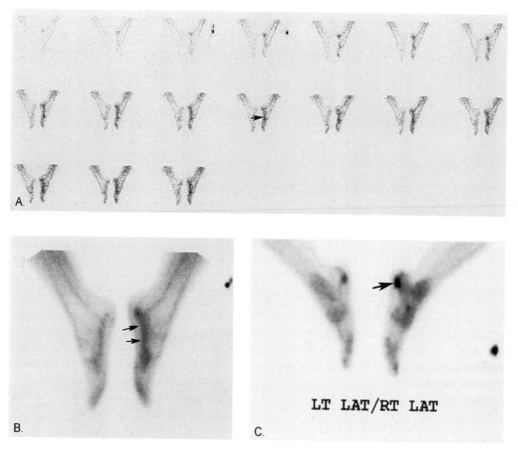

Figure 7–20. Plantar fasciitis pattern in a three-phase bone scan. There is linear increased radiotracer uptake along the fascia on the flow and blood pool phase images. Delayed images show focal increased radiotracer uptake at the plantar fascial insertion site. Without having the earlier views it is difficult to differentiate plantar fasciitis from calcaneal stress fracture.

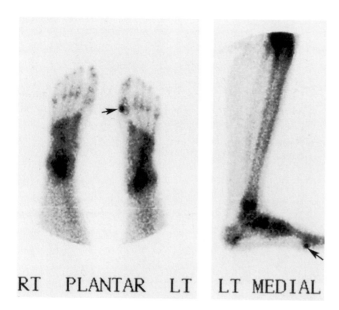

Figure 7–21. Bone scan of a runner demonstrating focal tracer uptake in the medial sesamoid bone of the left first metatarsophalangeal joint consistent with sesamoiditis.

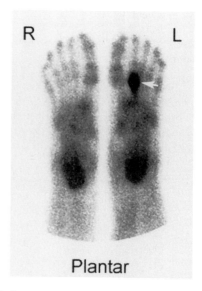

Figure 7–22. Bone scan of a jogger showing intense tracer uptake in the left second metatarsal consistent with a metatarsal stress fracture.

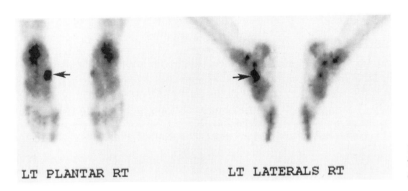

LT PLANTAR RT   LT LATERALS RT

Figure 7–23. Bone scan demonstrating intense focal uptake in the left navicular region consistent with a navicular stress fracture.

forceful and/or repetitive plantar flexion, such as downhill running and in soccer players. These actions can cause direct trauma to the os trigonum or ossicular impingement between the calcaneus and the posterior rim of the distal tibia with or without concurrent tenosynovitis of the adjacent flexor hallucis longus.

Radiographs of the ankle and foot can reveal the presence of an accessory ossicle, but may not be able to differentiate a clinically relevant pathologic process from a normal variant or inactive lesion. A technetium bone scan or MRI are very useful in diagnosing symptomatic tarsal bones or accessory ossicles within the foot by demonstrating increased focal radiotracer uptake or edema in bone marrow and surrounding soft tissues, respectively.[56]

REFERENCES

1. Van Mechelen W: Running injuries: A review of the epidemiological literature. *Sports Med* 1992:14, 320.

2. O'Toole ML: Prevention and treatment of injuries to runners. *Med Sci Sports Exerc* 1992:24(9, suppl), S360.

3. Fredericson M: Common injuries in runners: Diagnosis, rehabilitation and prevention. *Sports Med* 1996:21, 49.

4. Ballas MT, Tytko J, Mannarino F: Commonly missed orthopedic problems. *Am Fam Physician* 1998:52, 267.

5. Tung GA, Brody JM: Contemporary imaging of athletic injuries. *Clin Sports Med* 1997:16, 393.

6. Kneeland JB, Scheff A: Basic principles of medical imaging: Applications to sports medicine, in Halpren B, Herring SA, Altchek D, Herzog R (eds.), *Imaging in Musculoskeletal and Sports Medicine,* Malden, Mass, Blackwell Scientific, 1997:8.

7. Potok PS, Hopper KD, Umlauf MJ: Fractures of the acetabulum: Imaging, classification, and understanding. *Radiographics* 1995:15, 7.

8. Brossmann J, Preidler KW, Daenen B, et al.: Imaging of osseous and cartilaginous intraarticular bodies in the knee: Comparison of MRI imaging and MR arthroscopy with CT and CT arthrography in cadavers. *Radiology* 1996:200, 509.

9. Fishman EK: Spiral CT evaluation of the musculoskeletal system, in Fisherman EK, Jeffrey RB (eds.), *Spiral CT: Principles, Techniques, and Clinical Applications,* New York, Raven Press, 1995:141.

10. Obermann WR: Optimizing joint-imaging: CT arthrography. *Eur Radiol* 1996:6, 275.

11. Farooki S, Seeger LL: Magnetic resonance imaging in the evaluation of ligamentous injuries. *Skeletal Radiol* 1999:28, 61.

12. Irizarry JM, Recht MP: MR imaging of knee ligament injuries. *Semin Musculoskeletal Radiol* 1997:1, 83.

13. Curl LA, Potter HG, Wickiewicz T: Thigh and knee injuries, in Halpren B, Herring SA, Altchek D, Herzog R (eds.), *Imaging in Musculoskeletal and Sports Medicine,* Malden, Mass, Blackwell Scientific, 1997:209.

14. Adler RS: Future and new developments in musculoskeletal ultrasound. *Radiol Clin North Am* 1999:37, 623.

15. Nielsen PT, Hedeboe J, Thommsesen P: Bone scintigraphy in the evaluation of fracture of the carpal scaphoid bone. *Acta Orthop Scand* 1983:54, 303.

16. Jimenez CE: Advantages of diagnostic nuclear medicine: Musculoskeletal disorders. *Phys Sportsmed* 1999:27, 45.

17. Martiere JR: Differentiating stress fracture from periostitis. *Phys Sportsmed* 1994:22, 71.

18. Intenzo CM, Wapner KL, Park CH, et al.: Evaluation of plantar fasciitis by three-phase bone scintigraphy. *Clin Nucl Med* 1991:16, 325.

19. Karl RD, Yedinak MA, Hartshorne MF, et al.: Scintigraphic appearance of the piriformis muscle syndrome. *Clin Nucl Med* 1985:10, 361.

20. Shah S, Achong DM: The painful accessory navicular bone: Scintigraphic and radiographic correlation. *Clin Nucl Med* 1999:24, 125.

21. Rockett JF, Magill HL, Moinuddin M, Buchignani JS: Scintigraphic manifestation of iliotibial band injury in an endurance athlete. *Clin Nucl Med* 1991:16, 836.

22. Jimenez CJ, Pacheco EJ, Moreno AJ, Carpenter AL: A soldier's neck and shoulder pain. *Phys Sports Med* 1996:24, 81.

23. Leitha T, Staudenhers A, Korpan M, et al.: Pattern recognition in five-phase bone scintigraphy: Diagnostic patterns of reflex sympathetic dystrophy in adults. *Eur J Nucl Med* 1996:23, 256.

24. Hough DA, Pearson R, Tryciecky E: Pelvic injuries, in Halpren B, Herring SA, Altchek D, Herzog R, (eds.),

Imaging in Musculoskeletal and Sports Medicine, Malden, Mass, Blackwell Scientific, 1997:196.

25. Pavlov H: Roentgen examination of groin and hip pain in the athlete. *Clin Sports Med* 1987:6, 829.

26. Noakes TD, Smith JA, Lindenberg G: Pelvic stress fractures in long distance runners. *Am J Sports Med* 1985:13, 120.

27. De Paulis F, Cacchio A, Michelini O, et al.: Sports injuries in the pelvis and hip: Diagnostic imaging. *Eur J Radiol* 1998:27, S49.

28. Burke G, Joe C, Levine M, et al.: Tc-99m bone scan in unilateral osteitis pubis. *Clin Nucl Med* 1994:19, 535.

29. Kneeland JB: MR imaging of sports injuries of the hip. *Magn Reson Imaging Clin North Am* 1999:7, 105.

30. Metzmaker JN, Pappas AM: Avulsion fractures of the pelvis. *Am J Sports Med* 1985:13, 349.

31. Fernandez-Ulloa M, Klostermeier TT, Lancaster KT: Orthopedic nuclear medicine: The pelvis and hip. *Semin Nucl Med* 1998:25, 25.

32. Egol KA, Koval KJ, Kummer F, et al.: Stress fracture of the femoral neck. *Clin Orthop* 1998:348, 72.

33. Devas MB: Stress fracture of the femoral neck. *J Bone Joint Surg* 1965:47B, 728.

34. Knapp TP, Garrett WE: Stress fractures: General concepts. *Clin Sports Med* 1997:16, 339.

35. Nattiv A, Armsey TD: Stress injury to bone in the female athlete. *Clin Sports Med* 1997:16, 197.

36. McBryde AM: Stress fracture in runners. *Clin Sports Med* 1985:4, 737.

37. McBryde AM Jr: Stress fractures, in Baxter DE, (ed) *The Foot and Ankle in Sports,* St. Louis, Mosby Year Book, 1995:81.

38. Etchebehere EC, Etchebehere M, Gamba R, et al.: Orthopedic pathology of the lower extremities: Scintigraphic evaluation of the thigh, knee, and leg. *Semin Nucl Med* 1998:28, 41.

39. Zwas ST, Frank G: The role of bone scintigraphy in stress and overuse injuries, in Freeman LM, Weissman HS, (eds.), *Nuclear Medicine Annual,* New York, Raven Press, 1989:109.

40. Zwas ST, Elkanovitch R, Frank G: Interpretation and classification of bone scintigraphic findings in stress fractures. *J Nucl Med* 1989:28, 452.

41. Stiell IG, Greenberg GH, Wells GA, et al.: Prospective validation of a decision rule for the use of radiograph in acute knee injuries. *JAMA* 1996:275, 611.

42. Stiell IG, Greenberg GH, Wells GA, et al.: Derivation of a decision rule for the use of radiograph in acute knee injuries. *Ann Emerg Med* 1995:26, 405.

43. Kaye JJ, Nance EP: Pain in the athlete's knee. *Clin Sports Med* 1987:6, 873.

44. Geschickter CF, Maseritz IH: Myositis ossificans. *J Bone Joint Surg* 1938:20, 674.

45. Gilmer WS, Anderson LD: Reactions of soft somatic tissue which may proceed to The thigh,bone formation: Circumscribed (traumatic) myositis ossificans. *South Med J* 1959:52, 1432.

46. Michaelsson JE, Granroth G, Anderson LC: Myositis ossificans following forcible manipulation of the leg. *J Bone Joint Surg* 1980:62A, 811.

47. Shellock FG, Fleckenstein JL: The thigh, in Stoller DW, (ed.), *Magnetic Resonance Imaging in Orthopedics and Sports Medicine,* 2nd ed., Philadelphia, Lippincott-Raven, 1997: 1345.

48. Lipscomb AB, Thomas ED, Johnson RK: Treatment of myositis ossificans traumatica in athletes. *Am J Sports Med* 1976:4, 111.

49. Orzel JA, Rudd TG: Heterotopic bone formation: Clinical laboratory imaging correlation. *J Nucl Med* 1984:26, 125.

50. Stiell IG, McKnight RD, Greenberg GH, et al.: Implementation of the Ottawa ankle rules. *JAMA* 1994:271, 827.

51. Plint AC, Bulloch B, Osmond MH, et al.: Validation of the Ottawa ankle rules in children with ankle injuries. *Acad Emerg Med* 1999:6, 1005.

52. Hollister MC, De Smet AA: MR imaging of the foot and ankle in sports medicine. *Semin Musculoskeletal Radiol* 1997:1, 105.

53. Weinfeld SB, Haddad SL, Myerson MS: Metatarsal stress fractures. *Clin Sports Med* 1997:16, 319.

54. Maitra RS, Johnson DL: Stress fractures. *Clin Sports Med* 1997:16, 259.

55. Groshar D, Gorenberg M, Ben-Haim S: Lower extremity scintigraphy: The foot and ankle. *Semin Nucl Med* 1998:28, 62.

56. Jimenez CA, Torres E: Posterior ankle pain in a recreational athlete. *Phys Sports Med* 1998:26, 59.

Chapter 8

ELECTRODIAGNOSTIC TESTING

Venu Akuthota, Larry H. Chou, and Joel M. Press

INTRODUCTION

Electrodiagnostic (EDX) testing can be an important tool in the evaluation of runners with neurologic problems. The thorough EDX consultation integrates the history, physical examination, and selected nerve conduction or needle electromyographic studies into a meaningful diagnostic conclusion.[1] In essence, EDX studies are an extension of the clinical examination. Whereas imaging studies identify structural abnormalities, EDX studies evaluate the physiology and function of the peripheral nervous system. The EDX examination, however, only evaluates the physiology of nerves and muscles studied *at that time*. That is, some electrophysiologic abnormalities might not yet have appeared whereas other findings may have resolved and left no detectable residual deficit. Furthermore, a negative EDX examination does not rule out the possibility of pathology because electrophysiologic studies are time- and severity-dependent.[2] In this light, the EDX impression must be based on the entire clinical picture. Clinical judgment needs to be used summarily in EDX consultations, and therefore EDX studies are highly dependent on the quality of the electromyographer.[1]

This chapter will describe the pathophysiology of nerve injury and associated chronology of electro-physiologic findings. Subsequently, a description of the components of an EDX evaluation will be provided. Typically, electrodiagnostics are divided into nerve conduction studies (NCS) and needle examination (NE). The NE is also referred to as electromyography (EMG). Many clinicians, unfortunately, use the term "electromyography" for all components of the electrodiagnostic evaluation. This misuse in terminology should be abandoned. The chapter will go on to list the usefulness and limitations of the various aspects of electrophysiologic testing. A special section will be included on dynamic EDX studies because these tests are often requested in runners whose symptoms only manifest during or after running. The purpose of the information presented in this chapter will be to provide the clinician a basis of ordering and understanding proper EDX reports.

ANATOMY

EDX studies evaluate the integrity of the peripheral nerve system or lower motor neuron pathway. A clear understanding of peripheral nerve and motor unit anatomy is necessary for understanding and performing EDX tests. The peripheral nervous system includes both the afferent sensory pathway and the efferent motor pathway. The sensory pathway begins with cutaneous receptors forming sensory axons. These sensory axons coalesce in either pure sensory or mixed nerves. The sensory fibers travel through specific portions of nerve plexuses (e.g., brachial plexus, lumbosacral plexus) and house their cell bodies in the dorsal root ganglion, usually located within intervertebral foramina. The sensory fibers then form dorsal roots as they synapse in the dorsolateral spinal cord. NCS of pure sensory and mixed nerves are used to evaluate this aspect of the peripheral nervous system.

The efferent motor pathway starts at the level of the spinal cord with anterior horn cells. The motor axons, originating from the cell bodies of their anterior horn cells, exit the spinal canal as spinal nerves and divide into ventral and dorsal rami. The motor fibers in the ventral rami traverse their respective plexuses ending as peripheral motor nerves.[1] Peripheral motor nerves synapse at specific muscles through individual neuromuscular junctions, where acetylcholine is transported to the muscle membrane to induce an all-or none action potential. An anterior horn cell, its axon (within limb plexuses and multiple peripheral nerve branches), and the muscle fibers innervated are known as a motor unit. NCS of the pure motor and mixed nerves are used to evaluate this aspect of the peripheral nervous system from the point of stimulation to the recording site. Motor units can be evaluated during needle EMG with voluntary muscle activation.

PATHOPHYSIOLOGY OF NERVE INJURY

Peripheral nerves can either be myelinated or unmyelinated. Myelinated fibers are interspersed with nodes of Ranvier, which facilitate saltatory ("jumping") conduction along the nerve fiber. NCS evaluate the fastest conducting fibers within nerve funiculi. Typically these are the A alpha myelinated fibers.

Peripheral nerve injury is categorized by injury to the myelin alone or to the axon. Seddon divides peripheral nerve injury into neurapraxia, axonotmesis, and neurotmesis (Table 8–1). Neurapraxia refers to focal conduction slowing or focal conduction block. Though myelin is injured, the nerve fibers remain in axonal continuity. This results in impaired conduction across the demyelinated segment. However, impulse conduction is normal in the segments proximal and distal to the injury. While demyelination is mostly seen with focal nerve entrapments (e.g., carpal tunnel syndrome), demyelination may also occur in peripheral polyneuropathies as either a patchy process (e.g., Guillain-Barré syndrome) or a diffuse process (e.g., diabetic peripheral neuropathy). Runners often experience neurapraxic injury of the tibial nerve branches with putative tarsal tunnel syndrome, possibly due to repeated traction injury with the foot in pronation.[3] Axonotmesis and neurotmesis refer to axonal injury with wallerian degeneration of nerve fibers disconnected to their cell bodies. There is a loss of nerve conduction at the injury site and distally. Axonotmetic injuries involve damage to the axon with preservation of the endoneurium whereas neurotmetic injuries imply a complete disruption of the enveloping nerve sheath.[4] EDX studies typically cannot separate axonotmesis from neurotmesis. Runners can often experience axonal injury with conditions such as a radiculopathy.

SPECIFIC ELECTRODIAGNOSTIC STUDIES

Nerve Conduction Studies

NCS may be performed on motor, sensory, or mixed nerves. There are numerous pitfalls with NCS (Table 8–2); therefore it is imperative that a well-trained consultant performs EDX studies.[1] Both motor and sensory nerve conduction studies test only the fastest, myelinated axons of a nerve, thus the lightly myelinated or

TABLE 8–1. CLASSIFICATION OF NERVE PATHOPHYSIOLOGY

Type	Pathology	EDX Correlation	Prognosis
Neurapraxia	Myelin injury	CV slowing across segment DL prolonged across segment Loss of amplitude proximal but not distal NE normal	Recovery in weeks
Axonotmeses	Axonal injury with endoneurium intact	Loss of amplitude distal and proximal NE shows spontaneous activity NE shows abnormal voluntary motor units	Longer recovery
Neurotmeses	Severance of entire nerve	No waveform with proximal or distal stimulation NE shows spontaneous activity NE shows no recruitable motor units	Poor recovery

CV = conduction velocity; DL = distal latency; NE = needle examination.

TABLE 8–2. SOURCES OF ERROR IN NERVE CONDUCTION STUDIES

- Temperature
- Inadequate or excessive stimulation
- Improper placement of electrodes
- Tape measurement error
- Age
- Anomalous innervation
- Volume conduction of impulse to nearby nerve
- Improper filter settings
- Improper electrode montage setup
- Involuntary muscle contractions

unmyelinated fibers (C pain fibers) are not examined with EDX.[5] Motor nerves are stimulated at accessible sites, and the compound muscle action potential (CMAP) is recorded over the motor points of innervated muscles (Fig. 8–1). Deep motor nerves and deep proximal muscles are more difficult to study and interpret.[6] Sensory nerves can be studied along the physiologic direction of the nerve impulse (orthodromic) or opposite the physiologic direction of the afferent input (antidromic). Stimulated and recorded sensory nerves produce a sensory nerve action potential (SNAP) (Fig. 8–2). Frequently, sensory axons are tested within mixed nerves, such as the plantar nerves, and produce a mixed nerve action potential (MNAP) (Fig. 8–3).

CMAP, SNAP, and MNAP waveforms are analyzed and interpreted by the clinician. Waveform parameters include amplitude, latency, and conduction velocity. In general, amplitude measurement evaluates the number of functioning axons in a given nerve and, for motor studies, the number of muscle fibers

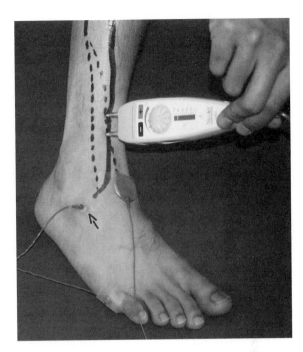

Figure 8–1. Compound motor action potential (CMAP). Electrical stimulation of the deep peroneal nerve (solid line) is recorded at the motor point over the extensor digitorum brevis (arrow).

activated. Latency refers to the time from the stimulus to the recorded action potential. With motor NCS, latency takes into account the peripheral nerve conduction (distal to the site of stimulation), neuromuscular junction transmission time, and muscle fiber activation time.[1] With sensory nerves, latency measures only the conduction of the segment of nerve stimulated. Conduction velocity across a segment of nerve can also be

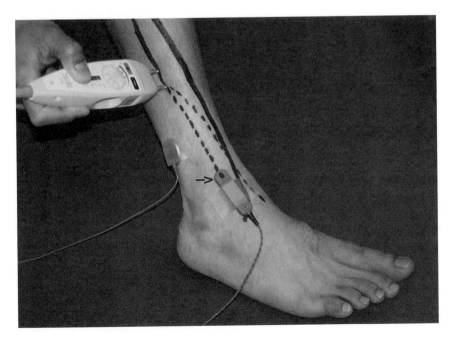

Figure 8–2. Sensory nerve action potential (SNAP). The superficial peroneal nerve is stimulated proximally while a bar electrode is used distally to record an antidromic sensory action potential (arrow) from the lateral branch of the superficial peroneal nerve.

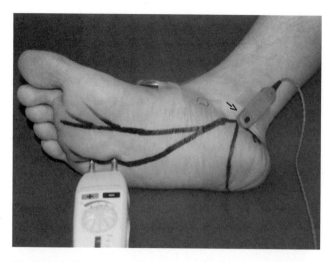

Figure 8–3. Mixed nerve action potential (MNAP). The mixed sensory and motor lateral plantar nerve is stimulated in the foot and recorded from the tibial nerve (arrow). Similarly, the medial plantar nerve can also be stimulated with pickup at the same location on the tibial nerve.

calculated when nerves are stimulated at a distal and proximal site.

Late Responses

The H reflex is the electrophysiologic analog to the ankle stretch reflex. It measures afferent and efferent conduction mainly along the S1 nerve root pathway.[7] A latency difference of at least 1.5 msec is significant in most laboratories. Amplitude of <50% compared with the uninvolved side is also significant. However, since the amplitude of this reflex is sensitive to contraction of the plantar flexor muscles, amplitude changes without significant latency abnormalities should be interpreted with caution.[8] The H reflex is able to look at the afferent and efferent pathways, thus it gives information about the sensory pathway that is not tested by standard needle EMG. The S1 nerve injury can be due to S1 radiculopathy from a herniated lumbar disc or lumbar stenosis; peripheral neuropathy (usually with bilaterally abnormal H reflexes); or sciatic/tibial nerve injuries. Therefore evaluation of other peripheral nerves through standard NCS may be helpful to sort out the differential diagnosis.

The F wave is a late muscle potential that results from a motor nerve volley created by supramaximally stimulated anterior horn cells.[9] Unlike the H reflex, the F wave can be elicited at many spinal levels and from any muscle. F wave studies, like H reflexes, look at a long pathway. Consequently, small focal abnormalities tend to be obscured by the longer segments. Abnormalities with F wave values may be due to nerve injury anywhere along the long pathway evaluated.

Needle Examination

The NE evaluates the entire motor unit (lower motor neuron pathway), but not the sensory pathway. This component of the EDX evaluation includes needle EMG of muscles at rest (to detect axonal injury) and with volitional activity (to evaluate voluntary motor unit morphology and recruitment). The NE needs to be timed such that abnormalities are optimally detected. If the NE is performed too early (i.e., less than 2 to 3 weeks after the initial injury), spontaneous muscle fiber discharges (denervation potentials) may not have had time to develop. If the NE is performed too late (i.e., more than 6 months after the initial injury), reinnervation via collateral sprouting may have halted spontaneous muscle fiber discharges.[8]

When muscles are studied at rest, the electromyographer studies the electrical activity of selected muscles for abnormal waveforms. Of these abnormal waveforms, the most common abnormal finding is the presence of fibrillations and positive waves. They are found when the muscle tested has been denervated.[4] Fibrillations and positive sharp waves are graded on a scale from 0 to 4+ (Table 8–3). Complex repetitive discharges (CRDs) are also common. They represent a group of single muscle fibers that are time-linked because of crosstalk between neighboring muscle fibers. Fasciculation potentials can be found in a variety of benign and malignant conditions. They represent spontaneous discharges of an entire motor unit; thus they are much larger than fibrillations and positive waves. Sometimes fasciculations can be grossly observed as muscle twitches. Benign fasciculations may be found in runners following heavy exercise, dehydration, anxiety, fatigue, coffee consumption, or smoking. When muscles are studied with activation, motor units may be analyzed. Motor unit analysis offers a good opportunity to distinguish between neuropathic and myopathic processes.[1]

NE also may help differentiate acute from chronic neuropathic conditions. The amplitude of fibrillations can grade nerve injury as occurring for less than or more than 1 year.[10] This can be particularly helpful in distinguishing a runner's acute on chronic

TABLE 8–3. GRADING OF FIBRILLATIONS AND POSITIVE WAVES

Grading	Characteristics
0	No activity
1+	Persistent (longer than 1 second) in 2 muscle regions
2+	Persistent in 3 or more muscle regions
3+	Persistent in all muscle regions
4+	Continuous in all muscle regions

nerve injury. Chronic nerve injuries, without significant ongoing denervation, will additionally show large-amplitude, long-duration, polyphasic motor unit potentials.[8]

Dynamic Electrodiagnostics

Some authors advocate performing EDX after exercise or with the limbs in provocative positions. These techniques have not been validated with sound research and are subject to measurement error. Anecdotally, however, they appear to have a limited use. Leach and colleagues[11] describe peroneal nerve entrapment in runners which was detected only with EDX testing following exercise. Runners diagnosed with compartment syndrome and potential nerve entrapment (e.g., superficial peroneal nerve entrapment as it exits the fascia of the lateral compartment) have also been postulated as needing EDX testing following exercise.[12] Fishman and Zybert[13] have suggested that electrophysiologic evidence of piriformis syndrome is more apparent when an H reflex is performed with the sciatic nerve on stretch (hip flexed to 90 degrees, maximally adducted, and knee flexed to 90 degrees). These techniques need to be interpreted with caution as many "abnormal" readings occur based on measurement error alone.

Quantitative Electromyography

Numerous studies have employed electrophysiologic techniques to demonstrate sequence of muscle recruitment and muscle force. Quantitative EMG does not constitute a diagnostic test and is only available in specialized gait laboratories. Quantitative EMG employs surface or needle electrodes placed into muscles to record EMG signals through multiple channels. Often fine wire electrodes are used to record signal in deeper muscles. Caution should be used in correlating EMG signal amplitude with muscle force because the relationship is not consistently linear.[14] Quantitative EMG has also been used to assess the degree of muscle fatigue and biomechanics of sports activities.[6] The kinesiology of the running gait has been elucidated with EMG. The gluteal muscles and hamstrings are more active in running than in walking, particularly at the termination of the swing phase in preparation for foot strike. The quadriceps and posterior calf group also work during a greater percentage of the swing and stance phase during running than in walking. The calf muscle group in particular becomes much more active as the speed of gait increases.[15] Surface EMG can be used as a biofeedback technique in runners to improve their running biomechanics. For instance, the use of hip extensors may be trained with the use of surface EMG.

INDICATIONS FOR ELECTRODIAGNOSTIC TESTING

The utility of EDX testing in a given runner may be estimated following a thorough history and physical examination, by a review of supplemental information (e.g., imaging studies), and through an appreciation for the chronology of the electrophysiologic changes that occur following nerve injury. Some useful generalizations about the indications for EDX studies are worthy of review and are discussed below[8]:

1. *Establish and/or confirm a clinical diagnosis* A thorough electrophysiologic examination can rule in a suspected diagnosis or rule out a competing diagnosis. Nerve injury localization often needs to be objectively confirmed prior to contemplating invasive or surgical treatment. Additionally, EDX studies may alert the examiner to the possibility of an unsuspected concomitant pathologic process, such as a runner with tarsal tunnel syndrome with superimposed radiculopathy.

2. *Localize Nerve Lesions* In order for nerve injuries to be precisely treated, the exact location of nerve injury needs to be elucidated. For example, a runner presenting with plantar foot numbness and tingling may have a sciatic nerve lesion anywhere along the course of the nerve or its branches. EDX studies can then be used to determine if the sciatic nerve injury is occurring at the piriformis or at its terminal branches.

3. *Determine the Extent and Chronicity of Nerve Injury* Properly timed EDX studies can differentiate a neurapraxic injury from axonal degeneration. This information may have a significant impact on the aggressiveness of treatment for nerve injury. The acuteness and chronicity of a nerve lesion may also be assessed using fibrillation amplitude measurement and motor unit analysis, as well as clinical history.[1,10]

4. *Correlate Findings of Anatomic Studies* When so-called abnormal findings are found on imaging tests, EDX studies are useful to correlate nerve function to anatomic abnormalities. This may be particularly useful in the spine because disc herniations effacing nerve roots can be seen in asymptomatic individuals.[16]

5. *Assist in Prognosis and Return to Play* By determining the degree of nerve injury, the clinician can predict nerve function recovery. In general,

neurapraxic injuries recover sooner than axonal injuries. CMAP amplitude measurements of weak muscles (compared with asymptomatic contralateral amplitude) can give an idea of the extent of neurapraxia and of potential recovery. A side-to-side amplitude difference of greater than 50% is probably significant. However, EDX studies should not be the sine qua non for return to play because they may lag behind clinical recovery. The best determination of return to play remains the athlete's functional performance in simulated sports activities.[6]

LIMITATIONS OF ELECTRODIAGNOSTIC TESTING

EDX is not a perfect test and should not be performed in every athlete with neurologic signs or symptoms. Some diagnoses are unequivocal and treatment should be initiated without delay. If the athlete has progressive neurologic deficits, such as after a traumatic posterior knee dislocation, the results of the EDX studies will be unimportant, as the patient will require emergent care. When ordering EDX studies, the timing of findings should be kept in mind (Table 8–4). For example, NE findings can take from 2 to 6 weeks to become manifest. With traumatic injuries, serial EDX studies, including an immediate study, may be helpful

to thoroughly determine the degree of nerve injury. Relative contraindications to EDX include pacemaker (no Erb's point stimulation), arteriovenous fistula, open wound, coagulopathy, lymphedema, anasarca, and pending muscle biopsy.[2]

SPECIFIC CONDITIONS

Many pain complaints in runners present as neurologic signs and symptoms. Runners most frequently complain of numbness or tingling and focal weakness in the foot. Dyck and coworkers[17] found that although most long distance runners do not complain of symptoms of neuropathy, they do appear to have subclinical changes in quantitative sensory thresholds and nerve conduction velocities. However, rarely runners may present with focal nerve entrapments (Table 8–5). Runners with nerve pain describe a burning, shooting, tingling, numb, and/or electric quality to their pain. Runners may commonly present with tibial and peroneal nerve problems which can be evaluated by EDX techniques.

Park and Del Toro[18] have outlined EDX techniques to evaluate the tibial nerve and its terminal branches. The tibial nerve has four terminal branches: a) medial plantar nerve, b) lateral plantar nerve, c) inferior calcaneal nerve, and d) medial calcaneal nerve (Fig. 8–4). The medial plantar nerve is easily tested as

TABLE 8–4. TIMING OF EDX FINDINGS WITH AXONAL INJURY

Time	NCS	NE
Day 0	Decreased CMAP/SNAP amplitudes proximally Normal distal to lesion	Decreased recruitment
Day 1–3	Decreased CMAP/SNAP amplitudes proximally Normal distal to lesion	
Day 3–7	Decreasing CMAP then SNAP amplitudes, proximally and distally	
Day 7–9	Decreased or absent CMAP amplitudes, proximally and distally	Increased insertional activity in proximal muscle
Day 10–14	Decreased or absent SNAP amplitudes	Large PSW/Fibs in proximal denervated muscles
Week 3–6		Large PSW/Fibs in distal denervated muscles
Week 6–8	Increasing amplitude w/recovery	Nascent reinnervation of proximal muscles (VMUP = polyphasic, low amplitude, increased duration)
Month 3–4	Increasing amplitude w/recovery Proximal CV 80% normal	
Month 4		Nascent reinnervation of distal muscles Maturing reinnervation of proximal muscles (VMUP = polyphasic, high amplitude, increased duration)
Month 4–5		Maturing reinnervation of distal muscles
Year 1		Smaller PSW/Fibs

PSW = positive sharp waves; Fibs = fibrillations; SNAP = sensory nerve action potential; CMAP = compound muscle action potential; VMUP = voluntary motor unit potentials; CV = conduction velocity.

TABLE 8–5. FOCAL ENTRAPMENT NEUROPATHIES SEEN IN RUNNERS

Syndrome/nerve	Symptoms	Entrapment Site
Tarsal tunnel syndrome (tibial nerve proper)	Plantar pain/paresthesias, worse at night and with prolonged standing or walking	Under flexor retinaculum
Medial calcaneal neuritis	Medial heel pain	At medial heel
Inferior calcaneal nerve (first branch of lateral plantar nerve)	Chronic heel pain No numbness Weakness of ADM	Between AH and QP or calcaneal heel spur
Medial plantar nerve (jogger's foot)	Medial arch pain	At master knot of Henry (hypertrophy of AH)
Morton's toe (interdigital nerve)	N/T in toes	At intermetatarsal ligament
Superficial peroneal nerve	Lateral ankle pain Fascial herniation	At deep crural fascia as exits lateral compartment
Deep peroneal nerve	Dorsum of foot pain Tightly laced shoes	At inferior extensor retinaculum
Common peroneal nerve	N/T in lateral leg, dorsum of foot	Compression in fibular tunnel by fibrous edge of peroneus longus Traction from ankle sprains

N/T = numbness/tingling; AH = abductor hallucis; QP = quadratus plantae; ADM = abductor digiti minimi

a motor nerve conduction study, stimulating at the tibial nerve proximal to the medial malleolus and recording over the abductor hallucis (Fig. 8–5). The lateral plantar motor nerve study is performed by stimulating the tibial nerve proximal to medial malleolus and recording over the flexor digiti minimi brevis (Fig. 8–6). The inferior calcaneal motor nerve study is performed to the abductor digiti minimi pedis (Fig. 8–7). The medial calcaneal nerve can be studied as a sensory nerve antidromic study, where the recording electrode is placed over the skin of the medial calcaneus (Fig. 8–8). The sensory components of the medial and lateral plantar nerves may be practically tested with an antidromic

mixed nerve study. The medial and lateral plantar nerves are stimulated individually at the plantar aspect of the foot and the sensory nerve action potential is recorded under the medial malleolus (Fig. 8–3).

The peroneal nerve's motor and sensory components can be consistently studied with nerve conduction studies. The motor nerve study is performed by stimulating the peroneal nerve at multiple sites, including the anterior ankle, the fibular head, and the popliteal fossa. Recording is usually over the extensor digitorum brevis; however, the anterior tibialis can be used as an alternative muscle (Fig. 8–1). The sensory nerve study is performed by stimulating the

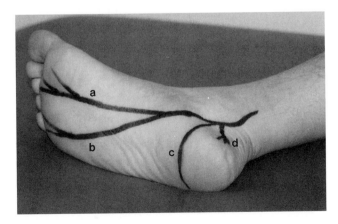

Figure 8–4. Terminal branches of the tibial nerve: (a) medial plantar nerve, (b) lateral plantar nerve, (c) inferior calcaneal nerve, and (d) medial calcaneal nerve.

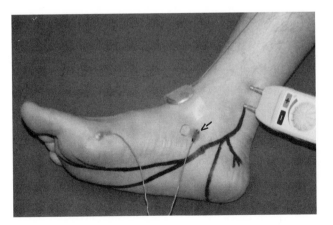

Figure 8–5. Recording over the abductor hallucis (arrow), the tibial nerve is stimulated behind the medial malleolus. Note the placement of the recording electrode slightly posterior to the tubercle of the navicular.

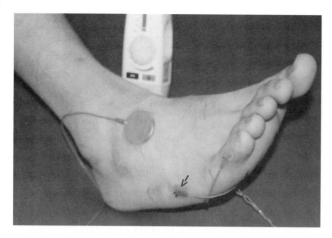

Figure 8–6. Recording from the flexor digiti minimi brevis (arrow) which is deep to the tendon of the abductor digiti minimi pedis and inferior to the fifth metatarsal, the tibial nerve is stimulated behind the medial malleolus.

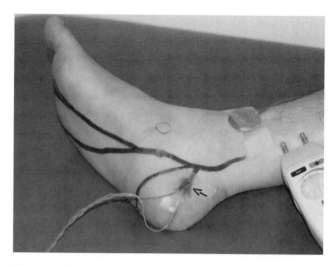

Figure 8–8. Medial calcaneal nerve recordings are made (arrow) by stimulating the tibial nerve behind the medial malleolus.

superficial peroneal branch as it exits the lateral compartment and recording over the ankle (Fig. 8–2).

ELECTROMYOGRAPHY REPORT

The electrophysiologic report should include a number of important pieces of data for the referring physician. The electrophysiologic findings should correlate with physical findings and any discrepancies identified. Inconsistencies may have as much importance in the clinical treatment of the patient as consistent results. Also, the degree of definitiveness of findings needs to be conveyed to the referring physician. A diagnosis of S1 radiculopathy by H reflex changes alone will carry different weight than abundant spontaneous activity in the S1 myotomal distribution. Electrodiagnostic examiners

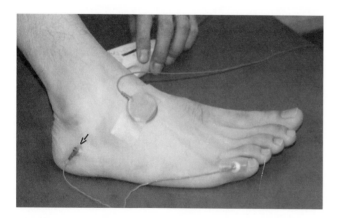

Figure 8–7. The tibial nerve is stimulated behind the medial malleolus, and a recording electrode is placed over the abductor digiti minimi pedis (arrow), just distal the lateral malleolus along the shaft of the fifth metatarsal.

and referring physicians need to remember that one abnormal finding does not make the diagnosis if all other evidence is pointing to a different diagnosis.[2] There should also be sufficient evidence to rule out alternative possibilities and to identify superimposed conditions. The electromyographic interpretation should mention the degree of injury and chronicity, if possible. Prognosis is critical for referring physicians to know, if a prognosis is obtainable. Finally, comparison with previous EDX data should be done whenever possible. Table 8–6 provides a checklist for referring physicians to use when evaluating an EDX report for its technical and practical usefulness.

SUMMARY

The effectiveness and reliability of EDX in detecting pathology in runners is high, but it must always be understood in light of its capabilities and limitations.

TABLE 8–6. CHECKLIST FOR EVALUATING THE EDX REPORT

- Specific question answered?
- Clinical findings consistent with your evaluation?
- Limb temperatures monitored and recorded?
- Cool limbs warmed?
- Individual measures reported?
- Presence of partial or complete conduction block described?
- Normal values provided?
- Sufficient evaluation to document problem?
- Sufficient data to rule out alternative diagnoses?
- Appropriate negative findings described?
- Interpretation consistent with clinical findings?

Source: From Albers.[19]

Indiscriminate use of this or any testing procedure should be avoided. EDX studies are examiner-dependent and, when possible, should be performed by a physician who is a specialist in EDX medicine. EDX studies evaluate the degree and location of nerve injury but do not measure pain. When performed at the appropriate time, runners with neurologic symptoms may be aided by EDX studies.

REFERENCES

1. Robinson LR, Stolp-Smith KA: Paresthesiae and focal weakness: The diagnosis of nerve entrapment, in AAEM Annual Assembly, 1999, Vancouver, Johnson Printing Company.

2. Rogers CJ: *Electrodiagnostic Medicine Handbook,* San Antonio, University of Texas Health Science Center-San Antonio, 1996.

3. Jackson DL, Haglund B: Tarsal tunnel syndrome in athletes. Case reports and literature review. *Am J Sports Med* 1991:19, 61.

4. Dimitru D: *Electrodiagnostic Medicine.* Philadelphia, Hanley and Belfus, 1995.

5. Wilbourn AJ, Shields RW: Generalized polyneuropathies and other nonsurgical peripheral nervous system disorders, in Omer GE, Spinner M, Beek ALV (eds.), *Management of Peripheral Nerve Problems,* Philadelphia, Saunders, 1998:648.

6. Feinberg JH: The role of electrodiagnostics in the study of muscle kinesiology, muscle fatigue and peripheral nerve injuries in sports medicine. *J Back Musculoskel Med* 1999:12, 73.

7. Fisher MA: AAEM Minimonograph: 13: H reflexes and F waves: Physiology and clinical indications. *Muscle Nerve* 1992:15, 1223.

8. Press JM, Young JL: Electrodiagnostic evaluation of spine problems, in *The Nonsurgical Management of Acute Low Back Pain,* Gonzalez G, Materson RS (eds.), New York, Demos Vermande, 1997:191.

9. Fisher MA: The contemporary role of F-wave studies. F-wave studies: Clinical utility [see comments]. *Muscle Nerve* 1998:21, 1098; discussion 1105.

10. Kraft GH: Fibrillation potential amplitude and muscle atrophy following peripheral nerve injury. *Muscle Nerve* 1990:13, 814.

11. Leach RE, Purnell MB, Saito A: Peroneal nerve entrapment in runners. *Am J Sports Med* 1989:17, 287.

12. Bachner EJ, Friedman MJ: Injuries to the leg, in Nicholas JA, Hershman EB (eds.), *The Lower Extremity and Spine in Sports Medicine,* St. Louis, Mosby, 1995.

13. Fishman LM, Zybert PA: Electrophysiologic evidence of piriformis syndrome. *Arch Phys Med Rehabil* 1992:73, 359.

14. Basmajian JV, DeLuca CJ: *Muscles Alive: Their Functions Revealed by Electromyography,* 5th ed., Baltimore, Williams & Wilkins, 1988.

15. Mann RA: Biomechanics of running, in Nicholas JA, Hershman EB, (eds.), *The Lower Extremity and Spine in Sports Medicine,* St . Louis, Mosby, 1995:335.

16. Jensen MC, Brant-Zawadzki MN, Obuchowski N, et al.: Magnetic resonance imaging of the lumbar spine in people without back pain. *N Engl J Med* 1994: 331, 69.

17. Dyck PJ, Classen SM, Stevens JC, O'Brien PC: Assessment of nerve damage in the feet of long-distance runners. *Mayo Clin Proc* 1987:62, 568.

18. Park TA, Del Toro DR: Electrodiagnostic evaluation of the foot. *Phys Med Rehabil Clin North Am* 1998:9, 87, vii.

19. Albers JW: Numbness, tingling, and weakness, in AAEM Annual Assembly, 1999. Vancouver, Johnson Printing Company.

Chapter 9

COMPARTMENT SYNDROME TESTING

John E. Glorioso, Jr. and
John H. Wilckens

INDICATIONS FOR MEASUREMENT OF COMPARTMENT PRESSURES

Exertional leg pain is a common complaint in the running athlete. Chronic exertional compartment syndrome is defined as reversible ischemia secondary to a noncompliant osseofascial compartment that is unresponsive to the expansion of muscle volume that occurs with exercise. It presents as recurrent episodes of leg discomfort experienced at a given distance or intensity of run. Though a characteristic history is highly suggestive of exertional compartment syndrome, no physical examination finding can firmly establish the diagnosis.[1] Diagnosis based solely on clinical presentation can lead to misdiagnosis and inappropriate therapy or delay of proper therapy.[2] An exercise challenge and documentation of elevated compartment pressure in one or more of the compartments of the leg is essential to confirm the diagnosis.

Indications for compartment pressure measurement include any patient with clinical evidence of chronic exertional compartment syndrome. Significant historical features include recurrent, exercise-induced leg discomfort which increases as the training session continues. The quality of pain is usually described as a tight, cramp-like, or squeezing ache over a specific compartment of the leg. The complaint of paresthesias of the leg or foot with exertion may be described.

ASSESSMENT

Because the physical examination is often normal at rest, some clinicians may prefer to exercise challenge the athlete prior to a decision to perform invasive compartment pressure measurements. There is no doubt that an exercise challenge with detailed physical examination immediately after reproduction of symptoms will lead to a more judicious use of invasive techniques. After reproduction of discomfort, the athlete should be assessed for tenderness, tightness, and swelling over the involved compartments. The tenderness noted should involve the muscle mass and not the bone or muscle-tendon junction. Strength of the muscles of the compartment should be assessed in order to detect any specific muscle involvement and weakness induced by the transient ischemia. Measurement of leg girth before and after exercise may be helpful in detecting increased volume or hypertrophy of the muscle induced by exertion.[3] The measurements should be compared with those of the unaffected limb, because some degree of swelling is expected as a normal response to activity.

A neurologic and vascular examination should also be performed with reproduction of the symptoms. Understanding the distribution of nerves and functions of muscles in relation to symptoms can help identify the affected compartment in cases where the pain is not well localized to one specific compartment, or it may help determine which compartments are more severely affected in cases where more than one compartment is involved. If the anterior compartment is affected, the patient may display weakness of dorsiflexion or toe extension and paresthesias over the dorsum of the foot, numbness in the first web space, or even transient or persistent foot drop.[4] Paresthesias in the plantar aspect of the foot and weakness of toe flexion and foot inversion may be revealed when the deep posterior compartment is involved, whereas dorsolateral foot hypoesthesia and plantar flexion weakness may be present if the superficial posterior compartment is affected. Lateral compartment pressure elevation with compression of the superficial peroneal nerve can induce sensory changes over the anterolateral aspect of the leg and weakness of ankle eversion. An inversion as well as equinus deformity may also be present.[5]

The patient should have normal dorsalis pedis and posterior tibialis pulses with reproduction of symptoms. If pulses are diminished or absent compared with baseline, a vascular etiology such as popliteal artery entrapment should be sought.

If a suspicion of chronic exertional compartment syndrome exists and the athlete meets the criteria above, compartment pressure testing should be scheduled. In the diagnostic evaluation and work-up of athletes with chronic exertional ischemia, it is important to note that the athlete may have bilateral symptoms as well as more than one compartment affected simultaneously. Since multiple compartments may be involved, any compartment that is symptomatic warrants measurement.

The amount of time necessary to perform compartmental pressure measurements is variable. The time needed depends on how much experience the clinician has performing the procedure, how long it takes to set up the equipment and prep the athlete, and the number of compartments to be measured. The rate limiting step, however, is the amount of time it takes the athlete to reproduce symptoms. In general, at least $\frac{1}{2}$ hr should be allotted for the technical aspects of the procedure, 15 min for prep and measurement of resting pressures, and 15 min for postexertional measurement and review of the results with the athlete.

TESTING METHODS

Several techniques have been described in the literature for measuring both static and dynamic intramuscular pressures. These techniques include the needle manometer,[6] the wick catheter,[7] slit catheter,[8] continuous infusion,[9] and a solid-state transducer

intracompartmental catheter.[10] Each of these techniques offers several advantages and disadvantages. However, all are time-consuming and require some degree of skill and experience to set up and perform.

The authors' preferred method for measurement of compartment pressures is with a battery-operated, hand-held, digital, fluid pressure monitor. The Stryker Intracompartmental Pressure Monitor (Stryker Corporation, Kalamazoo, Mich) is a convenient and easy-to-use measuring device for use in the clinical setting.[11] This device has been found to be more accurate, versatile, convenient, and much less time-consuming to use than the needle manometer method.[12] Measurements were also found to be more reproducible among different examiners with the Stryker instrument.

The usefulness of pressure measurement and maintenance of patient safety with this invasive technique relies upon a thorough knowledge of the anatomy of the leg. Prior to attempting to measure compartment pressures the physician should thoroughly study the anatomical structures in each compartment in order to avoid damaging neurovascular structures (see Chapter 16).

EQUIPMENT

Equipment needed includes the Stryker pressure monitor and a disposable packet designed for use in conjunction with it (Fig. 9–1). Each disposable packet contains a sterile 18-gauge needle for static measurements, a diaphragm chamber, and a syringe filled with 3 cc of normal saline. A slit catheter can also be attached to

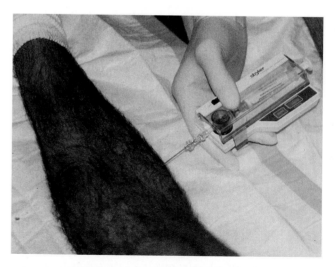

Figure 9–1. Compartment pressure measurement with a battery operated, hand-held, digital fluid pressure monitor, the Stryker Intracompartmental Pressure Monitor. (*Source: Photo published with permission of Stryker Instruments, Kalamazoo, Mich*).

the monitor if dynamic measurements are desired. Other necessary equipment includes Betadine solution, alcohol prep pads, gauze, and a 25- or 27-gauge needle and syringe for local anesthesia. Lidocaine 1% solution without epinephrine and bupivacaine 0.5% should be used for local anesthesia. The bupivacaine solution is particularly important to avoid reanesthetizing the skin in athletes who may require considerable time to reproduce symptoms.

THE PROCEDURE

Prior to the procedure, the athlete must be made aware of the indications for the procedure, how the procedure is performed, and its risks. Consent should be obtained and the athlete counseled on the risk of infection, scarring, damage to nerve and vascular structures, and reaction to local anesthesia.

The Stryker monitor should be assembled as detailed in the directions contained in each disposable packet; key points include snug fit of the syringe to the diaphragm and the diaphragm to either the straight needle or slit catheter. Saline should be carefully infused through the system and one should make sure that no air bubbles are in the diaphragm. The system must be calibrated prior to each use by zeroing the instrument.

Prior to the resting measurement, the examiner must decide whether static or dynamic measurements are to be obtained. The Stryker system is compatible with either continuous or intermittent monitoring during exercise challenge. The straight needle is used for intermittent static measurements. The slit catheter can be taped to the athlete's leg for dynamic continuous measurements.

There is controversy about the use of dynamic testing. Though some believe that the pressure measurements obtained during running are most significant in the diagnosis of exertional compartment syndrome,[10] the general consensus is that the results are inconsistent and difficult to obtain and interpret.[13,14] Problems with dynamic measurements include maintaining the placement of catheter, attachment of the system to the athlete, and restrictions of the athlete's gait as he or she runs to reproduce symptoms. In addition, it is impossible for athletes being tested to run outdoors on their usual training surface while measuring pressure changes; however, the system does work on a treadmill. Another limitation is that only one compartment can be measured at a time, and pressures cannot be compared with those in the contralateral leg.

The authors prefer the use of the straight needle and static measurements prior to exertion, immediately after (1 min) the reproduction of symptoms, and 5 to 10 min into rest. The downside to this technique compared with dynamic measurement is that repeated sticks are necessary. Though there is much debate as to which pressure measurement method is most reliable in assessing exertional compartment syndrome, most agree that the most important measurement is the resting pressure taken immediately after the exercise challenge.[13,15]

Though attempts may be made to reproduce symptoms in the office by repetitive resisted ankle movements and jogging in place, some patients will be unable to reproduce their symptoms. The optimal way for the athlete to display symptoms is to perform the specific activity that produces discomfort. This is best accomplished by having the patient run on a treadmill or outside the office if a running space is available. The athlete should be instructed to run to the point at which they usually cease activity secondary to discomfort (exercise until pain or fatigue limits further activity). Immediately after the run the patient should have his or her compartmental pressures measured.

MAINTAINING TESTING ACCURACY

Three important factors may lead to inaccurate pressure readings. First, it is important to always zero the monitor at the same angle that will be used to penetrate the skin. With repeat sticks, one must maintain the same angle as that used when the device was initially calibrated. This is most efficiently performed by placing the needle just away from the skin over the compartment to be measured at an angle of 90 degrees perpendicular to the skin. Just prior to insertion into the epidermis, the monitor should be zeroed. This should be repeated prior to each measurement.

Second, it has been determined that both knee and ankle positioning affect pressure readings.[16] Therefore the joint position of the knee and ankle should be standardized when obtaining serial measurements of intracompartmental pressures.

Finally, while attempting to stabilize the leg with one hand while holding the monitor in the other, care must be taken not to squeeze the leg. It has been observed that externally applied pressure raises the pressure level within the compartment.[9]

ANATOMY AND APPROACH

Each compartment should be approached with an understanding of its anatomical contents in order to avoid injury to neurovascular structures.

The approach to the anterior compartment is most easily accomplished by palpating the muscle belly of the anterior tibialis just lateral to the anterior tibial border at the level of the mild-third of the tibia. The neurovascular bundle containing the deep peroneal nerve and anterior tibial artery and veins is deep to the anterior tibialis muscle sitting just above the interosseous membrane.

The muscle bellies of the peroneus longus and brevis in the lateral compartment are accessible on the lateral surface of the leg just superficial to the shaft of the fibula. Our technique to enter this compartment first involves palpation of the head of the fibula and lateral malleolus and palpating the muscle bellies at the midpoint between these two bony landmarks.

Another landmark helpful in distinguishing the anterior and lateral compartments is the intermuscular septum. The intermuscular septum lies halfway between the tibial crest and the fibula and can be palpated between these two sites. The anterior compartment is anterior to the intermuscular septum and the lateral compartment is posterior to it.

The posterior superficial compartment is easily penetrated after palpation of the muscle bellies of the gastrocnemius and soleus muscles. We prefer to approach this compartment just medial to the midline to avoid the small saphenous vein and the medial and lateral sural cutaneous nerves.

The approach to the posterior deep compartment is technically more difficult than those previously mentioned. Many physicians are reluctant to attempt to measure compartment pressures in this compartment due to the proximity of neurovascular structures. The posterior deep compartment has two bundles with which one should be familiar prior to attempting to penetrate the fascia with a needle. A vascular bundle consisting of the peroneal artery and veins lies medial to the posterior aspect of the fibula. A neurovascular bundle containing the tibial nerve and posterior tibial artery and veins lies in the posterior aspect of this compartment behind the mass of the tibialis posterior muscle. Our technique to enter this compartment is to first palpate the posterior medial aspect of the mid-tibia. The needle is then inserted just posterior to the tibia, closely approximating the posterior border of the bone. The needle will first enter the flexor digitorum longus muscle and if guided deeper will enter the posterior tibialis muscle. This approach will keep the needle anterior and medial to the described neurovascular structures as long as it is not driven too deeply.

CONFIRMING THE DIAGNOSIS

Generally accepted criteria for the diagnosis of chronic exertional compartment syndrome are described by Pedowitz and colleagues.[2] One or more of the following pressure criteria must be met in addition to a history and physical examination that is consistant with the diagnosis of CECS. Pre exercise pressure ≥15 mm Hg; 1 min postexercise pressure ≥30 mm Hg; or 5 min postexercise pressure ≥20 mm Hg.

Recent interest has focused on the use of the triple phase bone scan in the diagnosis of exertional compartment syndrome.[17] The dynamic bone scan may support the diagnosis based on specific tracer uptake patterns. The characteristic appearance is that of decreased radionuclide concentration in the vicinity of the area of increased pressure with increased soft tissue concentration both superior and inferior to the abnormality. The area of decreased uptake is believed to be due to the increased pressure and decreased blood flow to the region.[18] The triple phase bone scan offers an alternative to direct intracompartmental pressure measurements in cases in which the athlete is averse to repeated needle sticks or where the results of pressure monitoring may be borderline.

SUMMARY OF THE PROCEDURE

1. If historical and physical examination findings support the diagnosis, the procedure should be discussed with the patient and consent obtained.
2. Assemble the Stryker monitor per manufacturer directions. Each disposable kit contains a sterile needle, diaphragm transducer, and a syringe filled with 3.0 cc of 0.9% saline. The diaphragm transducer should be connected to the syringe on one end and the needle on the other. Next, prime the diaphragm by slowly pressing on the plunger of the syringe. Watch the fluid as it fills the diaphragm and continue to slowly press until fluid drips from the needle tip. Visually inspect the diaphragm to ensure no air bubbles are within it. The system should then be placed securely into the monitor. The monitor should be turned on to be sure that the battery has power.
3. Identify the compartments to be measured and have a thorough understanding of the anatomical structures to be avoided. Sterilize the skin surrounding the site to be penetrated with alcohol and Betadine.
4. Anesthetize the area by infiltrating the subcutaneous tissue with 0.5 to 1.0 cc of a mixture of 1% lidocaine without epinephrine and bupivacaine. If the fascia is to be anesthetized and penetrated, only a small volume

of anesthetic should be used. No anesthetic should be injected into the compartment, as this may alter pressure measurements.

5. Wear sterile gloves and keep one hand sterile to guide the needle and use the other to hold the monitor.

6. Standardize the position of the knee and leg on the examination table. Zero the monitor at a 90-degree angle just off the skin. Once zeroed, penetrate skin and subcutaneous tissue. As the needle contacts the fascia, resistance will be noted. Upon penetrating through the fascia, a "pop" should be felt. Care should be taken to control the depth of the needle insertion once penetration through the fascia has occurred.

7. Infuse a small amount of saline into the muscular compartment to ensure a rapid rise in the pressure on the digital display. Release the plunger on the syringe and follow the pressure on the digital display as it falls. The pressure should initially show a rapid decline followed by a slower decrease. Once the pressure is equilibrated (indicated by minor pressure fluctuations on the display), record the pressure and withdraw the needle from the compartment. Cover the puncture wound with sterile gauze and tape. Measure the other compartments in a similar manner.

8. Have the athlete run to reproduce symptoms. The athlete should return to the examination room still jogging in place and symptomatic. Have the athlete sit on the examination table in the same position as that used for the prior measurements. Remove the dressing and reprep the site(s) with alcohol before betadine. Obtain measurements within 1 min of stopping activity. Zero the monitor and enter each compartment through the same needle hole. Obtain the pressure measurement as before.

9. Cover needle penetration site with a sterile bandage. Dispose of the needles in a biohazard container.

10. Advise the patient on postprocedure care, including an immediate return for treatment of any bleeding, neurologic complaints, signs of infection, or other sequelae. The patient should be advised to rest after the procedure and not perform strenuous physical activity involving the lower extremity for the rest of the day.

REFERENCES

1. Styf JR, Korner LM: Diagnosis of chronic anterior compartment syndrome in the lower leg. *Acta Orthop Scand* 1987:58, 139.

2. Pedowitz RA, Hargens AR, Mubarak SJ, et al.: Modified criteria for the objective diagnosis of chronic compartment syndrome of the leg. *Am J Sports Med* 1990:18, 35.

3. Styf J: Chronic exercise-induced pain in the anterior aspect of the lower leg: An overview of diagnosis. *Sports Med* 1989:7, 331.

4. Detmer DE, Sharpe K, Sufit RL, et al.: Chronic compartment syndrome: Diagnosis, management, and outcomes. *Am J Sports Med* 1985:13, 162.

5. Gordon G: Leg pains in athletes. *J Foot Surg* 1979:18, 55.

6. Whitesides TE, Haney TC, Harada H, et al.: A simple method for tissue pressure determination. *Arch Surg* 1975:110, 1311.

7. Mubarak SJ, Hargens AR, Owen CA, et al.: The wick catheter technique for measurement of intramuscular pressure. *J Bone Joint Surg* 1976:58-A, 1016.

8. Rorabeck CH, Castle GSP, Hardie R, et al.: Compartmental pressure measurements: An experimental investigation using the slit catheter. *J Trauma* 1981:21, 446.

9. Matsen FA, Mayo KA, Sheridan GW, et al.: Monitoring of intramuscular pressure. *Surgery* 1976:79, 702.

10. McDermott AGP, Marble AE, Yabsley RH, et al.: Monitoring dynamic anterior compartment pressures during exercise—A new technique using the STIC catheter. *Am J Sports Med* 1982:10, 83.

11. Hutchinson MR, Ireland ML: Chronic exertional compartment syndrome—gauging pressure. *Physician Sports Med* 1999:27, 101.

12. Awbrey BJ, Sienkiewicz PS, Mankin HJ: Chronic exercise induced compartment pressure elevation measured with a miniaturized fluid pressure monitor: A laboratory and clinical study. *Am J Sports Med* 1988:16, 610.

13. Rorabeck CH, Bourne RB, Fowler PJ, et al.: The role of tissue pressure measurement in diagnosing chronic anterior compartment syndrome. *Am J Sports Med* 1988:16, 143.

14. Rorabeck CH, Fowler PJ, Nott L: The results of fasciotomy in the management of chronic exertional compartment syndrome. *Am J Sports Med* 1988:16, 224.

15. Bourne RB, Rorabeck CH: Compartment syndromes of the lower leg. *Clin Orthopaed Related Res* 1989:240, 97.

16. Gershuni DH, Yaru NC, Hargens AR, et al.: Ankle and knee position as a factor modifying intracompartmental pressure in the human leg. *J Bone Joint Surg* 1984:66-A, 1415.

17. Samuelson DR, Cram RL: The three phase bone scan and exercise induced lower leg pain: The tibial stress test. *Clin Nucl Med* 1996:21, 89.

18. Matin P: Basic principles of nuclear medicine techniques for detection and evaluation of trauma and sports medicine injuries. *Semin Nucl Med* 1988:18, 90.

Chapter 10

EXERCISE-INDUCED ASTHMA TESTING

Fred H. Brennan, Jr.

INTRODUCTION

Exercise-induced asthma (EIA) is a common medical condition that affects 10% to 15% of athletes. It is often characterized by coughing, wheezing, and/or chest tightness during or shortly after exercise.[1] Running has been recognized as an asthmagenic exercise that may present with those symptoms. However, occasionally runners with EIA will complain of fatigue, "being out of shape," or simply "feeling stale." As a clinician it is important for you to listen to your patient's history and to recognize those subtle signs of EIA. Formal testing for EIA can then be performed to document the presence or absence of this condition. Testing can also be useful to differentiate EIA alone from EIA with underlying chronic asthma, which may alter the patient's therapy.

TESTING FOR EXERCISE-INDUCED ASTHMA

There have been many studies done evaluating different techniques for diagnosing EIA.[2] Three basic techniques will be discussed in this chapter: the exercise challenge, the methacholine challenge, and the eucapnic voluntary hyperventilation (EVH) test. All of these tests require baseline pulmonary function testing (PFT/spirometry) or peak flow (PF) measurements, followed by a challenge or provocative test with subsequent measurements.

Pulmonary Function Test

In evaluating a runner for EIA with pulmonary function tests, the most commonly used measurement is the change in FEV_1 from baseline values.[3] FEV_1 is the forced expiratory volume, measured in liters, exhaled by the athlete in the first second of exhalation. Three to five trials should be performed each time and the three best FEV_1 measurements averaged and recorded. A drop in the FEV_1 of 10% to 15% from baseline values during and/or after provocative testing is considered diagnostic of EIA.[4] Another spirometric value that can be assessed is the forced expiratory flow ($FEF_{25\%-75\%}$). This is the measurement, in liters, of the amount of air expired in the middle 50% of the exhalation cycle. A decrease of 20% after provocative testing is considered diagnostic for EIA.[5] Finally, a Wright peak flow meter can be used to assess the peak expiratory flow rate (PEFR). This is the maximum rate that air is expired, measured in liters per second. The best PEFR value of three attempts should be used as the baseline PEFR. A decrease of 15% to 25% in PEFR from baseline after provocative testing is considered diagnostic of EIA.[3,6] Some authors debate the reliability of peak flow testing for EIA; however, this method is still considered a viable testing option. It must be mentioned that, although the percentages of change in pulmonary function test values appear concrete, the patient's history and symptoms must also always be considered. For example, if a runner, especially an elite runner, has a decrease in FEV_1 of only 8% after provocative testing but is symptomatic with classic symptoms, this may still be considered a positive test for EIA.

Provocative Testing/Challenge for Exercise-Induced Asthma

Exercise Challenge

This type of provocative testing is commonly used to evaluate athletes for EIA. Although its reliability as a diagnostic test is debated, clinicians often use this as a first-line test.[3] When exercise challenging an athlete it is imperative that you test the athlete sport-specifically in the environment in which the symptoms typically occur. For example, a runner should be challenged outside on a track and not indoors on a treadmill if his or her symptoms tend to occur outside. An athlete may not be exposed to allergens, temperatures, and pollutants that may be triggering their asthma if they are tested in an indoor environment.

Conducting an Exercise Challenge Test on a Runner

1. Allow the athlete to stretch but do not let him or her warm up. Warming up may cause a false-negative test.
2. Obtain baseline PFT with spirometry or PEFR using the best effort of three attempts. Record FEV_1, $FEF_{25\%-75\%}$, and/or PEFR.
3. Have the athlete run for 8 to 10 minutes at a heart rate of 85% to 90% of their maximum predicted heart rate (which equals 220 minus the patient's age in years). This is very important.
4. After 10 minutes, stop the athlete and give a 1-minute cool-down. Then check PFTs or peak

flows three times and record the best of the three attempts.
5. Repeat these tests at 3, 5, 10, 15, and 20 minutes postexercise and record these values (Table 10–1). Some athletes' values will drop 15 to 20 minutes postexercise. As mentioned earlier, a decrease in FEV_1 of >10% or a decrease in $FEF_{25\%-75\%}$ of 20% is diagnostic for EIA. A decrease in PEFR of >15% is also suggestive of EIA.
6. A bronchodilator may be administered with repeat testing to verify reversibility of the findings, thus demonstrating bronchospasm consistent with EIA.

See Table 10–2 for reference values of peak expiratory flow rates.

Methacholine Challenge

Another technique that is used to assess a runner with potential EIA is the methacholine challenge test. Methacholine seems to stimulate muscarinic receptors located in the airway smooth muscle.[7] A baseline pulmonary function test is conducted first with the best of three FEV_1 trials being recorded. Methacholine solutions are then prepared in the following concentrations: 0.025, 0.25, 2.5, 10, and 25 mg/ml. The athlete then inhales five breaths of the lowest concentration of nebulized solution and in 3 minutes PFTs are repeated as they were for baseline testing. The cycle is continued every 3 to 5 minutes, gradually increasing the nebulized methacholine solution concentration for each trial. The test is concluded when a drop in FEV_1 of 20% is noted *or* the maximum concentration of 25 mg/ml is administered.[2] A positive methacholine challenge is a drop in FEV_1 of at least 20%. It does not matter what concentration of methacholine is used; however, the concentration should be noted because it may give some indication of bronchial sensitivity to stimuli. A positive response at a lower concentration of methacholine may indicate airways that are more prone to bronchospasm. Figures 10–1 and 10–2

TABLE 10–1. EXERCISE SPIROMETRY WORKSHEET

Conditions	FVC	FEV$_1$	FEF$_{25\%-75\%}$	FEV$_1$/FVC	FEV$_1$ % Baseline
Baseline					
1 minute					
3 minutes					
5 minutes					
10 minutes					
15 minutes					
20 minutes					

Max heart rate = 220 − age (years)
Target heart rate = _____ (90% of max heart rate)
85% of FEV$_1$ (15% decrease) = _____

TABLE 10–2. NORMAL PREDICTED AVERAGE PEAK EXPIRATORY FLOW (LITERS PER MINUTE)

Males						Females						Children and Adolescents			
Age (Years)	Height 60"	65"	70"	75"	80"	Age (Years)	Height 55"	60"	65"	70"	75"	Height (Inches)	Males & Females	Height (Inches)	Males & Females
20	554	602	649	693	740	20	390	423	460	496	529	43	147	55	307
25	543	590	636	679	725	25	385	418	454	490	523	44	160	56	320
30	532	577	622	664	710	30	380	413	448	483	516	45	173	57	334
35	521	565	609	651	695	35	375	408	442	476	509	46	187	58	347
40	509	552	596	636	680	40	370	402	436	470	502	47	200	59	360
45	498	540	583	622	665	45	365	397	430	464	495	48	214	60	373
50	486	527	569	607	649	50	360	391	424	457	488	49	227	61	387
55	475	515	556	593	634	55	355	386	418	451	482	50	240	62	400
60	463	502	542	578	618	60	350	380	412	445	475	51	254	63	413
65	452	490	529	564	603	65	345	375	406	439	468	52	267	64	427
70	440	477	515	550	587	70	340	369	400	432	461	53	280	65	440
												54	293	66	454

The National Asthma Education Program recommends that a patient's "personal best" be used as his/her baseline peak flow. "Personal best" is the maximum peak flow that the patient can obtain when his or her asthma is stable or under control. This table is intended to be used a guideline only. This table was modified and reproduced with the permission of the W.B. Saunders Co. (publishing).

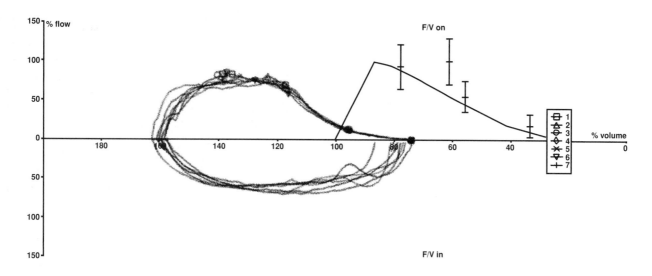

	FVC		FEV 1	MMEF	FEV1%F
Pred	3.16		2.46	2.33	77.35
BASE	3.46		2.72	2.36	78.41
0.025 METH	3.49		2.68	2.32	76.73
0.25 METH	3.56		2.73	2.36	76.71
2.5 METH	3.44		2.65	2.27	77.22
10.0 METH	3.42		2.64	1.99	76.99
25.0 METH	3.39		2.53	1.94	74.72
POST/ALB	3.38		2.64	2.11	78.19

Figure 10–1. Normal methacholine challenge. Patient was given all five increasing doses of methacholine and never fell below 95% of predicted value. Four puffs of albuterol were given after methacholine challenge with no significant change in FEV_1.

demonstrate normal and abnormal methacholine challenge tests.

Upon completion of a positive methacholine challenge test, albuterol may be administered and repeat PFTs performed 3 minutes later to document reversibility of airway obstruction and to help the patient recover. Respiratory therapists typically perform this test under physician supervision.

Eucapnic Voluntary Hyperventilation (EVH)

This provocative test is not commonly used but is considered to be as effective for diagnosing EIA as the methacholine challenge.[2] It can be performed with dry gas or cold air. The athlete has baseline PFTs calculated and is then asked to inhale a 5% carbon dioxide/air mixture at 80% of a predetermined maximal voluntary ventilation rate. The athlete will voluntarily hyperventilate at this rate for 5 to 6 minutes. PFTs are then performed immediately after and at 5-minute intervals for 15 to 20 minutes. A documented decrease of 10% in the FEV_1 is considered diagnostic for airway hyperresponsiveness/EIA.[2]

RECOMMENDATIONS FOR EXERCISE-INDUCED ASTHMA TESTING

If an athlete presents with a history suspicious for exercise-induced asthma, formal EIA testing should be performed (Fig. 10–3). I recommend an exercise challenge in the same environment or one similar to the one that tends to provoke the athlete's symptoms.

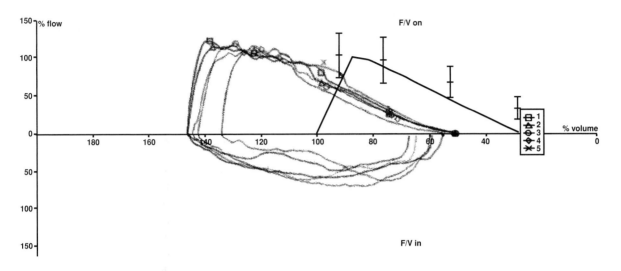

	FVC	FEV 1	MMEF	FEV1%F
Pred	3.13	2.85	3.85	90.77
BASE	4.15	3.53	3.88	84.95
0.025 METH	4.14	3.51	3.58	84.67
0.25 METH	4.01	3.33	3.27	83.09
2.5 METH	3.43	2.79	2.65	81.17
10.0 METH	4.06	3.60	4.26	88.57
25.0 METH				
POST/ALB				

Figure 10–2. Abnormal methacholine challenge. The patient demonstrated good effort on all tests, and had a greater than 20% drop in FEV_1 on a 2.5 mg/ml methacholine concentration. Six puffs of albuterol were administered to bring the patient back up to his baseline FEV_1.

Remember that the athlete must exercise for at least 8 to 10 minutes at a heart rate of 85% to 90% of their maximum predicted rate (220 − age in years). A bronchodilator given after a positive test can also help demonstrate reversibility of the airway obstruction consistent with asthma.

If this challenge is inconclusive but the clinical suspicion is still high, a methacholine challenge should be performed. If both provocative tests are negative for EIA then it is unlikely that the athlete is experiencing true bronchoconstriction. Another diagnosis such as vocal cord dysfunction should be considered.[8]

In summary, avoid the temptation to treat an athlete with a bronchodilator such as albuterol without formal spirometric and provocative testing. The baseline PFTs will give the clinician insight into whether the athlete has chronic asthma requiring antiinflamma-

tory treatment along with preexercise bronchodilators. Preexercise bronchodilators are much more effective if the chronic asthmatic condition is controlled with appropriate anti-inflammatory medications like inhaled corticosteroids. Formal provocative testing is necessary to document true bronchospasm. I recommend starting with an exercise challenge test as described in this chapter. If one provocative test is negative and clinical suspicion is still high, perform a different provocative test to rule EIA in or out. A methacholine challenge test is my next choice. If the decrease in FEV_1 or PEFR does not quite meet diagnostic criteria but the athlete is markedly symptomatic with respiratory problems, especially an elite athlete, the diagnosis may still be EIA. Remember that not all asthma wheezes and everything that wheezes is not necessarily asthma.

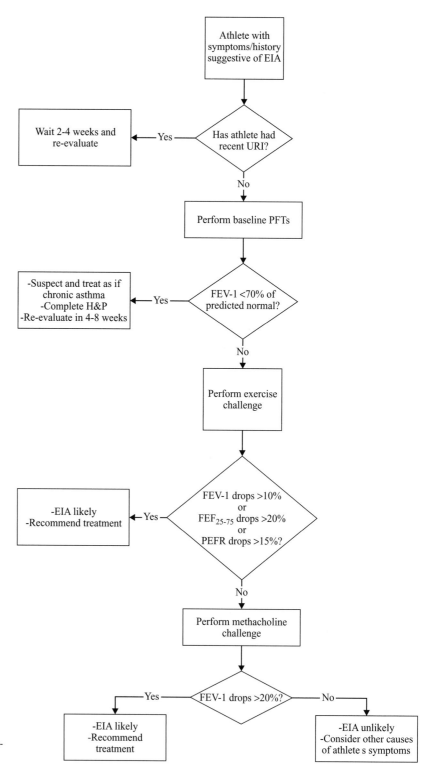

Figure 10–3. Exercise-induced asthma testing algorithm.

REFERENCES

1. Mahler DA: Exercise induced asthma. *Med Sci Sports Exerc* 1993:25, 554.
2. Eliasson AH, Phillips YY, Rajagopal KR: Sensitivity and specificity of bronchial provocation testing. An evaluation of four techniques in exercise-induced bronchospasm. *Chest* 1992:102, 347.
3. Storms WW: Exercise-induced asthma: Diagnosis and treatment for the recreational or elite athlete. *Med Sci Sports Exerc* 1999:31, S33.

4. Mannix ET, Manfredi F, Farber MO: A comparison of two challenge tests for identifying exercise-induced bronchospasm in figure skaters. *Chest* 1999:115, 649.

5. Provost CM, Arbour KS, Sestili DC, et al.: The incidence of exercise-induced bronchospasm in competitive figure skaters. *J Asthma* 1996:33, 67.

6. Virant FS: Exercise-induced bronchospasm: Epidemiology, pathophysiology, and therapy. *Med Sci Sports Exerc* 1992:24, 851.

7. Lin CC, Wu JL, Huang WC, et al.: A bronchial response comparison of exercise and methacholine in asthmatic subjects. *J Asthma* 1991:28, 31.

8. Lacroix VJ: Exercise-induced asthma. *Physician Sportsmedicine* 1999:27, 75.

Chapter 11

TESTING FOR MAXIMAL AEROBIC POWER

Patricia A. Deuster and
Bryant R. Martin

INTRODUCTION

Maximal aerobic power, or maximal oxygen uptake ($\dot{V}O_2max$), is defined as the greatest amount of oxygen a person can take in during physical exercise. It is an important measure because it serves as an index of maximal cardiovascular and pulmonary function; it is a useful single measurement for characterizing the functional capacity of the oxygen transport system; and it is a limiting factor in endurance performance. Thus, its measurement serves multiple roles.

The term maximal aerobic power is appropriate because running on a treadmill results in mechanical movement, or work (force × distance) and involves a time component, or work per unit of time. Maximal aerobic power is typically expressed as L/min or ml/kg/min. An individual's maximal aerobic power, or $\dot{V}O_2max$, can be measured or estimated by a variety of techniques including treadmill running, cycle ergometry, arm cranking, stair stepping, rowing, or walking. However, the gold standard is progressive treadmill testing by running to exhaustion. The objectives of this chapter are to present (1) an historical overview of how the concept of maximal aerobic power evolved; (2) an overview of maximal and submaximal exercise testing; (3) selected criteria for documenting that a true maximal value was achieved; (4) different ways of measuring and estimating maximal aerobic power; (5) controversial issues with respect to maximal testing and factors that both affect and limit maximal values; and finally, (6) terms that should be familiar to those interested in training.

HISTORICAL PERSPECTIVE

As early as 1923, Hill and Lupton were studying the respiration of muscle tissues and the oxygen requirements during exercise, in particular running.[1] They demonstrated that during moderate exercise, oxygen intake ($\dot{V}O_2$) would rise from resting values to a constant or steady-state value and that the time for this steady state to be achieved was typically within 2 to 3 minutes. The term *steady-state exercise* was coined, and the same authors demonstrated that during such exercise, a dynamic equilibrium was achieved when the oxygen supply was adequate to meet the demands of exercise. Under such conditions, the rate of lactate production was balanced by its oxidative removal.[1] They also noted that the actual oxygen requirement during exercise could easily exceed availability, as long as the debt was repaid at a later time. They coined the term *oxygen debt* to describe the total amount of oxygen used to recover from a bout of strenuous exercise.[1]

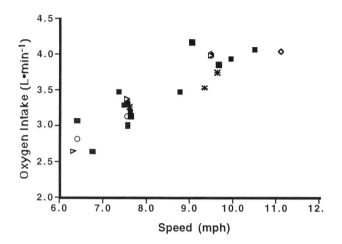

Figure 11–1. Plot of data obtained by Hill and Lupton[1] for running at various speeds on a track. Note that speeds have been converted to mph, whereas Hill and Lupton used m/min. Each set of points represents one individual running at different speeds.

Further investigation led to the use of the term *maximum oxygen intake.*[1] These investigators used running on a flat surface at increasing speeds to study $\dot{V}O_2$. Upon examination of their data, they concluded that $\dot{V}O_2$ increased with increasing speed; however, a point was reached when further increases in speed no longer resulted in increases in $\dot{V}O_2$. They concluded that "the heart, lungs, circulation, and diffusion of oxygen to the active muscle-fibres have attained their maximum activity," or $\dot{V}O_2$max. Figure 11–1 presents the data reported by Hill and Lupton, and although the number of data points are limited, one can see how the concept of $\dot{V}O_2$max evolved.

In 1933 investigators at the Harvard Fatigue Laboratory demonstrated that when individuals were exercised at a work rate in excess of their maximal aerobic capacity, their $\dot{V}O_2$ peaked within the second to third minute of exhausting work.[2] From this observation they developed a standard exercise test that consisted of walking 3.5 mph at an 8.6% grade for 15 minutes followed by running 7 mph at an 8.6% grade. This work rate was considered a maximal effort for most individuals, since few individuals exceeded 5 minutes, and typically resulted in the attainment of $\dot{V}O_2$max values after 3 minutes. This particular speed and grade should elicit a $\dot{V}O_2$ of approximately 55.5 ml/kg/min if one uses the metabolic calculation formulas in the *Guidelines for Exercise Testing and Prescription* of the American College of Sports Medicine (ACSM).[3] Thus, although most people would achieve their $\dot{V}O_2$max in a short period, a higher work rate would be required for highly trained, endurance athletes with $\dot{V}O_2$max values in excess of 55.5 ml/kg/min, as discussed below.

MAXIMAL AND SUBMAXIMAL TESTING

Expected Values for Exercise Testing

By definition, *maximal aerobic power* is the highest $\dot{V}O_2$ achieved during exercise, and the absolute value provides an indication of cardiovascular function because it is highly correlated with cardiac output and stroke volume.[4] Absolute values, typically expressed in liters per minute ($L \cdot min^{-1}$), may range from as low as 1.0 L/min (or lower in cardiovascular disease) up to $6\ L \cdot min^{-1}$ (or even higher in large, well-trained individuals). Because two individuals of quite different sizes may have the same absolute value, $\dot{V}O_2$max is often normalized for body weight to allow for between-subject comparisons. For example, if two men both have absolute values of $4.2\ L \cdot min^{-1}$ and one weighs 70 kg and the other 95 kg, then their $\dot{V}O_2$max values relative to body weight would be 60 ml/kg/min for the 70-kg man and 44.2 ml/kg/min for the 90-kg man. This relative $\dot{V}O_2$max provides an indication of an individual's potential for work, particularly running and climbing, and overall endurance. Clearly the man who weighs only 70 kg is in better shape for physical work because he could work with less relative effort at $40\ ml \cdot kg^{-1} \cdot min^{-1}$ than the 90-kg man (66% vs. 90% of $\dot{V}O_2$max). Table 11–1

TABLE 11–1. NORMATIVE MAXIMAL AEROBIC POWER RANGES FOR MEN AND WOMEN BY AGE[a]

Sex	Age	Poor to Very Poor	Fair	Good	Excellent	Superior
Men						
	<30	<34	34–41	42–47	48–54	55+
	30–39	<32	32–38	39–45	46–52	53+
	40–49	<30	30–35	36–41	42–47	48+
	>49	<28	28–31	32–36	37–42	43+
Women						
	<30	<27	27–35	36–42	43–48	49+
	30–39	<26	26–33	34–38	39–40	41+
	40–49	<26	26–30	31–36	37–40	41+
	>49	<23	23–25	26–30	31–34	35+

[a]Air Force Fitness Standards for men and women.

presents normative data by age and gender from the Air Force Fitness Standards so that $\dot{V}O_2$max values can be interpreted in light of the general population. These particular standards are comparable to others, such as those published by the Institute for Aerobics Research.[3]

Principles of Exercise Testing

When the concept of exercise testing for maximal aerobic power emerged, it soon became clear that certain requirements must be met in order to obtain a valid measure of $\dot{V}O_2$max. Importantly, Åstrand[5] reported that the exercise must involve large muscle groups, and the rate of work must be measurable and reproducible. He recommended that test conditions be standardized and that the mode of exercise should be tolerated by most people. Furthermore, all maximal exercise tests should begin with a warm-up so the individual is adapted to submaximal levels prior to undergoing maximal exercise.[6] Finally, Taylor et al.[7] recognized the importance of a test being independent of the motivation or specific skill sets of the individual. For these reasons, the primary modes for exercise testing include the treadmill and the cycle ergometer. Although stair-stepping tests, which do not require specific skills, have been used for many years, they are not among the preferred tests when direct measures of $\dot{V}O_2$ are to be made. The reason is that it is difficult to "drive" a subject to his/her maximum with stair stepping because it is uncomfortable and requires self-motivation.[5] However, it is useful in the field and/or under conditions in which large numbers of persons need to be tested.

Types of Exercise Tests

Over the years, a variety of test methodologies have emerged to either measure or estimate maximal aerobic power. These methodologies include steady-state tests, discontinuous progressive tests, continuous progressive tests with 2- to 3-minute stages, or continuous progressive tests with less than 2-minute stages, often referred to as ramp tests.[5] Figure 11–2 provides a graphic view of these various test methodologies. Whereas the steady-state protocols are always submaximal, the progressive test can be either submaximal or maximal. When submaximal progressive tests are conducted, only an estimate of maximal aerobic power can be obtained. Further discussion on estimating $\dot{V}O_2$max is presented later.

Significant efforts have been spent examining the maximal values obtained with various exercise paradigms to ascertain the most suitable way of achieving $\dot{V}O_2$max. In particular, comparisons of values attained by treadmill, cycle ergometer, stair stepping, arm, and combined arm and leg protocols have been made.[4,8,9–14]

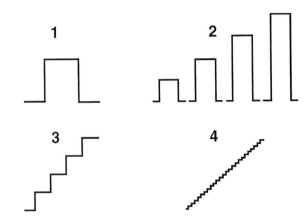

Figure 11–2. Various types of exercise testing methodologies: 1, steady state; 2, progressive, discontinuous; 3, progressive multi-stage; and 4, ramp test.

Table 11–2 provides a comparison of these efforts and shows that treadmill running with a grade is the preferred form of exercise.

In many instances the magnitude of the differences across tests depends on the sports preference of the subject being tested. For example, a $\dot{V}O_2$max approaching 80% of the value during arm and leg work combined was noted during arm cranking, but only in a trained canoeist.[9] Similarly, the upper range for upright cycling applies primarily to those who are trained cyclists.[4,5]

Treadmill Tests for Maximal Aerobic Power

By the time exercise testing had become an accepted tool for assessing cardiopulmonary function, a variety of test protocols had been described and compared.[5–7,15–19] Most of these tests are widely used and, depending on the setting and specific requirements, all are excellent tests. One of the first tests was a constant grade test with increments in speed.[1] However, many subjects other than athletes find this very difficult, and most data suggest that a true $\dot{V}O_2$max cannot be achieved. Other tests use a constant speed and impose incremental grade changes; these include the Balke,[15]

TABLE 11–2. MAXIMAL VALUES ACHIEVED DURING VARIOUS TYPES OF MAXIMAL EXERCISE TESTS

Type of Exercise	% of $\dot{V}O_2$max
Uphill running	100
Horizontal running	95–98
Upright cycling	90–96
Supine cycling	82–85
Arm cranking	62–80
Arms and legs	100–104
Step test	97
Swimming	85

Taylor,[7] and Stanford[3] tests. In 1989 Kyle et al.[20] described a continuous version of the Taylor test: the choice of the constant speed (6 to 8 mph) was determined by heart rate after a 10-minute warm-up, and the grade was increased from 0% by 2.5% every 2 minutes. This is an excellent test, which can be used with the criteria described below.

In addition, there are protocols that change both grades and speeds. The most commonly used test is the one described by Bruce et al.[6] Although the time to complete the Bruce protocol is minimal, this test was modified because it imposed marked increases in both speed and grade, which many people found very difficult. In contrast, the original Balke protocol, which uses 2% increments in grade and 3-minute stages, takes a long time to achieve $\dot{V}O_2$max. Modified versions of both protocols have been offered and can be used, depending on the population of interest. Clearly, smaller grade increments and a slow speed are preferred for older and/or deconditioned subjects, whereas larger work increments and higher speeds are suitable for the younger and highly active populations. Figure 11–3 provides a range of relative $\dot{V}O_2$ values expected for various speeds and grades. This information can provide the tester with at least an estimate of what to expect, despite significant individual variation due to biomechanics, body composition, and other such characteristics. Importantly, the individual to be tested should be assessed in terms of expectations so that an appropriate protocol is selected.

Interestingly, many of the standard treadmill exercise tests have been compared over the years, with respect to differences in grade and speed changes, type of test (i.e., ramp and different times for multistage tests), and reliability of repeated tests. Although there may be some small differences in the final $\dot{V}O_2$max values achieved across different test protocols, if the test is conducted in a standardized manner, the subject has been familiarized with the test procedures, and the testing personnel are well trained, these differences are minimal.[18,19,21–23] In terms of repeatability, if multiple tests are conducted with the same protocol over a short period, the within-subject variability has been reported to average about 4%, regardless of the training status of the persons tested.[20,24] This is certainly an acceptable variability and indicates that the measure of $\dot{V}O_2$max is reliable. However, it is important to recognize that subjects need to be familiar with the equipment and protocol for this to hold true.

Cycle Ergometer Tests for Maximal Aerobic Power

Although similar principles can be applied to cycle ergometer tests, the cycle ergometer is different from the treadmill in that work rates are weight independent, and the two primary variables are cycling rate and resistance. These factors determine the power, or work per unit of time, which is expressed in watts (W). With cycling, if $\dot{V}O_2$ is measured during steady state at various work rates, a linear relation between work rate (W) and $\dot{V}O_2$ is noted, with a range of 9 to 11 ml of O_2 per W[25,26]; Figure 11–4 depicts this relation for cycling exercise. Although there is some variability, the relationship is used to estimate $\dot{V}O_2$ when actual measurements are not possible. For cycle ergometer tests, a cycling rate of 50 revolutions/rotations per minute (rpm) is often used, although some subjects find this too slow at the lower work rates. In all cases, the subject should have

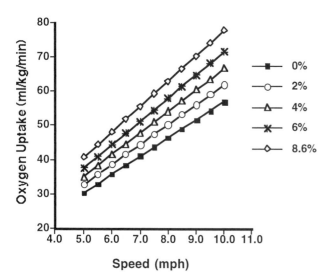

Figure 11–3. Oxygen uptake values expected for various speeds and grades as determined by the ACSM's formulas for metabolic calculations.[3]

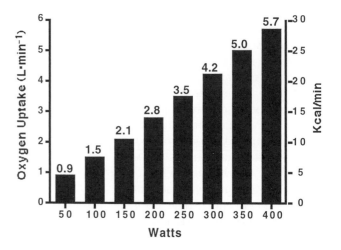

Figure 11–4. Predicted $\dot{V}O_2$ requirements for various power outputs (W) on a cycle ergometer. Note: these requirements are independent of body weight.

a warm-up with either no load or minimal load (25 W) prior to any progressive increase in resistance. Each progressive stage should be between 1 and 3 minutes, and the step increments in W can range from 25 to 60, depending on the subject popu-lation. For a detailed description of cycle and treadmill exercise test protocols, the reader should consult the ACSM's *Guidelines for Exercise Testing and Prescription*.[3]

Documenting Attainment of Maximal Aerobic Power

When a maximal aerobic power test is to be conducted, it is important to document whether a true $\dot{V}O_2$max has been achieved. Such a determination begins with a basic understanding of the physiologic responses to severe exercise and assessment of selected parameters that have been designated as criteria for making this determination. The current parameters considered as criteria include the primary measure of a plateau in $\dot{V}O_2$ and the secondary measures of blood (or plasma) lactate, respiratory exchange ratio (RER), heart rate, and perceived exertion.[3,28,29]

CRITERIA FOR MAXIMAL AEROBIC POWER

A Plateau in Oxygen Uptake

A plateau in oxygen intake, despite increasing work rates, emerged through the work of Hill and Lupton and was taken up by other investigators during the late 1920s and 1930s.[7,27] However, it was not until 1955 that Taylor et al.[7] undertook efforts to define precise criteria for attaining a plateau. They evaluated a variety of factors that could influence the quantification of $\dot{V}O_2$max, including within-subject variability and the roles of increases in grade and speed on plateau of $\dot{V}O_2$. Objectifying that $\dot{V}O_2$max is associated with a plateau in $\dot{V}O_2$ as workload continued to rise was considered of primary importance. Using a discontinuous protocol, subjects ran at 7 mph at a given grade (0% to 12.5%) for 3 minutes with grade increases of 2.5% until the subject could go no longer; increasing grades were typically done on different days or after a period of rest. With this protocol, Taylor et al.[7] showed that a 2.5% grade increase typically resulted in a rise in $\dot{V}O_2$ of approximately 300 ml·min^{-1}. However, at a certain point, higher levels of exercise, which were different for each person, did not elicit the 300 ml·min^{-1} increase. Based on this information, it was determined that an increase of less than 150 ml/min or 2.1 ml/kg/min in $\dot{V}O_2$ for a higher work rate marked a plateau in $\dot{V}O_2$. They concluded that a grade increase was preferable to speed increases for achieving a plateau, and further, they

demonstrated that 108 of 115, or 93.9%, of subjects achieved the designated plateau.

Despite some controversy, the first criterion proposed for demonstrating a true $\dot{V}O_2$max (<150 ml/min or 2.1 ml/kg/min) is still used today as the primary criterion, or the gold standard.[28,29] Some critics state that 150 ml/min is too large a value and causes $\dot{V}O_2$max to be underestimated. More conservative numbers have been suggested, such as an increase of <50 ml·min^{-1},[30] 80 ml·min^{-1},[8] or 100 ml/min.[31] Meyer et al.[32] suggested that a plateau phenomenon is not always seen with various protocols today because of the sampling interval selected (e.g., breath-by-breath, 5-, 10-, or 15-second averages) and the magnitude of the work increments for each exercise stage. However, other investigators have demonstrated attainment of the plateau criteria according to Taylor's criteria. Kyle et al.,[20] who used a slight modification of the Taylor protocol, showed that 100% of subjects achieved the designated plateau in at least one of three treadmill tests. Similarly, Stachenfeld et al.,[33] who used a cycle ergometer, reported that 88% of subjects met the criteria on their first test; the remaining subjects met the criteria on the second or third tests. Because no consensus has been reached, values between 50 and 150 ml·min^{-1} are currently acceptable for verification. Importantly, a plateau will not be seen in all people, due to various factors such as physical restrictions, age of the individual, or motivation. Thus the secondary criteria described below have evolved.

Blood Lactate Levels

In the absence of a true plateau in $\dot{V}O_2$, a rise in blood lactate has been used to demonstrate a maximal effort.[4,5,8] As the workload continues to rise and the person moves toward a maximal effort, blood lactate levels increase due to an acceleration in glycogen breakdown in muscle, an increased recruitment of fast-twitch muscle fibers, a reduction in liver blood flow, and an elevation in plasma epinephrine concentration.[4,5,8,34] These observations were first made by Åstrand, who noted that in the absence of a visible plateau, lactate values, along with a subject-reported stress level, could be used to document that the subject had attained a true $\dot{V}O_2$max.[4,5,8]

Although identifying a standard cutoff for blood lactate levels has been difficult, the data from Åstrand's earliest studies suggested a cutoff of 7.9 mM to 8.4 mM.[4,5,8] Subsequent investigators have noted that 8 mM is a reasonable value for use as a criterion.[28–30,33] Cumming and Borysyk[30] and Stachenfeld et al.[33] found that 78% of their subjects achieved levels greater than 8 mM. Moreover, 8 mM was the best criterion in terms of specificity and positive predictive value compared with other secondary criteria.[33]

Although current standards vary, a value greater than 8 mM appears to be consistent with research studies and is well accepted by researchers in general.

Respiratory Exchange Ratio

The respiratory quotient (RQ) and RER are both calculated as the ratio of CO_2 volume produced to O_2 volume used, or $\dot{V}CO_2/\dot{V}O_2$, and typically range between 0.7 and 1.0. The RQ, which is an indicator of metabolic fuel or substrate utilization in tissues, must be calculated under resting and steady-state conditions; a ratio of 0.7 is indicative of mixed fat utilization and a ratio of 1.0 of carbohydrate utilization exclusivity.[31] Thus, during low-intensity, steady-state exercise, when fatty acids are the primary fuel, the RQ and RER are typically between 0.80 and 0.88. As the intensity of the exercise increases, and carbohydrates become the dominant or primary fuel, the RQ and RER increase to between 0.9 and 1.0. Whereas the RQ cannot exceed 1.0 because it reflects tissue substrate utilization, the RER, which reflects respiratory exchange of CO_2 and O_2, commonly exceeds 1.0 during strenuous exercise. During non–steady-state, strenuous exercise, individuals typically hyperventilate, which results in an increased unloading of CO_2 and increases in muscle lactic acid: additional CO_2 evolves in the buffering of lactic acid, and RER is no longer indicative of substrate usage. Thus, RER becomes reflective of both hyperventilation and blood lactate.[4,28,29,31]

Because the RER reproducibly increases during exercise, it is considered a potential parameter for documenting maximal effort. Issekutz et al.,[31] the first to propose the use of RER as a criterion for $\dot{V}O_2$max, noted that it must be in excess of 1.15 the higher the value, the more accurate the assessment of $\dot{V}O_2$max. The 1.15 value appears to be reasonable, although not all subjects are able to achieve it. Recent studies have used values of 1.00, 1.05, 1.10, and 1.13 as criteria for maximal performance,[28,29] but at present there is no clear consensus.

Age-Predicted Maximal Heart Rate

The widely recognized linear relationship between heart rate and $\dot{V}o2$ has encouraged the use of maximal heart rate as a criterion. In fact, attaining a target percentage of the age-predicted maximal heart rate (220 · age or 210 − 0.5 × age) is one of the most widely recognized criterion.[28,29] Unfortunately, this criterion is very difficult to meet because of the wide variability in the measure, with one standard deviation of ±10 to 12 bpm.[3] As such, a maximal effort may rarely be documented if heart rate is used as the sole criterion. For this reason, the ACSM and others have recommended that heart rate should not be used alone, but rather in conjunction with other secondary criteria.[3,28,29]

Borg Scale, or Rating of Perceived Exertion

Dr. Gunnar Borg, a Swedish physiologist, has long been the advocate of using perceived exertion as a measure of stress and performance. Borg[35,36] declared that an individual is the best rater of his/her own "degree of physical strain" and believed that individuals can monitor or evaluate a decrease or increase in their physical work capacity independent of physiological methods. Subjectively rated perceived exertion only becomes an issue when one is trying to quantify it as a measure of actual exertion and when comparing the perceptions of individuals. Thus, he developed the Borg Scale or rating of perceived exertion (RPE).

The Borg Scale, the most widely used method of quantifying perceived exertion, was designed to increase in a linear fashion as exercise intensity increased and to parallel the apparent linearity of $\dot{V}O_2$ and heart rate with workload.[35,36] The original scale ranged from 6 to 20, with each number anchored by a simple and understandable verbal expression. The specific numbers of the scale were intended to be a general representation of actual heart rate, such that when a person was exercising at 130 bpm, a perceived exertion of 13 should be reported. Similarly, if a perceived exertion of 19 were reported, a heart rate of 190 might be expected. The scale was not intended to be exact, but rather as a way to aid in the interpretation of perceived exertion.

Further studies have demonstrated a good correlation between RPE and $\dot{V}O_2$.[37,38] Eston et al.[37] obtained RPE values during a graded exercise test and reported a good correlation between heart rates and $\dot{V}O_2$ when the reported RPE was between 13 and 17. In terms of establishing RPE as a criterion for assessing the arrival of $\dot{V}O_2$max, a value of 17 or greater should be accepted as a positive indicator.

Since the initial scale was developed, a variant scale using 0 to 10 as the numeric ratio has been proposed. This scale, which has not been widely accepted, is suitable for examining subjective symptoms such as breathing difficulties.[36] However, for the purposes of criteria for $\dot{V}O_2$max, the original 15-point RPE scale remains the standard. Table 11–3 provides the ratings for the original and new Borg Scales.

Recommended Criteria for Testing

It must be noted that there are problems associated with the criteria for documenting $\dot{V}O_2$max. Specifically, because no guidelines have been established, the criteria used across studies are inconsistent.[28,29] Moreover, the criterion for $\dot{V}O_2$ was initially established for a discontinuous treadmill test with 2.5% increases in grade. To date, the criterion for a plateau

TABLE 11–3. THE ORIGINAL AND NEW BORG SCALES FOR RATING OF PERCEIVED EXERTION

Original Scale		New Scale	
6	No exertion at all	0	Nothing at all
7	Extremely light	0.5	Very, very weak
8		1	Very weak
9	Very light	2	Weak
10		3	Moderate
11	Light	4	Somewhat strong
12		5	Strong
13	Somewhat hard	6	
14		7	Very strong
15	Hard (heavy)	8	
16		9	
17	Very hard	10	Very, very strong
18		*	Maximal
19	Extremely hard		
20	Maximal exertion		

TABLE 11–4. CRITERIA FOR DOCUMENTING A MAXIMAL EFFORT TEST[a]

Increase in $\dot{V}O_2$ <150 ml/min or 2.1 ml/kg/min with a 2.5% grade increase
Blood lactate ≥ 8 mM
RER ≥ 1.15
Increase in HR to maximal estimated for age ±10
Borg Scale >17

[a]If the first criterion is not met, then at least two of the remaining four should be met. RER, respiratory exchange rate; HR, heart rate.

has not been redefined for other specific tests, and thus the 150 ml · min^{-1} increase continues to be used. Figure 11–5 depicts typical data obtained during a maximal effort test for a 29-year-old man who weighed 109 kg. He did not meet the criterion of <150 ml/min increase in $\dot{V}O_2$ with an increase in grade, and he did not come within 10 beats of his estimated maximal heart rate. However, his postexercise lactate was 13.6 mM, and his RER was 1.15. Furthermore, his Borg Scale score was 19. Thus, he met three of the secondary criteria, and we are certain he achieved his $\dot{V}O_2$max. In summary, we believe that attainment of a true plateau is not an absolute prerequisite and that some combination of secondary criteria is preferable. We offer the criteria presented in Table 11–4 as a guide

and suggest that at least two, but preferably three, of the criteria be met. If a true plateau is noted, then this would be adequate for establishing a true $\dot{V}O_2$max.

PREDICTING MAXIMAL AEROBIC POWER

Although laboratory measurements are the only way to quantify $\dot{V}O_2$max accurately, this procedure does pose limitations, the first being that the equipment required for direct sampling of oxygen is very expensive to purchase and maintain. In addition, the subject must wear a cumbersome/uncomfortable apparatus, the individual performing the test must be well trained, and the nature of a maximal test itself can be limiting to some subjects. In particular, the elderly, children, and people with physical impairments, such as cardiovascular/pulmonary disease and/or musculoskeletal restrictions, cannot tolerate maximal exercise tests. Finally, large groups cannot be efficiently tested within a reasonable period. All these factors have led to the development of multiple "prediction" tests that can be

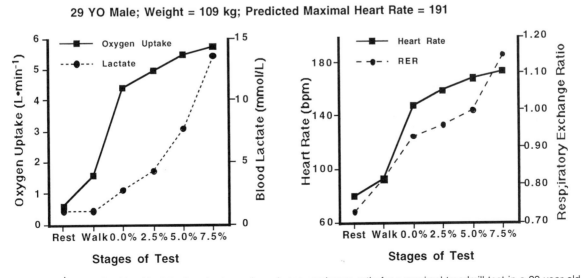

Figure 11–5. $\dot{V}O_2$ uptake, blood lactate, heart rate, and respiratory exchange ratio for a maximal treadmill test in a 29-year-old, 109-kg man.

conducted in clinical, commercial, and/or outdoor arenas. Current prediction tests can be divided into three types, depending on the situation: maximal effort prediction tests, submaximal effort prediction tests, and nonexercise prediction tests. Understanding the advantages, disadvantages, and limitations of each test can be important for determining the most appropriate test for a given environment, a specific population, and a particular need.

Maximal Prediction Tests

Maximal prediction tests, although designed to reduce the problems associated with "true" $\dot{V}O_2$max tests, do require the subject to perform a given protocol to maximal effort. Some aspect of performance is then used to predict $\dot{V}O_2$max based on the values collected from a sample study. Although cycling and arm ergometry can also be used, the most common maximal prediction tests involve running, because the tests can be performed in a variety of ways:

- Run a required distance as quickly as possible.
- Run as far as possible within a set time.
- Perform a shuttle/track run.
- Use time on treadmill from a standard maximal treadmill test.

One of the best known examples of a prediction test is the Cooper 12-minute field performance test.[39] Subjects are required to run on a level surface (usually a measured track) for 12 minutes, and the distance (D = meters covered) is recorded. Cooper found that $\dot{V}O_2$max could be predicted based on a regression equation with a considerable reliability ($r = 0.897$); as a result, this test has been used by many health professionals. Correlation coefficients (r) between this test and actual $\dot{V}O_2$max measures are typically around 0.87 to 0.89.[39,40] The following regression equation can be used to estimate $\dot{V}O_2$max from the distance covered in 12 minutes[3]:

$$\dot{V}O_2\text{max in ml/kg/min} = D \times 0.02233 - 11.3.$$

Another commonly used walking/running test is the 1.5-mile run: subjects must complete 1.5 miles in as short a time as possible; the time (T) required to complete the distance is used to predict the aerobic capacity of the individual.[3,40,41] Correlations between this test and actual $\dot{V}O_2$max measures have been reported to range from 0.73 to 0.92.[39,40,42] The equation for the 1.5-mile run is as follows:

$$\dot{V}O_2\text{max in ml/kg/min} = (483/T) + 3.5$$

Other variations of the 1.5-mile run have been developed, and these tests often include variables other than time.[3,42,43] For example, the Rockport 1-mile walk test uses body weight, age, gender, and heart rate.[3,42,43] Fortunately, all these tests yield essentially comparable values, and it is incumbent on the tester to determine which test will be easier and most feasible to conduct.

Other types of tests that are useful for runners in training are the shuttle/track run tests. The individual starts running at a certain speed and covers a fixed distance (20 to 400 ms) multiple times for a specified time.[44–47] After each distance, the speed is increased, or the time allotted to complete each shuttle is reduced. This reduction in time (or increase in speed) is continued until the subject can no longer keep pace. The speed achieved can then be used to predict the individual's aerobic capacity from regression formulas. Correlations between values obtained from these tests and actual measurements range from 0.83 to 0.98.[44–47] The formula for estimating $\dot{V}O_2$max from the 20-m shuttle, where S = speed in km/hr is as follows[46]:

$$\dot{V}O_2\text{max in ml/kg/min} = 5.857 \times S - 19.458.$$

One other way to estimate $\dot{V}O_2$max is by using the time a person stays on the treadmill for a standardized maximal exercise test. For each of the major maximal effort treadmill protocols, regression equations to predict $\dot{V}O_2$max from time have been developed. For example, for the Bruce protocol, regression equations with correlations between 0.86 and 0.92 have been developed for active men, sedentary men, men with coronary heart disease, and healthy adults.[6,17–19] One of the more general equations for predicting $\dot{V}O_2$max from time to complete the Bruce protocol was reported by Pollack et al.[18] The equation, where T = time in minutes, is as follows:

$$\dot{V}O_2\text{max in ml/kg/min} = 4.326 \times T - 4.66.$$

In addition to the Bruce protocol, regression equations have been developed for the Balke and Ellestad protocols, all with a reasonable degree of accuracy.[6,17–19] Such equations can be developed within any test facility from a particular standardized protocol. However, it must be remembered that prediction equations are typically specific for a certain population and should, therefore, be used with caution. Other variables, including gender, age, and perceived functional ability, may be important in such prediction equations.

The above-mentioned tests are all examples of prediction tests that involve maximal effort. The first three tests can be performed without the restrictions of the $\dot{V}O_2$max tests done in the laboratory, whereas the fourth test must be conducted on a treadmill, but without the expensive metabolic equipment. Each has a specific utility, depending on the goals and the population of interest, but each also has the inherent problems and/or errors that come with any prediction equation.

Submaximal Prediction Tests

Individuals who are just starting an exercise program and are less fit or individuals recovering from medical conditions often cannot tolerate a maximal effort. In response to this need, submaximal effort prediction tests have been developed, as either constant load, steady state, or progressive. Submaximal prediction tests have at least four advantages over maximal exertion tests: they are physically less demanding, take less time to perform, are safer to conduct, and can often be performed with large groups. However, to accomplish this, a degree of accuracy is sacrificed.

Virtually all submaximal tests use heart rate in the estimation of $\dot{V}O_2$max. Åstrand and Ryhming[48] were among the first to report a linear relationship between heart rate and $\dot{V}O_2$; they recommended the use of heart rate in the prediction of $\dot{V}O_2$max. Thus, heart rate provides the theoretical basis behind most submaximal tests: when a subject works at submaximal levels, heart rate can be used to predict a maximal performance, either by extrapolation to maximal heart rate or from heart rate at a known workload.

The relation between heart rate and workload is particularly important for progressive, submaximal cycle ergometer protocols. One typical progressive cycle ergometer protocol, in which the initial workload is based on the body weight of the subject and a self-reported activity level, utilizes four incremental 2-minute stages.[49] For example, a 95-kg, physically active subject would complete the four-stage protocol at workloads of 50, 100, 150, and 200 W, respectively, while pedalling at 50 rpm. Heart rates at the four work rates are then plotted, and the line is extrapolated to maximal heart rate; the point on the line that coincides with maximal heart rate then provides an estimate of $\dot{V}O_2$max (Fig. 11–6). Other progressive tests with known workloads have been used in a similar manner; such tests have included devices such as stair-steppers,[50] treadmills, and seated rowing machines.[51]

Steady-state submaximal effort tests are also commonly used for prediction of $\dot{V}O_2$max. Treadmills, track walking/running, stair-steppers, cycle ergometers, bench steps, rowing machines, and squat repetitions have all been used.[3,41–43,48,50,52–54] Although different, each of these tests maintains a few points in common. All require a steady-state workload and a measure of the subject's heart rate upon completion of the test. From there, heart rate may be used alone to predict $\dot{V}O_2$max from a nomogram[48,54] or in conjunction with other variables, such as age, weight, gender, and other variables from a regression equation.[42,43,52,53] One of the first nomograms for predicting $\dot{V}O_2$max from heart rate at submaximal workloads was derived by Åstrand and Ryhming[48] from cycle, stair-stepping, and treadmill-running data. Although

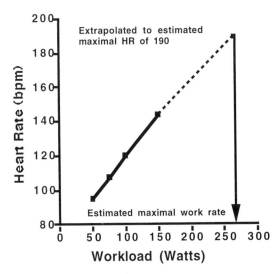

Figure 11–6. Extrapolation of $\dot{V}O_2$max from heart rate and workload on a cycle ergometer test.

their nomogram is still used, it was later modified for use with other populations.[54]

In addition to nomograms, regression equations have been developed to predict $\dot{V}O_2$max based on walking/jogging on a treadmill at submaximal levels,[52] stepping up and down stairs for a set time,[41] and/or jogging 1 mile on a track.[42] Although these equations can be useful, care must be taken because they are typically derived from results from a particular population. Thus the equation may not apply to a different population with regard to age, gender, and fitness level.

In summary, although submaximal prediction tests do not provide the same physiological data as a true maximal $\dot{V}O_2$max test, they do serve an important role in estimating aerobic capacity. In addition, it should be noted that these tests have shown strong retest accuracies and are, therefore, excellent for tracking performance over time.[39] However, all submaximal tests have proved to be somewhat variable in their accuracy because the predictive value of a test relies on an accurate estimate of maximal heart rate. Unfortunately, there is inherent error in estimating maximal heart rate. As noted previously, maximal heart rate can be estimated as 220 − age (as a low estimate) or as 210 − 0.5 × age (as a higher estimate), but despite these equations, the actual maximal heart rate can still be higher or lower by as much as 20 to 30 bpm (one standard deviation = ±10 to 12), depending on age and training.[3,49] Moreover, these equations assume that the decline in maximal heart rate for a given age is uniform. Clearly, an erroneous estimate of maximal heart rate can markedly affect the estimate. For example, if the estimated maximal heart rate is 183 (Fig. 11–6), then the estimated $\dot{V}O_2$max is 3500 ml/kg;

however, if the true maximal heart rate was only 170, then the $\dot{V}O_2$max would be only 3010 ml/kg. Finally, it must be recognized that regression equations developed from particular submaximal tests may have been derived from a selected age group and gender and may not, therefore, be generalizable to the population of interest. Thus, understanding the limitations of the subject and the tests and knowing the goals of the test will allow for the clinician or health provider to select the most appropriate test for estimating aerobic capacity.

Nonexercise Prediction Tests

The value of cardiorespiratory fitness as an indicator of all-cause mortality has been reported,[55] and thus the need to estimate $\dot{V}O_2$max noninvasively has increased. Prediction equations that use nonexercise parameters such as age, body composition, gender, level of physical activity, and the subject's perceived functional ability to walk, jog, or run given distances have emerged.[56,57] Although new to the arena of prediction tests, the reliability studies do show promise. For example, George et al.[56] found that a questionnaire-based regression equation predicted $\dot{V}O_2$max with a correlation of 0.85 in a sample of physically active college students. Similarly, Heil et al.[57] developed an equation for men and women aged 20 to 79 years and noted a correlation of 0.88 for the generalized equation (men and women together). Their equation included percent body fat, age, gender, and an activity code derived from personal statements about activity level. Although this equation may be useful because of its wide age range, very few of the subjects were highly fit, and thus it may be best for a fairly sedentary population. Overall, the nonexercise prediction tests have one significant advantage—such tests can be administered during an office visit without the requirements of equipment, supervision, or any inconvenience to the subject. However, as with all regression equations, their generalization to populations, other than the one from which they were derived, remains questionable.

FACTORS AFFECTING MAXIMAL AEROBIC POWER

An individual's $\dot{V}O_2$max is determined by a variety of intrinsic and extrinsic factors, as indicated in Table 11–5. Genetics is a dominant intrinsic factor in determining $\dot{V}O_2$max and may account for 25% to more than 70% of an individual's inherent $\dot{V}O_2$max.[4,58] However, many other intervening factors, including age, gender, heart structure and function, and properties of skeletal muscle are certainly important intrinsic factors.[58] Åstrand and Rodahl[4] elegantly depicted age- and gender-related influences when they showed that maximal values are comparable in boys and girls prior to puberty

TABLE 11–5. SELECTED FACTORS KNOWN TO INFLUENCE $\dot{V}O_2$max

Genetics	Activity levels
Gender	Nutritional status
Age	Environmental conditions
Body composition	Medications
Heart structure and function	Presence of disease
Skeletal muscle characteristics	

and that they continue to rise in both genders until they peak, often between 18 and 20 years.[4] Thereafter, a gradual decline in $\dot{V}O_2$max, which reflects both changes in activity levels and changes in body composition, is noted.[4]

The differences between girls and boys, and men and women, can largely be accounted for by differences in body composition. Typical values for men are 25% to 50% higher than values for women, when expressed in absolute terms or relative to body weight. However, if the absolute values are normalized for lean body mass, instead of body weight, the differences between men and women are minimal. Thus, body composition, in particular lean muscle mass, is an important factor influencing $\dot{V}O_2$max.

The primary extrinsic factor that influences $\dot{V}O_2$max is physical activity; training alone can improve[58] and inactivity can markedly compromise $\dot{V}O_2$max.[4,59] Whereas exercise training can increase the $\dot{V}O_2$max of sedentary individuals by 25% over several months,[58] physical inactivity, as characterized by bed rest, can decrease $\dot{V}O_2$max by as much as 26% after only 21 days.[59] Typically, the magnitudes of the increase or decrease are related to the duration of activity/inactivity, initial fitness, and health. With respect to bed rest, those with higher initial fitness levels appear to demonstrate greater declines than those who are less fit, over a comparable period.[59] Figure 11–7 provides an estimate of

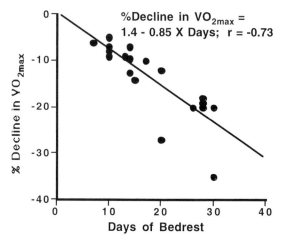

Figure 11–7. Estimated declines in $\dot{V}O_2$max with increasing days of bed rest. (*Source: From permission: VA Convertino.[59]*)

the decrease in $\dot{V}O_2$max as a function of bed rest over time. Other factors that can affect $\dot{V}O_2$max include the environmental extremes of altitude, heat, cold, and air pollution, overall health (in terms of disease processes and nutritional), status, sleep habits, and other behaviors.[4,7] It is clear that the only real approach toward effecting a change in $\dot{V}O_2$max is participation in physical activity.

TERMS AND CONCEPTS ASSOCIATED WITH MAXIMAL AEROBIC POWER AND TRAINING

With their sustained interest in factors that affect performance, exercise physiologists are always searching for clues as to why individuals with comparable $\dot{V}O_2$max values perform in disparate ways. In other words, although $\dot{V}O_2$max is a good predictor of athletic performance in a sample from a mixed population, it does not do well when the performance of a runner requires prediction. Thus, over the years a number of terms and concepts have emerged out of a search for both knowledge and explanations for individual differences. Those that seem to be important for predicting and improving running performance include the following:

- Lactate threshold, maximal lactate at steady state, and critical power
- Exercise intensity domains
- Economy of movement
- Velocity at maximal aerobic power
- Training heart rate

Lactate Threshold, Maximal Lactate at Steady State, and Critical Power

Lactate Threshold

Although there are several definitions for the lactate threshold (LT), it is defined here as the intensity of exercise at which blood lactate concentration rises 1 mM above baseline.[25,60–62] Typically, LT is determined by measuring blood lactate at the end of each stage during a progressive exercise test. Once obtained, the lactate values can be plotted as a function of $\dot{V}O_2$, W, or velocity, and the 1-mM increase can be ascertained from the graph (Fig. 11–8). Once determined, the LT can be expressed as a function of $\dot{V}O_2$max (i.e., 65% of $\dot{V}O_2$max), velocity (i.e., 7.5 mph), or power output (i.e., 150 W). The LT is often characterized as the exercise intensity that athletes are able to maintain during prolonged exercise, such as a marathon,[60,62] and it is believed to be a function of $\dot{V}O_2$max, aerobic enzyme activity, and muscle fiber composition.[25,62] The LT has been shown to be highly predictive of distance running

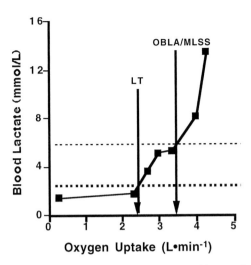

Figure 11–8. Characterization of the concepts of lactate threshold (LT) and maximal lactate at steady state (MLSS) or onset of blood lactate accumulation (OBLA).

performance for various distances.[60,62] As such, the LT can be extremely useful for setting a training pace.

Maximal Lactate at Steady State

Technically, the maximal lactate at steady state (MLSS) is defined as the highest exercise intensity for which blood lactate level increases less than 1.0 mM between the 10th and 30th (or 5th and 20th) minutes of steady-state exercise.[60,61] In other words, MLSS is the upper limit of blood lactate concentration that can be maintained at a new steady-state level of exercise (Fig. 11–8).[25,51,60,61] Previously, the MLSS was identified/ defined by the work rate that elicited a 4.0 mM blood lactate value[51,60,61]; however, this fixed value could not be justified in that some athletes are able sustain lactate values between 6 and 10 mM for over an hour.[62] Thus, the work rate associated with this MLSS value may be different in every individual. Other terms have also been used to describe the point at, or above, the MLSS, including anaerobic threshold (AT), onset of blood lactate accumulation (OBLA), and onset of plasma lactate accumulation (OPLA).[25,51,60,61] These differences in terminology can be confusing, particularly the term AT, which has been used for many years. Despite some disagreement, the AT, OBLA, OPLA, and MLSS probably describe the same relative work intensity. However, since lactate production may not be due to lack of oxygen, the term "anaerobic" may not be appropriate.[27,62]

Like the LT, the MLSS work rate can be determined. Although there are approaches to determining MLSS by heart rate, it is best if one has access to a lactate analyzer. Preferably, a maximal exercise test with lactate measures at each successive work rate has been conducted previously so that the LT and $\dot{V}O_2$max are known. One way to determine MLSS is to have the subject exercise for 20 minutes at two intensities (one below and one above the expected MLSS, e.g., 65% and 80% of $\dot{V}O_2$max), with 40 minutes of rest between the two tests.[60,61] During the two tests, blood lactate values should be obtained at 5 and 20 minutes after the start of exercise and the differences calculated between the two values ($D_{Lactate} = Time_{20} - Time_5$) within each test. The lower intensity should result in a steady-state lactate, and the higher intensity should be above the MLSS. From this information the work rate or relative intensity for the MLSS can be calculated as

$$MLSS = (Work_1 \times D_{Lactate2} - Work_2 \times D_{Lactate1})/ (D_{Lactate2} - D_{Lactate1})$$

where $Work_1/Work_2$ are either the velocities, relative intensities, or W during the two tests, and $D_{Lactate1}/D_{Lactate2}$ are the differences in blood lactates at 5 and 20 minutes for the each of the two exercise bouts. Table 11–6 provides an example of how MLSS can be calculated from such a test. One concern should be mentioned with this method: it may not work if the individual's MLSS is well above 80% of $\dot{V}O_2$max, and it may be better to choose a higher intensity for the second test, between 85% and 90%. Finally, two important points should be noted for the LT and the MLSS: both parameters can be shifted to the right with training, and both are sport specific.[25,51,60,61] In other words, the LT and MLSS for running may be quite different from the LT and MLSS for cycling or rowing within the same individual.[25,51,60,61] Much still remains to be learned about this and related terms.

Critical Power

The term *critical power* was derived from strength literature, subsequently adapted to cycling, and more recently adapted to other sports, such as running, rowing, kayaking, and swimming.[63,64] The critical power

concept is based on the hyperbolic relation between power output and time to exhaustion: with increasing power output, the shorter the time to exhaustion. The critical power point is the maximum work rate that can be sustained for a very long time without fatigue.[64] Thus, if the imposed power were below the critical power output, fatigue should theoretically not occur. However, the critical power point as defined in the literature is at or above the LT; thus, it cannot be sustained indefinitely because other factors, such as energy stores, could become limiting. Work below the critical power can be sustained for extended periods, such as a marathon race.[63,64] Critical power is considered an inherent characteristic of the aerobic energy system, and as such it has been examined for its association with other parameters. To date, investigators who have examined critical power in relation to LT have found it to be 13% to 28% higher than the LT.[64]

Actual determinations of critical power are difficult to obtain because multiple, high-intensity efforts to exhaustion must be conducted to evaluate the power–time-to-exhaustion relationship. With respect to running, the term power is often substituted for velocity.[64] The term "critical velocity," which is also used, typically represents the highest speed or fastest pace a runner can sustain without exhaustion; as with critical power, critical velocity probably lies between the LT and $\dot{V}O_2$max. Critical velocity has been characterized as the speed that can be maintained during a 10-km race, and as such, it may coincide with the MLSS boundary and/or the AT.[60] Further work is required to document this possibility.

Exercise Intensity Domains

During a progressive or a constant work rate exercise test, the metabolic, respiratory, and cardiovascular responses are determined by the absolute and relative intensity of the work imposed.[25,26] Accordingly, Poole et al.[25,26] have

TABLE 11–6. CALCULATING MLSS AS A VELOCITY AND PERCENT OF $\dot{V}O_2$max FROM TWO EXERCISE BOUTS OF 20 MINUTES EACH[a]

	Exercise Bout 1	Exercise Bout 2
	65% $\dot{V}O_2$max 7 mph	80% $\dot{V}O_2$max 9 mph
Lactate (mm)		
5 min	2.4	4.2
20 min	2.0	6.5
DLactate	2.0 − 2.4 = −0.4 mM	6.5 − 4.2 = 2.3 mM
MLSS=	$\dfrac{[7 \times 2.3 - 9 \times (-0.4)]}{2.3 - (-0.4)} = 7.3$ mph	$\dfrac{[65 \times 2.3 - 80 \times (-0.4)]}{2.3 - (-0.4)} = 67.2\%$

[a]Blood lactate was sampled at 5 and 20 minutes of exercise. MLSS, maximal lactate at steady state.

defined three specific exercise domains characterized by their $\dot{V}O_2$ and metabolic profiles. The three domains consist of moderate, heavy, and severe exercise.[25,26]

Moderate exercise, which comprises all work rates below the LT, is typified by a stabilization of both $\dot{V}O_2$ and blood lactate, usually within a 3-minute time period.[25,26] The second exercise domain is that of heavy exercise and is described by its upper and lower boundaries.[25,26] The lower boundary is the work rate at the LT, whereas the upper boundary is the highest work rate at which blood lactate can be stabilized or for which lactate can attain a new MLSS value. The work rate at the upper boundary of heavy exercise is also believed to be comparable to critical power on a cycle ergometer[64] and critical velocity during running.[61,63,65] Finally, because of different uses of terminology, some consider the work rate at the upper boundary to be the AT.[25,26] The third exercise domain, that of severe exercise, is characterized by an instability in both $\dot{V}O_2$ and lactate: both will continue to rise until maximal values are achieved at the point of fatigue.[25,26] Clearly, exercise within this domain is typically not tolerated for long.

One important aspect of both the heavy and severe exercise domains is the slow component of $\dot{V}O_2$.[25,26] The slow component is only seen with work rates above the LT, and it is characterized by a slow increase in $\dot{V}O_2$, above steady state predicted from submaximal work rates.[25,26,65,66] This additional increase in $\dot{V}O_2$ represents a supplemental energetic component, which can be greater than $1.5\ L \cdot min^{-1}$.[23,25,26,65–67] As the intensity of the exercise increases progressively above the LT, the magnitude of the slow component increases; at work rates above the MLSS, the work rate will drive $\dot{V}O_2$ to its maximum, even during "submaximal" exercise.[25,26,65–67] It also appears that the magnitude of the slow component is much greater for

cycling than running.[65] Figure 11–9 provides a graphic representation of the three exercise domains, the slow components of $\dot{V}O_2$ associated with each domain, and what is expected with respect to blood lactate.

This model has tremendous utility in terms of setting up training programs: one goal could be to shift $\dot{V}O_2$ kinetics to the left, and another to shift the LT and MLSS to the right. The more rapidly an individual achieves steady-state $\dot{V}O_2$ or can accelerate $\dot{V}O_2$ kinetics, the lower the reliance on intramuscular energy stores and the greater the reliance on aerobic metabolism.[23,25,26] Training will result in such adaptations,[23,25,26] which should be evidenced by marked improvements in running performance.

Economy of Movement

The term *economy of movement* reflects an individual's work efficiency. It is a measure of the energy required to produce a certain power output or to cover a certain distance. The term has been used for many years and is now being recognized as a factor for predicting endurance performance. Its importance was first noted by Costill and Winrow,[68] who observed that the oxygen cost at a given speed was lower in the faster of two runners with comparable values for $\dot{V}O_2$max. As an example, if three runners had $\dot{V}O_2$max values of 63 ml/kg/min and $\dot{V}O_2$ values of 51.7, 55.4, and 47.4 ml/kg/min while running at 9 mph, then their running economies would be quite different, with values of 345, 372, and 318 ml/kg/mile, respectively. Theoretically, the most efficient individual, or the one with the economy of 318 ml of $O_2 \cdot kg^{-1} \cdot mile^{-1}$, should be the better runner. It is important to note that these values are simply determined by multiplying $\dot{V}O_2$ by 60 to obtain units as ml/kg/hr, and then dividing $\dot{V}O_2$ by the velocity, in this case, 9 mph. Thus, if the $\dot{V}O_2$

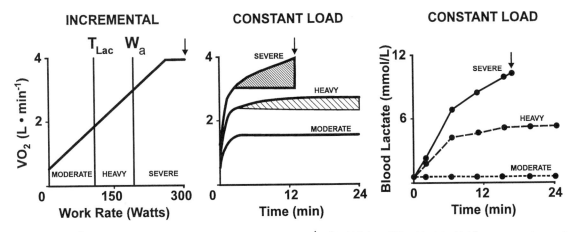

Figure 11–9. The $\dot{V}O_2$ responses to incremental exercise (left) and the $\dot{V}O_2^1$ (middle) and blood lactate (right) responses to constant load exercise as a function of exercise intensity domains. T_{Lac} represents the lactate threshold, and W_a represents the critical power or work rate where maximal lactate steady, state occurs. (*Source: From permission: Poole and Richardson[25] and Gaesser and Poole.[26]*)

were 51.7 ml/kg/min, then the hourly units would be 3102 ml/kg/hr (51.4 ml/kg/min × 60); when divided by 9 mph, one obtains 345 ml/kg/mile, or the running economy at 9 mph. Similar calculations could be used for cycling, except that economy for cycling is defined as "W produced per liter of O_2 uptake per minute."[62] The issue of economy of movement has also been discussed by Noakes,[27] who believes that although it is useful, other parameters for predicting running performance may be preferable.

Velocity at Maximal Aerobic Power

One term that has evolved and appears to be important with respect to running/endurance performance is the velocity at $\dot{V}O_2$max, or $v\dot{V}O_2$max. Strictly speaking, this is the velocity associated with or that elicits $\dot{V}O_2$max,[63,69,70] yet a number of investigators have calculated the value in different ways. Thus, the use of the term, $v\dot{V}O_2$max, is not always consistent.[63,69] Hill and Rowell[69] carefully examined the various definitions in the literature for $v\dot{V}O_2$max and concluded that some have an anaerobic component and some do not. Thus, in some cases, the term *maximal aerobic speed* may be more appropriate.

The five most frequently cited laboratory methods of determining $v\dot{V}O_2$max include those of Daniels et al.,[71] Billat et al.,[61] Lacour et al.,[70] diPrampero et al.,[72] and Noakes.[27] Each one calculated the $v\dot{V}O_2$max from treadmill running without an increase in slope, but their approaches differed, as can be seen in Table 11–7. Figure 11–10 provides a graphical representation of a velocity/heart rate, and $\dot{V}O_2$ relationship from a female runner with a $\dot{V}O_2$max of 60 ml/kg/min and a maximal heart rate of 195 bpm. These data were then used to calculate $v\dot{V}O_2$max according to Daniels et al.,[71] who used the velocity/$\dot{V}O_2$ relationship at submaximal work rates to develop a regression equation and then predict $v\dot{V}O_2$max by using the predetermined $\dot{V}O_2$max. The equation $\dot{V}O_2$max = 5.2837 × Velocity + 6.3949 was obtained from the data in Fig. 11–10 and from the known $\dot{V}O_2$max (60 ml/kg/min), the $v\dot{V}O_2$max was calculated to yield a value of 10.1 mph (or 16.3 km/hr). Running economy, or net oxygen cost of running, for the same subject was also calculated from $\dot{V}O_2$ and velocity at three different speeds and then averaged; it was found to be 335 ml/kg/mile. To calculate $v\dot{V}O_2$max values as defined by Lacour et al.[70] and diPrampero et al.,[72] an estimate of running economy is required. As noted by Billat et al.[63] and others,[44,69] the least anaerobic velocities are derived from the methods of Lacour and diPrampero.

These methodologies, although somewhat technical, can be used by coaches to establish a peak running velocity and from that, set a training velocity; it is

TABLE 11–7. COMPARISON OF VARIOUS PROTOCOLS FOR ESTIMATING $v\dot{V}O_2$max

Investigator	Methodology
Daniels et al.[71]	$v\dot{V}O_2$max extrapolated from submaximal velocities up to predetermined $\dot{V}O_2$max
Billat et al.[73]	Evaluated as the velocity/$\dot{V}O_2$ relationship: lowest velocity that elicited $\dot{V}O_2$max
Lacour et al.[70]	Calculated as ($\dot{V}O_2$max − $\dot{V}O_2$rest)/net O_2 cost of running (running economy)
diPrampero et al.[72]	Calculated as $\dot{V}O_2$max/running economy
Noakes[27]	Peak running velocity reached at exhaustion and maintained for 1 min
Léger and Boucher[45]	On track with continuous stages of 2-min and 1-km/hr velocity increases

useful for marathon, half-marathon, 10-km, and 1500- to 5000-m runners.[70] In the absence of metabolic measurements, the easiest way to determine maximal velocity is to measure heart rate and velocity while runners run on a treadmill or track at increasing velocities. Two such tests have been described.[63,73,74] The first was described by Léger and Boucher and is known as the Université Montréal Track Test (Table 11–7). The last velocity sustained for at least 1 minute can be considered the $v\dot{V}O_2$max. A similar type of speed and heart rate test, first described by Conconi et al.[74] in 1982, has been used on a large number of athletes, ranging from marathon runners and sprinters to cyclists and rugby players. Their calculation of "maximal aerobic speed" revealed higher values in endurance runners compared with sprinters, and they concluded that maximal aerobic speed could be improved by endurance training. Importantly, Noakes[27] has suggested that

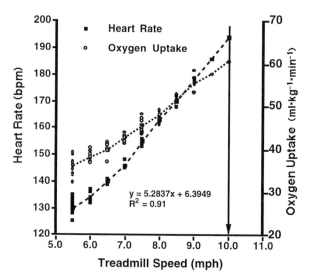

Figure 11–10. Progressive increases in heart rate and $\dot{V}O_2$ plotted as a function of speed of treadmill (mph). Note: the velocity that elicited $\dot{V}O_2$max is designated by the arrow, or around 10.1 mph.

peak treadmill running velocity and the running velocity at the LT may be the best predictors of running performance. Thus, using one of the aforementioned methods to evaluate some form of $v\dot{V}O_2max$ should be an important aspect of any running program.

Target Heart Rate

Although many different types of exercise programs can be prescribed, one of the key issues for any training program is defining a target heart rate range. Several basic methods for estimating the target heart rate range for an exercise program have been proposed.[3] The two most common ways of calculating a target heart rate range are using maximal heart rate and heart rate reserve.[3] For the first way, one simply takes 60% and 90% of maximal heart rate, either estimated or measured, and then uses those two heart rates for the lower and upper end of the range within which to exercise.[3] Thus, if the maximal heart rate were 190 bpm, then the target heart rate range would be between 114 (190 × 0.6) and 171 (190 × 0.9) bpm.

The second approach, known as the Karvonen method, involves determining the heart rate reserve; this is simply the difference between the resting and maximal heart rate. Next, a percentage of the heart rate reserve (usually 50% to 85%) is taken and added back to the resting heart rate. For example, if the $\dot{V}O_2max$ of a 25-year-old was 60.0 ml/kg/min, and the resting and maximal heart rates were 65 and 190 bpm, respectively, then the heart rate reserve would be 190 − 65, or 125 bpm. The target heart rate range would then be between 128 (125 × 0.5 + 65) and 171 (125 × 0.85 + 65) bpm. Both ways are acceptable, but what must be considered is the actual relative exercise intensity that results from exercising within the specified target heart rate range. Table 11–8 provides an indication of how the two methods differ with respect to heart rate and the actual exercise intensity as a percentage of $\dot{V}O_2max$.

A third way to determine a target heart rate range is to undergo a maximal exercise test and then create a plot or graph of heart rate and $\dot{V}O_2$. This allows for a clear representation of the actual heart rate/$\dot{V}O_2$

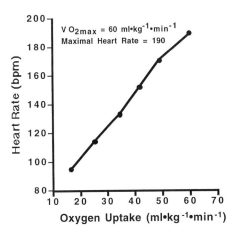

Figure 11–11. A plot of heart rate VS. $\dot{V}O_2$ for a maximal exercise test.

relationship and allows one to monitor exercise intensity carefully. Figure 11–11 provides an example of the results of an exercise test, with heart rate plotted against $\dot{V}O_2$. Whichever method is chosen, records of changes over time are useful for documenting training and performance improvements.

Finally, although there is wide variability among individuals of the same age in terms of maximal heart rate, the use of an individual's heart rate during training is an extremely stable and valuable marker: individual variability in heart rate across days at the same intensity has been reported to be less than 2%, regardless of intensity.[20] Thus, heart rate during training can be used as an indicator of overtraining or "staleness." For example, if one frequently runs a known route in a specified time and has determined the "usual" training heart rate during that run, any type of elevation in heart rate can be used to indicate a need for self-evaluation—the presence or onset of illness, tiredness or unexplained fatigue, loss of appetite, heat illness, and other such symptoms. Fortunately, heart rate monitors are widely available and can be purchased at very reasonable prices.

SUMMARY

In summary, maximal aerobic power, or $\dot{V}O_2max$, is an extremely valuable measure of cardiovascular and pulmonary function, work capacity, and endurance performance. It can be directly measured by using a standardized maximal treadmill or cycle ergometer protocol, or it can be predicted by using either a maximal or submaximal protocol. A variety of protocols for predicting $\dot{V}O_2max$ are readily available, and many are extremely easy to administer. All tests have certain advantages and limitations that should be considered by the test administrator.

TABLE 11–8. RELATIVE EXERCISE INTENSITIES ACCORDING TO HEART RATES CALCULATED AS A PERCENTAGE OF MAXIMAL HEART RATE (MHR) AND HEART RATE RESERVE (HRR) FOR AN MHR OF 190 AND RESTING HR OF 65

%	% of MHR	% $\dot{V}O_2max$	% of HRR	% $\dot{V}O_2max$
90	171	84	178	89
80	152	70	165	80
70	133	55	152	70
60	114	41	140	61
50	95	27	128	52

Although $\dot{V}O_2$max is certainly an important determinant of running performance, other factors including lactate threshold, running economy, maximal lactate at steady state, and the velocity associated with $\dot{V}O_2$max are also important and should be considered when embarking on a training program to improve performance over a specific distance.

REFERENCES

1. Hill AV, Lupton H: Muscular exercise, lactic acid, and the supply and utilization of oxygen. *Q J Med* 1923:16, 136.
2. Margaria R, Edwards HT, Dill DB: The possible mechanisms of contracting and paying the oxygen debt and the role of lactic acid in muscular contraction. *Am J Physiol* 1933:106, 689.
3. American College of Sports Medicine: *Guidelines for Exercise Testing and Prescription,* 5th ed. Baltimore, Williams & Wilkins, 1995:277.
4. Åstrand P-O, Rodahl K: *Textbook of Work Physiology.: Physiological Bases of Exercise,* 3rd ed. New York, McGraw-Hill, 1986.
5. Åstrand P-O: Quantification of exercise capability and evaluation of physical capacity in man. *Prog Cardiovasc Dis* 1976:19, 51.
6. Bruce RA, Kusumi F, Hosmer D: Maximal oxygen intake and nomographic assessment of functional aerobic impairment in cardiovascular disease. *Am Heart J* 1973:85, 546.
7. Taylor HL, Burskirk E, Henschel A: Maximal oxygen intake as an objective measure of cardio-respiratory performance. *J Appl Physiol* 1955:8, 73.
8. Åstrand P-O, Saltin B: Maximal oxygen uptake and heart rate in various types of muscular activity. *J Appl Physiol* 1961:16, 977.
9. Bergh U, Kanstrup I-L, Ekblom B: Maximal oxygen uptake during exercise with various combinations of arm and leg work. *J Appl Physiol* 1976:41, 191.
10. Brahler CJ, Blank SE: VersaClimbing elicits higher $\dot{V}O_2$max than does treadmill running or rowing ergometry. *Med Sci Sports Exerc* 1995:27, 249.
11. Gleser MA, Horstman DH, Mello RP: The effect on $\dot{V}O_2$max of adding arm work to maximal leg work. *Med Sci Sports Exerc* 1974:6, 104.
12. Kasch FW, Phillips WH, Ross WD, et al.: A comparison of maximal oxygen uptake treadmill and step-test procedures. *J Appl Physiol* 1966:21, 1387.
13. Nagle FJ, Richie JP, Geise MD: $\dot{V}O_2$max responses in separate and combined arm and leg air-braked ergometer exercise. *Med Sci Sports Exerc* 1984:16, 563.
14. Secher NH, Ruberg-Larsen N, Binkhorst RA: Maximal oxygen uptake during arm cranking and combined arm plus leg exercise. *J Appl Physiol* 1974:36, 515.
15. Balke B, Ware R: An experimental study of physical fitness of Air Force personnel. *US Armed Forces Med J* 1959:10, 675.
16. Ellestad MH, Allen W, Wan MCK, Kemp G: Maximal treadmill stress testing for cardiovascular evaluation. *Circulation.* 1969:39, 517.
17. Froelicher VF, Brammell H, Davis G, et al.: A comparison of three maximal treadmill exercise protocols. *J Appl Physiol* 1974:36, 720.
18. Pollock Ml, Bohannon RL, Cooper KH, et al.: A comparative analysis of four protocols for maximal treadmill stress testing. *Am Heart J* 1976:92, 39.
19. Pollock ML, Foster V, Schmidt D, et al.: Comparative analysis of physiologic responses to three different maximal graded exercise test protocols in healthy women. *Am Heart J* 1982:103, 363.
20. Kyle SB, Smoak BL, Douglass LW, et al.: Variability of responses across training levels to maximal treadmill exercise. *J Appl Physiol* 1989:67, 160.
21. Foster C, Crowe AJ, Daines E, et al.: Predicting functional capacity during treadmill testing independent of exercise protocol. *Med Sci Sports Exerc* 1996:28, 752.
22. Gibson ASC, Lambert MI, Hawley JA, et al.: Measurement of maximal oxygen uptake from two different laboratory protocols in runners and squash players. *Med Sci Sports Exerc* 1999:31, 1226.
23. Zhang Y-Y, Johnson MC, Chow N, et al.: The role of fitness on $\dot{V}O_2$ and $\dot{V}CO_2$ kinetics in response to proportional step increases in work rate. *J Appl Physiol* 1991:63, 94.
24. Bingisser R, Kaplan V, Scherer T, et al.: Effect of training on repeatability of cardiopulmonary exercise performance in normal men and women. *Med Sci Sports Exerc* 1997:29, 1499.
25. Poole DC, Richardson RS: Determinants of oxygen uptake: Implications for exercise testing. *Sports Med* 1997:24, 308.
26. Gaesser GA, Poole DC: The slow component of oxygen uptake kinetics in humans, in Holloszy JO (ed.), *Exercise and Sport Science Reviews.* vol. 24, Baltimore, Williams & Wilkins, 1996:35.
27. Noakes TD: Implications of exercise testing for prediction of athletic performance: A contemporary perspective. *Med Sci Sports Exerc* 1988:20, 319.
28. Duncan GE, Howley ET, Johnson BN: Applicability of $\dot{V}O_2$max criteria: Discontinuous versus continuous protocols. *Med Sci Sports Exerc* 1997:29, 273.
29. Howeley ET, Bassett DR, Welch HG: Criteria for maximal oxygen uptake: Review and commentary. *Med Sci Sports Exerc* 1995:27, 1292.
30. Cumming CG, Borysyk ML: Criteria for maximum oxygen uptake in men over 40 in a population survey. *Med Sci Sports Exerc* 1972:14, 18.
31. Issekutz R, Birkhead NC, Rodahl K: Use of respiratory quotient in assessment of aerobic work capacity. *J Appl Physiol* 1962:17, 47.
32. Myers J, Walsh D, Sullivan M: Effect of sampling on variability and plateau in oxygen uptake. *J Appl Physiol* 1990:68, 404.
33. Stachenfeld NS, Eskenazi M, Gleim GW, et al.: Predictive accuracy of criteria used to assess maximal oxygen consumption. *Am Heart J* 1992:123, 922.
34. Stallknecht B, Vessing J, Galbo H: Lactate production and clearance in exercise. Effects of training. *Med Sci Sports Exerc* 1998:8, 127.
35. Borg, G. and B. Noble. Perceived exertion, in Wilmore JH (ed.), *Exercise and Sport Science Reviews,* New York, Academic Press, 1974:131.

36. Borg GAV: Psychophysical bases of perceived exertion. *Med Sci Sports Exerc* 1982:14, 377.

37. Eston, RG, BL Davies, JG Williams: Use of perceived effort ratings to control exercise intensity in young healthy adults. *Eur J Appl Physiol* 1987:56, 222.

38. Glass SC, Knowlton RG, Becque MD: Accuracy of RPE from graded exercise to establish exercise training intensity. *Med Sci Sports Exerc* 1992:24, 1303.

39. Cooper KH: A means of assessing maximal oxygen intake. *JAMA* 1968:203, 135.

40. McNaughton L, Hall P, Cooley D: Validation of several methods of estimating maximal oxygen uptake in young men. *Percept Motor Skills* 1998:87, 575.

41. Zwiren, LD, Freedson PS, Ward A, et al.: Estimation of $\dot{V}O_2$max: A comparative analysis of five exercise tests. *Res Q Exerc Sport* 1991:62, 73.

42. George JD, Vehrs PR, Allsen PE, et al.: V.$\dot{V}O_2$max estimation from a submaximal 1-mile track jog for fit college-age individuals. *Med Sci Sports Exerc* 1993:25, 401.

43. Kline GM, Porcari JP, Intermeister R, et al.: Estimation of $\dot{V}O_2$max from a one-mile track walk, gender, age, and body weight. *Med Sci Sports Exerc* 1987:19, 253.

44. Berthoin S, Pelayo P, Lensel-Corbeil G, et al.: Comparison of maximal aerobic speed as assessed with laboratory and field measurements in moderately trained subjects. *Int J Sports Med* 1996:17, 525.

45. Léger L, Boucher R: An indirect continuous running multistage field test: The Université de Montreal track test. *Can J Appl Sports Sci* 1980:5, 77.

46. Léger LA, Lambert J: A maximal multistage 20-m shuttle run test to predict $\dot{V}O_2$max *Eur J Appl Physiol* 1982:49, 1.

47. McNaughton L, Cooley D, Kearney V, Smith S: A comparison of two different shuttle run tests for the estimation of $\dot{V}O_2$max. *J Sport Med Phys Fitness* 1996:36, 85.

48. Åstrand P-O, Ryhming I: A nomogram for calculation of aerobic capacity (physical fitness) from pulse rate during submaximal work. *Med Sci Sports Exerc* 1954:7, 218.

49. Lockwood PA, Yoder JE, Deuster PA: Comparison and cross-validation of cycle ergometry estimates of $\dot{V}O_2$max. *Med Sci Sports Exerc* 1997:29, 1513.

50. Holland GJ, Hoffman JJ, Vincent W, et al.: Treadmill vs. steptreadmill ergometry. *Physician Sportsmed* 1990:18, 79.

51. Beneke R: Anaerobic threshold, individual anaerobic threshold, and maximal lactate steady state in rowing. *Med Sci Sports Exerc* 1995:27, 863.

52. Ebbeling CB, Ward A, Puleo EM, et al.: Development of a single-stage submaximal treadmill walking test. *Med Sci Sports Exerc* 1991:23, 966.

53. Inoue Y, Nakao M: Prediction of maximal oxygen uptake by squat test in men and women. *Kobe J Med Sci* 1996:42, 119.

54. Teraslinna P, Ismail AH, MacLeod DF: Nomogram by Åstrand and Ryhming as a predictor of maximum oxygen intake. *J Appl Physiol* 1966:21, 513.

55. Blair, SN, Kohl HW, Paffenbarger RS et al.: Physical fitness and all-cause mortality: A prospective study of healthy men and women. *JAMA* 1989:262, 2395.

56. George JD, Stone WJ, Burkett LN: Non-exercise $\dot{V}O_2$max estimation for physically active college students. *Med Sci Sports Exerc* 1997:29, 415.

57. Heil DP, Freedson PS, Ahlquist LE, et al.: Nonexercise regression models to estimate peak oxygen consumption. *Med Sci Sports Exerc* 1995:27, 599.

58. Bouchard C, Dionne FT, Simoneau J-A, Boulay MR: Genetics of aerobic and anaerobic performances, in Holloszy JO (ed.), *Exercise and Sport Science Reviews*, vol. 20, Baltimore, Williams & Wilkins, 1992:27.

59. Convertino VA: Cardiovascular consequences of bed rest: Effect on maximal oxygen uptake. *Med Sci Sports Exerc* 1997:29, 191.

60. Billat LV: Use of blood lactate measurements for prediction of exercise performance and for control of training. *Sports Med*, 1996:22, 157.

61. Billat V, Dalmay F, Antonini MT, Chassain AP: A method for determining the maximal steady state of blood lactate concentration from two levels of submaximal exercise. *Eur J Appl Physiol* 1994:69, 196.

62. Coyle EF: Integration of the physiological factors determining endurance performance ability, in Holloszy JO (ed.), *Exercise and Sport Science Reviews*, vol. 23, Baltimore, Williams & Wilkins, 1995:25.

63. Billat LV, Koralsztein JP: Significance of the velocity at $\dot{V}O_2$max and time to exhaustion at this velocity. *Sports Med* 1996:22, 90.

64. Hill DW: The critical power concept: A review. *Sports Med* 1993:16, 237.

65. Billat LV, Richard R, Binsse VM: The $\dot{V}O_2$ slow component for severe exercise depends on the type of exercise and is not correlated with time to fatigue. *J Appl Physiol* 1998:85, 2118.

66. Sloniger MA, Cureton KJ, Carrasco DI, et al.: Effect of the slow-component rise in oxygen uptake on $\dot{V}O_2$max. *Med Sci Sports Exerc* 1996:28, 72.

67. Jones AM, Carter H, Doust JH: A disproportionate increase in $\dot{V}O_2$ coincident with lactate threshold during treadmill exercise. *Med Sci Sports Exerc* 1999:31, 1299.

68. Costill DL, Winrow E: A comparison of two middle-aged ultramarathon runners. *Res Q Exerc. Sport* 1970:41, 135.

69. Hill DW, Rowell AL: Running velocity at $\dot{V}O_2$ max. *Med Sci Sports Exerc* 1996:28, 114.

70. Lacour JR, Padilla-Magunacelaya S, Chatard JC, et al.: Assessment of running velocity at maximal oxygen uptake. *Eur J Appl Physiol* 1991:62, 77.

71. Daniels J, Scardina N, Hayes J, et al.: Elite and subelite female middle- and long-distance runners, in Landers DM (ed.), *Sport and Elite Performers*, vol. 3, *Human Kinetics*, Champaign, IL, 1984:57.

72. di Prampero PE, Atchou G, Brückner JC, Moia C: The energetics of endurance running. *Eur J Appl Physiol* 1986:55, 259.

73. Billat V, Binsse V, Petit B, Koralsztein JP: High level runners are able to maintain a $\dot{V}O_2$ steady-state below $\dot{V}O_2$ max in an all-out run over their critical velocity. *Arch Physiol Biochem* 1998:106, 38.

74. Conconi F, Grazzi G, Casoni I, et al.: The Conconi test: Methodology after 12 years of application. *Int J Sports Med* 1996:17, 509.

Part III

COMMON RUNNING INJURIES

Chapter 12

THE SPINE

Carolyn M. Ruan, Andrew J. Cole, and Cary Bucko

INTRODUCTION

Low back pain can occur following a variety of athletic activities. Although lumbar spine pain is one of the less-common etiologies of running injuries, the impact can be debilitating. When establishing a diagnosis and treatment plan for a runner with spinal pain it is important to know that many running injuries are multifactorial. Understanding the lower extremity kinetic chain and its ultimate convergence on the lumbar spine is imperative because lower extremity mechanical dysfunction can cause secondary mechanical adaptations and spinal pain. Similarly, spinal injury can cause secondary peripheral joint injury. Knowledge of lumbar spine anatomy, biomechanics, and kinesiology is necessary to determine a specific diagnosis and to formulate a rehabilitation program. Changes in strength, balance, flexibility, and proprioception may result from the stresses of running. A rehabilitation program should include acute and subacute phases. Acute treatment considerations include athlete education, physical modalities, medication, manual therapy, and therapeutic exercise. Subacute rehabilitation for runners is an extension of the acute phase with optimization of strength, flexibility, endurance, and coordination, as well as prevention of recurrence or further injury. Spinal injections or surgery may need to be considered for some types of spinal dysfunction and pain.

EPIDEMIOLOGY

Low back pain in the general population has a lifetime prevalence of 60% to 90% and an annual incidence of 5%.[1] The natural history of low back pain can be self-limited but recurrence of symptoms can be as high as 70% to 90%.[2] Back pain can be problematic in a variety of sports. Sports that commonly involve back injuries include gymnastics, ballet, football, weightlifting, golf, and baseball. The etiology of pain often involves a combination of repetitive lumbar extension, rotation, and compression.[3]

The majority of running injuries are attributable to overuse. The incidence of injury ranges from 37% to 56% per year.[4] Spine injuries in runners are not as common as lower extremity injuries and their incidence can range from 5% to 19%.[5-8] Koplan and colleagues[7] followed a group of recreational runners over a period of 10 years and found that 53% had sustained an injury in that period and 31% had sought medical care. The percentage of back injuries did not change over the 10-year period and remained at about 9%, compared with the most commonly injured site, the knee, at 30%.

Wen and coworkers[8] studied issues of alignment and risk of specific injuries in a group of 304 runners in a training program for marathoners. There were several statistically significant findings in the back-injured group compared with the group without back injury.

The back-injured group spent a lower percentage of time training on concrete or asphalt than did the non-injured back group (49.2% versus 71.6%). Since this was a retrospective study, it is not certain whether the actual running surface was the cause of low back pain or whether those with low back pain modified the surface they trained on because of their pain. Most other reviews of running injuries in relation to surface types have been inconclusive. However, one study reported that women who run on concrete are at higher risk of injury.[9] Leg length discrepancies were divided into terciles in the study by Wen and colleagues. Back pain had a statistically significant association with both the lowest and highest terciles suggesting that those without a leg length discrepancy and those with the greatest leg length discrepancy had more back pain. This contradictory evidence makes the significance of this finding questionable. This and many epidemiologic studies of running injuries are retrospective. The data were collected by questionnaire and were subject to recall and self-report bias. There have been no prospective studies that evaluate the risk factors and epidemiology of spinal injuries in runners. Prospective research studies of running injuries and their relationship to mechanical alignment or training techniques are sorely needed.

FUNCTIONAL ANATOMY

Rehabilitation of runners' spine injuries requires a thorough understanding of the functional anatomy and biomechanics of the spine. This allows a specific diagnosis to be made so that a comprehensive and appropriate rehabilitation program can be prescribed. A detailed review of spinal anatomy is beyond the scope of this chapter. The reader should refer to the listed references for more detail. Since the lumbar spine is the most commonly injured portion of the spinal axis, this discussion will focus on that region.

The lumbar spine is made up of five lumbar vertebrae. The basic kinematic unit, called a motion segment, consists of one intervertebral disc positioned between the hyaline cartilage endplates of a superior and inferior vertebral body, and a pair of zygapophysial joints formed by the articular processes of the superior and inferior vertebrae[10] (Fig. 12–1).

Each lumbar vertebra is made of a vertebral body, pedicle, and the posterior elements. The vertebral body is a shell of cortical bone surrounding a cancellous cavity. The cortical bone consists of reinforced thin rods of bone called trabeculae that run in vertical and transverse directions. This provides weightbearing strength and load-bearing capacity to the vertebrae.

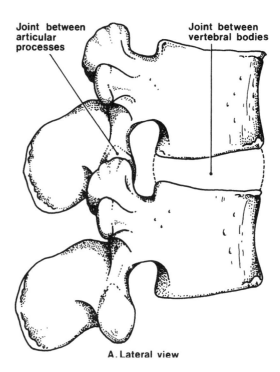

Figure 12–1. The three-joint complex (*Source: From Bogduk.*[10])

The lumbar nerve roots exit below the pedicle of each vertebra.

The disc is made up of an outer annulus fibrosus and a central nucleus pulposus. The nucleus pulposus is a semifluid structure. The surrounding annulus fibrosus is composed of 10 to 20 circumferential collagenous layers called lamellae. The fibers in each lamella run parallel to one another, but the direction of inclination alternates with each layer. The outer half of the annulus consists primarily of type I collagen and has great tensile strength. The inner half of the annulus consists primarily of type II collagen that is more elastic and best accommodates pressure changes. The annulus and nucleus pulposus are involved in weightbearing.

The zygapophysial joints (Z-joints) are formed by the articulations of the inferior and superior articular processes of two adjacent vertebrae. The joint is covered by articular cartilage that is bridged by a synovial membrane. The orientation of the joint changes from a parasagittal plane in the proximal lumbar spine to a more coronal plane in the distal spine. The proximal Z-joints, because of their sagittal orientation, help resist rotation and the lower Z-joints, because of their coronal orientation, primarily limit forward displacement[11] (Fig. 12–2).

The pars interarticularis can develop a defect known as spondylolysis. In the athlete, this is thought to be due to repetitive microtrauma aggravated by repetitive hyperextension and/or rotation of the spine.

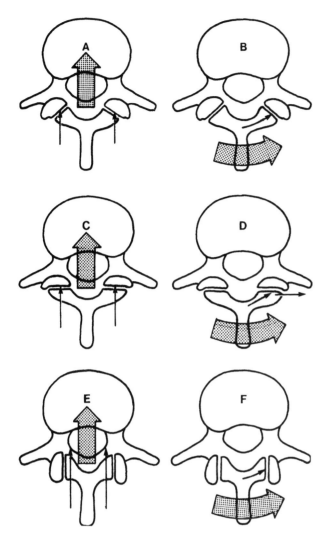

Figure 12–2. The mechanics of flat lumbar zygapophysial joints. A flat joint at 60° to the sagittal plane affords resistance to both forward displacement (A) and rotation (B). A flat joint at 90° to the sagittal plane strongly resists forward displacement (C), but during rotation (D) the inferior articular facet can glance off the superior articular facet. A flat joint parallel to the sagittal plane offers no resistance to forward displacement (E) but strongly resists rotation (F). (*Source: From Bogduk.[10]*)

Spondylolisthesis is the slipping of one vertebra on another due to a structural defect of the pars interarticularis.[12,13]

PAIN INNERVATION

The outer third of the intervertebral disc is innervated with both encapsulated and free nerve endings.[14] The greatest concentration of these nerve endings is in the posterolateral portion of the disk. The sinu-vertebral nerve supplies the posterior margin of the annulus and the posterior longitudinal ligament. The ventral rami

and the gray ramus communicans supply the anterior annulus and anterior longitudinal ligament. The zygapophysial joints are supplied by the medial branches of the dorsal primary rami. These nerve endings are located in the zygapophysial joint capsule and contiguous ligamentum flavum, muscles, and tendons. The lateral, intermediate, and medial branches of the primary dorsal rami innervate the muscles and ligaments that support the lumbar spine.[15]

Mechanical, vascular, and neurochemical factors may all contribute to the production of low back pain and radicular symptoms. Mechanical impingement of a disc against a nerve does not always cause pain. Herniated discs have been found in asymptomatic individuals.[16] Herniated discs release inflammatory mediators such as phospholipase A_2.[17,18] This may act directly on neural membranes or increase production of prostaglandins and leukotrienes. Symptomatic disc herniation has also been shown to produce matrix metalloproteinase, nitric oxide, interleukin-6, and prostaglandins.[19] Neuropeptides such as substance P, vasoactive intestinal polypeptide (VIP), and calcitonin gene-related peptide (CGRP) occur in primary afferent neurons and the dorsal root ganglion. These can contribute to the inflammatory cascade when released in response to tissue injury or inflammation by lowering the firing threshold of mechanical fibers, increasing sensitization of pain fibers, or influencing vasodilation, plasma extravasation, and histamine release.[20] This sensitization can result in pain responses to spinal movement or stress that would not normally cause a noxious event (Fig. 12–3).

BIOMECHANICS OF THE SPINE

Combined forces are transmitted through the lumbar spine during movements of flexion/extension, torsion, and lateral bending. A center of movement known as the instantaneous axis of rotation (IAR) must be maintained within a very small radius at any fixed point in the joint's overall range of motion to maintain joint stability. A line connecting the IARs of a specific motion segment during movement is termed a centrode. The centrodes of normal lumbar discs are short and tightly clustered while degenerative segments have longer and displaced centrodes[21] (Fig. 12–4).

Three common mechanisms of injury include 1) excessive compression or axial loading of the spine, 2) torque, which causes rotation, and 3) shear, which causes translation. Normally, axial compression is distributed via the semifluid nucleus pulposus to the surrounding circumferential annular fibers. This helps the spine rapidly adapt to a variety of forces by temporally

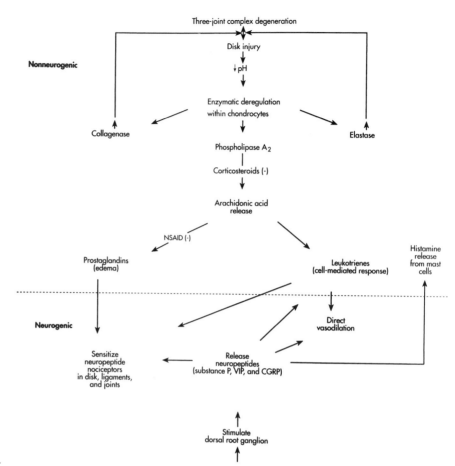

Figure 12–3. Hypothesized interaction between nonneurogenic and neurogenic inflammatory pain mediators. (*Source: Herring et al.[32]*)

dispersing and attenuating the speed with which a force is transmitted to its neighboring motion segment. Any derangement or degeneration of the annulus may change the biomechanics of a motion segment, making it unable to distribute an axial load and this may result in injury.[10] Recent studies also suggest that the vertebral endplate may play a critical role in distributing applied forces and minimizing the chance of injury.[22]

Torsional stresses may also result in injury to the annulus, resulting in circumferential or radial tears. Microtears of the outer annulus occur between 3 and 12 degrees of rotation, and frank failure of the annulus can occur beyond 12 degrees of rotation. Resistance to torsion is achieved 65% from the ipsilateral Z-joint and 35% from the annulus. Only 2 to 3 degrees of pure rotation are allowed by the 90-degree orientation of the lumbar Z-joints, thus keeping the annulus in a safe range.[23] Circumferential tears resulting from torsional stresses on the annulus tend to concentrate in the posterolateral corners of the disc. These annular fibers, located the farthest from the centrode, are tightly curved as they wrap around the disc, and this therefore

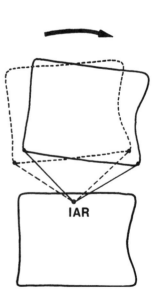

Figure 12–4. During flexion-extension, each lumbar vertebra exhibits an arcuate motion in relation to the vertebra below. The center of this arc lies below the moving vertebra and is known as the instantaneous axis of rotation (IAR). (*Source: Bogduk.[10]*)

becomes a site of stress concentration, known as a stress riser.[24]

DEGENERATIVE CASCADE

Before applying spinal biomechanics to the evaluation of running injuries, a review of the degenerative cascade is required. A complete understanding of the normal changes that occur in a spine as it ages is helpful in determining the source of injury as well as formulating a rehabilitation program. Kirkaldy-Willis[25] divides the spectrum of degenerative changes into three phases: 1) segmental dysfunction, 2) segmental instability, and 3) segmental stabilization. In phase 1, an alteration in the normal biomechanics of a motion segment can result in injury. The disc develops annular laxity with disorganization of its annular lamellae. Small circumferential tears ensue and ultimately progress to radial tears that can invade the nucleus pulposus. Radial annular tears are more likely to progress to a herniation than are circumferential tears. Z-joint degeneration accompanies disc degeneration. Progressive motion of the Z-joint allows excessive rotational and compressive strain, resulting in joint synovitis and capsular inflammation. An individual will often have pain with activities that cause anterior shear or translation (flexion), torsional shear (twisting or rotation), or a Valsalva maneuver. The segmental posterior muscles are often hypertonic, with restriction of normal movement in one or more directions.

During the instability phase the disc dehydrates with progressive loss of disc height. Multiple annular tears can result in internal disc disruption. Increased movement within the affected motion segment occurs. With further degeneration, the disc space narrows and the vertebral bodies on either side become dense and sclerotic. The Z-joints develop increasing capsular laxity and excessive joint motion may occur. Compensatory abnormal increased movement may develop in a segment adjacent to a hypomobile dysfunctional segment.

In the stabilization phase, the disc develops progressive fibrosis and osteophytosis resulting in progressive loss of disc space height. The Z-joints lose articular cartilage and develop enlargement secondary to osteophytosis. The changes in these structures result in a more stable segment with reduced movement. This may result in central, lateral recess or foraminal stenosis.

KINEMATICS OF RUNNING

The reader should refer to Chapter 2 for a full review of the running gait cycle. Issues that directly impact the lumbar spine will be briefly reviewed. In running, the ground reaction force can be two to four times as great as that of walking. The initial impact is absorbed through the lower extremities until forces are ultimately distributed through the pelvis, lumbar spine, and supporting trunk musculature. Any abnormal stress or mechanical dysfunction in the kinetic chain may injure the lumbar spine. An altered gait cycle due to a lower extremity injury or due to poor running mechanics such as a larger amplitude arm swing may cause excessive torsion of lumbar motion segments. Injuries may also occur to the pelvic structures and manifest themselves as lumbo-pelvic pain. Repetitive loading of the annulus beyond the limit of its safe range can lead to circumferential tears and resultant low back pain. In a study by Saamanen and colleagues,[26] 55-week-old beagle dogs were made to run 20 km daily for 15 weeks on a treadmill with a 15-degree uphill inclination. A decreased proteoglycan/collagen ratio in the annulus fibrosus was documented and was thought to represent tissue adaptation to increased lumbar motion and stress. This decreased proteoglycan/collagen ratio could also alter the mechanical properties of annular tissue.

When running, less time is spent in the stance and swing phase and more time is spent in the float phase than in walking, but the number of times the foot impacts the ground can occur twice as often in running as in walking.[27,28] In order for the runner to continue running in a straight line, motion segments in the lumbar spine must adapt to repetitive and rapid changes in motion. Thurston and coworkers[29] found that below the T7 level (vertebrae which remained relatively neutral), the thoracic spine rotated approximately 8 degrees in one direction and the lumbar spine rotated approximately 8 degrees in the opposite direction. When the pelvis and lumbar spine rotated clockwise, the upper torso would rotate counterclockwise. This would cause the facet joints to come into tight contact with each spinal rotation in the gait cycle. These excessive rotational forces may cause a higher risk of injury in an aging runner with normal degeneration of discs or Z-joints.

Additional mechanical stresses on the spine should be considered in uphill and downhill running. Running uphill requires a combination of rotation and additional flexion. An increase in relative flexion should increase intradiscal loads due to the additional compressive loads applied to the disc by the action of the back muscles that control flexion.[30] Runners with a history of an annular tear or herniated disc would theoretically place the involved segment at increased risk with a great deal of uphill running.[31]

Running downhill can result in increased extension of the lumbar spine. Additional hyperextension of the lumbar spine occurs as the trailing leg leaves the ground and the hyperextension will increase as running speed increases.[5] Increased lumbar extension in older runners can cause back or leg pain due to narrowing of the central canal in spinal stenosis or excessive force through the posterior elements in degenerative spondylolisthesis. Leg pain may also be caused by narrowing of the neural foramen in runners with pre-existing foraminal stenosis. Younger runners may develop discomfort from spondylolysis, spondylolisthesis, or a foraminal disc herniation as their lower lumbar foramina narrow during extension.[31] Leg symptoms may be more noticeable during stance phase at heel strike, when the impact load is the greatest.

EVALUATION

History

A comprehensive rehabilitation program requires an accurate and complete diagnosis. A careful history should include the onset and etiology of symptoms and mechanism of injury. Activities that increase or exacerbate symptoms may give insight into an anatomic diagnosis. As mentioned previously, increased pain with uphill running may suggest a discogenic source. Pain distribution patterns obtained by history or a pain diagram may be helpful. Pain referred below the knee may be radicular pain from a herniated nucleus pulposus. Discogenic pain that does not cause nerve root compression may be in a sclerotomal pattern and radiate into the buttock, hip, or thigh. Other symptoms that may suggest discogenic pain include discomfort with sitting, coughing, or a Valsalva maneuver. Posterior element pain from zygapophysial joints or spondylolysis may be exacerbated with extension during downhill running. Pain distribution may include the low back, buttocks, or thighs. Since athletes do not usually develop spondylolysis directly from running, awareness of involvement in other activities (such as weightlifting) that put an athlete at high risk for that particular type of injury is important.[13] Aging runners with central spinal stenosis may complain of neurogenic claudication, which may include back and/or leg pain, and paresthesias that occur during running and are relieved by flexing the spine, sitting, or lying down.

Training methods must be reviewed since most running injuries are due to overuse. Determining whether an injury is acute, chronic, an acute exacerbation of a chronic injury, or a subclinical functional alteration will influence the rehabilitation approach.[32]

Physical Examination

The physical examination of an injured runner should include a thorough and directed musculoskeletal and

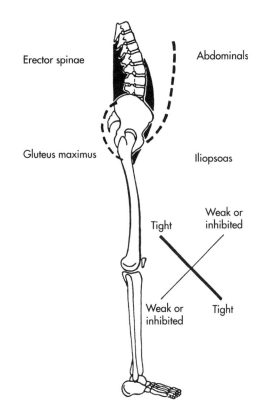

Figure 12–5. Pelvic crossed syndrome. (*Source: Jull G et al.*[34])

neurological examination of the spine, pelvis, and lower extremities. Changes in sensation, strength, or reflexes in a dermatomal pattern are suggestive of a discogenic source. Special attention in evaluating a runner with spinal pain should be given to spine and trunk flexibility, posture, and trunk strength.[3] A hyperlordotic posture, tight hamstrings, and increased pain with hyperextension are often present with a pars defect.[12] Many runners with mechanical low back pain can be treated with vigorous stretching exercises.[33] The iliopsoas, hamstrings, and spine extensor muscles tend to be areas of tightness. Abdominal muscles in runners tend to be weak, as there is no specific mechanism of strengthening them with running. This pattern of muscle imbalance and weakness is similar to those Jull and Janda[34] describe in the pelvic crossed syndrome, in which the erector spinae and iliopsoas are shortened and tight, and the abdominal and gluteal muscles are relatively weak. The combined forces of these muscle imbalances affect the dynamic functioning of the lumbo-pelvic-hip region (Fig. 12–5).

Diagnostic Testing

Diagnostic imaging may be considered early when diagnosing some cases of low back pain in runners. X-rays are often obtained initially because of easy availability, speed, cost, and the wealth of information they offer. Patients that are under the age of 20 with back pain for more than 3 weeks should be imaged to rule out a stress fracture or spondylitic defect. Other more unusual findings may include osteoid osteoma or infection.[33,35] A history of trauma or corticosteroid use may predispose to fracture, therefore imaging is needed in these cases. X-rays may be necessary to help rule out a malignancy in some cases: 1) runners over the age of 50; 2) those who have pain at night; 3) those with unexplained weight loss; or 4) runners with a history of cancer.

At a minimum, a basic lumbar x-ray series should include anteroposterior and lateral films. Oblique views are necessary to visualize details of the facets and pars interarticularis. A coned-down lateral view provides more accurate information about the L5-S1 interspace. Lateral flexion and extension views may be helpful to rule out lumbar instability.

Advanced imaging techniques provide additional details. Bone scan or single photon emission computed tomography (SPECT) have increased sensitivity and specificity for detection of pars stress fractures and acute fractures compared with plain films.[35] A computed tomography (CT) scan provides detailed imaging of bone, including pars defects, fractures, osteophytes, and bony destruction due to tumor. Myelography may be used in conjunction with CT to further evaluate nerve root compression in patients in which MRI is contraindicated or results are equivocal. MRI is more useful to detect soft-tissue injury including annular tears. MRI also provides more detail of the thecal sac, epidural space, spinous ligaments, and bone marrow.[36] Caution should be maintained when correlating imaging studies to the patient's history and clinical examination. Boden and Kavis[16] discovered abnormal disc findings in the lumbar MRIs of approximately one third of asymptomatic volunteers.

REHABILITATION

The goal of a rehabilitation program is restoration of function. The absence of symptoms does not necessarily mean that full recovery has occurred, especially in an athlete. The presence of subclinical maladaptations and biomechanical deficits that have not been adequately and thoroughly rehabilitated may result in higher risk of repeat injury. Suboptimal retraining may result in suboptimal athletic performance. The sports medicine physician must also recognize the unique physiological and psychological needs of a runner. A rehabilitation program will differ significantly for a highly competitive athlete compared with that for a recreational jogger. The aggressiveness of treatment and need for cross-training needs to be individualized for each athlete. A lumbar rehabilitation program should include 1) correction of soft-tissue injuries;

2) optimization of spinal segmental motion; 3) improvement in trunk and lower extremity strength, endurance, and power; 4) education and training for posture, body mechanics, and proprioception; and 5) a safe return to sporting activity.[31,33]

The initial goals of rehabilitation are to control pain and inflammation. The athlete must be instructed in proper body mechanics to help minimize additional stress to the injured segment. Medication, manual therapy, modalities, and therapeutic exercise may be initiated early in the rehabilitation phase. During the subacute phase, pain-free range of motion of the injured and adjacent motion segments of the lumbar spine, pelvis, and lower extremities must be achieved. As the runner's condition improves, a gradual progression from passive mobilization techniques to active flexibility, strength, and endurance training is provided. Running-specific rehabilitation should be incorporated into the subacute phase.

Medications

There are a variety of medications that can be helpful in the acute phase. Nonsteroidal anti-inflammatory drugs (NSAIDs) can be prescribed for a reduction in both pain and inflammation. NSAIDs work by inhibiting cyclooxygenase with subsequent inhibition of prostaglandin formation. NSAIDs have also been found to modify nonprostaglandin cellular and inflammatory processes.[37]

There are few data comparing the efficacy of different NSAIDs, and dosing is often determined by the physician's exposure and experience. There is a ceiling effect to the analgesic response in NSAIDs beyond which additional dosing increments yield no additional analgesia.[38] Potential adverse reactions most commonly include gastrointestinal tract irritation, inhibition of platelet aggregation, increased bleeding time, and renal toxicity. Caution should be maintained in chronic usage and in the aging athlete, and appropriate monitoring should include renal and liver function tests, complete blood count, and urinalysis.[37] Acetaminophen can provide analgesia in those who cannot tolerate NSAIDs. There are limited trials of acetaminophen use in back pain, but comparisons of acetaminophen and NSAIDs in the treatment of knee osteoarthritis found similar therapeutic benefits.[39]

Narcotics may be used for severe acute pain on a time-limited basis. Medication should be titrated to achieve pain relief on a time-contingent schedule. Narcotics should only be used on a short-term basis to avoid tolerance and long-term physical dependence. The use of muscle relaxants to treat spinal pain is controversial and their efficacy is questionable.[40] Muscle relaxants have no direct effect on muscle and actually exert their effect via central nerve pathways. Muscular pain is reduced through depression of central nerve pathways.[41] Sedation, a common side effect that is also caused by central nervous system depression, may limit a runner's ability to participate in a rehabilitation program. However, muscle relaxants may improve sleep hygiene.

Corticosteroids have greater anti-inflammatory effects than NSAIDs because they inhibit phospholipase A_2, an enzyme that involves the production of inflammatory mediators by cyclooxygenase and lipoxygenase pathways. Fluoroscopically guided, contrast-enhanced lumbar spinal injections can be used for both diagnostic and therapeutic purposes.[42]

Modalities

Modalities may also help reduce pain and inflammation. Therapeutic cold or cryotherapy diminishes arteriolar and capillary blood flow, decreases capillary permeability, and increases pain threshold.[43,44] The time to cool an injured structure varies from 10 to 30 minutes and is dependent on the depth of intervening fat.[44] Heat application results in increased blood flow, increased capillary permeability, and increased extensibility of collagen tissue.[43,44] Ultrasound can be an effective deep-heating modality for soft-tissue problems. Ultrasound can increase blood flow to damaged tissue to provide needed nutrients to healing tissue and aid in the removal of inflammatory by-products.[45,46] Electrical stimulation techniques including transcutaneous electrical nerve stimulation (TENS), high-voltage pulsed galvanic stimulation (HVPGS), interferential electrical stimulation, and minimal electrical noninvasive stimulation (MENS) have been reported to promote analgesia, muscle relaxation, and reduction of edema and inflammation.[47]

Bracing

Bracing may be necessary in the athlete with a spondylitic defect. There are a number of protocols available.[12,13,48] Specifics of the athlete's age, skeletal maturity, degree of competitiveness, and acuity of injury must be considered. A lumbosacral corset or Boston brace (an antilordotic orthosis) can be used.[49]

Determining acuity with plain x-rays and SPECT scans can be helpful in determining bracing needs. Hambly and colleagues[13] developed general guidelines for use of radiographs and bracing. In athletes with x-rays that are negative or show a possible pars defect but have a positive bone scan, a brace is needed and the patient should be taken off athletics for at least 3 months. Repeat x-rays are recommended at 3 months and a repeat bone scan at 6 months. Immobilization and time off athletics should continue until the bone scan shows healing. A typical time to healing may be

6 to 9 months. While braced, the athlete can participate in gentle spine-neutral rehabilitation and cross-training. Prognosis for healing is good for negative x-ray findings and fair for x-rays with a possible pars defect.

The same time course for immobilization and bracing is also used for x-rays with a definite pars fracture and with positive bone scan. Bracing continues until the bone scan and x-rays show healing or until there is continuing evidence that the fracture is not going to heal. Prognosis is more guarded for healing. Fractures that appear old on x-rays and a negative or mildly positive bone scan can be treated symptomatically. Rehabilitation and bracing may be helpful, but full healing is very unlikely. A surgical consultation may be warranted in fractures that do not respond to conservative treatment.

Therapy Techniques

A variety of rehabilitation techniques have been employed to treat low back pain. A combination of therapy techniques that are individualized to a runner's specific needs is usually the most effective.

Manual therapy encompasses a wide variety of techniques to treat soft tissue and osseous restrictions. Manipulation or mobilization techniques involve taking a joint complex through all or part of its physiologic range of motion. Mobilization involves repetitive passive movements which allow effective synovial fluid distribution over and through the articular cartilage.[50] Passive joint motion has been shown to stretch joint capsules, lubricate tissues, and improve vertebral motion restriction.[50,51] Manipulation involves low-amplitude, high-velocity thrusts that reestablish normal physiologic range of motion. Shekelle[52] reviews four hypotheses for lesions that respond to manipulation: 1) release of entrapped synovial folds or plica, 2) relaxation of hypertonic muscle by sudden stretching, 3) disruption of articular or periarticular adhesions, and 4) unbuckling of motion segments that have undergone disproportionate displacements. Manual therapy techniques may be helpful to decrease pain and restore segmental mobility in a runner's spine during the initial stages of a rehabilitation program. Abnormal motion in one or more segments usually causes a compensatory change in mobility in another segment. Correction of these abnormal motion segments is an important step before advancing the runner to a more active phase in a rehabilitation program.

Therapeutic exercise may be initiated as the runner becomes less symptomatic. The exercise program should be customized to each runner's specific dysfunction. Runners with acute discogenic pain may benefit from exercises that attempt to centralize leg pain and decrease lumbar pain as in the McKenzie approach.[53] This involves a mechanical assessment of a patient's low-back pain and uses end-range lumbar test movements to help centralize leg pain. This often, but not always, involves extension-based exercises. Some conditions, however, may be exacerbated in extension, such as large central disc herniations, internal disc disruption, foraminal herniations, as well as lateral and recess stenosis.

Williams' flexion exercises were initially thought to relieve symptoms by decreasing the load of the posterior aspect of the disc and widening the neural foramen. However, these exercises can often exacerbate symptoms in acute disc herniations by increasing intradiscal pressure.[54] Patients with posterior element pain or central spinal stenosis may benefit from flexion-based exercises.

Lumbar stabilization techniques are widely used to successfully rehabilitate athletes with low-back pain[55,56] (Fig. 12–6). The cornerstone of treatment is the concept of "neutral spine." This is defined as the position of the spine that is the least painful and that minimizes biomechanical stresses. This position minimizes tension on ligaments and joints and helps balance forces equally between the disc and zygapophysial joints. Inflexibility of pelvic and lower extremity muscles contributes to alterations in lumbo-pelvic posture and secondary spinal dysfunction. Muscle flexibility must be incorporated as part of the stabilization program to allow the runner to assume his or her unique neutral spine position so that strength is developed to maintain this position. Runners tend to have tight hamstrings and hip flexors. Aggressive stretching of these muscles and strengthening of the antagonist muscles, hip extensors, and knee extensors can often alleviate back pain.[3]

The progressive development of flexibility, trunk strength, balance, and coordination involves training the muscular stabilizers of the lumbar spine, including the abdominal muscles, latissimus dorsi, spinal intersegmental muscles, iliopsoas, erector spinae, and quadratus lumborum. A stepwise program begins with learning the neutral position in a supine position. The level of difficulty is increased by adding additional arm and leg movements, first while supine, and then in progressively more challenging positions such as bridging, prone lying, and quadruped. Once these exercises are perfected, additional challenges can be added by exercising on a Swiss ball. This develops

---

Exercise Training for Lumbar Disc Disorder

Soft Tissue Flexibility
- Hamstring musculotendinous unit
- Quadriceps musculotendinous unit
- Iliopsoas musculotendinous unit
- Gastrocsoleus musculotendinous unit
- External and internal hip rotators

Joint Mobility
- Lumbar spine segmental mobility
- Hip ROM
- Thoracic segmental mobiliy

Stabilization Program
- Finding neutral position
  (standing, sitting,
  jumping, prone)
- Prone gluteal squeezes with
  arm raises
  alternate arm raises
  leg raises
  alternate leg raises
  arm and leg raises
  alternate arm and leg raises
- Supine pelvic bracing
- Bridging progression
  basic position
  one leg raises with ankle weights
  stepping
  balancing on gym ball

- Quadruped (with alternating arm and leg
  movements with ankle and wrist weights)
- Kneeling stabilization (double knee, single
  knee, lunges with and without weight)
- Wall slide quadriceps strengthening
- Position transition with postural control

Abdominal Program
- Curl-ups
- Dead bugs (supported, nonsupported)
- Diagonal curl-ups
- Diagonal curl-ups on incline board
- Straight leg lowering

Gym Program
- Latissimus pull downs
- Angled leg press
- Lunges
- Hyperextension bench
- General upper-body weight exercises
- Pulley exercises to stress postural control °

Aerobic Program
- Progressive walking
- Swimming
- Stationary bicycling
- Cross-country ski machine
- Running (initially supervised on
  a treadmill)

Figure 12–6. Lumbar stabilization program. (*Source: Saal.[55]*)

strength and coordination of the smaller intersegmental spinal muscles such as the multifidi. This program can be particularly useful in runners, as they tend to have weakness of the abdomen and trunk muscles. A lumbar stabilization program is useful because correction of a runner's postural dysfunction requires good isometric trunk strength. For example, a runner with a forward head and decreased lumbar lordosis will have a flexed trunk posture. This requires that a greater force be generated through the resisting trunk extensors and ligamentous structures of the lumbar spine, creating increased shear forces through the lumbar spine and intervertebral discs. Once the runner learns to maintain a spine-neutral position in static situations, increasing challenges in both static and dynamic situations can then be incorporated. The final portion of training should include sport-specific running with emphasis on neutral spine mechanics.

Cross-Training

Cross-training should be part of a runner's program to maintain cardiovascular fitness. Runners with discogenic pain may begin with water walking, water running, swimming, or unloaded walking on a treadmill by using an overhead harness[57] (Fig. 12–7). Runners with posterior element pain may tolerate a more

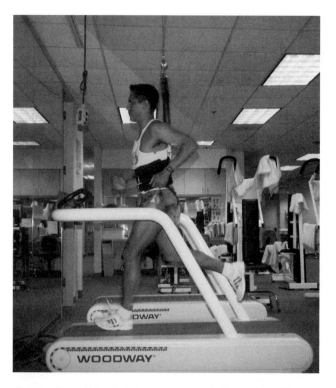

Figure 12–7. Unloaded harnessed treadmill running. (*Source: Courtesy of Aquatechnics Consulting Group, Inc., Aptos, Calif, used with permission.*)

flexion-based program with water walking, stationary bike riding, supine swimming, or stair stepping. As a runner advances, open-chain deep water running can be useful for cardiovascular fitness, proprioceptive awareness, and optimizing running mechanics.[57] Training can occur in progressively more shallow water before transitioning to land. Using an overhead harness for unloaded treadmill running can be an excellent alternative to water. A reintroduction to impact-loading exercises can include a trampoline, jumping rope, or indoor track running.[58] As the runner progresses, transitioning to a treadmill, indoor track, and ultimately back to a regular running program occurs.

SURGERY

Conservative treatment for a lumbar herniated nucleus pulposus generally has a favorable prognosis.[59] Saal noted that even neurologic motor deficit (not including cauda equina syndrome and progressive neurologic loss) could have a favorable natural history, although surgical intervention should also be considered in patients with motor loss that does not improve in 6 weeks. McCulloch[60] reviewed surgical outcomes of micro- and macrodiscectomy with an initial success rate of 80% to 96%. Outcome was more reliant on appropriate patient selection than surgical technique. In addition, long-term studies have not shown a significant difference between those treated surgically and nonsurgically. Wang and colleagues[61] followed 14 elite college athletes who had undergone lumbar disc surgery for radiculopathy that was refractory to conservative treatment. All 14 were followed an average of 3.1 years postoperatively and were pain free in activities of daily living. Nine of 10 athletes who underwent microdiscectomy returned to varsity athletics. Of the five athletes that retired, three required two-level discectomies, one had a single-level open discectomy, and one had a single-level microdiscectomy. However, these five athletes were able to participate in several activities at a recreational level. Postoperative rehabilitation strategies for runners is beyond the scope of this chapter.

CONCLUSIONS

The incidence of spine injuries may be a small proportion of overall injuries from running, but they can result in substantial disability and loss of training time. A thorough understanding of spinal anatomy and biomechanics in relation to the overall effects on the runner's kinetic chain is important in the diagnosis and management of spine injuries in runners. A comprehensive rehabilitation program that focuses on flexibility, strength, endurance, and coordination of the lumbar spine and lower extremities must be customized for each runner. An aggressive rehabilitation program should begin soon after an injury to minimize time lost from training. A progressive and stepwise rehabilitation program should help a runner return to full function and help prevent future injury.

REFERENCES

1. Frymoyer JW: Back pain and sciatica. *N Engl J Med* 1988:318, 291.
2. Von Korff M, Saunders K: The course of back pain in primary care. *Spine* 1996:21, 2833.
3. Watkins RG: Lumbar spine injuries, in Watkins RG (ed.), *The Spine and Sports*, St. Louis, Mosby, 1996:137.
4. Van Mechelen W: Running injuries: A review of the epidemiological literature. *Sports Med* 1992:14, 320.
5. Brody DM: Running injuries: Prevention and management. *Ciba Clinical Symposia* 1987:2.
6. Rendall EO, Mogtadi GH: Survey of competitive distance runners in Alberta: Satisfaction with health care services with respect to running injuries. *Clin J Sports Med* 1997:7, 104.
7. Koplan JP, Rothenberg RB, Jones EL: The natural history of exercise: A 10-year follow-up of a cohort of runners. *Med Sci Sports Exerc* 1995:27, 1180.
8. Wen DY, Puffer JC, Schmalzried TP: Lower extremity alignment and risk of overuse injuries in runners. *Med Sci Sports Exerc* 1997:29, 1291.
9. Brill PA, Macera CA: The influence of running patterns on running injuries. *Sports Med* 1995:20, 365.
10. Bogduk N: The lumbar vertebrae, in Bogduk N (ed.), *Clinical Anatomy of the Lumbar Spine and Sacrum*, 3rd ed., Edinburgh, Churchill Livingstone, 1997:1.
11. Bogduk N: The zygapophysial joints, in Bogduk N (ed.), *Clinical Anatomy of the Lumbar Spine and Sacrum*, 3rd ed., Edinburgh, Churchill Livingstone, 1997:33.
12. Flemming JE: Spondylolysis and spondylolisthesis in the athlete. *State of the Art Rev* 1990:4, 339.
13. Hambly MI, Wiltse LL, Peek RD: Spondylolisthesis, in Watkins RG (ed.), *The Spine and Sports*, St. Louis, Mosby, 1996:157.
14. Malinsky J: The ontogenetic development of nerve terminations in the intervertebral discs of man. *Acta Anat* 1959:38, 96.
15. Bogduk N: Nerves of the lumbar *Spine*, in Bogduk N (ed.), *Clinical Anatomy of the Lumbar Spine and Sacrum*, 3rd ed., Edinburgh, Churchill Livingstone, 1997:127.
16. Boden SD, Kavis DO: Abnormal magnetic resonance scans of the lumbar spine in asymptomatic subjects: A prospective investigation. *J Bone Joint Surg* 1990:72A, 403.
17. Saal JS, Franson RC, Dobrow R, et al.: High levels of inflammatory phospholipase A₂ activity in lumbar disc herniations. *Spine* 1990:15, 674.
18. Piperno M, Hellio Lebraverand MP, Reboui P, et al.: Phospholipase A₂ activity in herniated lumbar discs. *Spine* 1997:22, 2061.
19. Kang JD, Georgescu HI, McIntyre-Larkin L, et al.: Herniated cervical intervertebral discs spontaneously produce matrix metalloproteinase, nitric oxide, interleukin 6 and prostaglandin E2. *Spine* 1995:20, 2373.
20. Cavanaugh JM: Neural mechanisms of lumbar pain. *Spine* 1995:20, 1804.
21. Gertzbein SD, Seligman J, Holtby R, et al.: Centrode patterns and segmental instability in degenerative disc disease. *Spine* 1985:10, 257.
22. McGill SM: The scientific foundation for low back exercise. Lecture. American Academy of Physical Medicine & Rehabilitation annual meeting, Washington DC, November 11, 1999.
23. Farfan JF, Cossetle JW, Robertson GH, et al.: The effects of torsion on the lumbar intervertebral joints: The role of torsion in the production of disc degeneration. *J Bone Joint Surg (Am)* 1970:52A, 468.
24. Farfan HF, Gracovdgsky S: The nature of instability. *Spine* 1984:9, 714.
25. Kirkaldy-Willis WH: Pathology and pathogenesis of low back pain, in Kirkaldy-Willis WH, Burton CV (eds.), *Managing Low Back Pain*, 3rd ed., New York, Churchill Livingstone, 1992:49.
26. Saamanen AM, Puustjarvi K, Ilues K, et al.: Effect of running exercise on proteoglycans and collagen content in the intervertebral discs of young dogs. *Int J Sports Med* 1993:14, 48.
27. Thordson DB: Running biomechanics. *Clin Sports Med* 1997:16, 239.
28. Uppal GS, O'Toole M, Dillin WH: Running, in Watkins RG (ed.), *The Spine and Sports*, St. Louis, Mosby, 1996:475.
29. Thurston A, Harris J: Normal kinematics of the lumbar spine and pelvis. *Spine* 1983:8, 199.
30. Andersson GBJ, Ortengren R, Nachemson A: Intradiscal pressure, intra-abdominal pressure and myoelectric back muscle activity related to posture and loading. *Clin Orthop* 1977:129, 156.
31. Cole AJ, Herring SA, Stratton SA, et al.: Spine injuries in runners: A functional approach. *J Back Musculoskel Rehab* 1995:5, 317.
32. Herring SA, Weinstein SM: Assessment and nonsurgical management of athletic low back injury, in Nicholas JA, Hershman EB (eds.), *The Lower Extremity and Spine in Sports Medicine*, 2nd ed., New York, Mosby, 1995: 1171.
33. Watkins RG, Dillin WH: Lumbar spine injury in the athlete. *Clin Sports Med* 1990:9, 419.
34. Jull G, Janda V: Muscles and motor control in low back pain, in Twomey LT, Tayor JR (eds.), *Physical Therapy for the Low Back: Clinics in Physical Therapy*, New York, Churchill Livingstone, 1987.
35. Micheli LF: Back injuries in gymnastics. *Clin Sports Med* 1985:4, 85.
36. Cole AJ, Herzog RJ: The lumbar spine: Imaging options, in Cole AJ, Herring SA (eds.), *The Low Back Pain Handbook*, Philadelphia, Hanley & Belfus, 1996:169.

37. Honig SM: Nonsteroidal anti-inflammatory drugs, in Tollison CD, et al. (eds.), *Handbook of Pain Management,* 2nd ed., Baltimore, Williams & Wilkins, 1994:165.

38. Portenoy RK: Drug treatment of pain syndromes. *Semin Neurol* 1987:7, 139.

39. Bradley JD, Brandt KD, Katz BP, et al.: Comparison of an anti-inflammatory dose of ibuprofen and acetaminophen in the treatment of patients with osteoarthritis of the knee. *N Engl J Med* 1991:325, 87.

40. Deyo RA: Drug therapy for back pain: Which drugs help which patients? *Spine* 1996:21, 2840.

41. Gallagher RM: Muscle relaxant medications, in Tollison CD, et al. (eds.), *Handbook of Pain Management,* 2nd ed., Baltimore, Williams & Wilkins, 1994:173.

42. Woodward JL, Weinstein SM: Epidural injections for the diagnosis and management of axial and radicular pain syndromes. *Phys Med Rehab Clin North Am* 1995:6, 691.

43. Ohnmeiss DD: Nonsurgical treatment of sports-related spine injures: I. Modalities, in Hochschuler SH (ed.), *Spine State of the Art Rev: Spinal Injuries in Sports,* 1990:4, 442.

44. Lehmann JS, Watten CG, Scham SM: Therapeutic heat and cold. *Clin Orthop* 1974:99, 207.

45. Gann N: Ultrasound current concepts. *Clin Manage* 1991:2, 64.

46. Cole AJ, Eagleston RA: The benefits of deep heat-ultrasound and electromagnetic diathermy. *Phys Sportsmed* 1994:22, 77.

47. Windsor RE, Lester JP, Herring SA: Electrical stimulation in clinical practice. *Phys Sports Med* 1993:21, 85.

48. Blanda J, Bethem D, Moats W, Lew M: Defect of pars interarticularis in athletics, a protocol for nonoperative treatment. *J Spinal Disord* 1993:6, 406.

49. Micheli LJ, Hare JE, Miller ME: Use of modified Boston brace for back injuries in athletes. *Am Sports Med* 1980:8, 1980.

50. Twomey L, Taylor J: Exercise and spinal manipulation in the treatment of low back pain. *Spine* 1995:20, 615.

51. Farrell JP: Cervical passive mobilization techniques: The Australian approach. *Phys Med Rehab: State of the Art Rev* 1993:4, 309.

52. Shekelle PG. Spine update: Spinal manipulation. *Spine* 1994:19, 858.

53. McKenzie RA: *The Lumbar Spine: Mechanical Diagnosis and Therapy,* Waikanae, New Zealand, Spinal Publications, 1981.

54. Nachemson A: Disc pressure measurements. *Spine* 1981:6, 93.

55. Saal JA: Dynamic muscular stabilization in the nonoperative treatment of lumbar pain syndromes. *Orthop Rev* 1991:19, 691.

56. Watkins RG: Spinal exercise program, in Watkins RG (ed.), *The Spine and Sports,* St. Louis, Mosby, 1996:282.

57. Wilder R, Brennan D: Physiological responses to deep water running in athletes. *Sports Med* 1993:16, 374.

58. Regan JJ: Back problems in the runner, in Hochschuler SH (ed.), *State of the Art Rev: Spinal Injuries in Sports* 1990:4, 346.

59. Saal JA: Natural history and nonoperative treatment of lumbar disc herniations. *Spine* 1996:21, 2S.

60. McCulloch JA: Focus issue on lumbar disc herniation: Macro- and microdiscectomy. *Spine* 1996:21, 45S.

61. Wang JC, Shapiro MS, Hatch JD, et al: The outcome of lumbar discectomy in elite athletes. *Spine* 1999:24, 570.

Chapter 13

HIP AND PELVIS INJURIES

Robert P. Wilder, William J. Barrish, and Joseph A. Volpe

INTRODUCTION

Thirty percent to 50% of all sports injuries are caused by overuse.[1-3] In the primary care setting, overuse injuries account for the majority of athletic injuries seen by physicians.[4] For example, overuse accounted for more than 80% of hip and pelvis injuries presenting to a general sports medicine clinic.[5] However, the etiology and management of pelvis and hip disorders have not been documented as well as those for the more common injuries to the knee, lower leg, and foot. Understanding the basic anatomy and the etiology and treatment of overuse injuries in general, with special attention paid to common injuries of the hip and pelvis, aids the sports medicine clinician in treating patients who have sports-related musculoskeletal injuries.

ANATOMY

The bony pelvis is formed by the two paired innominate bones, the sacrum, and the coccyx. Each innominate bone consists of the fused ilium superiorly and the ischium and pubis inferiorly. The upper edge of the ilium, the iliac crest, ends anteriorly in the anterior superior iliac spine (ASIS) and posteriorly in the posterior superior iliac spine (PSIS). Other important ilial landmarks include the anterior inferior iliac spine (AIIS) anteriorly and the posterior inferior iliac spine (PIIS)

posteriorly. The ASIS and PSIS are located at the ends of the iliac crest and can be easily palpated. The PIIS sits just above the sciatic notch.[6-12]

The inferior aspect of the innominate bone is formed by the ischium posteriorly and the pubis anteriorly. The two innominate bones are firmly attached to the sacrum posteriorly through the sacroiliac joints (SIJs). The SIJs are classified as synovial joints surrounded by a fibrous capsule that is well formed anteriorly, but posteriorly may have tears and rents.[6-8] Primary ligamentous support is provided by the relatively weak anterior sacroiliac ligament, the stronger posterior iliosacral ligament, and the interosseous ligaments. Accessory ligaments provide additional support and include the iliolumbar, sacrotuberous, and sacrospinous ligaments.[6,9] The SIJ receives innervation from the L3–S3 nerves, with S1 providing the primary contribution.[6,10] Shear, compressive, and other moment loads are created in the SIJ by a number of muscles including the erector spinae, quadratus lumborum, psoas major and minor, piriformis, latissimus dorsi, obliquus internus, externus abdominis, and gluteus maximus, medius, and minimus. The pelvis is attached anteriorly at the pubic symphis.

The hip joint is a ball and socket formed by the pelvic acetabulum and the femoral head. The superior, anterior, and posterior margins of the acetabulum form its articular surface. The inferior margin, known as the acetabular notch, is a nonweightbearing surface. A fibrocartilaginous labrum surrounds the acetabulum, encasing the femoral head and thus contributing to the joint's stability.[11,12]

The femoral neck bridges the femoral head to the shaft, angled medially approximately 125 degrees. Coxa vara exists when the angle of the neck to the shaft is decreased, and this may contribute to increased shearing and torsional forces. Coxa valga exists when the angle is increased. Increased compressive forces may contribute to accelerated degeneration.[11] The femur is also angled in the anteroposterior plane in approximately 15 degrees of anteversion (medial femoral torsion).

The capsule of the hip joint is reinforced along the anterior and posterior surfaces by the iliofemoral, pubofemoral, and ischiofemoral ligaments. The iliofemoral ligament (Y ligament of Bigelow) resembles an inverted Y arising from the AIIS, subsequently dividing and inserting into the femur at the greater trochanter and on the anterior aspect of the femur inferior to the intertrochanteric line. The iliofemoral ligament restrains hyperextension at the hip. The pubofemoral ligament primarily limits abduction and extension; the ischiofemoral ligament primarily limits extension.

With the ligaments functioning as a group, the greatest stability is provided in extension, abduction, and external rotation. Therefore, the hip joint is least stable in flexion, adduction, and internal rotation, the most frequent position of hip dislocation.[12]

Dual vascular supply is provided to the hip by a small artery to the femoral head in the ligamentum teres and by the medial and lateral circumflex arteries, which pierce the capsule. Muscular action at the hip is summarized in Table 13–1.[11,13]

CONCEPTS OF OVERUSE INJURY

Overuse injuries result from repetitive microtrauma that leads to inflammation and local tissue damage in the form of cellular and extracellular degeneration.[14] This tissue damage can be cumulative, resulting in myositis, bursitis, ligament sprains, joint synovitis, cartilaginous degeneration, stress fractures, neurapraxic or axonal nerve injury, and tendinitis or tendinosis.[1,14] The musculotendinous unit appears to be particularly susceptible to injury resulting from microtrauma caused by excessive eccentric loading.[4,15] Acute injury results

TABLE 13–1. MUSCULAR ACTION AT THE HIP

Hip Action	Muscles: Prime Movers	Muscles: Assistant Movers
Flexors	Psoas Iliacus Pectineus Rectus femoris	Sartorius Tensor fasciae latae Gracilis Adductor brevis Adductor longus
Extensors	Gluteus maximus Semitendinosus Semimembranosus Biceps femoris (long head)	
Abductors	Gluteus medius	Gluteus minimus Tensor fasciae latae Sartorius Rectus femoris
Adductors	Adductor magnus Adductor longus Adductor brevis Gracilis Pectineus	
External rotators	Gluteus maximus Gemellus inferior Gemellus superior Obturator externus Obturator internus Quadratus femoris Piriformis	Adductor longus Adductor brevis Biceps femoris (long head) Sartorius Pectineus
Internal rotators	Tensor fasciae latae Gluteus minimus	Semitendinosus Semimembranosus Gracilis

TABLE 13–2. RISK FACTORS THAT CONTRIBUTE TO OVERUSE INJURIES

Intrinsic	Extrinsic
Malalignment	Training errors
Muscle imbalance	Equipment
Inflexibility	Environment
Muscle weakness	Technique
Instability	Sport-imposed deficiencies

in the development of an inflammatory response. As inflammation becomes chronic, tissue changes occur, characterized by the development of new vascular elements with fibroblastic proliferation (angiofibroblastic hyperplasia), ultimately leading to tendon degeneration.[4,16] The most common etiology of overuse injuries is repetitive trauma that overwhelms the tissue's ability to repair itself.

Both intrinsic and extrinsic factors contribute to overuse injuries (Table 13–2).[1,14,15] Intrinsic factors are biomechanical and physiologic abnormalities unique to a particular athlete; extrinsic factors are primarily related to training errors. In addition to injury-specific management, the management of overuse injuries addresses these risk factors. The interaction of such intrinsic and extrinsic factors with repetitive overuse leading to tissue injury and kinetic chain adaptations is also illustrated by the vicious overload cycle. According to Kibler and colleagues,[17] there are five complexes associated with the vicious cycle. The *tissue injury complex* describes the group of anatomic structures that have sustained damage. The *clinical symptom complex* comprises those symptoms and signs that manifest themselves due to the injury. The *tissue overload complex* encompasses the group of tissues subject to tensile overload. The *functional biomechanical deficit complex* includes the constellations of inflexibilities and muscle strength imbalances that can then alter normal biomechanics. Finally, the *subclinical adaptation complex* describes all of the adaptive means that are used to compensate for the altered biomechanics. Kibler's cycle underscores the necessity to address deficits throughout the kinetic chain in addition to injury-specific management in order to produce the most successful treatment.

REHABILITATIVE MANAGEMENT OF OVERUSE INJURIES

The diagnosis and management of overuse injuries requires a multidisciplinary approach. The clinician's principal responsibilities are to establish a correct pathoanatomic diagnosis and direct rehabilitation, which often involves enlisting the help of physical therapists, orthotists, athletic trainers, and coaches.

A comprehensive rehabilitation program following overuse injuries of the hip and pelvis comprises a series of stages leading to a return to participation in sports. The steps build on one another yet overlap considerably. In addition, these basic management principles can be applied to the management of overuse injuries in general, although different tissues have unique characteristics and vary somewhat in response to treatment.[14-21] These concepts are fully developed in Chapter 40.

DIAGNOSIS AND TREATMENT OF SPECIFIC DISORDERS

Overuse injuries of the hip and pelvis in sports are classified according to their anatomic location (i.e., anterior, posterior, or lateral) (Table 13–3). Treatment discussions detail rehabilitative exercises directed specifically at the hip and pelvis. However, it must be emphasized again that imbalances and abnormalities at each level of the kinetic chain (i.e., lumbar spine, knee, foot, and ankle) must also be identified and corrected.

Anterior Overuse Injuries

Quadriceps Strain

Strains of the quadriceps most commonly involve the rectus femoris and occur during sports involving sprinting, jumping, or kicking. Strains are graded as mild (grade I), moderate (grade II), or severe (grade III)[22-28] (Table 13–4). Factors that can increase the risk of quadriceps strain include tightness (especially the

TABLE 13–3. COMMON OVERUSE INJURIES OF THE HIP AND PELVIS IN SPORTS

Anterior	Posterior	Lateral
Quadricep strain/ contusion	Hamstring strain	Greater trochanter bursitis
Adductor strain	Piriformis syndrome	Gluteus medius bursitis
Femoral stress fracture	Ischial bursitis	External snapping hip
Osteitis pubis	Sacroiliac joint dysfunction	Lateral hip pointer
Anterior hip pointer		Tensor fasciae latae syndrome
Internal snapping hip		Meralgia paresthetica

TABLE 13–4. QUADRICEP STRAINS

Grade	Severity	Description
I	Mild	Overstretch with minimal disruption of musculotendinous unit integrity. There is probably less than 5% fiber disruption. Patient experiences soreness with motion, but only minimal strength loss.
II	Moderate	Incomplete muscle tear. There is intramuscular bleeding with hematoma formation. Muscle strength is clearly compromised.
III	Severe	Complete rupture. Muscle function is essentially lost. Avulsion injuries are included in this category.

rectus femoris) or weakness (especially the vasti) of the quadriceps musculature, hamstring tightness, lack of sufficient warm-up or stretching prior to exercise, previous injury without rehabilitation, and overtraining.[12]

The functional adaptations that persist when return to activity is too early include greater reliance on the unaffected leg for upward propulsion in jumping, shortened running stride with reduced hip flexion, and reduced running velocity. Occasionally the athlete tries to maintain an externally rotated femur so the adductor group can be used to advance the thigh.[12] Quadriceps strains must be distinguished from quadriceps contusions that result from impact trauma with secondary hematoma formation.

DIAGNOSIS. The athlete complains of local pain and tenderness in the anterior aspect of the thigh. Pain may be gradual in onset or may occur suddenly during an explosive muscle contraction. Grade I strains result in pain with resisted active contraction and with passive stretching. Local spasm may be present. Athletes with grade I strains generally are able to continue sport activity. Grade II strains cause significant pain with passive and unopposed active stretching. Athletes with grade II strains generally are unable to continue sport activity. Complete tears of the rectus femoris are rare and are associated with a sudden violent contraction; a defect is palpable when the muscle is contracted. Radiographic studies rule out associated avulsion of the AIIS, especially in children. Myositis ossificans can be a complication of quadriceps strain and contusion and is identified by swelling, erythema, and a palpable hard mass. Confirmation is made by plain films or bone scans.

TREATMENT. Ice and nonsteroidal anti-inflammatory drugs (NSAIDs) are useful in limiting pain and inflammation. Pain-free stretching is instituted early to preserve range of motion. Associated tightness in the hamstrings and hip flexors and inhibition of the gluteus maximus must be corrected. Soft-tissue mobilization may assist with motion. Special emphasis is placed on strengthening exercises, because loss of strength may be marked and is actually considered to be a major predisposing factor to injury. Straight-leg raises are initiated with the patient in the supine position and progress to long sitting (i.e., sitting on a floor or mat with the knees extended). Short-arc quadriceps sets in pain-free ranges are expanded to full range as tolerated. Both concentric and eccentric exercises are performed. Attention is given to hip flexor and hamstring strength and flexibility to ensure muscular balance. Closed kinetic chain exercises at submaximal weight (i.e., leg press, partial squats) are initiated in short arcs and progress to full range. The stair-climber and bicycle are very effective, but isolated restrengthening of the injured leg is essential. Sport-specific functional retraining is completed before a return to sport.

Following a quadriceps contusion, loss of motion can be significant; therefore, special emphasis is placed on early maintenance of range of motion, particularly in flexion.[29,30] Ryan and colleagues[29] advocate maintenance of the hip and knee in pain-free flexion with the use of elastic wrap for 24 to 48 hours to minimize hematoma formation and preserve flexion range. Ice is applied several times daily. Active stretching is then performed in pain-free ranges only during the next 7 to 10 days. Soft-tissue therapy and electrical stimulation also are useful but are avoided during the first few days. Ultrasound is avoided as it has been implicated in the development of myositis ossificans.[12] Multiangle isometric quadriceps contractions and isotonic exercises without weights in pain-free ranges are expanded to full range with weights as tolerated. Biking is used for strengthening and general fitness. When flexion of more than 120 degrees and strength of more than 85% of the uninjured side are attained, functional retraining should begin. Myositis ossificans, if present, is treated by the principles of PRICEMM (protection, relative rest, ice, compression, elevation, modalities, medication). Prophylactic use of diphosphonates does not seem warranted. The use of NSAIDs such as indomethacin is common among clinicians, but has not been conclusively shown to halt the progression of the lesion.[12] Follow-up radiographs and "cold" bone scans are useful in determining whether the lesion has become "mature."[12] Physical activity is gradually increased after maturity has been reached. On rare occasions, surgical excision of a mature lesion is necessary. This should generally be reserved for patients with pain and loss of range of motion persisting for 6 to 12 months after the lesion has matured.[12]

Adductor Strain

Adductor or groin strain can result from an acute strain or from chronic angiofibroblastic tendinosis of the hip adductor group, particularly the adductor longus at the proximal musculotendinous junction, tendoosseous insertion to the inferior pubic rami, or the muscle belly itself.[31–35] Eccentric overload, such as that experienced during quick changes in direction from a stretched-out lunge position, is thought to be especially contributive.[32–35] Ballistic stretching, which is advised in many exercise tapes and aerobics classes, often leads to groin strain.

DIAGNOSIS. The clinical symptom complex presents as pain in the groin region worsened with passive abduction or active adduction and flexion against resistance. Primary muscle involvement can be established by reproducing the symptoms during resisted adduction in three positions of hip rotation: external rotation (adductor magnus), neutral (adductor longus), and internal rotation (pectineus).[22] Acute cases may be accompanied by swelling and ecchymosis. A palpable defect may be present, representing a tear. Also commonly seen is ipsilateral pelvic and hip pain, worse with walking or running. The functional biomechanical deficits center around tightness of the ipsilateral adductors and contralateral tensor fasciae latae. The ipsilateral gluteus medius and gluteus minimus will then become inhibited or weak, as will the lower abdominal muscles. The functional adaptation complex includes an increase in lateral tilt of the pelvis where the contralateral side of the pelvis drops in the swing phase of gait. An ipsilateral inferior pubic rami dysfunction is often associated. The tissue overload complex is exhibited by excessive strain and inflammation of the lateral pelvic and hip structures, including the gluteus medius and gluteus minimus, as well as the trochanteric bursa. Along the kinetic chain, the tensor fasciae latae and iliotibial band as well as lateral knee structures and lumbar region of the spine have increased overload. The knee, in particular the patellofemoral joint, are overloaded, as well as distal structures such as the shoulder, owing to altered pelvic stability. The abdominals are considered overloaded due to the position of the pubic rami inferiorly, which stretches the abdominals, placing them at risk for tears. Finally, the adductors inhibit the contraction of the glutei after the propulsion phase of running.[31]

TREATMENT. In acute cases, ice and NSAIDs are used to limit pain and inflammation. Elastic spica wrapping or compressive shorts helps control swelling and minimize pain during ambulation and sport activity. Rehabilitative exercise emphasizes full motion strengthening of the hip adductor group and improving flexibility. Functional deficits in the glutei, tensor fasciae latae, and pelvis are corrected. Strengthening involves both concentric and eccentric loading. Proprioceptive neuromuscular facilitation (PNF) diagonal motions effectively exercise the muscles to promote balanced strength and flexibility around the joint. Soft-tissue mobilization and electrical stimulation are useful adjunctive treatments. In more chronic adductor strains, ultrasound is a useful modality to precede mobilization. Five or six treatments of deep friction massage to break up scar tissue before stretching may also be necessary. Flexibility and strength of the abductor group ensure muscular balance. Sport-specific activities should include the slide board (for side-to-side gliding) and lateral sprints.

Femoral Stress Fractures

Stress fractures of the hip or pelvis are uncommon, with incidence ranging from 0.05% to 0.22% of all running injuries and 3.2% to 4.0% of all stress fractures in athletes.[5,36,37] Femoral stress fractures are more common, accounting for up to 10% of all stress fractures in runners.[38] The majority of femoral stress fractures occur at the femoral neck. Femoral shaft stress fractures are less common and generally occur in the subtrochanteric region but can occur in the midshaft and distal regions as well.[39,40]

Stress fractures result from accelerated bone remodeling in response to repeated stress.[36,38,40,41] Several factors contribute to this excessive stress: repetitive microloads from pounding (which does not allow the bone time to heal with its normal reparative process),[38,42,43] the transmission of excessive force loads to bone secondary to surrounding muscle fatigue,[38,44] and the repetitive action of muscular traction on bone.[38,45,46] Specifically, Butler and co-workers[39] speculated that subtrochanteric fractures are caused by excessive traction at the origin of the vastus medialis or adductor brevis, producing tension on bone. Femoral stress fractures should be included in the differential diagnosis of hip pain in all athletes, particularly in those with persistent pain, because of the risk of displacement or avascular necrosis of the femoral head.

DIAGNOSIS. The athlete generally complains of non-specific deep thigh or groin pain that is aggravated by activity and relieved by rest.[36,38–40,47,48] Onset is often associated with a recent change in training (particularly an increase in distance or intensity) or a change in training surface. Physical examination may reveal normal hip motion and strength. Advanced cases will be associated with decreased strength and motion with pain on end rotation. Direct palpation over the involved bony area may elicit pain in patients with femoral shaft fractures, as will stressing the femur over the edge of the examining table, distal to the site of pain. Hopping on one leg may reproduce pain.

Initial x-ray findings are often negative, and as many as one-third of femoral stress fractures never show radiologic changes on plain films. Bone scans or MRI should be ordered if suspicion is high, particularly if pain has persisted for more than 2 weeks.[12]

With femoral neck fractures, the type of fracture must be differentiated. Compression-type injuries occur at the lower border of the femoral neck, and displacement is rare. Distraction-type fractures occur in the superior part of the neck; displacement is more common, thus necessitating internal fixation.[40,49]

TREATMENT. Patients with nondisplaced femoral neck fractures are generally placed on crutches with partial weightbearing status until pain is absent and radiologic follow-up indicates sufficient callus formation (3 to 8 weeks). During this time, the athlete should continue conditioning with nonweightbearing activity (deep-water running, swimming, biking) as well as upper-extremity strengthening. Rehabilitative exercise restores muscle flexibility, strength, and balance. The stair-climber and stationary cross-country skiing machines are then useful for further conditioning. A gradual walking, jogging, and running program is followed before a return to sport activity. Correction of foot and leg malalignments and running gait pattern may help limit intrinsic stress. Displaced fractures require internal fixation. Most early femoral neck stress fractures (x-ray negative, bone scan positive) will heal conservatively. Femoral neck stress fractures evident on x-ray are usually an indication for orthopedic referral. Femoral shaft and pelvic fractures typically respond to a protracted period of weightbearing rest (2 to 4 months).

Osteitis Pubis

Osteitis pubis represents a chronic inflammatory and overuse condition of the pubic symphysis and adjacent ischial rami.[50–61] Most commonly associated with urologic procedures, prostatectomy, and childbirth, osteitis pubis also can occur in athletes and appears to be related to repetitive shear forces transmitted to the pubic symphysis during running and repetitive adductor contractions during kicking sports.

DIAGNOSIS. The athlete typically complains of the gradual onset of discomfort in the lower abdomen or groin area that is worsened by sport activity and relieved by rest. Physical examination reveals point tenderness at the pubic tubercles, rectus abdominis insertion, adductor origin, and inferior pubic rami. Pain is intensified with sit-ups and resisted hip adduction. Range of motion is maintained. Radiographic studies may reveal a fraying or roughening of the periosteum of the pubic symphysis. However, x-ray signs may be delayed for as long as 4 weeks after the onset of symptoms; a bone scan is needed to assist diagnosis in early stages.

TREATMENT. Almost all patients with osteitis pubis will respond to a period of relative rest (up to $1^1/_2$ to 2 months) and anti-inflammatory medications, with a gradual return to sport activity. Soft-tissue flexibility and strength deficits and pelvic and SIJ dysfunction are corrected. Nonpainful fitness exercises such as swimming and deep-water running are undertaken as tolerated during this phase. Leg-length discrepancies and excessive pronation can be corrected with orthotic devices. Abdominal and adductor strengthening and adductor stretching should be performed in moderation. A corticosteroid injection into the pubic symphysis can be useful in refractory cases.

Anterior Hip Pointer

Anterior hip pointer refers to pain localized to the ASIS that may result from a direct blow in contact sports or from repetitive overuse strain of the sartorius (common in runners and gymnasts).[62,63]

DIAGNOSIS. Pain and tenderness are localized at the ASIS. Passive hip extension increases symptoms, as do resisted hip flexion, external rotation, and abduction. Radiographic studies should be performed to rule out an avulsion of the ASIS.

TREATMENT. Early treatment emphasizes ice, NSAIDs, relative rest, ultrasound, and electrical stimulation. Subsequent management includes flexibility training and strengthening, most specifically of the hip flexors, abductors, and external rotators. Especially effective exercises include long-sitting and straight-leg raises with the hip externally rotated, as well as the PNF leg-diagonal flexion adduction, external rotation to extension, abduction, and internal rotation.

Internal Snapping Hip Syndrome

Internal snapping hip syndrome is most often caused by friction of the iliopsoas tendon over an osseous ridge on the lesser trochanter or the iliopectineal eminence.[50,64] Less commonly, loose bodies, labral tears, and osteochondritis dissecans can be intra-articular sources of the snap.[12]

DIAGNOSIS. Patients complain of diffuse, aching pain in the anteromedial hip or groin region. A discrete area of tenderness to palpation generally is not present. An audible snap typically occurs with extension of the flexed, abducted, and externally rotated hip.

TREATMENT. Ice, NSAIDs, and electrical stimulation are used in acute cases. Superficial heating is followed by prolonged stretching of the hip flexors. Re-education of the antagonistic gluteus maximus helps restore proper balance. Soft-tissue mobilization assists flexibility and motion. Strengthening of the hamstrings promotes muscular balance. All hip motions should be evaluated for flexibility and strength deficits and appropriately exercised.[31]

Refractory Groin Pain

In athletes with persistent groin pain for whom conservative measures fail, a broader differential diagnosis should be entertained (Table 13–5). Athletes with bursitis, nerve syndromes, and enthesopathy may respond to steroid injections in addition to physical therapy.[32,33,35,65–69]

A small subset of athletes will experience longstanding groin pain despite aggressive conservative measures (medications, rest, physical therapy, massage, flexibility, strengthening).[66–75] Myers describes pubalgia in athletes chronic exertional lower abdominal/inguinal pain near the pubic insertion, which is not explainable by a demonstrable hernia or other medical diagnosis.[73]

The pain progresses to involve the adductor longus tendon as well as the contralateral inguinal and adductor regions. The location of pain suggests injury to both the rectus abdominis and adductor longus muscles. Paramount to the diagnosis of athletic pubalgia is the exclusion of other causes of groin pain. Athletes who fail to respond to conservative management, including flexibility and strengthening of the core abdominal and hip musculature, may benefit from surgical remediation, which includes attachment of the abdominal muscle firmly to the anterior pelvis and, in those cases with adductor pain, a partial adductor release also.[72,73]

Other proposed etiologies for chronic groin pain seen in the literature have included (A) Deficiency of the transversalis fascia, with a weakening and bulging of the posterior wall of the inguinal canal ("sportsman's hernia"),[70,71] either alone or in combination with splitting of the conjoint tendon and/or dilation of the internal inguinal ring[71]; and (B) attenuation or laddering of the external oblique in conjunction with separation of the conjoint tendon from the inguinal ligament and laxity of the transversalis fascia (Gilmore's groin).[74]

Surgical procedures described to correct the above include For (A), repair of the posterior wall of the inguinal canal by plication of the transversalis fascia,[70,71] as well as repair of the deficit in the conjoint tendon, if present; and for (B), reinforcement of the weakened transversalis fascia and reattachment of the conjoint tendon to the ilioinguinal ligament.[74]

As with pubalgia as described by Myers, athletes considered for surgical remediation must have failed conservative care, including strengthening of the core pubic and abdominal muscles, and should be referred to surgeons with experience treating athletes with chronic groin pain. In the authors' experience, it can take several (6–8) months of regular strengthening and stabilization before significant results occur, but many athletes have returned to sports following conservative treatment. No studies exist comparing the different surgical procedures, but all appear to surgically provide stability to the lower abdominal core stabilizing muscles.

Posterior Overuse Injuries

Hamstring Strain

Hamstring strains are a common cause of posterior thigh pain in athletes and may present as acute, subacute, or chronic injury. These strains commonly occur in sprinters, hurdlers, jumpers, and athletes in other sports involving sudden sprinting such as soccer, football, tennis, and hockey. Excessive eccentric muscle force appears related to hamstring injury; many hamstring strains occur during the last part of the swing phase or at foot strike, during which time the hamstrings work maximally eccentrically to decelerate the

TABLE 13–5. DIFFERENTIAL DIAGNOSIS OF GROIN PAIN IN ATHLETES

Tendinitis (adductor, flexor, abdominal)
Pelvic/femoral stress fracture
Osteitis pubis
Snapping hip syndrome
Bursitis (iliopsoas)
Nerve entrapment (ilioinguinal, obturator)
Enthesopathy (inguinal ligament)
Pubalgia/Sports hernia/Gilmore's groin
Degenerative joint disease
Avascular necrosis of the hip
Lumbar-referred pain
Genitourinary disease
Inguinal hernia
Systemic disease (rheumatologic, other)

leg. Factors related to hamstring injury include poor hamstring flexibility, strength, and endurance; muscular imbalance (such as a hamstring to quadriceps strength ratio <0.6 or compared with the contralateral hamstring group); lumbar degenerative joint disease; lumbar and SIJ dysfunction; increased neural tension; biomechanical inadequacies (i.e., excessive anterior pelvic tilt); and inadequate warm-up.[22,76–79] The tissue injury complex can include all hamstring muscles, most commonly the short head of the biceps femoris.

DIAGNOSIS. The clinical symptom complex includes pain in the posterior region of the thigh. The athlete with an acute strain may report a "pop" or a tearing sensation. Tenderness to palpation can be located throughout the muscle, including the origin at the ischial tuberosity, as well as the muscle belly and distal insertions. Pain is intensified with resisted knee flexion. Functional biomechanical deficits are identified. Flexibility is often decreased, and weakness of the involved hamstring group may be identified with manual muscle testing or more formal isokinetic testing. Tightness in the hip flexors and inhibition of the glutei may be identified; anterior pelvic tilting is not uncommon. Examination of the lumbar region of the spine is important, because muscle injury may be related to referred pain with subsequent muscle inhibition and weakness.[22,35] Radiographic studies may be performed to rule out avulsion of the ischial tuberosity if suspected, particularly in younger athletes. Lumbar referred pain should also be considered in the athlete with posterior thigh pain, especially when a clear injury history is not present.

TREATMENT. Treatment of acute or subacute injuries follows the principles of PRICEMM, emphasizing ice, electrical stimulation, and pulsed ultrasound to minimize the extent of tissue damage. A neoprene thigh sleeve provides comfort and a possible counterforce effect. Active exercises within pain-free ranges of motion are begun soon after injury, as is stretching, ensuring proper orientation with collagen deposition. Strengthening of the hamstrings is advanced as tolerated and incorporates isometric, isotonic, and isokinetic exercise of both knee and hip actions. Special emphasis ultimately is placed on eccentric loading. Isokinetic testing at 60 degrees/sec should demonstrate hamstring strength of at least 60% of quadriceps strength and no more than 10% deficit when compared with the uninjured leg. Soft-tissue therapy (transverse friction, transverse gliding, and myofascial release) is useful for increasing mobility and decreasing pain in the patient with chronic injury but is often unnecessary for acute injury if strengthening and flexibility are initiated early. Flexibility of the rectus femoris and hip flexors,

and facilitation and strengthening of the vasti and glutei are important to provide muscular balance. Biomechanical factors, particularly excessive anterior tilt of the pelvis and leg-length discrepancies, should be corrected. Hypomobility and dysfunction of the lumbar region of the spine and SIJ must be corrected if present.[22,35,77] Neuromobilization to mobilize the connective tissue of the sciatic nerve may also be effective. This on-off stretching technique helps stretch supporting neural and muscle connective tissue. Running is resumed at low speeds on flat terrain, with an emphasis on adequate warm-up and stretching before running and stretching and icing afterward. Trampoline and bounding drills are useful transition exercises. Athletes must demonstrate adequate sport-specific function before returning to competition.

Other reported causes of posterior thigh pain have included ischial stress fractures[80] and posterior compartment syndrome.[81,82] Healing of stress fractures of the ischium will require a prolonged period of activity modification (no running for 6 to 8 weeks) after which rehabilitation following the hamstring strain protocol above commences. Posterior compartment syndrome is less common than the compartment syndromes of the lower leg and presents with chronic exertional posterior thigh pain refractory to rehabilitative measures. Intracompartmental pressure testing is diagnostic and fasciotomy is curative.

Piriformis Syndrome

The piriformis muscle originates on the anterolateral aspect of the sacrum and passes posterolaterally through the sciatic notch, inserting into the upper border of the greater trochanter. The sciatic nerve typically exits the pelvis through the sciatic notch anterior to the piriformis muscle. In approximately 15% of the population, however, the sciatic nerve passes through the piriformis muscle itself. Pain may result from a strain or overload of the piriformis muscle or from pressure on the sciatic nerve, most commonly in patients in whom the sciatic nerve courses through the piriformis muscle.[22,50,83,84] A common cause of piriformis overload is a tight hip adductor with hip abductor inhibition. This leads to the piriformis acting as an abductor.[31]

DIAGNOSIS. The clinical symptom complex consists of buttock and hip pain that may radiate down the posterior aspect of the leg. Passive internal rotation of the affected hip is limited and may increase pain (Freiberg sign).[85] Pain and weakness are present with resisted abduction or external rotation of the hip. Rectal examination will reveal distinct tenderness on the lateral pelvic wall that reproduces symptoms. Examination of the lumbar spine is important to rule out lumbar dysfunction. The structures within the tissue overload complex are the piriformis, gluteal muscles, gemelli, quadratus lumborum, sacroiliac ligaments, and the sciatic nerve. The functional biomechanical deficits include tight piriformis, external rotators, and adductors; hip abductor weakness; SIJ hypermobility; and lower lumbar spine dysfunction. Functional adaptations consist of ambulating with an externally rotated thigh, shortened stride length, and functional limb-length shortening.[12] Any runner who develops buttock and varying lower-extremity paresthesias without evidence of radiculopathy should be considered to have piriformis syndrome.[31]

TREATMENT. Treatment includes correcting dysfunction of the SIJ and pelvis. Prior to stretching of the piriformis or iliopsoas muscles, the hip joint capsule in its anterior and posterior portion should be mobilized, which will allow for more effective stretching of these muscles. Prolonged stretching includes hip flexion, adduction, and internal rotation in supine and standing positions. Soft-tissue therapy of the piriformis muscle, including longitudinal gliding combined with passive internal hip rotation, as well as transverse gliding and sustained longitudinal release with the patient lying on one side, may be useful.[22] Effective exercises include the knee-to-chest stretch in adduction, internal rotation in which the knee of the involved lower extremity is brought toward the opposite shoulder, and the adduction/external rotation stretches. Ultrasound or phonophoresis may be useful modalities. Local trigger point or corticosteroid injections may be useful for more recalcitrant cases.[83,84] Correction of lumbar spine and SIJ dysfunction and hypomobility is important, particularly in patients in whom piriformis irritability and pain are related to lumbar disorders. Any strength or flexibility deficit at the hip is corrected with appropriate exercise.

Ischial Bursitis

Ischial bursitis, an inflammation of the ischial bursa, is often associated with proximal hamstring strains. It is not uncommon in cyclists (probably caused by prolonged sitting). It can also be seen in adolescent runners, often in conjunction with traction apophysitis.

DIAGNOSIS. Tenderness is localized to the ischium. Isolated ischial bursitis can be differentiated from hamstring strains, because patients with isolated ischial bursitis generally will not complain of pain in the posterior thigh or demonstrate hamstring flexibility and strength deficiencies.

TREATMENT. Most patients with ischial bursitis respond to ice, NSAIDs, soft-tissue massage, relative rest, and avoidance of prolonged sitting. Hamstring strength and flexibility deficits are corrected as needed. When the cause is prolonged sitting, the patient's workstation should be modified to allow for activities to be conducted in a standing position and a cushion should be used when sitting. Physical therapy for ultrasound, phonophoresis, and massage can augment exercise. Corticosteroid injections can be helpful for persistent bursitis.[12]

Sacroiliac Joint Dysfunction

The SIJ has been reported to be responsible for approximately 20% of cases of low-back pain and referred pain.[6,86] Pain at the SIJ can result from primary pain at the joint and the overlying soft tissues (sacral hilum and iliofibrocartilage, supporting ligaments, and joint capsule), or may be the result of referred pain.[6] SIJ dysfunction resulting from a biomechanical imbalance at the SIJ is by far the most common painful condition affecting this joint. Up to 14 different patterns of imbalance have been reported, the most common being right anterior innominate rotation, followed in frequency by left posterior innominate rotation.[31] Differential diagnoses include fracture, infections, inflammatory conditions (ankylosing spondylitis, psoriatic arthritis, Reiter's disease), degenerative joint disease, metabolic disease (gout, calcium pyrophosphate disease), tumor, osteitis condensans ilia, reactive sacroiliitis as a late sequela of pelvic inflammatory disease, and referred pain (from lumbar disk or facet disease, radiculopathy, hip disease, or gluteal/multifidi trigger points). Pregnancy also results in relative hypermobility of the SIJ, which may predispose to ligamentous sprain.[6]

DIAGNOSIS. Patients with SIJ pain can complain of pain that is sharp, aching, or dull, and generally localize the pain to the involved SIJ or PSIS[6,87] (Fortin JD, Personal observations, 1993). Due to a wide range of segmental innervation of the SIJ, pain can also be referred to the buttocks, groin, posterior thigh, or distally beyond the knee and even into the foot.[6,86] Patients may give a history of trauma. Symptoms generally increase with joint motion, especially when changing from a sitting to standing position or during rotational movements. Pain is usually unilateral and tends to have a right-sided bias, with 45% right, 35% left, and 20% bilateral.[6,7] Tenderness to palpation may be localized over the sacral sulcus and just medial to the PSIS.[7] Asymmetry and pelvic rotation may be appreciated by palpation of the iliac crest and iliac spines. A variety of additional physical examination test categories have been recommended by various authors to clinically predict SIJ dysfunction, as follows: 1) soft-tissue examination for zones of hyperirritability; 2) evaluation of fascial and musculotendinous restrictions; 3) determination of length-strength muscle relationships; 4) postural analysis; 5) true leg-length determination; 6) functional leg-length determination[88–90]; 7) osteopathic evaluation, including static and dynamic osseous landmark evaluation (structural testing)[6]; 8) dynamic osteopathic screening tests[89,91–94]; 9) evaluation of regional tissue texture changes; 10) provocative testing, including traditional orthopedic tests such as the Gaenslen or Patrick test; 11) motion demand (articular spring) tests[95]; 12) ligament tension tests[89]; and 13) hip rotation testing.[7] No test or combination of tests has been found to be pathognomonic for SIJ pain and dysfunction.[6]

The absence of neurologic findings helps differentiate SIJ pain from lumbar-referred pain.[22] Radiographic testing is generally unrevealing in isolated SIJ dysfunction, but may be useful in ruling out fracture, infection, and inflammatory conditions, as well as associated lumbar disease. In recalcitrant cases or confusing presentations, a fluoroscopically guided, contrast-enhanced, intra-articular SIJ injection can be used for diagnostic as well as therapeutic purposes.[6]

TREATMENT. Treatment of SIJ dysfunction must include the entire lumbopelvic complex and lower extremity kinetic chain. A number of treatment techniques from various philosophies, including osteopathic, manual, and chiropractic, have evolved to help rehabilitate SIJ dysfunction. At this point, no research has recognized one treatment protocol as superior and the most successful rehabilitation programs may integrate aspects of each of these schools of thought.[6]

The acute phase of rehabilitation addresses the tissue injury complex and clinical symptom complex. In SIJ dysfunction, the tissue injury complex involves the SIJ, including the sacral hyaline cartilage and iliofibrocartilage, supporting ligaments, and joint capsule. The clinical symptom complex involves the patient's primary complaint of local sacroiliac, buttock, and posterior thigh pain, as well as referred pain to the groin, hip, and lower extremity. Pain and inflammation are controlled with NSAIDs and modalities including therapeutic cold and electrical stimulation. SIJ belts may help proprioception and decrease motion and pain.[88,96] Patient education and a home exercise program are initiated early and built upon throughout rehabilitation. Subsequent phases continue to address tissue overload complex, as well as functional biomechanical deficits and subclinical adaptation complex. Functional biomechanical deficits include associated soft-tissue dysfunction. In right anterior dysfunction, these include tightness in the ipsilateral adductors, rectus femoris, iliopsoas, quadratus lumborum, latissimus dorsi, and tensor fasciae latae. Weaknesses or inhibitions

are identified in the ipsilateral glutei, lumbosacral paraspinal, and abdominal muscles.[31] The subclinical adaptation complex includes pelvic rotation and subsequent lumbar dysfunctions. Various manual approaches include inhibitive techniques including positional release; functional techniques; general muscle stretching; and mobilization including muscle energy and direct oscillation. Manipulation using a high-velocity, low-amplitude, short-lever arm thrust technique can be employed if needed. Following mobilization or manipulation, a maintenance exercise program is imperative to prevent recurrences.[6,97,98] Leg-length discrepancies greater than $1/2$ inch should be corrected.[99] Manual therapy techniques also eliminate associated restriction in lumbar and pelvic motion. Flexibility and strength of soft tissues about the lumbar-pelvic-hip complex are enhanced. Aerobic conditioning is important throughout the rehabilitation program as tolerated. A home exercise program to maintain flexibility and strength is continued after rehabilitation is completed. In refractory cases, a fluoroscopically guided, contrast-enhanced injection may aid in decreasing pain and promote subsequent mobilization and rehabilitation. Injections may also be made in the overlying muscles or ligaments.[6]

Other, more invasive techniques have also been proposed for the treatment of SIJ pain. Prolotherapy or sclerotherapy has been employed to treat SIJ pain due to presumed laxity of the SIJ ligamentous complex. If followed by proper stretching, it is theorized that collagen will be laid down in an orderly fashion to help stabilize the joint. No controlled clinical study has proved the efficacy of these techniques for SIJ pain, however, and therefore it should be considered only in refractory cases of hypermobility and performed only by clinicians with extensive experience with them.[6] Fusion techniques for the SIJ exist, but they should be considered only in patients with SIJ pain proven by diagnostic anesthetic blocks, with severe disabling symptoms that have failed to respond to all attempts at aggressive conservative care.[6] Any SIJ fusion should be bilateral, as unilateral fusion could cause significant biomechanical dysfunction.

Lateral Overuse Injuries

Trochanteric Bursitis

Trochanteric bursitis is an inflammation of the greater trochanteric bursa, often related to friction of the iliotibial tract as it crosses the greater trochanter.

DIAGNOSIS. The clinical symptom complex includes pain and tenderness localized to the greater trochanter. Pain is reproduced with flexion of the hip from an extended position and resisted hip abduction as well as by stretching of the iliotibial tract. Functional biomechanical deficits consist of shortening of the tensor fasciae latae, rectus femoris, and hamstrings and weakness of the abductors. Functional adaptations include increased hip external rotation with an altered gait or running pattern.[12,20]

TREATMENT. Early treatment includes relative rest, ice, NSAIDs, electrical stimulation, phonophoresis, and soft-tissue massage. A steroid injection at the area of tenderness over the greater trochanter may be useful for particularly intense or recalcitrant bursitis. Stretching of the iliotibial tract is emphasized, as well as flexibility of the external rotators, quadriceps, and h[...] Strengthening of the hip abductors and esta[...] of muscular balance between the adduc[...] abductors is also important. All motions at th[...] evaluated for strength and flexibility, and exer[...] prescribed to establish balanced motion.

Gluteus Medius Bursitis
Gluteus medius bursitis results from inflammat[...] the gluteus medius bursa and often occurs in conjunction with gluteus medius tendinitis or tendinosis. This condition is often associated with excessive lateral tilt of the pelvis.[22]

DIAGNOSIS. Tenderness is localized immediately above the greater trochanter and is intensified by stretching the gluteus medius. Functional biomechanical deficits may include tight adductors and inhibited gluteus medius and minimus.[31]

TREATMENT. Treatment includes relative rest, ice, NSAIDs, electrical stimulation, soft-tissue massage, re-education of the inhibited gluteus medius and minimus, and stretching of the adductors and abductors. If the pain is particularly severe, a steroid injection may be placed into the area of maximal tenderness above and behind the greater trochanter. Pelvic stability exercises are important in patients with bursitis associated with excessive lateral tilt.

External Snapping Hip Syndrome
The external snapping hip syndrome is caused by friction of the iliotibial band or the anterior border of the gluteus maximus on the greater trochanter.

DIAGNOSIS. Pain is localized to the lateral part of the hip over the greater trochanter. An audible snap is heard during repetitive hip motion.

TREATMENT. Patients generally are markedly relieved by reassurance that this is not an intra-articular condition.

Early treatment follows the principles of PRICEMM. Stretching of the iliotibial band and gluteus maximus is emphasized. Flexibility of the external rotators, hip flexors, and quadriceps is also addressed. Flexibility is enhanced by soft-tissue mobilization. Any deficit in strength or flexibility at the hip is addressed to provide balanced motions.

Lateral Hip Pointer
A lateral hip pointer consists of pain localized to the lateral iliac crest that usually represents a contusion resulting [from a] direct blow to the iliac crest in contact [sports such as fo]otball and rugby. A lateral hip pointer [may also result fr]om acute strain or chronic overuse of [the hip abductors (gl]uteus medius and minimus) and external [ob]dominal muscles.

[Pain an]d tenderness are localized to the [iliac crest. S]welling and ecchymosis may accompany [acut]e injuries. Truncal side bending [away fr]om the affected hip increases pain, as does resisted abduction of the affected hip. Radiographic studies should be performed to rule out an iliac crest fracture.[100–102]

TREATMENT. Initial treatment emphasizes ice, NSAIDs, electrical stimulation, and relative rest. Compression can be used for traumatic hip pointers; if a hematoma is present, aspiration may be useful. Management of overuse injuries emphasizes flexibility and strength of the hip abductors and external oblique muscles followed by balanced hip flexibility and strengthening. Soft-tissue mobilization is useful in regaining motion but should be avoided in the first 2 to 3 days following traumatic injury. Adequate hip padding is mandatory in contact sports.

Tensor Fasciae Latae Strain
Inflammation and ultimately angiofibroblastic changes can occur in the tensor fasciae latae, particularly where it passes over the greater trochanter. This overuse injury is common in runners and cyclists.[50] Overload of the tensor fasciae latae is often seen with inhibition of the gluteus medius and minimus. This may be from tight hip adductors reciprocally inhibiting these abductors or simply as a response to painful stimuli.

DIAGNOSIS. The onset of lateral hip pain is generally gradual and localized to the greater trochanter and distally along the tensor fasciae latae. There is often a history of a recent change in training regimen. The Ober test result is positive, revealing a tight iliotibial band. A snapping of the tensor fasciae latae as it passes over the greater trochanter and greater trochanteric bursitis also may be associated. Radiographic studies and bone scanning are performed if a femoral neck stress fracture is suspected.

TREATMENT. Initial treatment follows the principles of PRICEMM. Rehabilitative management is similar to that described for the external snapping hip syndrome and emphasizes flexibility of the iliotibial band, external rotators, hip flexors, and quadriceps followed by balanced flexibility and strengthening throughout the hip. Soft-tissue mobilization is a useful adjunctive treatment. Re-education of the inhibited hip abductors is also important.

Meralgia Paresthetica
This syndrome consists of pain and paresthesias in the lateral region of the thigh caused by irritation of the lateral femoral cutaneous nerve. Injury may occur by violent hip extension or by compression, most commonly at the inguinal ligament. Compression may be caused by a tight belt or clothing, obesity, or pregnancy.

DIAGNOSIS. Decreased sensation is limited to the distribution of the lateral femoral cutaneous nerve. As this is a purely sensory nerve, motor deficits are not observed.

TREATMENT. Treatment includes correction of contributing factors such as weight loss or eliminating tight clothing and restrictive equipment. Neuroleptic medicines such as neurontin, amitriptyline or carbamazepine may be useful. Refractory cases may respond to corticosteroid injections.

Special Concerns in the Pediatric Athlete

APOPHYSITIS AND APOPHYSEAL AVULSIONS
In younger athletes, the apophyseal attachment of tendons may be more likely injured than the myotendinous junction, as in adults. Common sites of injuries of apophyses about the hip and pelvis involve the hamstring origin at the ischial tuberosity, the sartorius origin at the ASIS, the rectus femoris origin at the AIIS, the iliopsous at the lesser trochanter, and the abdominal insertions at the iliac crest. Mild displacements are treated as are their respective related soft-tissue injuries, although they may require a longer period of activity modification. More severe displacement may require orthopedic surgical intervention.[22]

Legg-Calvé-Perthes Disease
Legg-Calvé-Perthes disease is an idiopathic avascular necrosis of the proximal femoral epiphysis. It occurs in children between the ages of 3 and 12 years, most commonly between 5 and 7 years. Boys are affected three to five times more frequently than girls and both hips are involved in 10% to 20% of patients.[103,104]

DIAGNOSIS. The affected athlete presents with a limp and vague pain in the groin, hip, thigh, or knee (any child with a vague knee pain should have a hip evaluation). Physical examination reveals variable shortening of the involved leg, which may accentuate a limp. Almost all affected children will have limited hip abduction and internal rotation when tested in both hip flexion and extension, even in early stages of the disease. Anteroposterior and frog-leg radiographs should be carefully scrutinized in suspected cases. Early disease is characterized by a dense epiphysis that is patchy, more distal, and uneven at the margins. A bone scan may be useful if x-ray findings are negative and clinical suspicion is high. Later stages show more involvement of the femoral head with cystic changes and fragmentation.[103]

TREATMENT. Initial treatment is directed toward regaining range of motion and may include traction, range-of-motion exercises, and limited weightbearing.

Containment of the femoral head within the acetabulum is usually accomplished with an abduction orthosis; however, osteotomy may be necessary. If the physiatrist has not had experience treating this condition, orthopedic referral is mandated. In general, children diagnosed before the age of 5 years have a more favorable prognosis while those diagnosed after the age of 8 years have a less favorable outcome.[103–105]

Slipped Capital Femoral Epiphysis
Both acute and chronic slips result in displacement of the capital femoral epiphysis through the growth plate relative to the femoral neck. Posterior medial slips are the most common and they are bilateral in approximately 60% of patients.[103,106] The periods of highest risk for developing a slipped epiphysis is during periods of peak height velocity (10 to 13 years old for girls and 12 to 15 years old for boys).[103,107] Children large for their age or maturity are at higher risk.[103]

DIAGNOSIS. Children with a chronic slipped epiphysis may have a mild limp and complain of vague groin, hip, or knee pain. Medial knee pain, referred from the hip via the obturator nerve, may be the only complaint. As the slip develops, the affected child develops progressive out-toeing and a worsening limp. Acute slipped epiphyses result in severe pain and are more likely to be identified early. Physical examination reveals a decreased range of motion, especially in flexion, internal rotation, and abduction. The classic finding is a hip that externally rotates as it is passively flexed.[103]

In normal hips, a line drawn through the center of the femoral neck should bisect the epiphysis on both the anteroposterior and frog-leg lateral radiographs.[103,106] Comparison views are of questionable help as most slips are bilateral.

TREATMENT. Slipped epiphyses are considered a relative orthopedic emergency once the diagnosis is made. Even minimally displaced chronic slips are prone to sudden progression with a misstep or twist of the leg. Patients should be placed on nonweightbearing crutches or bed rest pending orthopedic management.[103]

CONCLUSIONS

The majority of athletic injuries of the hip and pelvis are caused by overuse. Most of these injuries will respond to adequate rehabilitative management, including correction of intrinsic and extrinsic risk factors and control of the abusive force loads that may have contributed to injury. In addition to injury-specific rehabilitation, imbalances and abnormalities at each level of the kinetic chain must be corrected to ensure optimal healing.

REFERENCES

1. Herring SA, Nilson KL: Introduction to overuse injuries. *Clin Sports Med* 1987:6, 225.
2. Orava S: Exertion injuries due to sports and physical exercise: A clinical and statistical study of nontraumatic overuse injuries of the musculoskeletal system of athletes and keep-fit athletes. Thesis. University of Ouler, Finland, 1980.
3. Renstrom P, Johnson RJ: Overuse injuries in sports: A review. *Sports Med* 1985:2, 316.
4. Puffer JC, Zachazewski JE: Management of overuse injuries. *Am Fam Physician* 1988:38, 225.
5. Lloyd-Smith R, Clement DB, McKenzie DC, et al.: A survey of overuse and traumatic hip and pelvis injuries in athletes. *Phys Sportsmed* 1985:13, 131.
6. Cole AJ, Dreyfuss P, Stratton SA: The sacroiliac joint: A functional approach. *Crit Rev Phys Med Rehabil Med* 1996:8, 125.
7. Bernard TN, Cassidy JD: The sacroiliac joint syndrome: Pathophysiology, diagnosis, and management, in Frymoyer JW (ed.), *The Adult Spine: Principles and Practice*, New York, Raven Press, 1991:2107.
8. Lavignolle B, Vital JM, Senegas J, et al.: An approach to the functional anatomy of the sacroiliac joints in vivo. *Anat Clin* 1983:5, 169.
9. Weisl H: Ligaments of sacroiliac joint examined with particular reference to their function. *Acta Anat* 1954:20, 201.
10. Bradley KC: The anatomy of the backache. *Aust N Z J Surg* 1974:44, 227.
11. Anderson LC, Blake DJ: The anatomy and biomechanics of the hip joint. *J Back Musculoskel Rehabil* 1994:4, 145.
12. Young JL, Olsen NK, Press JM: Musculoskeletal disorders of the lower limbs, in Braddom RL (ed.), *Physical Medicine and Rehabilitation*, Philadephia, Saunders, 1996:783.
13. Rasch PJ, Burke RK. *Kinesiology and Applied Anatomy*, 4th ed., Philadelphia, Lea & Febiger, 1971.
14. O'Connor FG, Sobel JR, Nirschl RP: Five-step treatment for overuse injuries. *Phys Sportsmed* 1992:20, 128.
15. Hess GP, Cappiello WL, Poole RM: Prevention and treatment of overuse tendon injuries. *Sports Med* 1989:8, 371.
16. Nirschl RP: The etiology and treatment of tennis elbow. *J Sports Med* 1974:2, 308.
17. Kibler BW, Chandler TJ, Pace BK: Principles of rehabilitation after chronic tendon injuries. *Clin Sports Med* 1992:11, 661.
18. Ekstrand J, Gillquist J: Soccer injuries and their mechanisms: A prospective study. *Med Sci Sports Exerc* 1983:15, 267.
19. Kibler WB, McQueen C, Uhl T: Fitness evaluations and fitness findings in competitive junior tennis players. *Clin Sports Med* 1988:7, 403.
20. Press JM, Herring SA, Kibler WB: Rehabilitation of the combatant with musculoskeletal disorders, in Zajtchuk R (ed.), *Textbook of Military Medicine*, Washington, DC, Office of the Surgeon General, 1998:353.
21. McKeag DB: Criteria for return to competition after musculoskeletal injury, in Cantu RC, Micheli LJ (eds.), *ACSM's Guidelines for the Team Physician*, Philadelphia, Lea & Febiger, 1991:196.
22. Brukner P, Khan K: *Clinical Sports Medicine*, Sydney, McGraw-Hill, 1993.
23. Jarvinen M: Muscle injuries, in Renstrom PAFH (ed.), *Clinical Practice of Sports Injury Prevention and Care*, London, Blackwell, 1994:115.
24. Young JL, Laskowski ER, Rock M: Thigh injuries in athletes. *Mayo Clin Proc* 1993:68, 1099.
25. Zarins B, Ciullo JV: Acute muscle and tendon injuries in athletes. *Clin Sports Med* 1983:3, 167.
26. Loosli AR, Quick J: Thigh strains in competitive breaststroke swimmers. *J Sport Rehabil* 1992:1, 49.
27. Parker MG: Characteristics of skeletal muscle during rehabilitation: Quadriceps femoris. *Athletic Training* 1981:18, 122.
28. Ryan AJ: Quadriceps strain, rupture and charley horse. *Med Sci Sports* 1969:1, 106.
29. Ryan JB, Wheeler JH, Hopkinson WJ, et al.: Quadriceps contusions. *Am J Sports Med* 1991:19, 299.
30. Aronen JG, Chromister RD: Quadricep contusions—hastening the return to play. *Phys Sportsmed* 1992:20, 130.
31. Geraci MC. Overuse injuries of the hip and pelvis. *J Back Musculoskel Rehabil* 1996:6, 5.
32. Estwanik JJ, Sloane B, Rosenberg MA: Groin strain and other possible causes of groin pain. *Phys Sportsmed* 1990:18, 54.
33. Smodlaka VN: Groin pain in soccer players. *Phys Sportsmed* 1980:8, 57.
34. Martens MA, Hansen L, Mulier JC: Adductor tendinitis and muscular rectus abdominis tendopathy. *Am J Sports Med* 1987:15, 353.

35. Muckle DS: Associated factors in recurrent groin and hamstring injuries. *Br J Sports Med* 1982:16, 37.

36. Taunton JE, Clement DB, Webber D: Lower extremity stress fractures in athletes. *Phys Sportsmed* 1981:9, 77.

37. Orava S: Stress fractures. *Br J Sports Med* 1980:14, 40.

38. Jackson DL: Stress fracture of the femur. *Phys Sportsmed* 1991:19, 39.

39. Butler JE, Brown SL, McConnell BG: Subtrochanteric stress fractures in runners. *Am J Sports Med* 1982:10, 228.

40. Lombardo SJ, Douglas WB: Stress fractures of the femur in runners. *Phys Sportsmed* 1982:10, 219.

41. McBryde AM: Stress fracture in athletes. *J Sports Med* 1975: 3, 212.

42. Branch HE: March fractures of the femur. *J Bone Joint Surg* 1944:26, 387.

43. Walter NE, Wolf MD: Stress fractures in young athletes. *Am J Sports Med* 1977:5, 165.

44. Blat DJ: Bilateral femoral and tibial stress fractures in a runner. *Am J Sports Med* 1981:9, 322.

45. Stanitski CL, McMaster JH, Scranton PE: On the nature of stress fractures. *Am J Sports Med* 1978:6, 391.

46. Devas MB: Stress fractures in athletes. *J Sports Med* 1973:1, 49.

47. Belkin SC: Stress fractures in athletes. *Orthop Clin North Am* 1980:11, 735.

48. Hershman EB, Mailly T: Stress fractures. *Clin Sports Med* 1990:9, 183.

49. Devas MB: Stress fractures of the femoral neck. *J Bone Joint Surg [Br]* 1965:47, 728.

50. Flynn TW: Pelvis and thigh injuries, in Lillegard WA, Rucker KS (eds.), *Handbook of Sports Medicine*, Boston, Andover Medical, 1993:123.

51. Hanson PG, Angevine M, Juhl JH: Osteitis pubis in sports activities. *Phys Sportsmed* 1978:4, 111.

52. Pearson RL: Osteitis pubis in a basketball player. *Phys Sportsmed* 1988:16, 69.

53. Koch RA, Jackson DW: Pubis symphysitis in runners. *Am J Sports Med* 1981:9, 62.

54. Harris NH, Murray RO: Lesions of the symphysis in athletes. *BMJ* 1974:4, 211.

55. Cochrane GM: Osteitis pubis in athletes. *Br J Sport Med* 1971:5, 233.

56. Fricker PA, Taunton JE, Ammann W: Osteitis pubis in athletes: Infection, inflammation or injury? *Sports Med* 1991:12, 266.

57. Howse AJG. Osteitis pubis in an Olympic road walker. *Proc R Soc Med* 1964:57, 88.

58. McMurtry CT, Avioli LV: Osteitis pubis in an athlete. *Calcif Tissue Int* 1986:38, 76.

59. Pyle LA: Osteitis pubis in an athlete. *J Am Coll Health Assoc* 1975:23, 238.

60. Wiley JJ: Traumatic osteitis pubis: The gracilis syndrome. *Am J Sports Med* 1983:11, 360.

61. Williams JG: Limitation of hip-joint movement as a factor in traumatic osteitis pubis. *Br J Sports Med* 1978:12, 129.

62. Reider B, Belniak R, Miller DW: Football, in Reider B (ed.), Sports Medicine: *The School-Age Athlete*, Philadelphia, Saunders, 1991:559.

63. Clancy WG: Running, in Reider B (ed.), *The School-Age Athlete,* Philadelphia, Saunders, 1991:632.

64. Schaberg JE, Harper MC, Allen WC: The snapping hip syndrome. *Am J Sports Med* 1984:12, 361.

65. Ashby EC: Chronic obscure groin pain is commonly caused by enthesopathy: Tennis elbow of the groin. *Br J Surg* 1994:81, 1632.

66. Ekberg O, Persson NH, Abrahamsson P, et al.: Long-standing groin pain in athletes. A multi-disciplinary approach. *Sports Med* 1988:6, 56.

67. Lovell G: The diagnosis of chronic groin pain in athletes: A review of 189 cases. *Aust J Sport* 1995:27, 76.

68. Merrifield HH, Cowan RFJ: Groin strain injuries in ice hockey. *J Sports Med* 1973:1, 41.

69. Renstrom P, Peterson L: Groin injuries in athletes. *Br J Sports Med* 1980:14, 30.

70. Malycha P, Lovell G: Inguinal surgery in athletes: The "sports-man's" hernia. *Aust N Z J Surg* 1992:62, 123.

71. Polglase AL, Frydman GM, Farmer KC: Inguinal surgery for debilitating chronic groin pain in athletes. *Med J Aust* 1993:155, 674.

72. Taylor DC, Meyers WC, Moylan JA, et al.: Abdominal musculature abnormalities as a cause of groin pain in athletes. *Am J Sports Med* 1991:13, 239.

73. Myers WC, Foley DP, Garrett WE, et al.: Management of severe lower abdominal or inguinal pain in high-performance athletes. *Am J Sports Med* 2000:28, 2.

74. Brannigan AE, Kerin MJ, McEntee GP: Gilmore's groin repair in athletes. *J Orthop Sports Phys Ther* 2000:30, 329.

75. Thomas JM: Groin strain versus occult hernia: Uncomfortable alternatives or rivals? *Lancet* 1995:345, 1522.

76. Agre JC: Hamstring injuries: Proposed etiological factors, prevention and treatment. *Sports Med* 1985:2, 28.

77. Heiser TM, Weber J, Sullivan G, et al.: Prophylaxis and management of hamstring muscle injuries in intercollegiate football players. *Am J Sports Med* 1984:12, 368.

78. Liemohn W: Factors related to hamstring strains. *J Sports Med* 1978:18, 71.

79. Paranen J, Orara S: The hamstring syndrome: A new diagnosis of gluteal sciatic pain. *Am J Sports Med* 1988:16, 517.

80. Mowat AG, Kay VJ: Ischial stress fracture. *Br J Sports Med* 1983:17, 94.

81. Raether PM, Lutter LD: Recurrent compartment syndrome in the posterior thigh. Report of a case. *Am J Sports Med* 1982:10, 40.

82. Orava S, Rantanen J, Kujala UM: Fasciotomy of the posterior femoral muscle compartment in athletes. *Int J Sports Med* 1998:19, 71.

83. Pace JB, Nagle D: Piriformis syndrome. *West J Med* 1976:124, 435.

84. Barton PM: Piriformis syndrome: A rational approach to management. *Pain* 1991:47, 345.

85. Freiberg AH: Sciatica pain and its relief by operation on muscle and fascia. *Arch Surg* 1937:34, 377.

86. Schwarzer AC, Aprill CN, Bogduk N: The sacroiliac joint in chronic low back pain. *Spine* 1995:20, 31.

87. Fortin JD: Sacroiliac joint dysfunction—a new perspective. *J Back Musculoskel Rehabil* 1993:3, 31.

88. Vleeming A, Stoeckart R, Snijders CJ: General introduction, in Vleeming A, Mooney V, Dorman T, Snijders CJ (eds.), *The Integrated Function of the Lumbar Spine and Sacroiliac Joint*, Rotterdam, Eco, 1992:3.

89. Beal MC: The sacroiliac problem: Review of anatomy, mechanics, and diagnosis. *J Am Osteopath Assoc* 1982:81, 667.

90. Lee D: The relationship between the lumbar spine, pelvic girdle, and hip, in Vleeming A, Mooney V, Dorman T, Snijders CJ (eds.), *The Integrated Function of the Lumbar Spine and Sacroiliac Joint*, Rotterdam, Eco, 1992:464.

91. Bourdillon JF: *Spinal Manipulation*, 3rd ed., London, Heinemann Medical, 1982.

92. Mitchell FL Jr, Moran PS, Pruzzo NA: An evaluation and treatment manual of osteopathic muscle energy techniques. Valley Park, MO, Mitchell, Moran, and Pruzzo Associates, 1979:49, 109.

93. Bernard TN Jr, Kirkaldy-Willis WH: Recognizing specific characteristics of non-specific low back pain. *Clin Orthop* 1987:217, 266.

94. Dreyfuss P, Dreyer S, Griffin J, et al.: Positive sacroiliac joint screening tests in asymptomatic adults. *Spine* 1994:19, 1138.

95. Hesch J, Aisenbray JA, Guerino J: Manual therapy evaluation of the pelvic joints using palpatory and articular spring tests, in Vleeming A, Mooney V, Dorman T, Snijders CJ (eds.), *The Integrated Function of the Lumbar Spine and Sacroiliac Joint*, Rotterdam, Eco, 1992:435.

96. Vlemming A, Buyruk HM, Stoekart R, et al.: Towards an integrated therapy for peripartum pelvic instability: A study based on the biomechanical effects of pelvic belts. *Am J Obstet Gynecol* 1992:166, 1243.

97. Cassidy JD, Kirkaldy-Willis WH, McGregor M: Spinal manipulation for the treatment of chronic low back and leg pain: An observational study, in Buerger AA, Greenman PE (eds.), *Empirical Approaches to the Validation of Spinal Manipulation*, Springfield, Ill, Charles C Thomas, 1985:119.

98. Kirkaldy-Willis WH, Cassidy JD: Spinal manipulation in the treatment of low back pain. *Can Fam Phys* 1985:31, 535.

99. Cibulka MT, Koldehoff RM: Leg length disparity and its effect on sacroiliac joint dysfunction. *Clin Manage* 1986:6, 10.

100. Butler JE, Eggert AW: Fracture of the iliac crest apophysis: An unusual hip pointer. *Sports Med* 1975:3, 192.

101. Godshall RW, Hansen CA: Incomplete avulsion of a portion of the iliac crest epiphysis: An injury of young athletes. *J Bone Joint Surg [Am]* 1973:6, 1301.

102. Clancy WG, Foltz AS: Iliac apophysitis and stress fractures in adolescent runners. *Am J Sports Med* 1976:4, 214.

103. Zukowski CW, Lillegard WA: Special considerations for the pediatric running population. *J Back Musculoskel Rehabil* 1996:6, 21.

104. Wenger DR, Ward WT, Herring JA: Current concepts review: Legg-Calvé-Perthes disease. *J Bone Joint Surg [Am]* 1991:73, 778.

105. Gross ML, Nasser S, Finerman GA: Hip and pelvis, in De Lee JC, Drez D (eds.) *Orthopedic Sports Medicine*, Philadelphia, Saunders, 1994:1063.

106. Hagglund G, Hansson LI, Ordeberg G, Sandstrom S: Bilaterality in slipped upper femoral epiphysis. *J Bone Joint Surg [Br]* 1988:70, 179.

107. Kendig RJ, Field L, Fischer LC: Slipped capital femoral epiphysis, a problem of diagnosis. *J Miss State Med Assoc* 1993:34, 147.

Chapter 14

THE KNEE

Michael Fredericson

INTRODUCTION

This chapter discusses other causes of knee pain in runners not specifically addressed in Chapter 15, Patellofemoral Pain Syndrome. The more common overuse injuries are discussed with their associated differential diagnoses including patellar and quadriceps tendinopathy, Osgood-Schlatter disease, Sinding-Larsen-Johannson disease, plica syndrome, pes anserine bursitis, iliotibial band syndrome, and popliteal tenosynovitis. Intraarticular knee injuries are only briefly mentioned here, but are addressed more thoroughly in Chapter 52, Surgical Considerations of the Knee.

ANTERIOR KNEE PAIN

Patellar Tendinopathy (Jumper's Knee)

Change due to overuse in the patellar tendon at or near its insertion into the lower pole of the patella is frequently seen in athletes who participate in sports involving jumping, cutting, or rapid acceleration/deceleration; however, it is also sometimes encountered in runners.[1] At ground contact the knee extensor moment is five times greater in running than it is in walking.[2] At the time the knee extensor moment is greatest, there is also twice the amount of knee flexion than occurs in walking. This increased flexion puts a large amount of stress on the extensor mechanism, and over time the repetitive overload of running can cause chronic inflammation at the patellar tendon-bone attachment.

The pain related to patellar tendinitis or tendinosis is often associated with a diffuse ache distally along the path of the tendon. On examination, tenderness is noted at the distal pole of the patella. This is facilitated by pressing down on the proximal pole of the patella, causing the patella to tilt its distal pole anteriorly, making the proximal attachment of the patellar tendon more accessible.

Radiographic findings are typically normal; however, the distal pole of the patella may have an elongated or fragmented tip. Occasionally, ectopic bone or calcific deposits are noted in the tendon. Ultrasound is an inexpensive imaging study that can help define patellar tendon pathology, but sensitivity is dependent on the experience of the examiner. Classic findings are paratenon changes, hypoechoic zones, or pathologic tendon thickness. The presence of a focal hypoechoic lesion that corresponds to the site of tenderness on the tendon is indicative of tendon degeneration.[3]

Magnetic resonance imaging (MRI) usually shows eccentric thickening of the involved portion of the tendon and occasionally associated edema of adjacent soft tissues. There is often a focus of intermediate signal on T1-weighted and high signal on T2-weighted images, typically located within the substance of the upper third of the patellar tendon, at the site of the attachment of the tendon to the patellar apex (Figure 14–1). This abnormal signal is also consistent with tendon degeneration.[4]

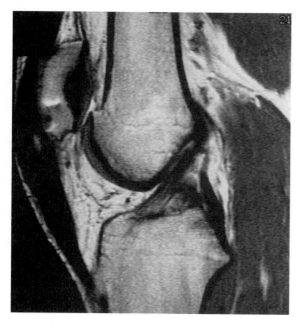

Figure 14–1. MR image of patellar tendinopathy. Sagittal T2 weighted images show thickening and a focal area of hyperintense signal within the proximal aspect of the tendon.

The key to treating patellar tendinopathy is to recognize that in chronic conditions, normal fibrous-connective tissue is replaced by mucinous degeneration and fibrinoid necrosis within the proximal aspect of the tendon, related to repetitive microtears within the tendon substance.[4,5] Consistent with a chronic tendinopathy there is also an absence of inflammatory cells,[5] indicating that antiinflammatory medications would be ineffective. Because this is a degenerative condition, it will often take several months before results of a physical therapy program can be evaluated.

The therapy program should focus on correction of any hamstring, quadriceps, or gastrocsoleus muscle tightness along with the same muscle re-education and strengthening and patellar taping techniques as described for patellofemoral syndrome.[6] Patellar straps or stabilizing braces may also be useful. Surgical debridement is reserved for those patients who have failed an extensive rehabilitation program. Arthroscopic treatment was reported to allow a quicker return to full activity versus an open procedure.[7]

Quadriceps Tendinopathy

Quadriceps tendinopathy is less common than that of the patellar tendon. It is associated with pain at the proximal pole of the patella. The tenderness is over the central portion of the tendon's insertion onto the patella, usually more lateral than medial. Pain can typically be provoked with resisted knee extension or passive hyperflexion of the knee.

X-rays are usually negative. In chronic cases a prominent lateral epicondylar ridge or an osteophyte from degenerative changes in the patellofemoral joint is present.[1] In the adolescent runner x-rays are helpful to evaluate for a multipartite patella, which often presents with pain at the superolateral patellar margin. MRI may occasionally prove helpful to better define the lesion or distinguish it from other pathology in the area, such as a suprapatellar plica.

Treatment is also similar to that for patellar tendinopathy. In recalcitrant cases, surgery can help to debride degenerative tissue or excise heterotopic calcifications or osteophytes.[8]

Hoffa's Fat Pad Impingement

A less well recognized cause of infrapatellar pain in runners is impingement of Hoffa's fat pad. This can occur in isolation or in conjunction with patellar tendon pathology. The patellar tendon is attached to the nonarticular part of the retropatellar surface and is separated in most cases from the femoral surface by the fat pad. This is a richly vascularized tissue with significant potential for inflammation when injured by direct compression or repetitive microtrauma.

These patients typically experience pain with knee hyperextension. On examination the fat pad is inflamed and tender, unlike in patellar tendinopathy, in which the inferior pole of the patella is tender; however the differentiation between these two conditions is not always clear. It has been suggested that Hoffa's fat pad impingement is related to an abnormal longitudinal tilt of the patella, with the inferior pole buried in the infrapatellar fat pad. The patella may also be described as having an inferior-posterior tilt, with the inferior pole posterior to the superior pole in the coronal plane.[9] This can be checked dynamically during a maximal quadriceps contraction. If the inferior pole disappears leaving a dimple, then the test is positive. To verify whether the infrapatellar fat pad is the culprit, the clinician should shorten the fat pad by lifting it toward the patella. If symptoms are relieved with this technique and worsened by performing passive extension of the knee, then the diagnosis of fat pad irritation is confirmed. Treatment with McConnell taping to correct the anterior-posterior tilt and fat pad impingement is indicated. If the pain persists, then the patient has patellar tendinitis. Adjunctive treatment includes ice and nonsteroidal anti-inflammatory drugs (NSAIDs). Surgical debridement is rarely necessary. MRI in symptomatic individuals characteristically shows a region of fat pad edema, usually limited to the proximal and lateral aspects of the infrapatellar fat pad.

Symptomatic Synovial Plica

A symptomatic synovial plica is another possible cause of knee pain in runners. The classic presentation is anteromedial knee pain with running or other activities requiring repetitive flexion and extension of the knee. This syndrome is more frequent in teenagers, in whom meniscal and ligamentous lesions are less common. Symptoms also include snapping, buckling, and pain with prolonged sitting. Swelling is usually not a significant complaint.

A plica is a synovial septum that is a remnant from the embryologic knee, which was divided into three compartments: medial, lateral, and suprapatellar. A medial plica occurs in up to 30% of the population, and is the most frequent of the four types of knee plicas to be associated with symptoms (Figure 14–2). It originates proximally and medially and is attached distally to the medial patellar fat pad. The suprapatellar type is the second most common, while the infrapatellar and lateral plicas are rarely of clinical significance. If a normal medial plica is chronically inflamed and turns fibrotic, it may bow-string over the medial femoral condyle during knee motion and cause chronic irritation and often a snapping sensation.[10] Even chondral fissuring and thinning can be caused by a fibrotic plica.

On physical examination the findings are limited. The medial plica usually reveals a point of local tenderness over the femoral condyle adjacent to the medial border of the patella. In this area, one may also feel a small fibrous band rolling beneath the palpating finger as the leg is held in internal rotation, the patella displaced slightly medially, with the knee passively extended.[10] Occasionally, this is associated with a pop between 45 and 60 degrees of flexion. If the suprapatellar plica is involved, there may be tenderness and sometimes crepitus on compression of the patella and quadriceps tendon.

Four grades of plica have been identified. Type A is a thin elevation of synovium under the medial retinaculum, type B is a narrow pleat that does not impinge on the medial condyle (Figure 14–3), type C is a larger structure that partially covers the medial condyle, and type D is a fenestrated type C, or band-like plica.[12] Cadaver studies have shown no strict correlation between the rigidity and fibrotic aspect of the plicae and their width; narrow plicae could be rigid, and large plicae were sometimes soft.[13]

Most patients will respond to conservative treatment, similar in outline to that for patellofemoral pain syndrome (see Chapter 15). Attempts to decrease inflammation, especially in the more acute cases, can be tried with iontophoresis, phonophoresis, or intraplical steroid injection. Rovere and Adair[14] studied 31 knees in 30 patients and found that 73% experienced complete relief of symptoms with return to activity following injection of the plica with local anesthetic and steroid. Of the group they defined as competitive athletes, most had symptoms for only 1 to 3 weeks. In my experience, once symptoms are chronic and the plica has become fibrotic, it is unlikely for a steroid injection to offer long-term relief. Thus, when conservative treatment fails, definitive treatment can be obtained with arthroscopic resection. This will usually entail little downtime for the runner, especially if laser

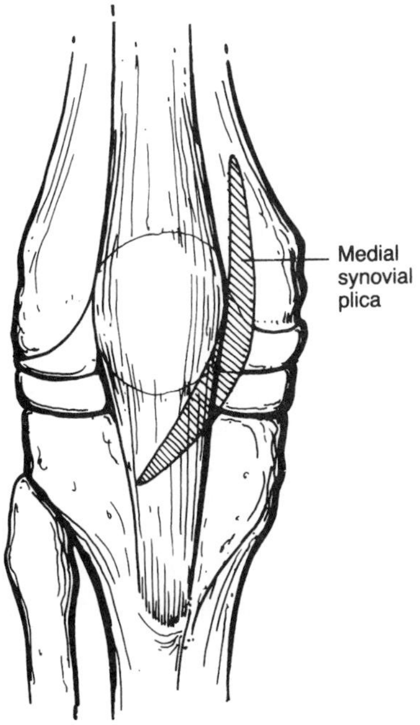

Figure 14–2. Medial patellar plica. (*Source: DeLee JC, Drez D, (eds.),* Orthopaedic Sports Medicine, *Vol. 2, Philadelphia, Saunders, 1994:1255.*)

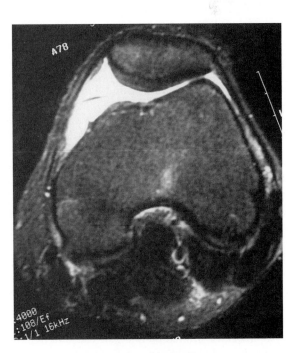

Figure 14–3. MR image of a medial plica, type B on axial T2 weighted fat-saturated image outlined by joint effusion.

ablation is used, with its decreased bleeding and post-operative swelling. The medial plica does have a static, medializing effect on the patella, and the excision of a medial plica can have an effect on patellar tracking.[9]

Traction Apophysitis

In the adolescent runner, traction apophysitis can cause pain at the proximal (Sinding-Larsen-Johannson disease) and distal (Osgood-Schlatter disease) patellar tendon insertions. Symptoms typically manifest during or after a rapid growth spurt and are present bilaterally in 20% to 30% of patients.[15] Girls tend to be involved earlier (age 11 to 13 years versus 12 to 15 years for boys), reflecting their earlier maturity.[16]

Sinding-Larsen-Johannson disease is similar in presentation to patellar tendinitis, with pain and tenderness localized to the inferior pole of the patella, whereas runners with Osgood-Schlatter disease present with pain localized to the tibial tuberosity. Occasionally, these conditions present concomitantly. There may also be stigmata of malalignment (i.e., patella alta) or external tibial torsion, both of which can create increased tension in the patellar tendon.[17,18]

Treatment involves moderation of activity, a knee brace (patellar strap or stabilizing sleeve), ice massage, and antiinflammatory medication. In severe cases a brief 1- to 2-week period of knee immobilization is recommended. Stretching exercises are indicated for any tightness present in the quadriceps, hamstrings, or Achilles tendon, along with quadriceps strengthening. Both these conditions typically resolve spontaneously within 12 to 18 months.[16,19]

Chronic or recurrent symptoms into adulthood may be related to a symptomatic unfused ossicle, or even a fracture through an ossicle.[19,20] In these cases surgical removal of the ossicle may be indicated. One case series found that a true joint can form between an ossicle in the patellar ligament and a facet on the tibia, also requiring surgical treatment.[21]

MEDIAL KNEE PAIN

Pes Anserine Bursitis

Due to the prominent role of the hamstrings during running, the large bursa located deep to the three medial tendons, the sartorius, gracilis, and semitendinosus, are occasionally affected in runners. The bursa lies between the aponeurosis of these tendons and the medial collateral ligament approximately 2 inches below the anteromedial joint line. This can sometimes be confused with Voshell's bursitis, deep to the superficial portion of the medial collateral ligament. The tenderness associated with Voshell's bursitis is located immediately below the joint line deep to the medial collateral ligament. Pes anserine bursitis is associated with tenderness in a more distal location.[1,10]

Treatment involves addressing biomechanical factors that may increase stress to the medial knee (such as excessive subtalar pronation), antiinflammatory medications, ultrasound, and corticosteroid injections. Flexibility and closed kinetic chain strengthening exercises are also an important part of the rehabilitation program.

When there is direct bone tenderness along the anteromedial aspect of the proximal tibia just below the medial joint line or into the tibial diaphysis, it is prudent to consider a stress fracture of the medial tibial plateau or proximal tibia. If radiographs are negative, a bone scan or MRI should be obtained before proceeding with further treatment.[22]

Other conditions to consider in the differential diagnosis include patellofemoral pain syndrome, medial collateral ligament sprain, semimembranosus tendinitis, osteoarthritis of the medial compartment (especially in the older runner), medial meniscal tears, juxtaarticular bone cysts, referred pain from intraarticular hip pathology, or saphenous nerve entrapment.

LATERAL KNEE PAIN

Iliotibial Band Syndrome

Iliotibial band syndrome (ITBS) is the most common cause of lateral knee pain in runners, with an incidence as high as 12% of all running-related overuse injuries.[23–25] It is believed to result from recurrent friction of the iliotibial band (ITB) sliding over the lateral femoral epicondyle.

The distal part of the ITB is free from bony attachment between the superior aspect of the lateral femoral epicondyle and Gerdy's tubercle,[26] moving anteriorly to the epicondyle as the knee extends and posteriorly as the knee flexes. One study found the posterior edge of the band impinging against the lateral epicondyle just after foot strike in the gait cycle, when the knee flexes to around 30 degrees.[27] This can produce irritation and subsequent inflammatory reaction, especially in the region beneath the posterior fibers of the ITB, which are tighter against the lateral femoral condyle than the anterior fibers.[28] Histopathologic studies in patients with chronic ITBS show that the tissue under the ITB consists of a synovium that is a lateral extension and invagination of the actual knee joint capsule, and not a separate bursae as previously described in the literature.[29] One MRI study also found that patients with ITBS have significantly thicker bands than those without symptoms.[30]

Messier and colleagues[31] retrospectively examined specific training and biomechanical factors between 56 runners with ITBS and 70 runners in a noninjured control group. They found the injured runners were less experienced, their weekly mileage was significantly greater, and they spent a greater percentage of time training on the track compared with noninjured runners. Additionally, the injured runners were weaker bilaterally in knee flexion and knee extension and exhibited lower maximal normalized braking forces.

James observes that alignment in runners with ITBS often shows genu varum and/or tibia vara, heel varus, forefoot supination, and compensatory pronation.[1] Evaluation with high-speed videography, however, has shown that runners with ITBS in comparison to a control group showed little difference in rearfoot motion. If anything, there was a tendency for the injured group to pronate less relative to the control group. Others postulate leg-length discrepancies contribute to ITBS. This can be secondary to a true anatomic discrepancy or environmentally induced by training on crowned roads.[23,24,32]

A recent study at our institution[33] that examined 24 distance runners (14 females, 10 males) with ITBS versus a similar control group of noninjured runners found that runners with ITBS had significant weakness in their hip abductors in their affected limb in comparison to their noninjured limb and the limbs of noninjured control runners. Electromyographic studies of joggers[34] have shown that in order to control coronal plane motion during stance phase, a continuous hip abductor moment is needed by the gluteus medius, and to a lesser extent the tensor fascia lata. While the gluteus medius and tensor fascia lata are both hip abductors, the gluteus medius (especially the posterior aspect) is an external rotator of the hip, whereas the tensor fascia lata is an internal rotator of the hip.[35] Consequently, with fatigue or weakness the runner may demonstrate increased thigh adduction and internal

rotation at midstance, with an increased valgus vector at the knee. It is postulated[33] that this places the iliotibial band under increased tension and makes it more prone to impingement upon the lateral epicondyle of the femur, especially during the early stance phase of gait (foot contact) when maximal deceleration occurs to absorb ground reaction forces.

The main symptom associated with ITBS is a sharp pain or burning sensation on the lateral aspect of the knee. Runners will often note that they start out running pain-free, but after a reproducible time or distance they become symptomatic. Early on, the symptoms will subside shortly after a run is over, but will return with the next run. If allowed to progress, the pain can persist even when walking, and particularly when ascending or descending stairs.

The knee examination reveals localized tenderness and occasionally swelling over the distal ITB where the band moves over the lateral femoral condyle. Pain or paresthesias sometimes extend along the length of the band. Crepitation, snapping, or mild pitting edema can also occur over the affected area. Pain can be elicited with the patient lying on his or her side with the affected knee up and flexed up to 90 degrees. Pressure is then applied to the ITB over the lateral femoral condyle, and as the knee approaches 30 degrees of flexion, pain is elicited as the tensed ITB rubs directly over the lateral femoral condyle (Noble compression test).[25]

For all suspected cases of ITBS it is also important to perform the modified Thomas test to evaluate for flexibility deficits in the iliopsoas, rectus femoris, and tensor fascia lata/iliotibial band as well evaluate for strength deficits in the gluteus medius muscle[36] (Figure 14–4).

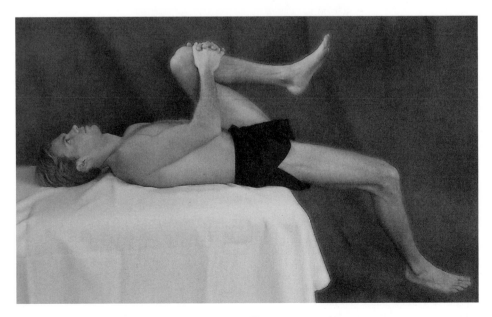

Figure 14–4. Modified Thomas test position.

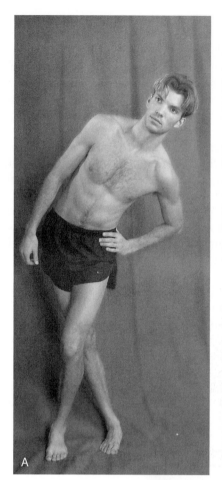

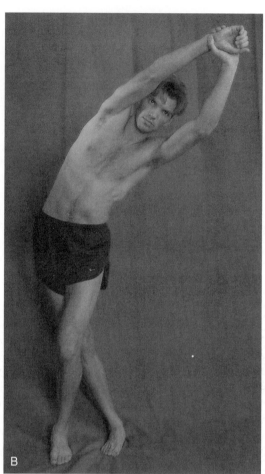

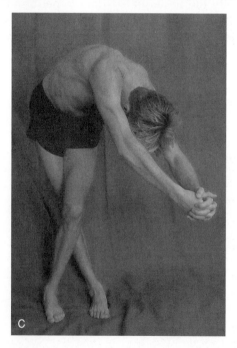

Figure 14–5. (*A*) ITB standing stretch. Stand upright, using a wall for balance if needed. Extend and adduct the leg being stretched across the noninvolved side. Exhale, and slowly flex your trunk laterally to the opposite side until a stretch is felt on the side of the hip. Extending or tucking the pelvis can vary the area being stretched. (*B*) Progression of initial stretch by grasping your arm to accentuate the lateral trunk flexion. (*C*) Further progression of stretch by bending downward and diagonally, while reaching out and extending with hands clasped.

Myofascial restrictions not directly associated with the friction of the ITB sliding over the lateral femoral epicondyle may contribute to the severe lateral knee pain associated with ITBS.[36] Evaluation often reveals tender areas in the vastus lateralis, more proximally along the ITB in the gluteus minimus, and in the distal biceps femoris muscles. Within these tender areas are often discrete trigger points with pain referral zones along the lateral thigh to the knee or even to the lateral lower leg. The examination consists of thorough and very firm palpation of the suspected trigger points. This is best performed with the patient in a relaxed side-lying position with the hip on the symptomatic side flexed to about 45 degrees and the knees slightly flexed. If the indicated areas are sensitive, and particularly if the patient reports feeling sensations in the referral zones, myofascial treatment is strongly indicated.

Initial treatment includes local application of ice and phonophoresis to reduce the acute inflammatory process. Activity modification is necessary to reduce the repetitive mechanical stress at the site of the lateral femoral condyle. Oral NSAIDs may also prove beneficial at this stage. If there is grossly visible swelling in the area that does not subside after 3 days of treatment, a local injection of a corticosteroid is indicated.

Stretching exercises (Figs. 14–5 and 14–6) and deep massage to release myofascial restrictions should be started after the acute inflammation has subsided. Self-massage using an epifoam roller is a valuable part of the home therapy program (Fig. 14–7).

Strengthening is initiated once range-of-motion restrictions and any myofascial restrictions are resolved.

The initial exercise recommended is the side-lying leg lift to help the athlete learn to isolate the gluteus medius muscle (Fig. 14–8).

Because training is specific to limb position, it is essential that the athlete be transitioned to weight-bearing exercise. Initially, the athlete is asked to stand in front of a full length mirror and perform the step-down exercise (see Chapter 15). Maintenance of pure sagittal plane motion is encouraged by asking the athlete to squat with the knee progressing over the second toe while maintaining a stable pelvis and avoiding any excessive hip adduction or internal rotation. Once this is mastered the athlete is started on the pelvic-drop exercise (Fig. 14–9). For all strength exercises, start with one set of 20 repetitions and gradually build up to three sets of 20 repetitions done per day.

Most athletes are fully recovered by 6 weeks. As a general rule, once the runner can perform the full regimen of strength exercises without flare of symptoms, he or she can return to running. We recommend running every other day for the first week starting with easy sprints on level ground. Biomechanical studies have shown faster-paced running is less likely to aggravate ITBS because at foot strike the knee is flexed beyond the angles at which friction occurs.[27] Then over a 3- to 4-week period, a gradual increase in distance and frequency is permitted.

Various surgical techniques are described to decrease the impingement of the ITB on the lateral femoral condyle, although with an aggressive rehabilitation program surgery is rarely necessary. The most common procedure involves releasing the posterior

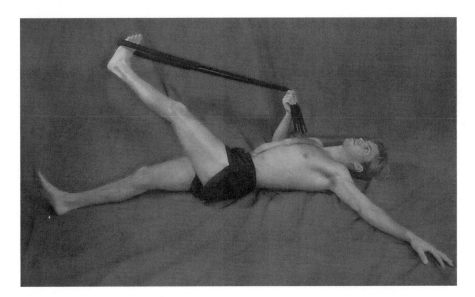

Figure 14–6. ITB supine rope stretch. Lying on back with strap or rope around ankle of involved leg; hold rope in opposite hand and pull across other leg keeping pelvis level on the ground.

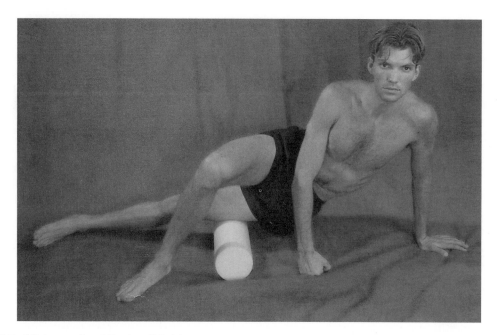

Figure 14–7. ITB foam roll mobilization. Side-lying on a 3" to 6" foam roll with side of involved leg; cross uninvolved leg over straight one and oscillate up and down from hip to knee, emphasizing tight areas. Support upper body with hand on floor.

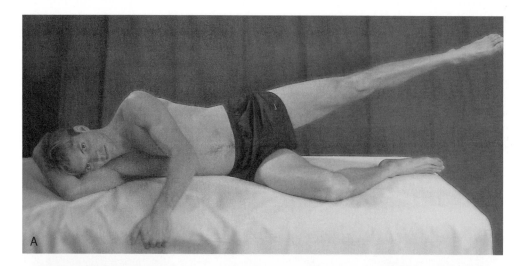

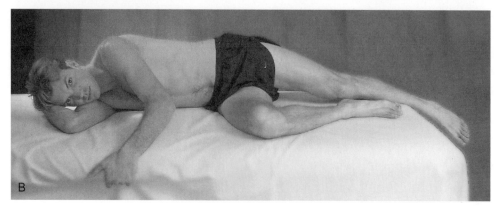

Figure 14–8. Side-lying leg lifts. (*A*) The lower leg is flexed for balance, the abdominals braced, and the upper leg in slight hip extension and external rotation, with an arc of movement of 30 degrees and with each repetition held for 1 sec at extremes of motion. (*B*) The leg is then slowly lowered into maximal adduction and the exercise repeated.

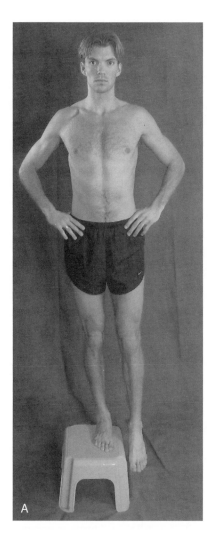

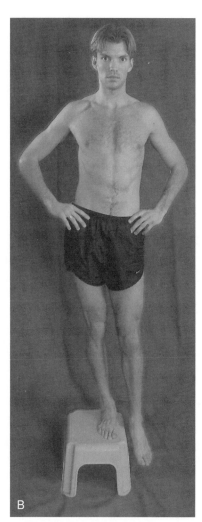

Figure 14–9. Pelvic drop exercise. (*A*) This involves standing on a step with the involved leg, and holding on to a wall or stick if necessary for support. (*B*) With both knees locked, the opposite, noninvolved pelvis is lowered towards the floor, shifting the body weight to the inside part of the foot and involved leg, creating a swivel action at the hip. Then, by contracting the gluteus medius on the involved side, the pelvis is brought back to a level position. A mirror is used during the initial stages to provide visual feedback until the exercise is performed correctly.

2 cm of the ITB at the level of the lateral condyle, where it appears to create the most tension over the femoral condyle.[23,37]

The differential diagnosis for other causes of lateral knee pain includes lateral patellofemoral compression syndrome, early degenerative joint disease, lateral meniscal pathology, superior tibiofibular joint sprain, biceps femoris tendinitis, common peroneal nerve injury, or referred pain from the lumbar spine. In most cases these other entities can be easily differentiated by a careful history and examination. A diagnostic local anesthetic injection is a simple office technique to differentiate local soft tissue pain from possible intraarticular or referred pain.

POSTERIOR KNEE PAIN

Popliteal Tendinitis

Pain in the posterior to posterolateral aspect of the knee may be due to popliteus tenosynovitis.[38] Pain is often associated with downhill running. Banked surfaces may also produce rotatory stress and traction on the popliteus muscle. Occasionally there are complaints of snapping.[39] The popliteus tendon arises from the lateral femoral condyle with aponeurotic attachments from the posterior lateral meniscus, knee capsule, and fibula, to form a conjoined structure that passes distally and medially deep to the fibular collateral ligament and inserts on the tibia and fibula just anterior to the fibular collateral ligament[40] (Fig. 14–10).

The popliteus derotates the knee joint at the initiation of flexion and assists the posterior cruciate ligament in preventing forward displacement of the femur on the relatively fixed tibia during stance phase, especially when running downhill.[10,38] The most prominent finding on physical examination is tenderness directly over the popliteal tendon just posterior to the fibular collateral ligament. This area is easiest to palpate with the lower extremity in a "figure of four" position (Fig. 14–11). A less consistent finding is pain on external rotation of the tibia on the fixed femur when the patient is not bearing weight, or by full weightbearing on

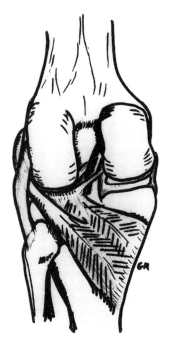

Figure 14–10. Popliteus tendon anatomy. (*Source: Permission pending. Mayfield GW. Popliteus tendon tenosynovitis. Am J Sports Med 1977:5, 33.*)

the affected side, while rotating the femur internally on the fixed tibia with the knee flexed to 30 degrees.[38]

Radiographs may show radiodensities in the area of the popliteus tendon while MR images usually show

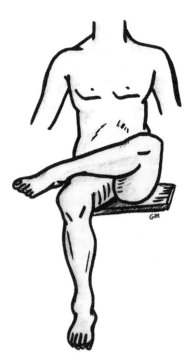

Figure 14–11. Testing position for popliteus tendon. (*Source: Permission pending. Mayfield GW. Popliteus tendon tenosynovitis. Am J Sports Med 1977:5, 33.*)

fluid around the popliteal tendon, but this may not be specific because fluid in the popliteal bursa is not rare if a joint effusion is present.[41] MRI may also show other pathology of the popliteal tendon such as a ganglion of the sheath of the popliteus tendon, which has been reported as a cause of chronic posterior knee pain.[11]

The treatment should emphasize a decrease or modification of the running program (i.e., no running downhill or on banked surfaces). Anti-inflammatory medication and physical therapy modalities can be helpful. In persistent cases a corticosteroid injection into the tendon sheath is a reasonable treatment approach. Arthroscopy can be helpful for cases of suspected tendon rupture or meniscal pathology. In cases of a snapping popliteal tendon, excision of the prominent portion of the articular ridge below the sulcus popliteus on the lateral femoral condyle is curative.[39]

Other considerations in the differential of posterior knee pain in runners include gastrocnemius tendinitis (especially the medial side at the origin of the posterior femoral condyle), hamstring tendinitis, Baker's cyst (often with associated intra-articular knee damage), lumbar radiculopathy, tibial nerve entrapment, or deep vein thrombosis.

OSTEOCHONDRITIS DISSECANS OF THE KNEE

Osteochondritis dissecans is a lesion of bone and articular cartilage that results in delamination of subchondral bone with or without articular cartilage mantle involvement. This may result in partial or complete separation of the fragment with significant effects on joint mechanics. A variety of possible etiologies have been proposed including abnormal trauma, avascular necrosis and normal joint variant.[42] This often is seen in the lateral aspect of the medial femoral condyle or in the patella.

The athlete presents with vague knee pain and intermittent swelling worsened with activity. Physical examination is often non-specific and may include antalgia, tenderness to palpation, and decreased range of motion. Osteochondritis of the patella may mimic patellofemoral syndrome. X-rays, including a tunnel view are usually diagnostic, however CT and MRI are often used to further delineate the lesion. Conservative treatment may include immobilization, however orthopaedic referral is recommended for consideration for surgical debridement or fixation when indicated.

ACKNOWLEDGMENT

Special acknowledgment to Joseph Handler, Ph.D. for editorial assistance.

REFERENCES

1. James SL: Running injuries to the knee. *J Am Acad Orthop Surg* 1995:3, 309.
2. Cavanagh PR, LaFortune MA: Ground reaction forces in distance running. *J Biomech* 1980:13, 397.
3. Duri ZA, Aichroth PM, Wilkins R: Patellar tendonitis and anterior knee pain. *Am J Knee Surg* 1999:12:99.
4. Yu JS, Popp JE, Kaeding CC: Correlation of MR imaging and pathologic findings in athletes undergoing surgery for chronic patellar tendonitis. *Am J Roentgenol* 1995:165, 115.
5. Khan KM, Bonar F, Desmond PM, et al.: Patellar tendinosis (jumper's knee): Findings at histopathologic exam, US, and MR imaging. *Radiology* 1996;200, 821.
6. Lian O, Engebretsen L, Ovrebo RV, et al.: Characteristics of the leg extensors in male volleyball players with jumper's knee. *Am J Sports Med* 1996:24, 380.
7. Romeo AA, Larson RV: Arthroscopic treatment of infrapatellar tendonitis. *Arthroscopy* 1999:15, 341.
8. Walsh WM: Patellofemoral joint, In DeLee JC, Drez D, (eds.), *Orthopaedic Sports Medicine,* Vol. 2, Philadelphia, Saunders, 1994:1163.
9. Grelsamer RP, McConnell J: *The Patella,* Gaithersburg, Md, Aspen, 1998.
10. Cox JS, Blanda JB: Peripatellar pathologies, In DeLee JC, Drez D, (eds.), *Orthopaedic Sports Medicine,* Vol. 2, Philadelphia, Saunders, 1994:1249.
11. Weber D, Friederich NF, Nidecker A, et al.: Deep posterior knee pain caused by a ganglion of the popliteus tendon—a case report. *Knee Surg Sports Traumatol Arthrosc* 1996:4, 157.
12. Nakanishi K, Inoue M, et al.: MR evaluation of mediopatellar plica. *Acta Radiol* 1996:37, 567.
13. Dupont JV: Synovial plicae of the knee: Controversies and review. *Clin Sports Med* 1997:16, 87.
14. Rovere GD, Adair DM: Medial synovial shelf plica syndrome. Treatment by intraplical steroid injection. *Am J Sports Med* 1985:13, 382.
15. Mital MA, Matza RA, Cohen J: The so-called unresolved Osgood Schlatter's lesion. *J Bone Joint Surg* 1980:62A, 732.
16. Stanitski CL: Patellofemoral mechanism: Osgood-Schlatter disease, in Stanitski CL, DeLee JC, Drez D, (eds.), *Pediatric and Adolescent Sports Medicine,* 1st ed., Philadelphia, Saunders, 1994:320.
17. Jakob RP, von Gumppenberg S, Engelhardt P: Does Osgood-Schlatter disease influence the position of the patella? *J Bone Joint Surg [Br]* 1981:63B, 579.
18. Turner MS, Smillie IS: The effect of tibial torsion on the pathology of the knee. *J Bone Joint Surg [Br]* 1981:63B, 396.
19. Krause BL, Williams JP, Catterall A: Natural history of Osgood Schlatter disease. *J Pediatr Orthop* 1990:10, 65.
20. Konsens RM, Seitz WH: Bilateral fractures through "giant" patellar tendon ossicles: A late sequela of Osgood-Schlatter disease. *Orthop Rev* 1988:17, 797.
21. Hogh J, Lund B: The sequelae of Osgood-Schlatter's disease in adults. *Int Orthop* 1988:12, 213.
22. Fredericson M, Bergman AG, Hoffman KL, et al.: Tibial stress reaction in runners: Correlation of clinical symptoms and scintigraphy with a new magnetic imaging grading system. *Am J Sports Med* 1995:23, 472.
23. Barber FA, Sutker AN: Iliotibial band syndrome. *Sports Med* 1992:14, 144.
24. Linderburg G, Pinshaw R, Noakes TD: Iliotibial band syndrome in runners. *Phys Sportsmed* 1984:12, 118.
25. Noble CA: Iliotibial band friction syndrome in runners. *Am J Sports Med* 1980:8, 232.
26. Terry GC, Hughston JC, Norwood LA: The anatomy of the iliopatellar band and the iliotibia tract. *Am J Sports Med* 1986:14, 39.
27. Orchard JW, Fricker PA, Abud AT, et al.: Biomechanics of iliotibial band friction syndrome in runners. *Am J Sports Med* 1996:24, 375.
28. Nishimura G, Yamato M, Tamai K, et al.: MR findings in iliotibial band syndrome. *Skeletal Radiol* 1997:26, 533.
29. Nemeth WC, Sanders BL: The lateral synovial recess of the knee: Anatomy and role in chronic iliotibial band friction syndrome. *Arthroscopy* 1996:12, 574.
30. Ekman EF, Pope T, Martin DF, et al.: Magnetic resonance imaging of iliotibial band syndrome. *Am J Sports Med* 1994:22, 851.
31. Messier SP, Edwards DG, Martin DF, et al.: Etiology of iliotibial band friction syndrome in distance runners. *Med Sci Sports Exer* 1995:27, 951.
32. Schwellnus MP: Lower limb biomechanics in runners with the iliotibial band friction syndrome (abstract). *Med Sci Sports Exer* 1993:25, S67.
33. Fredericson M, Cookingham CC, Chaudhari AM, Dowdell BC, Oestreicher N, Sahrmann SA: Hip abductor weakness in distance runners with iliotibial band syndrome. *Clin J Sports Med* 2000:10, 169.
34. Mann RA, Moran GT, Dougherty SE: Comparative electromyography of the lower extremity in jogging, running, and sprinting. *Am J Sports Med* 1986:14, 501.
35. Hollingshead WH, Jenkins DB: *Functional Anatomy of the Limbs and Back,* Philadelphia, Saunders, 1982:265.
36. Fredericson M, Guillet M, DeBenedictis L: Quick solutions for iliotibial band syndrome. *Phys Sportsmed* 2000:28, 53.
37. Martens M, Libbrecht P, Burssens A: Surgical treatment of iliotibial band friction syndrome. *Am J Sports Med* 1989:17, 651.
38. Mayfield GW: Popliteus tendon tenosynovitis. *Am J Sports Med* 1977:5, 31.
39. Crites BM, Lohnes J, Garrett WEJ: Snapping popliteal tendon as a source of lateral knee pain. *Scand J Med Sci Sports* 1998:8, 243.
40. Reis FP, de Carvalho CA: Anatomical study on the proximal attachments of the human popliteus muscle. *Rev Bras Pesqui Med Biol* 1975:8, 373.
41. Bergman AG, Fredericson M: MR imaging of stress reactions, muscle injuries, and other overuse injuries. *MRI Clinics NA* 1999:7, 151.
42. Stanitski CL: Osteochondritis dissecans of the knee, in Stanitski CL, DeLee JC, Drez D, (eds.), *Pediatric and Adolescent Sports Medicine,* 1st ed., Philadelphia, Saunders, 1994:387.

Chapter 15

PATELLOFEMORAL PAIN SYNDROME

Michael Fredericson

INTRODUCTION

The average recreational runner has a 37% to 56% incidence of injury during the course of a year's training.[1] Knee injuries comprise approximately 30% to 50% of these injuries, and the majority of these involve the patellofemoral joint.[1,2] In many runners with patellofemoral pain there are factors contributing to malalignment of the patella in the intercondylar groove. The malalignment, in conjunction with excessive mileage or other training errors, can cause a runner's symptoms.[3]

CLASSIFICATION SYSTEMS

There are many classification systems for patellofemoral pain. Most of these are based on radiographic findings, grading the extent of chondral injury, or patellar position. These are typically devised to help in surgical planning, but are not easily applicable in the clinical setting. A newer classification system by Holmes and Clancy[4] (Table 15–1) has tried to address this shortcoming. I have found it helpful in classifying the variety of patellofemoral pathology seen in a sports medicine clinic, particularly in clarifying patellofemoral pain or instability related to malalignment.

PREDISPOSING FACTORS FOR PATELLAR MALALIGNMENT AND INSTABILITY

Patellar Anatomy

As the knee begins to flex, the articular surface of the patella comes into contact with the lateral femoral condyle, and the patella then follows an S-shaped curve through the trochlea. Part of the patellar surface remains in contact with the trochlea throughout the remainder of the flexion arc. This contact between the femur and patella progresses from a distal to a proximal position on the patella.[5] Helping to keep the patella centered in the trochlear groove is the V-shaped anatomy of the patella and the configuration of the femoral condyles. In normal knees the lateral condyle is higher than the medial one. There may be various degrees of true dysplasia of the medial or lateral portions of the trochlear groove leading to decreased stability of the patellofemoral joint.[6] This can be due either to excessive thickness of the floor of the trochlea or insufficient height of one or both femoral condyles. Asymmetry of patellar facets also affects patellar congruity. The normal ratio of the lateral to medial facet is 3:2, such that the lateral facet is longer and more sloped, matching the higher and wider lateral femoral condyle.[7]

TABLE 15–1. CLASSIFICATION OF PATELLOFEMORAL PAIN AND DYSFUNCTION

Patellofemoral instability
  A. Subluxation or dislocation, single episode
  B. Subluxation or dislocation, recurrent
    1. Lateral subluxation or dislocation
      a. Normal functional Q-angle
      b. Increased functional Q-angle
      c. Dysplastic trochlea
      d. Grossly inadequate medial stabilizers
      e. Patella alta
      f. Tight lateral retinaculum
    1. Medial subluxation or dislocation
      a. Iatrogenic
  C. Chronic dislocation of patella
    1. Congenital
    2. Acquired
  D. Associated fractures
    1. Osteochondral
    2. Avulsion

Patellofemoral pain and malalignment
  A. Increased functional Q-angle
    1. Femoral anteversion
    2. External tibial torsion
    3. Genu valgum
    4. Foot hyperpronation
  B. Tight lateral retinaculum (lateral patellar compression syndrome)
  C. Grossly inadequate medial stabilizers
  D. Electrical dissociation
  E. Patella alta
  F. Patella baja
  G. Dysplastic femoral trochlea

Patellofemoral pain without malalignment
  A. Tight medial and lateral retinacula
  B. Plica
  C. Osteochondritis dissecans
    1. Patella
    2. Femoral trochlea
  D. Traumatic patellar chondromalacia
  E. Fat pad syndrome
  F. Patellofemoral osteoarthritis
    1. Posttraumatic
    2. Idiopathic
  G. Patellar tendinitis
  H. Quadriceps tendinitis
  I. Prepatellar bursitis
  J. Apophysitis
    1. Osgood-Schlatter
    2. Sinding-Larsen-Johansson
  K. Symptomatic bipartite patella
  L. Other trauma
    1. Quadriceps tendon rupture
    2. Patellar tendon rupture
    3. Patella fracture
    4. Proximal tibial epiphysis (tubercle) fracture
    5. Contusion
    6. Turf knee/wrestler's knee
    7. Cruciate ligament instability
  M. Reflex sympathetic dystrophy

Source: Permission from Holmes WS, Clancy WG: Clinical classification of patellofemoral pain and dysfunction. Journal Orthopedic Sports Physical Therapy *28:300, 1998.*

Lower Extremity Malalignment

Torsional or angular malalignment of the lower extremity has a significant influence on patellofemoral joint mechanics, which may result in patellofemoral knee pain. For example, anteversion of the femoral neck is frequently associated with external torsion of the tibia, and frequently, compensatory pronation of the foot. Conversely, intrinsic pathology in the foot, such as forefoot varus, subtalar varus, or ankle joint equinus, can be the cause of excessive subtalar joint pronation.[8] Pronation is considered excessive if it occurs too far into midstance when the foot should be supinating in preparation for efficient push-off.

The tibia internally rotates with pronation and externally rotates during supination. If excessive pronation is evident in midstance, then internal tibial rotation is increased or prolonged and there is an increased valgus force at the knee and a constant lateral force on the patella every time the quadriceps fire.

Muscle and Soft Tissue Imbalances

Probably the most important anatomic factor proposed for affecting dynamic patellar stabilization is the balance between the medial and lateral quadriceps muscles. It is felt that the vastus medialis oblique (VMO), the primary active medial stabilizer of the patella,[9] is often overpowered by the lateral forces acting on the patella, which include the iliotibial tract, the lateral retinaculum, and the vastus lateralis.[10] Decreased timing or intensity differences between the vastus medialis and vastus lateralis on EMG studies, however, is not consistently seen in patients with patellofemoral pain and further research is necessary to clearly define the role of the VMO in contributing to patellar kinematics.[11,12]

Abnormal soft tissue length can also affect patellofemoral mechanics. For example, tightness in the quadriceps muscle can directly increase the contact pressure between the articular surfaces of the femur and patella, whereas tightness in the hamstrings and gastrocnemius can indirectly increase patellofemoral joint reaction forces by producing a constant flexion moment to the patella.[13] Tightness in the hamstrings or gastrocnemius will also restrict talocrural dorsiflexion, producing compensatory pronation in the subtalar joint[8] and an increase in the dynamic Q-angle. The talocrural joint requires 10 degrees of dorsiflexion for walking and 15 to 25 degrees for running. If this motion is not available, compensatory pronation occurs to allow dorsiflexion of the midfoot on the rearfoot.[14]

One of the most common findings in the runner with patellofemoral pain is tightness along the iliotibial band (ITB). The distal ITB fibers blend with the superficial and deep fibers of the lateral retinaculum and tightness in the ITB can contribute to lateral patellar tilt and excessive pressure on the lateral patella.

PATHOPHYSIOLOGY

The pathophysiology of patellofemoral pain is not well understood. Although chondromalacia (articular cartilage softening or fibrillation) is sometimes associated with patellofemoral pain, arthroscopy often shows no gross evidence of pathology in many young patients who have patellofemoral pain. This is in sharp contrast to older patients, in whom chondromalacia or patellar osteoarthrosis (progressive articular degeneration) can be more often be arthroscopically proven; however, the degree of involvement of the articular surface correlates poorly with the severity of symptoms.[7]

Insall and colleagues[15] believe that the etiology of pain is abnormal stress resulting from patellofemoral malalignment. They describe the vertical crest of the patella as a convex bony surface covered by a thick layer of relatively soft cartilage. Excessive stress or normal stress applied in an abnormal direction to the cartilage, with resultant deformation, might transmit abnormal shear stress to the subchondral bone. Nerves are associated with the blood supply to the subchondral bone, and the increase in pressure between the patella and femur caused by running is likely transmitted to these nerve receptors and perceived as patellar pain.

Fulkerson and co-workers[16] and more recently Sanchis and colleagues,[13] postulated that the lateral retinaculum also plays an important role in patellofemoral pain. They propose that chronic lateral subluxation of the patella can lead to shortening of the retinaculum with secondary nerve damage, resembling the histopathogic picture of a Morton's neuroma. Substantiating this theory was a clear correlation between the severity of pain and the tendency to generate neuromas.

CLINICAL PRESENTATION

One of the difficulties in evaluating runners with patellofemoral pain is the vague nature of the pain. Runners typically note the insidious onset of an ill-defined ache localized to the anterior knee, behind the knee cap. Occasionally the pain may be centered along the medial or lateral patellofemoral joint and retinaculum. The pain may vary throughout the run and is particularly aggravated by hills, when the patellofemoral joint reaction force may increase up to six times that found during level walking.[17] Symptoms may also

occur when the runner must sit with the knee flexed for a long period of time, as in a movie theater or when traveling in a small car. There may be occasional complaints of mild swelling, but it is rare for there to be a gross effusion seen with a traumatic knee injury. A complaint of giving way may also be reported, and is believed secondary to reflex inhibition of the quadriceps muscle. In the subset of patients with patellar instability, there is often a sensation of patellar slippage, or a feeling of actual bony subluxation, particularly with twisting, cutting, or pivoting. Only rarely, however, will a runner turn sharply enough to sustain a dynamic force sufficient to cause an acute dislocation of the patella.

PHYSICAL EXAMINATION

The positive findings in patellofemoral pain are often subtle and it is not always clear if they correlate with the patient's symptoms. Clinical studies have not been able to consistently demonstrate biomechanical or alignment differences between patients with patellofemoral pain and healthy individuals.[3,18,19] Some of this relates to the difficulty in defining where the range of normal alignment ends and malalignment begins. Given this, I still believe that the physical examination, when systematically performed, can highlight factors predisposing to patellofemoral malalignment that are important to address in the design of an individualized treatment program.

Standing Examination

Alignment of the lower extremity is evaluated by noting evidence of femoral anteversion, knee position (genu varum, valgum, or recurvatum), external tibial rotation, and foot and ankle weightbearing alignment. The functional Q-angle, when the patient is in a weightbearing position, is also a useful measurement. It is a way to assess the degree of valgus stress on the knee and laterally-directed force on the patella. Meisser and colleagues[3] studied 36 male and female runners between 16 and 50 years of age and found that a Q-angle greater than 16 degrees was a discriminator between runners with patellofemoral pain syndrome (>16 degrees) and symptom-free runners (<16 degrees). Assessment of the true Q-angle requires the patella to be centered. This is important to remember; if the patella is subluxed laterally out of the trochlea, the Q-angle will be falsely normal.

Dynamic alignment can be tested by having the runner step slowly up and down a 6-inch stool or perform single-leg squats. In patients with patellofemoral pain, there may be a reduction in eccentric muscular control with altered symmetry and smoothness of the movement. The hip should be in line with the knee and the knee with the foot. The presence of any abnormal movements of the patella as it engages and disengages the trochlea is noted, as well as any body shifting, trunk rotation, or loss of hip control. Normally the patella travels smoothly through the trochlear groove and follows a straight or slightly curved path. An abrupt or sudden lateral movement of the patella as the knee nears full extension is considered abnormal. Called a positive J sign, this movement is due to excessive lateral forces as the patella exits the femoral trochlea at 10 to 30 degrees of flexion[7,16] and is seen in a small number of patients with patellar malalignment, and a majority of those with frank patellofemoral instability.

Sitting Examination

The muscle bulk of the VMO is observed and compared with the other side, looking for the level of insertion and presence of atrophy. When the patient holds both knees actively at 45 degrees of flexion, the VMO should normally be present as a substantial muscle arising from the adductor tubercle and medial intermuscular septum, inserting into the upper ⅓ to ½ of the patella. In general, the lower the VMO's insertion, the greater its biomechanical advantage in stabilizing the patella against lateral forces.[20]

In the sitting position one can also assess patellar height for signs of alta or baja position. In cases of patella alta, the patella may have a "grasshopper eye" appearance with the patella pointed toward the ceiling and slightly tilted laterally. A prominent infrapatellar fat pad often accompanies patella alta, as does genu recurvatum. Patella alta is more frequently seen in females and is a common finding in a congenitally subluxing patella because it causes the patella to enter the femoral sulcus late in knee flexion. Patella baja is more rare and is sometimes seen as a complication of anterior cruciate ligament reconstruction. The path of the patellar tendon insertion into the tibial tuberosity is also noted. When the tibial tubercle is situated more laterally than normal, so the patellar tendon descends at an angle rather than directly downward, proximal external tibial torsion is present.

Supine Examination

Leg-length discrepancies can be screened by measuring the distance from the anterior superior iliac spine to the highest point of the medial malleolus. The knee joint is then observed and palpated for any swelling. As little as 20 to 30 cc of fluid in the knee joint can inhibit VMO function.[21] It is unusual, however, to have any more than a mild synovitis of the knee with chronic extensor mechanism problems.

The examination then focuses on palpation of the patella and peripatellar soft tissues for tenderness. The lateral retinaculum interdigitates with fibers from the vastus lateralis and iliotibial band, and tenderness in this area related to the chronic recurrent stress of a maligned patella is frequently palpated.[16,22] This is often associated with tenderness along the medial patellar facet, and less often the lateral patellar facet. These are best palpated by curling the fingers around the border of the patella. The examiner next palpates along the patellar tendon, specifically at its attachment to the distal pole of the patella. Patellar tendinitis is demonstrated by tenderness to palpation in this area. Examination of the patellar tendon is facilitated by pressing down on the proximal pole of the patella. This causes the patella to tilt its distal pole anteriorly, making the proximal attachment of the patellar tendon easily palpable. Less commonly, tenderness is located at the proximal pole of the patella at the quadriceps insertion, indicating quadriceps tendinitis. Additionally, there may be a positive compression test with downward pressure on the patella producing pain; however, this is often positive in asymptomatic individuals.

Close observation of the patella in relation to the femur is continued. McConnell[10] describes four components that are believed to affect patellar position statically or dynamically: Glide, tilt, rotation, and anterior-posterior position. The glide test is an assessment of lateral/medial displacement of the patella and measures the distance from the midpole of the patella to the medial and lateral femoral epicondyles with the knee flexed to 20 degrees. The patella may sit equidistant to the condyles, but moves laterally when the quadriceps contracts, indicating a dynamic problem. Although it is common for patients with patellofemoral pain to have some degree of lateral displacement, these clinical measurements should be interpreted with caution, since they may not be a true reflection of anatomic position. A recent study[23] found that the clinical assessment of patellar glide (medial/lateral displacement) overestimated the true amount of lateral displacement on MRI.

Patellar tilt compares the height of the anterior aspect of the medial patellar border with the height of the anterior aspect of the lateral patellar border. This is considered normal when the two borders are level in the frontal plane. Mild tilt is present when greater than 50% of the depth of the lateral border can be palpated but the posterior surface is not palpable, and tilt is more severe when palpation of the lateral border reveals that less than 50% of its depth can be palpated. To determine the presence of a dynamic tilt problem, simulate an active contraction by passively moving the patella medially. If the depth of the lateral border

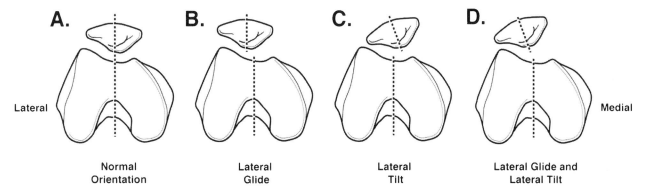

Figure 15–1. Example of patellar orientation with a lateral glide and/or tilt component.

becomes more difficult to palpate, then a dynamic tilt is present. If lateral tilt is severe, it can lead to lateral patellar compression syndrome, sometimes requiring surgical release (Fig. 15–1).

Rotational measurements help to determine if there is any deviation of the long axis of the patella from the long axis of the femur, and if present is believed to be another indication that a particular part of the retinaculum is tight and a potential source of symptoms. In my experience this is somewhat difficult to assess and has greater potential for miscalculation. Normal rotation is present when a line connecting the superior and inferior poles of the patella is parallel to the long axis of the femur. If the inferior pole is medial to the long axis of the femur, this signifies internal rotation; if the inferior pole of the patella is lateral to the long axis of the femur, this signifies external rotation.

The evaluation of anteroposterior (AP) alignment assesses if the inferior pole is tilted posteriorly compared with the superior pole. Such tilting can irritate the fat pad and is common in patients who have pain on extension or hyperextension of the knee, since the inferior pole gets buried in the fat pad. These patients are often diagnosed as having patellar tendinitis and usually have pain with quad sets and straight-leg raises. AP tilt occurs when the distal third of the patella, or the inferior pole of the patella, is not as easy to palpate as the superior third and superior pole. Patients with this condition often present with a dimple in their knee. Dynamically, AP tilt can be determined during a maximal quadriceps contraction. If the inferior pole disappears and becomes a dimple, then the test is positive.

Also important is assessment of patellar mobility.[24] The knee is supported in 20 to 30 degrees of flexion and the quadriceps is relaxed. The patella is divided into four longitudinal quadrants and it is displaced medially and laterally with the examiner's

thumb and index finger to determine the amount of patellar tightness (Fig. 15–2). A lateral displacement of three quadrants suggests an incompetent medial restraint. A lateral displacement of four quadrants defines a dislocatable patella. A medial displacement of only one quadrant indicates a tight lateral retinaculum and usually correlates with an abnormal passive patellar tilt test. Medial displacement of three or four quadrants suggests a more globally hypermobile patella without tightness of the lateral restraints, and is often seen in patients with other stigmata of generalized ligamentous laxity. During these maneuvers one is looking not only for patellar mobility but also for any associated apprehension. When positive this is a very specific test for patellar instability.

The ligamentous stability of both knees is assessed, particularly if there is a previous history of

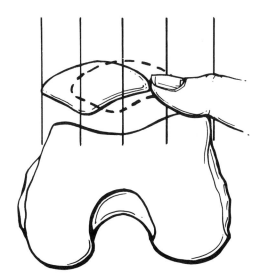

Figure 15–2. Assessment of patellar mobility medially and laterally. (*Source: RB: Permission from DeLee JC, Drez D, (eds.)*, Orthopaedic Sports Medicine, *Vol. 2, Philadelphia, Saunders, 1994: 1179.*)

knee injury. Both anterior and posterior cruciate deficiencies are associated with peripatellar pain. Careful evaluation for meniscal pathology is noted by palpation of the medial and lateral joint lines and McMurray testing. Joint line tenderness can be present with patellar pathology and is not necessarily indicative of meniscal injury or femorotibial arthritis.[10] Identification of a symptomatic synovial plica is equally important.

Hip range of motion and Faber's maneuver should be thoroughly assessed to help rule out pain referred to the knee from intra-articular hip pathology. Internal rotation that exceeds external rotation is suggestive of femoral anteversion. Following this, soft tissue length should be measured in the hamstrings and hip flexors.

Side-Lying Examination

In the side-lying position, with the knee flexed at 20 degrees, the lateral retinaculum can be evaluated for excessive tightness by passively moving the patella in a medial direction.[10] The superficial retinacular fibers are thought to be tight if the femoral condyle is not easily exposed. To test the deep fibers, the hand is placed on the middle of the patella, the slack of any lateral glide is removed, and an anteroposterior pressure on the medial border of the patella is applied. The lateral patellar border should move freely away from the femur, and on palpation the tension in the retinacular fibers should be similar.

In this position ITB tightness can be evaluated with Ober's test and the gluteus medius can be tested for strength deficits.

Prone Examination

This position allows a more accurate assessment of rearfoot and forefoot alignment, subtalar position, and gastrocsoleus and quadriceps muscle flexibility.

Observational Gait Analysis

This is one of the most important aspects of the examination, designed to evaluate dynamic function by observing the runner's angle of gait while walking and running. In more complicated cases, it may be helpful to utilize treadmill running or even videotaping to analyze the runner's gait (See Chapter 6).

DIAGNOSTIC STUDIES

It is important to obtain x-rays in the runner who has apparent patellofemoral pain not demonstrating improvement after several weeks of conservative treatment, or if there has been a history of recent trauma or dislocation.

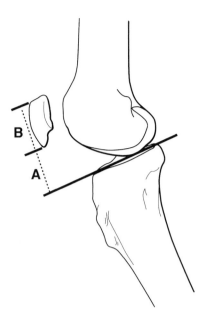

Figure 15–3. Technique of Blackburne and Peel to assess patella alta on lateral x-rays of the knee.

On standard anteroposterior (AP) x-rays of the knee, one can identify accessory ossification centers, degenerative joint disease, and other unrelated diagnoses such as bone tumors.[25]

The lateral view is most helpful for assessing patellar height. There are a plethora of measurement techniques described in the literature for this purpose.[10] The Blackburne-Peel technique[26] is one that is easy to use and fairly reliable. It measures the distance from the tibial plateau to the inferior pole, which should equal the length of the patellar articular surface (Fig. 15–3). Normal values are approximately 1.0, with higher values indicative of patella alta. It should be used with caution in adolescent patients with a skeletally immature proximal tibial epiphysis, certain patellar morphotypes with a short articular surface, or when there is an abnormal slope of the tibial plateau.[10]

Axial views of the patellofemoral joint are recommended with the knee flexed 30 degrees.[10] Some subluxation can be detected at 30 degrees that could be missed at 45 degrees. This view allows evaluation of degenerative changes in the patellofemoral joint, osteochondritis dissecans of the patella, patellar morphology, dysplasia of the trochlear groove, and accessory ossification centers and ectopic calcifications in the retinaculum. The position and orientation of the patella relative to the trochlear groove are also evaluated with the sulcus angle, congruence angle, and the patellar tilt angle.

The sulcus angle measures the angle of the bony trochlea. With the knee flexed at 30 to 45 degrees, the normal sulcus angle is approximately 140 degrees.[27]

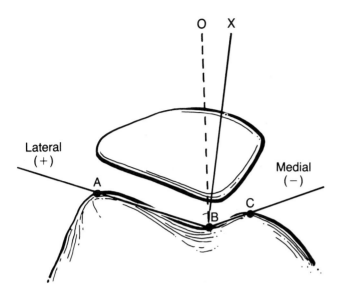

Figure 15–4. Congruence angle of Merchant. Line BO is the bisector of angle ABC. Line BX passes through the lowest point on the median ridge of the patella. Angle OBX is the congruence angle. If line BX falls to the medial side of line BO, the angle is expressed in negative degrees. If it falls to the lateral side of line BO, it is expressed in positive degrees. (*Source: Permission from DeLee JC, Drez D, (eds.),* Orthopaedic Sports Medicine, *Vol. 2, Philadelphia, Saunders, 1994:1186.*)

Patellar instability is associated with a more shallow trochlea, whereas too steep a trochlea is associated with patellar pain without instability.[28]

The congruence angle is an index of medial/lateral subluxation of the patella within the trochlear groove, similar to the assessment on physical examination of patellar glide, and in nondislocators the average angle is −6 (SD 11 degrees)[22] This means that a congruence angle of greater than +16 degrees is abnormal at the 95th percentile (Fig. 15–4).

The patellar tilt angle is an index of the medial/lateral tilt of the plane of the patella relative to the femur (Fig. 15–5). In the normal patellofemoral

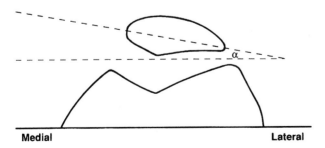

Figure 15–5. Patellar tilt angle. The tilt angle is measured by a line joining the corners of the patella and any horizontal line. (*Source: Permission from Grelsamer RP, McConnell J:* The Patella, *Gaithersburg, Md, Aspen, 1998:68.*)

joint, the angle formed by the lateral patellar facet and any horizontal line should open laterally, whereas in patients with patellar subluxation, the lines used to define the angle are parallel or open medially.[29] For this to be accurate and repeatable, the radiograph must be taken with the foot vertical and the cassette maintained parallel to the ground. If the patient exhibits external tibial torsion, the natural position of the feet is maintained. A tilt angle between 0 and 5 degrees is normal, 5 to 10 degrees is borderline, and an angle greater than 10 degrees is considered abnormal. In a study by Grelsamer,[30] abnormal tilt was detected in 85% of patients suffering from malalignment pain. The 15% of patients whose malalignment was not detected exhibited either abnormal tilt that became normal at 30 degrees of flexion or malalignment not related to tilt (i.e., patella alta or lateral displacement).

Because the patella usually becomes unstable as it nears extension, a lateralized patella may not be detected by a Merchant view that requires the knee be flexed to at least 30 degrees. Thus if surgery is contemplated and plain films are negative an MRI or CT scan should be used to further evaluate patellar tracking. Serial CT scans taken at knee flexion angles in the range of 0 to 30 degrees can provide even greater information about the tracking of the patella in the trochlear groove. Measurements of sulcus angle, congruence angle, and patellar tilt angle can be carried out on CT scans just as they can on conventional axial radiographs and may be helpful in understanding the patient with a difficult patellofemoral problem.[31] Three patterns of malalignment can be characterized by the congruence angle and patellar tilt angle: lateral subluxation without lateral tilt, subluxation with tilt, and tilt without subluxation. More recently, kinematic CT of the patellofemoral joint during active flexion and extension was found even more useful than serial images.[32]

Kinematic studies can also be accomplished with MRI[33,34] without exposure to radiation, though still obviously involving considerable expense. In addition to defining tracking abnormalities, MRI is particularly helpful in detecting any degenerative joint changes such as cartilage fissuring or thinning, subchondral bone marrow edema, subchondral cysts, and other pathologic entities such as synovial plica and patellar tendinitis. At our institution, we are now using an MR unit in which the patient can stand upright in a weight-bearing position while performing continuous slow flexion and extension, using an MR tracker device to more accurately define patellar motion abnormalities (Fig. 15–6).

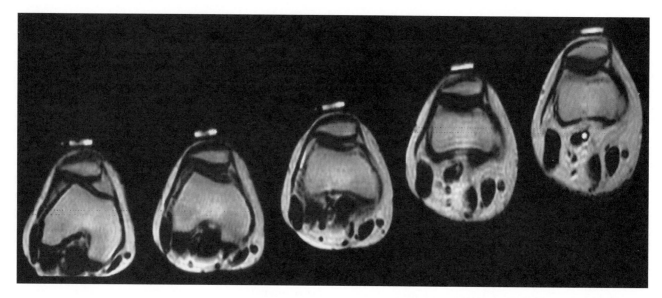

Figure 15–6. A sequence of axial MR images obtained during active knee flexion with the patient upright and weightbearing demonstrates dynamic patellar subluxation. An open magnet was used, with an MR tracker assuring consecutive images were obtained in a constant location relative to the patella.

REHABILITATION

Some form of training modification is often necessary to resolve the pain. Sometimes all that is necessary is for the runner to do less hill work or decrease total weekly mileage. Oral anti-inflammatory agents are rarely useful unless there is an associated effusion present.

Whether or not patellofemoral tracking abnormalities can be found, most patients have clinical weakness in the quadriceps.[11,35,36] Two prospective studies have found that restoration of quadriceps strength and function was the main factor contributing to good recovery.[18,37] Additionally, a lack of bilateral symptoms at follow-up, low body weight, and young age were associated with good long-term outcome. Neither radiologic nor MRI changes of the affected knee had a clear association with outcome.

Correcting abnormal patella posture utilizing the McConnell taping technique[10] is one way of optimizing the entry of the patella into the trochlea and is a transitional step in the rehabilitation process in those patients unable to perform strengthening exercises due to their pain. Taping the patella of symptomatic individuals during stair ascent and descent exercises, so that the symptoms were diminished by 50%, led to earlier activation of the VMO, increased quadriceps activity, and increased loading of the knee joint.[38,39]

Isometrics and open kinetic chain exercises, such as knee extensions, are recommended if there is significant quadriceps weakness or pain with weightbearing.[40] As quickly as possible, however, patients should progress to the core of the rehabilitation program, which includes a closed kinetic chain quadriceps strengthening regimen that has shown to be more effective than isokinetic joint isolation and open chain exercises in improving function.[41,42] Closed chain exercises more closely mimic the physiologic demands of running and produce less patellofemoral joint reaction forces than an open chain exercise such as knee extensions, in the important range of 0 to 45 degrees of knee flexion.[40,43] Isolated recruitment of the VMO as proposed by many therapists has not been proven to occur with exercises that are commonly prescribed for the treatment of patellofemoral pain. One electromyographic study examined nine commonly used strengthening exercises and found that the activity of the vastus medialis oblique was not significantly greater than that of the vastus lateralis, the vastus intermedius, and the vastus medialis longus, suggesting that most exercises likely translate into a general quadriceps-strengthening effect.[44]

Examples of closed chain exercises include lunges, wall slides, and use of leg press machines, emphasizing improved quadriceps endurance, with more repetitions at lower loads. To improve eccentric control the athlete should also include exercises done while standing on one leg. In this position the pelvis is kept level and the lower abdominals and the glutei are working together while the other leg is swinging back and forward, simulating the activity of the stance phase of gait.[10] Activation of the lower abdominal and oblique muscles helps to decrease the anterior rotation

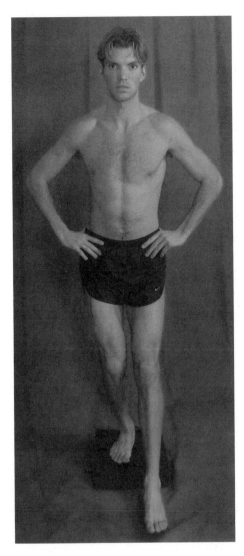

Figure 15–7. Step-down exercise. The pelvis should remain parallel with the floor; the hip, knee, and foot should be aligned, avoiding excessive hip adduction or internal rotation. The goal is to activate the gluteal and quadriceps muscles by maintaining erect posture, and avoiding forward body lean as one steps down. Start on a step only a few inches off the ground and increase the distance as stability improves.

of the pelvis and resultant internal rotation of the femur.

Step-down exercises are also helpful (Fig. 15–7). When done, the pelvis must remain parallel with the floor; the hip, knee, and foot should be aligned. The aim is to achieve a carryover from these functional exercises to the single-leg stability required with running.

Soft-tissue inflexibilities, particularly in the hamstrings and the ITB, can also affect normal patella excursion and should be addressed.[45] Soft-tissue mobilization and stretching techniques are also important to address tight retinaculum structures contributing to abnormal patellar tracking.

Excessive pronation, whether secondary to abnormal compensation as a result of abnormal structure in the trunk or lower extremity, or secondary to pathology in the foot itself, should also be addressed. Excessive pronation can increase the Q-angle, causing a dynamic abduction moment at the knee and a consequent increase in the laterally directed force on the patella. Over-the-counter arch supports may work for mild cases, but many runners will come to need a custom-molded orthotic for maximal biomechanical control. Traditionally, orthotic devices have been designed to address primary control of rearfoot motion. Three-dimensional studies, however, have shown that forefoot stability may play an integral role in rearfoot stability.[46] These studies indicate that instability in the forefoot at push-off may create instability in the rearfoot. For this reason an orthotic that extends all the way to the sulcus or web space of the toes is considered crucial for control of forefoot instability in runners.[10]

Finally, runners with patellar malalignment may find relief from pain by wearing a properly-fitted dynamic patellar stabilization brace. Powers[47] found 50% of subjects experienced an improvement in symptoms with use of the Bauerfeind Genutrain P3 Brace. Further study[48] evaluating the same brace, however, found it was unable to correct patellar tracking patterns as measured quantitatively by kinematic MRI. This suggests that the improvement with bracing may be related to a more subtle effect on patellofemoral joint mechanics. Powers and colleagues hypothesize that the effectiveness of braces may be related to contact area (personal communication). By increasing contact area (through compression) and thereby dispersing the joint reaction force over a greater surface, joint stress may be decreased.

The vast majority of runners with patellofemoral pain and malalignment, including those with minor instability problems, will respond to nonoperative treatment. The lateral retinacular release is perhaps the most frequently performed operation, but is only indicated if a major contributor to malalignment is a tight lateral retinaculum causing isolated patellar tilt.[24] A common complication of lateral retinacular release is an incomplete release. This is most commonly the failure to release the patellar tibial portion of the lateral retinaculum along with the patellofemoral portion. Conversely, an overzealous release can lead to medial subluxation or dislocation. A lateral release will not correct more global patellar hypermobility, or an abnormal anatomic Q-angle. In these cases, more extensive realignment surgery may be contemplated, but it is unlikely to permit a return to serious running.[8,22]

REFERENCES

1. Van Mechelen W: Running injuries: A review of the epidemiologic literature. *Sports Med* 1992:14, 320.
2. O'Toole ML: Prevention and treatment of injuries to runners. *Med Sci Sports Exerc* 1992:24, 360.
3. Meisser SP, Davis SE, Curl WW, et al.: Etiologic factors associated with patellofemoral pain in runners. *Med Sci Sports Exerc* 1991:23, 1008.
4. Holmes WS, Clancy WG: Clinical classification of patellofemoral pain and dysfunction. *Journal Orthopedics Sports Physical Therapy* 1998:28, 299.
5. Goodfellow J, Hungerford DS, Zindel M: Patellofemoral joint mechanics and pathology. 1. Functional anatomy of the patellofemoral joint. *J Bone Joint Surg* 1976:58B, 287.
6. Walsh WM: Patellofemoral joint, in DeLee JC, Drez D, (eds.), *Orthopaedic Sports Medicine,* Vol. 2, Philadelphia, Saunders, 1994:1163.
7. Hughston JC, Walsh WM, Puddu G: *Patellar Subluxation and Dislocation,* Philadelphia, Saunders, 1984.
8. James SL, Jones DC: Biomechanical aspects of distance running injuries, in Cavanagh PR (ed.), *Biomechanics of Distance Running,* Champaign, Ill, Human Kinetics, 1990:249.
9. Bose K, Kanagasuntherum R, Osman M: Vastus medialis oblique: An anatomical and physiologic study. *Orthopedics* 1980:3, 880.
10. Grelsamer RP, McConnell J: *The Patella,* Gaithersburg, Md, Aspen, 1998.
11. Powers CM: Rehabilitation of patellofemoral joint disorders: A critical review. *J Orthop Sports Phys Ther* 1998:28, 3453.
12. Powers CM, Landel R, Perry J: Timing and intensity of vastus muscle activity during functional activities in subjects with and without patellofemoral pain. *Phys Ther* 1996:76, 946.
13. Sanchis-Alfonso V, Rosello-Sastre E, Martinez-Sanjuan V: Pathogenesis of anterior knee pain syndrome and functional patellofemoral instability in the active young. *Am J Knee Surg* 1999:12, 29.
14. Root M, Orien W, Weed J: *Clinical Biomechanics,* Vol. 11, Los Angeles, Clinical Biomechanics Corp, 1977.
15. Insall J, Goldberg V, Salvati E: Recurrent dislocation and the high-riding patella. *Clin Orthop* 1972:88, 67.
16. Fulkerson JP, Kalenak A, Rosenberg TD, et al.: Patellofemoral Pain. AAOS Instructional Course Outlines. 1994:57.
17. Scott SH, Winter DA: Internal forces at chronic running injury sites. *Med Sci Sports Exerc* 1990:22, 357.
18. Kannus P, Nittymaki S: Which factors predict outcome in the nonoperative treatment of patellofemoral pain syndrome? A prospective follow-up study. *Med Sci Sports Exerc* 1994:26, 289.
19. Thomee R, Renstrom P, Karlsson J, et al.: Patellofemoral pain syndrome in young women. I. A clinical analysis of alignment, pain, parameters, common symptoms and functional activity level. *Scand J Med Sci Sports* 1995:5, 237.
20. Outerbridge RE, Dunnlop J: The problem of chondromalacia patellae. *Clin Orthop* 1975:110, 177.
21. de Andrade JR, Grant C, Dixon AS: Joint distention and reflex muscle inhibition in the knee. *J Bone Joint Surg* 1965:47A, 313.
22. Merchant AC: Patellofemoral malalignment and instabilities, in Ewing JW, (ed.), *Articular Cartilage and Knee Joint Function: Basic Science and Arthroscopy,* New York, Raven Press, 1990:79.
23. Powers CM, Mortenson S, Nishimoto D, et al.: Criterion-related validity of a clinical measurement to determine the medial/lateral component of patellar orientation. *J Orthop Sports Phys Ther* 1999:29, 372.
24. Kolowich PA, Paulos LE, Rosenberg TD, Farnsworth S: Lateral release of the patella: Indications and contraindications. *Am J Sports Med* 1990:18, 359.
25. Bergman AG, Fredericson M: MR imaging of stress reactions, muscle injuries, and other overuse injuries in runners. *MRI Clin North Am* 1999:7, 151.
26. Blackburne JS, Peel TE: A new method of measuring patellar height. *J Bone Joint Surg* 1977:59B, 241.
27. Brattström H: The picture of the femoro-patellar joint in recurrent dislocation of the patella. *Acta Orthop Scand* 1963:33, 373.
28. Buard J, Benoit J, Lortat-Jacob A, et al.: Les trochlées fémorales creuses. *Rev Chir Orthop* 1981:67, 721.
29. Laurin CA, Levesque HP, Dussault R, Labelle H, et al.: The abnormal lateral patellofemoral angle. *J Bone Joint Surg* 1978:60A, 55.
30. Grelsamer RP, Bazos AN, Proctor CS: A roentgenographic analysis of patellar tilt. *J Bone Joint Surg* 1993:75B. 822.
31. Schutzer SF, Rasby GR, Fulkerson JP: Computed tomographic classification of patellofemoral pain patients. *Orthop Clin North Am* 1986:17, 235.
32. Dupuy DE, Hangen DH, Zachazewski JE, et al.: Kinematic CT of the patellofemoral joint. *Am J Roentgenol* 1997:169, 211.
33. Brossman J, Muhle C, Schroder C, et al.: Motion-triggered MR imaging: Evaluation of patellar tracking patterns during active and passive knee extension. *Radiology* 1993:187, 205.
34. Shellock FG, Stone KR, Crues JV: Development and clinical application of kinematic MRI of the patellofemoral joint using an extremity MR system. *Med Sci Sports Exerc* 1999:31, 788.
35. Thomee R, Renstrom P, Karlsson J, et al.: Patellofemoral pain syndrome in young women. II. Muscle function in patients and healthy controls. *Scand J Med Sci Sports* 1995:5, 245.
36. Werner S: An evaluation of knee extensor and knee flexor torques and EMGs in patients with patellofemoral pain syndrome in comparison with matched controls. *Knee Surg Sports Traumatol Arthrosc* 1995:3, 89.
37. Natri A, Kannus P, Jarvinen M: Which factors predict the long term outcome in chronic patellofemoral pain syndrome? A 7-yr prospective follow-up study. *Med Sci Sports Exerc* 1998:30, 1572.
38. Gilleard W, McConnell J, Parsons D: The effect of taping on the onset of vastus medialis obliquus and vastus lateralis muscle activity in persons with patellofemoral pain. *Phys Ther* 1998:78, 25.

39. Powers CM, Landel R, Sosnick T, et al.: The effect of patellar taping on stride characteristics and joint motion in subjects with patellofemoral pain. *J Orthop Sports Phys Ther* 1997:26, 286.
40. Escamilla RF, Fleisig GS, Zheng N, et al.: Biomechanics of the knee during closed kinetic chain and open kinetic chain exercises. *Med Sci Sports Exerc* 1998:30, 556.
41. Doucette SA, Child DD: The effect of open and closed chain exercise and knee joint position on patellar tracking in lateral patellar compression syndrome. *J Orthop Sports Phys Ther* 1996:23, 104.
42. Steine HA, Brosky T, Reinking MF, et al.: A comparison of closed kinetic chain and isokinetic isolation exercise in patients with patellofemoral dysfunction. *J Orthop Sports Phys Ther* 1996:24, 136.
43. Steinkamp LA, Dillingham MF, Markels MD, Hill JA, Kaufman KR: Biomechanical considerations in patellofemoral joint rehabilitation. *Am J Sports Med* 1993:21, 438.
44. Mirzabeigi E, Jordan C, Gronley JK: Isolation of the vastus medialis oblique muscle during exercise. *Am J Sports Med* 1999:27, 50.
45. Doucette SA, Goble EM: The effect of exercise on patellar tracking in lateral patellar compression syndrome. *Am J Sports Med* 1992:20, 434.
46. Engsberg JR, Andrews JG: Kinematic analysis of the talocalcaneal/talocrural joint during running support. *Med Sci Sports Exerc* 1987:19, 275.
47. Powers CM: The effects of patellar bracing on clinical changes and gait characteristics in subjects with patellofemoral pain (Abstract). *Phys Ther* 1998:30, S48.
48. Powers CM, Shellock FG, Beering TV: Effect of bracing on patellar kinematics in patients with patellofemoral joint pain. *Med Sci Sports Exerc* 1999:31, 1714.

Chapter 16

EXERTIONAL LEG PAIN

John E. Glorioso, Jr. and
John H. Wilckens

INTRODUCTION

Exertional leg pain is a commonly encountered complaint in the running athlete. In studies of overuse injuries seen in athletes, 18% were located in the area of the shin.[1] Clinically, pains in and around the leg may present with very similar complaints and historical findings despite variable pathoanatomy. Determination of a specific diagnosis for the leg pain and initiation of the proper therapy is not always clearly evident. Often, the discomfort and frustration experienced by the athlete can only be paralleled by the diagnostic dilemma and challenge faced by the physician in determining the specific etiology so as to initiate appropriate therapy and return the athlete to running.

Multiple etiologies have been identified as the cause of exertional leg pain. In the running athlete, the most common diagnoses are tendinitis, periostitis, chronic exertional compartment syndrome, and stress fracture. However, the frequency of occurrence of each of these diagnoses has not been established. The true incidence of these disorders has been obscured by the inconsistent use of definitions (or rather a lack of standardization of definitions) for these specific entities in the literature and in studies examining their occurrence.

Much of the confusion in the medical literature stems from the use of the term "shin splints." This classical term is used to describe any exertional leg pain from the knee to the ankle, yet it designates no specific pathoanatomic diagnosis. Use of the term shin splints is descriptive, not diagnostic, and gives no indication of the location or etiology of the pain.[2–4]

Although there are many specific causes of exertional leg pain in the runner, the underlying pathogenesis is often related to overuse in association with training errors. The incidence of running injuries has been associated with the distance run per week. Distance runners have a higher incidence of injury compared with joggers and sprinters.[1,5]

It is important to note that the diagnostic groups are not mutually exclusive, as more than one etiology of leg pain may coexist.[6] Detmer[7] has shown coexistent periostitis and compartment syndrome as well as stress fracture and periostitis. In addition, the initial disorder may induce a secondary pathology. The athlete with an injury may continue with his or her routine, responding with biomechanical maladaptation and development of a second injury. An example would be medial tibial stress fracture with a secondary stress fracture from alterations in gait to accommodate for the initial discomfort. It must also be appreciated that various etiologies may occur in a progressive fashion and present a continuum of progressive disorder if no intervention is taken. As an illustration of this progression, Matin[8] has proposed a five-stage description of skeletal injury from minimal periosteal reaction through adaptive bone reaction (early stress fracture) and finally complete full-thickness stress fracture.

ANATOMY OF THE LEG

A thorough understanding of the anatomy of the leg is essential in establishing the etiology of leg pain. The anatomic boundaries of the "leg" extend from the knee to the ankle. The leg contains four anatomically distinct muscle compartments with structural support provided by the tibia and fibula. The tough interosseous membrane connects the tibia and fibula. Each compartment is covered by a tight fascia.

The anterior compartment is formed by the lateral surface of the tibia, the anterior crural fascia, the interosseous membrane, the anterior intermuscular septum, and the anterior surface of the fibula. It houses four muscles used for extension of the toes and dorsiflexion of the ankle. The tibialis anterior arises from the upper two-thirds of the tibia and is a dorsiflexor of the ankle and inverter of the foot. The extensor hallucis longus extends the great toe; the extensor digitorum longus extends the other toes and assists in eversion. The peroneus tertius, a portion of the extensor digitorum longus, assists in eversion. Blood supply to the anterior compartment is from the anterior tibial artery. The muscles are innervated by the deep peroneal nerve as it passes through the compartment. Occasionally, a branch of the common peroneal nerve innervates the tibialis anterior and the extensor digitorum longus. Lesions of the deep peroneal nerve can cause foot drop and sensory loss to the dorsum of the first and second toes (web space between great and second toe).

The lateral compartment contains the evertors of the foot, the peroneus longus and the peroneus brevis. This compartment lies between the anterior and posterior intermuscular septum, with the medial boarder being the fibula. Nerve supply is via the superficial peroneal nerve, which provides sensation to the greater part of the dorsum of the foot. Blood supply is from branches of the peroneal artery but does not by itself run through the lateral compartment.

The posterior compartment is divided into superficial and deep by the deep transverse crural fascia. The superficial posterior compartment contains the plantarflexors of the foot, the gastrocnemius, soleus, and plantaris. These muscles are supplied by branches of the tibial nerve. The sural nerve, a cutaneous nerve, supplies sensation to the calf and the lateral side of the foot and little toe.

The deep posterior compartment contains the muscles of toe flexion, ankle plantarflexion, and inversion. The flexor hallucis longus is the flexor of the great toe, and the flexor digitorum longus is the flexor of the lesser toes. Both of these muscles also contribute to plantarflexion of the ankle. The tibialis posterior arises from the tibia, fibula, and interosseous membrane. Its role is as a plantarflexor and inverter of the foot. These muscles are supplied by the tibial nerve and posterior tibial artery. The peroneal artery, arising from the posterior tibial artery, runs through the deep posterior compartment.

It should be noted that the fascia surrounding the posterior tibialis has been described as a separate and distinct compartment, the fifth compartment.[9] Isolated exertional compartment syndrome has been described in this compartment. Patients may present with pain along the posteromedial border of the lower third of the tibia. However, involvement of this area may mimic symptoms of other compartments or account for symptoms that are difficult to examine in one of the classical compartments.

GENERALIZED CLINICAL ASSESSMENT

Because the clinical presentations of exertional leg pain often overlap, a detailed history and physical examination are needed to establish a specific diagnosis or guide further ancillary studies.[10] A standardized approach to the runner presenting with exertional leg pain should be performed. The history and physical examination should emphasize particular extrinsic and intrinsic risk factors that may play a significant role in the development of running-related leg injuries.

History

A complete and thorough history should focus on the onset and duration of complaints, association with activity, location and quality of discomfort, and changes in the training regimen.

The onset of pain reported by the athlete can be classified as acute or chronic. Acute pain usually implies macrotrauma, often in a single event or episode that the athlete can recall. In chronic injuries the patient cannot recall a specific injury or mechanism, rather they state that the symptoms have gradually evolved over time. Gradual onset with chronic progression of symptoms is most often due to accumulated microtrauma and overuse.

The association of discomfort with activity should also be sought. Specifically, the athlete should be asked at what point in the run the discomfort occurs. It should be determined whether the pain is present at rest, early on in the run, at a predictable point, after the run, or at night.

Location of discomfort and the quality of the pain will provide diagnostic clues. It should be established whether the discomfort is focal or diffuse and which structures are involved (bone, muscle, tendon, or muscle-bone interface). The athlete should be questioned as to whether pain is present in the ankle, knee, hip, or back, which may indicate referred pain. Neurologic findings also point to specific anatomic areas.

Because overuse injury is the most frequent cause of exercise-related leg pain, additional history should focus on the training routine and extrinsic risk factors. Questions regarding initiation of the training program, pretraining fitness level, and changes in frequency, duration, and intensity should be asked. The concept of "too much, too fast, and too soon," especially in a deconditioned athlete, is frequently identified as an etiology of overuse injuries.[11]

Additionally, the physician should inquire about possible training errors. It has been shown that training errors are associated with 60% of injuries, of which 29% are due to excessive mileage.[5] These include intensity of workout, changes in surface, running course, changes in incline or decline, and equipment. Changing from a soft surface such as a cushioned running track or off-road trail to pavement running increases muscle and bone stress applied to the leg from the impact forces due to decreased shock absorption. Similarly, running over the identical course and surface applies constant forces repetitively to the lower extremity. Altering the running course not only decreases monotony but also allows adaptive responses to occur as different forces and loads are applied.

Changes in equipment relate to running shoes and their role in shock absorption and resultant impact stress or reaction force on the lower extremity. The athlete should be questioned as to the age of the running shoes, their condition, the number of miles on the shoes, or a recent change in running shoe. The type of shoe should also be examined in that the footwear may be inadequate for the running athlete, e.g., a recent change for a distance runner into racing flats or a novice runner into cross-training or basketball shoes. The body type should also be matched to the shoe. Heavy runners should have shoes with more shock absorption capacity.

Female athletes should be questioned in regard to menstrual cycle, caloric intake, and use of oral contraceptives as well as history of stress fracture or overuse injuries. This questioning may elicit a female athlete at risk for the female athlete triad.

Physical Examination

The physical examination should begin as soon as the patient enters the examination room. The athlete's gait should be examined to determine the presence of a limp or any obvious biomechanical imbalances.

Next, inspection of the athlete's lower extremity should be performed with the athlete in shorts. Inspection should include the back and the entire lower extremity to determine possible etiologies of the leg pain, including the hip, knee, and ankle joints.

The athlete should be asked to point to the area of maximal tenderness and say whether the tenderness is generalized or diffuse. Palpation of the lower extremity should follow, with emphasis on any abnormalities noted by inspection. Each of the compartments of the leg should be individually palpated for tenderness or defects such as a muscle tear or fascial hernia. The course of the tibia and fibula should be palpated for tenderness or abnormal nodular densities. If pain is present on palpation, it should be determined whether the pain is over the bone, the muscle, the tendon, or the interface of muscle attachment onto bone.

Range of motion of each joint should be tested. The ankle should be examined in plantarflexion, dorsiflexion, inversion, and eversion. Passive and active range of motion, as well as performance against resistance, should be tested with palpation of the muscles and muscle tendon junctions. In addition, muscles that span two joints should be examined with both joints in stretch (i.e., the knee extended and the ankle dorsiflexed). A careful neurologic and vascular examination of the leg and foot should be included.

Provocative maneuvers such as impact or resistance of plantar- and dorsiflexion may be helpful. If the athlete is free of discomfort at the time of examination, an attempt to produce symptoms should be included as part of the physical examination. An exercise challenge should be initiated by which the athlete is encouraged to reproduce the symptoms. The specific activities that cause symptoms or induce impact load stress should be performed and the examination repeated with onset of symptoms.

In addition, a search for anatomic variants and faulty biomechanics should be performed and attempts to correct abnormalities should be initiated early in the rehabilitation phase (see Chapters 5 and 6). Such intrinsic variables include structural and functional abnormalities in the foot and ankle,[12] leg length discrepancy, lower extremity malalignment, and running gait. Imbalances in muscle strength, fatigue, and flexibility also play a significant role. Due to the high mileage and chronic repetitive motion in running, even with mild variation in biomechanics, the deleterious effects are magnified.[5] Just as faulty biomechanics play a significant role in the etiology of overuse injury of the lower extremity, so too can they slow or inhibit rehabilitation. The foot should be evaluated as well as the running shoe. The muscles of the leg are intimately involved in foot movements, and any abnormality of foot motion can cause pathology in the shins where the muscles attach.[4] Pronation of the foot, pes planus, and pes cavus have all been associated with an increased risk of exertional leg pain; these respond to appropriate shoe orthotics. The running shoe should be inspected for any patterns of abnormal wear, which can be indicative of faulty biomechanics (see Chapter 46).[13,14]

Ancillary Studies

Additional studies can be utilized to confirm or rule out specific entities. Their use should be dictated by the history and physical examination (see Chapter 7).

Radiographs in the anteroposterior, lateral, and oblique views can be used to rule out bony etiology to the leg pain. Fracture, stress fracture, periosteal reaction, or endosteal reaction may be identified by radiographs. In addition, bone tumors and osteomyelitis can be ruled out. Stress fractures and stress reactions of bone, however, may not be appreciated on initial radiographs and may require several weeks and a healing response before the radiograph is "positive."

Triple-phase bone scan or scintigraphy is a highly sensitive method for evaluating disorders of the leg. This study can be used to differentiate periosteal injuries, stress fractures, delayed union or nonunion of stress fractures or fractures, compartment syndrome, myositis ossificans, connective tissue abnormalities, muscle injury, and rhabdomyolysis.[8]

Magnetic resonance imaging (MRI) can be used to quantify stress fractures or muscle tendon injuries. Information obtained from the MRI can often aid in establishing a diagnosis.

Compartment pressures are needed when the diagnosis of chronic exertional compartment syndrome is suspected. Measurements done before and after exercise should be obtained for comparison (see Chapter 9).

Angiography, nerve conduction studies, and electromyography (EMG) should be obtained as needed or dictated by history, physical examination, or failure to respond to treatment (see Chapter 8).

Treatment

Although specific treatment guidelines exist for each specific etiology of exercise-induced leg pain, a general principle of treatment of overuse injuries is common to all. In treatment, removing the athlete from the inducing insult is the hallmark of therapy. Rest should be prescribed as relative or absolute. Initially absolute rest or removing the athlete from all impact activity should be initiated so as to allow adaptive and reparative processes to begin. Additionally, the athlete should avoid any activity that causes pain or discomfort. If the patient is experiencing pain with weightbearing, crutches should be used for a brief period until ambulation can be performed pain free.

After the patient is pain free, he or she should initiate a program of "relative rest." Here, low-impact activity cross training such as water running, swimming, cross-country skiing, or stationary bike riding is initiated to maintain cardiorespiratory fitness and aerobic capacity. A flexibility program should be instituted. Resistance training is also believed to be beneficial in that stronger muscles fatigue less and absorb more shock. Depending on the diagnosis, a progressive running program can be initiated when there is no longer tenderness to digital palpation or impact activity.

Early in the rehabilitation process, correction of any biomechanical factors identified should be made, including orthotics and proper running shoes. Video gait analysis may prove to be beneficial in some athletes. The athlete should also be educated on any training errors that may have contributed to injury. If these factors are not corrected or identified, the injury will recur.

Close follow-up and reexamination are important in the therapy of exertional leg pain. If athletes are not responsive to an initial period of rest, the initial diagnosis should be questioned, and a more thorough investigation into an alternate diagnosis should be made.

"NORMAL" AND BENIGN CAUSES OF LEG PAIN

Many individuals will experience leg discomfort when beginning an exercise program from a deconditioned state. Similarly, conditioned athletes may experience leg pain when they exert themselves beyond a previously conditioned level. The natural response to abrupt onset or changes in training may appear immediately or be delayed. A metabolic origin is experienced during and immediately after intense exercise. The immediate response is believed to be caused by the biochemical end products of metabolism or temporary hypoxia due to muscle ischemia.[15] This discomfort is believed to be caused by mechanical and/or biochemical stimulation of nociceptors, with pain being due to the accumulation of noxious metabolites (bradykinin, hydrogen ion, prostaglandins, substance P, and lactate). Leg pain produced by these metabolites decreases rapidly during the first 3 minutes of recovery, followed by a slower secondary decline.[16] This is believed to be due to the removal of metabolites from the leg muscles during recovery. The naturally occurring discomfort experienced in the lower extremities with initiation of an exercise program shows a physiologic adaptation to exercise with continued training (training response). As conditioning improves, the athlete experiences less discomfort and can exercise for longer times and distances before the occurrence of discomfort (trained vs. untrained).

Delayed-onset muscle soreness (DOMS) is muscle discomfort and stiffness felt after unaccustomed exercise or muscular activity as a delayed response. The degree of discomfort is related to both the intensity of the muscular contraction and the duration of the activity. This disorder is highly associated with eccentric muscle contractions such as downhill running. In the unconditioned athlete, it is usually attributed to a single episode of unaccustomed activity. In the advanced or trained runner, it is caused by a sudden increase or change in training, especially in regard to intensity or volume (adding speed work or hills), after resuming training after an extended break, or addition of an activity that incorporates muscle groups not normally used.[17]

After a bout of exercise, serum enzymes peak at 8 to 24 hours, and peak soreness occurs 24 to 48 hours after exercise.[18] By 5 to 7 days after exercise, the symptoms are resolved.[15,19] The prevalence is unknown, since this is a temporary discomfort and those affected usually do not seek medical attention.

The etiology and pathophysiology of this entity is not completely understood. Possible mechanisms that have been proposed include metabolic stress (changes in cellular metabolism and metabolic waste products), mechanical factors (damage to contractile and connective tissue), thermal insult, and disturbed microcirculation.[15,20] These initial events may lead to a secondary response, including an inflammatory reaction.[17,20] This inflammatory response may be responsible for initiating, amplifying, and/or resolving the muscle injury.[21]

The characteristic presentation includes the complaint of a dull, aching muscular pain with stiffness of the involved muscles. Physical examination is significant for swelling, strength loss, decreased range of motion, and localized, tender muscles. Initially, the soreness is most evident at the muscle-tendon junction. This is followed by generalized tenderness throughout the muscle.[21]

Although multiple therapies may provide symptomatic relief, delayed-onset muscle soreness is a transient and self-limited response that usually requires no treatment. Nonsteroidal anti-inflammatory agents may be prescribed, but special care should be taken to ensure that the patient has no renal impairment or that a much more severe form of muscle damage, such as rhabdomyolysis, does not exist.

STRESS FRACTURE OF THE TIBIA AND FIBULA

Stress fracture of the lower extremity is a common overuse injury that should always be considered in the running athlete who presents with exertional leg pain. Running is the most common sport associated with stress fractures in athletes, with the most frequent anatomic site being the tibia.[22,23] The fibula has also consistently been shown to be a frequent site of stress fracture in athletes, especially in running events.[24]

Stress fracture is the ultimate response to an overuse injury, indicating that the body's ability to adapt to stress has been overloaded. Impact forces to the lower extremity that are generated during running are absorbed by muscle, bone, and joint mechanics (i.e., subtalar motion). Bone responds to this stress by remodeling. The initial (radiologically silent) response is resorption by osteoclasts, followed by new bone deposition by osteoblasts. Radiologically, the repair process is evidenced by cortical hypertrophy (the stress reaction). A "rest" period is required for this reparative and adaptive response. If the athlete continues to stress the bone, osteoclastic activity exceeds osteoblastic activity and results in a weakened bone in which individual trabeculae collapse, causing "microfractures" or stress fracture.[8]

Etiology

The etiology of stress fracture is multifactorial. Race, gender, and age have been identified as nonmodifiable risk factors. Intrinsic factors include subtalar/foot anatomy (pes planus or pes cavus) and cross-sectional area of the tibia (nonmodifiable). Factors that are highly associated with the development of stress fracture include initial fitness level, an abrupt change in the training regimen, running surface, or shoes, and inappropriate technique or gait. Factors related to calcium metabolism and the bony response to stress include menstrual irregularity, disordered eating, diet and caloric deprivation, and hormonal factors. Inadequate absorption of shock by fatigued or weakened muscle may also play a role.[25]

Clinical Assessment

Athletes with stress fracture usually present with a history of insidious onset of symptoms characteristic and highly suggestive of this pathology. Patients describe a gradual onset or progression of symptoms that initially begins as pain during or after exercise and progresses to pain during nonsport activities. Pain then occurs at rest and ultimately leads to reduced activity or none at all. The quality of pain is described as an initial focal and dull ache over the tibia or fibula. Over time, the pain becomes sharp and penetrating. Patients with fibular stress fractures will describe lateral leg pain or even ankle pain.

A properly conducted physical examination is highly suggestive of stress fracture. Patients often enter the examination room with an altered gait, in an attempt to limit the impact placed on the affected limb. Patients may have tenderness over the involved bone or soft tissue, but maximal tenderness is well localized. If a patient has had the complaint for some time, a palpable lump may be appreciated over the site, indicating periosteal reaction with local cortical thickening or callus formation.

An attempt to reproduce the pain with activity may also be conducted in the examination room. Having the patient apply impact to the bone by jumping up and down or jogging in place often elicits the characteristic pain. Bowing the tibia by applying pressure proximal and distal across a fulcrum may indicate stress fracture. In this "fulcrum" or "springing" test, the stress applied across the fracture plane should induce pain if the area is weakened.[25,26]

Two additional simple tests have been described that may assist in supporting the diagnosis of stress fracture may be performed using a tuning fork or an ultrasound machine.[10,27,28] The tuning fork test is performed by placing a vibrating tuning fork over the area of maximal tenderness. Exquisite pain is suggestive of a fracture. Similarly, continuous ultrasound passed over the suspected area of stress fracture may elicit pain. The reliability of these two test, however, has not been firmly established.

If stress fracture is suspected, radiographs should be obtained. Multiple views should be ordered, and a radioopaque marker placed at the site of maximal tenderness may be helpful. Radiographs have a high specificity but low sensitivity. Initial radiographs are often negative, as it may take several weeks to show radiologic evidence of fracture healing. The earliest radiographic evidence is cortical hyperostosis with occasional periosteal or endosteal reaction. Late signs include the fracture plane and callus, which confirm the diagnosis. The "dreaded black line" is a radiolucent line indicative of delayed healing or a nonunion of the anterior cortical surface of the tibia. Negative radiographs should not rule out the diagnosis of stress fracture.

If no radiographic evidence of stress fracture is noted, two possible courses of action may be taken based on the presence of symptoms and the level of the athlete. In the recreational athlete or when there is no doubt as to the diagnosis, the athlete should be treated for stress fracture and removed from training with close follow-up. When the diagnosis leaves some doubt or the athlete cannot afford a period of rest and a conclusive

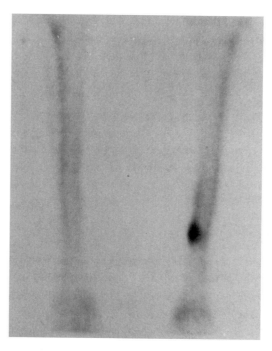

Figure 16–1. Focal fusiform uptake is noted in the posteromedial aspect of the distal left tibia. This image displays the typical scintigraphic finding of a stress fracture.

diagnosis must be made, a bone scan or MRI can be obtained.

Scintigraphy is currently the accepted gold standard for diagnosis of stress fracture and will usually be positive 3 to 5 days after the onset of pain. A bone scan is very reliable, with a characteristic focal uptake, high sensitivity, and the ability to distinguish stress reaction from stress fracture (Fig. 16–1). A bone scan may reveal radionuclide uptake at asymptomatic sites corresponding to painless remodeling of bone in response to stress (bone strain).[22]

MRI and computed tomography are also effective in identifying a stress fracture. MRI is highly sensitive and specific and can help determine other etiologies of exertional leg pain.

Treatment

The mainstay of treatment for stress fracture is cessation of the offending activity and rest, to allow adaptive cortical hypertrophy. Close follow-up is essential. The patient should be removed from any impact or activity that causes discomfort. Impact loading across the bone should be limited by use of crutches until the athlete can ambulate without discomfort. Limiting impact loading across the fracture site by splinting or use of a pneumatic leg brace may also be beneficial and may speed return to activity.[29] Cast immobilization should be considered if pain cannot be relieved by the lack of weightbearing. This complaint may suggest that a completion of the fracture is imminent. Women with menstrual irregularity should be advised on the importance of menstrual function and the role of hormones is stress fracture pathogenesis. Female athletes may even desire regulation of their menstrual cycle with oral contraceptives. Adequate caloric intake and supplemental calcium may also be recommended. Additional studies may include bone density monitoring. If the female athlete triad is suspected, the athlete should be referred to counseling for evaluation and treatment of any existing eating disorder (see Chapter 34).

Athletes should be encouraged to maintain aerobic fitness during the bony response phase. Rehabilitation with nonimpact activities such as swimming, pool jogging, or stationary bike riding is encouraged as long as no pain is elicited with these activities. A stretching and flexibility program should also be initiated. A resistive weight-training program may also be beneficial to the athlete. Strengthening the muscle will increase muscle endurance, decrease fatigue, and increase the ability to absorb shock.

The athlete should return for reevaluation at 2 weeks. Repeat radiographs should be obtained if the athlete notes continued pain. This is especially important if a question of compliance exists, as, again, the patient may have attempted to return to running with completion of the fracture.

Most stress fractures heal within 4 to 6 weeks. When the athlete can perform impact activities without pain and has no pain on digital palpation at the fracture site, and when radiographic evidence of healing is evident, he or she can return to a slowly progressive running program. Any risk factors should be modified. Specifically, foot anatomic variants should be corrected with orthotics. If no anatomic abnormalities are identified, an over-the-counter shock-absorbing insole can still be helpful. The athlete should begin running on a soft surface before running on pavement. Pain should be used as an indicator of progression of training. If at any point the athlete experiences discomfort, he or she should back off from the running program and seek consultation.

Special attention should be paid to stress fractures of the anterior cortex of the middle third of the tibia due to the high risk of nonunion and progression to a complete fracture.[25,30,31] These stress fractures require rest and a prolonged healing time. External electrical stimulation may assist in healing in some patients.[32] If pain recurs or a fracture is resistant to healing, as evidenced by the dreaded black line on follow-up radiographs, consultation with an orthopedic surgeon should be sought, as these stress fractures usually require intramedullary fixation and bone grafting (see

Chapter 53). Stress fracture of the medial malleolus also carries the potential for delayed union.[33]

TENDON INJURY

Tendon injury is a frequent cause of exertional leg pain in the running athlete. The clinical spectrum of tendon injury can range from inflammation (tendinitis, tendinosis, tenosynovitis) to partial disruptions (strains) or complete tears of the muscle tendon unit. Muscle-tendon injuries can occur in any of the muscles of the leg.

Acute tendon injury is often localized to the muscle tendon unit and is commonly attributed to poor preparticipation stretching or conditioning. In contrast, chronic injury often involves the entire course of the tendon and is attributed to repetitive microtrauma, presenting as a gradual progression of symptoms. In both the chronic and acute presentations, the patient will display pain with resistance of the specific motor group as well as discomfort when the inflamed tendons are stretched.[10] Swelling and crepitation over the involved tendon may be noted as the tendon is moved within its sheath (tenosynovitis).

Etiology

The contributing etiologic factors include the same extrinsic and intrinsic factors previously discussed. The most common etiologic factors, however, are poor preparticipation conditioning and muscle tendon inflexibility. Posterior tibialis and peroneal tendonitis may be secondary to ankle instability.

Clinical Assessment

Patients with tendinitis usually present with symptoms occurring during normal daily activities. Patients will complain of stiffness or weakness with any stress of the involved muscles. Specific muscle testing in passive, active, and resisted range of motion will determine the involved muscles. To distinguish which muscles are involved, first determine which compartment is involved, anterior, posterior, or lateral. After the compartment has been isolated, then the specific muscle-tendon unit can be determined by manual muscle testing of each muscle of the compartment. Posterior tibialis tendinitis has presenting symptoms like medial tibial stress syndrome and chronic exertional compartment syndrome of the deep posterior compartment. As part of a complete physical examination, muscle tendon flexibility should be examined over the entire lower extremity, including the hip, knee, and ankle. The diagnosis is based on history and physical examination. Radiologic and other ancillary studies described earlier may be used to rule out other etiologies.

A muscle strain or tear of the medial head of the gastrocnemius at the muscle-tendon junction has been termed *tennis leg*. This syndrome is most often acute but can be chronic.[34] Athletes complain of a sudden, intense pain in the calf while running and may or may not experience pain with normal ambulation. Range of motion testing will reveal decreased dorsiflexion of the foot and decreased pain in the extremes of motion (extension or full dorsiflexion). Patients also display pain with toe raises and with toe-off in a walk or run cycle. The Thompson test (passive test) should also be performed to test the integrity of the gastrocnemius-soleus complex. Clinically, the patient may also have a Homan's sign, suggesting a deep vein thrombosis.

Treatment

Treatment principles depend on the degree to which the muscle-tendon unit is injured. Mild strains are injuries without muscle dysfunction, evidenced only by an inflammatory response and discomfort. These are treated according to the PRICEMM principle (protection, rest, ice, compression, elevation, medication, and modalities). A stretching and strengthening program should be included in the rehabilitation of the athlete, and normal flexibility and strength should be present prior to the return to activity.

A decreased range of motion or decreased strength indicates more severe injury with damage to the muscle-tendon unit. In addition to the PRICEMM principles, these strains may necessitate a short period of immobilization to allow initiation of healing. If a defect is palpable, indicating a tear of the muscle-tendon unit to any degree, a severe strain is present. Here, there exists some degree of loss of muscle function. Orthopedic consultation should be obtained as these injuries may require surgical intervention.

Prevention includes a program of regular stretching and lower extremity flexibility.

COMPARTMENT SYNDROMES

Compartment syndromes in the running athlete can occur in two forms, acute and chronic. The distinction between the two is in the reversibility of the ischemic insult. In acute compartment syndrome, the ischemia is irreversible and rapidly leads to tissue necrosis unless emergency decompression is performed. In chronic exertional related compartment syndrome, the ischemia is reversible and subsides with rest or discontinuation of the offending activity.

Acute Compartment Syndrome

Acute compartment syndrome usually occurs in association with trauma. However, it has been reported following minor athletic injury.[35] It is rare in previously active patients. In athletics, it is most commonly seen in an individual unaccustomed to intense physical activity who engages in a prolonged event or with gross overexertion.[36] In the trained or elite runner, acute compartment syndrome may occur along with a history of chronic exertional compartment syndrome, which may progress to the acute form, especially if an attempt is made to run through the pain.[37]

Although one must maintain a high index of suspicion based on the history of the injury, some characteristic findings include pain out of proportion to injury, presence of paresthesias and sensory deficits, tense and swollen compartment on palpation, decreased or loss of active motion, and severe pain with passive stretch. The treatment for acute compartment syndrome is emergency surgical decompression via fasciotomy.

Chronic Exertional Compartment Syndrome

Much more commonly experienced in athletes is chronic exertional compartment syndrome. This is the development of recurrent episodes of reversible ischemia due to a transient elevation in the intracompartmental pressure, which subsides with rest or cessation of activity. Although thought to be uncommon in relation to other exertional leg complaints, this etiology is probably more prevalent than expected, with the diagnosis often being missed and patients treated with inappropriate therapy.[36,38] Although any athlete can develop these symptoms, runners are most commonly affected.[37–39]

Etiology

Four factors are believed to contribute to an increase in intracompartmental pressure during exercise.[40] These are enclosure of compartmental contents in an inelastic fascial sheath, increased volume of the skeletal muscle with exertion due to blood flow and edema, muscle hypertrophy as a response to exercise, and dynamic contraction factors due to the gait cycle. It has been noted that the development of symptoms may be more common at the beginning of running season due to muscle hypertrophy, which decreases the volume in the compartment.[36] Rapid increases in muscle size due to fluid retention are also believed to play a role in the development of chronic exertional compartment syndrome in athletes taking the popular supplement creatine.

Whether due to the increased volume of the compartments with exercise, the abnormally small or inelastic compartment, or both, the end result is an increase in pressure within the myofascial compartment to the point that blood flow is compromised. When tissue perfusion is not adequate to meet the metabolic demands, the result is traversing neurologic and muscular ischemia, pain, and impairment of muscular function.

Clinical Assessment

The characteristic presenting complaint of patients with chronic exertional compartment syndrome is recurrent exercise-induced leg discomfort that occurs at a well-defined and reproducible point in the run and increases if the training persists. The quality of pain is usually described as a tight, cramp-like, or squeezing ache over a specific compartment of the leg. Athletes can reliably predict at what intensity or what distances the discomfort will occur as well as how long pain will last, depending on the intensity and distance run. Relief of symptoms only occurs with discontinuation of activity.

Most say that the discomfort developed gradually with increased conditioning, with progressive worsening over time. The time to result in performance decline is variable and has been described over weeks or months.[40] One theory that may explain the progressive nature of this disorder is that of an evolving vicious cycle of response to continued insult by repeated bouts of exertion despite clinical symptoms. It is thought that fascia exposed to stretch respond by thickening and increased tensile strength.[7] This is thought to account for both the progressive increase of symptoms seen in patients over time as their exercise routine is continued and the thickened fascial tissue noted on biopsy.[38]

Other historical factors that may indicate chronic exertional compartment syndrome include foot numbness, muscle weakness, or a sense of ankle instability or fatigue.[41] The complaint of paresthesias of the leg or foot with exertion may be described and indicates involvement of the nerve traversing the compartment. The athlete may have bilateral symptoms, and more than one compartment may be affected simultaneously.

Additional historical inquiry should focus on the use of ergogenic supplements such as creatine. We have seen chronic exertional compartment syndrome symptoms resolve in athletes after they have stopped taking creatine.

Nerve entrapment syndromes of the lower extremity as well as the intermittent claudication of atherosclerosis present with similar manifestations and should be included in the differential diagnosis.

Although some athletes experience persistent, unrelenting tightness, most athletes with exertional compartment syndrome will usually present with a normal gait and a normal lower extremity examination. The only abnormality that may be noted at rest is a muscle hernia through a fascial defect.[42] The patient can often localize symptoms to the involved compartment.

If the history is strongly suggestive of exertional compartment syndrome, after a normal resting examination is established, the athlete should undergo an exercise challenge and a complete postexercise examination as detailed in Chapter 9. Although a classic history may suggest the diagnosis of chronic exertional compartment syndrome, an exercise challenge and measurement of compartmental pressures are essential to confirm the diagnosis.

Radiographs are not beneficial in the diagnosis of chronic exertional compartment syndrome, but they may be used to rule out other etiologies.

Treatment

To date, the only conservative symptom-relieving therapy is cessation of the insulting activity, participating at an intensity that does not induce symptoms or, ultimately, a change in sport. Athletes who want to continue aerobic conditioning but who do not desire surgical intervention should consider cycling as an alternative exercise. Cycling does not induce compartment pressure elevations as high as those seen with running.[43]

Fasciotomy is indicated if the athlete is unwilling to decrease the level of activity or experiences severe symptoms or restrictions with any activity (see Chapter 53).

Although the ischemia of chronic exertional compartment syndrome is generally considered reversible, chronic and repetitive recurrence of elevated pressures can induce irreversible injury to the muscles and the nerves within the affected compartment. Abnormal muscle and fascial biopsies taken at the time of fasciotomy have been described.[38] In addition, in athletes with chronic exertional ischemia, the risk of progression exists from reversible deficits to irreversible acute compartment syndrome.[41] Athletes who do not desire fasciotomy should be advised that continued symptoms or attempts to perform through the pain can result in acute compartment syndrome.

TIBIAL STRESS REACTION: PERIOSTITIS AND THE MEDIAL TIBIAL STRESS SYNDROME

Pain along the tibial shaft with exertion that is not focal but generalized is often produced by a traction periostitis at the muscle attachment site to bone. Periostitis is believed to be more common than both stress fractures and chronic compartment syndrome.[36] Again, runners are the athletes most frequently encountered with this disorder.[44]

Periostalgia is most commonly seen over the anterolateral or posteromedial aspects of the tibia and has been described as "anterior periostitis" and "medial periostitis."[27] Anterior periostitis is due to overuse and traction of the periosteum of the anterior tibialis muscle and peroneus tertius. Medial periostitis affects the posterior compartment muscles and induces pain in the posteromedial aspect of the distal tibia. The medial variant, frequently referred to in the literature as "medial tibial stress syndrome," is believed to be more common and has been shown to occur in 13% of all running injuries.[5] Although most commonly attributed to the posterior tibialis muscle, the soleus muscle has also been implicated as the cause of the pain in this location.[45]

Etiology

The development of periosteal inflammation is believed to be part of a continuum of tibial stress reaction due to repetitive impact loading forces on the lower extremity and overuse of the muscles of the anterior or posterior compartment. The traction forces applied to the periosteum result in a traction periostitis. In an attempt to adapt to the chronic insult, the periosteum produces osteoblasts in response to the stress on bone. Periosteal thickening and cortical hypertrophy occur. If rest is implemented and a progressive exercise program is implemented, the muscle-bone interface has time to adapt, and periosteal thickening and cortical hypertrophy occur. If the athlete continues to work through the discomfort or does not decrease the current exercise regime, a stress fracture may develop. With triple-phase bone scans, Matin[8] has proposed a five-stage description of stress response of the tibia (stages of skeletal injury) from minimal periosteal reaction through adaptive bone reaction (early stress fracture), to complete full-thickness stress fracture (Fig. 16–2).[8] A similar progressive staging system has been proposed using MRI.[46] It is not uncommon to see tibial cortical hypertrophy on radiographs in runners who present with the complaint of generalized discomfort over the tibial shaft with exertion. This subperiosteal new bone and cortical hypertrophy represent radiologic evidence of functional adaptation.[2]

Periostitis often imitates other pathologic conditions in that it is variable in its clinical presentation and by history can often be confused with stress fracture, tendinitis, and chronic exertional compartment syndrome. With the notion that periostitis is one point in a continuum, the diagnosis should be one of exclusion. Attempts must be made to rule out stress fracture, tendinitis of the posterior or anterior compartment muscles, or chronic compartment syndrome. It is important to note that the diagnosis of stress fracture or chronic exertional compartment syndrome does not necessarily rule out the coexistence of periostitis. These

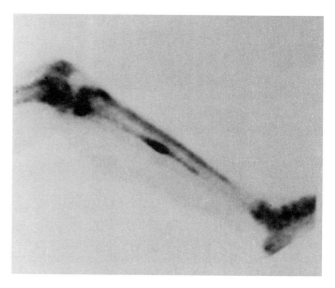

Figure 16–2. This image displays the appearance of a stress fracture with coexisting periostitis on bone scan. A fusiform area of intense uptake is noted in the posteromedial cortex of the midshaft. In addition, a more diffuse linear uptake is noted that is consistent with periostitis.

etiologies may exist with a concomitant periosteal reaction as a possible contributing factor or a direct result of the associated pathology.

The development of periostitis is multifactorial, often with both extrinsic and intrinsic factors contributing in combination. Abrupt changes in training, running on hard surfaces, inadequate arch support, and poor running shoes are commonly seen in the patient with periostitis. Biomechanical factors that have been shown to correlate highly with the development of periostalgia include muscle fatigue, muscle-tendon inflexibility, pes planus, subtalar joint mobility, and greater Achilles' tendon angle.[12] Overpronation is a well-documented cause of periostitis.[45,47,48] The influence of prior training is also important, with periostitis commonly occurring in the unconditioned athlete who initiates a vigorous training program compared with a conditioned athlete.[11,36] It has been shown that periostitis is more common early in the sporting season or when workouts are intensified.[26]

Clinical Assessment

Athletes with periostalgia characteristically complain of recurrent dull ache along the tibial shaft, most commonly along the anterolateral or posterior medial aspect of the distal tibia, that may occur at any point in the workout. The description of the quality and occurrence of discomfort with exertion is variable. The quality of pain ranges from a dull, aching soreness to a sharp, persistent pain. The athlete will note that the pain initially occurs with exertion but then may resolve with continued running (ability to run through the pain). During the run or activity, the discomfort may recur or occur after the workout, at rest, or with walking. Like chronic exertional compartment syndrome, the pain may impair or limit participation in the event or may progress to nonsport activities. Fifty percent of patients complain of bilateral symptoms.[7]

Athletes with periostalgia present with the finding of diffuse tenderness to palpation along the tibial shaft at rest and after activity. Patients with involvement of the anterior compartment muscles will present with pain over the anterolateral aspect of the tibia, whereas those with involvement of the posterior compartments will complain of pain along the posteromedial border of the distal third of the tibia. Pain can usually be elicited by manual muscle testing, which will also indicate the muscles involved. This can easily be accomplished by active resisted plantarflexion or having the patient stand on the toes. Pain will be generalized over the tibial shaft and will not involve the muscle-tendon junction or the muscle bellies themselves. The athlete will have a normal neurologic as well as vascular examination.

It is extremely important to include an examination for biomechanical deficiencies in the initial and subsequent evaluations.

Initial studies should include radiographs to rule out stress fracture. However, since the clinical presentation of generalized, diffuse tenderness is distinctly different that that of the focal tenderness seen with stress fracture, radiographs may be reserved for those who fail to respond to a short period of rest and in whom symptoms persist at follow-up examination. Radiographs in athletes with periostalgia will usually be normal but can occasionally show stress reactions such as endosteal thickening, periosteal new bone formation, or cortical thickening of the tibia, as described earlier (Fig. 16–3).[45,47]

In highly competitive athletes for whom a brief trial of rest or decrease in training regimen is not acceptable and in whom the differentiation from periostitis and stress fracture must be made, bone scan has become invaluable for this distinction. Bone scans are also useful if the patient is not responding or slowly responding to therapy or when confirmation of the diagnosis is desired.

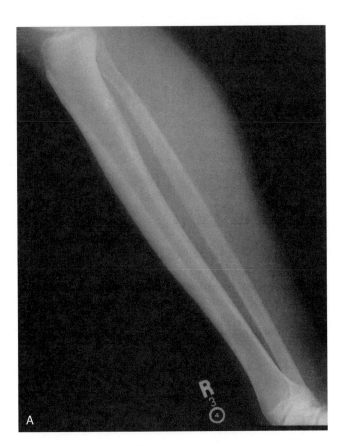 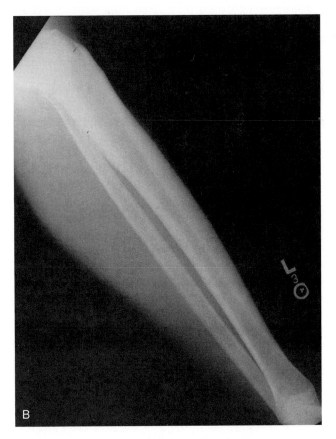

Figure 16–3. (*a, b*) Radiographs from a patient with chronic periostitis. Note cortical thickening of each tibia and irregularity of the anterior cortex. On palpation, the patient had multiple nodular densities over the anterior tibia, which was consistent with callus at sites of healed stress fractures. These "speed bumps" can be appreciated at close inspection of the radiographs.

Periostitis has a distinctive scintigraphic appearance. The triple-phase bone scan will identify periostitis as diffuse cortical hypertrophy seen as diffuse periosteal uptake. Tracer uptake will display a longitudinally oriented lesion involving one-third or more of the length of the bone that is specific to periostitis. Histologically, the increased metabolic activity seen on the bone scan is due to a periostitis with new bone formation.[45]

MRI can also be used to grade the severity of the stress injury and differentiate periostitis from stress fracture.[46]

In the patient with exertional leg pain, compartment pressure readings can help differentiate between periostitis and chronic exertional compartment syndrome. A diagnostic injection may also be useful to differentiate periostitis from compartment syndrome and stress fracture. Injection of a local anesthetic into the area has been shown to relieve the pain and allow the patient to exercise without discomfort.[47]

Treatment

The most important aspect in the treatment for periostalgia is rest, allowing the traction response of the muscle-bone connection to occur with adaptive cortical bone hypertrophy. The most important aspect in the prevention of future recurrence is correction of training errors, determined by history, as well as biomechanical deficiencies identified on physical examination. If biomechanical deficiencies are not identified and corrected, the athlete can expect recurrence.

Whether the rest is absolute or relative depends on the severity of the presentation, the limitations imposed on the athlete, and the athlete's level of participation. Relative activity modification guidelines should be followed, e.g., aqua jogging for cross training (see Chapter 40). The clinician should additionally focus on prevention of recurrence and a gradual, slowly progressive programmed return to activity. Athletes with excessive pronation should be considered for prescription orthotics. Athletes should run on compliant surfaces that absorb impact prior to returning to hard, unyielding terrain, as well as ensuring that they wear a shock-absorbing, well-fitted shoe. A strengthening and flexibility program should be initiated with the goal of correcting any muscle imbalances. As a minimum, flexibility of the gastrocsoleus should be emphasized, as well as strengthening, including the foot intrinsics, dorsiflexors, plantarflexors, invertors, evertors, and gluteals. All deficits within the kinetic chain should be corrected.

Additional forms of therapy that have been utilized include nonsteroidal anti-inflammatory agents (NSAIDs) and cryotherapy before and after exertion. Compression with an elastic bandage may provide relief to some athletes. The thought here is that uniform compression stabilizes the muscles and decreases the tension and sheer forces applied to the muscle-tendon junction and/or periosteum. A commercially available sleeve is available that has been shown anecdotally to assist some athletes with more rapid return to their running program.

Operative therapy has been described for the athlete with severe limitations of physical activity, frequent recurrence, or no response to available therapy.[7,44] Surgical treatment for periostalgia has not been uniformly successful and should be reserved for recalcitrant symptoms that have not responded to a well-documented treatment program of at least 6 months.

NEUROLOGIC ETIOLOGIES

Nerve Entrapment and Compression

Nerve entrapment and compression are less frequent causes of exertional leg pain. This diagnosis should be entertained in any athlete who is suspected of having exertional compartment syndrome but is noted to have normal intracompartmental pressures.

In the lower extremity, the nerve most commonly subject to compression or entrapment is the peroneal nerve. In the leg, the common peroneal nerve leaves the popliteal fossa and winds forward around the lateral aspect of the neck of the fibula. Here, in the lateral compartment, it divides into a deep and a superficial peroneal nerve. The deep peroneal nerve enters the anterior compartment, and the superficial nerve remains in the lateral compartment.

Entrapment of the common peroneal nerve presents as activity-related pain, paresthesias, and/or numbness during running in the anterolateral aspect of the leg.[49,50] Patients may have tenderness to palpation over the nerve at the fibular neck, a positive Tinel's sign, motor weakness, or a foot drop. Athletes may also display a diminished muscle mass in the anterolateral aspect of the leg.[51]

Superficial peroneal nerve injury is most commonly seen in runners.[52,53] Athletes with entrapment of the superficial peroneal nerve present with a history very similar to that of chronic exertional compartment syndrome of the lateral compartment. Most commonly, the complaint is of a burning, superficial pain with alterations in sensation over the nerve's distribution over the dorsum of the foot associated with activity and relieved by rest. A muscle herniation associated with a fascial defect may be noted over the anterolateral aspect of the leg approximately 10 cm above the lateral malleolus at the site where the nerve is entrapped.[54]

Athletes are often asymptomatic at the time of initial examination, and an exercise challenge is often needed to reproduce symptoms. EMG and nerve conduction studies are useful in the confirmation of the diagnosis. The test should be conducted after exertion, as the athlete may have a normal nerve conduction test if it is performed at rest.[55]

Saphenous nerve entrapment presents as medial knee and medial leg pain. This syndrome is usually seen after localized medial knee trauma. A classic example would be a track athlete who strikes her medial knee while jumping a hurdle and sustains mild soft tissue injury but notes persistent pain and irritation on the medial aspect of the knee or leg. Here, a diagnostic lidocaine block can assist in making the diagnosis.

Entrapment of the sural nerve will present with posterior calf symptoms and can be almost indistinguishable from chronic exertional compartment syndrome of the superficial posterior compartment.

The proximal tibial nerve may be compressed at the popliteal fossa, by the head of the gastrocnemius, or by a baker's cyst. The differential diagnosis should include scarring after gastrocnemius rupture, posterior compartment syndrome, dynamic popliteal artery compression, and medial tibial stress syndrome.[56]

Mild cases of nerve entrapment syndromes of the lower extremity can usually be effectively treated with NSAIDs, relative rest, and biomechanical correction with orthotics if necessary. Recalcitrant cases or those involving denervation may require surgical release at the site of compression.

Lumbosacral Radiculopathy

A herniated lumbar disc should be suspected in any runner with the complaint of leg pain, especially if it is associated with back or buttock discomfort.[57] Physical examination findings may include a positive straight leg raise test or neurologic deficits. Tests that can help confirm the diagnosis include radiography, EMG, and MRI (see Chapter 12 for detailed therapeutic recommendations).

Neurogenic Claudication

Lumbar spinal stenosis can be the cause of both back and leg pain in the older athlete. Although the most common complaint is back pain with radiation into the buttocks and thighs, neurogenic intermittent claudication may present with symptoms limited to the lower legs and feet.[58] Symptoms include leg fatigue, paresthesias, and weakness that occur in association with physical activity and remain present until activity ceases. CT or MRI will demonstrate lumbar canal and foraminal narrowing. Conservative treatment includes anti-inflammatory measures and rehabilitative exercise. Surgical decompression/stabilization is required in refractory cases and those with progressive neurologic deficits.

VASCULAR ETIOLOGIES

Vascular etiologies are rarely involved in exertional leg pain. Symptoms of claudication in the runner can be caused by arterial vascular diseases, including popliteal artery entrapment, adventitial cystic disease, adductor canal outlet syndrome, systemic arteritis (vasculitis), or Buerger's disease.[59,60] A venous etiology such as deep venous thrombosis should also be considered.

Popliteal artery entrapment should be included in the differential in the running athlete with exertional calf and upper leg pain.[61,62] This syndrome has classically been attributed to a congenitally abnormal relationship between the popliteal artery and the medial head of the gastrocnemius, which causes intermittent claudication during exertion.[36,63] However, a "functional" popliteal entrapment has been described in which no anatomic abnormalities are noted in the popliteal fossa and entrapment has been attributed to compression from the soleus and plantaris muscles,[64] as well as muscle hypertrophy of the gastrocnemius.[65] Popliteal artery entrapment is often misdiagnosed as chronic posterior exertional compartment syndrome, due to the ischemic etiology in the pathogenesis of symptoms in both syndromes. Not only is proper diagnosis important to return the athlete to activity, but, more importantly, repeated popliteal artery compression is believed to initiate changes in the arterial wall leading to premature localized atherosclerosis.

Symptoms include cramping, calf pain, and coolness and/or paresthesias of the foot that occur with exertion and are relieved with rest. Physical examination at rest is normal, and an exercise challenge is often required to produce symptoms. Popliteal, posterior tibial, and dorsalis pedis pulses should be checked before and after the exercise challenge. Specific in-office clinical testing that may elicit a decrease in pedal pulses includes active plantarflexion or passive dorsiflexion of the ankle with the knee extended.[59,61]

The diagnosis of popliteal artery entrapment can be established with careful selection of diagnostic studies.[66] Noninvasive studies such as Doppler ultrasonography should be used as initial screening tests. An ankle/brachial index should be performed both before and after an exercise challenge.[67,68] MRI and dynamic magnetic resonance angiography may be beneficial in the evaluation for anatomic etiologies of entrapment. Arteriography with provocative maneuvers is needed to confirm the diagnosis.

Nonoperative treatment is avoidance of the offending or exacerbating activities. This often entails discontinuation of the current level of the running program. If this option is not acceptable to the athlete, the definitive option is surgery.

The *adductor canal syndrome* or *adductor hiatus syndrome* is a rare cause of leg claudication. The etiology of this syndrome is thrombosis of the superficial femoral artery at the level of the adductor hiatus due to constriction from the vastus medialis or adductor magnus tendon.[59] Symptoms include calf pain, numbness, paresthesias, and coolness of the foot. Decreased distal pulses are noted on physical examination due to the occluding thrombus. Angiography is diagnostic, and the treatment is surgical.

Effort-induced venous thrombosis has been reported in the literature in running athletes.[69–71] This syndrome may present in some ways like periostitis.[69] Typical complaints from the athlete include pain and swelling of the leg. Physical examination may reveal calf tenderness with a positive Homan's sign and superficial venous distention. Dehydration, hemoconcentration, and a hypercoagulable state have all been identified as potential etiologies. Doppler ultrasonography may detect this condition, but venography is not infrequently required for equivocal cases. The treatment is anticoagulation.

Adventitial cystic disease is a rare cause of intermittent claudication. In this entity, myxomatous degeneration of the adventitial layer of the popliteal artery occurs, forming a cystic structure that can induce ischemia.[59] These patients present with calf claudication and absent or diminished popliteal and pedal pulses. Arterial ultrasound and/or angiography are used for diagnosis, and the treatment is surgical.

Buerger's disease, also known as thrombangitis obliterans, occurs most commonly in young adult males and involves segmental inflammatory occlusion of small and medium-sized arteries of the extremities.[59] This etiology should be suspected in athletes who use tobacco products and complain of claudication of the calf or foot, as well as coolness, numbness, or cyanosis of the feet or hands. Arterial ultrasound and/or angiography are used for diagnosis, and the mainstay of therapy involves discontinuation of tobacco use.

MUSCULAR ETIOLOGIES

Muscle cramps are painful involuntary muscle contractions that occur most commonly in the gastrocnemius. The exact mechanism or etiology of the contraction is uncertain. Possible origins include dehydration and electrolyte disturbances (hyponatremia, hypokalemia, and hypocalcemia). Cramps may be evident clinically by muscle twitches or fasciculations. Treatment involves active stretching, passive stretching, and massage as well as adequate hydration. Although quinine has been used as a treatment for muscle cramps, its efficacy for this use has not been firmly established.[72] The nutritional supplement creatine has also been found to be associated with cramps.

Exertional rhabdomyolysis is an acute, rapidly progressive, and potentially lethal response to severe exertion. It is often difficult to distinguish this entity clinically from delayed-onset muscle soreness, and it may actually be the extreme form of this latter condition.[19] Rhabdomyolysis presents with diffuse muscle pain, decreased range of motion, weakness, swelling, and tenderness to palpation of the involved muscle group. It may also be recognized by the presence of dark brown urine due to the myoglobinuria. Characteristic laboratory abnormalities include elevations of creatine phosphokinase, lactate dehydrogenase, blood urea nitrogen, creatinine, and myoglobinuria.[73] Compartment pressures may be elevated. Risk factors for the development of rhabdomyolysis include excessive exertion, poor level of fitness, dehydration, hot weather, and sickle cell trait.

Early identification and aggressive intervention is essential. Potential complications of this disorder include compartment syndrome, acute renal failure due to myoglobin in the kidneys, cardiac arrhythmias due to increased plasma potassium, and death. The triplephase bone scan may aid in the diagnosis as well as localization of muscle necrosis.[8]

Treatment is hospitalization with intravenous hydration. Close monitoring of urine output and lab values should be performed. Alkalinization of the urine may also be necessary to prevent myoglobin deposition in the kidney.

Myositis is due to overuse of muscle. In the leg, the anterior tibialis and posterior tibialis are commonly affected, but any muscle of the leg may be involved. The presentation and history are very similar to those of periostitis and tendinitis. Tenderness is located over the muscle and muscle-tendon junction rather than along the tibia. Like periostitis, symptoms are most common early in the season in unconditioned athletes.[74] The treatment is rest, anti-inflamatory medications, and a rehabilitation program of stretching and strengthening.

Myositis ossificans is heterotopic ossification of muscle tissue that occasionally complicates healing of a muscular contusion. In the lower extremity, the most common sites are the quadriceps and the gastrocnemius. Typical complaints include swelling, tenderness to palpation, muscle pain, and stiffness following an incident of blunt trauma. Chronic pain or muscle dysfunction may also be presenting complaints. The athlete may note crepitus or a cracking sensation if the ectopic bone has fractured within the muscle. On physical examination, the ossification may be appreciated with deep palpation. Athletes may also have loss of strength in the affected muscle group.[75]

Radiographs are needed to make the diagnosis. However, early after the injury the calcification cannot be identified by radiographs. Bone scan and MRI, however, can detect early development of this phenomenon. Scintigraphy is also useful to evaluate maturity if surgical excision is considered. Laboratory findings may also be present and include increased erythrocyte sedimentation rate and serum alkaline phosphatase.[73]

Treatment should initially begin with the muscular contusion. Immediate gentle passive stretching of the involved muscle limits the zone of injury and decreases the formation of hematoma and subsequent scarring. This early stretching may limit the chance of heterotopic ossification and maintain muscle length as well as decrease contracture.

Surgical excision should not be performed unless deficits are noted and maturity of lesion is evidenced by bone scan.

Interesting variants have been described in the literature. The involvement of the entire anterior and part of the deep posterior compartments has been reported after compartment syndrome in a patient who presented with limitation of ankle movements and pain with walking.[76] Chronic interosseous membrane sprain causing myositis ossificans of the interosseous tibiofibular ligament has also been described.[26] Here, tearing of the anterior and posterior tibiofibular ligament and lower third of the interosseous membrane occurs with the spreading of the fibula away from the tibia. Bone develops as an exostosis or across the interspace, causing a synostosis. The athlete complains of a spasm-like feeling in the leg and instability of the ankle with activity.[26]

OTHER ETIOLOGIES

Several other less common etiologies should be considered in the differential diagnosis of exertional leg pain. Infectious etiologies such as *cellulitis* or *osteomyelitis* should not be excluded. Similarly, *neoplastic* processes always deserve consideration. Osteoid osteoma, a benign bone tumor, may also be associated with exertional leg pain. Typically, patients complain of night pain that is relieved by aspirin. A bone scan and CT scan will help differentiate this condition from a stress fracture.

SUMMARY

Exertional leg pain is a common complaint in the running athlete. Though multiple etiologies exist, the underlying pathogenesis is often related to overuse in association with training errors. A detailed history, physical examination, and proper use of ancillary studies are essential to establish a specific pathoanatomic diagnosis. Treatment and rehabilitation should include identification and correction of biomechanical deficiencies and modifiable risk factors as well as ensure full strength and flexibility prior to the return of the athlete to their running program.

REFERENCES

1. Orava S, Puranen J: Athletes' leg pains. *Br J Sports Med* 1979:13, 92.
2. Batt ME: Shin splints—a review of terminology. *Clin J Sport Med* 1995:5, 53.
3. Briner WW: Shinsplints. *Am Fam Physician* 1988:37, 155.
4. Bates P: Shin splints—a literature review. *Br J Sports Med* 1985:19, 132.
5. James SL, Bates BT, Osternig LR: Injuries to runners. *Am J Sports Med* 1978:6, 40.
6. Allen MJ, Barnes MR: Exercise pain in the lower leg: Chronic compartment syndrome and medial tibial syndrome. *J Bone Joint Surg Br* 1986:68-B, 818.
7. Detmer DE: Chronic shin splints—classification and management of medial tibial stress syndrome. *Sports Med* 1986:3, 436.
8. Matin P: Basic principles of nuclear medicine techniques for detection and evaluation of trauma and sports medicine injuries. *Semin Nucl Med* 1988:18, 90.
9. Davey JR, Rorabeck CH, Fowler PJ: The tibialis posterior muscle compartment—an urecognized cause of exertional compartment syndrome. *Am J Sports Med* 1984:12, 391.
10. Hutchinson MR, Cahoon S, Atkins T: Chronic leg pain: Putting the diagnostic pieces together. *Physician Sportsmed* 1998:26, 37.
11. Andrish JT, Bergfeld JA, Walheim J: A prospective study on the management of shin splints. *J Bone Joint Surg Am* 1974:56-A, 1697.
12. Viitasalo JT, Kvist M: Some biomechanical aspects of the foot and ankle in athletes with and without shin splints. *Am J Sports Med* 1983:11, 125.
13. Cook SD, Brinker MR, Poche M: Running shoes—their relationship to running injuries. *Sports Med* 1990:10, 1.
14. Drez D: Running footwear: Examination of the training shoe, the foot, and functional orthotic devices. *Am J Sports Med* 1980:8, 140.
15. Cleak MJ, Eston RG: Delayed onset muscle soreness: Mechanisms and management. *J Sports Sciences* 1992:10, 325.
16. Cook DB, O'Connor PJ, Eubanks SA, et al.: Naturally occurring muscle pain during exercise: Assessment and experimental evidence. *Med Sci Sports Exerc* 1997:29, 999.

17. Pyne DB: Exercise-induced muscle damage and inflammation: A review. *Aust J Sci Med Sport* 1994:26, 49.

18. Tiidus PM, Ianuzzo CD: Effects of intensity and duration of muscular exercise on delayed soreness and serum enzyme activities. *Med Sci Sports Exerc* 1983:15, 461.

19. Armstrong RB: Mechanisms of exercise induced delayed onset muscular soreness: A brief review. *Med Sci Sports Exerc* 1984:16, 529.

20. Kuipers H: Exercise-induced muscle damage. *Int J Sports Med* 1994:15, 132.

21. MacIntyre DL, Reid WD, McKenzie DC: Delayed muscle soreness: The inflammatory response to muscle injury and its clinical implications. *Sports Med* 1995:20, 24.

22. Matheson GO, Clement DB, McKenzie DC, et al.: Stress fractures in athletes: A study of 320 cases. *Am J Sports Med* 1987:15, 46.

23. Hulkko A, Orava S: Stress fractures in athletes. *Int J Sports Med* 1987:8, 221.

24. Brukner P, Bradshaw C, Khan KM, et al.: Stress fractures: A review of 180 cases. *Clin J Sport Med* 1996:6, 85.

25. Monteleone GP: Stress fractures in the athlete. *Orthop Clin North Am* 1995:26, 423.

26. Gordon G: Leg pains in athletes. *J Foot Surg* 1979:18, 55.

27. Rzonca EC, Baylis WJ: Common sports injuries to the foot and leg. *Clin Podiatr Med Surg* 1988:5, 591.

28. Giladi M, Ziv Y, Aharonson Z: Comparison between radiography, bone scan, and ultrasound in the diagnosis of stress fractures. *Milit Med* 1984:149, 459.

29. Swenson EJ, DeHaven KE, Sebastianelli WJ, et al.: The effect of a pneumatic leg brace on return to play in athletes with tibial stress fractures. *Am J Sports Med* 1997:25, 322.

30. Green NE, Rogers RA, Lipscomb AB: Nonunions of stress fractures of the tibia. *Am J Sports Med* 1985:13, 171.

31. Orava S, Karpakka J, Hulkko A, et al.: Diagnosis and treatment of stress fractures located at the mid-tibial shaft in athletes. *Int J Sports Med* 1991:12, 419.

32. Rettig AC, Shelbourne KD, McCarroll JR, et al.: The natural history and treatment of delayed union stress fractures of the anterior cortex of the tibia. *Am J Sports Med* 1988:16, 250.

33. Andrish JT: The leg, in DeLee JC, Drez D (eds.), *Orthopaedic Sports Medicine: Principles and Practice.* Philadelphia, WB Saunders, 1994:1603.

34. Schon LC, Clanton TO: Chronic leg pain, in Baxter DE (ed.); *The Foot and Ankle in Sport,* St. Louis, Mo, Mosby, 1995:265.

35. Egan TD, Joyce SM: Acute compartment syndrome following a minor athletic injury. *J Emerg Med* 1989:7, 353.

36. Detmer DE: Chronic leg pain. *Am J Sports Med* 1980:8,141.

37. Martens MA, Moeyersoons JP: Acute and recurrent effort-related compartment syndrome in sports. *Sports Med* 1990:9, 62.

38. Detmer DE, Sharpe K, Sufit RL, et al.: Chronic compartment syndrome: Diagnosis, management, and outcomes. *Am J Sports Med* 1985:13, 162.

39. Pedowitz RA, Hargens AR, Mubarak SJ, et al.: Modified criteria for the objective diagnosis of chronic compartment syndrome of the leg. *Am J Sports Med* 1990:18, 35.

40. McDermott AGP, Marble AE, Yabsley RH, et al.: Monitoring dynamic anterior compartment pressures during

exercise—a new technique using the STIC catheter. *Am J Sports Med* 1982:10, 83.

41. Martens MA, Backaert M, Vermaut G, et al.: Chronic leg pain in athletes due to a recurrent compartment syndrome. *Am J Sports Med* 1984:12, 148.

42. Hoover JA: Exertional anterior compartment syndrome with fascial hernias. *J Foot Surg* 1983:22, 271.

43. Beckham SG, Grana WA, Buckley P, et al.: A comparison of anterior compartment pressures in competitive runners and cyclists. *Am J Sports Med* 1993:21, 36.

44. Wallensten R: Results of fasciotomy in patients with medial tibial syndrome or chronic anterior compartment syndrome. *J Bone Joint Surg Am* 1983:65-A, 1252.

45. Michael RH, Holder LE: The soleus syndrome: A cause of medial tibial stress (shin splints). *Am J Sports Med* 1985: 13, 87.

46. Fredericson M, Bergman AG, Hoffman KL, et al.: Tibial stress reaction in runners: Correlation of clinical symptoms and scintigraphy with a new magnetic resonance imaging grading system. *Am J Sports Med* 1995:23, 472.

47. Mubarak SJ, Gould RN, Lee YF, et al.: The medial tibial stress syndrome: A cause of shin splints. *Am J Sports Med* 1982:10, 201.

48. Holder LE, Michael RH: The specific scintigraphic pattern of "shin splints in the lower leg": Concise communication. *J Nucl Med* 1984:25, 865.

49. Moller BN, Kadin S: Entrapment of the common peroneal nerve. *Am J Sports Med* 1987:15, 90.

50. Leach RE, Purnell MB, Saito A: Peroneal nerve entrapment in runners. *Am J Sports Med* 1989:17, 287.

51. Mitra A, Stern JD, Perrotta VJ, et al.: Peroneal nerve entrapment in athletes. *Ann Plast Surg* 1995:35, 366.

52. Fallon KE: Neurology, in Fields KB, Fricker PA (eds.), *Medical Problems in Athletes,* Malden, MA, Blackwell Science, 1997:186.

53. Schon LC, Baxter DE: Neuropathies of the foot and ankle in athletes. *Clin Sports Med* 1990:9, 489.

54. Sridhara CR, Izzo KL: Terminal sensory branches of the superficial peroneal nerve: An entrapment syndrome. *Archi Physi Med Rehabili* 1985:66, 789.

55. Styf J, Morberg P: The superficial peroneal tunnel syndrome: Results of treatment by decompression. *J Bone Joint Surgery Br* 1997:79-B, 801.

56. Schon LC: Nerve entrapment, neuropathy, and nerve dysfunction in athletes. *Orthop Clin North Am* 1994:25, 47.

57. Guten G: Herniated lumbar disc associated with running: A review of 10 cases. *Am J Sports Med* 1981:9, 155.

58. Alvarez JA, Hardy RH: Lumbar spine stenosis: A common cause of back and leg pain. *Am Fam Physician* 1998: 57, 1825.

59. Cohn SL, Taylor WC: Vascular problems of the lower extremity in athletes. *Clin Sports Med* 1990:9, 449.

60. Rudo ND, Noble HB, Conn J, et al.: Popliteal artery entrapment syndrome in athletes. *Physician Sportsmed,* 1982:10, 105.

61. Darling RC, Buckley CJ, Abbott WM, et al.: Intermittent claudication in young athletes: Popliteal artery entrapment syndrome. *J Trauma* 1974:14, 543.

62. Duwelius PJ, Kelbel JM, Jardon OM, et al.: Popliteal artery entrapment in a high school athlete: A case report. *Am J Sports Med* 1987:15, 371.

63. Lysens RJ, Renson LM, Ostyn MS, et al.: Intermittent claudication in young athletes: Popliteal artery entrapment syndrome. *Am J Sports Med* 1983:11, 177.

64. Turnipseed WD, Pozniak M: Popliteal entrapment as a result of neurovascular compression by the soleus and plantaris muscles. *J Vasc Surg* 1992:15, 285.

65. Rignault DP, Pailler JL, Lunel F: The "functional" popliteal entrapment syndrome. *Int Angiol* 1985:4, 341.

66. Stager A, Clement D: Popliteal artery entrapment syndrome. *Sports Med* 1999:28, 61.

67. Collins PS, McDonald PT, Lim RC: Popliteal artery entrapment: An evolving syndrome. *J Vasc Surg* 1989:10, 484.

68. McDonald PT, Easterbrook JA, Rich NM, et al.: Popliteal artery entrapment syndrome: Clinical, noninvasive and angiographic diagnosis. *Am J Surg* 1980:139, 318.

69. Harvey JS: Effort thrombosis in the lower extremity of a runner. *Am J Sports Med* 1978:6, 400.

70. Ali MS, Kutty MS, Corea JR: Deep vein thrombosis in a jogger. *Am J Sports Med* 1984:12, 169.

71. Gorard DA: Effort thrombosis in an American football player. *Br J Sports Med* 1990:24, 15.

72. McGee SR: Muscle cramps. *Arch Intern Med* 1990:150, 511.

73. Arrington ED, Miller MD: Skeletal muscle injuries. *Orthop Clin North Am* 1995:26, 411.

74. Brown DE: Ankle and leg injuries, in Mellion MB, Walsh WM, Shelton GL (eds.), *The Team Physician's Handbook,* 2nd ed., Philadelphia, Hanley and Belfus, 1997:579.

75. King JB: Post-traumatic ectopic calcification in the muscles of athletes: A review. *Br J Sports Med* 1998:32, 287.

76. Hyder N, Shaw DL, Bollen SR: Myositis ossificans: Calcification of the entire tibialis anterior after ischaemic injury (compartment syndrome). *J Bone Joint Surg Br* 1996: 78-B, 318.

Chapter 17

ANKLE INJURIES

Arlon H. Jahnke, Jr. and
Mark T. Messenger

INTRODUCTION

Millions of Americans have become more committed to maintaining physical fitness during the past several decades. Jogging and running have become very popular means of obtaining and maintaining physical fitness. Most individuals who participate in this type of physical activity will at some time sustain a running-related injury. Most of the injuries associated with running or jogging involve the lower extremity and spine. The majority of these injuries are secondary to overuse and consist of tendinopathies. Runners, however, also experience traumatic injuries including sprains or strains of muscles, tendons, or ligaments.[1] Ankle injuries are endemic to all sports that involve running, jumping, cutting, or kicking. The health care professional involved with the care of the acutely injured athlete must be proficient in diagnosing and treating common injuries to the ankle, as well as recognizing signs and symptoms of more significant injuries that require referral to specialty care. Ankle injuries are among the most common afflictions seen at all levels of athletic participation and account for approximately 15% of all athletic injuries.[2] In this chapter, a brief review of anatomy is presented, followed by a discussion of various injuries that may involve the ankle joint. A symptom-oriented approach is presented to familiarize the practitioner with the diagnosis and treatment of each of these injuries.

ANATOMY AND BIOMECHANICS

An understanding of the anatomy of the tendons, ligaments, and osseous structures about the ankle is necessary to adequately diagnose and treat injuries that occur to this joint. The ankle joint consists of the close anatomic relationship between the distal tibia and fibula proximally, and the talus bone distally. The osseous anatomy of the ankle joint is unique and creates a mortise between the talus and distal tibia/fibula. The articular surface of the talus is in the shape of a truncated cone (the width of the talus is narrower posteriorly). This bony anatomy results in stability of the ankle with the foot in a neutral position. In this position, the ankle resembles a mortise and tenon with the talus locking tightly within the distal tibia and fibula. As the foot goes into plantar flexion, the ankle has less bony stability as the narrower posterior portion of the talus rides into the wider area between the medial and lateral malleoli. As the bony stability decreases with plantar flexion, stability of the ankle depends more and more on the ligamentous structures about the ankle joint.

The ligaments of the ankle joint can be divided into three anatomic areas: The distal tibiofibular ligaments (syndesmotic ligaments), the lateral ligaments, and the medial ligaments. The lateral ligaments consist of the anterior talofibular ligament (ATFL), the calcaneofibular ligament (CFL), and the posterior talofibular ligament (PTFL) (Fig. 17–1). The ATFL is a

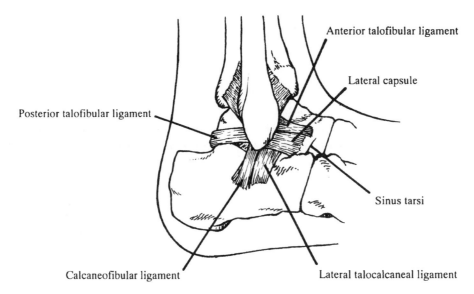

Figure 17–1. Ligamentous anatomy of the lateral side of the ankle joint. (*Reproduced with permission from* WA Lillegard, JO Butcher, KS Rucker. A Symptom-Oriented Approach. *Handbook of Sports Medicine 2nd ed.* Butterworth-Heinmann publishers, 1999.)

broad, flat ligament that courses from the anterior border of the distal fibula to the anterolateral aspect of the talus. With the foot flat on the ground, the ligament courses relatively parallel to the floor. This ligament's primary function is to prevent anterior translation of the talus in the mortise of the distal tibia and fibula. As the foot goes into plantar flexion, the ligament fibers become more perpendicular to the floor and it therefore becomes more of a collateral ligament that prevents inversion of the talus within the ankle mortise. The CFL is a more tubular structure that courses from the tip of the distal fibula to a small tubercle on the lateral wall of the calcaneus. The CFL lies deep to the peroneal tendons and courses nearly perpendicular to the floor with the foot in a neutral position. The CFL crosses two joints and acts to prevent inversion of both the ankle and subtalar joints. The PTFL is the strongest of the three lateral ligaments of the ankle and the least frequently injured. It also is a fairly broad, stout ligament that courses relatively horizontal to the floor from the posterior aspect of the lateral malleolus to the talus, posterior and lateral to the articular surface of the talus. This strong ligament prevents forward dislocation of the leg on the foot.

The medial ankle ligaments, or "deltoid ligament," is a very strong, fan-shaped structure that consists of superficial and deep components (Fig. 17–2). The medial ligaments of the ankle are much stronger than the lateral and syndesmotic ligaments and are less commonly injured. The superficial portion of the deltoid ligament courses from the medial malleolus to the navicular anteriorly, and to the sustentaculum tali posteriorly. This

portion of the ligament prevents eversion of the ankle. The deep portion courses relatively horizontal from the deep, posterior surface of the medial malleolus to the medial aspect of the talus. Its relatively horizontal orientation results in its ability to prevent lateral displacement of the talus within the ankle mortise.

The syndesmotic ligaments consist of the anterior inferior tibiofibular ligament (AITFL), the posterior inferior tibiofibular ligament (PITFL), and the interosseous membrane (IOM). The syndesmotic ligaments are responsible for maintaining the relationship of the distal tibia and fibula. These ligaments hold the distal fibula snug in a small groove on the distal lateral aspect of the tibia. Disruption of this ligamentous complex results in widening of the bony ankle mortise.

LATERAL ANKLE PAIN

Ligamentous Sprains

Injuries to the lateral ligamentous structures of the ankle are among the most common injuries seen in sports.[1–3] The running athlete is at risk for sudden twisting injuries to the ankle joint. Most commonly, these episodes result in injuries to the ligaments and soft tissues on the lateral side of the ankle joint. The majority of these injuries occur in persons under 35 years of age, most commonly in runners aged 15 to 19 years old.[3] The treatment of these injuries depends on the severity of the injury. An accurate diagnosis will enable the physician to direct and implement the proper treatment and rehabilitation regimen.

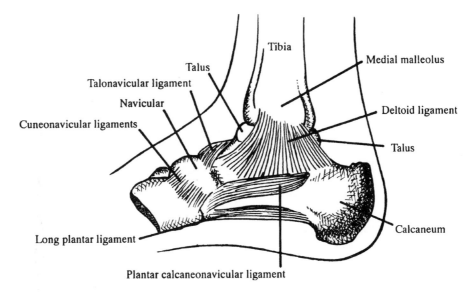

Figure 17–2. Ligamentous anatomy of the medial side of the ankle joint. (*Reproduced with permission from* WA Lillegard, JO Butcher, KS Rucker. A Symptom-Oriented Approach. *Handbook of Sports Medicine 2nd ed.* Butterworth-Heinmann publishers, 1999.)

Injuries to the lateral ligamentous structures occur with inversion of the tibiotalar joint and hindfoot. In jumping-type sports, the foot is often in a plantarflexed position at the time of injury, resulting in strain to the anterior talofibular ligament (ATFL). With the foot plantarflexed, the ATFL is the primary stabilizer to inversion stress, because the bony architecture is not as inherently stable. Injuries also occur in cutting-type sports. Again, the primary stress is inversion; however, the ankle is in a neutral position or dorsiflexion. More severe injuries may occur in this position because more stress is placed on ligaments other than just the ATFL.

Traditionally, sprains of the ankle ligaments have been classified in clinical practice as grade I (mild), grade II (moderate), or grade III (severe) injuries.[4] Grade I injuries involve ligament stretching without macroscopic tearing. Clinically, there is little swelling and mild tenderness, minimal functional loss, and no instability symptoms. A grade II injury is a moderate injury involving partial macroscopic tearing of the ligamentous structures. Clinically, there is moderate swelling and tenderness over the lateral ligamentous structures. There is slight loss of motion and mild-to-moderate joint instability. A grade III injury is a complete ligament rupture. Clinically, the patient has severe swelling, ecchymosis, and inability to bear weight on the extremity. There is marked functional limitation and joint instability. The diagnosis of grade I, II, or III lateral ligamentous injuries requires a careful clinical evaluation consisting of an accurate history, thorough physical examination, and radiographic evaluation.

The athlete can usually describe the mechanism of injury quite well, and from this information the physician may be able to predict which structures have been injured. It is important to determine whether the injury is a first-time injury or a recurrent event. A precise history should include questions regarding previous injuries to the ankle, history of recurrent sprains, mechanism of injuries, presence of a "pop" or "snap" at the time of injury, ability to bear weight after the injury, initial treatment given, and presence and time to development of swelling and ecchymoses. After an injury to the lateral ligaments of the ankle, the patient often experiences a sudden, intense pain localized on the lateral side of the ankle. The pain often improves after a few minutes only to return as the ankle swells. Most patients experience pain and discomfort when they try to bear weight on the injured extremity. Swelling occurs in minutes to hours depending on the severity of the ligamentous tearing. Ecchymosis appears in 24 to 48 hours as the hematoma develops over and dependent to the site of injury.

The correct diagnosis relies on the ability to perform a thorough and accurate physical examination. The ability to examine the ankle within the first hour or two after injury is advantageous. Initially, the point of maximal tenderness will be localized to the injured structures on the lateral side of the ankle. This is most commonly over the ATFL and/or the CFL. If the patient is not seen until several hours after the injury, generalized swelling and pain make the examination more difficult and unreliable. The physical examination begins with inspection of the joint for any deformity, swelling, or discoloration. The entire lower extremity should be undressed to fully evaluate the injury. Examine the skin for abrasions or breaks. The location of abrasions or lacerations will help the clinician understand the extent of the trauma to the ankle. Palpation should be performed in a systematic manner beginning with structures you believe are not injured. Laterally, palpate the distal fibula, the ATFL, the CFL, the posterior talofibular ligament (PTFL), and the base of the fifth metatarsal. Medially, it is important to palpate the medial malleolus, the deltoid ligament, and the navicular bone. For completeness, the proximal fibula and the insertion of the Achilles tendon should be palpated for tenderness. Range of motion of the ankles should be evaluated, both actively and passively. Normal range of motion for the ankle joint is 20 degrees of dorsiflexion and 50 degrees of plantarflexion.

Several tests have been described to determine the integrity of the ligaments about the ankle. The anterior drawer test is performed with the patient sitting on the edge of the examining table with his/her legs dangling (Fig. 17–3). The injured foot is placed in a few degrees of plantarflexion. The examiner places one hand on the anterior aspect of the lower tibia and the calcaneus is grasped with the other hand. The calcaneus is gently drawn anteriorly while stabilizing the distal tibia with the other hand. Normally, the ATFL is tight in all positions of ankle joint motion and there should be minimal forward movement of the talus. With injury to the ATFL, either acutely or chronically, the test results in abnormal translation of the talus relative to the distal tibia. This is noted as a positive anterior drawer sign. The second test to determine lateral ligament stability of the ankle is the talar tilt test (Fig. 17–4). This test is performed by gently inverting the talus within the ankle mortise while the ankle is in both neutral dorsiflexion and slight plantarflexion. If the talus gaps and rocks open while the ankle is in plantarflexion, this indicates laxity of the ATFL. If there is lateral tilt with the ankle in neutral dorsiflexion, then there is laxity of both the CFL and ATFL.

The physical examination is continued with a neurovascular examination. The dorsalis pedis and posterior tibial pulses should be palpated. Capillary refill to all of the digits should be brisk. A brief sensory examination completes the physical examination. Radiographic evaluation may not be required in relatively

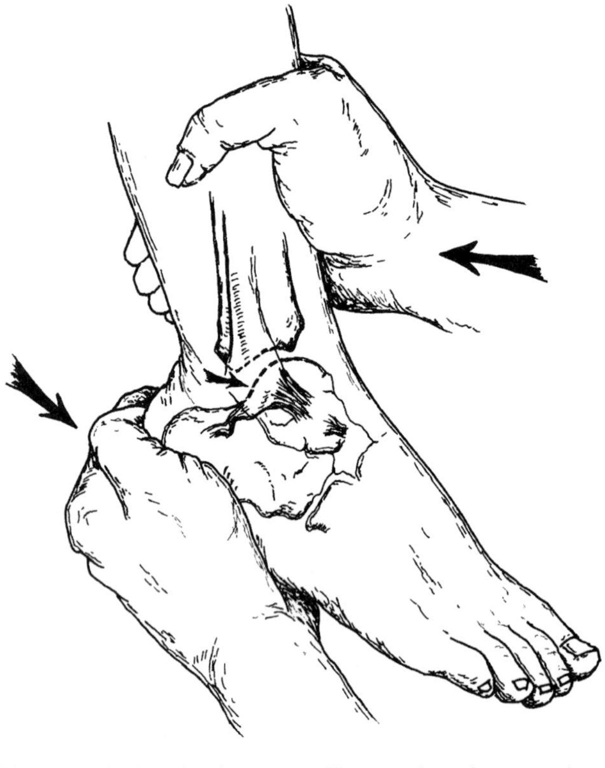

Figure 17–3. Anterior drawer test. The examiner places one hand on the anterior aspect of the patient's lower tibia and grasps the calcaneus with his or her other hand. The patient's calcaneus is gently drawn anteriorly while the examiner stabilizes the patient's distal tibia with his or her other hand. Increased translation compared with the contralateral ankle indicates laxity or rupture of the anterior talofibular ligament. (*Reproduced with permission from* WA Lillegard, JO Butcher, KS Rucker. A Symptom-Oriented Approach. *Handbook of Sports Medicine 2nd ed.* Butterworth-Heinmann publishers, 1999.)

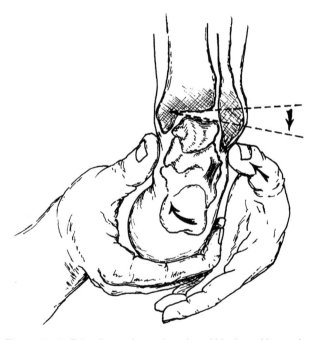

Figure 17–4. Talar tilt test. Invert the talus within the ankle mortise. If the talus gaps and rocks open while the ankle is in slight plantarflexion, this indicates laxity of the anterior talofibular ligament. Increased talar tilt with the ankle in neutral position indicates laxity of the calcaneofibular ligament as well. (*Reproduced with permission from* WA Lillegard, JO Butcher, KS Rucker. A Symptom-Oriented Approach. *Handbook of Sports Medicine 2nd ed.* Butterworth-Heinmann publishers, 1999.)

minor injuries to the ankle. If there is significant swelling, ecchymosis, or pain present about the ankle, radiographs of the ankle should be obtained. Routine radiographic series of the ankle should include an anteroposterior (AP), lateral, and mortise views. The mortise view is an AP radiograph taken with the leg internally rotated 15 to 30 degrees. With symptoms of chronic instability, specialized stress radiographs may be required. Both AP and lateral stress views should be obtained if stress radiographs are needed. The lateral stress view is a lateral radiograph obtained with an anteriorly applied force to the talus/calcaneus (Fig. 17–5). On the lateral stress view, the shortest distance from the posterior lip of the distal tibia to the talar dome is measured. A distance of more than 10 mm

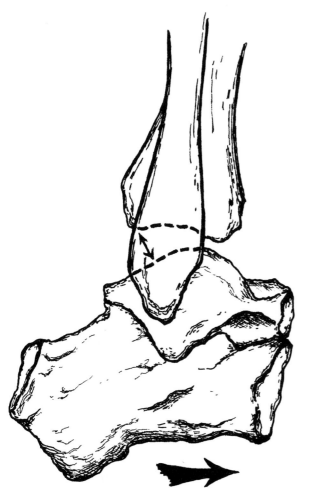

Figure 17–5. Lateral stress view. With the talus stressed anteriorly, the shortest distance from the posterior lip of the distal fibula to the talar dome is measured. If this distance is greater than 10 mm or 3 mm greater than the asymptomatic ankle, abnormal laxity exists in the anterior talofibular ligament. (*Reproduced with permission from* WA Lillegard, JO Butcher, KS Rucker. A Symptom-Oriented Approach. *Handbook of Sports Medicine 2ⁿᵈ ed.* Butterworth-Heinmann publishers, 1999.)

or 3 mm more than the asymptomatic ankle indicates abnormal laxity of the ATFL.[5] The AP stress radiograph is performed while applying an inversion stress to the talus/calcaneus. An angle is measured between lines drawn parallel to the tibial plafond and the talar dome. The stress radiograph is abnormal if the angle measured is greater than 20 degrees, or 10 degrees more than the asymptomatic ankle.[6,7] Other specialized studies including bone scans, arthrography, computerized tomography, and magnetic resonance imaging are rarely needed to evaluate lateral ligament injuries.

Treatment of acute lateral ligamentous ankle injuries depends on the severity of the injury. Most injuries can be treated initially with rest, ice, compression, elevation, and early range-of-motion exercises. Immobilization has not been shown to be superior to functional protected early range-of-motion exercises in severe sprains, but can be considered on a short-term basis if symptomatically required. Weightbearing can begin after the initial swelling resolves. The use of functional braces such as stirrup braces, elastic sleeves, and laced ankle supports may be beneficial during the patient's rehabilitation from these injuries. The rehabilitation program should emphasize range-of-motion exercises early followed by proprioceptive training and global ankle strengthening with emphasis on the peroneal muscles. Surgery is reserved for more severe injuries, those associated with fractures, and chronic or recurrent lateral ligament insufficiency.

Peroneus Tendon Subluxation

Traumatic dislocation or subluxation of the peroneal tendons, either acute or chronic, is an uncommon injury. The injury most commonly occurs in skiers, but also can occur in the running athlete who sustains a sudden, forceful, passive dorsiflexion force to the ankle while the foot is in slight eversion. This results in powerful reflex contraction of the peronei, which are the dynamic lateral stabilizers of the ankle. The injury results in tearing of the peroneal retinaculum and subsequent anterior subluxation or dislocation of the peroneal tendons anterior to the lateral malleolus. Tenderness is usually located posterior to the lateral malleolus; however, swelling can be quite severe and this may obscure the diagnosis. You can stress the retinaculum by eliciting active eversion of the foot with the ankle held in dorsiflexion. In patients with an acute subluxation, this test will produce severe pain and is diagnostic of the problem. Because of the rapid resolution of symptoms and the difficulty of establishing the diagnosis in the acute stage, the patient most commonly seeks medical evaluation when chronic subluxation is established. Patients with recurrent subluxation complain of lateral ankle pain and instability.

Treatment of this condition if diagnosed acutely consists of a well-molded, nonweightbearing cast that includes a stabilizing horseshoe, for 5 to 6 weeks. Patients with chronic instability usually require surgical reconstruction to prevent recurrent subluxation.

Subtalar Ligament Injury

Injury to the subtalar ligamentous complex results from mechanisms similar to those causing lateral ankle ligament injuries. Patients complain of pain along the lateral aspect of the foot localized to the sinus tarsi region. With chronic strains, the symptoms may be identical to those of chronic lateral instability with recurrent inversion instability and lateral pain. Often with isolated subtalar instability, the stress radiographs for ankle instability are normal. Specialized radiographs (Broden's views) are necessary to evaluate the subtalar joint.[8] Often this becomes a diagnosis of exclusion after lateral ankle ligament instability has been eliminated. Acute injuries are treated similar to those of lateral ankle ligament sprains, with rest, ice, compression, elevation, early range-of-motion, and peroneal muscle strengthening. Chronic subtalar instability may require surgical reconstruction.

LATERAL SOFT-TISSUE IMPINGEMENT

Soft-tissue impingement occurs when a soft-tissue lesion forms over the anterior aspect of the ankle and impinges between the talus and anterolateral tibia or distal fibula with dorsiflexion of the foot. The soft tissue causing the symptoms is most commonly scar, or hypertrophic synovium that becomes pathologic after an injury to the ankle. Other causes of impingement include a "meniscoid lesion" on the inferior border of the distal anterior tibiofibular ligament. Injury to the anterolateral ankle capsule and synovium results in hemorrhage and synovitis, which may cause the formation of a mass of fibrocartilage or scar. Patients most commonly present with chronic anterolateral ankle pain after an inversion injury. They may have symptoms of catching and giving way, although physical examination will detect no evidence of instability. Pain is often reproduced with forced dorsiflexion of the ankle.

Initial treatment includes rest, activity modification, ice, nonsteroidal anti-inflammatory medications (NSAIDs), and physical therapy modalities including stretching, strengthening, and proprioceptive exercises. If such conservative measures fail to bring relief of symptoms, further evaluation should be instituted. Stress radiographs should be obtained to rule out instability, and a bone scan and/or MRI should rule out occult osseous injury. An injection of corticosteroid combined with a local anesthetic into the joint should relieve the patient's symptoms if a soft-tissue impingement lesion is present. Repeat injections of corticosteroids into the ankle joint should be avoided. Persistent symptoms despite conservative treatment for 4 to 6 months may warrant surgical consultation.

PERONEUS TENDINITIS

Tendinitis of the peroneal tendons without subluxation over the fibula can be due to friction between the peroneal tendons within their sheath, partial or intrasubstance tears, accessory slips of tendon in which friction develops, association with avulsion fractures of the CFL, or posttraumatic conditions that narrow the fibulocalcaneal space (enlargement of the peroneal tubercle, old calcaneal fractures, or lateral displacement of the subtalar joint). Initial treatment of this condition is with ice, NSAIDs, a lateral heel wedge for calcaneal varus, physical therapy modalities, and rehabilitation. Ankle bracing may also provide symptomatic improvement. In resistant cases, CT or MRI may identify the aforementioned causes, and surgery may be indicated.

Tarsal Coalitions

Tarsal coalition is a bony, fibrous, or cartilaginous connection of two or more tarsal bones. The cause of the anomaly is unknown but it occurs in 1% to 3% of the population. The most common coalitions of the tarsal bones are the talocalcaneal and the calcaneonavicular. A more unusual coalition is the talonavicular coalition. Patients usually present in adolescence, when the cartilaginous or fibrous coalition tends to ossify and become less compliant. The patient usually complains of vague lateral or diffuse foot pain that may or may not be associated with trauma. Physical findings include localized pain over the subtalar joint, spastic flatfeet, and/or limited subtalar joint motion. The diagnosis can be made with plain radiographs or CT. The oblique radiograph of the foot should reveal the calcaneonavicular coalition. The talocalcaneal coalition is often difficult to see on plain radiographs and CT is necessary to make the diagnosis.

The initial treatment of these conditions should be conservative measures to relieve the patient's pain. This includes immobilization with casting or orthotics, NSAIDs, and activity modifications. Patients who continue to complain of pain despite conservative treatment should be considered for surgical treatment. Surgical treatment consists of resection of the bar and placement of fat or muscle into the resulting defect to prevent recurrence. For patients with large coalitions and secondary degenerative changes in the subtalar joints, arthrodesis of the joints may be necessary.

Distal Fibula Stress Fracture

The distal fibula is the fifth most common site of stress fracture seen in the running population.[9] The overall incidence of stress fractures in an athletic population has been reported to be 0.12%.[10] By far, the vast majority of stress fractures occur in running athletes. Women have been found to be up to 12 times more susceptible to the development of a stress fracture at some point during their running career than their male counterparts.[10]

Clinically, the patient with a stress reaction or fracture will complain of pain along the distal fibula that occurs only after running. As the condition advances, the pain begins to occur during the running activity as well. With time, the pain may be present with activities of daily living. Tenderness is usually well localized to the distal fibula. A high index of suspicion is needed to accurately diagnose this problem. Radiographic findings are variable and will often lag behind the patient's symptoms by several weeks. A patient with a suspected stress reaction or fracture to the distal fibula should undergo evaluation with a technetium 99 bone scan. This diagnostic study is very sensitive for identifying occult stress reactions or fractures.

The great majority of fibular stress fractures heal with conservative treatment. This treatment includes simply restricting running activities until the individual is pain free. The average length of time of rest for the fibular stress fracture is 4 to 6 weeks. Structural support with removable braces is often helpful symptomatically. Special consideration should be given to the female patient who develops stress fractures. Investigation into dietary habits and menstrual history may be important in the treatment of a stress fracture in the female athlete.

Other Causes

Lateral ankle pain in the running athlete can also be caused by osteochondral fracture of the talus and lateral calcaneal nerve compression. Osteochondral fractures and osteochondritis dessicans will be discussed later in this chapter. Conditions and injuries involving the foot are discussed elsewhere in this text.

ANTERIOR ANKLE PAIN

Tibiofibular Ligament and Syndesmosis Sprain

Diastasis of the syndesmosis occurs with partial or complete rupture of the syndesmosis ligament com-

plex. These injuries are often seen with fractures about the ankle. Isolated injuries to the syndesmosis are relatively rare. The injury is caused by sudden external rotation of the ankle which causes the talus to press against the fibula, thus opening the distal tibiofibular articulation.

An isolated syndesmosis tear can be very difficult to diagnose. Pain and tenderness are located principally on the anterior aspect of the syndesmotic ligaments and the interosseous membrane. Active external rotation of the foot is painful. The patient usually cannot bear weight on the ankle due to pain. In patients with complete tears, the diagnosis may easily be made through a simple squeeze test. The squeeze test is performed by compressing the fibula to the tibia proximal to the midpoint of the calf. This proximal compression results in pain along the interosseous membrane and its supporting structures. The external rotation stress test is performed by stabilizing the distal tibia with one hand and applying an external rotational force to the foot with the other hand (Fig. 17–6). This maneuver will reproduce pain localized to the area of the syndesmosis.

Routine radiographs including AP, lateral, and mortise views should be obtained. The diagnosis of syndesmosis disruption is made with widening of the medial space between the medial malleolus and medial

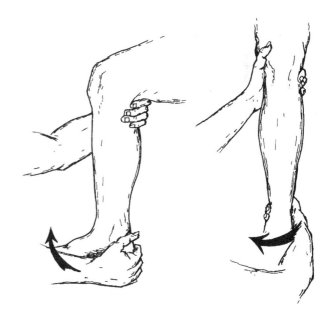

Figure 17–6. External rotation stress test. The patient's distal tibia is stabilized with one hand and an external rotation force is applied to the foot with the other hand. If this maneuver reproduces pain in the syndesmosis, it is suggestive of an anterior ankle sprain or syndesmotic ligament sprain. (*Reproduced with permission from WA Lillegard, JO Butcher, KS Rucker. A Symptom-Oriented Approach. Handbook of Sports Medicine 2*nd *ed.* Butterworth-Heinmann publishers, 1999.)

talar dome greater than 5 mm. When widening of the medial "clear space" is present, it is important to obtain radiographs of the entire fibula to rule out the possibility of a proximal fibular fracture, or Maisonneuve fracture. If there is no widening of the clear space on the routine radiographs, stress radiographs should be obtained to ensure integrity of the syndesmotic ligaments. A mortise radiograph is obtained while applying an external rotational force to the foot. An injection of xylocaine into the syndesmosis prior to this examination may improve the sensitivity of the test. Finally, the diagnosis can also be made from evaluating the routine AP radiographs.[11] A measurement is made from the lateral border of the posterior tibial malleolus to the medial border of the fibula. This measurement should be less than 5 mm. Similarly, measurement from the medial border of the fibula to the lateral border of the anterior tibial prominence (tibia-fibula overlap) should be greater than or equal to 10 mm.

The treatment of syndesmosis sprains depends on the severity of the injury. Less-severe sprains without complete disruption and no objective widening on radiographic studies should be treated initially with RICE principles (rest, ice, compression, and elevation). Taping or bimalleolar semirigid orthoses can help stabilize the ankle during healing. Once the initial pain and inflammation of the injury subside, normal ambulation is encouraged. The patient then does active resistive and proprioceptive exercises in physical therapy. Gradual return to activity is allowed as symptoms permit. For complete tears of the syndesmosis, indicated by widening of the medial clear space on radiographs, referral to an orthopedic surgeon is necessary. The syndesmosis can be stabilized by either cast immobilization or operatively through the use of sutures or a syndesmosis screw.

Anterior Tibialis Tendinitis or Rupture

Anterior tibialis tendinitis can occur in the running athlete and results in irritation over the anterior ankle. On physical examination, there is tenderness over the extensor retinaculum and along the course of the tibialis anterior tendon. There is often pain with forced dorsiflexion of the ankle. This condition is typically an overuse problem and responds to rest, physical therapy modalities, and NSAIDs. Plantarflexion stretching exercises of the ankle are also beneficial.

Rupture of the tibialis anterior tendon is an extremely unusual injury caused by forced plantarflexion of the foot and ankle. The patient complains of loss of strength in dorsiflexion and has difficulty walking due to an unsteady gait (drop foot). Physical examination reveals swelling or a mass (pseudotumor) and a palpable defect of the normal anterior prominence of the tendon

with resistive dorsiflexion of the ankle. If the diagnosis is made acutely, direct repair of the tendon may be possible. However, these injuries often present late and require more complex reconstructive surgical procedures.

MEDIAL ANKLE PAIN

Deltoid Ligament Sprain

Isolated injuries to the deltoid ligament are very rare. Most injuries to this ligament complex occur in conjunction with fractures of the lateral malleolus or proximal fibula (Maisonneuve fracture). These injuries to the deltoid ligament occur as a result of an external rotational force to the planted foot in athletics. Clinical examination reveals the majority of tenderness to be located on the medial aspect of the ankle. With medial tenderness and suspected injury to the deltoid ligament, it is important to rule out fractures of the lateral malleolus or proximal fibula, and injuries to the syndesmosis. Similarly, the proximal aspect of the fibula should be palpated to rule out proximal fracture. On radiographic examination, widening of the medial clear space greater than 5 mm on the mortise view is significant for deltoid ligament injury. Most clinicians agree that partial deltoid ligament ruptures should be treated nonoperatively. The treatment is similar to that for lateral ankle ligament injuries. There remains disagreement with respect to the best treatment of complete tears. Most agree that operative repair with stabilization of accompanying fractures is appropriate.[12,13] Still others believe excellent results can be obtained with cast immobilization and rehabilitation.[14,15]

Posterior Tibialis Tendon Injury

Posterior tibialis tendon injuries range from minor sprains with subsequent tendinitis symptoms to complete rupture and acquired flatfoot deformities. Sprains to the posterior tibial tendon occur in all age groups and are usually associated with athletic activities including running. In contrast, nearly all complete ruptures of this tendon are associated with degenerative changes within the tendon and subsequently occur in older patients.

Acutely, patients complain of severe pain along the posterior tibial tendon sheath, posterior to the medial malleolus. Symptoms usually resolve shortly after the injury. Patients may then develop symptoms secondary to the flatfoot deformity that ensues over months to years. Chronic symptoms may consist of pain along the posterior aspect of the medial malleolus or laterally secondary to impingement of the calcaneus on the lateral talar process or fibula. Patients may or may not notice gradual development of a flatfoot deformity. Physical examination may reveal tenderness, swelling, inversion weakness, deformity with standing, or pain with attempted heel rise. A patient with a posterior tibial tendon rupture will usually be unable to perform a single-leg toe raise on the affected extremity. This maneuver is performed by asking the patient to lift the asymptomatic extremity off the ground, thereby bearing all his or her weight on the symptomatic foot. Then ask the patient to raise up on his toes. It is important to stabilize the patient by holding his or her hands during this test because the patient is often quite unstable. With weightbearing on the symptomatic extremity, the foot maintains a position of hindfoot valgus, talar plantarflexion, and forefoot abduction. If observed from behind, the foot will appear to have "too many toes" (Fig. 17–7).

Radiographs in patients with suspected posterior tibial tendon ruptures should be taken while bearing weight on the extremity. These should reveal the flatfoot deformity. There may be degenerative changes recognized in the subtalar, calcaneocuboid, and talonavicular joints in patients with chronic ruptures. MRI is the imaging study of choice for imaging the posterior tibial tendon. Treatment of acute sprains of the posterior tibial tendon can consist of a short period of immobilization followed by rehabilitation and strengthening. Complete ruptures with secondary flatfoot deformities may require surgical reconstruction with tendon transfers or arthrodesis of the peritalar joints.

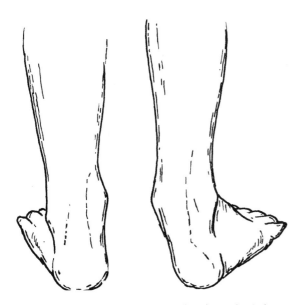

Figure 17–7. Too-many-toes sign. Viewing the patient's lower extremities from behind will reveal "too many toes" in the patient with chronic posterior tibialis tendon dysfunction and a planovalgus foot. (*Reproduced with permission from* WA Lillegard, JO Butcher, KS Rucker. A Symptom-Oriented Approach. *Handbook of Sports Medicine 2nd ed.* Butterworth-Heinemann publishers, 1999.)

Tarsal Tunnel Syndrome

Tarsal tunnel syndrome is caused by entrapment of the posterior tibial nerve within the tarsal tunnel. The tarsal tunnel is formed by the flexor retinaculum over the posterior medial malleolus. The tendons of the posterior tibialis, flexor digitorum longus, and flexor hallucis course through the tunnel along with the posterior tibial nerve. Tendinitis from any of these tendons, a tight retinaculum, or overpronation of the forefoot can compress or stretch the nerve and cause symptoms. Clinical symptoms often consist of a burning dysesthesia in the plantar aspect of the foot that is aggravated by repetitive use.

Physical examination may reveal hypesthesia over the plantar foot, tenderness posterior to the medial malleolus, and a positive Tinel's sign over the tarsal tunnel. Associated tendinopathies as discussed in preceding sections should be addressed. Electromyographs (EMGs) and nerve conduction studies are often useful to assess the severity of nerve compression. Treatment consists of orthotics to relieve pressure, physical therapy modalities, NSAIDs, and occasional localized injections with corticosteroids. Surgical release and exploration is indicated if these measures fail.

Flexor Hallucis Longus Tendinitis

The flexor hallucis longus tendon is responsible for flexion of the interphalangeal and metatarsophalangeal joints of the great toe. It is very important in push-off during most athletic endeavors. Overuse injury and partial tears of this tendon can occur with running and long-distance walking activities. Physical examination reveals tenderness along the posteromedial ankle, approximately 1 to 2 cm posterior to the medial malleolus, and just posterior to the tibial artery. There may be a more distal tenderness medially over the course of the tendon or pain on standing on tiptoe. Passive dorsiflexion or active flexion of the great toe may aggravate the pain. Conservative treatment includes relative rest, physical therapy emphasizing stretching of these structures, modalities (iontophoresis, electrical stimulation, moist heat, etc.), NSAIDs, and functional orthotics (to decrease stress on the tendon). A short period of immobilization may be necessary to allow the tendon to rest. Tenolysis is occasionally needed if these measures fail. If an athlete experiences "triggering" of the great toe, partial rupture of the flexor hallucis longus tendon at the ankle should be considered and orthopedic consultation obtained.

Other Causes

Stress fractures of the sustentaculum tali and medial malleolus can be a cause of chronic medial ankle pain. If radiographic changes are not apparent, further investigation should be undertaken with a technetium 99 bone scan. Subtle osteochondral injuries may also cause medial ankle pain and these are discussed later in this chapter.

POSTERIOR ANKLE PAIN

Achilles' Tendon Injury

Injuries to the Achilles' tendon include peritendinitis, tendinosis, and partial or complete ruptures. Peritendinitis or tendinitis of the Achilles' tendon is one of the more common overuse injuries seen in running athletes. These injuries result from cumulative impact loading and repetitive microtrauma to the tendon. Complete ruptures result from a combination of intrasubstance degeneration of the tendon and excessive mechanical forces. Ruptures most commonly occur 3 to 4 cm proximal to the tendon's insertion on the calcaneus. The precipitating event in nearly all patients who sustain this injury is an active, forceful, sometimes unexpected, plantarflexion of the foot.

The predominant symptom of Achilles' tendinitis is pain that is localized to the tendon. Initially, the patient may complain of pain only with prolonged activity. The pain usually subsides with rest but may be exacerbated by climbing stairs. As the tendinitis progresses, the patient will have pain earlier in the activity being performed. In the later stages of tendinitis or partial rupture of the tendon, the patient will be unable to perform the activity and will complain of pain at rest. In chronic tendinitis, the patient will complain of more diffuse pain throughout the tendon substance. Often there is development of nodularity and fusiform swelling of the tendon. Patients who sustain spontaneous ruptures of the Achilles' tendon note a sudden "snap" in the heel region at the time of injury and subsequent pain with active or passive flexion of the foot. Many patients do not seek immediate treatment because they can still plantarflex their ankles. Patients may complain of a moderate limp and weakness in the ankle. Physical examination should provide the diagnosis in most patients.

Physical findings in patients with tendinitis include soft-tissue swelling, localized tenderness to palpation, and crepitus with movement of the ankle. Nodularity and diffuse, fusiform swelling should make the examiner suspicious of tendinosis or a partial rupture of the tendon. With complete ruptures of the tendon, a palpable depression over the area of the rupture will be recognized. The patient will have weakness and pain with active plantarflexion of the ankle. The Thompson's test is performed with the patient prone on the examination table and the patient's feet extending over the end of the table. The calf musculature is gently squeezed in the middle third of the muscle belly, just distal to the place of widest girth. Normally, with this maneuver there is passive plantar movement of the foot. A positive test is indicated by a lack of plantar movement of the foot and indicates a complete rupture of the tendon. Standard radiographs are useful to rule out osseous conditions. The lateral radiograph may rarely show calcification of the soft tissues around the tendon or in the tendon itself.

Most cases of tendinitis are successfully managed nonoperatively. Treatment principles are directed at temporarily decreasing the athlete's activities. A stretching program is often beneficial. Other modalities include the use of a $1/4$- to $3/8$-inch heel lift, oral NSAIDs, physical therapy modalities, ice, and the use of orthotics to correct excessive pronation of the foot. Total rest may not be required, but the intensity of training should be decreased or modified (see Chapter 40). For example, a runner should avoid hill work or interval training. Patients with chronic symptoms or more severe acute symptoms may benefit from a short period of immobilization. This usually involves casting for 1 to 3 weeks. The use of corticosteroid injections for the treatment of tendinitis should be discouraged. If an injection is used, it should be placed by an experienced individual and only into the retrocalcaneal bursa. Surgery may be considered for chronic cases of tendinitis that have failed all conservative treatment regimens. Treatment of complete ruptures is certainly controversial. Both operative[16,17] and nonoperative[18,19] approaches have been advocated with excellent results reported in the literature. Nonoperative approaches involve a period of casting with the foot in a relative equinus position followed by extensive rehabilitation. Surgical treatment consists of repair of the torn tendon followed by rehabilitation. The results of these treatment methods are similar. There may be a higher rate of recurrence in patients treated with nonoperative care.[20] Accordingly, surgical repair is generally recommended to the athletic population.

Posterior Impingement (Os Trigonum Syndrome)

The os trigonum is the nonunited lateral tubercle of the posterior aspect of the talus. Its incidence is estimated to be between 8% and 13% in the general population. In the majority of cases this bone is considered an asymptomatic finding. However, in certain athletic endeavors such as ballet dancing and kicking sports such as soccer and football, this bone may impinge on the posterior tibia in plantarflexion of the foot. This type of inflammatory process can also result from overuse in long distance running. In these activities acute or chronic pain can develop along the posterolateral aspect of the ankle.

The clues to the correct diagnosis of posterior impingement on the os trigonum are the location of the pain behind the peroneal tendons and reproduction of the pain with forced plantarflexion of the ankle. Routine radiographs will reveal the os trigonum. An additional lateral radiograph taken with the ankle in maximum plantarflexion may also be beneficial and may show the impingement of the posterior tibia on the posterolateral talus.

As with most conditions affecting the ankle joint, treatment of posterior impingement or os trigonum syndrome should initially be conservative. Antiinflammatory medications, rest, ice, and physical therapy modalities should be tried first. It is also important to avoid positioning the ankle in maximum plantarflexion. Taping techniques or orthotics may be useful to prevent the ankle from plantarflexing. If symptoms persist despite these conservative measures, the patient may be a candidate for surgical excision of the os trigonum.

DIFFUSE ANKLE PAIN

Osteochondral Lesions of the Talus

Osteochondral lesions of the talus are disruptions of the normal articular surface of the talar dome. This condition is also known as osteochondritis dessicans of the talus. Two types of osteochondral lesions of the talus can be seen. Lesions that occur laterally are usually related to trauma, cause more symptoms, rarely heal spontaneously, and are more likely to require early surgical treatment. The lateral lesions are usually thin and wafer-like, with a very thin piece of bone present. Medial lesions are less likely to be associated with trauma and may occur insidiously. These lesions are also less likely to be symptomatic, may heal spontaneously, and usually require surgery only when the lesion becomes displaced from the talus and becomes a loose body in the ankle joint. Morphologically, the medial lesions are more cup-shaped, deeper, and tend to stay in the crater. These two broad categories of osteochondral lesions can be remembered using the acronyms DIAL (Dorsiflexion, Inversion, Anterior, Lateral) for lateral lesions and PIMP (Plantarflexion, Inversion, Medial, Posterior) for medial lesions.

When the symptoms associated with a routine ankle sprain do not resolve, an osteochondral lesion of the talus should be considered. Symptoms of persistent pain, effusion, locking, or giving way after 5 to 6 weeks should prompt further investigation. Specialized radiographs, including a mortise view with the ankle in maximum plantarflexion, should be made in an attempt to see a fragment from the talus. Bone scintigraphy using a pinhole collimator is very sensitive for detecting these lesions. If a bone scan is negative, it is unlikely that there is significant osteochondral injury. If the bone scan is positive, further investigation with CT or MRI will better delineate the morphology and anatomic location of the lesion. This information is often necessary to direct the treatment of this injury.

The treatment of osteochondral lesions depends on the size and severity of the lesion. Small lesions that are not completely detached from the articular surface can be treated conservatively. This usually involves a period of nonweightbearing ambulation and immobilization. Larger areas of injury, and lesions that are completely detached from the articular surface, usually require surgical treatment. Surgical principles include repair of the lesion if the fragment is large enough, or excision of the fragment and attempts to induce fibrocartilaginous growth into the remaining defect if the lesion is smaller. Lesions on the anterior $\frac{1}{2}$ to $\frac{2}{3}$ of the talus can usually be approached arthroscopically. Lesions on the posterior half of the talus are more difficult to treat arthroscopically and usually require open surgical treatment.

Posttraumatic Arthritis

Posttraumatic arthritis of the ankle can occur after any ankle injury. At the time of the acute injury, the cartilage surfaces may be damaged microscopically and gross injury to the articular surface may go unrecognized. An intraarticular fracture may result in joint incongruities, which over time results in cartilage wear and degeneration. An intraarticular fracture that is reduced anatomically, with no subsequent joint incongruity, may also develop posttraumatic arthritis due to injury to the articular surface at the cellular level (Fig. 17–8). Posttraumatic arthritis may develop after repetitive minor injuries to the ankle (repeated ankle sprains). Finally, posttraumatic arthritis can develop as a result of altered biomechanics of the ankle due to soft-tissue injuries (i.e., posterior tibialis tendon ruptures, contractures about the ankle, etc.).

Clinically, patients with posttraumatic arthritis of the ankle present primarily with progressive pain and limited motion of the ankle. A common complaint is pain or inability to fully dorsiflex the ankle. Initially, the pain occurs only with strenuous activities, but may progress to pain with activities of daily living, and even pain at rest.

Patients with early or mild posttraumatic arthritis can be treated with activity modifications and NSAIDs. With more severe symptoms and pathology,

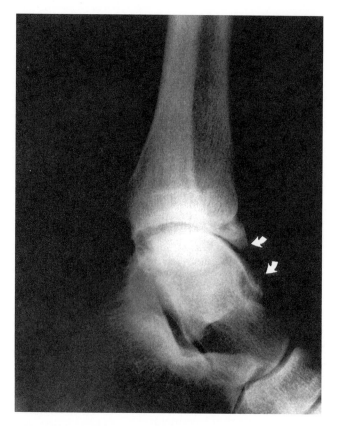

Figure 17–8. Anterior ankle bony impingement due to posttraumatic arthritis of the ankle joint. Radiograph demonstrates anterior talar and anterior tibial osteophytes ("spurs"). (*Reproduced with permission from* WA Lillegard, JO Butcher, KS Rucker. A Symptom-Oriented Approach. *Handbook of Sports Medicine 2nd ed.* Butterworth-Heinmann publishers, 1999.)

the patient may benefit from orthotics to limit motion in the ankle. Intraarticular injections of steroid preparations should be used cautiously. Surgical intervention may be required for severe symptoms and pathology that do not respond to conservative measures. Surgical treatment consists of arthroscopic debridement and excision of osteophytes or arthrodesis of the tibiotalar joint.

Other Causes of Diffuse Ankle Pain

Other causes of diffuse ankle pain include sympathetic-mediated pain syndromes, neoplasms or tumors involving the soft tissue or osseous structures about the ankle, and inflammatory arthropathies. The pain of sympathetic-mediated pain syndromes (i.e., reflex sympathetic dystrophy, complex regional pain syndromes) is noted by the persistence of pain despite prolonged conservative therapy. Vascular changes including swelling and discoloration may be present. A triple phase bone scan may demonstrate diffuse asymmetry when compared with the asymptomatic side. In addition

to rehabilitation, treatment may include the placement of transcutaneous electrical nerve stimulation (TENS) electrodes over the vascular channels of the lower extremity, and in recalcitrant cases sympathetic blockade.

The pain of a neoplastic process may be atypical and is often associated with rest or night pain. Inflammatory arthropathies such as rheumatoid arthritis, gouty arthritis, Reiter's syndrome, psoriatic arthritis, and ankylosing spondylitis can all affect the ankle joint. Serologic and radiographic studies are often needed to make these diagnoses. Finally, septic processes can involve the ankle joint. Unexplained ankle joint effusions should be aspirated and the synovial fluid sent for analysis and cultures.

SUMMARY

Injuries to the ankle joint continue to be some of the most common problems seen in running athletes. The majority of injuries can be accurately diagnosed with a thorough history and complete physical examination. Judicious use of imaging studies is often necessary to confirm a diagnosis. Most ankle injuries and overuse conditions can be treated nonoperatively. Persistent symptoms despite conservative treatment may warrant referral for specialized treatment. Attention to the principles outlined in this chapter will allow individuals with disorders of the ankle to return to regular activities in the shortest possible time.

REFERENCES

1. Clanton TO, Schon LC: Athletic injuries to the soft tissues of the foot and ankle, in Mann RA, Coughlin MJ (eds.), *Surgery of the Foot and Ankle*, 6th ed., Vol. 2, St. Louis, Mosby, 1993:1095.
2. Garrick JG, Requa RK: The epidemiology of foot and ankle injuries in sports. *Clin Sports Med* 1988:7, 29.
3. Smith RW, Reischl SF: Treatment of ankle sprains in young athletes. *Am J Sports Med* 1986:14, 465.
4. Lassiter TE, Malone TR, Garrett WE: Injury to the lateral ligaments of the ankle. *Orthop Clin North Am* 1989:20, 629.
5. Karlsson J, Bergsten T, Lasinger O, et al.: Surgical treatment of chronic lateral instability of the ankle joint. *Am J Sports Med* 1989:17, 26.
6. Renstrom PA, Kannus P: Injuries of the foot and ankle, in DeLee JC, Drez D (eds.), *Orthopaedic Sports Medicine*, Vol. 2, Philadelphia, Saunders, 1994:1705.
7. Ryan JB, Hopkinson WJ, Wheeler JH, et al.: Office management of the acute ankle sprain. *Clin Sports Med* 1989:8, 477.
8. Brantigan JW, Pedegana LR, Lippert FG: Instability of the subtalar joint. Diagnosis by stress tomography in three cases. *J Bone Joint Surg* 1977:59A, 321.

9. Matheson GO, Clements DB, McKenzie DC, et al.: Stress fractures in athletes. A study of 320 cases. *Am J Sports Med* 1987:15, 46.

10. Orava S, Hulkko A: Stress fractures in athletes. *Int J Sports Med* 1987:8, 221.

11. Stiehl JB: Complex ankle fracture dislocations with syndesmotic diastasis. *Orthop Rev* 1990:14, 499.

12. DeSouza LJ, Gustilo RB, Meyer TJ: Results of operative treatment of displaced external rotation-abduction fractures of the ankle. *J Bone Joint Surg* 1985:67A, 1066.

13. Yablon IG, Heller FG, Shouse L: The key of the lateral malleolus in displaced fractures of the ankle. *J Bone Joint Surg* 1977:59A, 169.

14. Harper MC: The deltoid ligament. An evaluation of need for surgical repair. *Clin Orthop* 1988:226, 156.

15. Chapman MW: Sprains of the ankle. *Instr Course Lect* 1975:24, 294.

16. Beskin JL, Sanders RA, Hunter SC, et al.: Surgical repair of Achilles tendon ruptures. *Am J Sports Med* 1987:15, 1.

17. Nistor L: Surgical and non-surgical treatment of Achilles tendon rupture. *J Bone Joint Surg* 1981:63A, 394.

18. Stein SR, Luekens CA: Methods and rationale for closed treatment of Achilles tendon ruptures. *Am J Sports Med* 1976:4, 162.

19. Jacobs D, Martens M, Audekercke RV, et al.: Comparison of conservative and operative treatment of Achilles tendon rupture. *Am J Sports Med* 1978:6, 107.

20. Inglis AE, Scott WN, Sculco TP, et al.: Ruptures of the tendon Achilles. *J Bone Joint Surg* 1976:58A, 990.

Chapter 18

FOOT INJURIES IN THE RUNNER

Stephen M. Simons

INTRODUCTION

Evolutionary adaptive changes to the human foot allowed upright, bipedal posture that liberated the hands to make tools. These anatomic changes and habitual bipedalism predate the expansion of the human brain. Expanding the calcaneus, closing the first intermetatarsal angle, reducing the first-ray mobility, and dorsiflexing the toes all contribute to allowing substantial single-limb support. These modifications produce three distinct arches helpful for shock absorption on impact followed by a rigid foot for muscular force transmission during propulsion. Mankind benefited greatly from the structural changes allowing bipedalism, but the foot also became vulnerable with this highly adaptable yet propulsive function. Single-limb support while running places great demands on the foot because three times body weight is transmitted through the force-transducing foot. The changes to the primate foot remarkably changed the course of human evolution.[1]

EPIDEMIOLOGY OF FOOT INJURIES

The foot and ankle are often cited as the most common sites for running-related injuries. Epidemiologic studies specifically identifying foot injuries are sparse. Definition of "injury" varies by author and these studies

rely on patient-driven reporting of their injuries. An "injury" may be as trivial as blisters or as career-ending as certain stress fractures or tendon ruptures. Runner injury rates are often gleaned from lists of race entrants and records from health care clinics. These methods exclude the recreational runner who drops running as an activity and therefore does not present to racing events or clinics. This "healthy-runner effect" introduces a self-selection bias that underestimates the risk of running injury.[2] Table 18–1 summarizes a few epidemiologic studies of runners. Included is a calculation of stress fractures of the foot as a percentage of total stress fractures in nine different studies (Bennell and Brukner).

ANATOMY

Knowledge of anatomy and biomechanics are fundamental to understanding the injuries that can occur to the runner's foot. This discussion of anatomy and biomechanics is provided as elementary background for understanding foot injuries. A more detailed discussion of biomechanics can be found in Chapter 2. Foot injuries will be anatomically described as forefoot, midfoot, or rearfoot injuries. The forefoot consists of structures distal to the tarsometatarsal joints, also known as LisFranc's joint. Skeletally this includes the metatarsals and phalanges. The midfoot includes the

TABLE 18–1.

Study	Setting	Percentage Injured Sufficient to Temporarily Cease Running	Foot Injuries as % of Total Injuries
Marti et al.[66]	Race participants; injuries in year before race.	45.8% of 4358 runners	10.2%
Jacobs and Berson[67]	Race participants; injuries in the preceeding two years.	66% of 451 runners	11% (plantar fasciitis)
Walter et al.[68]	Race participants; injuries in year following race.	48% of 1680 runners	19%
Bennell and Brukner[69]	Of 790 stress fractures in nine studies of runners or track and field athletes.		29.4% of all stress fractures were metatarsals or navicular

navicular, cuboid, and cuneiforms, and associated soft tissue. The rearfoot is the talus and calcaneus as well as the soft tissues that traverse this area.

The relevant forefoot bones include the metatarsals, phalanges, and sesamoids. The first metatarsal articulates proximally with the first cuneiform and the second metatarsal. The cuneiform in turn articulates more proximally with the navicular. This collective chain of navicular, medial cuneiform, and first metatarsal is often referred to as the *first ray*. The shape of the medial cuneiform determines the tarsometatarsal mobility of the first ray. The second and third metatarsals articulate proximally, also with the associated cuneiform. It is important to recognize the recessed position of the second metatarsal base. This makes the second metatarsal inherently more rigid than its neighbors. The fourth metatarsal articulates proximally with the cuboid and is also quite stable. The fifth metatarsal proximally articulates also with the cuboid and enjoys more mobility than the other lesser metatarsals. The sesamoids are positioned at midstance below the first metatarsal head. As the heel is lifted during propulsion, the sesamoids remain relatively fixed to the proximal phalanx while the metatarsal rotates to a position on top of the sesamoids. This functionally lengthens the metatarsal as weight is transferred from lateral to medial across the metatarsal heads.

The midfoot contains the "keystones" of the arches. The navicular provides stability to the medial longitudinal arch. The cuboid is the keystone for the lateral longitudinal arch. The cuneiforms form a transverse arch across the midfoot.

The calcaneus and talus form the rearfoot. Critical to the function of the rearfoot is the subtalar joint, consisting of three facets. The subtalar joint functions similar to a universal joint, allowing motions in several planes at once. This capability allows the foot to adapt to terrain of different slopes while maintaining the extremity in a relatively vertical position.

BIOMECHANICS

The gait cycle is defined as the movements involved from heel strike of one foot until the second heel strike of that same foot. The gait cycle is subdivided into stance phase and swing phase. Discussion of running foot biomechanics focuses on the stance phase, which is further subdivided into heel strike, midstance, and propulsion. Heel strike begins with heel contact and ends with forefoot loading. Midstance begins with forefoot loading and then ends when the heel lifts from the ground. Propulsion begins with heel lift and ends with toe-off. The stance phase consumes about 60% of the walking gait cycle with a periodicity of approximately one second. The running gait cycle differs from that of walking in that a single running gait cycle adds two float phases with both feet off the ground. Also, as the speed of gait increases the stance phase consumes proportionately less time than in walking. These two changes dramatically decrease the absolute and the relative amount of time the foot spends in stance phase. Newton's laws dictate that greater accelerative forces are imparted to the foot and up the kinetic chain.

The foot must perform as an accommodative mobile adapter at heel strike and then passively transition to a rigid lever for muscular propulsion by toe-off. The subtalar joint, beginning in a supinated position and proceeding to pronation assists the ankle, knee, and hip with impact shock absorption. Further mobility is provided by the midtarsal joints, which allow motion around longitudinal and oblique axes. As the body above crosses over the foot, external tibial rotation directs the foot into supination. Excessive or delayed resupination of the foot contributes to a poorly propulsive foot.

FOREFOOT PROBLEMS

Tendinitis

Extensor Tendinitis

Extensor tendinitis is a common problem in runners. The runner presents with dorsal foot pain and perhaps diffuse forefoot swelling. The history requires a search for changes in training and terrain changes. Introducing hill running may add new stresses to the extensor tendons. Uphill running forces the foot to dorsiflex more during swing phase to avoid striking the ground or pavement. Downhill running stresses the extensor tendons eccentrically during stance phase. Improperly fitting shoes or excessively tight lacing can also compress and impair normal tendon function. I have also seen this injury as a result of running on snowy or icy surfaces. The stride length is shortened as the runner prematurely lifts the foot into dorsiflexion to avoid the unstable sensation of slipping when the ground contact foot is well behind the center of gravity. Examination may reveal very little tenderness or may reveal swelling, crepitus, and pain with passive stretch to the tendons. Metatarsal stress fractures are the other common forefoot problem that must be considered. I find pain on passive stretch of the tendons suggestive of tendinitis, while pain with an axially directed load to the metatarsal head, away from the site of swelling, suggests stress fracture. Traumatic rupture of these tendons is quite rare. Treatment consists of ice, brief use of nonsteroidal anti-inflammatory drugs (NSAIDs), tongue pads, and an alternative lacing technique to remove pressure on the tendons. Rehabilitative exercise includes extensor strengthening and gastrocsoleus flexibility, as well as addressing other kinetic chain deficits identified during the examination.

Flexor Tendinitis

Flexor tendinitis is less common but can be more painful and disabling. Flexor hallucis longus tendinitis is more common in dancers but may occur in runners as well.[3] Examination for tenderness along the course of the tendon and pain with resisted great toe flexion suggests tendinitis. Treatment consists of attention to biomechanical issues, training modification with relative rest, examination of shoes, icing, and NSAIDs. Flexor muscle strengthening can be achieved by pleating a towel with toe curls.

The flexor hallucis longus (FHL) tendon can exhibit a stenosing tenosynovitis, which can mimic tendinitis, tarsal tunnel syndrome, and plantar fasciitis. Posterior medial ankle pain, arch pain, or a positive Tinel's sign was present in 19 dancers or runners undergoing MRI or tenography. Conservative measures were not helpful in these cases. Surgical tenolysis successfully returned these athletes to sport in 9 weeks.[4]

FHL tendon rupture has reportedly occurred during a half marathon.[5] This patient experienced a feeling "as though something was rolled up in his shoe." This runner was subsequently running 25 miles per week 6 months postoperatively. The site of FHL rupture is critical to the examination findings. There is a fibrous slip between the FHL and the flexor digitorum longus (FDL) tendon. If tendon rupture occurs distal to this slip the great toe lacks active flexion. But if the rupture occurs proximal to this connecting slip the FHL tendon recoils into the calf and there can be active great toe flexion, albeit weak, transmitted through the FDL tendon.

METATARSALGIA

History and Examination

Pain in the region of the metatarsal heads is generically known as metatarsalgia. A search for a specific source of the pain is necessary to direct management. Table 18–2 lists common causes of metatarsalgia.[6] Mechanically-induced metatarsal head pain results when vertical ground reaction forces are not properly distributed through the forefoot. Certain foot structures are predisposed to painful plantar keratoses. A rigid cavus foot with plantarflexed first or second ray should be suspected in patients that have thick, painful calluses under the first or second ray. Conversely, the hypermobile first ray excessively dorsiflexes in late stance phase. This flexible first ray fails to accept the transfer of weight to the first ray late in stance phase.

TABLE 18–2. CAUSES OF METATARSALGIA

Interdigital neuroma
Idiopathic MTPJ synovitis
Freiberg's disease
Inflammatory arthritis of MTPJs
Cavus foot with plantarflexed first and
   second rays
Morton's foot (long second ray)
Hypermobile first ray
Prominent lateral plantar condyle of
   metatarsal head
Tight Achilles' tendon
High-heeled shoes

MTPJ, metatarsophalangeal joint.

Consequently the second metatarsal head undergoes undue stress and is subject to metatarsal head pain or even stress fracture. I typically find a comma-shaped callus under the second metatarsal head when the first ray is hypermobile. The convex side of this callus points to the first metatarsal head. The hypermobile first ray is probably caused by a curved or rounded medial cuneiform first metatarsal joint. This allows for a greater dynamic first intermetatarsal angle and drift of the metatarsal head medially.[7] I explain to patients that this structure forces the first ray to behave more like a thumb than it would in a stable foot.

Some patients will develop an intractable plantar keratosis under a prominent lateral metatarsal head condyle. These are frequently confused with plantar warts. One clinical clue is the pinch test. Pinching a wart is often more painful than direct pressure, whereas direct pressure on an intractable plantar keratosis is more painful than pinching. Trimming this callus tissue will reveal a conical-shaped, deep callus lacking the soft, friable material of a typical plantar wart. It also lacks the typical punctate hemorrhages of warts.

Treatment

Metatarsalgia is first managed conservatively with accommodative padding to redirect vertical and frictional forces away from the painful lesions. A metatarsal pad placed proximal to the metatarsal heads may relieve pressure directly on the ends of the metatarsals and spread the forces over a broader area throughout the metatarsal. A custom orthotic that provides some plantar support to the hypermobile first ray or utilizes accommodative padding such as a horseshoe cutout around a specific metatarsal head can be helpful. The cavus foot with a plantarflexed first ray may benefit from the orthotic that unloads the high forces on the heel and metatarsal heads by moving the vertical loads a little more proximal. Other conservative measures include improving the flexibility to the gastroachilles complex, strengthening the foot intrinsics, running shoes with improved forefoot cushion, and avoidance of high-heeled shoes.

INTERDIGITAL NEUROMA

Etiology

Interdigital neuromas can afflict runners. Not a true neurologic tumor, an interdigital neuroma pathologically consists of perineural fibrosis, fibrinoid degeneration, demyelination, and endoneural fibrosis.[8] These neuromas are associated with wearing narrow shoes and extreme toe dorsiflexion as occurs with uphill or downhill running. The traction on the interdigital nerves with repeated

dorsiflexion probably contributes to neural or connective tissue injury. I describe these changes to patients as analogous to a callus around the nerve.

History and Examination

Common symptoms include burning-type pain radiating to the toes, pain increased with walking, plantar pain, and pain relieved by rest or removing the shoe. Only 40% of patients experience frank numbness in the toes.[9] Symptoms most commonly occur in the third interspace, although the first and fourth interdigital nerves may be involved.[10] Normal anatomy predisposes to the risk for third interdigital nerve involvement. This nerve is an "anastomosis," or a shared perineural sheath with branches from the medial and lateral plantar nerves. The third nerve has a larger cross-sectional diameter than the first, second, and fourth.[11]

Diagnosis is suspected by history and supported by examination. Squeezing the forefoot and compressing the metatarsal heads together aggravates tenderness to the web space. This compression test accompanied by a snapping sensation is known as Mulder's sign.[12] Other diagnoses should be included in the differential. These include local bone or joint pathology such as stress fracture, and Freiberg's infarction.

Treatment

Treatment first consists of attempts to widen the intermetatarsal space. Shoes with a wider toebox and more forefoot cushioning should be tried. A metatarsal pad placed in the shoe or incorporated into an orthotic device can widen the metatarsal heads. Nonathletic shoes with a firm rocker bottom–type sole such as a hiking boot may reduce the need for toe dorsiflexion in late stance phase.

Corticosteroid injection through a dorsal approach may provide complete or sufficient pain relief to return to activity. I usually inject a mixture of 1 ml triamcinolone, 1 ml xylocaine, and 1 ml bupivacaine. Recalcitrant and intolerable pain should prompt surgical consideration. There is controversy regarding the best operative management. Options include excising the interdigital nerve alone, transecting the intermetatarsal ligament alone, or performing both procedures.[10]

HALLUCAL SESAMOIDS

Anatomy

The hallucal sesamoids are located directly inferior to the head of the first metatarsal. These constant accessory bones are contained within the flexor hallucis brevis tendon. They assist the first metatarsal to accept weight during late stance phase. They elevate the first metatarsal head while the metatarsal rolls on top of the sesamoids to functionally lengthen the metatarsal during late stance phase. The tibial (medial) sesamoid bears the majority of the weight transfer. The abductor hallucis inserts onto the tibial sesamoid, and the adductor hallucis inserts onto the fibular (lateral) sesamoid. The flexor hallucis longus tendon traverses the plantar aspect of the joint, passing between the two sesamoids. A bony ridge on the plantar first metatarsal head also serves to separate the sesamoids. A bipartite or multipartite sesamoid occurs in 5% to 33% of the population.[6]

Injuries

Most sesamoid injuries are due to overuse. They occur in runners, dancers, shot-putters, marching band members, and any sport that involves running. The precise tissue pathology causing the pain can be elusive. Sesamoid injuries include stress fracture (40%), sesamoiditis (chondromalacia) (30%), acute fracture (10%), osteochondritis (10%), osteoarthritis (5%), and bursitis (5%).[13]

Clinical and Radiologic Findings

Clinically, the athlete presents with pain and swelling under the sesamoid. Sometimes a fluid-filled bursa can be appreciated. Plain radiographs are taken in the anteroposterior (AP), lateral, and axial (Lewis) views. This latter view places the great toe into maximum dorsiflexion while the x-ray beam is tangential to the metatarsal.[14] This is similar to the Merchant view of the knee. A tibial sesamoid view profiles the tibial sesamoid.[6] Plain radiography is often normal with pathologic changes delayed. Technetium bone scans can be quite sensitive but lack specificity. The bone scan is particularly helpful for demonstrating bone metabolic activity because it can clarify an anatomically abnormal x-ray or computed tomography (CT) scan. A CT scan performed in two planes visualizes the anatomy of the sesamoid quite well.[15]

As indicated above, stress fractures are the most common reason for sesamoid pain. A stress fracture that proceeds to frank fracture and then fracture nonunion can be difficult to differentiate from a bipartite sesamoid. Both will have rounded margins to the bone. It is also possible to have a chondral fracture through the bipartite sesamoid. Sesamoid osteochondritis will behave clinically similar to stress fractures. Early bone scan will show positive changes and there will be eventual changes on x-ray, showing mottling and fragmentation. This latter appearance, suggesting aseptic necrosis of the sesamoid, is usually indication for surgical resection. Sesamoiditis is a somewhat perplexing diagnosis, defined as pain and swelling of the peritendinous structures around the sesamoids. There

may be a degenerative chondromalacia of the articular cartilage around the sesamoid. Radiographs are often normal, but bone scan will show diffuse uptake.

Treatment

Precise tissue diagnosis is elusive, but fortunately treatment for all of these sesamoid conditions is essentially the same. Sesamoid injury can be quite debilitating. The athlete must first halt the offending activity. Determination of the degree of rest and immobilization needed requires clinical judgment. This can range from as little as prohibiting sports activity while allowing normal ambulation, to cast immobilization for 6 weeks. Using a stiff-soled shoe is a compromise measure. Plantar padding with a sesamoid cut-out pad to unload or distribute pressure away from the sesamoid can be incorporated into the shoe. This padding can also be incorporated into a custom-molded orthotic. Surgical excision of the sesamoid is considered only after all conservative efforts are exhausted. Surgical treatment should not be undertaken without concern for the biomechanical consequences.

FIRST METATARSOPHALANGEAL JOINT CONDITIONS

Hallux Rigidus

Hallux valgus and hallux rigidus are common conditions affecting the first metatarsophalangeal (MTP) joint. Running may not cause these problems but runners often have to deal with them. Hallux rigidus is characterized by restricted range of motion of the first MTP joint. Particularly problematic is the lack of dorsiflexion needed for normal walking or running. This problem is exaggerated with climbing hills or stairs or anything requiring greater dorsiflexion at the MTP. This is a degenerative condition, probably a consequence of some former trauma. Clinically, the patient will have pain in the MTP, numbness or tingling from compression of the dorsal cutaneous nerves, and altered biomechanics possibly predisposing to some other overuse injury. Irritation from shoes rubbing on the dorsal bunion caused by metatarsal head osteophytes may cause abrasion or frank ulceration. Running likely will accelerate this condition, but if the runner insists on running, a few conservative measures are indicated. These include use of stiff-soled shoes, training reduction, avoidance of hills, NSAIDs, passive joint mobilization efforts, and possibly a custom orthotic with a Morton's extension, limiting the need for MTP dorsiflexion. If these measures are not successful, the runner may need to consider alternative training and eventually surgical management.

Hallux Valgus

Development of hallux valgus is unrelated to running activities, but can nonetheless interfere with the ability to run. Commonly known as a bunion, hallux valgus is evident as a sometimes painful first MTP manifest with the great toe deviated in a valgus position while the first metatarsal drifts medially. The sesamoids are gradually subluxed laterally and the laterally deviating great toe encroaches the second toe. Painful plantar keratoses can develop under the second metatarsal head because weight transfer to the great toe is compromised. The asymptomatic hallux valgus deformity need not be treated. I caution the runner to seek professional advice at the first sign of symptoms related to the bunion. For the mildly symptomatic bunion, conservative care should first be attempted. A simple toe spacer between the first and second toes may be helpful. Silicone bunion padding over the MTP can alleviate direct pressure symptoms. A custom orthotic with a Morton's extension is worth trying. Shoe choice can be quite a challenge in an advanced case of hallux valgus. A wider toebox is necessary to accommodate the wider forefoot, but this may be hard to find. A wider shoe for the forefoot often comes with the price of a wider heel, allowing the runner's heel to slip. I often suggest using a soft heel cup in this situation simply to take up space in the rear of the shoe and reduce heel slippage. The intolerably painful hallux valgus can be eventually managed surgically.

METATARSAL STRESS FRACTURES

Middle Metatarsal Stress Fractures

Etiology

The original "march fracture" described in 1855 by Briethaupt aptly identified the common metatarsal stress fracture. The incidence of metatarsal stress fractures is second only to tibial stress fractures in incidence in the athletic population. Stress fractures of the second, third, and fourth metatarsals encompass 90% of metatarsal stress fractures. Ground reactive forces and the associated bending strain on the second metatarsal are 6.9 times greater than the force applied to the first metatarsal.[16] The base of the second metatarsal is recessed and more rigidly encompassed by the cuneiforms than the other metatarsals; this probably allows less sagittal plane motion producing more bending stress. Muscular fatigue of the long flexors of the toes also contributes to the high loading forces on the second metatarsal.[17] Metatarsal stress fractures are more frequently associated with pes planus, compared with tibial stress fractures that are associated with a pes cavus foot structure. A short first metatarsal or a Morton's foot was thought to contribute to a greater risk for second metatarsal stress fracture, but this anecdotal wisdom has been challenged. I suspect the biomechanical culprit is not the short first metatarsal, but the first metatarsal, which is hypermobile in the sagittal plane.

Presentation

Stress fractures of the lesser metatarsals, except for the base of the second or fifth metatarsals, usually present with poorly defined forefoot pain. The pain is aggravated by running and improved with rest. Often beginning as an intermittent pain, with continued running the fracture pain eventually becomes relentless and occurs during activities of daily living. There can be sudden pain escalation after a single, more intense run. The usual presentation appears 4 to 5 weeks after a sudden training change.[18]

Examination

The foot with a lesser metatarsal stress fracture may demonstrate dorsal swelling that can be focal or diffuse, often obliterating the usually visible extensor tendons. Careful palpation of each metatarsal shaft can delineate a bony origin to the tenderness. Advanced cases of metatarsal stress fracture may reveal a palpable bony callus. A clinical clue to differentiate the stress fracture from tendinitis is to request active extension of the toes against resistance. This maneuver often is not painful with a metatarsal stress fracture, whereas in tendinitis it is. I find that placing a thumb on the end of the metatarsal head while the proximal phalanx is dorsiflexed, and then applying an axially directed force along the shaft of the metatarsal may elicit pain at the fracture site and distant from the palpation site.

Radiographs

Radiographs of the foot will often remain normal for 3 to 6 weeks after symptom onset. Subperiosteal bone formation will appear along the diaphyseal shaft. Radiographs can remain normal in many confirmed cases of metatarsal stress fracture.[19] Technetium bone scan is positive within 48 to 72 hr of symptom onset. A triple phase scan positive in all three phases is most specific for a stress fracture.

Treatment

Reduction or cessation of running activities is usually adequate conservative treatment for a metatarsal stress fracture. Nonweightbearing training during this relative rest period will maintain cardiovascular and some muscular fitness to hasten return to activity once the fracture is healed. Temporary crutch use followed by wearing a stiff-soled shoe can be helpful for the particularly painful stress fracture. Intrinsic foot muscle strengthening with toe curls and extensions may be helpful. Four to 6 weeks' rest is usually sufficient for these common stress fractures. Clinical healing time was 7 weeks in one study of 19 metatarsal stress fractures in 51 runners.[20] Careful review of the training regimen used prior to injury can prevent repeating obvious training errors.

Prevention

A gradual return to training is required to avoid a recurrence of stress fracture. Certain foot structures may benefit from the use of a custom orthotic. Although theoretical empirical use of an orthotic is mechanically compelling, hard evidence for injury prevention is lacking. The foot exhibiting a hypermobile first ray can excessively load the second metatarsal. An orthotic with a Morton's extension will help unload the second metatarsal. I routinely examine the transverse arch across the metatarsal heads. It is my distinct clinical impression that some people will have an excessively long or rigidly plantarflexed lesser metatarsal when compared with its neighbors. A callus under the metatarsal head supports this assertion. I believe these patients benefit from a custom orthotic with a metatarsal head cutout under the injured metatarsal. This allows the metatarsal head to ride lower and directs vertical ground reaction forces to the adjacent metatarsals.

First Metatarsal

Stress fractures of the first metatarsal are rare. When they occur, it is usually at the junction of the metaphysis and diaphysis proximally. These fractures are frequently not apparent on radiography. Treatment is directed to restricted weightbearing while wearing a wooden-soled shoe. The period of rest is similar to that for fracture of the lesser metatarsals.[21] I once managed one of these stress fractures that improved only after 6 weeks in a removable boot cast.

Fifth Metatarsal

Fifth metatarsal stress fractures rarely occur in runners. These difficult fractures are more common in cutting-type sports. An extensive discussion of this complicated problem is covered in Chapter 19. The clinician should be aware of the types of fractures that affect the fifth metatarsal. Diaphyseal, shaft stress fractures should be managed much the same as the other lesser metatarsal shaft stress fractures. Avulsion fractures that accompany an inversion ankle sprain involve the proximal 1 cm of the metatarsal base and do not include the cubometatarsal joint. These fractures are managed symptomatically using activity modification

and a stiff-soled shoe or boot. Fractures occurring at the metaphyseal-diaphyseal junction are notorious for poor healing and fracture nonunion. Traumatically caused acute fractures with no antecedent pain history and no radiographic evidence of stress injury to the bone can be managed with nonweightbearing cast immobilization for 6 to 8 weeks. Seventy-two percent of athletes will return to sport in 7 to 21 weeks.[22] Proximal fractures at this metaphyseal-diaphyseal junction with radiographic evidence of prior stress injury may require internal fixation and are best managed by a practitioner familiar with this problem.[23]

MIDFOOT INJURIES

The most common midfoot injuries in runners are tendinopathies and stress fractures. Posterior tibial tendinitis and rupture is more common than its counterpart, peroneal tendinitis on the lateral side of the foot. Navicular stress fracture, discussed here and in Chapter 19, is an underappreciated injury.

Posterior Tibial Tendon (PTT)

Etiology

The posterior tibial tendon is subject to significant eccentric forces with each stance phase of the gait cycle. As a secondary, muscular restraint to the medial longitudinal arch, the posterior tibial muscle resists descent of the arch on contact and into midstance. Tendinitis can ensue following the common runner errors of overly rapid training changes or using worn or inadequate shoes, or in a structurally poor foot that allows excessive pronation. The left foot is particularly susceptible to this tendinitis when training on a track due to the added dynamic pronation from continuously turning left.

Clinical Presentation and Treatment

Clinically, the patient presents with pain along the course of the tendon, usually in the interval between the medial malleolus and the insertion at the base of the first metatarsal. Examination reveals tenderness along the course of the tendon and increased pain with resisted inversion of the foot. This condition usually resolves with ice, NSAIDs, relative rest, and attention to biomechanical factors that stress the longitudinal arch. A rehabilitative exercise program should emphasize foot intrinsic strengthening as well as eccentric strengthening of the posterior tibialis.

Rupture

Posterior tibial tendon rupture occurs rarely in runners. Previous corticosteroid injections probably predispose this tendon to rupture.[24,25] Relative hypovascularity of the tendon posterior and distal to the medial malleolus also predisposes this tendon to degenerative changes and rupture.[26] Collapse of the medial longitudinal arch and difficulty with single limb, standing on the tip toes, are clinical clues to this rare malady. Nonoperative treatment of posterior tibial tendon rupture is considered in the relatively inactive older individual. Immobilization in a nonweightbearing cast is followed by over-the-counter or custom orthoses to support the medial side of the foot. The younger, more active individual is best advised to have a ruptured posterior tibial tendon surgically repaired to minimize the development of a painful flat foot.

Peroneal Tendons

The peroneal tendons are also subject to tendinitis and occasional rupture. As on the medial side, symptoms are focused between the lateral malleolus and the tendon insertions. Peroneus longus involvement can create pain on the lateral side of the foot as well as on its plantar aspect. Examination reveals tenderness along the course of the tendon and increased pain with resisted foot eversion and plantarflexion. Treatment consists of rest, ice, gentle stretching, and seeking unusual biomechanical causes both intrinsic to the patient and dynamically related to the runner's training. In my own clinical experience caring for runners with peroneal tendinitis, I have noted that though these patients can have severe acute pain, it resolves relatively quickly and they are unlikely to experience chronic pain. Strengthening exercises, initially nonweightbearing, should emphasize foot plantarflexion and eversion against resistance using stretch bands.

Navicular Stress Fractures

Etiology

Navicular stress fractures, previously thought to be quite rare, are now appreciated as a very common stress fracture in track and field athletes with a propensity to afflict middle-distance runners.[27] These fractures frequently go undiagnosed for several months.[28] The etiology of these stress fractures is speculative. Impingement or bending forces exerted by the proximal and distal tarsal bones, combined with a relatively avascular segment are thought to be contributory.[29,30] Poor ankle dorsiflexion has been associated with this fracture. It routinely occurs in the middle segment of the navicular, oriented in the sagittal plane.

History and Examination

The patient presents with vague dorsal, medial midfoot pain. I have had at least two of these cases present as "ankle pain." This pain begins insidiously during exertion and slowly progresses to periods of forced inactivity. Examination is usually unremarkable except for tenderness directly over the apex of the navicular, a location coined the "N" spot by Khan and colleagues.[28] This spot is identified by finding the talon-avicular joint medially while pronating and supinating the foot, moving slightly distal to this joint, palpating the navicular tuberosity, and then moving up to the dorsum of the navicular. This is usually directly under the anterior tibial tendon. Another examination technique is to apply a high compressive force by hopping on the involved side with the foot held in equinus.[31]

Imaging

Imaging with plain radiography is quite insensitive, because the vast majority of x-rays are normal.[32] Continued clinical suspicion directs the clinician to proceed to bone scan or CT scan. Technetium bone scans are quite sensitive and may be most appropriate to identify bone pathology. The tarsal navicular stress fracture is usually revealed as diffuse uptake through the entire navicular. CT scan has supplanted the linear tomogram for clarifying the exact nature of this fracture. The proximal articular surface of the navicular is routinely densely sclerotic, appearing as a rim in true axial images. The fracture typically occurs in this sclerotic rim on the dorsal surface. Most fractures are curvilinear.[33]

Treatment

Treatment for tarsal navicular stress fractures is usually successfully done conservatively. Khan and coworkers reported that 89% of patients healed with nonweightbearing for 6 weeks.[28] Quirk, writing as president of the American Orthopaedic Foot and Ankle Society, outlines the following treatment protocol:[31]

1. Six weeks on crutches with a below-the-knee nonweightbearing cast, even patients who have previously failed surgery.
2. Remove cast and examine "N" spot. If it is still tender, treat with a similar cast for another 2 weeks.
3. When the cast is removed permanently, a very gradual closely supervised training program is designed.

Repeat imaging is not very helpful because CT and bone scans can remain abnormal long after the fracture is clinically ready to receive stress.

Return to sport is painstakingly slow, with an average time to return of 5.6 months. The patient is best forewarned about this lengthy recovery so as to avoid unrealistic expectations based on experience with other types of stress fractures. Preventive strategies have focused on improving gastroachilles flexibility and using custom molded orthotic management. I have had good personal experience with frequently changing to new shoes. Three to four hundred miles per pair of shoes would seem prudent. Rotating multiple pairs of shoes can minimize repeating the same biomechanical stresses daily.

Cuboid Stress Fractures

Cuboid stress fractures are relatively rare.[34] Presentation may mimic that of peroneal tendinitis. Persistent lateral foot pain merits evaluation; bone scan is most helpful. MRI may show bone edema in the asymptomatic runner.[35] Treat cuboid stress fractures with rest until pain-free for 2 weeks, then gradually resume training. Prevention should focus on evaluation of biomechanical issues. I have seen one cuboid stress fracture possibly caused by a custom orthotic made with an inappropriate valgus forefoot post in a track athlete with forefoot varus.

REARFOOT INJURIES

Stress Fractures

Talus

The talus, so named for its rocky, irregular shape, transmits all ground reactive forces to the lower leg. Considering this conduit's burden, it is surprising that the talus does not suffer more stress fractures. Only one talar neck stress fracture has been reported in runners.[36] This was in a 58-year-old runner described as having a mobile-type foot with excessive rearfoot motion. The patient presented with a painful swollen ankle and tenderness over the anterior talofibular and calcaneofibular ligaments. He was successfully treated with a nonweightbearing cast and gradual rehabilitation to return to running.

Talar stress fractures through the lateral process are reported in runners as well as other athletes.[37–39] Insidious onset of lateral ankle pain directs attention to the subtalar joint. These stress fractures can be mistakenly diagnosed as a sinus tarsi syndrome. Plain radiographs are routinely normal. Bone scan shows a "hot" talus adjacent to a "cold" calcaneus. A vertically oriented fracture through the lateral process is seen on CT scan.[39] These cases have been associated with an excessively pronating foot structure. Conservative care with nonweightbearing immobilization can be tried,

but return to sport has been relatively poor. Early diagnosis may improve the outcome, and surgical resection can also be successful.[39]

These talar stress fractures were identified with bone scan followed by CT scan to clarify the exact nature of the fracture. It should be noted that MRI can be exquisitely and overly sensitive to stress. In a series of 20 asymptomatic runners, 16 had some degree of edema seen on STIR (Short Tau Inversion Recovery) images in three to four bones of the foot.[35]

Calcaneus

Calcaneal stress fractures must be considered in the runner with heel pain. These patients will present with heel pain while running that is typically relieved by nonweightbearing. Examination is relatively nonspecific, but the examiner may be able to elicit pain when squeezing the calcaneus side to side simultaneously. A lateral projection radiograph may show a linear sclerosis parallel to the posterior margin of the calcaneus and perpendicular to the trabecular lines. Bone scan can confirm the clinical suspicions. Treatment consists of nonweightbearing using crutches until pain relief is achieved. Six to 8 weeks' rest is usually sufficient healing time prior to a gradual return to training. Attention to heel cushioning, calf stretches, and plantar fascia stretch are important.

Retrocalcaneal Bursitis

Presentation

Retrocalcaneal heel pain can be a difficult and recalcitrant problem. The examiner must first differentiate retrocalcaneal pain from Achilles' pain. Achilles'-generated pain is typically 2 to 3 cm proximal to the tendon's insertion on the calcaneus. Achilles' injuries are discussed in another chapter. The anatomy of the retrocalcaneal space includes the Achilles' tendon, which inserts into the middle third of the posterior calcaneus, the retrocalcaneal bursa intercedes between the calcaneus and the Achilles', and the adventitial bursa, located superficial to the Achilles' but underneath the skin. MRI was used recently to describe the normal retrocalcaneal bursa. A bursa larger than 1 mm anteroposterior, 11 mm transverse, or 7 mm craniocaudad is abnormal.[40] The superior posterior calcaneal tuberosity can be hyperconvex, normal, or hypoconvex. The more protuberant this tuberosity the greater chance for bursal irritation.

Examination

Examination will show swelling, erythema, and sometimes exquisite tenderness posterior to the calcaneus. It is important to distinguish this from the more proximal tenderness of Achilles' tendinitis and the more distal tenderness of a calcaneal stress fracture. Dorsiflexing the foot will usually aggravate the pain of a retrocalcaneal bursa by squeezing the bursa between the Achilles' tendon and the calcaneus. This may not be diagnostic, because a simple stretch of Achilles' tendinitis can cause similar pain.

Imaging

Imaging is usually not necessary before beginning conservative management of this common problem. A weightbearing lateral radiograph can assess the posterior calcaneal angle and view the sometimes-prominent posterior superior beak of the calcaneus. A bony prominence of the posterior superior calcaneus is known as a Haglund's deformity. Many authors have described various techniques for measuring the calcaneus. One such measurement is the Philip and Fowler Angle. This angle, as viewed on a lateral radiograph, is the angle formed by intersecting lines along the plantar surface and the posterior aspect of the calcaneus.[41] The upper limit of normal for this angle is 69 degrees. However, there are several other techniques described to assess the calcaneus as a potential source of retrocalcaneal pain. These efforts are probably not necessary unless surgical management is being considered.

Treatment

Treatment of retrocalcaneal bursitis is initially conservative with ice, NSAIDs, and perhaps topically applied nonsteroidal medicines and some accommodative padding. Schepsis and Leach reported that most runners responded to a regimen of (1) cessation or decreased weekly mileage, (2) halting interval or hill training, (3) softer running surfaces, (4) heel lift in or out of the shoe, and (5) stretching and strengthening the calf.[42] The runner can try wearing an open-backed shoe during nonathletic activities. Next, padding the heel of the shoe with a horseshoe-shaped pad or using a viscoelastic heel cup can be helpful. Attention to shoe fit is critical. The shoe must fit well enough to raise with the heel in late stance phase. A loose shoe or heel counter will drag and cause friction on the heel. The tight shoe will squeeze the bursa, contributing to an ischemic zone. Corticosteroid injections have been advocated but should be cautiously applied to avoid Achilles' tendon exposure. The runner suffering chronic heel pain not responding to these measures should be referred for possible surgical management.

Plantar Fasciitis

Heel pain may be the most problematic foot injury for the runner. Of all the causes for heel pain, plantar fasciitis is most common.

Anatomy

The plantar fascia is a nonelastic fibrous band of tissue originating on the tuberosities of the calcaneus. The largest central slip of the plantar fascia starts on the medial tuberosity. Smaller and thinner slips of the fascia begin medial and lateral to this central slip. The lateral portion begins on the lateral calcaneal tuberosity and covers the abductor digiti minimi; the medial portion covers the abductor hallucis muscle. The fascia fans out as it proceeds distally to insert on each of the proximal phalanges. Innervation to this area is the subject of some controversy. A recent anatomic study identified medial calcaneal branches arising from either the tibial nerve or the lateral plantar nerve. These branches supply the medial side of the posterior heel and terminate in the inferior fat pad. The inferior calcaneal nerve usually arises from the lateral plantar nerve and lies between the abductor hallucis muscle and the anterior tubercle of the calcaneus.[43]

Biomechanics

As was discussed earlier, the foot transforms from a mobile adapter on heel strike to a rigid lever during propulsion. The plantar fascia assists formation of a rigid arch from heel lift until toe-off. Minimal or no muscular support is needed to form an arch.[44] After midstance and during propulsion the tibia is externally rotating, thereby positioning the foot in heel varus. The subtalar and midtarsal joints are then positioned to form a locking mechanism, which resists arch collapse. The toes dorsiflex as the heel lifts from the ground. The plantar fascia, lacking elastic tissue, passively pulls the heel towards the toes, shortening this distance and lifting the longitudinal arch as a result. Its function has been likened to that of a windlass used in sailing or bridge building.[45]

Etiology

Several etiologies are proposed for plantar fasciitis. The plantar fascia undergoes histologic changes suggesting direct tissue necrosis.[46] Any proposed etiologies must therefore include mechanical and functional deficits that stress the plantar fascia. Ankle ranges of motion and strength deficits are associated with plantar fasciitis.[47] Anatomic foot configurations have also been associated with plantar fasciitis. Both the excessively pronated pes planus foot and the supinated pes cavus foot are implicated with differing pathomechanical explanations.[48,49] Training issues, height, weight, and age are also independent variables associated with plantar fasciitis.

Nerve entrapment has been implicated as a source of pain in this region; the medial calcaneal nerves are blamed in one study and the first branch of the lateral plantar nerve in others.[44] One recent study of recalcitrant heel pain syndrome asserted a 90% cure with tenolysis of the first branch of the lateral plantar nerve.[50]

History

Patients complain of an insidious onset of inferior heel pain often described as a burning sensation. Morning pain or pain with the first few steps after sitting in a chair, standing, or riding in a car is commonly cited. I speculate that the subtle accumulation of edema and inflammatory debris during inactivity is responsible for the pain with the first few steps. Walking pushes the edema into the venous and lymphatic drainage, temporarily alleviating the pain. The pain can progress to worsen as the day proceeds, as fatigue causes failure of secondary muscular assistance to foot function. Eventually the pain can interfere with athletic activity. Runners often describe pain present at the beginning of a run that improves and even abates, only to recur after the run. Climbing stairs, walking barefoot without support, and going up on tiptoes can all aggravate the pain of plantar fasciitis.

Examination

Swelling is often not visibly appreciated, but can be present in severe cases. There are rarely any skin changes such as ecchymoses present. Such signs suggest the possibility of a plantar fascia rupture. There is localized tenderness at the medial tuberosity of the calcaneus. Tenderness may also be present all along the plantar fascia through the arch, particularly on the medial side. The plantar fascia may be quite taut. Passive dorsiflexion of the toes with the foot held in a neutral position can increase the pain. I usually assess the dorsiflexion range of motion to the great toe with the foot in a relaxed plantarflexed position and with a forefoot-loaded subtalar neutral position. If dorsiflexion of the toe is greatly reduced when the forefoot is loaded (tethered by the medial slip of the plantar fascia) compared with the relaxed foot (assessing the MTP intrinsic joint dorsiflexion), it suggests an inordinately tight or short plantar fascia. Biomechanical examination in both stance and nonweightbearing positions will identify suggestive predisposing conditions. Ankle dorsiflexion is particularly important to assess.[47] If the patient lacks ankle dorsiflexion, he or she will modify their gait or stress adjacent structures to maintain stride length. Neurologic examination including Phalen's and Tinel's signs can be helpful when considering nerve entrapment.[50]

Imaging

Plain radiography can be most useful at ruling out other conditions such as bone cyst or stress fracture. Radiographic findings of plantar fasciitis are usually normal or show the presence of a small horizontal bone spur. Although somewhat controversial, most authors contend the bone spur is not the source of or associated with heel pain.[44] Bone scan is not routinely helpful unless calcaneal stress fracture is suspected. Ultrasonography is getting some attention as a noninvasive means of assessing the plantar fascia. Cardinal and colleagues[51] found that the symptomatic plantar fascia averaged 5.2 mm in sagittal thickness compared with 2.9 mm in patients with asymptomatic plantar fascia and 2.6 mm in a control group. The plantar fascia was diffusely hypoechoic in the symptomatic cases. Gibbon and Long[52] also confirmed plantar fascial thickening and abnormal echogenicity in plantar fasciitis. This study also identified peritendinous edema, subcalcaneal erosion and intratendinous calcification in a very few cases. It remains to be seen how ultrasonography may prove clinically valuable. Heel pain after plantar fasciotomy can be diagnostically challenging. MRI has proven helpful at determining the exact etiology of this postoperative pain.[53]

Treatment

Conservative, nonsurgical treatment for plantar fasciitis is successful 80% to 90% of the time.[54–57] Most runners have tried a variety of their own treatments before presenting to the health care professional.

Treating plantar fasciitis in the runner can be both frustrating and quite rewarding. Treatment strategies focus on acute phase pain relief efforts followed by stretching and strengthening, addressing biomechanical and functional deficits, foot support with orthotics, corticosteroid injections, night splints, and eventually surgical management.

Relative rest is the mainstay of treatment during the acute phase. For some this may mean avoiding weightbearing activity altogether, and for others a substantial diminution of the usual training regimen. NSAIDs used judiciously for a brief period may help relieve pain. Ice applied for 20 to 30 minutes after exercise may limit the inflammatory response. Physical therapy modalities, though successful in some cases, are more often disappointing for plantar fasciitis. Gentle range of motion exercises and isometric contractions using stretchable tubing are initiated during the acute phase of treatment. During this early treatment the runner can also focus on using well-supported lace-up shoes and over-the-counter soft insoles, and minimizing time spent walking barefoot.

Kibler and colleagues[47] and others identified dorsiflexion range-of-motion deficits and plantar flexor muscle–strength deficits associated with plantar fasciitis. It would be prudent for the runner with plantar fasciitis to concentrate on these deficits during the rehabilitative treatment period and as preventive strategies before making significant training changes. Kibler et al. suggest attention to strength and flexibility balance, plyometrics, and functional progressions from walking to running to jumping. Kwong and coworkers[49] recommend isolating the soleus by stretching the Achilles' tendon with the knee flexed. The runner should pay particular attention to local strength, coupled with work on the entire kinetic chain.

Heel cups or pads with an accommodative cutout are frequently recommended for plantar fasciitis. The heel cup theoretically works by restraining the subcalcaneal fat from splaying at heel contact. A viscoelastic heel pad provides extrinsic cushioning to the heel. These provide limited benefit to a few people because they do not reduce the tensile force applied to the plantar fascia origin. Turgut and colleagues[58] recently demonstrated that heel pad elasticity was not reliably associated with heel pain.

Posterior night splints place the foot in a passively dorsiflexed position while at rest. Batt et al.[59] and others added tension night splints to a treatment regimen of nonsteroidal drugs, a viscoelastic heel, and a stretching program. A control group received the same protocols without the night splints. All members of the study group improved by 12.5 weeks of treatment. Eleven of 17 in the control group failed treatment and were then crossed over to night splint treatment. Eight of these 11 improved by 13 weeks of night splint treatment.[59] Stretching of the plantar fascia is proposed by some as an explanation for the night splint benefit. The splints seem to have their greatest utility for relieving early morning pain. I propose that when the plantar fascia is taut, the tissue tamponades subtle swelling and the pain associated with the first few morning steps is alleviated.

Corticosteroid injections continue to be a popular treatment modality for the patient with recalcitrant heel pain.[60] A medial, lateral, or inferior approach varies by practitioner. I prefer a medial approach, placing the needle between the plantar fascia and the calcaneus. Pain relief can be significant, though it is most often temporary.[61] Corticosteroid injections predispose the plantar fascia to rupture. Acevedo and Beskin[60] evaluated 765 patients diagnosed with plantar fasciitis. There were 51 cases of plantar fascia rupture, of which 44 were associated with corticosteroid injection. The mean age was 51 and the rupture occurred an average of 10 weeks following injection. The authors had injected 122 of the 765 patients, resulting in 12 of the 44 ruptures of this cohort. Approximate risk for corticosteroid injection–caused rupture is not available, although it would appear from this study that the risk

is about 10%. Sellman[62] reported another cohort of 37 patients with plantar fascia rupture previously treated with corticosteroid injection. Plantar fascia rupture is associated with long-term consequences. In cadavers, plantar fascia release causes a drop in the medial and lateral columns of the foot.[63] Biomechanical models predict the plantar fascia carries 14% of the total weightbearing load on the foot.[64] Clinically, the patient with a plantar fascia rupture can suffer longitudinal arch strain, lateral and dorsal midfoot strain, lateral plantar nerve dysfunction, stress fracture, hammertoe deformity, swelling, and antalgia.[60]

Custom-molded orthoses have long been a recommended treatment for plantar fasciitis. The critical evaluation of custom-molded orthoses is daunting. Numerous nonbiomechanical variables such as training changes, weight, shoes, and others contribute to the perplexing etiology of plantar fasciitis. To this already confusing picture the practitioner must add multiple biomechanical variables. Kwong and colleagues[49] recommend a custom-molded semirigid orthosis with attention paid to supporting the first metatarsal late in the propulsive phase of gait. The foot with a hypermobile first ray lacks stability during propulsion. Disregarding this phenomenon will result in many custom orthotic failures. A firmly constructed heel counter to the shoe must assist the orthoses. Lacking this rearfoot control by the shoe, the foot will continue to pronate on top of the orthosis. The need for a custom made orthosis is challenged by Pfeffer and coworkers[65] in a recent prospective trial from 15 orthopedic centers treating foot and ankle problems. They conclude a prefabricated shoe insert is more likely to reduce symptoms than a custom polypropylene orthotic device. Most studies of plantar fasciitis do not focus strictly on the runner, particularly the younger runner. It is quite possible that the younger runner suffers from a form of plantar fasciitis that behaves differently from the usual process that often affects middle-aged women. Suffice it to say that recommending, prescribing, fabricating, and modifying custom orthoses remains more an art than a science.

REFERENCES

1. Bordelon RL: Foot first—evolution of man. *Foot Ankle* 1987:8, 125.
2. Wen DY: Injuries in runners: Is lower extremity alignment a risk factor? *Am J Med Sports* 1999:1, 126.
3. Omey ML, Micheli LJ: Foot and ankle problems in the young athlete. *Med Sci Sports Exerc* 1999:31, S470.
4. Oloff LM, Schulhofer SD: Flexor hallucis longus dysfunction. *J Foot Ankle Surg* 1998:37, 101.

5. Coghlan BA, Clarke NMP: Traumatic rupture of the flexor hallucis longus tendon in a marathon runner. *Am J Sports Med* 1993:21, 617.

6. Hockenberry RT: Forefoot problems in athletes. *Med Sci Sports Exerc* 1999:31, S448.

7. Mann RA, Coughlin MJ: Hallux valgus—etiology, anatomy, treatment and surgical considerations. *Clin Orthop Rel Res* 1981:157, 31.

8. Graham CE, Graham DM: Morton's neuroma: A microscopic evaluation. *Foot Ankle* 1984:5, 150.

9. Mann RA, Reynolds JC: Interdigital neuroma—a critical clinical analysis. *Foot Ankle* 1983:3, 238.

10. Wu KK: Morton's interdigital neuroma: A clinical review of its etiology, treatment, and results. *J Foot Ankle Surg* 1996:35, 112.

11. Graham CE, Johnson KA, Ilstrup DM: The intermetatarsal nerve: A microscopic evaluation. *Foot Ankle* 1981:2, 150.

12. Teasdell RD, Saltzman CL, Johnson KA: A practical approach to Morton's neuroma. *J Musculoskel Med* 1993:10, 39.

13. McBryde AM, Anderson RB: Sesamoid foot problems in the athlete. *Clin Sports Med* 1988:7, 51.

14. Lillich JS, Baxter DE: Common forefoot problems in runners. *Foot Ankle* 1986:7, 145.

15. Biedert R: Which investigations are required in stress fracture of the great toe sesamoids? *Arch Orthop Trauma Surg* 1993:112, 94.

16. Gross TS, Bunch RP: A mechanical model of metatarsal stress fracture during distance running. *Am J Sports Med* 1989:17, 669.

17. Sharkey NA, Ferris L, Smith TS, Matthews DK: Strain and loading of the second metatarsal during heel-lift. *J Bone Joint Surg* 1995:77-A, 1050.

18. Montelone GP: Stress fractures in the athlete. *Orthop Clin North Am* 1995:26, 423.

19. Hockenberry RT: Forefoot problems in athletes. *Med Sci Sports Exerc* 1999:31, S448.

20. Sullivan D, Warren RF, Pavlov H, et al.: Stress fractures in 51 runners. *Clin Orthop* 1984:187, 188.

21. Weinfeld SB, Haddad SL, Myerson MS: Metatarsal stress fractures. *Clin Sports Med* 1997:16, 319.

22. Clapper MF, O'Brien TJ, Lyons PM: Fractures of the fifth metatarsal—analysis of a fracture registry. *Clin Orthop Rel Res* 1995:315, 238.

23. Torg JS, Balduini FC, Zelko RR, et al.: Fractures of the base of the fifth metatarsal distal to the tuberosity. *J Bone Joint Surg* 1984:66A, 209.

24. Woods L, Leach RE: Posterior tibial tendon rupture in athletic people. *Am J Sports Med* 1991:19, 495.

25. Simpson RR, Gudas CJ: Posterior tibial tendon rupture in a world class runner. *J Foot Surg* 1983:22, 74.

26. Frey C, Shereff M, Greenidge N: Vascularity of the posterior tibial tendon. *J Bone Joint Surg* 1990:72-A, 884.

27. Brukner P, Bradshaw C, Khan KM: Stress fractures: A review of 180 cases. *Clin J Sport Med* 1996:6, 85.

28. Khan KM, Fuller PJ, Brukner PD: Outcome of conservative and surgical management of navicular stress fracture in athletes. *Am J Sport Med* 1992:20, 657.

29. Orava S, Karpakka J, Hulkko A, et al.: Stress avulsion fracture of the tarsal navicular: An uncommon sports-related overuse injury. *Am J Sports Med* 1991:19, 392.

30. Torg JS, Pavlov H, Cooley LH, et al.: Stress fractures of the tarsal navicular. A retrospective review of twenty-one cases. *J Bone Joint Surg* 1982:64A, 700.

31. Quirk R: President's guest lecture. Stress fractures of the navicular. *Foot Ankle Int* 1998:19, 494.

32. Khan KM, Brukner PD, Kearney C: Tarsal navicular stress fracture in athletes. *Sports Med* 1994:17, 65.

33. Kiss ZS, Khan KM, Fuller PJ: Stress fractures of the tarsal navicular bone: CT findings in 55 cases. *Am J Radiol* 1993:160, 111.

34. Beaman DN, Roeser WM, Holmes JR, et al.: Cuboid stress fractures: A report of two cases. *Foot Ankle* 1993:14, 525.

35. Lazzarini KM, Troiano RN, Smith RC: Can running cause the appearance of marrow edema on MR images of the foot and ankle? *Radiology* 1997:202, 540.

36. Cambell G, Warnekros W: Tarsal stress fracture in a long-distance runner: A case report. *J Am Podiatr Assn* 1983:72, 532.

37. Black KP, Ehlert KJ: A stress fracture of the lateral process of the talus in a runner. *J Bone Joint Surg* 1994:76A, 441.

38. Motto SG: Stress fracture of the lateral process of the talus—a case report. *Br J Sports Med* 1993:27, 275.

39. Bradshaw C, Khan K, Brukner P: Stress fracture of the body of the talus in athletes demonstrated with computer tomography. *Clin J Sport Med* 1996:6, 48.

40. Bottger BA, Schweitzer ME, El-Noueam KI, Desai M: MR imaging of the normal and abnormal retrocalcaneal bursae. *Am J Radiol* 1998:170, 1239.

41. Fowler A, Philip JF: Abnormality of the calcaneus as a cause of painful heel: Its diagnosis and operative treatment. *Br J Surg* 1945:32, 494.

42. Schepsis AA, Leach RE: Surgical management of Achilles tendinitis. *Am J Sports Med* 1987:15, 308.

43. Louisia S, Masquelet AC: The medial and inferior calcaneal nerves: An anatomic study. *Surg Radiol Anat* 1999:21, 169.

44. Schepsis AA, Leach RE, Gorzyca J: Plantar fasciitis: Etiology, treatment, surgical results, and review of the literature. *Clin Orthop Rel Res* 1991:266, 185.

45. Hicks JH: The mechanics of the foot. *J Anat* 1954:88, 25.

46. Snider MP, Clancy WG, McBeath AA: Plantar fascia release for chronic plantar fasciitis in runners. *Am J Sports Med* 1983:11, 215.

47. Kibler WB, Goldberg C, Chandler TJ: Functional biomechanical deficits in running athletes with plantar fasciitis. *Am J Sports Med* 1991:19, 66.

48. Chandler TJ, Kibler WB: A biomechanical approach to the prevention, treatment and rehabilitation of plantar fasciitis. *Sports Med* 1993:15, 344.

49. Kwong PK, Kay D, Voner RT, et al.: Plantar fasciitis: Mechanics and pathomechanics of treatment. *Clin Sports Med* 1988:7, 119.

50. Hendrix CL, Jolly GP, Garbalosa JC, et al.: Entrapment neuropathy: The etiology of intractable chronic heel pain syndrome. *J Foot Ankle Surg* 1998:37, 273.

51. Cardinal CE, Chhem RK, Beauregard CG, et al.: *Radiology* 1996:201, 257.
52. Gibbon WW, Long G: Ultrasound of the plantar aponeurosis (fascia). *Skeletal Radiol* 1999:28, 21.
53. Yu JS, Spigos D, Tomczak R: Foot pain after a plantar fasciotomy: An MR analysis to determine potential causes. *J Comp Assist Tomogr* 1999:23, 707.
54. DeMaio M, Paine R, Mangine RE, et al.: Plantar fasciitis. *Orthopedics* 1993:16, 1153.
55. Gill LH: Plantar fasciitis: Diagnosis and conservative management. *J Am Acad Orthop* 1997:5, 109.
56. Pfeffer GB, Baxter DE, Graves S, et al.: Symposium: The management of plantar heel pain. *Contemp Orthop* 1996:32, 357.
57. Wolgin M, Cook C, Graham C, et al.: Conservative treatment of plantar heel pain: Long-term follow-up. *Foot Ankle* 1994:15, 97.
58. Turgut A, Gokturk E, Kose N, et al.: The relationship of heel pad elasticity and plantar heel pain. *Clin Orthop* 1999:Mar(360), 191.
59. Batt ME, Tanji JL, Skattum N: Plantar fasciitis: A prospective randomized clinical trial of the tension night splint. *Clin J Sport Med* 1996:6, 158.
60. Acevedo JI, Beskin JL: Complications of plantar fascia rupture associated with corticosteroid injection. *Foot Ankle Int* 1998:19, 91.
61. Miller RA, Torres J, McGuire M: Efficacy of first-time steroid injection for painful heel syndrome. *Foot Ankle Int* 1995:16, 610.
62. Sellman JR: Plantar fascia rupture associated with corticosteroid injection. *Foot Ankle Int* 1994:15, 376.
63. Murphy GA, Pneumaticos SG, Kamaric E, et al.: Biomechanical consequences of sequential plantar fascia release. *Foot Ankle Int* 1998:19, 149.
64. Kim W, Voloshin AS: Role of plantar fascia in the load bearing capacity of the human foot. *J Biomech* 1995:28, 1025.
65. Pfeffer G, Cooper P, Frey C, et al.: Comparison of custom and prefabricated orthoses in the initial treatment of proximal plantar fasciitis. *Foot Ankle Int* 1999:20, 214.
66. Marti B: On the epidemiology of running injuries. The 1984 Bern Grand-Prix study. *Am J Sports Med* 1988:16, 285.
67. Jacobs SJ, Berson BL: Injuries to runners: A study of entrants to a 10,000 meter race. *Am J Sports Med* 1986:14, 151.
68. Walter SD, Hart LE, McIntosh JM, Sutton JR: The Ontario Cohort Study of Running-Related Injuries. *Arch Intern Med* 1989:149, 2561.
69. Bennell KL, Brukner PD: Epidemiology and site specificity of stress fractures. *Clin Sports Med* 1997:16, 179.

Chapter 19

STRESS FRACTURES

Peter D. Brukner and
Kim L. Bennell

INTRODUCTION

Physical exercise has beneficial effects on a number of physiologic systems including the skeleton. However, unwise training practices combined with potential risk factors may harm these systems. A stress fracture represents one form of breakdown in the skeletal system.[1] It can be defined as a partial or complete fracture of bone that results from the repeated application of a stress lower than that required to fracture the bone in a single loading situation.[2]

Historical Perspective

Stress fractures were first described in 1855 by Briethaupt, a Prussian military physician who observed foot pain and swelling in young military recruits unaccustomed to the rigors of training. He considered it to be an inflammatory reaction in the tendon sheaths due to trauma and called the condition Fussgeschwulst. It was not until the advent of radiographs that the signs and symptoms were attributed to fractures in the metatarsals.[3] The condition then became known as a "march fracture" because of the close association between marching and the onset of symptoms. Stress fractures were first noticed in civilians in 1921 by Deutschlander,[4] who reported six cases in women. However, it was not until 1956, more than a century following identification in military recruits, that stress fractures were recognized in athletes.[5]

A variety of terms have been used for different time periods to describe stress fractures. These have included march fractures, Deutschlander's fractures, pied force, fatigue fractures, or crack fractures.[4,6–10] Virtually all these terms have been intended to describe some etiologic attribute of the stress injuries of bone. In recent years the most commonly used term has been stress fracture.

Following the radiographic description of metatarsal stress fractures, many theories were set forth to explain the etiology of this injury. Most of the reports were based on small series, and the theories proposed were concerned with either mechanical factors such as spasm of the interossei or flat feet[4,11,12] or with inflammatory reactions such as nonsuppurative osteomyelitis.[7,8]

Etiology

It is now recognized that the development of a stress fracture represents the end product of the failure of bone to adapt adequately to the mechanical loads experienced during physical activity. Ground reaction forces and muscular contraction result in bone strain. It is these repetitive strains that are thought to cause a stress fracture. Bone normally responds to strain by increasing the rate of remodeling. In this process lamellar bone is resorbed by osteoclasts, creating resorption cavities, which are subsequently replaced with denser bone by osteoblasts. Since there is a lag between increased activity of the osteoclasts and osteoblasts, bone is

227

weakened during this time.[13,14] If sufficient recovery time is allowed, bone mass eventually increases. However, if loading continues, microdamage may accumulate at the weakened region.[14,15] Remodeling is thought to repair normally occurring microdamage.[16,17] The processes of microdamage accumulation and bone remodeling, both resulting from bone strain, play an important part in the development of a stress fracture. If microdamage accumulates, repetitive loading continues, and remodeling cannot maintain the integrity of the bone, a stress fracture may result.[15,18,19] This may occur because the microdamage is too extensive to be repaired by normal remodeling, because depressed remodeling processes cannot adequately repair normally occurring microdamage or because of some combination of these factors.[18]

EPIDEMIOLOGY

Stress fractures have been reported to occur in association with a variety of sports and physical activities. Clinical impressions suggest that stress fractures are more common in weightbearing activities, particularly those with a running or jumping component. However, it is difficult to compare the incidence of stress fractures in different sports or to identify the sport or activity with the greatest risk due to a lack of sound epidemiologic data. This section reviews the descriptive epidemiology of stress fractures. Most of the literature in this area pertains to female runners and to male military populations. There is no information about stress fracture rates in the general community.

Injury Rates

Studies investigating stress fracture rates in athletes are shown in Table 19–1.[20–31] Of these, only two allow a direct comparison of annual stress fracture rates in different sporting populations.[28,29] Johnson et al.[28] conducted a 2-year prospective study to investigate sports-related injuries in collegiate male and female atheletes. In total, 34 stress fractures were diagnosed over the study period. Track accounted for 64% of stress fractures in women and 50% of stress fractures in men. The stress fracture incidence rate (expressed as a case rate) in males was highest for track (9.7%) followed by lacrosse (4.3%), crew (2.4%), and American football (1.1%). The stress fracture incidence rate in women was highest for track athletes (31.1%), followed by crew (8.2%), basketball (3.6%), lacrosse (3.1%), and soccer (2.6%). No athlete sustained a stress fracture in fencing, hockey, golf, softball, swimming, or tennis.

Goldberg and Pecora[29] reviewed medical records of stress fractures occurring in collegiate athletes over

a 3-year period. Approximate participant numbers were available to allow calculation of estimated incidence case rates in each sport. The greatest incidence occurred in softball (19%), followed by track (11%), basketball (9%), lacrosse (8%), baseball (8%), tennis (8%), and gymnastics (8%). However, participant numbers were small in some of these sports, which may have led to a bias in incidence rates.

Both studies suggest that track athletes are at one of the highest risks for stress fracture. However, since neither study expressed incidence in terms of exposure, it may not be strictly valid to compare the risk of stress fracture in such diverse sports. To our knowledge, there is only one athlete study that has expressed stress fracture incidence rates in terms of exposure.[24] This 12-month prospective study followed a cohort of 95 track and field athletes. Results showed an overall rate of 0.70 stress fractures per 1000 training hours. Further research is needed to quantify incidence rates in this manner to allow more valid comparison between studies.

Retrospective studies have measured stress fractures rates in specific sporting populations, mostly runners and ballet dancers.[20,21,23,25–27,29–32] Variations in reported rates reflect differences in methodology, particularly cohort demographics and method of data collection. A history of stress fracture has been reported by 13% to 52% of female runners. The lowest rate was found in one that included recreational as well as competitive runners. Ballet dancers are another population in which stress fracture rates appear high, with 22% to 45% of dancers reporting a history of stress fracture. However, most studies failed to confirm the accuracy of subject recall, which may introduce bias into the figures reported. Nevertheless, it is clear that a stress fracture is a relatively common athletic injury.

Recurrence Rates

Clinically, it seems that recurrence of stress fractures at new sites is common. In female track and field athletes, half of those who reported a history of stress fracture had had a stress fracture on more than one occasion.[23] However, few studies have reported recurrence rates in either athletes or the military. When male and female track and field athletes were followed prospectively for 1 year, 60% of those who sustained a stress fracture had a previous stress fracture history.[24] The athlete recurrence rate in this study was particularly high, at 12.6%.

Comparison of Rates in Men and Women

It is often suggested that women sustain a disproportionately higher number of stress fractures than men, particularly in military studies. These studies

TABLE 19–1. STRESS FRACTURE RATES IN ATHLETES

Reference	Study Design	Population	No. and Sex	Method of Data Collection	Response Rate of Questionnaire (%)	Observed by	Diagnosis of SF	SF Rate (%)[a]
Barrow and Saha, 1988 (20)	R	Collegiate athletes Distance runners	240,F	Self-administered questionnaire	24	Hx	x-ray or BS	37.0
Brunet et al., 1990 (21)	R	Recreational/competitive runners	375,F 1130,M	Self-administered questionnaire	NS	Hx	NS	13.2,F 8.3,M
Cameron et al., 1992 (22)	R	State/national athletes Level runners	263,F 287,M	Self-administered questionnaire	67	Hx	NS	26.6,F 28.0,M
Bennell et al., 1995 (23)	R	Track and field athletes	53,F	Self-administered questionnaire	100	Hx	x-ray, BS, or CT	51.5 84.9[b]
Bennell et al., 1996 (24)	P	Track and field athletes	46,F 49,M	Monitoring	NA	1 yr	BS + CT	21.7,F 20.4,M 30.4,F[b] 24.5,M[b]
Johnson et al., 1994 (28)	P	Collegiate athletes	321,F 593,M	Monitoring	NA	2 yr	x-ray or BS	6.9,F[b,c] 2.0,M[b,c]
Goldberg and Pecora, 1994 (29)	R	Collegiate athletes	≈1200,F ≈1800,M	Review of questionnaire medical records	NA	3 yr	x-ray or BS	2.7,F[b,c] 1.4,M[b,c]

NS = not stated; NA = not applicable; P = prospective cohort; R = retrospective cohort; BS = bone scan; CT = computed tomography; Hx = history; SF = stress fracture.

[a]Expressed as participant rates unless noted otherwise.

[b]Stress fracture rates expressed as case rates: number of fractures per 100 athletes.

[c]Annual incidence.

Source: From Bennell KL et al.[197]

consistently show that female recruits have a greater risk of stress fracture than male recruits, with relative risks ranging from 1.2 to 10.[33–38]

In contrast, a gender difference in stress fracture rates is not as evident in athletic populations.[21,24,28,29,31,32] Studies show either no difference between male and female athletes or a slightly increased risk for women, up to 3.5 times that of men. A possible confounding variable is that, unlike the military population, for which the amount and intensity of basic training is rigidly controlled, it is difficult to assume equivalence of training between men and women in most of these studies. However, Bennell et al.[24] found no significant difference between gender incidence rates even when they were expressed in terms of exposure. Women sustained 0.86 stress fractures per 1000 training hours compared with 0.54 in men. It is feasible that a gender difference in stress fracture risk is reduced in athletes, as female athletes may be more conditioned to exercise than female recruits, and hence the fitness levels of male and female atheletes may be closer.

SITES

Numerous studies have reported the anatomic distribution of series of stress fractures[20,24,27–29,32,39–50] (Table 19–2). While great variation exists in the percentage of stress fractures reported at each bony site,

the most common sites appear to be the tibia, metatarsals, navicular, and fibula. A number of factors may influence the reported distributions of stress fractures. These include type and level of activity, gender, age, and, in particular, method of diagnosis. For example, tarsal navicular stress fractures are rarely evident on radiographs. Thus, these will be underreported in comparison with stress fractures at other sites if diagnosis is confined to radiographs.

Stress fractures develop at skeletal sites that are subjected to repetitive mechanical loading during a particular activity. The site specificity of stress fractures was illustrated in a prospective study in 95 track and field athletes.[24] Although stress fracture incidence rates were similar in power and endurance athletes, the site distribution differed. Power athletes (sprinters, hurdlers, jumpers) sustained significantly more foot fractures, whereas endurance athletes (middle-distance and distance runners) sustained more long-bone and pelvic fractures.

RISK FACTORS

Risk factors are markers that can be used to identify athletes who are more likely to sustain a stress fracture. Preventative strategies can then be directed toward these individuals. Although the risk factors themselves may not be involved in stress fracture

TABLE 19–2. ANATOMIC DISTRIBUTION OF STRESS FRACTURES IN ATHLETES[a]

Reference	Sport	No. of SFs in Series	Diagnosis of SF	Tibia (%)	Fibula (%)	Metatarsal (%)	Navicular (%)
Brubaker and James, 1974 (39)	Running	17	NS	41.2	17.6	29.4	5.9
Orava, 1980 (40)	Variety	200	x-ray ± BS	53.5	12.5	18.0	2.0
Pagliano and Jackson, 1980 (41)	Running	99	Self report	20.2	15.2	37.4	NS
Taunton et al., 1981 (42)	Running	62	x-ray or BS	55.0	11.3	16.1	3.2
Clement et al., 1981 (43)	Running	87	NS	57.5	9.2	20.7	3.4
Sullivan et al., 1984 (44)	Running	57	x-ray or BS	43.9	21.0	14.0	0
Barrow and Saha, 1988 (20)	Running	140	Self-report	63.0	9.0	21.0	0.7
Hulkko and Orava, 1987 (45)	Variety	368	x-ray ± BS	49.5	12.0	19.8	2.5
Matheson et al., 1987 (46)	Variety	320	BS	49.1	6.6	8.8	NS
Courtenay and Bowers, 1990 (47)	Variety	108	x-ray or BS	38.0	29.6	18.5	4.6
Ha et al., 1991 (48)	Variety	169	x-ray or BS	31.5	10.7	7.1	4.7
Cameron et al., 1992 (22)	Running	253	Self-report	37.5	12.0	22.5	10.0
Benazzo et al., 1992 (49)	Track and field	49	x-ray, CT, or BS	26.5	12.2	14.3	28.6
Kadel et al., 1992 (27)	Ballet	27	Self-report	22.0	0	63.0	NS
Goldberg and Pecora 1994 (29)	Variety	58	x-ray or BS	18.9	12.1	25.9	NS
Johnson et al., 1994 (28)	Variety	34	x-ray ± BS	38.2	0	20.6	11.8
Bennell et al., 1996 (24)	Track and field	26	BS and CT	45.0	12.0	8.0	15.0
Brukner et al., 1996 (50)	Variety	180	x-ray, CT,or BS	20.0	16.7	23.3	20.0

BS = bone scan; CT = computed tomography; NS = not stated; SF = stress fracture.
[a]Expressed as a percentage of the total number of stress fractures in each series.
Source: From Bennell KL et al.[197]

pathogenesis, they directly or indirectly increase the chance of a stress fracture developing, by their influence on either the mechanical environment of bone or the remodeling process. Although numerous risk factors for stress fractures have been proposed, research is needed to confirm anecdotal observations. Presently, most studies in athletes are case series, are confined to injured groups only, or are cross-sectional designs that do not allow the temporal relationship between risk factor and injury to be assessed. Methodologic issues such as small subject numbers, different definitions of stress fractures, and failure to assess the independent contributions of risk factors also limit their usefulness. There are also few data on risk factors in male athletes. Results from large military epidemiologic studies cannot be readily generalized to athletes, given important differences in training, fitness levels, footwear, and surfaces. However, these may provide additional insights, especially given the deficiencies in the athletic literature.

Genetic Predisposition

A large component of the variation in bone mass can be attributed to genetic factors.[51] Not surprisingly, then, a family history of osteoporosis is considered to be a risk factor for low bone density and osteoporosis in both men and women.[52,53] Similarly, a significant relationship between a family history of osteoporosis and yearly change in bone density has been demonstrated in studies of runners and nonrunners.[54] It is therefore feasible that some individuals may be genetically predisposed to stress fractures when they are exposed to suitable environmental conditions, such as vigorous exercise. This was implied in a case report in which a pair of 18-year-old monozygotic twins undergoing basic military training sustained identical multiple stress fractures in the femoral and tarsal bones.[55] The authors proposed that identical environmental conditions served to unmask a genetically determined deficiency in the affected bones. Although Myburgh et al.[56] failed to find a difference in the incidence of a family history of osteoporosis in a group of 25 athletes with stress fractures and a group without stress fractures, this may reflect the small sample. At present, there is little evidence to show that genetic factors predispose an athlete to this injury.

Menstrual Disturbances

Since hypoestrogenic postmenopausal women are at an increased risk of developing osteoporotic fractures, it has been suggested that stress fractures may be more prevalent in female athletes with menstrual disturbances. Estrogen deficiency could feasibly promote stress fracture development by

- accelerating the process of bone remodeling, leading to weakened areas of bone due to the lag period between resorption and formation
- increasing calcium excretion, resulting in greater calcium requirements, which may not be adequately met by dietary intake
- causing premature bone loss and hence lower bone density

Although progesterone may be a promoter of bone formation, particularly in cortical bone,[57] and luteal phase deficiency in athletes is associated with lowered progesterone levels, a possible link between luteal phase deficiency and stress fracture risk has not been sought. Research to date has focused on the relationship between stress fracture incidence and menstrual irregularity (amenorrhea and oligomenorrhea), age of menarche, and use of the oral contraceptive pill.

The findings of numerous studies suggest that stress fractures are more common in athletes exhibiting menstrual disturbances[20,25–27,56,58–63] (Fig. 19–1). Although not all results were statistically significant, power may have been limited by relatively small samples in some studies. In general, athletes with menstrual disturbances had a relative risk for stress fracture that was between two and four times greater than that of their eumenorrheic counterparts. However, in ballet dancers, logistic regression analysis showed that amenorrhea for longer than 6 months' duration was an independent contributor to the risk of stress fracture, with the estimated risk being 93 times that of a dancer with regular menses.[27]

The risk of multiple stress fractures also seems to be increased in those with menstrual disturbances.[20,64] Clark et al.[64] found that while amenorrheic and eumenorrheic groups reported a similar prevalence of single stress fractures, 50% of the amenorrheic runners reported multiple stress fractures compared with only 9% of those regularly menstruating.

Grimston et al.[65] developed a menstrual index that summarized previous and present menstural status. They found no relationship between this menstrual index and the incidence of stress fractures in 16 female runners. Conversely, Barrow and Saha[20] found that lifetime menstrual history did affect the risk of stress fracture. They showed the incidence of stress fracture to be 29% in the regular group and 49% in the very irregular group. The results of a prospective study also demonstrated that those with a lower menstrual index were at greater risk of stress fracture. Myburgh et al.[56] found that although athletes with stress fractures had a higher frequency of current menstrual dysfunction than athletes without stress fractures, there was no difference in past menstrual status. This finding suggests

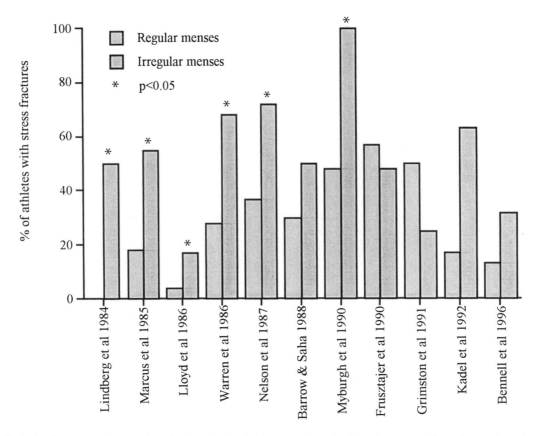

Figure 19–1. Studies comparing the percentage of female athletes with stress fractures in groups with and without regular menses.

that changes associated with menstrual dysfunction are reversible and do not impact on future stress fracture risk if regular menses return.

In summary, it would appear that there is a higher incidence of menstrual disturbances in female athletes with stress fracture than in those without. These findings have led some authors to assume that this is a direct result of decreased bone mineral density in athletes with menstrual disturbances. However, athletes with menstrual disturbances also exhibit other risk factors such as lower calcium intake,[66] greater training load,[67] and differences in soft-tissue composition.[68] Since these were not always controlled for in the studies discussed, it is difficult to ascertain which are the contributory factors.

The relationship between age of menarche and risk of stress fracture is uncertain. Some authors have found that athletes with stress fractures have a later age of menarche,[25,69,70] whereas others have found no difference.[26,27,56] In a prospective study, age of menarche was an independent risk factor for stress fracture, with the risk increasing by a factor of 4.1 for every additional year of age at menarche (Fig. 19–2).[63] However, the mechanism for this relationship is unclear, as a later age of menarche is also associated with an

increased likelihood of menstrual disturbance,[71] a lower energy intake,[72] decreased body fat or weight,[72] and excessive premenarcheal training,[71] all of which could influence stress fracture risk.

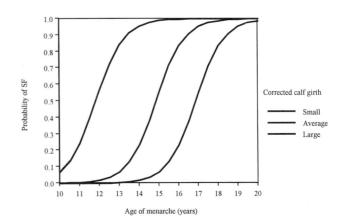

Figure 19–2. Plot of the probability of stress fracture at different ages of menarche for different corrected calf girths in female athletes. The plot for small corrected calf girth was calculated using the minimum value measured in the cohort, the average girth was calculated using the mean value, and the large girth was calculated using the maximum value. *(Source: From Bennell et al.[63])*

Some authors have claimed that the oral contraceptive pill (OCP) may protect against stress fracture development. Barrow and Saha[20] found that runners using the OCP for at least 1 year had significantly fewer stress fractures (12%) than nonusers (29%). This was supported by the findings of Myburgh et al.[56] Although no difference in OCP use was reported in ballet dancers with and without stress fractures,[27] few dancers were taking the OCP. Since these studies are cross-sectional or retrospective in nature, it is not known whether the athletes were taking the OCP prior to or following the stress fracture episode. In addition, athletes may or may not take the OCP for reasons that in themselves could influence stress fracture risk. A prospective study did not support a protective effect of OCP use on stress fracture development.[63] Nevertheless, it is not known whether the risk of stress fracture is decreased in athletes with menstrual disturbances who subsequently take the OCP. This is an important area for future research.

Low Bone Density

Theoretically, low bone mineral density (BMD) could contribute to the development of a stress fracture by decreasing the fatigue resistance of bone to loading and by increasing the accumulation of microdamage.[73,74] Results from a limited number of studies comparing regional bone density in military or athletic groups with and without stress fracture have been inconclusive[26,56,62,63,69,70,75–77] (Table 19–3). The discrepancy may reflect differences in populations, type of physical activity, measurement techniques, and bone regions. However, the findings of a 12-month prospective study using dual-energy x-ray absorptiometry (DXA) to measure bone mass indicate that low bone density is a risk factor for stress fractures in women and possibly in men.[63] Female athletes who sustained tibial stress fractures had 8.1% lower tibia/fibula BMD than athletes without stress fractures ($P < 0.01$). In the men, the tibial stress fracture group had 4.0% less tibia/fibula BMD than the non–stress-fracture group, although this was not significant ($P = 0.17$). However, it is important to note that in this study the athletes with stress fractures still had bone density levels that were similar to or greater than those of less-active control subjects. This implies that the level of bone density required by athletes for short-term bone health is greater than that required by the general population.

Bone Geometry

Bone geometry influences the ability of the bone to resist mechanical loads. A prospective study of 295 male Israeli military recruits assessed the influence of bone geometry on stress fracture risk.[78,79] Significantly fewer stress fractures were sustained by those with a greater mediolateral tibial width, measured using standard radiographs, than by those with a narrower tibia. This may be due to a greater area moment of inertia and hence increased ability of the bone to resist bending forces in the anteroposterior direction. However, the incidence of stress fractures did not correlate with cortical thickness. These findings were confirmed by a recent prospective study of 626 U.S. male recruits.[77] Using DXA to derive structural geometry, the authors found significantly smaller tibial cross-sectional area, smaller tibial section modules, and smaller tibial width in the stress fracture cases. These remained after adjusting for body weight differences between groups. There are no data on whether bone geometry predisposes to stress fractures in athletes.

Endocrine Factors

Alterations in calcium metabolism could affect bone remodeling and bone density and theoretically predispose to stress fracture. However, single measure-ments of serum calcium, parathyroid hormone, 25-OH-vitamin D, and 1,25-dihydroxyvitamin D have not been found to differ between stress fracture and non–stress-fracture groups in military recruits[80] or athletes.[25,56,69] This may reflect sampling procedures or the fact that many of these biochemical parameters are tightly regulated.

Nutritional Status

Low calcium intake may contribute to stress fracture development by directly influencing the processes of bone remodeling and bone mineralization or by indirectly affecting soft-tissue composition and ovarian function. Other dietary factors such as fiber, protein, and caffeine intake may play a role but have not been well studied.

There is limited evidence to suggest that low calcium intake may be associated with an increased risk for stress fracture.[56,81] Myburgh et al.[82] found a significantly lower intake of calcium in athletes with shin soreness compared with a matched control group. However, since exact diagnoses were not made, stress fracture may not have been the only pathology included in this group. A follow-up study in athletes with scintigraphically diagnosed stress fractures confirmed the original results.[56] Current calcium intake was significantly lower in the stress fracture group, being 87% of the recommended daily intake (RDI). This is consistent with their reduced consumption of dairy products. The authors claim that a calcium intake of greater than 800 mg/day protects against stress fracture development.

TABLE 19–3. SUMMARY OF STUDIES DIRECTLY INVESTIGATING THE RELATIONSHIP BETWEEN BONE DENSITY AND STRESS FRACTURES

Reference	Study Design	Subjects	Sex	Sample size	Technique	Sites	Results[a]
Pouilles et al., 1989 (75)	CS	Military	M	41 SF 48 NSF	DPA	Femoral neck Ward's triangle Trochanter	−5.7* −7.1* −7.4*
Carbon et al., 1990 (69)	CS	Various athletes	F	9 SF 9 NSF	DPA SPA	LSp Femoral neck Distal radius Ultradistal Radius	−4.0* −7.0 −7.7 0.0
Frusztajer et al., 1990 (26)	CS	Ballet dancers	F	10 SF 10 NSF	DPA SPA	LSp 1st metatarsal Radial shaft	−4.1 0.0 0.0
Myburgh et al., 1990 (56)	CS	Various athletes	M/F	25 SF 25 NSF (19 F, 6 M)	DXA	LSp Femoral neck Ward's triangle Trochanter Intertrochanter Proximal Femur	−8.5* −6.7* −9.0* −8.6* −5.5 −6.5*
Giladi et al., 1991 (76)	P	Military	M	91 SF 198 NSF	SPA	Tibial shaft	−6.0
Grimston et al., 1991 (62)	CS	Runners	F	6 SF 8 NSF	DPA	LSp Femoral neck Tibial shaft	8.2* 7.6* 9.7
Warren et al., 1991 (70)	CS	Ballet dancers	F	14 SF 34 NSF	DPA	LSp 1st metatarsal Distal radius	NS NS NS
Bennell et al., 1996 (63)	P	Track and field athletes	F	10 SF 36 NSF	DXA	Upper limb Thoracic spine LSp Femur Tibia/fibula Foot	−3.3 −6.7 −11.9* −2.2 −4.2 −6.6*
			M	10 SF 39 NSF	DXA	Upper limb Thoracic spine LSp Femur Tibia/fibula Foot	−4.9 −4.1 −0.8 −2.9 −4.0 −0.3
Beck et al., 1996 (77)	P	Military	M	23 SF 587 NSF	DXA	Femur Tibia Fibula	−3.9* −5.6* −5.2

CS = cross-sectional; DPA = dual photon absorptiometry; DXA = dual energy x-ray absorptiometry; LSp = lumbar spine; M = males; NS = not stated but not significantly different; P = prospective; SPA = single-photon absorptiometry.
[a]Results are given as the percent difference comparing stress fracture subjects (SF) with non-stress-fracture subjects (NSF).
*Statistically significant.

Conversely, other investigators have failed to confirm the relationship between stress fractures and dietary calcium.[26,27,63,69,70,83]

Many ballet dancers were found to consume less than the RDI for calcium regardless of their stress fracture status,[26,27] implying that other factors may be more important as risk factors in dancers. A calcium index, based on the variability in calcium intake during the ages of 12 to 23 years, did not differ in runners with and without stress fractures.[62] In a prospective study of track and field athletes, risk of stress fracture was not associated with current calcium intake, current intake of nutrients known to influence calcium bioavailability and bone mass, or calcium supplementation use. Since most athletes in this study were consuming more than the RDI for calcium, the results suggest that the relative risk of stress fracture is not influenced by daily intakes above this level. This is consistent with the concept of calcium as a threshold nutrient whereby effects on the skeleton are only apparent up to a certain level.[84] However, it does not rule out an association between calcium deficiency and a higher incidence of stress fracture.

There are no intervention studies assessing the effect of calcium supplementation on stress-fracture incidence in athletes. A randomized controlled study in male military recruits showed a similar incidence of stress fractures during a 9-week training program in 247 recruits taking 500 mg of calcium daily and in 1151 controls.[85] However, since both groups had a baseline dietary calcium intake greater than 800 mg/day, this may have been sufficient to provide protection against stress fracture. Alternatively, a longer duration of calcium intervention may be necessary for effects to become apparent, particularly at cortical bone sites.

Other factors such as protein, total energy, phosphorus, fiber, sodium, alcohol, and caffeine could potentially affect bone health and therefore stress fracture risk. At present, no associations have been found between these and the incidence of stress fractures in athletes.[26,56,63,69,70]

Dietary behaviors and eating patterns may differ in those with stress fractures. Ballet dancers with stress fractures were more likely to diet and restrict food intake, avoid high-fat dairy foods, consume low-calorie products, have a self-reported history of an eating disorder, and have weight fluctuations down to a lower percentage of ideal body weight than those without stress fractures.[26] However, scores on a validated test relating to dieting, bulimia, food preoccupation, and oral control (EAT-26) did not differ between ballet dancers or track and field athletes with and without stress fracture.[25,26,63]

Anthropometry and Soft-Tissue Composition

Anthropometric characteristics (such as height and weight) and soft-tissue composition (such as lean mass and fat mass) could theoretically affect stress-fracture risk directly by influencing the forces applied to bones[86] or indirectly via effects on bone density[87,88] and menstrual function.[68]

Unlike the military population, in which anthropometric characteristics appear to be related to stress-fracture incidence,[77] no study in athletes has reported a difference in height, weight, body mass index, or fat mass between those with and without stress fractures.[20,21,25,27,60,62,63,69] Failure to find a relationship in athletes may be due to the relative homogeneity in these characteristics, unlike the military population, in which a range of somatotypes would be expected.

Another explanation is that the relationship may be nonlinear.

Muscles could play a dual role in stress-fracture development. Some investigators consider that muscles act dynamically to cause stress fractures by increasing bone strain at sites of muscle attachment.[89,90] Greater muscle mass with greater ability to generate force would be associated with an increased risk for stress fracture. Others feel that since muscles act to attenuate and dissipate forces applied to bone,[91] muscle fatigue or muscle weakness would predispose to stress fracture by causing an increase and redistribution of stress to bone.[49,92] In the military, leg power was not associated with stress-fracture occurrence, although the testing method was relatively crude and nonspecific.[76] However, recruits with a larger calf muscle circumference developed significantly fewer stress fractures.[79] This finding was also evident in female athletes, in whom where every 1-cm decrease in calf girth was associated with a fourfold greater risk of stress fracture[63] (Fig. 19–2). Using a biomechanical model, Scott and Winter[93] calculated that during running, the tibia is subjected to a large forward bending moment as a result of ground reaction force. The calf muscles oppose this large bending moment by applying a backward moment as they contract to control the rotation of the tibia and the lowering of the foot to the ground. The total effect is a smaller bending moment. Extrapolating from this, a stress fracture could result if the calf muscles are unable to produce adequate force to counteract the loading at ground contact and to decrease excessive bone strain. The findings of a smaller calf girth in those with stress fractures tend to support the hypothesis that muscles act to protect against rather than cause stress fractures.

However, there have been no studies comparing muscle mass or muscle strength, particularly peak force production and fatigueability, in athletes with and without stress fractures. Grimston et al.[94] found that during the latter stages of a 45-minute run, females with a past history of stress fracture recorded increased ground reaction forces, whereas ground reaction forces did not vary during the run in the control group. The authors surmised that this may indicate differences in fatigue adaptation and muscle activity.

Training

Repetitive mechanical loading arising from athletic training contributes to stress fracture development. However, the contribution of each training component (volume, intensity, frequency, surface, and footwear) to the risk of stress fracture has not been elucidated. Training may also influence bone indirectly through changes in levels of circulating hormones, through effects on soft-tissue composition and associations with menstrual disturbances.

Large military studies have shown that various training modifications such as inclusion of rest periods,[95,96] elimination of running and marching on concrete,[34,97] use of running shoes rather than combat boots,[97,98] and reduction of high-impact activity[38,96,99] can decrease the incidence of stress fractures in recruits.

In contrast, there is little controlled research in athletes, most of which describes anecdotal observations or case series in which training parameters are examined only in those athletes with stress fractures. Surveys have reported that up to 86% of athletes can identify some change in their training prior to the onset of the stress fracture.[22,29,44] Other researchers have blamed training "errors" in a varying proportion of cases but do not adequately define these "errors."[30,42,47,100] Brunet et al.[21] surveyed 1505 runners and found that increasing mileage correlated with an increase in stress fractures in women but not men. An explanation for the apparent gender difference is unclear. Australian track athletes with a past history of stress fracture tended to report more weekly hours of training and running and greater weekly distances in the 5 years preceding the study compared with those who had never sustained a stress fracture.[32] In a study of ballet dancers, a dancer who trained for more than 5 hours a day had an estimated risk for stress fracture that was 16 times greater than that of a dancer who trained for less than 5 hours per day.[27] This supports a role for training volume as a risk factor for stress fracture but may be related to increased exposure to injury.

Training surface has long been considered to contribute to stress fracture development.[5] Anatomic and biomechanical problems can be accentuated by cambered or uneven surfaces, whereas ground reaction forces are increased by less compliant surfaces.[101,102] Zernicke et al.[81] in a study of female runners claimed that those who sustained stress fractures tended to train on harder surfaces but gave no further details. Other researchers have also implicated training surface or change in surface as a risk factor but do not provide substantial supportive evidence.[29,44]

Older or worn running shoes have been related to an increase in stress fractures,[103] which may be due to decreased shock absorption.[104] However, the use of a shock-absorbing viscoelastic insole made no difference to the incidence of tibial stress fractures in rabbits[105] or to the overall incidence of stress fractures in military recruits.[103,106,107] It is not clear why Milgrom et al.[106] found a significant insole effect limited to femoral stress fractures only. Another prospective study showed that a semirigid orthotic device significantly reduced the incidence of femoral stress fractures in recruits with high-arched feet and the incidence of metatarsal fractures in recruits with low-arched feet.[108] The incidence of tibial stress fractures was not affected by the use of this orthotic device. Since the device had a hindfoot post at 3 degrees varus altering the biomechanics of the foot, it is difficult to know whether the results of the study can be attributed to this feature or to the shock-absorption capability.

In track and field, clinical observation suggests that the use of running spikes may influence the likelihood of stress fracture. However, little research has focused on the kinetic and kinematic effects of this form of footwear or on the relationship of spikes to stress fracture.

Biomechanics

Biomechanical features may predispose to stress fractures by creating areas of stress concentration in bone or promoting muscle fatigue. Although various biomechanical features have been examined in military recruits, there are few data pertaining to athletes. Failure to report measurement reliability or to analyze data appropriately make results difficult to interpret.

High arches (pes cavus) may be associated with an increased risk for stress fracture, particularly at femoral and tibial sites in male military recruits.[108–110] In a prospective study, the overall incidence of stress fracture in the low-arched group was 10% as opposed to 40% in the high-arched group.[109] A similar trend was noted for tibial and femoral stress fractures. However, assessment of foot type was based on observation in a nonfunctional position, and recruits with extreme pes planus were excluded. Nevertheless, these findings were supported by a study using a contact pressure display method to provide foot-ground pressure patterns and derived stress-intensity parameters.[110] Although a relationship may exist between foot type and stress fracture, this may vary depending on the site of stress fracture. Using radiographs to assess foot type, femoral and tibial stress fractures were more prevalent in the presence of higher arches, whereas the incidence of metatarsal fractures was higher with lower arches.[108] The authors proposed that since a low-arched foot is more flexible, it reduces the forces transmitted proximally to the tibia and femur but concentrates the forces in the foot.

Limited observations in athletes tend to differ from military findings. Pes planus (pronated) was the most common foot type in athletes who presented to sports clinics with stress fractures.[42,44] However, the incidence of pes planus in noninjured athletes was not assessed. In another series of stress fractures, pes planus was more common in tibial and tarsal bone stress fractures and least common in metatarsal stress fractures.[46] This implies a possible heterogeneous effect of biomechanical features on stress-fracture risk depending on the anatomic location of the injured region.

A leg-length discrepancy is another feature that has been postulated as a potential risk factor due to resulting skeletal realignment and asymmetries in loading, bone torsion, and muscle contraction.[111] Using a radiologic method to assess leg length, Friberg[112] found that in 130 cases of stress fracture in military recruits, the longer leg was associated with 73% of tibial, metatarsal, and femoral fractures, whereas 60% of fibular fractures were found in the shorter leg. In a prospective analysis, he observed a positive correlation between the degree of leg-length inequality and the incidence of stress fractures. However, no statistical analyses were performed to assess the significance of these results. A leg-length discrepancy has also been found to be associated with a significant increase in the incidence of stress fractures in athletes.[21,63] Seventy percent of women who developed stress fractures displayed a leg-length difference of more than 0.5 cm compared with 36% of women without stress fractures.[63]

Large prospective studies in the Israeli military have included an orthopedic examination in addition to assessment of other risk factors for stress fractures.[76,113,114] Of the biomechanical variables, only range of hip external rotation was found to correlate with the incidence of stress fracture. Soldiers in whom hip external rotation was greater than 65 degrees were at a higher risk for tibial and total stress fractures than those with a range less than 65 degrees. The risk for tibial stress fracture increased 2% for every 1-degree increase in hip external rotation range.[113] However, a large prospective study in American recruits failed to confirm these findings.[115] Greater forefoot varus and restricted ankle joint dorsiflexion have also been associated with an increased risk of stress fracture in military recruits.[116] The only prospective study to examine a number of clinical biomechanical measurements in athletes (including range of hip rotation and ankle dorsiflexion, calf and hamstring flexibility, lower-limb alignment, and static foot posture) did not find any to be useful predictors of stress-fracture occurrence.[63]

Most studies have included static biomechanical measures that may not adequately reflect the dynamic situation.[117] Preliminary studies analyzing running gait and using a force platform suggest a possible role for external loading kinetics and load magnitude in the development of a stress fracture.[62,94] This is an important area for future research.

DIAGNOSIS

In the assessment of a patient presenting with a possible diagnosis of stress fracture, three questions need to be answered:

1. Is the pain bony in origin?
2. If so, which bone is involved?
3. At what stage in the continuum of bone stress is this injury?

To obtain an answer to these three questions, a thorough history, precise examination, and appropriate use of imaging techniques are used. In many cases the diagnosis of stress fracture will be relatively simple. In others, especially when the affected bone may lie deeply (e.g., femur) or the pattern of pain may be nonspecific (e.g., navicular), the diagnosis can present a challenge for the clinician.

History

The history of the patient with a stress fracture is typically one of insidious onset of activity-related pain. Initially the pain will usually be described as a mild ache occurring after a specific amount of exercise. If the patient continues to exercise, the pain may well become more severe or occur at an earlier stage of exercise. The pain may increase, eventually limiting the quality or quantity of the exercise performed or occasionally forcing cessation of all activity. In the early stages, pain will usually cease soon after exercise. However, with continued exercise and increased severity of symptoms, the pain may persist after exercise. Night pain may occasionally occur.

It is also important to determine the presence of predisposing factors. Therefore a training or activity history is essential. In particular, note should be taken of recent changes in activity level such as increased quantity of training, increased intensity of training, and changes in surface, equipment (especially shoes), and technique. It may be necessary to obtain information from the patient's coach or trainer. A full dietary history should be taken, and particular attention should be paid to the possible presence of eating disorders. In females a menstrual history should be taken, including age of menarche and subsequent menstrual status.

A history of previous similar injury or any other musculoskeletal injury should be obtained. It is essential to obtain a brief history of the patient's general health, medications, and personal habits to ensure that no factors are influencing bone health. It is also important to obtain from the history an understanding of the patient's work and sporting commitments. In particular, it is important to know the level, how serious the patient is about his or her sport, and what significant sporting commitments are ahead in the short and medium term.

Physical Examination

On physical examination the most obvious feature is localized bony tenderness. Obviously this is easier to determine in bones that are relatively superficial and may be absent in stress fractures of the shaft or neck of femur. It is important to be precise in the palpation of the affected areas, particularly in regions such as the foot, where a number of bones and joints in a relatively small area may be affected. Occasionally, redness and swelling may be present at the site of the stress fracture. Palpable periosteal thickening may also be found, especially in a long-standing fracture. Percussion of long bones may result in the production of pain at a point distant from the percussion.

Joint range of motion is usually unaffected except when the stress fracture is close to the joint surface such as a stress fracture of the neck or femur. Specific stress fractures may be associated with specific clinical tests. Examples of these are the hop test for stress fractures in the groin region, and hip extension while standing on the contralateral leg, used in the diagnosis of stress fractures of the pars interarticularis.

Some authors have suggested that the presence of pain when therapeutic ultrasound is applied over the area of the stress fracture is of potential use in detection.[118–120] Similarly, it is reported that application of a vibrating tuning fork to the affected bone and subsequent increase in pain are indicative of a stress fracture. Our own experience suggests that these methods are not particularly helpful.

The physical examination must also take into account the potential predisposing factors; in all stress fractures involving the lower limb, a full biomechanical examination must be performed. Any evidence of leg-length discrepancy, malalignment (especially excessive subtalar pronation), muscle imbalance, weakness, or lack of flexibility should be noted.

Imaging

Imaging plays an important role in supplementing clinical examination to determine the answers to the three questions mentioned above. In many cases a clinical diagnosis of stress fracture is sufficient. The classic history of exercise-associated bone pain and typical examination findings of localized bony tenderness have a high correlation with the diagnosis of stress fracture. However, if the diagnosis is uncertain, or in the case of the serious or elite athlete who wishes to continue training if at all possible and requires more

specific knowledge of his or her condition, various imaging techniques are available to the clinician.

Radiography

Radiography has poor sensitivity but high specificity in the diagnosis of stress fractures. The classic radiographic abnormalities seen in a stress fracture are new periosteal bone formation, a visible area of sclerosis, the presence of callus, or a visible fracture line. If any of these radiographic signs are present, the diagnosis of stress fracture can be confirmed.

Unfortunately, in most stress fractures there is no obvious radiographic abnormality. The abnormalities on radiography are unlikely to be seen unless symptoms have been present for at least 2 to 3 weeks. In certain cases they may not become evident for up to 3 months and in a percentage of cases never become abnormal.

Isotopic Bone Scan (Scintigraphy)

If plain radiography demonstrates the presence of a stress fracture, then there is seldom any need to perform further investigations. However, when there is a high index of suspicion of stress fracture and a negative bone radiograph, the triple-phase bone scan is the next line of investigation. The bone scan is highly sensitive but has low specificity. Prather et al.[121] found that the bone scan had a true-positive rate of 100%, and false-negative scans are relatively rare.[122,123]

Technetium-99 methylene diphosphonate (MDP) is the usual radionuclide substance. Other possibilities include gallium citrate (Ga 67) and indium 111-labeled leukocytes.[124] The advantage of technetium-99 MDP is its short half-life (6 hours), allowing a higher dose to be administered with improved resolution.[125]

In the first phase of the bone scan, flow images are obtained immediately after intravenous injection of the tracer. These initial images are usually taken every 2 seconds and correspond roughly to contrast angiography, albeit with much lower spatial and temporal resolution. This first phase of the bone scan evaluates perfusion to bone and soft tissues from the arterial to the venous circulation.

The second phase of the bone scan consists of a static blood pool image taken 1 minute after the injection and reflects the degree of hyperemia and capillary permeability of bone and soft tissue. Generally speaking, the more acute and severe the injury, the greater the degree of increased perfusion and blood pool activity.

The third phase of the bone scan is the delayed image, taken 3 to 4 hours after injection when approximately 50% of the tracer has concentrated in the bone matrix through the mechanism of chemisorption to the hydroxy-apatite crystals. On the 3-hour delayed image, the uptake of the tracer is proportional to the rate of osteoblastic activity, extraction, efficiency, and amount of tracer delivered per unit time or blood flow.[126] The inclusion of the first and second phases of the bone scan permits estimation of the age of stress-induced focal bony lesions and the severity of bony injuries, and helps to differentiate soft-tissue inflammation from bony injury.[127] As the bony lesion heals, the perfusion returns to normal first, followed by normalization of the blood pool image a few weeks later. Focal increased uptake on the delayed scan resolves last because of ongoing bony remodeling and generally lags well behind the disappearance of pain. As healing continues, the intensity of the uptake diminishes gradually over a 3- to 6-month period following an uncomplicated stress fracture, with a minimal degree of uptake persisting for up to 10 months[126] or even longer.

Changes on bone scan may be seen as early at 48 to 72 hours after the commencement of symptoms. The radionuclide scan may be positive as early as 7 hours after bone injury.[128]

The bone scan is virtually 100% sensitive, at least twice as sensitive as x-ray,[129] and consistently more sensitive than ultrasound,[130] thermography,[131] and computed tomography (CT).[132] In several studies, only 10% to 25% of bone scan–positive stress fractures had radiographic evidence of stress fracture.[46,133–135]

In the appropriate clinical setting, the scintigraphic diagnosis of a stress fracture is defined as focal increased uptake in the third phase of the bone scan. However, bone scintigraphy lacks specificity because other nontraumatic lesions such as tumor (especially osteoid osteoma), osteomyelitis, bony infarct, and bony dysplasias can also produce localized increased uptake. It is therefore vitally important to correlate the bone-scan appearance with the clinical features.

The radionuclide scan will detect evolving stress fractures at the stage of accelerated remodeling. At that stage, which may be asymptomatic, the uptake is usually of mild intensity, progressing to more intense and better defined uptake as microfractures develop.[13,136]

In stress fractures all three phases of the triple-phase bone scan are positive.[127,137] Other bony abnormalities such as periostitis (shin splints) are only positive on delayed images,[127,138] whereas certain other overuse soft-tissue injuries would only be positive in the angiogram and blood pool phase, thus allowing one to differentiate between bony and soft-tissue pathology. The characteristic bone-scan appearance of a stress fracture is of a sharply marginated or fusiform area of increased uptake involving one cortex or occasionally extending the width of the bone[13] (Fig. 19–3).

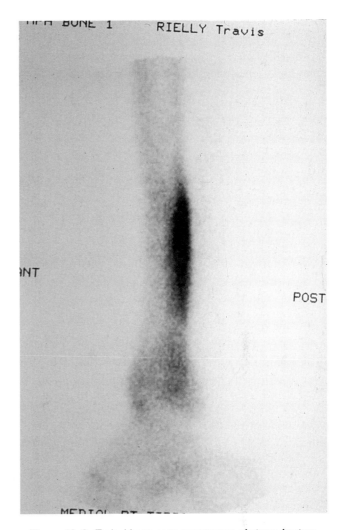

Figure 19–3. Typical bone scan appearance of stress fracture.

Increased radionuclide uptake is frequently found in asymptomatic sites.[97,139,140] Originally the presence of increased tracer uptake at nonpainful sites in athletes was interpreted as unrecognized stress fractures.[13,141,142] Other authors postulated that this may be nonspecific stress changes related to bone remodeling,[127] a false-positive finding,[143] and an uncertain finding.[144] Rosen et al.[142] found that asymptomatic uptake in 46% of cases with focal uptake was more common than diffuse uptake.

Matheson and his colleagues[145] in Vancouver proposed the concept of bone strain. They noted that the radionuclide bone scan, because of its sensitivity, was able to demonstrate the adaptive changes in bone at any point in the continuum from early remodeling to stress fracture. The term *bone strain* was coined to reflect the true dynamic response of bone to stress and allow the interpretation of bone changes along the continuum to be correlated with the wide range of presentations seen in clinical practice. They stated that excessive loading (from overuse, abnormal biomechanics, reduced shock absorption, or altered gait) produced a mechanical stress that is translated into bone remodeling via piezoelectric stimuli. The relative contribution of these factors as well as the athlete's activity pattern after the onset of remodeling determines the extent of bone strain seen clinically. Pain during activity may indicate small areas of remodeling that have low-intensity uptake on bone scan and negative x-rays. On the other hand, pain that persists after exercise and during rest may indicate more extensive remodeling, with intense uptake on scan and possibly abnormal radiographs.

This concept of a continuum of bone strain existing both clinically and scintigraphically is now widely accepted. It is now clear that bone stress can appear as an area of increased uptake on isotope bone scan before any symptoms occur. It is not clear what percentage of these cases progress to symptomatic bone stress and ultimately stress fracture if exercise is continued. It is also not clear what treatment is appropriate in these cases of asymptomatic bone stress. In many athletes and dancers in hard training, numerous areas of bone stress show up on an isotope bone scan. These are indicators of active remodeling and are not necessarily bone at risk for the development of stress fracture.

Attempts have been made to classify the bony continuum into "bone strain" or "asymptomatic stress reaction" and stress fracture. A summary of these features may be seen in Table 19–4. A scheme for grading bone scan appearance on the basis of severity has been proposed by Zwas et al.[135] and is shown in Table 19–5.

The sensitivity of bone scintigraphy can be further increased by the use of single-photon emission computed tomography (SPECT). Bone SPECT is most helpful in complex areas of the skeleton with overlapping structures that may obscure pathology such as the skull, pelvis, and spine. It is particularly useful in the detection of stress fractures of the pars interarticularis.

Computed Tomography

CT may be useful in differentiating those conditions with increased uptake on bone scan that may mimic stress fracture. These include osteoid osteoma, osteomyelitis with a Brodie's abscess, and other malignancies.

CT scans are also particularly valuable in imaging fractures when this may be important in treatment. In particular, CT scanning of the navicular bone is extremely helpful.[146,147] CT scanning may also be valuable in detecting fracture lines as evidence of stress fracture in long bones (e.g., metatarsal and tibia) where plain radiography is normal and isotope bone scan

TABLE 19–4. CONTINUUM OF BONY CHANGES WITH OVERUSE

Clinical Feature	Bone Strain	Stress Reaction	Stress Fracture
Local pain	Nil	Mild to moderate	Mild, moderate, or severe
Local tenderness	Nil	Mild to moderate	Moderate to severe
x-ray appearances	Normal	Normal	May show fracture after 10–14 days
Radiosotopic bone scan appearance	Increased uptake (mild)	Increased uptake (mild)	Increased uptake (severe)

Source: From Brukner PD et al.[177]

TABLE 19–5. GRADING OF TIBIAL OR LONG-BONE STRESS FRACTURES BY BONE SCAN OR MAGNETIC RESONANCE IMAGING (MRI) APPEARANCE

Grade	Bone Scan Appearance	MRI Appearance
I	Small, ill-defined cortical area of mildly increased activity	Periosteal edema: mild to moderate on T2-weighted images. Marrow edema: normal on T1 and T2-weighted images.
II	Better defined cortical area of moderately increased activity	Periosteal edema: moderate to severe on T2-weighted images. Marrow edema on T2-weighted images.
III	Wide fusiform cortical-medullary area of highly increased activity	Periosteal edema: moderate to severe on T2-weighted images. Marrow edema on T1- and T2-weighted images
IV	Transcortical area of increased activity	Periosteal edema: moderate to severe on T2-weighted images. Marrow edema on T1- and T2-weighted images; fracture line clearly visible.

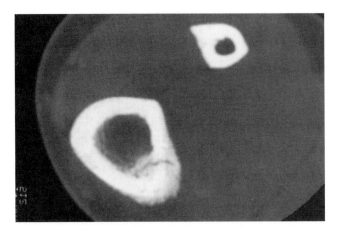

Figure 19–4. CT appearance of stress fracture of tibia.

shows increased uptake (Fig. 19–4). CT scanning will enable the clinician to differentiate between a stress fracture, which will be visible on CT scan, and a stress reaction. Particularly in the elite athlete, this may considerably affect rehabilitation and forthcoming competition programs.

Magnetic Resonance Imaging

Although magnetic resonance imaging (MRI) does not image cortical bone as well as CT scan, it has certain advantages in the imaging of stress fractures. Specific MRI characteristics of stress fracture include new bone formation and fracture lines appearing as very low-signal medullary bands that are contiguous with the cortex; surrounding marrow hemorrhage and edema seen as low-signal intensity on T1-weighted images and as high signal on T2-weighted and short T1 inversion recovery (STIR) images; and periosteal edema and hemorrhage appearing as high-signal intensity on T2-weighted and STIR images[148] (Fig. 19–5). These changes are best seen if the MRI is performed within 3 weeks of symptoms.[149] MRI is thought to be more sensitive than conventional radiography. MRI visualizes marrow hemorrhage and edema well, a characteristically difficult finding with CT. Although CT scan visualizes bone detail, another advantage of MRI is in distinguishing stress fractures from a suspected bone tumor or infectious process.[148]

Stafford et al.[150] reported findings of stress fractures in MRI. Zones of decreased signal of T1 images are seen in the affected region, whereas T2-weighted images show increased signal. A low-signal line may be seen running through the medullary cavity, presumably corresponding to the zone of localized fracture. Further advances in marrow imaging may be expected such as STIR sequences, which may help to identify such marrow pathology better.

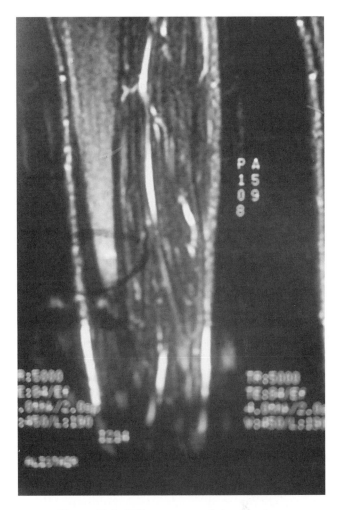

Figure 19–5. MRI appearance of stress fracture.

The appearance of a stress fracture on MRI is quite characteristic with intraosseous bands of very low signal intensity that are continuous with the cortex and surrounding areas of decreased signal intensity of the marrow space on T1-weighted images. T2 images show prominent intramedullary areas of high signal intensity as well as juxtacortical and/or subperiosteal areas of high signal intensity.[149,151]

Fredericson et al.[152] have proposed a grading scheme for MRI appearances of stress fractures based on fat-saturated images. They felt that their grades I to IV were equivalent to the bone-scan grading described by Zwas et al.[135] mentioned in the previous section. In this grading system grade I indicated mild to moderate periosteal edema on T2-weighted images only with no focal bone marrow abnormality. Grade II showed more severe periosteal edema as well as bone marrow edema on T2-weighted images only. Grade III showed moderate to severe edema of both the periosteum and marrow on both T1- and T2-weighted images. Grade

IV demonstrated a low-signal fracture line on all sequences with changes of severe marrow edema on both T1- and T2-weighted images. Grade IV may also show severe periosteal and moderate muscle edema. A comparison of stress-fracture grading between bone scan[135] and MRI[152] is shown in Table 19–5.

Fredericson et al.[152] examined runners with medial shin pain and compared the clinical findings, bone-scan appearances, and MRI appearances. In 14 of 18 symptomatic legs described in this study, MRI findings correlated with the established bone-scan grading system.[135] The authors felt that MRI more precisely defined the anatomic location and extent of injury. They also identified certain clinical symptoms such as pain with daily ambulation and physical examination findings including localized tibial tenderness and pain with direct repercussion that correlated with more severe grades of bony injuries, in this case, in the tibia. The authors recommended MRI over bone scan for grading of tibial stress lesions, stating that MRI is more accurate in correlating the degree of bone involvement with clinical symptoms. Additional advantages of MR bone imaging include lack of exposure to ionizing radiation and significantly less imaging time than triplephase bone scintigraphy. These authors suggest that periosteal edema represents the initial response of the tibia to nontraumatic, repetitive stress; although it can occur in the anterolateral portion of the tibia, it often appears in the same location as most tibial stress fractures, at the posterolateral cortex.

Steinbornn et al.[151] advocated the use of MRI in patients who have negative radiographs, a positive bone scan, and a less than firm diagnosis.

Differential Diagnosis

In the differential diagnosis of stress fracture, the causes can be nonbony or bony. Nonbony causes in particular relate to muscle or tendon injury (either muscle strain, hematoma, or delayed-onset muscle soreness or tendon inflammation) or degenerative change. Compartment syndrome, especially in the anterior and deep posterior compartments of the lower leg, may mimic a stress fracture as it also presents with exercise-related pain. Traction periostitis such as that previously termed shin splints or medial tibial stress syndrome may also mimic stress fractures, although the relationship of pain to exercise is different. Bone scan appearances of both compartment syndrome and periostitis differ from that of stress fracture.

Bony pathologies that can mimic stress fracture include tumor and infection. Osteoid osteoma is commonly mistaken for a stress fracture as it presents with pain and a discrete focal area of increased uptake on isotope bone scan. Two distinguishing features of osteoid osteoma are the presence of night pain and the relief of pain with the use of aspirin.

TREATMENT

The basis of treatment involves rest from the aggravating activity, a concept known as *relative rest*. The amount of time from a diagnosis of a stress fracture to full return to sport depends on a number of factors, including the site of the fracture, the length of the symptoms, and the stage in the spectrum of bone strain. Most stress fractures with a relatively brief history of symptoms will heal in a straightforward manner, and return to sport should occur within 6 to 8 weeks. However, there is a group of stress fractures that requires treatment additional to relative rest; these are considered later.

The primary aim of initial management of stress fracture is pain relief. This may involve the use of mild analgesics or nonsteroidal anti-inflammatory drugs (NSAIDs). Some times when activities of daily living are painful, nonweightbearing or partial weightbearing on crutches may be necessary for up to 7 to 10 days. In most cases this is not necessary, and merely avoidance of the aggravating activity will be sufficient.

The rate of resumption of activity should be modified according to symptoms and physical findings. Activity should always be pain free, and if any bony pain occurs then activity should cease for 1 to 2 days, resuming at a lower level. The patient should be clinically reassessed at regular intervals, in particular looking for bony tenderness.

When activities of daily living are pain free and there is no focal tenderness, then resumption of the aggravating activity can occur on a graduated basis. For lower-limb stress fractures for which running is the aggravating activity, we recommend a program that involves initial brisk walking increased by 5 to 10 minutes a day up to 45 minutes. Once this is achieved without pain, then we recommend an initial 5-minute period of slow jogging within the 45-minute walk. Assuming that this increase in activity does not reproduce the patient's symptoms, then the amount of jogging can be increased on a daily basis until the whole 45 minutes is completed at jogging pace. Once this is achieved, then strides can be introduced initially at half-pace and then gradually increasing to full pace. Once full sprinting is pain free, then gradual functional activities such as hopping, skipping and jumping, and twisting and turning can be introduced gradually. It is important that this process be graduated, and it is also important to err on the side of caution. For an uncomplicated lower-limb stress fracture, a typical program for resuming activity after a period of initial rest and activities of daily living is shown in Fig. 19–6.

	Day 1 (mins)	Day 2 (mins)	Day 3 (mins)	Day 4 (mins)	Day 5 (mins)	Day 6 (mins)	Day 7 (mins)
Week 1	Walk 5	Walk 10	Walk 15	Walk 20	Walk 25	Walk 30	Walk 35
Week 2	Walk 20 Jog 10 Walk 15	Walk 15 Jog 15 Walk 15	Walk 15 Jog 20 Walk 15	Walk 10 Jog 25 Walk 10	Walk 5 Jog 30 Walk 10	Walk 5 Jog 35 Walk 5	Jog 45
Week 3	Jog 35 Sprint 10	Jog 35 Sprint 10	Jog 30 Sprint 15	Jog 30 Sprint 15	Jog 25 Sprint 20	Jog 25 Sprint 20	Jog 20 Sprint 25
Week 4	Add functional activities	Gradually increase all week					
Week 5	RESUME FULL TRAINING						

Figure 19–6. Activity program for uncomplicated lower limb stress fracture following period of rest and activities of daily living.

Progress should be monitored clinically by the presence or absence of symptoms and local signs. It is not necessary to monitor progress by radiography, scintigraphy, CT, or MRI. Radiologic healing often lags behind clinical healing.

Fitness Maintenance

It is important that the athlete with a stress fracture be able to maintain strength and cardiovascular fitness while undergoing the appropriate rehabilitation program. It should be emphasized to the athlete that the rehabilitation program is not designed to maintain or improve fitness but rather to allow the damaged bone time to heal and gradually develop or regain full strength. Fitness should be maintained in other ways.

The most common means are biking, swimming, water running, and upper-body weight training. These workouts should mimic the athlete's normal training program as much as possible in both duration and intensity. Water running is particularly attractive to runners for this reason. Water running involves the use of a vest as a flotation device. Stretching should be performed to maintain flexibility during the rehabilitation process. Muscle strengthening is also an important component of the rehabilitation phase.

As well as maintenance of these parameters of physiologic fitness, it is possible in most cases for the athlete to maintain specific sports skills. In ball sports these can involve activities either seated or standing still. This active rest approach also greatly assists the athlete psychologically.

Modified Risk Factors

As with any overuse injury, it is not sufficient merely to treat the stress fracture. An essential component of the management of an athlete with an overuse injury involves identification of the factors that have contributed to the injury and, when possible, correction or modification of some of these factors to reduce the risk of injury recurrence. The fact that stress fractures have a high rate of recurrence is an indication that this part of the management program is often neglected.

The risk factors for the development of stress fractures have been discussed at length in a previous section. Although not yet supported by rigorous scientific evidence, one possible precipitating factor is training errors. Therefore it is important to identify these and to discuss them with the athlete and his or her coach when appropriate. Another important contributing factor may be inadequate equipment, especially running shoes. These shoes may be inappropriate for the particular foot type of the athlete, may have general inadequate support, or may be worn out.

TABLE 19–6. STRESS FRACTURES THAT REQUIRE SPECIFIC TREATMENT

Neck of femur
Anterior cortex, midshaft tibia
Navicular
Fifth metatarsal (base)
Sesamoid

Biomechanical abnormalities are also thought to be an important contributing factor to the development of overuse injuries in general and stress fractures in particular. Both excessively supinated and excessively pronated feet can be contributing factors to the development of stress fractures. Excessively supinated feet generally give poor shock absorption and require footwear that gives good absorption. Athletes with excessively pronated feet will require appropriate footwear for their foot type and possibly custom-made orthotics.

It is important that these risk factors be corrected by the time the athlete resumes training. When training resumes, it is important to allow adequate recovery time after hard sessions or hard weeks of training. In view of the history of stress fracture, it is advisable that some form of cross-training, e.g., swimming and cycling for a runner, be introduced to reduce both the stress on the previously injured area and the likelihood of a recurrence.

Stress Fractures Requiring Specific Treatment

Although most stress fractures will heal without complications in a relatively short time frame, some will require specific additional treatment. These are listed in Table 19–6 and described in detail in the next section.

AT-RISK STRESS FRACTURES

Femoral Neck

Stress fractures of the femoral neck were first described by Earnst,[153] who presented 13 cases. Subsequently Devas[154] described 25 cases and Blickenstaff and Morris[155] 36 cases. Fullerton and Snowdy[156] categorized the types of fractures, and Fullerton[157] has written an excellent review.

The patient usually presents with a history of anterior hip or groin pain aggravated by exercise. Occasionally night pain may be present. Physical examination usually shows pain and restriction at the end range of passive hip movement. There may occasionally be tenderness to deep palpation over the femoral neck.

In the athlete with exercise-related groin or hip pain, a plain radiograph should be taken. Fullerton and Snowdy,[156] however, showed that radiographs taken soon after symptoms began were positive in less than 20% of cases of femoral neck stress fracture. An isotope bone scan should be performed if there is any clinical suspicion of stress fracture. Although occasional cases of negative bone scan have been seen in athletes who subsequently developed radiographic evidence of stress fracture, most series indicate that isotope bone scan is the ultimate diagnostic test.[122] In most cases repeat radiographs will become positive in 1 to 2 weeks.[121]

Fullerton and Snowdy[156] developed a classification that combined the biomechanical factors and degree of displacement. The fractures may occur on the superior neck, the tension side, or the inferior aspect of the neck, the compression side. Both these sites show a spectrum of changes. The earliest stage is a normal radiograph with a positive isotope bone scan. The next stage is manifest with either endosteal or periosteal callus without a fracture. A cortical crack without displacement follows. The final stages are a widening of the cortical crack and then displacement.[157]

In the case of a normal radiograph with a positive bone scan or sclerosis only, bed rest is required until hip pain settles. The patient then progresses from partial to full weightbearing on crutches as symptoms permit. Once the patient is free of pain with crutches, he or she is allowed to progress to a cane and then to unprotected weightbearing. A progressive walking and then running program is prescribed, and the patient is returned over several months to full activity.[157] The patient with an undisplaced cortical crack on either the tension or compression side of the femoral neck is placed on immediate best rest, and serial radiographs are taken every 2 to 3 days for the first week or until rest pain is relieved.

Operative treatment is indicated if there is any widening of the fracture, if both cortices develop a defect, if bed rest is not feasible, or if the patient is unreliable or uncooperative. In any of these instances the fracture is stabilized on a semiemergent basis using multiple pins.[157] If there is no change in the serial radiographs once the patient is pain free at rest, he or she is allowed to progress activity as in the previous scenario.

In those fractures that present with any widening or with a defect in both cortices, immediate fixation is recommended. After radiographic fracture healing and resolution of hip pain with unsupported walking, consideration may be given to removal of the fixation. It is recommended that the patient's activity be restricted for at least 3 months after pin removal to allow filling of the pin tracks. During that period the patient may be allowed to progress to jogging but should not be involved in competitive running or sports. Once there is clinical and radiographic evidence that the postsurgical defects have healed, then the patient may resume a progressive controlled training program of gradual increase in activities such as running, walking, and jumping.[157]

Athletes who present with a displaced femoral neck stress fracture are treated surgically. Closed reduction and internal fixation with either multiple pins or a compression screw with a side plate should be used. After fracture healing, consideration should be given to implant removal, and a very gradual progression in athletic activity should be undertaken.

Fullerton and Snowdy[156] reported no problems with prolonged pain or subsequent progression in patients treated nonoperatively. Intermittent discomfort with activity for 6 months to 1 year can occur. Avascular necrosis and nonunion are two disastrous possible complications.[158]

Johansson et al.[159] followed 23 patients with stress fractures of the femoral neck for an average of 6.5 years after the injury. Sixteen of the patients had been treated with internal fixation, and the remaining seven were treated conservatively. Seven (30%) developed complications requiring major surgery. These complications were pseudo-arthrosis ($n = 1$), avascular necrosis ($n = 3$), and refracture ($n = 3$). Five of the complications occurred in patients with displaced fractures, and four of those were treated primarily by internal fixation; the two remaining patients had type 1 fractures with periosteal callus without a visible fracture line and were treated primarily with internal fixation or nonweightbearing. The three patients with avascular necrosis were treated with hip replacement ($n = 2$) or arthodesis ($n = 1$). Fifty percent of the patients with displaced fractures and 25% with type 1 fractures decreased their activity level as a consequence of the fracture, mainly due to the pain induced by activity. All the elite athletes in the study decreased their activity to recreational levels after the injury. The authors concluded that a displaced stress fracture of the femoral neck is a serious cause of major complications such as avascular necrosis, refracture, and pseudarthrosis. They speculated that early diagnosis and treatment may prevent displacement of the fracture and thus improve the prognosis. They emphasized the use of isotope bone scan when a patient, especially a runner, presents with a sudden onset of exertional groin pain and has pain at the extreme of hip movement.

Anterior Cortex of Tibia

Fractures of the anterior cortex of the midshaft of the tibia need to be considered separately from other stress fractures of the tibia as they are prone to delayed

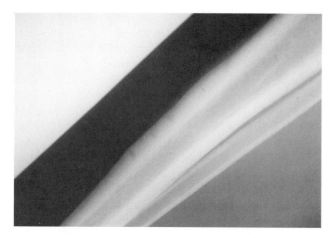

Figure 19–7. Multiple "dreaded black lines".

union, nonunion, and complete fracture. The appearance is described as the "dreaded black line" and is shown in Fig. 19–7.

These fractures were first described by Burrows[160] in 1956 in ballet dancers. In his series, four of the five dancers returned to activity at an average of 15 months after diagnosis; the fifth sustained a comminuted fracture of the midtibia 2 weeks after the onset of symptoms. This fracture healed after 14 months, with 8 months in a long-leg cast. Friedenberg[161] and Stanitski et al.[89] reported cases of nonunion of anterior tibial cortex stress fractures. Brahms et al.[162] presented a case report in which a spontaneous complete fracture through the stress-fracture area occurred.

Green et al.[163] presented six stress fractures of the anterior cortex of the middle third of the tibia that failed to unite with conservative management. The average age of the patients was 16.7 years, and five of the six stress fractures became complete fractures. The five patients who sustained a complete fracture were immobilized for an average of 6.6 months. One patient was treated with electromagnetic stimulation. Three underwent excision of the nonunion with the addition of iliac bone grafts at an average of 11 months after the stress fracture was first diagnosed. One patient underwent simple biopsy of the lesion, and the last patient underwent open reduction and internal fixation of his second complete fracture. They postulated that the reason for the high incidence of nonunion in their series and previous reports was that the particular area in the midshaft of the tibia was under tension rather than compression so that the fractures were more likely the result of tensile forces rather than compression forces. They recommended that initially these fractures, whether complete or not, should be treated with immobilization; then, after 4 to 6 months if there is no radiographic evidence of healing, serious consideration should be given to fixation with iliac bone grafting.

Blank[164] reported five cases of tibial transverse stress fractures of which three were in the anterior midthird. One patient developed a complete fracture line through the stress injury. Interestingly, bone scans in three of these cases showed no evidence of increased activity at the fracture site. Blank postulated that the lack of evidence of radionuclide activity was indicative of nonunion.

Rettig et al.[165] presented eight competitive basketballers with stress fracture of the anterolateral cortex of the tibial midshaft. All eight patients were treated with rest and/or pulsed electromagnetic field therapy. Although one of the patients required a bone grafting procedure, all eight of these patients showed complete healing and were able to return to full activity after an average of 8.7 months of treatment. The overall time from initial symptoms to return to competition averaged 12.5 months in this group of athletes. These authors suggested that the relative hypovascularity of the anterior tibial cortex due to its subcutaneous location may be a factor predisposing to delayed union.

Orava et al.[166] presented 17 patients (mean age 26 years) with this stress fracture. Six of the athletes were of international level and the rest of national level. All 17 cases were initially treated with rest from physical activity, and 8 of the 17 showed clinical healing in 3 to 10 months (average 6 months). Nine cases progressed to a delayed or nonunion requiring operational treatment. Surgery involved transverse drilling of the hypertrophied anterior cortex to enhance bone formation. In the surgically treated cases, the postoperative recovery time was, on average, 6 months.

Stress fracture of the anterior cortex of the medial third of the tibia presents with diffuse dull pain aggravated by physical activity. The bone is tender to palpation at the site of the fracture, and periosteal thickening may be present if the symptoms have been present for some time. Plain radiographs may be normal early on, although eventually periosteal thickening and callus will be seen in most cases. Isotope bone scan shows a discrete focal area of increased activity in the anterior cortex.

As with most stress fractures, it would appear that the less time from the onset of pain to the diagnosis and avoidance of activity, the more chance of healing. Some clinicians advocate the use of a cast in the treatment of these stress fractures; others recommend simple avoidance of the aggravating activity for a prolonged period, approximately 6 to 8 months. Monitoring of fracture healing should be both clinical and radiographic. Athletes should not return to activity until there is evidence of cortical bridging on radiography. If, after 4 to 6 months, there is no evidence of healing either clinically or radiologically, a diagnosis of nonunion can be made and bone grafting should be performed.

Medial Malleolus

Stress fractures of the medial malleolus were first described by Shelbourne et al.[167] These authors formulated the following criteria for the diagnosis of stress fracture of the medial malleolus. The patient presents with tenderness over the medial malleolus and ankle effusion, having experienced discomfort and pain during running and jumping activities for several weeks before an acute episode causes them to seek medical attention. The fracture line is frequently vertical from the junction of the tibial plafond and the medial malleolus, but it may arch obliquely from the junction to the distal tibial metaphysis. If clinical signs and history are present and the fracture line is not detected on radiographs, a bone scan should be performed. If there is increased uptake in the area of the medial malleolus on the bone scan, the injury fits the criteria for a stress fracture of the medial malleolus.

Shelbourne et al.[167] presented six case histories of patients with medial malleolar stress fractures. Three patients had a fracture line that could be seen on plain radiographs; they were treated by open reduction and internal fixation. The other three patients had normal radiographs, but bone scans showed increased uptake over the medial malleolus. These patients were treated with immobilization, either in a cast or in a pneumatic leg brace (Aircast).

Shelbourne and his coauthors[167] postulated that with forefoot pronation, the navicular bone moves into an abducted position relative to the talar head. This imposes an internal rotational force on the talus, which is subsequently transmitted to the medial malleolus. The rotation of the medial malleolus then causes tibial rotation. Thus there is a direct relationship between forefoot pronation and internal rotation of the tibia. This relationship is also noted when an athlete attempts to rotate the tibia externally while the forefoot is planted in pronation. External rotation of the tibia is then prevented by the talus, which distributes an opposing rotational force on to the medial malleolus. As a result of repetitive, overloading cyclic stress, a microfracture may develop at the junction of the medial malleolus and the tibial plafond.

The surgically treated patients of Shelbourne et al. began motion shortly after fixation and progressed to running activities within 6 weeks and full sports participation within 8 weeks. Nonsurgically treated patients were allowed unlimited ambulation in the pneumatic leg brace (Aircast) and also progressed to full participation in 6 to 8 weeks.

Rieder et al.[168] reported a case of nonunion of a medial malleolus stress fracture, noting that the rate of nonunion for acute fractures of the medial malleolus treated conservatively was as high as 10% to 15% due to inadequate closed reduction and interposition of periosteum. In this case the patient had had pain in the area for more than 2 years that had not been diagnosed correctly as a stress fracture.

Schils et al.[169] described seven patients with stress fracture of the medial malleolus and paid particular attention to the imaging features. Initially radiographic findings included one or two linear areas of hyperlucency 2 to 15 mm long. They originated at the medial malleolus-tibial plafond junction and were vertically oriented in five patients; the fissure arched obliquely through the medial malleolus in one patient, and one patient had normal radiographs. The fissure was best seen on the anteroposterior radiograph. Well-circumscribed lytic lesions surrounded the fissure in three patients. In two of these seven patients, a complete vertical fracture of the medial malleolus extending from the tibial plafond to the medial cortex occurred. Of the two patients who completely fractured the medial malleolus, one was treated with a cast for 8 weeks and returned to full athletic activities 5 months later; the other had a fracture while jogging 7 months after initial open reduction and internal fixation of the medial malleolus. Open reduction and internal fixation were again performed, and clinical and radiographic evidence of healing was seen 8 months later. Two of the other five patients were treated with open reduction and internal fixation of the medial malleolus; the remaining three were placed in a cast or pneumatic leg brace (Aircast) for 6 weeks.

Orava et al.[170] reported a series of eight patients with stress fracture of the medial malleolus. Initial radiographs revealed the fracture in only three patients. For the other patients, the diagnosis was made with isotope scans and confirmed with CT scans, MRI, or subsequent plain radiographs. One vertical fracture was treated initially by compression with AO screws. Two patients had delayed healing with symptoms for 8 and 12 months. These fracture sites were drilled, and the fractures healed 4 and 5 months after drilling. The five patients managed nonoperatively all healed within 5 months (average 4 months).

We recommend treating undisplaced or minimally displaced stress fractures of the medial malleolus conservatively in a pneumatic legbrace (Aircast) for 6 weeks. Displaced fractures or those that progress to nonunion should be treated operatively.

Navicular Bone

Stress fractures of the tarsal navicular bone were reviewed by Khan et al.[171] Navicular stress fractures are fractures in the sagittal plane involving the middle third of the bone. The central third of the navicular is thought to be particularly susceptible to stress fractures and subsequent delayed union because of the relative avascularity of the region of bone.[172]

The exact cause of navicular stress fractures is not clear. As with most stress fractures, a combination of overuse and training errors plays a significant role. It is thought that impingement of the navicular bone occurs between the proximal and distal tarsal bones with bending and compressive forces exerted by the muscles.[173] Fitch and colleagues[174] have proposed that there is a plane of maximum shear stress through the central portion of the navicular bone. Microangiographic studies of the blood supply show relative avascularity of the middle third of the bone.[172] A combination of these factors may result in fatigue failure in this portion of the bone, which is the consistent site of stress fractures within the navicular.

Navicular stress fractures have traditionally been regarded as a relatively unusual stress fracture; however, in recent years, various authors[146,172,174] have reported series of navicular stress fractures and suggested that with increased suspicion, these fractures are in fact far more common than earlier thought. Recent stress fractures series show a high percentage of navicular stress fractures.[46,49,50] They occur particularly in runners, usually sprinters, hurdlers, and long jumpers, but also middle distance runners. They are also seen in football, basketball, racquet sports, field hockey, ballet, gymnastics, and cricket.

The onset of symptoms is usually insidious, with increased foot pain after sprinting, jumping, or running.[174] Particularly in the early stages of the injury, pain is often ill defined. Most typically it radiates along the medial aspect of the longitudinal arch or along the dorsum of the foot.[172,175] Pain may also radiate distally along the first or second ray or laterally toward the cuboid. There is usually no swelling or discoloration. A limp may be present for a short time after exercise. Symptoms abate rapidly with rest, often allowing jogging within a week.[174–176] Occasionally there is an acute onset of injury without a history of previous pain.

Examination of the navicular bone requires precise knowledge of the anatomy of the midfoot and skilful palpation of the talonavicular joint. Having located this joint while inverting and everting the foot, the examiner palpates the proximal dorsal portion of the navicular bone. This has been described as the N-spot[146,177] and is shown in Fig. 19–8.

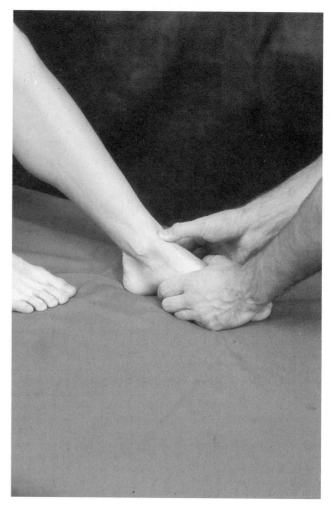

Figure 19–8. The N-spot.

Plain radiography has low sensitivity in the identification of navicular stress fracture, particularly partial fracture. In their review of the navicular stress fracture literature, Khan et al.[171] reported that 86 of the 128 feet radiographed had a false-negative result for fracture. Radioisotope bone scan is effective in demonstrating increased bony stress in the navicular. Plantar views have been more useful than the standard frontal, medial, and lateral views.[178] All 105 radioisotope scans reviewed[171] showed markedly increased focal uptake in the region of the navicular. Of these, 82 had previously had false-negative results on plain radiographic investigation. The characteristic appearance of a positive radioisotope scan outlines the entire navicular bone. CT scanning is a valuable tool in the assessment of navicular stress fracture. Precise radiologic technique is required to demonstrate the tiny navicular stress fractures. A bone algorithm must be used and the gantry angled to the plane of the talonavicular joint to take contiguous 1.5-mm slices.[147] Cuts should be

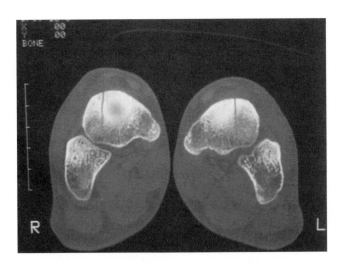

Figure 19–9. CT appearance of navicular stress fracture.

taken directly parallel to the talonavicular joint. On CT scan, the proximal articular rim of the normal navicular bone appears extremely dense, almost sclerotic, and is ring-like on true axial images. This apparent bone sclerosis may reflect the mechanical load normally borne by the relatively small concave articular surface of the navicular during weightbearing.[147] Most stress fractures are linear defects, some have associated bone fragments, and others appear as rim defects without a linear component.[147] The typical CT appearance of a navicular stress fracture is shown in Fig. 19–9.

Various treatments have been reported for navicular stress fracture. These include simple weightbearing rest, nonweightbearing cast immobilization for 2 weeks to 3 months, and surgery. Historically there has been a high incidence of delayed and nonunion injuries,[146,172,174,179] which has in some cases prevented the athlete from returning to his or her athletic career. Of the 131 cases in which the outcome was reported, 77 had a satisfactory result whereby the athlete returned to activity with no or minimal pain after the initial treatment.

Initial treatment of navicular stress fractures with weightbearing rest has met with a high rate of failure. Of 45 fractures initially treated in this manner, only 11 healed, albeit slowly, without complication. All five cases of refracture in the literature were initially treated with weightbearing rest. Decreased activity alone may alleviate the symptoms but will not allow osteoblastic activity to bridge the fracture site.[180,181] By contrast, navicular stress fractures treated with nonweightbearing cast immobilization had excellent results. Thirty-two of 36 patients were asymptomatic after treatment. Six complete navicular stress fractures treated initially with nonweightbearing cast immobilization recovered uneventfully.[146,172] Furthermore, 10 patients treated

initially with weightbearing rest continued to have symptoms and were subsequently treated with nonweightbearing cast immobilization. Nine of these patients (90%) recovered fully.[146,172] One patient who had internal fixation as the initial treatment but who had persisting symptoms also recovered fully with subsequent nonweightbearing cast immobilization.

In the reported cases, 22 of 27 fractures complicated by delayed union or displacement of fragments have been successfuly treated by surgery. Surgical methods used include internal fixation or curettage and grafting. The fracture is difficult to see at operation unless there is wide separation of the fragments because the dorsal surface of the navicular bone is rarely disrupted. It is frequently necessary to open the talonavicular joint and separate the articular surfaces by traction.[174] In another report, a Kirschner wire was inserted vertically into the estimated fracture site from above, and CT scanning was used during the operation to ascertain the position of the wire relative to the fracture and thus localize the fracture.[181] In most cases the postoperative treatment has involved 6 weeks of nonweightbearing with or without cast immobilization.

A patient presenting with persistent midfoot pain aggravated by activity and with a clinical finding of tenderness at the N-spot generally requires investigation with radionuclide scan since the sensitivity of radiography for navicular stress fracture is extremely low. If the radionuclide scan shows focal uptake in the navicular bone, fine-slice CT scan is required in the plane of the talonavicular joint to differentiate between a stress fracture and stress reaction since these would have different management.[146]

After diagnosis of partial or complete navicular stress fracture with plain radiography or CT scan, the patient must be treated with *strict* nonweightbearing cast immobilization for at least 6 weeks. With the advent of waterproof underwrap and casting material, it is possible for patients to shower and swim in the cast. Underwater running has not been shown to be safe in athletes with navicular stress fracture who are being treated in a cast.

Patients should be reviewed 3 weeks after they have been casted. This is an opportunity to assess the state of the cast, to reemphasize the importance of strict nonweightbearing, and to explain the rehabilitation program, which commences when the cast is removed. The cast should be removed after 6 weeks and healing assessed clinically. If still tender a further 2 weeks of nonweightbearing cast immobilization is recommended.

Athletes often feel some diffuse foot pain and paresthesia on first walking after nonweightbearing cast immobilization. However, it is usually different from their pain at presentation and it diminishes with passive joint mobilization and weightbearing activity. The pain is thought to be due to joint stiffness of the talocrural, subtalar, and midtarsal joints[182] as a result of the cast immobilization. As long as the navicular bone is not tender, such pain is not a contraindication to weightbearing rehabilitation.

The radiologic appearance after 6 weeks of cast immobilization is not a useful indicator of healing; therefore x-ray, radionuclide scan, and CT scan are not indicated at that stage.

If the fracture is clinically healed (no tenderness at the N-spot), a 6-week program of rehabilitation under the supervision of a sports physiotherapist is recommended. This includes a graduated return to activity, joint mobilization, soft-tissue therapy, and muscle strengthening.

For the initial 2 weeks of weightbearing, normal activities of daily living, swimming, and water running are all permitted. After this period the N-spot is reassessed, and if there is no increase in tenderness the athlete may begin jogging on grass for 5 minutes on alternate days. After three or four such sessions, the jogging time can be increased to 10 minutes. The athlete is reassessed after 2 weeks of jogging. If the N-spot is not tender, the athlete can begin "run-throughs" (faster running over 50 to 80 meters) with walk recovery on alternate days. The speed is gradually increased from half to three-quarters of maximum speed over another 2 weeks. After a total of 6 weeks of rehabilitation, the athlete is reassessed; if the N-spot is not tender, the athlete is permitted to continue to return to full training gradually.

At the time of cast removal, there will usually be associated stiffness of the talocrural, subtalar, and midtarsal joints. These should be treated during the rehabilitation period by passive joint mobilization.[177] There will also frequently be soft-tissue tightness, especially in the tibialis posterior and soleus muscles, which should be treated by active stretching and soft-tissue massage techniques including myofascial release.[177] Muscle weakness resulting from atrophy during the period of nonweightbearing needs to be corrected with a graded strengthening program before full activity is resumed.

As with any overuse injury, the possible contribution of abnormal biomechanics should be assessed. Although clinical research has not yet isolated any particular biomechanical abnormality common to all athletes with navicular stress fracture, we feel that any significant biomechanical abnormality (e.g., excessive subtalar joint pronation) should nevertheless be corrected with orthotics.

Navicular stress fractures are far more common than previously thought and require aggressive non-weightbearing cast immobilization as the first line of treatment. Those treated in this manner will have a high rate of healing.

Proximal Fifth Metatarsal

Fractures of the proximal third of the fifth metatarsal have caused considerable confusion among practitioners. The most common fracture seen is a simple avulsion fracture of the tuberosity at the base of the fifth metatarsal. This is caused by contraction of the peroneus brevis tendon as a result of an acute inversion injury. This is an uncomplicated fracture that usually heals well with a short period of immobilization for pain relief.

The fracture of most concern in this region is the fracture of the proximal diaphysis known as the Jones' fracture. In 1902, Sir Robert Jones[183] described a transverse fracture in the proximal diaphysis that he sustained himself while dancing around a tent pole at a military party. There are three main subtypes. The first is the acute fracture with no prior history of pain in the region of the fracture; x-ray confirms the presence of a fracture and shows no medullary scelorsis. These acute fractures have a good prognosis provided they are treated by immobilization in a short leg, nonweightbearing cast. We recommened placing the athlete in a cast initially for 6 weeks and at the time of removal assessing healing both clinically, by evidence of local tenderness, and radiologically. It may be necessary to place the patient back in a cast for a further period of up to 4 weeks. Occasionally nonunion may occur, and this can be treated surgically.

The second, and most common, type of Jones' fracture is an acute presentation of a stress fracture. The patient initially presents with what appears to be an acute fracture but when questioned describes a variable period of pain with activity in the region of the fracture. The x-ray shows a fracture line (Fig. 19–10) and, depending on the length of time of symptoms, possibly some evidence of medullary sclerosis. These fractures are prone to delayed union and nonunion, although most will heal eventually with conservative management. Most patients, however, are reluctant to spend a prolonged period in a cast, and we recommend surgical management for these cases of acute presentation of a fifth metatarsal stress fracture. In the case of a fracture without a considerable degree of medullary sclerosis, then a medullary compression screw fixation as described by Kavanaugh[184] and DeLee et al.[185] is performed. In athletes who have marked medullary sclerosis (frequently with a lengthy history of symptoms), open reduction and bone grafting is recommended.

The third type presents with an established nonunion radiographically or with a lengthy period

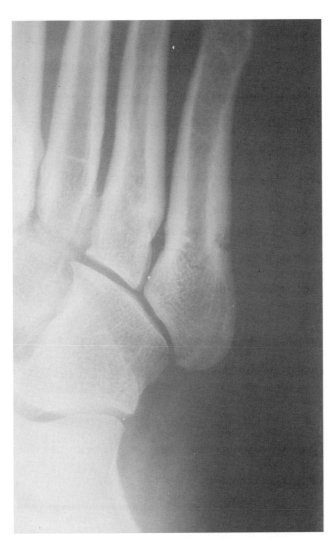

Figure 19–10. Jones' fracture.

of symptoms and evidence of intramedullary sclerosis on x-ray. These patients should be treated with bone grafting.

The anatomy of this region has been described by Dameron,[186] Torg et al.,[187] and Richli.[188] Jones himself[183] emphasized the very strong soft-tissue connections at the base of the fifth metatarsal as well as the strong connection between this metatarsal and the adjacent metatarsal and cuboid bone.

Stewart[189] suggests that there are up to seven structures inserting on the proximal fifth metatarsal. The joint capsule is probably the strongest; up to five muscles may also insert. The peroneus brevis and tertius, abductor digiti minimi, flexor digiti minimi, and interosseous muscles all insert in this region. There is also a band of plantar fascia that inserts into the most proximal tip of the fifth metatarsal. Richli[188] showed that the lateral cord of plantar fascia attaches proximally to

the other tendons. He also demonstrated that the force applied to this structure resulted in a transverse fracture through the tuberosity of the metatarsal posterior to most of the peroneus brevis insertion. Athletes whose sport involves repetitive pivoting inward and outward while weightbearing across the ball of the foot may be particularly susceptible to this condition.[190]

The Jones' fracture is one of the small group of stress fractures that require early recognition and aggressive treatment to maximize the possibility of complete healing.

Sesamoids

The medial and lateral sesamoid bones at the first metatarsophalangeal (MTP) joint act as a pulley for the flexor hallucis longus and brevis tendons and are necessary for stabilization of the joint. They may be injured in a number of ways, including traumatic fracture, stress fracture, and sprain of a bipartite sesamoid. Inflammatory changes and osteonecrosis around the sesamoid and the tendon are collectively known as sesamoiditis. The medial sesamoid is usually affected.

Van Hal et al.[191] first described stress fractures of the sesamoids, in one male and three female athletes with an average age of 21 years. All four patients experienced insidious onset of pain in the area of their first MTP joint during and/or after athletic activity. They had tenderness to palpation and pain on hyperdorsiflexion of their first MTP joint. In all four cases the stress fracture was demonstrated on plain radiograph, although three of the four previous radiographs had failed to demonstrate the fracture. Bone scan was also positive in all four cases. In this series, two of the stress fractures were in the medial sesamoid and two in the lateral. The authors advise that if standard radiographs suggest a multipartite rather than a fractured sesamoid, a bone scan should be performed. A multipartite sesamoid will be cold on scan. Bilateral foot radiographs are of little value since 75% of individuals with multipartite sesamoids have unilateral involvement.[192–194] None of the four patients in this study healed their fracture with 6 weeks of casting and/or 4 to 6 months of inactivity. All four patients eventually had their sesamoid excised. After surgery the patients were placed in short-leg casts for 3 weeks. At that point the cast was removed, and the patient was encouraged to increase activity as tolerated. The patients returned to their prefracture activities without symptoms within an average of 10 weeks of surgery and remained symptom free.

Clinically it is difficult to differentiate a stress fracture of the sesamoid from other causes of sesamoid pain. The patient complains of pain with forefoot weightbearing and will often walk with weight laterally to compensate. On examination there is marked tenderness and occasional swelling in the region of the sesamoid. X-ray or radiography may demonstrate the presence of a stress fracture but may be difficult to distinguish from bipartite or multipartite sesamoid bones. A radioisotopic bone scan should be performed if there is suspicion of a stress fracture.

Stress fractures of the sesamoid bones are prone to nonunion and may require an extended period of nonweightbearing. Davis and Alexander[195] recommend casting for 6 weeks as the initial treatment. If at that point clinical or radiographic healing is incomplete, recasting is recommended. Sesamoidectomy is then indicated in patients with persistent symptoms despite appropriate conservative management.

McBryde[196] recommends casting with full-length platform support and specific prevention of dorsiflexion. He advocates bone grafting for late union and nonunion, although selected partial or complete excision may be necessary.

We recommend treating these stress fractures symptomatically, that is, using nonweightbearing while monitoring progress clinically. Gradual weightbearing can be commenced when bony tenderness is no longer present. If nonunion occurs, excision of the sesamoid can be performed. Padding is used to distribute the weight away from the sesamoid bone.[197]

CONCLUSIONS

Stress fractures are a common injury, particularly in runners and in sports that involve a large amount of running. Various risk factors for the development of stress fractures have been proposed; however, the relative importance of these is still uncertain. The diagnosis is primarily on clinical grounds, but imaging can be used for confirmation or to assess the extent of injury. The treatment is straightforward in most cases, but a small group of stress fractures requires more specific management.

REFERENCES

1. Grimston SK, Zernicke RF: Exercise-related stress responses in bone. *J Appl Biomech* 1993:9, 2.
2. Martin AD, Bailey DA: Skeletal integrity in amenorrhoeic athletes. *Aust J Sci Med Sport* 1987: June, 3.
3. Stechow AW: Fussoedem und Roentgenstrahlen. *Dtsch Mil-Aerztl Zeitg* 1897:26, 465.
4. Deutschlander C: Ueber eine eigenartige Mittelfuszerkrankung. *Zentralbl f Chir* 1921:48, 1422.
5. Devas MB, Sweetnam R: Stress fractures of the fibula. A review of 50 cases in athletes. *J Bone Joint Surg Br* 1956:38B, 818.
6. Dodd H: Pied force or march foot. *Br J Surg* 1933:21, 131.
7. Roberts SM, Vogt EC: Pseudofracture of the tibia. *J Bone Joint Surg* 1939:21, 891.
8. Weaver JB, Francisco CB: Pseudofractures. A manifestation of non-suppurative osteomyelitis. *J Bone Joint Surg* 1940:22, 610.
9. Burrows HJ: Fatigue fractures of the fibula. *J Bone Joint Surg Br* 1948:30B, 266.
10. Hullinger CW: Insufficiency fracture of the calcaneus. Similar to march fracture of the metatarsal. *J Bone Joint Surg* 1944:26, 751.
11. Jansen M: March fractures. *J Bone Joint Surg* 1926:8, 262.
12. Sloane D, Sloane MF: March foot. *Am J Surg* 1936:31, 167.
13. Roub LW, Gumerman LW, Hanley EN, et al.: Bone stress: A radionuclide imaging perspective. *Radiology* 1979:132, 431.
14. Li G, Zhang S, Chen G, et al.: Radiographic and histologic analyses of stress fracture in rabbit tibias. *Am J Sports Med* 1985:13, 285.
15. Burr DB, Milgrom C, Boyd RD, et al.: Experimental stress fractures of the tibia. *J Bone Joint Surg* 1990:72, 370.
16. Martin RB, Burr DB: A hypothetical mechanism for the stimulation of osteonal remodelling by fatigue damage. *J Biomech* 1982:15, 137.
17. Mori S, Burr DB: Increased intracortical remodeling following fatigue damage. *Bone* 1993:14, 103.
18. Schaffler MB, Radin EL, Burr DB: Mechanical and morphological effects of strain rate on fatigue of compact bone. *Bone* 1989:10, 207.
19. Schaffler MB, Radin EL, Burr DB: Long-term fatigue behavior of compact bone at low strain magnitude and rate. *Bone* 1990:11, 321.
20. Barrow GW, Saha S: Menstrual irregularity and stress fractures in collegiate female distance runners. *Am J Sports Med* 1988:16, 209.
21. Brunet ME, Cook SD, Brinker MR, et al.: A survey of running injuries in 1505 competitive and recreational runners. *J Sports Med Phys Fitness* 1990:30, 307.
22. Cameron KR, Wark JD, Telford RD: Stress fractures and bone loss—the skeletal cost of intense athleticism. *Excel* 1992:8, 39.
23. Bennell KL, Malcolm SA, Thomas SA, et al.: Risk factors for stress fractures in female track-and-field athletes: A retrospective analysis. *Clin J Sport Med* 1995:5, 229.
24. Bennell KL, Malcolm SA, Thomas SA, et al.: The incidence and distribution of stress fractures in competitive track and field athletes. *Am J Sports Med* 1996:26, 211.
25. Warren MP, Brooks-Gunn J, Hamilton LH, et al.: Scoliosis and fractures in young ballet dancers: Relation to delayed menarche and secondary amenorrhea. *N Engl J Med* 1986:314, 1348.
26. Frusztajer NT, Dhuper S, Warren MP, et al.: Nutrition and the incidence of stress fractures in ballet dancers. *Am J Clin Nutr* 1990:51, 779.
27. Kadel NJ, Teitz CC, Kronmal RA: Stress fractures in ballet dancers. *Am J Sports Med* 1992:20, 445.

28. Johnson AW, Weiss CB, Wheeler DL: Stress fractures of the femoral shaft in athletes—more common than expected. A new clinical test. *Am J Sports Med* 1994:22, 248.

29. Goldberg B, Pecora C: Stress fractures. A risk of increased training in freshman. *Physician Sportsmed* 1994:22, 68.

30. Pecina M, Bojanic I, Dubravcic S: Stress fractures in figure skaters. *Am J Sports Med* 1990:18, 277.

31. Dixon M, Fricker P: Injuries to elite gymnasts over 10 yr. *Med Sci Sports Exerc* 1993:25, 1322.

32. Cameron KR, Telford RD, Wark JD, et al.: Stress fractures in Australian competitive runners, in *Australian Sports Medicine Federation Annual Scientific Conference in Sports Medicine,* 1992, Perth, Australia.

33. Protzman RR, Griffis CG: Stress fractures in men and women undergoing military training. *J Bone Joint Surg Am* 1977:59-A, 8.

34. Reinker KA, Ozburne S: A comparison of male and female orthopaedic pathology in basic training. *Milit Med* 1979:Aug, 532.

35. Brudvig TJS, Gudger TD, Oberinger L: Stress fractures in 295 trainees: A one-year study of incidence as related to age, sex, and race. *Milit Med* 1983:148, 666.

36. Jones H, Harris JM, Vinh TN, et al.: Exercise-induced stress fractures and stress reactions of bone: Epidemiology, etiology, and classification. *Exerc Sports Sci Rev* 1989:17, 379.

37. Jones BH, Bovee MW, Harris JM, et al.: Intrinsic risk factors for exercise-related injuries among male and female army trainees. *Am J Sports Med* 1993:21, 705.

38. Pester S, Smith PC: Stress fractures in the lower extremities of soldiers in basic training. *Orthop Rev* 1992:21, 297.

39. Brubaker CE, James SL: Injuries to runners. *J Sports Med* 1974:2, 189.

40. Orava S: Stress fractures. *Br J Sports Med* 1980:14, 40.

41. Pagliano J, Jackson D: The ultimate study of running injuries. *Runners World* 1980:November, 42.

42. Taunton JE, Clement DB, Webber D: Lower extremity stress fractures in athletes. *Physician Sportsmed* 1981:9, 77.

43. Clement DB, Taunton JE, Smart GW, et al.: A survey of overuse running injuries. *Physician Sportsmed* 1981:9, 47.

44. Sullivan D, Warren RF, Pavlov H, et al.: Stress fractures in 51 runners. *Clin Orthop* 1984:187, 188.

45. Hulkko A, Orava S: Stress fractures in athletes. *Int J Sports Med* 1987:8, 221.

46. Matheson GO, Clement DB, McKenzie DC, et al.: Stress fractures in athletes. A study of 320 cases. *Am J Sports Med* 1987:15, 46.

47. Courtenay BG, Bowers DM: Stress fractures: Clinical features and investigation. *Med J Aust* 1990:153, 155.

48. Ha KI, Hahn SH, Chung M, et al.: A clinical study of stress fractures in sports activities. *Orthopaedics* 1991:14, 1089.

49. Benazzo F, Barnabei G, Ferrario A, et al.: Stress fractures in track and field athletes. *J Sports Traumatol Rel Res* 1992:14, 51.

50. Brukner P, Bradshaw C, Khan K, et al.: Stress fractures: A series of 180 cases. *Clin J Sport Med* 1996:6, 85.

51. Pocock NA, Eisman JA, Hopper J, et al.: Genetic determinants of bone mass in adults. *J Clin Invest* 1987:80, 706.

52. Soroko SB, Barrett-Connor E, Edelstein SL, et al.: Family history of osteoporosis and bone mineral density at the axial skeleton: The Rancho Bernardo study. *J Bone Miner Res* 1994:9, 761.

53. Seeman E, Hopper JL, Bach LA, et al.: Reduced bone mass in daughters of women with osteoporosis. *N Engl J Med* 1989:320, 554.

54. Prior JC, Vigna YM, Schechter MT, et al.: Spinal bone loss and ovulatory disturbances. *N Engl J Med* 1990:323, 1221.

55. Singer A, Ben-Yehuda O, Bern-Ezra Z, et al.: Multiple identical stress fractures in monozygotic twins. *J Bone Joint Surg Am* 1990:72-A, 444.

56. Myburgh KH, Hutchins J, Fataar AB, et al.: Low bone density is an etiologic factor for stress fractures in athletes. *Ann Intern Med* 1990:113, 754.

57. Snow GR, Anderson C: The effects of continuous progestogen treatment on cortical bone remodelling activity in beagles. *Calcif Tissue Int* 1985:37, 282.

58. Lindberg JS, Fears WB, Hunt MM, et al.: Exercise-induced amenorrhea and bone density. *Ann Intern Med* 1984:101, 647.

59. Marcus R, Cann C, Madvig P, et al.: Menstrual function and bone mass in elite women distance runners. *Ann Intern Med* 1985:102, 158.

60. Lloyd T, Triantafyllou SJ, Baker ER, et al.: Women athletes with menstrual irregularity have increased musculoskeletal injuries. *Med Sci Sports Exerc* 1986:18, 374.

61. Nelson ME, Clark N, Otradovec C, et al.: Elite women runners: Association between menstrual status, weight history and stress fractures. *Med Sci Sports Exerc* 1987:19 (S13).

62. Grimston SK, Engsberg JR, Kloiber R, et al.: Bone mass, external loads, and stress fractures in female runners. *Int J Sport Biomech* 1991:7, 293.

63. Bennell KL, Malcolm SA, Thomas SA, et al.: Risk factors for stress fractures in track and field athletes: A 12 month prospective study. *Am J Sports Med* 1996:24, 810.

64. Clark N, Nelson M, Evans W: Nutrition education for elite female runners. *Physician Sportsmed* 1988:16, 124.

65. Grimston SK, Sanborn CF, Miller PD, et al.: The application of historical data for evaluation of osteopenia in female runners: the menstrual index. *Clin Sports Med* 1990:2, 108.

66. Kaiserauer S, Snyder AC, Sleeper M, et al.: Nutritional, physiological, and menstrual status of distance runners. *Med Sci Sports Exerc* 1989:21, 120.

67. Guler F, Hascelik Z: Menstrual dysfunction rate and delayed menarche in top athletes of team games. *Sports Med Training Rehabil* 1993:4, 99.

68. Wolman RL, Harries MG: Menstrual abnormalities in elite athletes. *Clin Sports Med* 1989:1, 95.

69. Carbon R, Sambrook PN, Deakin V, et al.: Bone density of elite female athletes with stress fractures. *Med J Aust* 1990:153, 373.

70. Warren MP, Brooks-Gunn J, Fox RP, et al.: Lack of bone accretion and amenorrhea: Evidence for a relative osteopenia in weight bearing bones. *J Clin Endocrinol Metab* 1991:72, 847.

71. Frisch RE, Gotz-Welbergen AV, McArthur JW, et al.: Delayed menarche and amenorrhea of college athletes in relation to age of onset of training. *JAMA* 1981:246, 1559.

72. Moisan J, Meyer F, Gingras S: A nested case-control study of the correlates of early menarche. *Am J Epidemiol* 1990:132, 953.

73. Carter DR, Hayes WC: Fatigue life of compact bone—1. Effects of stress amplitude, temperature and density. *J Biomech* 1976:9, 27.

74. Carter DR, Caler WE, Spengler DM, et al.: Fatigue behaviour of adult cortical bone: The influence of mean strain and strain range. *Acta Orthop Scand* 1981:52, 481.

75. Pouilles JM, Bernard J, Tremollieres F, et al.: Femoral bone density in young male adults with stress fractures. *Bone* 1989:10, 105.

76. Giladi M, Milgrom C, Simkin A, et al.: Stress fractures: Identifiable risk factors. *Am J Sports Med* 1991:19, 647.

77. Beck TJ, Ruff CB, Mourtada FA, et al.: Dual-energy x-ray absorptiometry derived structural geometry for stress fracture prediction in male U.S. marine corps recruits. *J Bone Miner Res* 1996:11, 645.

78. Giladi M, Milgrom C, Simkin A, et al.: Stress fractures and tibial bone width. A risk factor. *J Bone Joint Surg Br* 1987:69-B, 326.

79. Milgrom C, Giladi M, Simkin A, et al.: The area moment of inertia of the tibia: A risk factor for stress fractures. *J Biomech* 1989:22, 1243.

80. Mustajoki P, Laapio H, Meurman K: Calcium metabolism, physical activity, and stress fractures. *Lancet* 1983:2, 797.

81. Zernicke R, McNitt-Gray J, Otis C, et al.: Stress fracture risk assessment among elite collegiate women runners, in *International Society of Biomechanics XIVth Congress*, 1993.

82. Myburgh KH, Grobler N, Noakes TD: Factors associated with shin soreness in athletes. *Physician Sportsmed* 1988:16, 129.

83. Grimston SK, Engsberg JR, Kloiber R, et al.: Menstrual, calcium, and training history: Relationship to bone health in female runners. *Clin Sports Med* 1990:2, 119.

84. Matkovic V, Heaney RP: Calcium balance during human growth: Evidence for threshold behaviour. *Am J Clin Nutr* 1992:55, 992.

85. Schwellnus MP, Jordaan G: Does calcium supplementation prevent bone stress injuries? A clinical trial. *Int J Sport Nutr* 1992:2, 165.

86. Frederick EC, Hagy JL: Factors affecting peak vertical ground reaction forces in running. *Int J Sport Biomech* 1986:2, 41.

87. Lindsay R, Cosman F, Herrington BS, et al.: Bone mass and body composition in normal women. *J Bone Miner Res* 1992:7, 55.

88. Elliot JR, Gilchrist NL, Wells JE, et al.: Historical assessment of risk factors in screening for osteopenia in a normal Caucasian population. *Aust NZ J Med* 1993:23, 458.

89. Stanitski CL, McMaster JH, Scranton PE: On the nature of stress fractures. *Am J Sports Med* 1978:6, 391.

90. Meyer SA, Saltzman CL, Albright JP: Stress fractures of the foot and leg. *Clin Sports Med* 1993:12, 395.

91. Voloshin A, Wosk J: An in vivo study of low back pain and shock absorption in the human locomotor system. *J Biomech* 1982:15, 21.

92. Clement DB: Tibial stress syndrome in athletes. *J Sports Med* 1974:2, 81.

93. Scott SH, Winter DA: Internal forces at chronic running injury sites. *Med Sci Sports Exerc* 1990:22, 357.

94. Grimston SK, Nigg BM, Fisher V, et al.: External loads throughout a 45 minute run in stress fracture and non-stress fracture runners. *J Biomech* 1994:27, 668.

95. Worthen BM, Yanklowitz BAD: The pathophysiology and treatment of stress fractures in military personnel. *J Am Podiatr Med Assoc* 1978:68, 317.

96. Scully TJ, Besterman G: Stress fracture—a preventable training injury. *Milit Med* 1982:147, 285.

97. Greaney RB, Gerber RH, Laughlin RL, et al.: Distribution and natural history of stress fractures in U.S. marine recruits. *Radiology* 1983:146, 339.

98. Protzman RR: Physiologic performance of women compared to men. *Am J Sports Med* 1979:7, 191.

99. Taimela S, Kujala UM, Dahlstrom S, et al.: Risk factors for stress fractures during physical training programs. *Clin J Sport Med* 1992:2, 105.

100. McBryde AM: Stress fractures in runners. *Clin Sports Med* 1985:4, 737.

101. McMahon TA, Greene PR: The influence of track compliance on running. *J Biomech* 1979:1, 893.

102. Steele JR, Milburn PD: Effect of different synthetic sport surfaces on ground reactions forces at landing in netball. *Int J Sport Biomech* 1988:4, 130.

103. Gardner LI, Dziados JE, Jones BH, et al.: Prevention of lower extremity stress fractures: A controlled trial of a shock absorbent insole. *Am J Public Health* 1988:78, 1563.

104. Cook SD, Brinker MR, Poche M: Running shoes. *Sports Med* 1990:10, 1.

105. Milgrom C, Burr DB, Boyd RD, et al.: The effect of a viscoelastic orthotic on the incidence of tibial stress fractures in an animal model. *Foot Ankle* 1990:10, 276.

106. Milgrom C, Giladi M, Kashtan H, et al.: A prospective study of the effect of a shock-absorbing orthotic device on the incidence of stress fractures in military recruits. *Foot Ankle* 1985:6, 101.

107. Schwellnus MP, Jordaan G, Noakes TD: Prevention of common overuse injuries by the use of shock absorbing insoles. *Am J Sports Med* 1990:18, 636.

108. Simkin A, Leichter I, Giladi M, et al.: Combined effect of foot arch structure and an orthotic device on stress fractures. *Foot Ankle* 1989:10, 25.

109. Giladi M, Milgrom C, Stein M, et al.: The low arch, a protective factor in stress fractures. A prospective study of 295 military recruits. *Orthop Rev* 1985:14, 709.

110. Brosh T, Arcan M: Toward early detection of the tendency to stress fractures. *Clin Biomech* 1994:9, 111.

111. D'Amico JC, Dinowitz HD, Polchaninoff M: Limb length discrepancy: An electrodynographic analysis. *J Am Podiatr Med Assoc* 1985:75, 639.

112. Friberg O: Leg length asymmetry in stress fractures. A clinical and radiological study. *J Sports Med* 1982:22, 485.

113. Milgrom C, Finestone A, Shlamkovitch N, et al.: Youth is a risk factor for stress fracture. A study of 783 infantry recruits. *J Bone Joint Surg Br* 1994:76-B, 20.

114. Milgrom C: The Israeli elite infantry recruit: A model for understanding the biomechanics of stress fractures. *J R Coll Surg Edinburg* 1989:34, S18.

115. Montgomery LC, Nelson FRT, Norton JP, et al.: Orthopedic history and examination in the etiology of overuse injuries. *Med Sci Sports Exerc* 1989:21, 237.

116. Hughes LY: Biomechanical analysis of the foot and ankle for predisposition to developing stress fractures. *J Orthop Sports Phys Ther* 1985:7, 96.

117. Hamill J, Bates BT, Knutzen KM, Kirkpatrick GM: Relationship between selected static and dynamic lower extremity measures. *Clin Biomech* 1989:4, 217.

118. Cole JP, Gossman D: Ultrasonic stimulation of low lumbar nerve roots as a diagnostic procedure: A preliminary report. *Clin Orthop* 1979:153, 126.

119. Delacerda FG: A case study: application of ultrasound to determine a stress fracture of the fibula. *J Orthop Sports Phys Ther* 1981:2, 134.

120. Moss A, Mowat AG: Ultrasonic assessment of stress fractures. *BMJ* 1983:286, 1478.

121. Prather JL, Nusynowitz ML, Snowdy HA, et al.: Scintigraphic findings in stress fractures. *J Bone Joint Surg Am* 1977:59-A, 869.

122. Milgrom C, Chisin R, Giladi M, et al.: Negative bone scan and impending tibial stress fractures. A report of three cases. *Am J Sports Med* 1984:12, 488.

123. Keene JS, Lash EG: Negative bone scan in a femoral neck stress fracture. A case report. *Am J Sports Med* 1992:20, 234.

124. Monteleone G: Stress fractures in the athlete. *Orthop Clin North Am* 1995:26, 423.

125. Batillas J, Vasilas A, Pizzi WF, et al.: Bone scanning in the detection of occult fractures. *J Trauma* 1981:21, 564.

126. Ammann W, Matheson GO: Radionuclide bone imaging in the detection of stress fractures. *Clin J Sports Med* 1991:1, 115.

127. Rupani HD, Holder LE, Espinola DA, et al.: Three-phase radionuclide bone imaging in sports medicine. *Radiology* 1985:156, 187.

128. Rosenthall L, Hill RO, Chuang S: Observation on the use of ^{99m}Tc-phosphate imaging in peripheral bone trauma. *Radiology* 1976:119, 637.

129. Saunders AJS, Elsayed TF, Hilson AJW, et al.: Stress lesions of the lower leg and foot. *Clin Radiol* 1979:306, 49.

130. Giladi M, Ziv Y, Aharonson Z: Comparison between radiography, bone scan and ultrasound in the diagnosis of stress fractures. *Milit Med* 1984:149, 459.

131. Devereaux MD, Parr GR, Lachman SM, et al.: The diagnosis of the stress fractures in athletes. *JAMA* 1984:252, 531.

132. Somer K, Meurman KOA: Computed tomography of stress fractures. *J Comput Assist Tomogr* 1982:6, 109.

133. Clement DB, Ammann W, Taunton JE, et al.: Exercise-induced stress injuries to the femur. *Int J Sports Med* 1993:14, 347.

134. Prather JL, Nusynowitz ML, Snowdy HA, et al.: Scintigraphic findings in stress fractures. *J Bone Joint Surg Am* 1974:59-A, 869.

135. Zwas ST, Elkanovitch R, Frank G: Interpretation and classification of bone scintigraphic findings in stress fractures. *J Nucl Med* 1987:28, 452.

136. Wilcox JR, Moniot AL, Green JP: Bone scanning in the evaluation of exercise-related stress injuries. *Radiology* 1977:123, 699.

137. Martire JR: The role of nuclear medicine bone scan in evaluating pain in athletic injuries. *Clin Sports Med* 1987:6, 13.

138. Sterling JC, Edelstein DW, Calvo RD, et al.: Stress fractures in the athlete. Diagnosis and management. *Sports Med* 1992:14, 336.

139. Lombardo SJ, Benson DW: Stress fractures of the femur in runners. *Am J Sports Med* 1982:10, 219.

140. Meurman KOA, Elfving S: Stress fracture of the cuneiform bones. *Br J Radiol* 1980:53, 157.

141. Daffner RH, Martinez S, Gehweiler JA: Stress fractures in runners. *JAMA* 1982:247, 1039.

142. Rosen PR, Micheli LJ, Treves S: Early scintigraphic diagnosis of bone stress and fractures in athletic adolescents. *Pediatrics* 1982:70, 11.

143. Geslien GE, Thrawl JH, Espinosa JL, et al.: Early detection of stress fractures using 99mTc-polyphosphate. *Radiology* 1976:121, 683.

144. Butler JE, Brown SL, McConnell BG: Subtrochanteric stress fractures in runners. *Am J Sports Med* 1982:10, 228.

145. Matheson GO, Clement DB, McKenzie DC, et al.: Scintigraphic uptake of 99m Tc at non-painful sites in athletes with stress fractures. *Sports Med* 1987:4, 65.

146. Khan KM, Fuller PJ, Brukner PD, et al.: Outcome of conservative and surgical management of navicular stress fracture in athletes. Eighty-six cases proven with computerized tomography. *Am J Sports Med* 1992:20, 657.

147. Kiss ZA, Khan KM, Fuller PJ: Stress fractures of the tarsal navicular bone: CT findings in 55 cases. *AJR* 1993:160, 111.

148. Terrell PN, Davies AM: Magnetic resonance appearances of fatigue fractures of the long bones of the lower limb. *Br J Radiol* 1994:67, 332.

149. Lee JK, Yao L: Stress fractures: MR imaging. *Radiology* 1988:169, 217.

150. Stafford SA, Rosenthal DI, Gebhardt MC, et al.: MRI in stress fractures. *AJR* 1986:147, 553.

151. Steinbronn DJ, Bennett GL, Kay DB: The use of magnetic resonance imaging in the diagnosis of stress fractures of the foot and ankle: Four case reports. *Foot Ankle* 1994:15, 80.

152. Fredericson M, Bergman G, Hoffman KL, et al.: Tibial stress reaction in runners. Correlation of clinical symptoms and scintigraphy with a new magnetic resonance imaging grading system. *Am J Sports Med* 1995:23, 472.

153. Earnst J: Stress fracture of the neck of the femur. *J Trauma* 1964:4, 71.

154. Devas MB: Stress fractures of the femoral neck. *J Bone Joint Surg Br* 1965:47B, 728.

155. Blickenstaff LD, Morris JM: Fatigue fracture of the femoral neck. *J Bone Joint Surg Am* 1966:45-A or 48A,* 1031.

156. Fullerton LR, Snowdy HA: Femoral neck stress fractures. *Am J Sports Med* 1988:16, 365.

157. Fullerton LRJ: Femoral neck stress fractures. *Sports Med* 1990:9, 192.

158. Kaltsas D: Stress fractures of the femoral neck in young adults. *J Bone Joint Surg Br* 1981:63B, 33.

159. Johansson C, Ekenman I, Tornkvist H, et al.: Stress fractures of the femoral neck in athletes: The consequence of a delay in diagnosis. *Am J Sports Med* 1990:18, 524.

160. Burrows HJ: Fatigue in fracture of the middle of the tibia in ballet dancers. *J Bone Joint Surg Br* 1956:38-B, 83.

161. Friedenberg ZB: Fatigue fractures of the tibia. *Clin Orthop* 1971:76, 111.

162. Brahms MA, Fumich RM, Ippolita VD: Atypical stress fracture of tibia in a professional athlete. *Am J Sports Med* 1980:8, 131.

163. Green NE, Rogers RA, Lipscomb AB: Nonunions of stress fractures of the tibia. *Am J Sports Med* 1985:13, 171.

164. Blank S: Transverse tibial stress fractures. A special problem. *Am J Sports Med* 1987:15, 597.

165. Rettig AC, Shelbourne KD, McCarroll JR, et al.: The natural history and treatment of delayed union and nonunion stress fractures of the anterior cortex of the tibia. *Am J Sports Med* 1988:16, 250.

166. Orava S, Karpakka J, Hulkko A, et al.: Diagnosis and treatment of stress fractures located at the mid-tibial shaft in athletes. *Int J Sports Med* 1991:12, 419.

167. Shelbourne KD, Fisher DA, Rettig AC, et al.: Stress fractures of the medial melleolus. *Am J Sports Med* 1988:16, 60.

168. Rieder B, Falconier R, Yurkofsky J: Nonunion of a medial malleolus stress fracture. A case report. *Am J Sports Med* 1993:21, 478.

169. Schils JP, Andrish Jt, Piraino DW, et al.: Medial malleolar stress fractures in seven patients: Review of the clinical and imaging features. *Radiology* 1992:185, 219.

170. Orava S, Karpakka J, Taimela S, et al.: Stress fractures of the medial malleolus. *J Bone Joint Surg* 1995:77, 362.

171. Khan KM, Brukner PD, Kearney C, et al.: Tarsal navicular stress fracture in athletes. *Sports Med* 1994:17, 65.

172. Torg JS, Pavlov H, Cooley LH, et al.: Stress fractures of the tarsal navicular. A retrospective review of twenty-one cases. *J Bone Joint Surg Am* 1982:64-A, 700.

173. Orava S, Karpakka J, Hulkko A, et al.: Stress avulsion fracture of the tarsal navicular. An uncommon sports-related overuse injury. *Am J Sports Med* 1991:19, 392.

174. Fitch KD, Blackwell JB, Gilmour WN: Operation for non-union of stress fracture of the tarsal navicular. *J Bone Joint Surg Br* 1989:71B, 105.

175. Ting A, King W, Yocum L, et al.: Stress fractures of the tarsal navicular in long-distance runners. *Clin Sports Med* 1988:7, 89.

176. Hunter LY: Stress fracture of the tarsal navicular: More frequent than we realise? *Am J Sports Med* 1981:9, 217.

177. Brukner P, Khan K: *Clinical Sports Medicine,* Sydney, McGraw Hill, 1993.

178. Pavlov H, Torg JS, Freiberger RH: Tarsal navicular stress fractures: Radiographic evaluation. *Radiology* 1983:148, 641.

179. Orava S, Hulkko A: Delayed unions and nonunions of stress fractures in athletes. *Am J Sports Med* 1988:16, 378.

180. Gordon TG, Solar J: Tarsal navicular stress fractures. *J Am Podiatr Med Assoc* 1985:75, 363.

181. O'Connor K, Quirk R., Fricker P, et al.: Stress fracture of the tarsal navicular bone treated by bone grafting and internal fixation. Three cases studies and a literature review. *Excel* 1990:6, 16.

182. Maitland GD: *Peripheral Manipulation,* 3rd ed., London, Butterworths, 1986.

183. Jones R: Fractures of the base of the 5th metatarsal bone by indirect violence. *Ann Surg* 1902:34, 697.

184. Kavanaugh JH: The Jones fracture revisited. *J Bone Joint Surg Am* 1978:60-A, 776.

185. DeLee JC, Evans JP, Julian J: Stress fracture of the fifth metatarsal. *Am J Sports Med* 1983:11, 349.

186. Dameron TB: Fractures and anatomical variations of the proximal portion of the 5th metatarsal. *J Bone Joint Surg Am* 1975:57-A, 788.

187. Torg JS, Balduini FC, Zelko RR, et al.: Fractures of the base of the fifth metatarsal distal to the tuberosity. Classification and guidelines for non-surgical and surgical management. *J Bone Joint Surg Am* 1984:66A, 209.

188. Richli WR: Avulsion fractures of the 5th metatarsal. *AJR* 1984:143, 889.

189. Stewart IM: Jones' fractures: fracture of the base of the 5th metatarsal. *CORR* 1960:16, 190.

190. Sammarco GJ: Be alert for Jones fractures. *Physician Sportsmed* 1992:20, 101.

191. Van Hal ME, Keene JS, Lange TA, et al.: Stress fractures of the great toe sesamoids. *Am Sports Med* 1982:10, 122.

192. Golding C: Museum pages V: The sesamoids of the hallux. *Bone Joint Surg Br* 1960:42-B, 840.

193. Inge GAL, Ferguson AB: Surgery of the sesamoid bones of the great toe. *Archi Surg* 1933:27, 466.

194. Mann R: *DuVries Surgery of the Foot,* 4th ed., St. Louis, CV Mosby, 1978:122.

195. Davis AW, Alexander IJ: Problematic fractures and dislocations in the foot and ankle of athletes. *Clin Sports Med* 1990:9, 163.

196. McBryde AM: Stress fractures in athletes. *Am J Sports Med* 1975:3, 212.

197. Bennell KL, Brukner PD: Epidemiology and site specificity of stress fractures. *Clin Sports Med* 1997:16, 183.

Chapter 20

NERVE ENTRAPMENTS

Jay Smith and Diane L. Dahm

INTRODUCTION

Numerous conditions produce lower limb pain in runners, including muscle strains, tendinitis, stress-induced bone injury, compartment syndrome, vascular disease, fascial herniations, and nerve entrapment syndromes. Nerve entrapment is an uncommon source of lower limb pain, but it has received increasing attention since Massey and Pleet published a report of peroneal neuropathy (PN) and lateral femoral cutaneous neuropathy (LFCN) in runners.[1] Neurological conditions currently account for 10% to 15% of all exercise-induced leg pain among runners, representing the highest frequency of foot and ankle neurological conditions among all athletes.[2–4] Most nerve entrapments occur secondary to nonpenetrating trauma. Specific etiologies include contusion, compression, stretch, and iatrogenic injury from surgery.[4–9] The running motion produces complex, forceful, repetitive lower limb movements that may compress, stretch, or dislocate nerves as they traverse relatively unyielding musculotendinous compartments and tunnels. Repetitive trauma produces demyelination (neurapraxia), and potentially some degree of axonal loss (axonotmesis), with ensuing nerve dysfunction and neuropathic pain.[10] Neurological injury is discussed in detail in Chapter 8. Neurotmesis, complete nerve transection, does not occur in runners without major trauma.

Among runners, most nerve entrapments occur at or below the knee, although LFCN and radial neuropathy have been reported.[1] In order of decreasing frequency, common nerves affected include the interdigital nerve (interdigital or Morton's neuroma), the first branch of the lateral plantar nerve (FB-LPN), medial plantar nerve (MPN), tibial nerve (TN), peroneal nerve (deep and superficial portions; DPN and SPN), sural nerve (SN), and saphenous nerve.[4] This chapter will review the etiology, diagnosis, and treatment of entrapment neuropathies that might be encountered by clinicians caring for runners.

DIAGNOSTIC PRINCIPLES

Clinicians should bear in mind several general principles to facilitate the diagnosis and management of entrapment neuropathies: (1) maintain a high index of suspicion for neurological syndromes, (2) recognize common presentations of neuropathic pain, (3) perform a meticulous physical examination, including postexercise examination when necessary, (4) consider a broad differential diagnosis (neurological and non-neurological), (5) use diagnostic testing appropriately, and (6) make rational clinical decisions, including referral for second opinion when indicated.[4] When these principles are adhered to, diagnosis is simply a matter of applying anatomy and understanding some

---

TABLE 20–1. NEUROANATOMY OF THE LOWER LIMB: BRANCHING PATTERNS

Sciatic nerve (L4-S3 spinal segments)
  Tibial nerve (TN)[a]
    Medial contribution to sural nerve (MCSN)
    Medial calcaneal nerve (MCN)[b]
    Medial plantar nerve (MPN)
      Contribution to third interdigital nerve
      Medial hallucal nerve
    Lateral plantar nerve (LPN)
      First branch of LPN (FB-LPN)[c]
      Contribution to third interdigital nerve
    Common peroneal nerve (CPN)
      Lateral contribution to sural nerve (LCSN)
      Superficial peroneal nerve (SPN)
      Deep peroneal nerve (DPN)
Femoral nerve (FN; L2-L4 spinal segments)
  Saphenous nerve
Lateral femoral cutaneous nerve (LFCN; L2-L3 spinal segments)
Obturator nerve (ON; L2-L4 spinal segments)

---

[a]TN spinal segments at the tarsal tunnel are predominantly S1-S2.
[b]The MCN may arise from the LPN or MPN-LPN bifurcation.
[c]May arise directly from the TN; also called the inferior calcaneal nerve (ICN), Baxter's nerve, or the nerve to the abductor digiti quinti (NADQ).

specifics of each condition. Table 20–1 presents the neuroanatomic relations of nerves in the lower limb. Figures 20–1 to 20–7 depict the relevant neuroanatomy as it pertains to entrapment or injury sites. These figures form the foundation for the material presented in this chapter.

Nerve entrapment produces neuropathic pain, described as a diffuse, aching, burning discomfort, often accompanied by tingling and cramping. Numbness is less common. Neuropathic pain classically occurs in the nerve distribution distal to the injury site. Table 20–1 describes the neurological branching pattern of the lower limb. However, symptoms may affect only a portion of the distal nerve, and may also radiate proximally (called the Villeix phenomenon).[11] Symptoms usually occur during and shortly after running, although some syndromes include components of rest and nighttime pain (e.g., tarsal tunnel syndrome).

Examination should focus on identification of predisposing malalignments, symptom reproduction, and exclusion of alternative diagnoses. The most useful findings are tenderness over the affected site and a positive percussion sign.[6,9] The percussion sign, or Tinel's sign, involves percussion along the length of the nerve. Neuropathic pain reproduction with palpation or percussion suggests the possible level of the lesion.[12,13] Complete assessment of the spine and lower limb is necessary to exclude referred pain from neurologic and nonneurologic syndromes affecting the spine, hip, knee, ankle, and foot, as discussed elsewhere in this text.

Neurological differential diagnosis includes central nervous system disease (e.g., multiple sclerosis), radiculopathy, plexopathy, proximal neuropathy, polyneuropathy, and myopathy; assessment along the entire proximal and distal course of the nerve is necessary (Table 20–1 and Figs. 20–1 to 20–7).[1,12] "Double crush" injuries, in which a proximal nerve injury renders the distal portion of the nerve more susceptible to insult, have been reported in the lower limb.[14,15] Spine conditions, including radiculopathy, are reviewed in Chapter 12.

Diagnostic testing varies by condition. In general, the majority of entrapment neuropathies are diagnosed clinically, with supportive imaging and electrodiagnostic (EDX) testing. Radiographs are commonly obtained to exclude contributory osseous lesions. Magnetic resonance imaging (MRI) offers superior soft tissue imaging, particularly important in peroneal neuropathies or tarsal tunnel syndrome. Electrodiagnostic testing is only occasionally positive, but is useful to exclude alternative neurological conditions (see Chapter 8).[16]

Clinicians treating runners must recognize that symptoms, physical findings, and EDX abnormalities may only manifest during or immediately after running or with provocative examination maneuvers.[4] A post-treadmill running examination can be crucial in such cases. If the diagnosis remains elusive, the clinician should strongly consider obtaining a second opinion.

COMMON NERVE ENTRAPMENT SYNDROMES

Interdigital Neuroma (Morton's Neuroma)

Definition
Interdigital neuromas produce neuropathic pain in the distribution of the interdigital nerve (Fig. 20–1). The condition commonly affects the third web space, but may rarely affect the second or fourth web spaces. Multiple coexistent neuromas are uncommon and suggest an alternative diagnosis such as polyneuropathy. Interdigital neuromas typically affect runners in their 20s or older, exhibit a predilection for females (possibly secondary to wearing tight fitting and high-heeled dress shoes), and are thought to be caused by repetitive trauma and biomechanical factors.[4,6,9]

Anatomy, Pathophysiology, and Risk Factors
The plantar interdigital nerve in the third intermetatarsal space is composed of communicating branches from the lateral and medial plantar nerves (LPN, MPN) (Table 20–1, Fig. 20–2). At the level of the metatarsal heads, the interdigital nerve passes under (superficial)

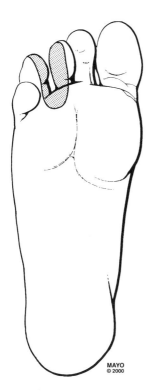

Figure 20–1. Interdigital neuroma. Shaded area demonstrates typical area of pain or sensory loss.

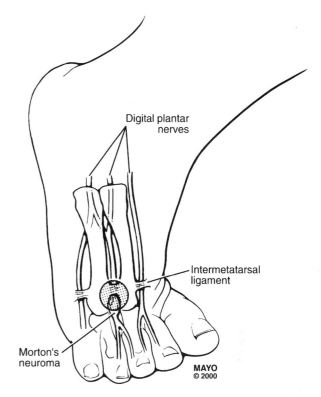

Figure 20–2. Interdigital neuroma. Interdigital nerve entrapment at the intermetatarsal ligament.

to the intermetatarsal ligament. During push-off, forceful toe dorsiflexion may compress and stretch the nerve beneath the intermetatarsal ligament, resulting in demyelination, scarring, and hypertrophy.[9] Subsequently, a tumorous mass may develop just distal to the intermetatarsal ligament, proximal to the interdigital nerve's bifurcation into the deep digital plantar nerves. Histologically, there is prominent peri-neural and endoneural fibrosis, with lesser degrees of demyelination.[6]

General risk factors include prolonged walking or running (especially during push-off), squatting, use of high-heeled shoes, or the demi-pointe in ballet. In runners, several contributing conditions may coexist. Hyperpronation dorsiflexes the third metatarsal relative to the fourth, exposing the nerve to injury during push-off.[4] Hallux valgus or a hypermobile first ray may lead to callus formation on the plantar aspects of the metatarsal heads, increasing intermetatarsal pressures. Idiopathic metatarsophalangeal joint (MTJ) synovitis may cause local edema and interdigital nerve compression.[6] Recent change to softer-soled footwear or a heel lift may precipitate symptoms due to increased toe dorsiflexion.

Symptoms and Signs
The athlete describes neuropathic pain radiating between the third and fourth toes, increased with running, standing, walking, toe dorsiflexion, and squatting. Burning and cramping are common, and night pain has been reported. Footwear removal and massaging the forefoot bring some relief.

Examination focuses on biomechanical assessment and provocative testing. The athlete is often tender in the affected intermetatarsal space. Provocative testing includes pressure application over the plantar aspect of the web space between the metatarsal heads, or squeezing the metatarsals together during palpation (metatarsal squeeze test); distal radiating neuropathic pain suggests the diagnosis. The squeeze test may also result in a click as the "neuroma" subluxes from between the metatarsals in a dorsal direction (Mulder's click).[4] A web space sensory deficit is occasionally seen, but no motor deficit is expected to occur along the purely sensory nerve. Palpation and motion testing of the MTJs may reveal subluxations or synovitis. Predisposing biomechanical factors should be determined.

Differential Diagnosis and Evaluation
Proximal tenderness or tenderness in all the intermetatarsal spaces are clues to consider alternative diagnoses. Differential diagnosis includes proximal and systemic neurological conditions; stress fractures; MTJ synovitis, instability or arthritis; and flexor-extensor tenosynovitis. Foot radiographs assist in excluding

articular or bony problems. Diagnostic interdigital nerve block of the affected interdigital nerve (usually the third) is confirmatory. MRI, EDX, and bone scans assist primarily in differential diagnosis, and are not universally indicated.

Treatment

Initial treatment includes activity modification, non-steroidal anti-inflammatory drugs (NSAIDs; especially if there is a local synovitis or tenosynovitis), footwear modifications, physical therapy, and treating underlying contributing conditions. The athlete may benefit from biomechanical interventions to reduce toe dorsiflexion, control hyperpronation, and maintain greater metatarsal separation. Options include a well-padded, supportive sole; wider shoe; metatarsal bar or pad ($^3/_{16}$ to $^1/_4$ inch); or orthosis. Achilles tendon flexibility is optimized. Some authors recommend up to three therapeutic corticosteroid injections.[10] Injection complications include MTJ capsular weakening and local adipose and subcutaneous tissue atrophy. Consequently, one author suggests avoiding any injections in athletic populations.[9]

Surgery is generally indicated in the presence of a firm clinical diagnosis (usually supported by a diagnostic anesthetic injection) with refractory symptoms. Universally accepted selection criteria do not exist. Neuroma excision is typically performed from a dorsal approach, with or without intermetatarsal ligament sectioning. Interdigital neuromas represent the most commonly resected neuroma in the foot.[12]

Tibial Nerve: Tarsal Tunnel Syndrome

Definition

Tarsal tunnel syndrome (TTS) represents a constellation of processes affecting the TN or its branches at the level of the ankle, producing neuropathic pain along the posteromedial ankle, medial foot, or plantar foot. Among runners, TN entrapment most commonly occurs at the level of the tarsal tunnel. There is a slight (56%) female predilection.[11]

Anatomy, Pathophysiology, and Risk Factors

The TN originates from the L4-S3 spinal segments and is the larger terminal branch of the sciatic nerve.[10] The TN supplies muscular innervation in the posterior thigh and leg, and a cutaneous contribution to the SN, prior to becoming superficial medial to the Achilles tendon and entering the tarsal tunnel posterior to the medial malleolus (Fig. 20–3).

The tarsal tunnel is a fibro-osseous space formed by the flexor retinaculum, medial calcaneus, posterior talus, distal tibia, and medial malleolus, and extends from the distal tibia to the navicular bone. Contents include the

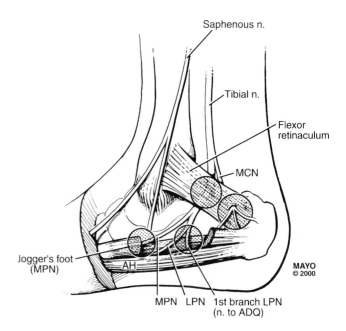

Figure 20–3. Tibial nerve and tarsal tunnel. Shaded areas indicate potential entrapment sites. (see Table 20–1 for abbreviations)

posterior tibialis (PT) tendon, flexor digitorum longus (FDL) tendon, flexor hallucis longus (FHL) tendon, and tibial neurovasular bundle. The flexor retinaculum spans a distance from 2 cm above to 2 cm below/distal to a line drawn from the center of the medial malleolus to the calcaneal tuberosity, the medial malleolar-calcaneal line.[11]

Over 90% of the time, the TN will divide into the MPN and LPN within the tarsal tunnel, typically at the medial malleolar-calcaneal line.[11] Within 1 to 2 cm below/distal to the medial malleolar-calcaneal line, the MPN and LPN enter separate fibro-osseous canals at the origin of the abductor hallucis muscle (AHM).[4,16] At this point, the LPN may be particularly vulnerable to injury due to its more proximal and oblique course.[11]

TTS can involve the TN, MPN, LPN, and at times the medial calcaneal nerve (MCN); consequently, a variety of distinct clinical syndromes may be possible. The common feature is a process arising within the tarsal tunnel. This section will review TTS in this context. Subsequent sections will review MPN, LPN, and MCN disorders separately.

Five broad etiologic categories for TTS exist: (1) trauma (contusion, ill-fitting footwear), (2) compression by space-occupying lesions (e.g., venous stasis, ganglion, tenosynovitis, os trigonum, tumor), (3) systemic disease, (4) biomechanical (excessive pronation, joint hypermobility), and (5) idiopathic.[16,17] Repetitive trauma in the setting of predisposing malalignments is most common in runners.[11] Hyperpronation will increase AHM tension and may entrap the TN or plantar nerves.[11] Compression from stiff orthoses or space-occupying lesions such as an os trigonum, tenosynovitis, tumor, or ganglion are less common. Nerve involvement may be axonal, demyelinative, or both. A specific etiology may be identified in 60% to 80% of cases.[11]

Symptoms and Signs

The athlete typically describes cramping, burning, and tingling at the medial ankle, medial foot, and/or plantar foot, beyond the limits of tendon and joint anatomical structures. Diffuse foot pain has been reported. Although proximal radiation may be seen in one third of cases, the medial heel is usually spared due to the proximal origin of the MCN (see subsequent section).[11] Symptoms increase with standing, walking, and running, and decrease with rest, elevation, and when wearing loose footwear. Running on a banked surface promotes hyperpronation and may particularly elicit symptoms.[10] Rest pain and night pain may occur in provocative positions, and shaking the foot or walking may provide relief, similar to carpal tunnel syndrome.[4,6] Weakness and sensory loss are uncommon, and TTS is rarely bilateral.

Examination includes inspection for malalignment, deformity, and muscular atrophy causing or resulting from TTS, such as forefoot pronation, claw toe, talipes calcaneus, or calcaneovalgus. Palpate all structures along the medial ankle and foot for ganglia, tenosynovitis, and neoplasms. Nerve palpation and percussion testing is completed over the TN and all its terminal branches; a Villeix phenomenon may be elicited.[18] Provocative maneuvers include sustained passive eversion or great toe dorsiflexion to stretch affected nerves, and postexercise examination. With palpation, percussion testing, or provocative maneuvers, symptom reproduction is crucial.

Intrinsic muscular atrophy may be observed, but weakness is difficult to test and uncommon. In severe cases, weakness of toe plantarflexion manifests by reduced push-off on the affected side.[10] Diminished sweat secretion or mild sensory loss may rarely occur on the sole. Ankle instability should be evaluated and could contribute to TTS in runners. A complete spine and lower limb examination is necessary to assist in differential diagnosis.

Differential Diagnosis and Evaluation

Differential diagnosis includes not only alternative diagnoses, but consideration of processes that produce nerve entrapment at the tarsal tunnel. Clinicians should consider polyneuropathy; proximal neuropathy (including "double crush" injuries from radiculopathy or sciatic neuropathy); distal neuropathy; deep posterior compartment syndrome; popliteal artery entrapment; vascular claudication; venous disease; tenosynovitis or ganglia; plantar fasciitis; tibiotalar or subtalar synovitis, instability or arthritis; and osseous compression.[15,19] Examination will help differentiate proximal TN injuries. Tibial nerve injury just distal to the SN contribution will spare lateral calcaneal and foot sensation and gastrocnemius-soleus function. Injury distal to the midportion of the leg will affect plantar sensation and result in claw toe deformity due to imbalance between the affected foot intrinsic and unaffected FDL and extensor digitorum brevis (EDB) muscles.[10] Prominent numbness and tingling, night pain, proximal radiation, and *reduced* pain during the first few steps in the morning differentiate TTS from plantar fasciitis, although the conditions can coexist.[20] Entrapment of the TN at the level of the medial gastrocnemius muscle has been reported ("high" TTS).[4,6,8,9]

TTS is primarily a clinical diagnosis, although treatment may be dictated by supportive diagnostic studies. Radiographs may reveal osseous compressive lesions or ankle-foot malalignments (weightbearing views). In the absence of bony anomalies, MRI is effective for examining the tarsal tunnel and reveals an inflammatory lesion or mass in up to 88% of patients with a firm clinical diagnosis of TTS.[21] In acute TTS or in failed nonoperative management, MRI is recommended to determine the presence of synovitis or a space-occupying lesion, and dictate further treatment. Laboratory testing is not universally necessary, but may assist in excluding systemic disease affecting nerves (e.g., diabetes, thyroid disease, pernicious anemia) and rheumatologic disorders. EDX studies assist in excluding alternative neurological disorders. They may be positive in up to 90% of patients with well-established TTS, but do not correlate with surgical findings or clinical outcome.[22]

Treatment

Authors have recently recommended that a firm diagnosis of TTS be made *only* when the following triad exists: (1) foot pain and paresthesias, (2) positive nerve percussion sign/Tinel's sign, and (3) positive EDX studies. If only two exist, the diagnosis of *probable* TTS is recommended, and if only one exists, the diagnosis should be reconsidered.[11]

Nonoperative treatment is initially warranted in almost all athletes, and is most successful in those with tenosynovitis or contributory flexible foot deformities. Treatment includes activity modification, NSAIDs, neuromodulatory medications (tricyclic and antiseizure medications), physical therapy, and biomechanical interventions. Physical therapy includes (1) strengthening the foot intrinsic and medial arch supporting muscles, (2) Achilles' stretching in subtalar neutral, (3) lower limb kinetic chain rehabilitation, and (4) proprioceptive enriched rehabilitation in cases of ankle or subtalar instability.[11]

Biomechanical management varies with clinical presentation. Pronation control may be assisted by use of a motion control shoe, medial heel wedge, medial sole wedge/medial buttress, ankle stirrup brace, or fixed ankle walking brace. If symptoms are reproduced by dorsiflexion, temporary use of a heel lift (in combination with appropriate stretching) may be useful. In severe deformities, medial wedges and arch supports may exacerbate symptoms and more rigid immobilization via a molded hindfoot orthosis, ankle-foot orthosis, or walking boot/cast is usually necessary to maintain the hindfoot in a neutral position. Temporary crutch-assisted weightbearing may be required. In runners with minor, recurrent symptoms, a change in running habits to reduce tibial nerve tension may be useful.[23]

Treatment should address contributing underlying systemic conditions, local tenosynovitis, venous congestion, or chronic edema. A well-placed corticosteroid injection at the entrapment site may produce excellent results, provided that the PT tendon is avoided and a period of postinjection protected weightbearing is implemented.[11]

Surgery may be indicated when the clinical diagnosis is probable or firm and the athlete has endured several months of debilitating symptoms unresponsive to appropriate nonoperative treatment.[11] Up to 65% of patients (not confined to runners) required surgical treatment in one study.[24] Surgery consists of a proximal medial incision, dissection progressing proximal to distal after identifying the TN, and release of the flexor retinaculum to decompress the TN and its branches as necessary. Postoperatively, neuropathic symptoms generally improve after 6 weeks, but maximal recovery may take 6 months or more.[6] Although authors traditionally reported good or excellent results in 79% to 95% of cases, a more recent, methodologically stringent study indicated only 44% of patients significantly benefited at a minimum 24-month follow-up.[11,18,25] The authors concluded that decompression should only be considered when an associated lesion is shown to be in or near the tarsal tunnel by MRI and/or EDX testing; patients with previous ankle-foot surgery, plantar fasciitis, or inflammatory systemic disease should be managed nonoperatively for extended time periods.[11,25] Endoscopic techniques are being developed, but concerns have been raised regarding the ability to adequately decompress the affected structures with this technique.[16] In cases where ankle or subtalar instability exists, reconstruction should be considered in addition to decompression.

First Branch of the Lateral Plantar Nerve

Definition

Isolated LPN entrapments are relatively rare. Baxter reported two cases, both of which occurred after plantar fascia release.[8,9] This syndrome appears to be uncommon among runners. More commonly, entrapment specifically affects the FB-LPN, sometimes called Baxter's nerve, the nerve to the abductor digiti quinti muscle (NADQ), or the inferior calcaneal nerve (ICN).

FB-LPN entrapment results in neuropathic pain along the medial heel, and less commonly the lateral foot. FB-LPN entrapment is reported to be the most common neurological cause of heel pain.[8] Up to 15% of athletes with chronic, unresolving heel pain may have FB-LPN entrapment, with runners and joggers accounting for the overwhelming majority of cases.[4] The average age of runners in the largest series to date was 38 years, and 88% were men.[8]

Anatomy, Pathophysiology, and Risk Factors

Within the tarsal tunnel, the FB-LPN usually arises from the LPN, but in 46% of cases it may originate directly from the TN (Fig. 20–3).[16] After penetrating the AHM and its fascia, the FB-LPN courses inferiorly, passing between the deep, taut fascia of the AHM medially and the medial, caudal margin of the medial head of the quadratus plantae muscle laterally.[8] The nerve then abruptly turns laterally, coursing towards the lateral foot between the flexor digitorum brevis and quadratus plantae muscles (Fig. 20–4). The FB-LPN ramifies into three terminal branches supplying the flexor digitorum brevis, the medial calcaneal periosteum, and abductor digiti quinti. The branch to the calcaneal periosteum often supplies branches to the long plantar ligament as well as an inconsistent branch to the quadratus plantae muscle.[4] There is no cutaneous innervation.

The actual site of FB-LPN entrapment remains controversial, but perhaps it most commonly occurs at the site of direction change from an inferior to lateral course deep to the AHM.[8] In this tight space, the FB-LPN may be compressed during pronation when the AHM and quadratus plantae muscle are forced together. Other authors propose that entrapment may occur in the osteomuscular canal between the calcaneus and the flexor digitorum brevis muscle at the level of the medial anterior corner of the calcaneus tuberosity, or at the plantar aspect of the long plantar ligament.[26] FB-LPN entrapment has also been reported secondary to AHM or quadratus plantae hypertrophy, accessory muscles, abnormal bursae, and venous varicosities.[8,9,26]

The FB-LPN origin lies deep (just superior) to the plantar fascia origin and the typical site of calcaneal spurs, which typically lie within the flexor digitorum

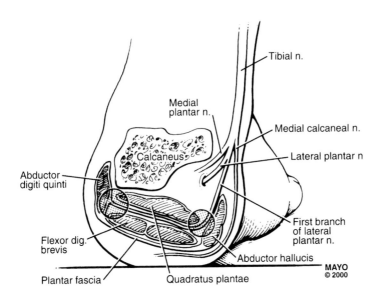

Tibial n.

Medial plantar n.

Medial calcaneal n.

Lateral plantar n

Calcaneus

Abductor digiti quinti

First branch of lateral plantar n.

Flexor dig. brevis

Abductor hallucis

MAYO © 2000

Plantar fascia

Quadratus plantae

Figure 20–4. First branch of lateral plantar nerve (FB-LPN). The FB-LPN courses laterally between the flexor digitorum brevis and quadratus plantae muscles. Shaded areas indicate entrapment sites.

brevis. Because of FB-LPN proximity to the plantar fascia, neural irritation is thought to occur in up to 15% to 20% of cases of chronic plantar fasciitis.[6,8–10,26] Patients who have proximal edema of the flexor digitorum brevis and edema or microtears in the plantar fascia may be more susceptible.[10] It must be emphasized that this represents only a small portion of the 5% to 10% of individuals with chronic refractory plantar fasciitis. Lying within 5 mm anterior to the calcaneus, the FB-LPN may be injured by a large or fractured calcaneal spur, or iatrogenically during spur removal.[5]

Symptoms and Signs

The diagnosis of FB-LPN entrapment is primarily clinical. The athlete typically complains of chronic, neuropathic, medial heel pain, often diagnosed as plantar fasciitis. Symptoms are precipitated by sports in 50% of cases.[8] Up to 25% of patients will have severe pain in the morning secondary to venous engorgement, but night pain is rare.[5]

According to Baxter and Pfeffer, the pathognomonic sign of FB-LPN entrapment is maximal pain elicited over the entrapment site on the medial heel, superior to the plantar fascia origin, along a line drawn parallel to the posterior tibia (Fig. 20–3).[8] In one study, 100% of patients exhibited maximal pain over this site, although 42% also had mild tenderness over the plantar fascia origin.[8] Positive percussion testing has been reported in only 17% of 53 patients (63 heels) in one study.[8] In severe cases, small toe abduction may be limited, or atrophy of the lateral foot muscles may be seen. There are no sensory or reflex deficits.

Differential Diagnosis and Evaluation

Differential diagnosis is similar to that for TTS, with the addition of local pathologies. Heel pain syndrome,

plantar fasciitis, and fat pad disorders are suggested by finding maximal tenderness in the plantar calcaneal region, anterior medial calcaneus, or the midmedial edge of the plantar fascia.[8] These conditions may coexist with FB-LPN entrapment. Sensory loss on the medial heel suggests a disorder affecting the MCN, L4 radiculopathy, plexopathy, or more diffuse neurological disease; FB-LPN entrapment does not cause sensory loss.

Diagnostic studies are not uniformly helpful. Radiographic bone spurs are seen in 50% of cases, but are not thought to cause entrapment in the majority of cases. MRI and EDX testing are not accurate enough to confirm or refute the clinical diagnosis of FB-LPN entrapment, but may assist in differential diagnosis. In 27 patients with 38 symptomatic heels from surgically documented FB-LPN entrapment, only 44% had some involvement of the lateral plantar nerve on EDX testing.[5]

Treatment

Most cases of FB-LPN entrapment respond to nonoperative measures following treatment principles used for insertional plantar fasciitis or primary heel pain syndrome.[26] Recommended interventions include activity modification, NSAIDs, and physical therapy and biomechanical management for pronation control. Success has been reported using heel cups with or without a lift, foot strappings, foot orthoses (flexible or rigid), padding, soft-soled shoes, and stretching exercises for the Achilles tendon and plantar fascia.[26] Physical therapy should focus on muscle rebalancing about the ankle-foot and the entire lower limb kinetic chain. Neuromodulatory medications (tricyclics and antiseizure medications) and local corticosteroid injections may be useful. One author recommends that no more than three injections at 2- to 4-week intervals be attempted.[10] Currently, no prospective trials exist to recommend one treatment or a combination of treatments over another.

Surgery is indicated for refractory cases and is often based on diagnosis by clinical examination and exclusion of alternative conditions. Most authors advocate at least 6 to 12 months of nonoperative care prior to considering surgery. Limited surgical approaches are utilized unless proximal tarsal tunnel entrapment is also suspected. Decompression includes the deep fascia of the AHM and a portion of the contiguous medial plantar fascia. Plantar spur removal is variable. Postoperative recovery typically takes 3 to 6 months, but may be longer if small toe abduction is weak preoperatively.[6] When athletes are carefully selected and the diagnosis is firm, good or excellent results may be seen in approximately 85% of patients.[8]

Medial Plantar Nerve: Jogger's Foot

Definition
Classically, "jogger's foot" describes a syndrome of neuropathic pain radiating along the medial heel and longitudinal arch, resulting from local entrapment of the MPN.[23] There is no age or gender predilection.[4]

Anatomy, Pathophysiology, and Risk Factors
After the MPN and LPN exit the tarsal tunnel, each nerve enters a fibro-osseous canal bounded superiorly by the calcaneonavicular or spring ligament and inferiorly by the attachment of the AHM to the navicular bone. The MPN then enters the sole of the foot, passes superficial to the traversing FDL tendon at the master knot of Henry, and continues distally along the FHL tendon to divide into terminal medial and lateral branches at the level of the base of the first metatarsal.[4] These branches ramify and terminate as three common plantar digital nerves within the medial three web spaces. The MPN is a mixed sensorimotor nerve providing sensation to the medial sole and plantar aspect of the first, second, third, and medial fourth toes, as well as motor innervation to the abductor hallucis, flexor hallucis brevis, flexor digitorum brevis, and first lumbrical muscles (Figs. 20–3 and 20–5).

MPN entrapment typically occurs at the AHM fibro-osseous canal or master knot of Henry.[9] The MPN may be compressed externally from orthoses or footwear, or internally by AHM tension.[23] Specific etiologies include AHM hypertrophy, a valgus running style, functional hyperpronation (e.g., calcaneovalgus), and high-arched orthoses.[9] A history of prior ankle injuries with instability is common. Jogger's foot has also been reported in association with hallux

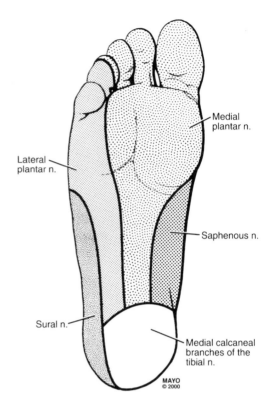

Figure 20–5. Cutaneous innervation of the plantar foot.

rigidus, in which it is hypothesized that AHM and flexor digitorum brevis muscle spasm resulted from an unconscious desire to splint the first MTJ from dorsiflexing.[4]

Symptoms and Signs
The athlete typically reports exercise-induced neuropathic pain radiating along the medial arch towards the plantar aspect of the first and second toes. Symptoms may coincide with implementation of new footwear or an orthosis. There is typically no rest or night pain.

Examination should follow general principles. The most useful palpatory finding is maximal tenderness at the superior aspect of the AHM at the navicular tuberosity, with distally radiating pain or tingling; this site is distinct from that described for FB-LPN entrapment (see above, and Fig. 20–3).[10,23] Provocative testing includes forceful passive heel eversion, standing on the balls of the feet, or percussion over the nerve. Sensory loss, weakness, or atrophy are rarely reported. Since symptoms may only be induced with exercise, examination may be completely normal unless the athlete is examined after running.[9] The athlete should be examined for ankle instabilities, malalignments, hallux rigidus, AHM hypertrophy, and a valgus running style.

Differential Diagnosis and Evaluation

For diagnostic purposes, the syndrome of MPN entrapment or jogger's foot consists of (1) burning medial heel pain, (2) longitudinal arch aching, and (3) medial sole paresthesias.[23] Differential diagnosis parallels that of TTS, with the exception of additional local pathological processes. Due to the proximity of the MPN to the FDL and FHL muscles, distinguishing neuropathic pain from tendinitis may be difficult, and the two conditions may coexist.[10] Resisted great toe plantarflexion or passive toe dorsiflexion will induce pain with flexor tendinitis, but not typically with nerve entrapment.[10] Hindfoot and midfoot synovitis and arthritis, as well as stress fractures, should be considered.

Evaluation is similar to that for TTS. Radiographs are commonly obtained, and bone scans are obtained as necessary. MRI has not been as useful for jogger's foot compared with TTS, but may reveal local midfoot arthritis or tendinopathies at the master knot of Henry. EDX testing aids in the differential diagnosis but sensitivity varies for detecting abnormalities. Diagnostic nerve block at the entrapment site can be useful.

Treatment

Initial nonoperative treatment is indicated and often successful. Treatment principles parallel those for TTS. Rigid orthoses should be modified, replaced, or removed to avoid MPN compression. Functional hyperpronation may be addressed by medial arch strengthening, kinetic chain rehabilitation, modifying running habits (less valgus) or terrain, or altering footwear.[23] Therapeutic injections should avoid direct nerve contact. Surgical release has been successful in refractory cases and is generally a distal extension of the surgery performed for TTS.

Common Peroneal Nerve (CPN)

Definition

Common peroneal nerve (CPN) entrapment typically occurs at the fibular head, proximal to the bifurcation into the SPN and DPN, and produces dorsiflexion weakness and possibly neuropathic pain extending over the anterolateral leg and foot dorsum. It is the most prevalent peroneal nerve injury seen in runners.[10,27,28]

Anatomy, Pathophysiology, and Risk Factors

The CPN consists of sensory and motor fibers from the L4-S2 segments and is the smaller terminal branch of the sciatic nerve (Figs. 20–5, 20–6, and 20–7). The CPN separates from the sciatic nerve just above the knee, where it supplies innervation to the short head of the biceps femoris (the only thigh muscle innervated by the peroneal nerve) and divides into the SPN, DPN, and lateral sural cutaneous nerve (LSCN) at the level of the fibular head (Table 20–1). The SPN innervates leg lateral compartment muscles, then emerges from the lateral compartment by penetrating the crural fascia 10.5 to 12.5 cm proximal to the tip of the lateral malleolus. It supplies sensation to the anterolateral leg, then divides into its terminal medial and intermediate cutaneous branches about 6 cm above the lateral malleolus (Figs. 20–6 and 20–7). These branches enter the foot dorsum *superficial* to the inferior extensor retinaculum and supply sensation to the foot dorsum, including the medial aspect of the first toe, and the adjacent sides of the third and fourth, and fourth and fifth toes (Fig. 20–7). The DPN traverses the leg anterior compartment, innervating all the muscles including the peroneus tertius, divides into medial and lateral branches 1 to 2 cm proximal to the ankle, and enters the foot *deep* to the inferior extensor retinaculum. Its medial branch supplies sensation to the first web space, and its lateral branch innervates the EDB as well as local joints. Up to 20% of individuals may have accessory innervation of the EDB from the SPN.[10]

The CPN is vulnerable to compression at the fibular head due to its superficial location and underlying bone. Reported etiologies of CPN injury include external compression (knee crossing, bed rest, casts, orthoses), aneurysms, tumors (e.g., neurofibroma), tibiofibular joint ganglion, fibular head dislocation, Baker's cyst, generalized ligamentous laxity, genu varum, genu recurvatum and compartment syndrome.[28–30] Repetitive combined plantarflexion and inversion while running downhill or on uneven surfaces may also produce stretching of the CPN at the fibular head.

Symptoms and Signs

The DPN is often more severely affected than the SPN. The athlete may report neuropathic symptoms affecting the anterior or anterolateral leg, extending into the dorsal foot and toe web spaces. However, the most common complaint is weakness, most often with ankle dorsiflexion given the propensity for DPN involvement.[10] Consequently, the athlete may complain of foot drop, steppage gait, foot slap, recurrent ankle sprains and/or an otherwise "funny sound" when running.

Physical examination may be unremarkable at rest, but palpation for masses, fascial defects, nerve sensitivity, pulses, and knee-tibiofibular problems should be performed. Knee lateral and posterolateral rotatory laxity or instability can produce stretch injury to the CPN or its branches at the fibular head. Leach and colleagues reported that postexercise percussion sensitivity or weakness was detected in all 7 patients with CPN injury who had normal baseline examinations.[27]

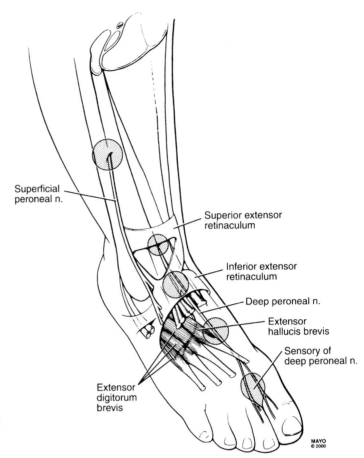

Superficial peroneal n.

Superior extensor retinaculum

Inferior extensor retinaculum

Deep peroneal n.

Extensor hallucis brevis

Sensory of deep peroneal n.

Extensor digitorum brevis

MAYO © 2000

Figure 20–6. Superficial and deep peroneal nerves. Shaded areas represent potential entrapment sites.

Differential Diagnosis and Evaluation

Differential diagnosis includes injury to all neurologic structures contributing to the CPN, compartment syndrome, and focal processes about the knee that can lead to CPN injury. A focal CPN injury would not involve the TN sensorimotor functions, or the cutaneous distribution of the saphenous nerve. Sciatic neuropathy, lumbosacral plexopathy, and L5 radiculopathy may also produce foot drop, but typically produce weakness in nonperoneal innervated muscles (e.g., posterior tibialis), nonperoneal territory sensory loss (e.g., plantar foot), and nonperoneal reflex loss (e.g., ankle reflex). Multiple sclerosis may present as exercise-induced foot drop, with relatively little pain.

Diagnostic studies may include radiographs and MRI to exclude compressive mass lesions. EDX studies may be extremely helpful for localization, prognostication, and differential diagnosis. However, EDX abnormalities may only occur postexercise.[27]

Treatment

CPN entrapments in runners are often self-limited provided the inciting factor is addressed.[27] If considerable axon loss occurs, recovery may be prolonged and incomplete. Treatment includes patient counseling; nerve protection; neuromodulatory medications and transcutaneous electrical nerve stimulation (TENS) for neuropathic pain; biomechanical interventions to reduce neural tension; dorsiflexion support (ankle brace, ankle foot orthosis, or high-top shoes); knee stabilization when necessary; change in running style to avoid excessive varus recurvatum knee moments; and observation. If recovery is prolonged and advanced imaging has not been obtained, strong consideration should be given to MRI evaluation with the site dictated by the history, physical examination, and EDX findings.[27]

Operative decompression usually provides satisfactory results if the clinical diagnosis is firm and significant axonal damage has not occurred. In one small study, 6 of 7 young and middle-aged runners returned to normal activities within 6 weeks of surgical treatment.[27]

Superficial Peroneal Nerve

Definition

SPN entrapment typically occurs as the nerve penetrates the crural fascia above the ankle, resulting in neuropathic pain in the SPN distribution. Among athletes, the mean age is 28 years, and men and women are equally affected.[4]

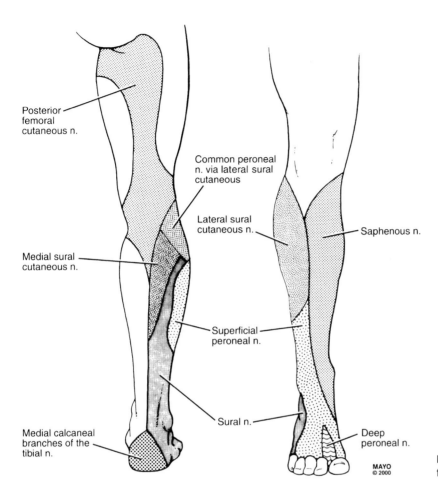

Figure 20–7. Cutaneous innervation of the thigh, leg, and foot dorsum.

Labels (left figure): Posterior femoral cutaneous n.; Common peroneal n. via lateral sural cutaneous; Lateral sural cutaneous n.; Medial sural cutaneous n.; Superficial peroneal n.; Sural n.; Medial calcaneal branches of the tibial n.

Labels (right figure): Saphenous n.; Deep peroneal n.

MAYO
© 2000

Anatomy, Pathophysiology, and Risk Factors

The relevant anatomy was discussed previously in the section above on the anatomy, pathophysiology, and risk factors of CPN nerve entrapment. SPN injury at the site of emergence from the lateral compartment may result from sharp fascial edges, chronic ankle sprains (25% of athletes have a history of trauma), muscular herniation, direct contusive trauma, fibular fracture, edema, varicose veins, wearing tight ski boots or rollerblades, biomechanical factors (see CPN entrapment, above), and space-occupying lesions such as nerve sheath tumors, lipomas, and ganglia. The nerve may be injured iatrogenically during anterior or lateral compartment release. Up to 10% of affected individuals may have chronic lateral compartment syndrome.[31] The medial branch, intermediate branch, or both may be affected. Since the terminal cutaneous branches enter the foot dorsal to the extensor retinaculum (Fig. 20–6), they are not entrapped beneath this tissue. However, tight footwear may externally compress the SPN or either of its two terminal branches at the level of the ankle or foot, resulting in distal radiating neuropathic pain.

Symptoms and Signs

The athlete typically reports a diffuse ache over the sinus tarsi or dorsolateral foot. One third will report numbness or tingling over the same areas.[4] Symptoms may be limited to a vague, achy distal anterolateral leg discomfort, and proximal radiation has been reported.[32] Symptoms typically worsen with weightbearing, are relieved by rest, and don't occur at night.

Examination may reveal percussion tenderness, a fascial defect (60% of patients), or muscular herniation at the exit site approximately 10 to 13 cm above the ankle. Provocative testing before and after exercise is the most useful clinical indicator of SPN entrapment and includes (1) pressure over the exit site during resisted ankle dorsiflexion-eversion, (2) pressure over the same area during passive plantarflexion combined with inversion, and (3) percussion over the SPN course while passive plantarflexion and inversion are maintained. Pain or paresthesias indicate a positive test and the presence of two positive tests strongly supports the diagnosis.[31,33] Sensation and EDB bulk may be diminished but are not common findings.[4] Ankle stability, biomechanical alignment, and dorsal footwear pressures should be examined in all athletes.

Differential Diagnosis and Evaluation

Differential diagnosis resembles that for CPN entrapment and should also consider the various etiologies of SPN injury specifically. Radiographs and EDX may help, but are often unremarkable. Normal nerve conduction studies recorded at rest do not exclude SPN, and postexercise testing has been advocated when necessary.[31] MRI can detect most mass lesions, but may not discern contributory fascial defects. Compartment testing is performed as clinically indicated.

Treatment

Treatment parallels that for CPN entrapment, but may also include corticosteroid injection at the site of emergence from the lateral compartment, ankle instability rehabilitation, myofascial release, and use of lateral wedges to decrease nerve stretch. Footwear modification may be necessary to reduce dorsal pressures at the ankle. In refractory confirmed cases, surgery typically consists of isolated release at the fascial exit site, reduction of muscular herniation, fat nodule resection, and fasciotomy if compartment syndrome is documented (see Chapter 16). Ankle reconstruction is performed as necessary. In isolated releases, athletes begin gradual return to activity at 2 weeks. In Styf's study,[33] up to 75% of patients remain improved at 18 months of follow-up; however, only 4 of 17 patients had unlimited activity, whereas 10 of 17 categorized their activity as improved but still limited.[31,33]

Deep Peroneal Nerve: Anterior Tarsal Tunnel Syndrome

Definition

DPN entrapment is also called anterior tarsal tunnel syndrome (ATTS), although all authors do not agree with this latter designation because there is no distinct fibro-osseous tunnel in this region. This syndrome results from DPN compression in the vicinity of the extensor retinaculum, resulting in neuropathic pain extending into the dorsomedial foot and first web space (Figs. 20–6 and 20–7).

Anatomy, Pathophysiology, and Risk Factors

The previous section on anatomy, pathophysiology, and risk factors discusses some of the relevant peroneal nerve anatomy. In the anterior leg compartment, the extensor hallucis longus (EHL) muscle courses in a medial, oblique direction. The DPN traverses deep to the EHL to course between the EHL and extensor digitorum

longus (EDL) at the level of the inferior aspect of the superior extensor retinaculum, approximately 3 to 5 cm above the ankle joint. At the level of the oblique superior band of the inferior extensor retinaculum, about 1 cm above the ankle joint, the DPN forms its terminal lateral and medial branches. The lateral branch innervates the EDB muscle. The medial branch courses distally with the dorsalis pedis artery, passing deep to the oblique inferior medial band of the inferior extensor retinaculum, where it may be entrapped by processes affecting the talonavicular joint.[4]

DPN entrapment may occur in several locations, including the inferior aspect of the superior extensor retinaculum where the EHL crosses over the DPN, the inferior extensor retinaculum (anterior TTS; most common site), and distally where the extensor hallucis brevis crosses the DPN in the first intermetatarsal space. In the latter two cases, an isolated sensory neuropathy of the medial branch occurs.

A variety of processes may entrap the DPN, including trauma (contusion, ankle sprain, or instability), shoe contact pressure ("boot top neuropathy"; wearing a key under the tongue of the shoe), osteophytic compression (tibiotalar, talonavicular, or first metatarsophalangeal), edema, and synovitis or ganglia arising from adjacent joints or tendons.[34]

Symptoms and Signs

Athletes typically report deep, aching, dorsal midfoot pain and neuropathic symptoms extending into the first web space. Symptoms are worse with activity, prolonged standing, and wearing tight-fitting or high-top or lace-up shoes, and are relieved by rest. Night pain can occur from pressure or prolonged plantarflexion.[16]

A detailed history will often direct attention to ill-fitting footwear as the probable etiologic factor in many, if not the majority, of cases.[16] Percussion along the course of the DPN starting at the fibular head may localize the entrapment site. Depending on the entrapment site, symptom provocation may occur with either plantarflexion or dorsiflexion of the foot.[9,16] EDB weakness is difficult to detect. Atrophy relative to the unaffected side may be seen, but should not be expected if only the medial branch is involved. Examination should also focus on revealing potential etiologic processes, as discussed below. Biomechanical factors are not as crucial in this nerve entrapment relative to those discussed previously.

Differential Diagnosis and Evaluation

Differential diagnosis parallels that for CPN and SPN entrapments, but also includes anterior compartment syndrome as well as an evaluation for treatable etiologies of DPN injury. Recall that CPN entrapments often preferentially affect the DPN fascicles, so CPN injury presenting as DPN injury should be excluded.[10] Involvement of the EDB localizes injury above the extensor retinaculum.

Radiographs may reveal dorsal midfoot osteophytes or accessory ossicles (e.g., os intermetatarseum) that may irritate terminal branches of the DPN.[17] EDX can assist in differential diagnosis and localization (e.g., involvement of the EDB or CPN). Compartment pressures and MRI are obtained as necessary.

Treatment

Nonoperative measures include footwear changes to avoid direct pressure, neuromodulatory and anti-inflammatory medications, TENS, edema control, ankle stability rehabilitation, and local corticosteroid injections. Local injections assist diagnostically and therapeutically. Treatable underlying etiologies are addressed. Surgery is sometimes necessary, is performed via a dorsomedial approach, and involves partial sectioning of the extensor retinaculum and osteophyte removal. Recovery may take 6 to 8 weeks.

MISCELLANEOUS NERVE ENTRAPMENT SYNDROMES

Although significantly less common among runners, several additional nerve entrapment syndromes merit consideration as they may be encountered by clinicians caring for runners.

Medial Calcaneal Nerve

MCN entrapment produces neuropathic pain at the medial heel secondary to entrapment in the vicinity of the tarsal tunnel. The MCN usually arises from the TN, but may arise from the LPN or at the MPN-LPN bifurcation; thus, the MCN may originate proximal to or within the tarsal tunnel. The MCN pierces the flexor retinaculum to provide cutaneous innervation to the posterior, medial, and plantar surfaces of the heel, providing no motor innervation (Figs. 20–3, 20–5, and 20–7). Entrapment usually occurs as the MCN pierces the flexor retinaculum. Excessive pronation may be contributory. Direct compression from external sources such as footwear or repetitive heel impact on hard surfaces may damage the MCN, and lead to fibrosis, thickening, and dysfunction. Neuropathic pain is limited to the medial heel and there is no motor or reflex deficit. Symptoms increase with activity. Rest pain or night pain is uncommon. The most useful clinical sign is percussion tenderness and paresthesias when palpating the MCN as it pierces the retinaculum posterior to

the TN (Fig. 20–3). Examination will less commonly reveal proximal radiation, or a "lamp cord sign" (a hypersensitive, tender thickening of the MCN along its oblique-posterior course).[35] Biomechanical and footwear evaluation may be helpful.

Differential diagnosis resembles that for TTS, but medial heel involvement suggests MCN entrapment. Radiographs are often obtained to exclude calcaneal stress fractures and to detect osseous abnormalities that may compress the MCN. EDX studies assist in the differential diagnosis, but are rarely useful in making the diagnosis. Nonoperative management follows general principles previously discussed and may also include measures to improve pronation control, corticosteroid injections, and cut-out pads and footwear alterations to reduce direct pressure on the MCN as necessary. The lamp cord sign is often a poor prognostic factor, and surgery is often recommended to remove this pseudoneuroma, often with excellent outcome.[35]

Sural Nerve

The SN is an uncommon area of neuropathy. There is no particular sex or age distribution, but the syndrome is reported most commonly in runners. The SN is formed by branches of the TN and CPN in the posterior calf, 11 to 20 cm proximal to the lateral malleolus. Two centimeters proximal to the malleolus, the SN provides a sensory branch to the lateral heel, then courses subcutaneously inferior to the peroneal tendons to the base of the fifth metatarsal, where it ramifies into distal sensory branches (Figs. 20–5 and 20–7).

Etiologies include recurrent ankle sprains, calcaneal or fifth metatarsal fractures, Achilles tendinopathy, space-occupying lesions such as ganglia (peroneal sheath, calcaneocuboid joint), direct contusion, footwear-induced pressure, or iatrogenic (postbiopsy neuroma). Symptoms consist of achy, posterolateral calf pain, with neuropathic pain in the SN distribution (Figs. 20–5 and 20–7). Examination should include percussion testing along the nerve and provocative testing by passive dorsiflexion and inversion. Diagnostic testing is not universally required, but may include radiographs, EDX, and diagnostic nerve blocks. Treatment emphasizes reduction of pressure from footwear, Achilles stretching, neuropathic pain treatment, edema control, and ankle stability rehabilitation. Etiologic conditions should be identified and treated. Surgery consists of exploration and decompression.

Saphenous Nerve

The saphenous nerve is the largest cutaneous branch of the femoral nerve. This purely sensory nerve arises from the femoral nerve in the femoral triangle and courses with the femoral artery to the medial knee, where its infrapatellar branch supplies cutaneous sensation to the medial knee. It then courses inferiorly with the saphenous vein to supply cutaneous sensation to the medial calf to the level of the ankle. At the ankle, a branch passes anterior to the medial malleolus to innervate the medial foot (Figs. 20–3 and 20–5). The saphenous nerve is most vulnerable at the medial knee, where it pierces the fascia and emerges from the distal subsartorial canal (Hunter's adductor canal). Etiologies of saphenous neuritis include entrapment at the adductor canal, pes anserine bursitis, contusion, and postsurgical (knee) iatrogenic injury. The athlete will typically report neuropathic pain and numbness in the area of the medial knee and/or calf, depending on whether there is isolated infrapatellar branch or complete saphenous nerve involvement. There should be no motor deficits. Examination includes percussion testing along the nerve starting at the adductor canal, and a search for underlying etiologies. Differential diagnosis includes all proximal femoral nerve, plexus, and root lesions, as well as musculoskeletal disorders about the knee. Diagnosis and treatment principles resemble those for SN entrapment, but focus upon different anatomical areas. Surgical release may be necessary.

Obturator Nerve

Obturator nerve (ON) entrapment has received increased attention as a potential source of groin pain in some athletes, but is probably rare in runners.[36] The ON arises from the L2-L4 spinal segments, and exits the pelvis via a fibro-osseous tunnel (obturator canal), in which it divides into terminal anterior and posterior branches.[36] These branches provide the predominant motor innervation to the thigh adductor group and sensory innervation to the distal $1/2$ to $2/3$ of the medial thigh. ON entrapment most commonly occurs at the exit of the obturator canal due to compressive fibrous bands located in this area.[36,37] Rarely, ON entrapment may occur secondary to the local inflammatory changes of osteitis pubis or from an obturator hernia.[36,38] The athlete will typically complain of activity-related groin pain of a deep, burning, achy quality. Pain radiation, numbness, tingling, and weakness are rare. Diagnosis is challenging. Examination is largely unremarkable, but assists in excluding more common causes of hip and groin pain among athletes (see Chapter 13). Radiographic imaging is not usually helpful. EDX studies may reveal fibrillation potentials in the adductor muscles in some cases, but is not uniformly helpful.[36,37] Local anesthetic and corticosteroid injections may assist in making the diagnosis,

and have successfully treated some cases when combined with rehabilitative efforts focused on improving hip flexibility and strength. Surgical treatment may become necessary, and is well described elsewhere.[37]

Lateral Femoral Cutaneous Nerve: Meralgia Paresthetica

LFCN injury has been reported in runners.[1] The LFCN arises from the L2-L3 spinal segments, and typically exits the pelvis via a small tunnel formed by a split in the lateral ilioinguinal ligament at its insertion into the anterior superior iliac spine (ASIS).[36] Just distal to the tunnel, the LFCN will split into two terminal branches supplying cutaneous innervation to the anterolateral thigh. There is no motor innervation. LFCN injury usually occurs at the level of the ilioinguinal ligament, where repetitive hip flexion-extension can injure the nerve, and the nerve is susceptible to local contusive trauma due to its superficial location. Specific etiologies include rapid weight change, compression from tight clothing or belts, and systemic disease affecting nerves such as thyroid disease and diabetes. In many cases, an inciting factor is not identified (idiopathic). The athlete will report burning, aching discomfort over the anterolateral thigh, with or without clear inciting factors. Examination is often normal, but may reveal percussion tenderness or a percussion sign approximately 1 cm anterior and inferior to the ASIS, or a sensory deficit in the cutaneous distribution. Differential diagnosis includes focal musculoskeletal pathologies (see Chapter 13), lesions affecting the lumbosacral plexus or L2-L3 nerve roots, and systemic disease such as hypothyroidism and diabetes. Local anesthetic and corticosteroid injections may not only be diagnostic, but therapeutic. Treatment involves removal of inciting factors, treatment of neuropathic pain, observation, and injections. Up to 90% of cases resolve with nonoperative management.[39] Surgical release is sometimes necessary.[36]

Medial Hallucal Nerve Entrapment

The medial hallucal nerve is a distal terminal branch of the MPN providing sensation to the medial aspect of the great toe. This nerve may rarely be entrapped as it exits the distal end of the AHM, producing medial first MTJ pain, and numbness and tingling extending along the medial great toe. Etiologies include pressure from hallux valgus, prominent tibial sesamoid, AHM tendinitis, and poorly-fitting footwear. Differential diagnosis includes medial tibial sesamoid disorders, MTJ disorders, and polyneuropathy. Diagnosis is clinical based on symptoms, percussion tenderness or a percussion sign over the nerve, and exclusion of alternative diagnoses with appropriate diagnostic testing. Nerve blocks may be useful when necessary. Treatment includes removal of inciting factors, and treatment of neuropathic pain as previously described.

SUMMARY

Nerve entrapment represents an uncommon but important cause of lower limb pain among runners. This chapter has reviewed the diagnosis and management of several nerve entrapment syndromes that may be encountered among runners, but clinicians must be aware that any peripheral nerve may be affected. Successful diagnosis and management are predicated upon several underlying principles: (1) maintain a high index of suspicion for neurological syndromes, (2) recognize common presentations of neuropathic pain, (3) perform a meticulous physical examination, including postexercise examination when necessary, (4) consider a broad differential diagnosis (neurological and nonneurological), (5) appropriately use diagnostic testing, and (6) make rational clinical decisions, including referral for a second opinion when indicated.[4] A thorough knowledge of neuroanatomy and running biomechanics will allow the clinician to successfully apply these principles to almost all clinical scenarios.

REFERENCES

1. Massey E, Pleet A: Neuropathy in joggers. *Am J Sports Med* 1978:6, 209.
2. Clanton T, Schon L: Athletic injuries to the soft tissues of the foot and ankle, in Mann R, Coughlin M (eds.), *Surgery of the Foot and Ankle*, 6th ed., St. Louis, Mosby, 1993: 1105.
3. Styf J: Chronic exercise induced pain in the anterior aspect of the lower leg: An overview of diagnosis. *Sports Med* 1989:7, 331.
4. Schon L, Baxter D: Neuropathies of the foot and ankle in athletes. *Clin Sports Med* 1990:9, 489.
5. Schon L, Glennon T, Baxter D: Heel pain syndrome: Electrodiagnostic support for nerve entrapment. *Foot Ankle* 1993:14, 129.
6. Schon L: Nerve entrapment, neuropathy, and nerve dysfunction in the athlete. *Orthop Clin North Am* 1994:25, 47.
7. Babcock J: Cervical spine injuries: Diagnosis and classification. *Arch Surg* 1976:111, 647.
8. Baxter D, Pfeffer G: Treatment of chronic heel pain by surgical release of the first branch of the lateral plantar nerve. *Clin Orthop Rel Res* 1992:279, 299.
9. Baxter D: Functional nerve disorders in the athlete's foot, ankle and leg. *Instructional Course Lectures* 1993:42, 185.
10. McCluskey L, Webb L: Compression and entrapment neuropathies of the lower extremity. *Clin Podiatr Med Surg* 1999:16, 96.
11. Lau J, Daniels T: Tarsal tunnel syndrome: A review of the literature. *Foot Ankle Int* 1999:20, 201.
12. Downey M, Barrett J: Peripheral nerve surgery of the foot and ankle: A review of current principles. *Clin Podiatr Med Surg* 1999:16, 175.
13. Henderson W: Clinical assessment of peripheral nerve injuries: Tinel's test. *Lancet* 1948:2, 801.
14. Upton A, McComas A: The double crush in nerve entrapment syndromes. *Lancet* 1973:2, 359.
15. Sammarco G, Chalk D, Feibel J: Tarsal tunnel syndrome and additional nerve lesions in the same limb. *Foot Ankle* 1993:14, 71.
16. Park T, DelToro D: Electrodiagnostic evaluation of the foot. *Phys Med Rehabil Clin North Am* 1998:9, 871.
17. Murphy P, Baxter D: Nerve entrapment of the foot and ankle in runners. *Clin Sports Med* 1985:4, 753.
18. Dumitru D: *Electrodiagnostic Medicine*, Philadelphia, Hanley & Belfus, 1995.
19. Turnipseed W, Pozniak M: Popliteal entrapment as a result of neurovascular compression by the soleus and plantaris muscles. *J Vasc Surg* 1992:15, 285.
20. Jackson D, Haglund B: Tarsal tunnel syndrome in runners. *Sports Med* 1992:13, 146.
21. Frey C, Kerr R: Magnetic resonance imaging and the evaluation of tarsal tunnel syndrome. *Foot Ankle* 1993:14, 153.
22. Galardi G, Amadio S, Maderna L, et al.: Electrophysiologic studies in tarsal tunnel syndrome: Diagnostic reliability of motor distal latency, mixed nerve and sensory nerve conduction studies. *Am J Phys Med* 1994:73, 193.
23. Rask M: Medial plantar neurapraxia (Jogger's foot). *Clin Orthop* 1978:181, 167.
24. Cimino W: Tarsal tunnel syndrome: Review of the literature. *Foot Ankle* 1990:11, 47.
25. Pfeiffer W, Cracchiolo A: Clinical results after tarsal tunnel decompression. *J Bone Joint Surg* 1994:76A, 1222.
26. Johnson M: Nerve entrapment causing heel pain. *Clin Podiatric Med Surg* 1994:11, 617.
27. Leach R, Purnell M, Saito A: Peroneal nerve entrapment in runners. *Am J Sports Med* 1989:17, 287.
28. Moller B, Kadin S: Entrapment of the common peroneal nerve. *Am J Sports Med* 1987:15, 90.
29. Di Risio D, Lazaro R, Popp A: Nerve entrapment and calf atrophy caused by a Baker's cyst: Case report. *Neurosurgery* 1994:35, 333.
30. Nagel A, Greenebaum E, Singson R, et al.: Foot drop in a long-distance runner. An unusual presentation of neurofibromatosis. *Orthop Rev* 1994:23, 526.
31. Styf J, Morberg P: The superficial peroneal tunnel syndrome: Results of treatment by decompression. *J Bone Joint Surg* 1997:79B, 801.
32. Lowdon I: Superficial peroneal nerve entrapment. *J Bone Joint Surg* 1985:67B, 58.
33. Styf J: Entrapment of the superficial peroneal nerve: Diagnosis and results of decompression. *J Bone Joint Surg* 1989:71B, 131.

34. Dellon A: Deep peroneal nerve entrapment on the dorsum of the foot. *Foot Ankle* 1990:11, 73.

35. Cohen S: Another consideration in the diagnosis of heel pain: Neuroma of the medial calcaneal nerve. *J Foot Ankle Surg* 1974:13, 128.

36. McCrory P, Bell S: Nerve entrapment syndromes as a cause of pain in the hip, groin, and buttock. *Sports Med* 1999:27, 261.

37. Bradshaw C, McCrory P, Bell S, et al.: Obturator nerve entrapment: A cause of groin pain in athletes. *Am J Sports Med* 1997:25, 402.

38. Kopell H, Thompson W: Peripheral nerve entrapments of the lower extremity. *N Engl J Med* 1962:266, 216.

39. Williams P, Trzil K: Management of meralgia paresthetica. *J Neurosurg* 1991:74, 76.

Part IV

MEDICAL PROBLEMS

Chapter 21

DERMATOLOGICAL DISORDERS

Mark S. Williams and Kenneth B. Batts

INTRODUCTION

In the last quarter century, physical fitness and competitive sports have become individualized and team oriented, with running remaining the mainstay for achieving aerobic fitness. A runner's performance may be adversely effected by a diversity of dermatological disorders.[1] Both the physical condition and the psychological mind-set of the runner may be hindered by a debilitating skin condition. The skin provides natural insulation from the cold, wind, and rain and serves as a corporeal thermostat in the heat. The skin is a protective barrier for fighting infection and preserving the integrity of the corpus against physical forces. Although the runner requires minimal equipment, long hours of training with improperly fitted clothing and shoes may produce skin irritation. As the largest organ in the body, the skin is predisposed to injury, infection, irritation, and exposure; these may produce common dermatological disorders that hamper the runner.

The health care provider must be able to render a definitive diagnosis, thus enabling the runner to resume safe activity and prevent further injury. This chapter discusses the common skin disorders of runners with treatment strategies to return the athlete to full participation. The specific disorders are divided into four major areas (mechanical injury, infection, irritation, and environmental exposure) with clear diagnostic descriptions and treatment options.

MECHANICAL INJURY

Abrasions/Contusions

Abrasions (road rash, strawberries, raspberries) are areas of denuded epidermis/dermis produced when the runner accidentally falls or strikes a rough surface or object. Contusions occur with blunt trauma, producing swelling and ecchymosis of the surrounding skin.

Copious irrigation and removal of denuded skin, necrotic material, and foreign debris with warm water and antibacterial soap is the first stage of treatment. Once the area is clean and bleeding is controlled, antibacterial ointments (e.g., bacitracin) are applied to promote wound healing in a moist environment. In more severe injuries, hydromembranes such as a hydrocolloid (DuoDerm) or a hydrogel (Geliperm) can be applied for 3 days to decrease the pH (inhibiting bacterial growth) and promote rapid healing. Oral antibiotics and tetanus immunization should be considered for puncture wounds to eliminate secondary infections.

Blisters

Blisters (Fig. 21–1) develop after separation of the epidermal layer from the dermis and present as vesicles or bullae on the prominent bony surfaces of the feet. The vesicular fluid is usually clear or serosanguinous, but it may become pustular, resulting in infection, if repeated pressure and friction are not alleviated. A moist environment can lead to maceration of the skin

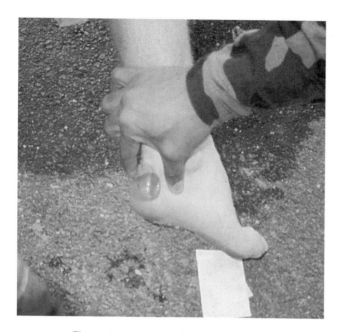

Figure 21–1. Hemorrhagic friction blisters.

and an increase in blister formation. The most common cause in the runner is the use of new shoes that may have been improperly fitted.[2]

Treatment of "hot spots," in which the epidermis is only inflamed, requires removal of the antecedent cause or relief with padding or moleskin. Large, painful blisters should be drained with an 18-gauge needle at the inferior border of the epidermis.[3] The roof of the blister should be preserved to provide protection over the inflamed dermis. If the blister reoccurs, it needs to be drained and tincture of benzoin applied to fuse the blister roof to the underlying dermis. To prevent blister formation, the runner may use petroleum jelly over bony prominences, nylon hose to decrease friction, talcum-powdered cotton socks to absorb perspiration, and properly fitted shoes. For long-distance runners, some advise use of a thin coating of antiperspirant spray over the foot to decrease moisture within the shoe. At least two or three layers of moleskin shaped like a donut with the hole over the de-roofed blister will protect the tissue from further injury. If the blister becomes unroofed, the underlying dermis can be protected with DuoDerm for 5 to 7 days. Antibiotic ointments (bacitracin, mupirocin) may prevent secondary infections.

Calluses

Calluses are the most common sports dermatosis.[4] Calluses large circumscribed areas of hyperkeratosis over bony prominences of the plantar feet. Calluses a compensatory protective reaction of the skin to chronic friction and normally are not painful.

Primary prevention includes metatarsal head cushions in runners with narrow, supinated, or high midarched (pes cavus) feet. Secondary prevention includes removal of the external friction by modifying the footwear with polysorbothane cushioning. If it is painful, the callus can be removed by paring with a scalpel blade, pumice stone, emery board, or application of a topical keratolytic agent. Keratolytic agents such as salicylic acid, lactic acid, or urea lotions should be used in amounts that will cover the lesion but not involve the surrounding normal epidermis.

Corns

Corns (clavus; Fig. 21–2) are cone-shaped, hyperkeratotic lesions with a characteristic translucent core. They are found overlying bony prominences of the foot and between the toes. These lesions are usually painful and need to be differentiated from calluses and plantar warts. Corns have a central clearing that is not noted in calluses or plantar warts and are painful with squeezing or application of pressure.

Treatment to remove the corn requires *** of the translucent core with a scalpel blade and application of keratolytic agents over the lesion. Treatment measures like those for calluses can be beneficial in relieving painful corns, but protection and prevention remain the mainstay of therapy.[5]

Piezogenic Papules

Piezogenic papules are painful, 2- to 5-mm skin-colored lesions on the lateral and medial surfaces of the heel. They result from herniation of subdermal fat into the dermis, producing multiple small protrusions around the heel.[6] These papules are more noticeable upon standing and are found in 20% of the general population.[7] Although they are mostly asymptomatic,

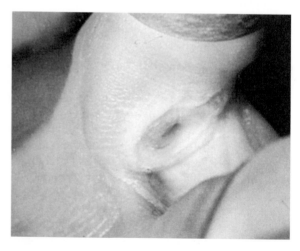

Figure 21–2. Corn.

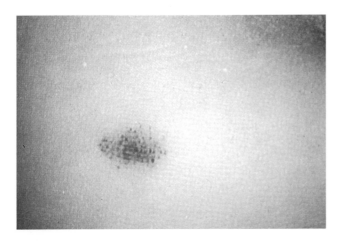

Figure 21–3. Black heel.

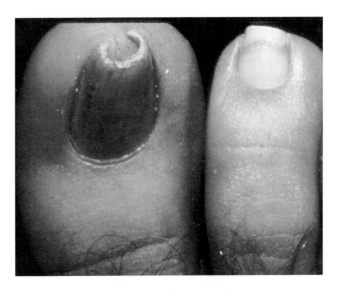

Figure 21–4. Black toenail.

long-distance runners may experience debilitating pain and may have to discontinue running.

No medical or surgical intervention has been shown to cure the condition totally. Relief may occur with the use of heel cups, orthotics, felt pads, or taping.

Black Heel

Black heel, or *talor noir* (Fig. 21–3), consists of horizontally arranged petechiae at the upper edge of the heel. It is a common complaint of young adult sprinters and hurdlers who are stopping and starting frequently, producing shearing forces of the epidermis over the papillary dermis. Although it is asymptomatic, hemorrhagic discoloration of the skin in this location may resemble melanoma. The diagnosis is confirmed by mixing scrapings of the stratum corneum with a few drops of water and then using an occult screening test to confirm the presence of blood.[2]

Treatment consists of primary prevention using heel cups, felt pads, or cushioned athletic socks. The hemorrhage will resolve spontaneously with rest in 2 to 3 weeks.

Ingrown Toenail

Ingrown toenails commonly occur in the great toes of runners and can produce debilitating pain on push-off. They occur from pressure along the nailbed, forcing the nail plate into the dermis of the lateral fold of the toe. As the lateral edge of the nail penetrates the dermis, it acts as a foreign body, producing inflammation in the lateral fold. Repeated pressure and lack of attention to the area is a setup for infection.

Primary prevention requires the runner to trim the distal nail plate properly, straight from one nail fold to the other. Filing the middle of the nail may decrease lateral pressure on the edges of the plate. Also, the condition can be avoided by wearing shoes with a wide

toe box. Oral first-generation cephalosporin antibiotics may be used in the acute condition, with warm Epsom salt soaks to reduce the inflammation. For recalcitrant cases, partial or total excision of the nail may be necessary to provide relief.[8]

Black Toenail

Subungual hemorrhage of the nailbed in a runner, "jogger's toe" (Fig. 21–4), occurs when shearing forces of the distal nail plate produce dyshesion of the plate from the nailbed. Uncut nails, dorsiflexion of the toes in the shoe, and short, narrow toe boxes in running shoes may predispose the runner to this disorder. The runner characteristically has minimal symptoms and after removing his or her shoes will notice blood on the socks. The pooled blood under the great toenail can elevate the nail plate from the nailbed.

Proper nail hygiene and a shoe with a wide toe box can prevent this disorder. Draining the blood acutely can preserve the nail plate and provide pain relief. A disposable electrocautery probe or an 18-gauge needle can be gently inserted into the nail plate on the dorsal surface to relieve pressure.[9] Proper shoes will allow for foot expansion and toe dorsiflexion; the shoe should be at least 2 cm longer than the length of the foot. Fitting the shoe at night, after normal daily expansion, will also help guarantee a proper fit.

INFECTION

Plantar Warts

Plantar warts (Fig. 21–5) are a common viral infection found on pressure points of the toes, metatarsal heads,

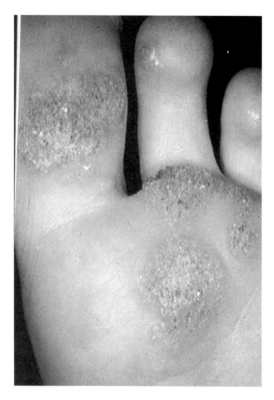

Figure 21–5. Plantar warts.

and heels. Recognition of small black dots of thrombosed capillaries within a hyperkeratotic plaque confirms the diagnosis. The papules will coalesce and commonly form a mosaic pattern on the sole of the foot. The thrombosed capillaries within the lesion differentiate it from the translucent core of the corn and the normal skin markings of a callus. The warts most commonly occur after exposure of the foot to the virus in locker rooms and public bathing areas.[10]

Asymptomatic lesions may disappear spontaneously. The goal of therapy is to ablate the virus through the epidermal layer without producing a scar. A conservative approach using 40% topical salicylic acid for 1 week, followed by salicylic acid-lactic acid compound applied diligently, may allow the runner to continue training during therapy. Other therapeutic options include cryosurgery, laser surgery, electrodessication, and curettage, which may lead to increased morbidity. Moleskin with a donut cutout placed over the wart will help relieve tenderness on ambulation and exercise. Using shower shoes and 20% aluminum chloride may prevent further infection.

Tinea

Tinea (Figs. 21–6 and 21–7) is a superficial fungal infection caused by dermatophytes and labeled by the specific portion of the body where it is most commonly

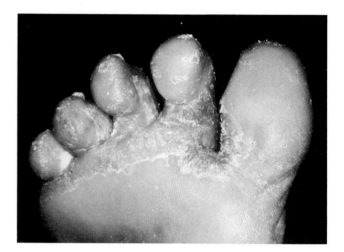

Figure 21–6. Tinea pedis.

found. These fungi are transmitted from person to person through fomites living in the warm, humid environments commonly found in communal bathing facilities.[11] The intertriginous areas (cruris), feet (pedis), and body (corporis) are predisposed to infection due to chronic perspiration, which produces maceration from occlusive footwear and clothes. Tinea cruris, or "jock itch," is a pruritic, scaling, erythematous plaque with sharply demarcated margins found on the inner thighs and usually sparing the scrotum in males. If the scrotum is involved, then candidiasis or moniliasis (yeast infection with satellite lesions) is the diagnosis and can be treated with topical nystatin or imadazole creams. Tinea pedis, or "athlete's foot," is a macerated red area with opaque white scales located in the third or fourth toe-web spaces or along the arch of the foot. A moccasin-type distribution of white scales may be

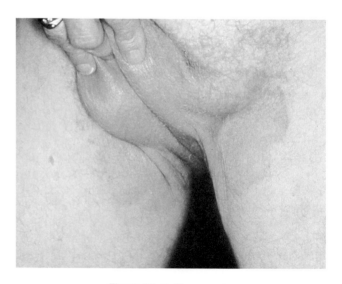

Figure 21–7. Tinea cruris.

seen along the lateral foot and heel in severe cases. Tinea corpora are small to large, erythematous, sharply demarcated plaques usually found on the neck and extremities. Tinea infections are confirmed when a skin scraping on a potassium hydroxide (KOH) slide exhibits septated hyphae or mycelia.

Primary prevention for the runner consists of using over-the-counter antifungal powders, avoiding constrictive clothing, proper air-drying of footwear, and immediate showering after exercise. Topical application of imidazole (clotrimazole, miconazole, ketoconazole) creams twice a day for 10 to 14 days will usually relieve the pruritus and clear the infection. For severe cases, either oral griseofulvin, 250 mg twice a day for 6 weeks, or oral terbinafine (Lamisil), 250 mg every day for the first week of 4 consecutive months, are most effective.[8]

Onychomycosis

Tinea unguium is the most common form of onychomycosis (Fig. 21–8). The dermatophyte infection of the nail plate manifests as an irregular thickening with a brownish yellow discoloration. Onychomycosis can be attributed to yeast or *Candida* species. As the condition worsens, the nail thickens, becomes more convex, furrowed, and ultimately brittle, and develops into a horny mass. All these changes result in an increased mechanical stress along the lateral edges of the nailbed that favor formation of ingrown toenails and paronychia. The diagnosis can be made by either a KOH preparation positive for hyphae of the nail plate or culture of the nail.

Treatment with topical antifungal agents is totally ineffective. Griseofulvin and ketoconazole are alternative therapeutic agents, but they carry the risk of liver toxicity. The mainstay of therapy is oral terbinafine (Lamisil) or itraconazole (Sporanox). The usual dose is 250 mg daily for Lamisil, or 200 to 400 mg daily, for the first week of 4 consecutive months, for Sporanox.[5]

Tinea Versicolor

Tinea versicolor (Fig. 21–9) is a chronic, asymptomatic fungal infection with either hypopigmented (white) or hyperpigmented (brown) macules located on the trunk, neck, and upper extremities. The diagnosis can be made either with a Wood's lamp, revealing yellow-green fluorescence of the skin scales, or with the characteristic "spaghetti and meatballs" of hyphae and spores on a KOH microscopic preparation. The condition is due to yeast, *Pityrosporum orbiculare*, found on the normal skin flora; the active form of the fungus is *Malassezia furfur*. It is not known whether the disorder is contagious. Increased sebaceous activity in environments with excessive heat and humidity predisposes the skin to fungus.

Treatment options vary with the extent of skin involvement. Mild or moderate rashes can be treated with selenium sulfide 2.5% shampoo (Selsun) for 30 minutes for 10 days, or the lotion may be applied once a week overnight for 4 consecutive weeks. In more severe forms, oral ketoconazole 200 mg daily for 15 days or one 400-mg dose once a month may be used, with close follow-up. After taking the ketoconazole, the patient should exercise and allow the sweat to dry on the skin overnight prior to showering. Griseofulvin is not effective against tinea versicolor. Encourage the runner to continue normal training to allow for the drug to collect in the sweat and act as a topical preparation over the skin lesions.[12]

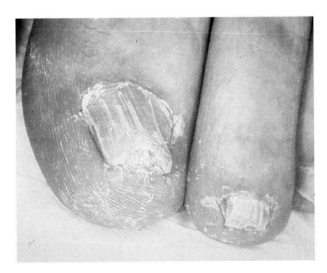

Figure 21–8. Onychomycosis.

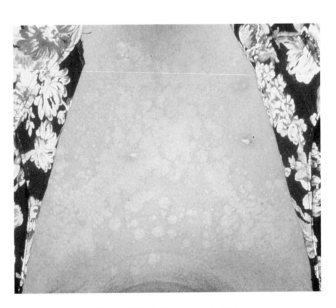

Figure 21–9. Tinea versicolor.

Acne

Acne vulgaris is a common skin disorder, especially among adolescents. Running may exacerbate or worsen an already existing form of the condition if proper hygiene is not judiciously performed.[5] Acne is characterized by inflammation and hyperkeratinization of the pilosebaceous unit. Excess formation of sebum and proliferation of the bacterium *Propionibacterium acnes* on the skin produce comedones. Acne is graded as mild, moderate, or severe based on the number and predominant type of lesions present. *Acne mechanica* is more commonly exhibited in runners wearing occlusive, tight-fitting clothing (nylon tights or spandex) with poor ventilation; this type of clothing is usually worn in cold weather.

Treatment is based on the grade of acne. In mild forms of the disease, topical benzoyl peroxide in 2.5%, 5%, or 10% gels can be applied twice a day to induce drying and peeling of the skin. A keratolytic agent, tretinoin (Retin-A), in various strengths and bases can be applied at night in combination with the benzoyl peroxide gels. The runner must be informed that dryness, redness, and photosensitivity from sun exposure can occur with these agents. Moderate acne with more erythematous papules requires the use of topical antibiotics such as clindamycin (Cleocin T) or erythromycin (A/T/S, EryDerm, T-Stat). If no improvement is seen and if pustules are present, then the use of oral antibiotics is warranted. A common oral agent is tetracycline 250 to 500 mg twice a day. The runner must be instructed to take the medication on an empty stomach to increase intestinal absorption and to avoid direct sunlight so as not to develop a photosensitivity reaction. Erythromycin can be taken with food in similar doses to decrease the inflammatory lesions. Minocycline or doxycycline, 50 to 100 mg twice a day, is another alternative but is more expensive than tetracycline. The use of isotretinoin (Accutane) is reserved for the most severe cystic forms of acne. All sexually active female runners need to be warned of the teratogenic potential of all retinoids, including isotretinoin, and they should be placed on oral contraceptives 1 month prior to starting the medication after obtaining a negative pregnancy test. Muscle and joint pain, as well as lethargy and fatigue, have been described as side effects of oral isotretinoin, which may inhibit the performance of some runners.[13]

Folliculitis

Folliculitis usually appears in the groin or on the legs of runners. *Staphylococcus* folliculitis produces small pustules at individual hair follicles due to irritation from nylon mesh clothing rubbing on the skin. In superficial folliculitis, a painless or tender red papule

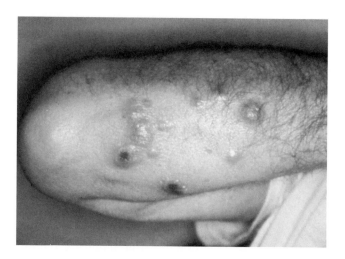

Figure 21–10. Furunculosis.

or pustule may manifest after irritation, injury, or abrasion.

The rash may subside spontaneously with only topical antibiotics such as mupirocin or bacitracin ointments. More severe cases will require wet Burow solution compresses applied three times a day and oral antibiotics (erythromycin, dicloxacillin, cephalexin) for 10 to 14 days.

Furunculosis

A furuncle, painful boil, or loculated abscess (Fig. 21–10) may appear in areas of friction on the buttocks, thighs, groin, axilla, and waist. Occlusive clothing over these areas in a runner with hyperhidrosis encourages bacterial overgrowth of *Staphylococcus aureus, Escherichia coli, Lactobacillus, Pseudomonas aeruginosa,* and *Peptostreptococcus* species. The athlete will often have comedones and moderate acne in the same areas, which suggests a diagnosis of hidradenitis suppurativa. Multiple furuncles may coalesce into a carbuncle.

Treatment consists of incision and drainage with culture of the pustular center. The mainstays of antibiotic therapy include dicloxacillin and erythromycin. Recurrent episodes of furunculosis can be treated with entire body scrubs using Betadine, Hibiclens, or pHisoHex soaps. A daily prophylatic dose of rifampin, 600 mg daily for 7 to 10 days, can be utilized for resistant cases.

Molluscum Contagiosum

Molluscum contagiosum (Fig. 21–11) is a highly contagious viral infection caused by a poxvirus. The lesions are discrete, skin-colored papules with an umbilicated center. They are usually found on the neck, thighs, groin, and trunk. Molluscum contagiosum is transmitted by direct person-to-person contact.

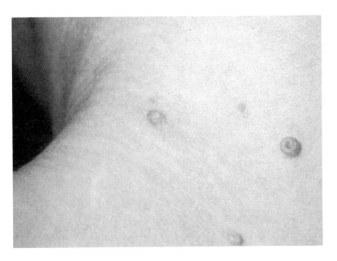

Figure 21–11. Molluscum contagiosum.

Treatment consists of simple curettage without local anesthesia if only a few papules persist. Cryosurgery can be offered using a liquid nitrogen applicator for a period of 5 to 10 seconds until a 1-mm halo develops around the lesion. Alternative therapies include use of cantharidin 0.7% applied over the papule and electrocautery or laser surgery for more extensive disease.

Erythrasma

Erythrasma (Fig. 21–12) is a bacterial (*Corynebacterium minutissimum*) infection involving the intertriginous areas of the inguinal folds and axilla. The examination reveals a well-demarcated reddish brown, scaly plaque that often resembles tinea cruris. When viewed with a Wood's lamp, erythrasma will fluoresce a coral-red compared with tinea cruris, which will not fluoresce.

Treatment consists of either oral erythromycin, 250 mg four times a day for 2 weeks or topical erythromycin twice a day for 2 weeks.

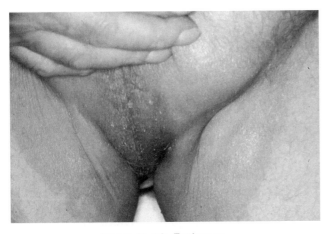

Figure 21–12. Erythrasma.

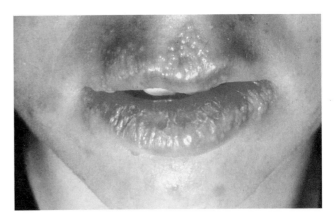

Figure 21–13. Herpes labialis.

Herpes Simplex

Herpes simplex virus (Fig. 21–13) presents as a painful group of small vesicles on a red base. The lesions are described as primary (first occurrence) or secondary (latent, recurrent) and labeled by their location on the oral-labial or genital areas of the body. Local trauma, sun exposure, chapping, menses, or fatigue may predispose the runner to a recurrence of this virus. The diagnosis is confirmed by either a viral culture or a Tzanck preparation that reveals multinucleate giant epidermal cells.

Current treatment guidelines recommend the use of acyclovir (Zovirax), famciclovir (Famvir), or valacyclovir (Valtrex). The first episode is treated with oral acyclovir, 200 mg five times a day for 7 to 10 days. Recurrent herpes simplex within 2 days of onset may benefit from oral acyclovir, 400 mg three times a day for 5 days. Daily suppressive therapy with acyclovir, 400 mg twice a day for 1 year, can be effective if the runner has had more than six recurrences. The runner must also use sunscreen and zinc oxide on the lips, wear a hat, and avoid the midday sun.

IRRITATIONS

Jogger's Nipple

Jogger's nipple is a painful irritation from friction of coarse, cotton fabrics rubbing against the breast nipple. The condition most commonly occurs in male marathon runners and triathletes, but it may even occur in women who wear padded support bras.[14] The nipple appears red, dry, scaly, and abraded by repeated irritation. The runner will often relate blood stains the size of a quarter on clothing after competition or training.

Multiple home remedies to reduce irritation include the use of Band-Aids or tape over the nipple, application of two coats of clear fingernail polish, or the use of small, round electrocardiographic lead pads over the areola. Runners are instructed to wear loose nylon or silk shirts and if irritation develops to apply lotions such as Lac-Hydrin twice a day.

Runner's Rump

Runner's rump is a hyperpigmented area in the superior portion of the gluteal cleft in marathon and ultra-marathon runners.[14] The condition is caused by continual contact/friction between the sides of the buttocks during the running stride. It is frequently diagnosed by presentation of gluteal ecchymosis at the sacral cleft in serious long distance runners.

The runner needs to be reassured that the skin changes will resolve with a temporary decrease in running and that aerobic conditioning can be achieved with alternative exercise. However, the runner may develop persistent post-inflammatory hyperpigmentation skin changes.

Dyshidrotic Eczema

Dyshidrotic eczema (pompholyx; Fig. 21–14) is a pruritic, vesicular eruption commonly found on the palms, fingers, and soles of the feet. Chronic infection results in more fissures, erosions, and scaling. The name implies an abnormality of sweating, but there is no dysfunction of the eccrine sweat glands. The etiology of this disorder is unknown. The differential diagnosis includes scabies, contact dermatitis, and dermatophytosis.

Treatment consists of cold, wet Burow's solution compresses, medium potency topical steroids, and oral erythromycin or dicloxicillin, 250 mg four times a day, to prevent a secondary bacterial infection in the chronic form of the disorder. The runner needs to be vigilant in wearing dry, clean white socks. A reduction in stress level, with changes in training and competition, may be effective.

Contact Dermatitis

Contact dermatitis is a localized reaction of the epidermis and dermis due to an external or allergic

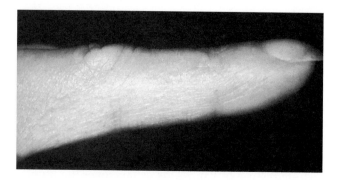

Figure 21–14. Dyshidrotic eczema.

irritant. The skin reveals patches of erythema, edema, and small vesicles with symptomatic burning and pruritus in the acute stage. Poison ivy, poison oak, rubber, sunscreens, nickel, and chromium may cause contact dermatitis. Allergy to the rubber in shoes and dyes in sportswear may produce a contact dermatitis.[2]

The primary prevention is avoidance of the irritant. Therapy includes medium- to high-potency topical steroids, cool wet Burow's solution dressings, antihistamines to control the pruritus, and a tapered dose of oral prednisone. If recurrence occurs without identifying the irritant, the runner may need to be evaluated by an allergist for patch testing.

Miliaria

Miliaria, commonly known as heat rash or prickly heat, occurs when sweat ducts or eccrine glands are occluded. During periods of excessive heat or exertion, an inflammatory response of erythema, papules, and vesicles occurs on the epidermis, and then the sweat ducts rupture into the surrounding tissues, producing a stinging or prickly sensation. Sparing of the palms and soles is a clue in making the diagnosis. This condition is more common in humid climates or during periods of heavy perspiration and may precede a heat injury.

Symptomatic relief may be obtained by removing the runner from the environment or avoiding humid, hot training periods. Hydrophilic ointments (Eucerin) and frequent changes of dry clothing can relieve symptoms by promoting sweating.

ENVIRONMENTAL EXPOSURES

Solar Urticaria

Solar urticaria is a sun-induced reaction to ultraviolet light that develops in minutes and disappears in an hour. Itching and burning are the first symptoms, followed by erythema and wheal formation on exposed skin. Skin that has not been exposed to the sun is more prone to developing this dermatitis, whereas tanned skin may not develop the condition.

Treatment includes use of sunblock, protective clothing, and gradual tanning while not training. The nonsedating antihistamines loratadine (Claritin) and fexofenadine (Allegra), used judiciously, can provide relief.

Cold Urticaria

Runners in cold climates may experience cold urticaria. A familial and acquired form of this condition exists. The urticarial reaction does not occur in the cold, but during the postexercise rewarming phase. The diagnosis can be confirmed by placing ice on the skin for 1 to 5 minutes and then noting whether wheals appear immediately on rewarming. The wheals usually occur only on the skin exposed to the cold.

Treatment includes avoiding cold, wearing protective clothing, and using cyproheptadine (Periactin), 2 mg once or twice a day, or doxepin (Sinequan), 10 mg two or three times daily.

Cholinergic Urticaria

Cholinergic urticaria is known as heat-induced or stress-induced urticaria. Distinctive round, red papular wheals are found during or shortly after exercise, heat, or emotional stress. The first symptoms are warmth, pruritus, and tingling of the skin followed by hives. The athlete will usually not experience systemic symptoms. The diagnosis can be made by having the runner perform 10 to 15 minutes of exercise on a bike or treadmill and then observing for the formation of hives.

The use of antihistamines may help some individuals, but avoiding heat and exercise may be the only relief for others. Hydroxyzine, 10 to 50 mg, may temporarily relieve the symptoms if given an hour prior to exercise.

Sunburn

Sunburn (Fig. 21–15) is very common among long-distance runners and is the most avoidable dermatitis. Sunburn varies in the acute presentation from mild erythema to intense blistering, edema, and pain. Long-term exposure to the sun leads to premalignant and malignant conditions. Sunburn most frequently develops in white or fair-skinned individuals.

Avoidance and common sense are the key to caring for this most preventable disease. Wearing sunscreen with a sun protection factor (SPF) greater than 15, protective white clothing, and not exercising in the sun between 10 AM and 2 PM are all measures to prevent sunburn. During excessive sweating, the sunscreen should be reapplied. During the acute phase, the individual should apply cool compresses or take frequent tepid showers. Nonsteroidal anti-inflammatory medications, bed rest, fluid replacement, and oral corticosteroids are also commonly used to decrease the inflammatory response.

Cold Injuries

Frostnip, chillblains (pernio), and frostbite (Fig. 21–16) characterize progressive changes to the skin from prolonged exposure to the cold. A cyclic physiological mechanism of vasoconstriction and vasodilation occurs to protect the acral regions of the body during prolonged cold exposure. The exposed surfaces of the body such as the face, ears, and shins will develop tender, erythematous nodules and papules. Frostnip develops over exposed areas, and the skin will appear firm, cold, and white. Days later, the skin will form blisters and peel. Both frostnip and pernio develop as the skin is exposed to temperatures below 50°F (10°C). Frostbite occurs as the tissue is cooled below 28°F. The thickness of frozen tissue determines the degree of frostbite. Initially the skin will be white and numb and display no vesicles. As the injury involves the dermis, the skin develops bullae with clear fluid. As the thickness of the injury increases, the skin develops hemorrhagic bullae and sloughs. Full-thickness frostbite displays the black carapace of gangrene.

The treatment of any type of cold injury is to evacuate the person expeditiously and prevent any further possibility of tissue injury due to refreezing. The affected areas need to be rewarmed with appropriately monitored water temperatures.[10] Runners should wear dry insulated clothing protecting the face and distal extremities. Properly layered clothing decreases the risk of cold exposure.

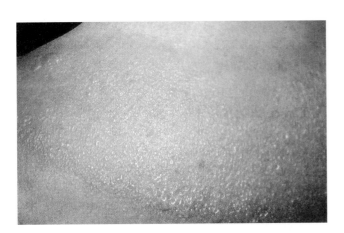

Figure 21–15. Sunburn.

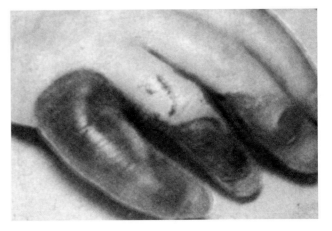

Figure 21–16. Frostbite.

CONCLUSIONS

The runner is prone to a diversity of dermatological disorders that can prevent the achievement of ultimate performance. These conditions are not specific to runners but are commonly found at all levels of athletic fitness. The runner deserves prompt diagnosis and treatment so as to return to the challenge within the sport of running.

REFERENCES

1. Bergfeld WF, Helm TN: The skin, in Strauss RH (ed.), *Sports Medicine*, 2nd ed., Toronto, WB Saunders, 1991:117.
2. Pharis DB, Teller C, Wolf JE: Cutaneous manifestations of sports participation. *J Am Acad Dermatol* 1997:36, 448.
3. Cortese TA, Fukayama K, Epstein WL, et al.: Treatment of friction blisters. *Arch Dermatol* 1968:97, 717.
4. Helm TN, Bergfeld WF: Sports dermatology. *Clin Dermatol* 1998:16, 159.
5. Crowe MA, Sorensen GW: Dermatologic problems in athletes, in Lillegard WA, Butcher JD, Rucker KS (eds.), *Handbook of Sports Medicine: A Symptom-Oriented Approach*, 2nd ed., Boston, Butterworth-Heinemann, 1999:367.
6. Shelly WB, Raunsley AM: Painful feet due to herniation of fat. *JAMA* 1968:205, 308.
7. Dover JS: Sports dermatology, in Fitzpatrick TB, Eisen AZ, Wolf K, et al. (eds.), *Dermatology in General Medicine*, New York, McGraw-Hill, 1991:1617.
8. Lillegard WA, Butcher JD, Fields KB: Dermatologic problems in athletes, in Fields KB, Fricker PA (eds.), *Medical Problems in Athletes*, Malden, Blackwell Science, 1997:234.
9. Kantor GR, Bergfeld WF: Common and uncommon dermatologic diseases related to sports activities. *Exerc Sport Sci Rev* 1988:16, 215.
10. Basler RS: Skin problems in athletes, in Mellion MS, Walsh WM, Shelton GL (eds.), *The Team Physician's Handbook*, 2nd ed., Philadelphia, Hanley & Belfus, 1997:341.
11. Ajello L, Getz ME: Recovery of dermatophytes from shoes and shower stalls. *J Invest Dermatol* 22:17–24, 1954.
12. Berger TG, Elias PM, Wintroub BU: *Manual of Therapy for Skin Disease*, New York, Churchill Livingstone, 1990.
13. Basler RSW: Sports-related skin injuries, in Callen JP, Dahl MV, Golitz LE, et al. (eds.), *Advances in Dermatology*, vol 4, Chicago, Year Book Medical Publishers, 1989:29.
14. Basler RS, Basler DL, Basler GC, et al.: Cutaneous injuries in women athletes. *Dermatol Nurs* 1998:10, 9.

Chapter 22

EXERCISE-INDUCED BRONCHOSPASM

C. Randall Clinch and
Koji D. Nishimura

DEFINITION

Exercise-induced bronchospasm (EIB) is the occurrence of acute airflow obstruction, typically following vigorous physical exertion. Classic symptoms, including dyspnea, cough, wheezing, chest tightness, fatigue, and/or chest pain, occur 5 to 20 min after exercise. Symptoms resolve over a 20- to 60-minute period following the cessation of exercise. Exercise-induced bronchospasm has been described by a variety of terms, including exercise-induced bronchoconstriction, exercise-induced airway narrowing, and exercise-induced asthma. Exercise-induced asthma is the least appropriate of these descriptors, because exercise does not induce the medical condition of asthma, and confusion between the diagnosis of exercise-induced anaphylaxis may result when using the abbreviation "EIA."

EPIDEMIOLOGY

EIB is the most common exercise-related pulmonary syndrome in the athlete. It occurs in up to 90% of asthmatics[1] and 35% to 40% of individuals with allergic rhinitis.[2] These are significant numbers given the self-reported prevalence rate for asthma in the United States of 13.7 million individuals.[3]

EIB can present at any age, but it is predominantly a disorder of children and young adults due to the increased levels of physical activity in these populations. Of United States athletes participating in the 1996 Summer Olympic Games in Atlanta, 117 out of 699 athletes (16.7%) had a history of asthma, took asthma medications, or both. Sixty-seven out of 597 athletes (11.2%) participating in the 1984 United States Summer Olympic Games in Los Angeles were described as having EIB. Thirty-five athletes in the 1996 and 41 athletes in the 1984 Summer Olympic Games won medals despite the diagnosis of asthma or EIB,[4,5] indicating the high level of performance attainable with these diagnoses.

The prevalence of EIB in middle-school, high-school, and collegiate athletes is poorly defined, varying according to the clinical definition of EIB and the study methodology. The prevalence of EIB in these athletes varies from 2.8% to 44%.[6–11]

PATHOPHYSIOLOGY

The chain of events leading to bronchoconstriction following exercise is multifactorial. Proposed mechanisms include hyperventilation, respiratory heat exchange within the airways, respiratory water loss, chemical mediator release, and rebound rewarming of the airways.[12] An understanding of these factors will enhance the management of EIB.

Hyperventilation

Vigorous exercise, which induces a four- to eightfold increase in pulmonary ventilation (tidal volume × respiratory rate), favors mouth breathing over nasal breathing. The typically effective air warming and humidification associated with nasal breathing is therefore reduced, forcing the deeper airways to warm and humidify the incoming air.

Voluntary hyperventilation under similar conditions of temperature and humidity produces identical degrees of bronchoconstriction, airway cooling, and response of the airways to various medications as does exercise-induced hyperventilation.[13,14] The specific sporting event is not as important as the degree of hyperventilation it produces in a given athlete and the environmental conditions under which sports participation occurs (e.g., cold, dry climate). Therefore exercise alone is insufficient to explain an episode of EIB. Rather, it is the recruitment of larger proportions of the airways to participate in heat exchange, the climatic/environmental conditions under which the exercise is performed, and the baseline irritability of an asthmatic's airways that influence the manifestation of EIB.

Respiratory Heat Exchange

A cold, dry environment is the most asthmogenic condition for exercise. Inspiration of cold air leads to greater convective heat loss from the airways. The colder the inspired air, the greater the respiratory heat exchange and the greater the resulting bronchoconstriction.[13] Inspiration of dry air leads to greater evaporative heat losses. The mechanisms of respiratory heat exchange are identical in asthmatic and nonasthmatic athletes.[15] The increased degree of baseline airway irritability in the asthmatic athlete, however, leads to greater bronchoconstriction.

Rebound Airway Rewarming

Rapid rewarming (reactive hyperemia) of the airways upon cessation of exercise leads to additional airflow obstruction.[16] Blood vessels in the airways play a major role in this process. Inhalation of a vasoconstrictor leads to a decrease in the mucosal blood supply, which has been demonstrated to cause a decrease in the reactive hyperemia and resultant bronchospasm.[17]

Additional Factors

An increase in the osmolarity of respiratory airway surface fluid, resulting from airway dehydration caused by hyperventilation, has been considered a cause of EIB. Studies in asthmatic and nonasthmatic individuals suggest, however, that major osmolar changes do not occur during hyperventilation either induced voluntarily or during exercise.[16] A variety of chemical mediators released from mast cells (including histamine and leukotrienes, among others) have been implicated in the pathophysiology of EIB. Controversy exists, however, as to the impact of these mediators on the development of bronchospasm. A typical mediator effect is difficult to accept as a cause of EIB given that the inhalation of either cold or warmed humidified air following the cessation of exercise can impact the bronchospastic response.[13] Other factors considered include a reflex lower airway bronchoconstriction from irritation of the upper airways, viral respiratory infections, airborne allergens and pollutants, stress, and overtraining.[18]

EVALUATION

Exercise-induced bronchospasm is often undiagnosed among all levels of athletes. An athlete's performance may be limited by undiagnosed symptoms of EIB. They may appear winded despite adequate conditioning or exhibit a cough noted by others on the field or in the locker room following practice. Typical symptoms of EIB are listed in Table 22–1. The preparticipation physical examination should allow for assessing risk factors for EIB. A remote history of asthma, wheezing, or atopy, and/or residence in an impoverished area have been shown to be significantly associated with the presence of EIB.[6,19] Historical risk factors are listed in Table 22–2.

Atopy, the genetically determined state of hypersensitivity to environmental allergens,[20] and type of sporting event have been demonstrated to be significant risk factors for EIB.[19] Atopy, as assessed by skin prick testing, was associated with increased bronchial responsiveness. The type of sporting event plays a role in the type of environmental allergens to which an atopic athlete is exposed and the duration of that exposure. As noted in the study of Helenius and

---

TABLE 22–1. TYPICAL SYMPTOMS OF EIB

Wheezing
Dyspnea
Chest tightness
Cough ("locker room coughing")
Winded sensation/appearance despite adequate
    conditioning
Excessive fatigue following exercise
Poor tolerance for prolonged exercise

TABLE 22–2. HISTORICAL RISK FACTORS FOR EXERCISE-INDUCED BRONCHOSPASM

Current or past history of asthma
Current or past history of wheezing
Current of past history of allergic rhinitis
History of atopy
Symptoms following strenuous exertion (dyspnea, wheeze, cough, chest tightness)
Medication use:
  Inhaled bronchodilators (short- or long-acting beta₂ agonists)
  Inhaled steroids or other inhaled anti-inflammatory agents
  Oral asthma medications (theophyllines, leukotriene receptor antagonists [Zafirlukast, Montelukast], 5-lipoxygenase inhibitors [Zileuton], beta₂ agonists, Nedocromil, corticosteroids)
  Antihistamine use (sedating or nonsedating)
History of allergy shots (immunotherapy) for environmental allergens
History of being restricted from sports participation secondary to above-mentioned symptoms

TABLE 22–3. DIFFERENTIAL DIAGNOSTIC POSSIBILITIES FOR EIB

Pulmonary conditions:
  Asthma (potentially unrecognized or undertreated)
  Acute/chronic pulmonary infectious process
  Laryngotracheobronchitis (croup)
  Cystic fibrosis
Cardiac conditions:
  Cardiac valvular defects
  Congestive heart failure
Other:
  Vocal cord dysfunction
  Gastroesophageal reflux disease
  Exercise-induced anaphylaxis
  Medication side effects (ACE inhibitor, beta blocker)

colleagues,[19] atopic speed/power athletes (limited exposures) had a relative risk for current or previously diagnosed asthma 25-fold greater than control subjects, whereas atopic long-distance runners exhibited a 42-fold relative risk and atopic swimmers a 97-fold relative risk.

The presenting symptoms of EIB are often nonspecific. The diagnosis can be confirmed through a history consistent with the onset of typical symptoms following vigorous exercise and the spontaneous resolution of symptoms over a 60-minute period following cessation of exercise. Objectively, a fall in the forced expiratory volume in 1 second (FEV_1) of 10% to 15% or a fall in the peak expiratory flow (PEF) rate of 10% to 25% from the pre-exercise baseline is considered diagnostic of EIB.[6,21,22] Please refer to Chapter 10 for a thorough review of the diagnostic testing related to EIB. The differential diagnosis of EIB is presented in Table 22–3. It is important to recognize when an athlete has symptoms that are not consistent with those typical for EIB, because a complete diagnostic evaluation should be pursued to identify the underlying medical condition.

Asthma is not synonymous with EIB. As mentioned previously, up to 90% of chronic asthmatics will experience EIB; however, EIB exists alone in some individuals with no other symptoms of asthma. A thorough history should be obtained from all athletes with suspected EIB to rule out underlying asthma. *The Practical Guide for the Diagnosis and Management of Asthma* (NIH Publication No. 97-4053) is a useful reference.

Gastroesophageal reflux disease (GERD) may also present with coughing and/or wheezing. However,

EIB is not associated with the retrosternal burning, acidic taste, or nonexertional symptoms associated with GERD. Asthma and GERD often coexist with up to 80% of asthmatics having an abnormal lower esophageal sphincter.[23,24] The athlete with symptoms suggestive of EIB and GERD should be evaluated for the presence of underlying asthma.

The athlete with an acute pulmonary infection may manifest some of the symptoms of EIB. Along with signs of acute infection (i.e., fever, productive cough), there should not be the typical resolution of symptoms within approximately 60 minutes following exertion. A chronic pulmonary process, infectious or otherwise, may be aggravated by the hyperventilation associated with strenuous exertion. However, there are likely to be other clinical signs and symptoms including cough unrelated to exercise, dyspnea, weight loss, hemoptysis, and/or sputum production.

Cardiac valvular defects with or without congestive heart failure may present with cough and/or "cardiac wheezing" from the presence of pulmonary edema. Symptoms related to cardiac conditions will not be limited to the period following exertion or resolve spontaneously, as with EIB. In all of these instances, again, the athlete requires a detailed history and evaluation due to the presence of symptoms atypical for EIB.

Vocal cord dysfunction resulting from abnormal adduction of the vocal cords can mimic EIB. Patients with vocal cord dysfunction may experience airflow obstruction sufficient to produce wheezing, chest tightness, dyspnea, and cough related to exercise. Additional symptoms may include throat tightness, a change in the quality of the voice, inspiratory stridor, and the abrupt onset and resolution of symptoms.[25,26] The diagnosis of vocal cord dysfunction is made with the use of flexible fiberoptic rhinolaryngoscopy while the patient is symptomatic, documenting the abnormal adduction of the cords upon inspiration. Accurate diagnosis is mandatory because management is dramatically different from that of EIB; speech therapy, breathing exercises, hypnosis, biofeedback, and psychotherapy have been utilized in the management of vocal cord dysfunction.[25,26]

Athletes often experience a "refractory period" of 2 to 4 hours following an episode of EIB, when subsequent strenuous exertion does not precipitate a fall in the FEV_1. Awareness of this phenomenon is an important aspect of patient education because the airways are "refractory" to bronchospasm with additional exercise but are still susceptible to other stimuli. A "late phase" period of bronchoconstriction has been described,[27] but controversy remains as to the possibility of it reflecting poor control of the athlete's underlying asthma.[18]

THERAPY

The therapy of EIB focuses on nonpharmacologic interventions, medications to prevent episodes of exercised-induced bronchospasm, and the control of any underlying asthma. The choice of medications used to treat EIB depends on the duration of exercise and the severity of the symptoms. An algorithm for the evaluation and treatment of EIB is presented in Fig. 22–1.

Nonpharmacologic Therapy

Nonpharmacologic interventions include short repeated warm-ups, generally consisting of five to eight short (30-second) runs with 1.5-minute rests between bouts of exercise,[28,29] a continuous warm-up (15 minutes of running at 60% $\dot{V}O_2max$),[28] gradual cool-downs,

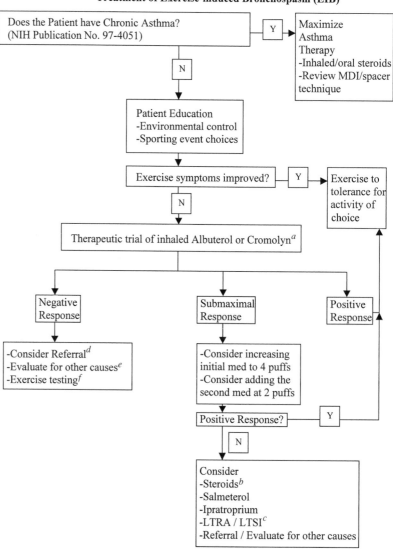

Figure 22–1. Treatment of Exercise-Induced Bronchospasm.
[a]Initial therapeutic options include 2 puffs of inhaled albuterol via a metered-dose inhaler with a spacer device, 15 to 30 minutes prior to the onset of exercise.
[b]Consider inhaled steroids if possible for the athlete; some may require oral steroids acutely or chronically (see Table 22–6 for USOC/NCAA-approved medications).
[c]LTRA, leukotriene receptor antagonist (montelukast [Singulair], zafirlukast [Accolate], etc.); LTSI, leukotriene synthesis inhibitor (zileuton [Zyflo]).
[d]Consider referral based on likely diagnostic possibilities (i.e., pulmonologist, cardiologist, allergist, gastroenterologist, etc.).
[e]See Table 22–3 for differential diagnostic possibilities for EIB.
[f]See Chapter 10 for a thorough review of exercise testing for EIB.

TABLE 22–4. SPORTING EVENT AS RISK FACTOR FOR EXERCISE-INDUCED BRONCHOSPASM

Level of Risk	Sporting Event
High-risk sports:[a]	Cross-country skiing
	Ice skating
	Ice hockey
	Basketball
	Running (middle- to long-distance)
	Soccer
	Cycling
	Rowing
Low-risk sports:[b]	Running sprints
	Football
	Tennis
	Volleyball
	Indoor swimming
	Gymnastics
	Baseball
	Riflery
	Archery
	Weightlifting

[a]High-risk sports are those requiring continuous exertion at a high percentage of aerobic capacity.
[b]Low-risk sports are those requiring only intermittent exertions at a low percentage of aerobic capacity.
Source: Modified with permission from Fuentes et al.[30]

and counseling as to what sports might expose the athlete to higher-risk conditions (Table 22–4).[30]

A customized aerobic exercise program for the asthmatic athlete can also improve cardiac output and muscle tissue oxygen transport at lower levels of hyperventilation, thereby increasing the amount of exercise an athlete can perform before onset of EIB symptoms.[30] Other options include use of a face mask to increase warmth and humidity of inspired air and counseling as to which sporting events place the athlete at increased risk for exposure to cold, dry air (Table 22–4). Despite the use of the above measures, most athletes will require medication to eliminate or attenuate episodes of EIB.

First-Line Medical Therapies (Table 22–5)

Beta$_2$ agonists have an 80% to 90% protective effect against exercise-induced symptoms and are first-line agents due to their rapid onset, ease of use, and availability. They exert their effects by causing relaxation of bronchial smooth muscle and bronchodilation of the airway.

Short-acting agents, such as albuterol (Proventil, Ventolin) are first-line medications for EIB. Albuterol is dosed as two puffs 15 to 30 minutes before exercise and its effects last up to 4 hours. Other useful short-acting agents include terbutaline (Brethaire, Bricanyl), pirbuterol (Maxair), or bitolterol (Tornalate). These agents are highly beta$_2$ selective, yielding fewer cardiovascular

side effects, and have a longer duration of action than the other agents listed in Table 22–5.[18] For athletes unable to use inhaled therapy, oral albuterol is an alternative. In this form, however, albuterol exhibits decreased efficacy, a slower onset of action (30 min), and increased systemic side effects (tremor, tachycardia).[18] Terbutaline in oral form has not been shown to be effective in EIB.[31]

Long-acting beta$_2$ agonists have a slower onset of action, but their duration of up to 12 hours allows for intermittent or unscheduled bouts of exercise with continued protective effects. Salmeterol (Serevent) is dosed as two puffs 30 to 60 minutes prior to exercise. Tolerance to the protective effects of salmeterol on EIB has been seen with long-term use (twice daily for a month). A decreased duration of action (no effect seen at 6 to 9 hours) may occur with as little as 2 weeks of continued use.[32] Formoterol, not currently available in the United States, is another long-acting beta$_2$ agonist effective in the prevention of EIB.[33,34]

Other Therapies for EIB

The khellin derivatives, cromolyn (Intal) and nedocromil (Tilade), are short-acting nonbronchodilator agents used to prevent EIB with a duration of effect of 2 hours. Cromolyn and nedocromil are dosed as two puffs 10 to 60 minutes prior to exercise. Both agents are equally protective against EIB,[35] and are effective in up to 70% to 85% of patients with EIB.[12,18] These agents may be a first-line choice in those with allergic rhinitis.

Anticholinergic medications such as ipratropium (Atrovent) have been used for treatment of EIB[36]; however, effectiveness is shown to vary widely between studies and between participants within a given study.[18] Ipratropium is a quaternary ammonium short-acting bronchodilator with a duration of effect of 3 to 5 hours. It is dosed as two puffs 15 minutes prior to exercise and is often used in conjunction with a beta$_2$ agonist. Consider ipratropium if a patient does not exhibit a good response to inhaled beta$_2$ agonists or khellin derivatives.

Leukotrienes are involved in the asthmatic inflammatory response and recent interest in EIB management has focused on medications that attenuate their inflammatory effects.[37] Leukotriene receptor antagonists (montelukast, zafirlukast, pranlukast, and cinalukast) act to block the action of the leukotrienes on the CysLT1 receptor. Leukotriene synthesis inhibitors (zileutin) act to prevent the transformation of arachidonic acid by 5-lipoxygenase to the cysteinyl leukotrienes (LTA4, LTB4, LTC4, LTD4, and LTE4).

Daily treatment with montelukast (Singulair) is effective in protection against exercise-induced asthma, and tolerance with long-term use does not appear to

TABLE 22–5. INHALED MEDICATIONS FOR EXERCISE-INDUCED BRONCHOSPASM

Generic Name	Trade Names	Formulation	Available Inhaler	Manufacturer's Recommended Dose	Onset	Peak	Duration
Beta₂ Agonists							
Albuterol (salbutamol)	Proventil	MDI 90 μg/puff	17 g (200 puffs)	2 puffs 15 min before exercise, 2 puffs q 4–6 h or prn	<5 min	1–2 h	3–4 h
	Ventolin	MDI 90 μg/puff	17 g (200 puffs)	2 puffs 15 min before exercise, 2 puffs q 4–6 h or prn			
	Ventolin rotacaps	DPI 200 μg	100 caps	1 cap 15 min before exercise, 1 cap q 4–6 h or prn			
Bitolterol	Tornalate	MDI 370 μg/puff	16.4 g (300 puffs)	2–3 puffs prn, 2 puffs q 8 h	3–5 min	0.5–2 h	4–8 h
Isoetharine	Bronkometer	MDI 340 μg/puff	10 mL (200 puffs)	1–2 puffs q 4 h	5 min	5–15 min	1–4 h
Isoproterenol	Isuprel Medihaler-iso	MDI 131 μg/puff MDI 80 μg/puff	11.2 g (200 puffs)	1–2 puffs q 3–4 h	2–5 min	5–30 min	1 h
Isoproterenol w/phenylephrine	Duo-medihaler	MDI 160 μg/puff w/ 240 μg/puff phenylephrine			2–5 min	5–30 min	>1 h
Metaproterenol (orciprenaline sulfate)	Alupent Metaprel	MDI 650 μg/ puff MDI 650 μg/puff	14 g (200 puffs) 14 g (200 puffs)	2–3 puffs q 3–4 h 2–3 puffs q 3–4 h	1 min	<1 h	2–3 h
Pirbuterol	Maxair inhaler	MDI 200 μg/puff	25.6 g (300 puffs)	2 puffs q 4–6 h	5 min	30–60 min	5 h
	Maxair autohaler	Breath actuated MDI 200 μg/puff	14 g (400 puffs)	1–2 puffs q 4–6 h			
Salmeterol	Serevent	MDI 21 μg/puff	13 g (120 puffs)	2 puffs 30–60 min before exercise or 2 puffs q 12	10–30 min		12 h
Terbutaline	Brethaire	MDI 200 μg/puff	7.5 g (200 puffs)	2 puffs q 4–6 h	<5 min	1–2 h	3–4 h
Khellin Derivatives							
Cromolyn sodium (disodium cromoglycate)	Intal Intal spinhaler	MDI 800 μg/puff DPI 20 mg	14.2 g (200 puffs)	2 puffs 10–15 min before exercise			2 h 2 h
Nedocromil	Tilade	MDI 1.75 μg/puff	16.2 g (112 puffs)	2 puffs 4×/day			2 h
Anticholinergics							
Ipratropium bromide	Atrovent	MDI 18 μg/puff	14 g (200 puffs)	2 puffs 4×/day	15 min	1–2 h	3–4 h
Leukotriene Receptor Antagonists							
Montelukast	Singulair	5 mg chewable; 10 mg tablet		5 mg PO hs (age 6–14) 10 mg PO hs (adult)			
Zafirlukast	Accolate	20 mg tablet		20 mg PO bid (children 12 and over)			
Leukotriene synthesis inhibitor							
Zileutin	Zyflo	600 mg tablet		600 mg PO qid (children 12 and over)			

MDI, metered-dose inhaler; DPI, daily permissible intake.
Source: Modified with permission from Smith et al.[18]

occur.[38] The effectiveness of montelukast may be greater than that of salmeterol.[39] Montelukast is currently approved for use in children as young as 6 years old.

Zafirlukast (Accolate) has been shown to be effective in limiting EIB in children (6 to 14 years old) for 4 hours after a single oral dose[40]; the dose is taken 2 hours before exercise. Additionally, regular treatment with zafirlukast has been proven effective for at least 8 hours following regular dosing in adults.[41] Zafirlukast is approved for use in children 12 years of age and older.

Theophylline and aminophylline are methylxanthines of moderate potency used at times in the treatment of underlying refractory asthma. Because of the narrow therapeutic window between minimum effective serum concentration and toxic serum levels (10 to 20 μg/ml), serum levels must be monitored closely. With the advent of longer-acting inhaled beta$_2$ agonists, the uses of these medications are limited.

Systemic and inhaled glucocorticoids are mainstays of therapy for patients with chronic asthma. Patients with well-controlled chronic asthma have fewer EIB symptoms.[49] There is no immediate prophylactic benefit of glucocorticoids; 2 to 4 weeks of use are often necessary to obtain benefit.

Experimental Therapies for EIB

Nebulized heparin is effective in EIB prophylaxis.[42] In this form, heparin was more effective than cromolyn at preventing EIB. The effect is maximal when given 1 hour prior to exercise, and the duration is at least 3 hours.[43] Delivery of heparin to the lower respiratory tract is maximal at a concentration of 20,000 IU/ml with an airflow of 10 L/min.[44] When inhaled, the low-molecular-weight heparin Enoxaparin appears to be as potent, if not more so, than unfractionated heparin in preventing EIB.[45] Neither agent is considered a first-line medication and they are not readily available for dosing with a nebulizer. Use of these medications should only occur under the supervision of an asthma specialist.

Furosemide (Lasix) in inhaled form is as effective as cromolyn in preventing EIB in children (dosing, 10 mg/m^2 body area).[46] Furosemide (frusemide) given via metered dose inhaler and spacer (20 mg) is also effective against EIB in children.[47] The mechanism of action of inhaled furosemide remains unknown. Dosing with 30 mg of furosemide in children leads to a longer duration of action, but has a significant diuretic effect.[48] Like the nebulized heparins, nebulized furosemide is not a first-line agent or readily available.

Table 22–6 provides information regarding medications approved by the US Olympic Committee and the National Collegiate Athletic Association (NCAA).

SUMMARY

The symptoms of EIB are well characterized and recurrent, yet the disorder is underdiagnosed at all levels of competitive athletics. When the diagnosis of EIB is considered, carefully review the differential diagnosis for reversible or coexistent conditions and test for EIB if the clinical presentation is not obvious. Evaluate every patient for the presence of underlying chronic asthma and treat appropriately. Therapy for EIB will not be as effective if the patient has poorly managed chronic asthma. Most patients will benefit from a trial of an inhaled short-acting beta$_2$ agonist such as albuterol, 15 to 30 minutes prior to exercise. In those who don't respond adequately, consider increasing the dosage (as limited by side effects), substituting another inhaled first-line medication (Table 22–5), reconsidering your original diagnosis, and/or referring to an asthma specialist. Athletes with EIB can be expected to attain a high level of performance with recognition and proper management of this common condition.

REFERENCES

1. Joint Task Force on Practice Parameters, representing the American Academy of Allergy Asthma and Immunology, the American College of Allergy, Asthma and Immunology, and the Joint Council of Allergy, Asthma and Immunology. Practice parameters for the diagnosis and treatment of asthma. *J Allergy Clin Immunol* 1995:96, 714.
2. Committee on Sports Medicine and Fitness. American Academy of Pediatrics. Metered-dose inhalers for young athletes with exercise-induced asthma. *Pediatrics* 1994:94, 129.
3. Centers for Disease Control and Prevention: Surveillance for asthma—United States, 1960–1995. *Morbid Mortal Weekly Rep* 1998:47, 1.
4. Weiler JM, Layton T, Hunt M: Asthma in United States Olympic athletes who participated in the 1996 Summer Games. *J Allergy Clin Immunol* 1998:102, 722.
5. Voy RO: The U.S. Olympic Committee experience with exercise-induced bronchospasm, 1984. *Med Sci Sports Exerc* 1986:18, 328.
6. Kukafka DS, Lang DM, Porter S, et al.: Exercise-induced bronchospasm in high school athletes via a free running test. *Chest* 1998:114, 1613.

TABLE 22–6. APPROVED MEDICATIONS

US Olympic Committee (USOC)[a]	National Collegiate Athletic Association (NCAA)
Inhaled beta$_2$ agonists	
Albuterol	Most *inhaled* prescription
Terbutaline	therapies[b]
Salmeterol	
Inhaled corticosteroids	
Beclomethasone	Examine over-the-counter
Budesonide	preparations for prohibited
Dexamethasone	substances (e.g., ephedrine)
Flunisolide	
Fluticasone	
Triamcinolone	

[a]The USOC approves only the medications listed here with medical notification prior to competition.
[b]The NCAA does not approve oral beta$_2$ agonists.

7. Rice SG, Bierman CW, Shapiro GG, et al.: Identification of exercise-induced asthma among intercollegiate athletes. *Ann Allergy* 1985:55, 790.

8. Rupp NT, Brudno DS, Guill MF: The value of screening for risk of exercise-induced asthma in high school athletes. *Ann Allergy* 1993:70, 339.

9. Rupp NT, Guill MF, Brudno DS: Unrecognized exercise-induced bronchospasm in adolescent athletes. *Am J Dis Child* 1992:146, 941.

10. Huftel MA, Gaddy JN, Busse WM: Finding and managing asthma in competitive athletes. *J Respir Dis* 1991:12, 1110.

11. Feinstein FA, LaRussa J, Wand-Dohlman A, et al.: Screening adolescent athletes for exercise-induced asthma. *J Clin Sports Med* 1996:6, 119.

12. Wilkerson LA: Exercise-induced asthma. *J Am Osteopath Assoc* 1998:98, 211.

13. McFadden ER Jr: Exercise-induced airway narrowing, in *Allergy Principles and Practice,* Middleton E Jr, Yunginger JW, Reed CE, et al., (eds.), St. Louis, Mosby-Year Book, 1998:953.

14. Gilbert IA, Fouke JM, McFadden ER Jr: Intraairway thermodynamics during exercise and hyperventilation in asthmatics. *J Appl Physiol* 1988:64, 2167.

15. Gilbert IA, Fouke JM, McFadden ER Jr: Heat and water flux in the intrathoracic airways and exercise-induced asthma. *J Appl Physiol* 1987:63, 1681.

16. McFadden ER Jr, Lenner KA, Strohl KP: Post-exercise airway rewarming and thermally-induced asthma. *J Clin Invest* 1986:78, 18.

17. Gilbert IA, McFadden ER Jr: Airway cooling and rewarming: The second reaction sequence in exercise induced asthma. *J Clin Invest* 1992:90, 699.

18. Smith BW, LaBotz M: Pharmacologic treatment of exercise-induced asthma. *Clin Sports Med* 1998:17, 343.

19. Helenius IJ, Tikkanen HO, Sarna S, et al.: Asthma and increased bronchial responsiveness in elite athletes: Atopy and sport event as risk factors. *J Allergy Clin Immunol* 1998:101, 646.

20. *Stedman's Medical Dictionary.* 1999 on-line dictionary, Lippincott Williams & Wilkins, access date 11/15/99, URL: www.pdr.net.

21. Jones COH, Qureshi S, Rona RJ, et al.: Exercise-induced bronchoconstriction by ethnicity and presence of asthma in British nine year olds. *Thorax* 1996:51, 1134.

22. Hofstra WB, Sont JK, Sterk PJ, et al.: Sample size estimation in studies monitoring exercise-induced bronchoconstriction in asthmatic children. *Thorax* 1997:52, 739.

23. Simpson WG: Gastroesophageal reflux disease and asthma: Diagnosis and management. *Arch Intern Med* 1995:155, 798.

24. Mujica VR, Rao SSC: Recognizing atypical manifestations of GERD: Asthma, chest pain, and otolaryngologic disorders may be due to reflux. *Postgrad Med* 1999:105, 53.

25. Kayani S, Shannon DC: Vocal cord dysfunction associated with exercise in adolescent girls. *Chest* 1998:113, 540.

26. Landwher LP, Wood RP 2nd, Blager FB, et al.: Vocal cord dysfunction mimicking exercise-induced bronchospasm in adolescents. *Pediatrics* 1996:98, 971.

27. Chhabra SK, Ojha UC: Late asthmatic response in exercise-induced asthma. *Ann Allergy Asthma Immunol* 1998: 80, 323.

28. McKenzie DC, McLuckie SL, Stirling DR: The protective effects of continuous and interval exercise in athletes with exercise-induced asthma. *Med Sci Sports Exerc* 1994:26, 951.

29. de Bisschop C, Guenard H, Desnot P, et al.: Reduction of exercise-induced asthma in children by short, repeated warm ups. *Br J Sports Med* 1999:33, 100.

30. Fuentes RJ, DiMeo M: Exercise-induced asthma and the athlete, in *Athletic Drug Reference '99,* Fuentes RJ, (ed.), Durham, NC, Clean Data, Inc., 1999:225.

31. Fuglsang G, Hertz B, Holm EB: No protection by oral terbutaline against exercise-induced asthma in children: A dose-response study. *Eur Respir J* 1993:6, 527.

32. Nelson JA, Strauss L, Skowronski M, et al.: Effect of long-term salmeterol treatment on exercise-induced asthma. *N Engl J Med* 1998:339, 141.

33. Bartow RA: Formoterol. An update of its pharmacological properties and therapeutic efficacy in the management of asthma. *Drugs* 1998:55, 517.

34. Pauwels RA, Lofdahl CG, Postma DS, et al.: Effect of inhaled formoterol and budesonide on exacerbations of asthma. Formoterol and Corticosteroids Establishing Therapy (FACET) International Study Group. *N Engl J Med* 1997:337, 1405.

35. de Benedictis FM, Tuteri G, Pazzelli P, et al.: Cromolyn versus nedocromil: Duration of action in exercise-induced asthma in children. *J Allergy Clin Immunol* 1995:96, 510.

36. Corren J: The impact of allergic rhinitis on bronchial asthma. *J Allergy Clin Immunol* 1998:101, S352.

37. Rachelefsky G: Childhood asthma and allergic rhinitis: The role of leukotrienes. *J Pediatrics* 1997:131, 348.

38. Leff JA, Busse WW, Pearlman D, et al.: Montelukast, a leukotriene-receptor antagonist, for the treatment of mild asthma and exercise-induced bronchoconstriction. *N Engl J Med* 1998:339, 147.

39. Villaran C, O'Neill SJ, Helbling A, et al.: Montelukast versus salmeterol in patients with asthma and exercise-induced bronchoconstriction. *J Allergy Clin Immunol* 1999:104, 547.

40. Pearlman DS, Ostrom NK, Bronsky EA, et al.: The leukotriene D4-receptor antagonist zafirlukast attenuates exercise-induced bronchoconstriction in children. *J Pediatrics* 1999:134, 273.

41. Dessanges J, Prefaut C, Taytard A, et al.: The effect of zafirlukast on repetitive exercise-induced bronchoconstriction: The possible role of leukotrienes in exercise-induced refractoriness. *J Allergy Clin Immunol* 1999:104, 1155.

42. Ahmed T, Garrigo J, Danta I: Preventing bronchoconstriction in exercise-induced asthma with inhaled heparin [see comments]. *N Engl J Med* 1993:329, 90.

43. Garrigo J, Danta I, Ahmed T: Time course of the protective effect of inhaled heparin on exercise-induced asthma. *Am J Respir Crit Care Med* 1996:153, 1702.

44. Bendstrup KE, Newhouse MT, Pedersen OF, et al.: Characterization of heparin aerosols in jet and ultrasonic nebulizers. *J Aerosol Med* 1999:12, 17.

45. Ahmed T, Gonzalez BJ, Danta I: Prevention of exercise-induced bronchoconstriction by inhaled low-molecular-weight heparin. *Am J Respir Crit Care Med* 1999:160, 576.

46. Melo RE, Sole D, Naspitz CK: Comparative efficacy of inhaled furosemide and disodium cromoglycate in the treatment of exercise-induced asthma in children. *J Allergy Clin Immunol* 1997:99, 204.

47. Munyard P, Chung KF, Bush A: Inhaled frusemide and exercise-induced bronchoconstriction in children with asthma. *Thorax* 1995:50, 677.

48. Novembre E, Frongia G, Lombardi E, et al.: The preventive effect and duration of action of two doses of inhaled furosemide on exercise-induced asthma in children. *J Allergy Clin Immunol* 1995:96, 906.

49. Freezer NJ, Croasdell H, Doull IJ, et al.: The effect of regular inhaled beclomethasone on exercise and methacholine airway responses in school children with recurrent wheeze. *Eur Respir J* 1995:8, 1488.

Chapter 23

EVALUATION AND MANAGEMENT OF HEADACHE IN RUNNERS

Seth John Stankus

INTRODUCTION

Headache is one of the most common complaints prompting patients to seek medical attention. Epidemiologic data reveal that headache is most common in the adolescent and adult populations. Therefore, virtually all physicians caring for athletes will encounter this problem.

Athletes may present with a history of headaches that occur sporadically and are not necessarily associated with exercise. Others will present with headaches that are precipitated or exacerbated by exercise. In either case, headaches have the potential to limit athletic performance or cause the athlete to stop exercising completely until the headache has passed.

Headaches, particularly exercise-induced headaches, may be a manifestation of serious or even life-threatening intracranial or systemic disease. Physicians caring for athletes should have a clear understanding of how to accurately diagnose and manage this common problem. Additionally, the physician needs to identify patients in need of more extensive diagnostic testing or specialty consultation.

This chapter will review the basic epidemiology, pathophysiology, diagnosis, and treatment of headache with regard to the athletic population. Special emphasis will be placed on identifying dangerous

headaches. Throughout this chapter headache classification will be based on criteria developed and published by the Headache Classification Committee of the International Headache Society.[1] Although the treatment of headache must be individualized for each patient, general principles of treatment will be presented that should decrease the headache burden while producing the least impact on athletic performance. Caring for the athlete with headaches can be both challenging and gratifying. Athletes tend to be highly motivated to control their headaches and it is truly the unusual patient that does not benefit from our intervention.

PREVALENCE OF HEADACHE

Headache is common in the general as well as athletic populations. In the general population, the prevalence of migraine headache alone is 17.6% for women and 6% for men.[2] The widespread impact of headache is even more clearly demonstrated by the fact that 99% of all women and 93% of all men report at least one severe headache in their lifetime.[3]

There are clear differences in migraine prevalence among racial groups in the United States. Among women, Caucasians have the highest prevalence (20.4%)

295

followed by African-Americans (16.2%) and Asian-Americans (9.2%).[4] This is strongly suggestive of a genetic component. Additionally, as many as 70% of migraine patients report a family history of headache.[5] There is a stronger familial relationship in those patients that report an aura with their migraine headache than those that do not.

Headache is at least as common in athletes as it is in the general population. One study conducted on male and female distance runners revealed the overall prevalence of migraine headache to be 32.6%.[6] Despite the frequency of migraine headaches in this group, only 5% had sought medical attention. Another study conducted on university-aged medical students and physical education majors revealed a 35% prevalence of exercise-induced headache.[7] A second part of this study revealed that the majority of exercise-induced headaches were effort-related migraine headaches or tension-type headaches.[8]

Headaches can adversely impact athletic performance. As many as 36% of athletes report moderate to severe headaches.[6] Many of these patients require complete cessation of strenuous activity in addition to taking medication or going to sleep to alleviate their headaches. The apprehension over developing an exercise-induced headache may prevent the athlete from performing at his or her maximum capability. In addition to the impact of headache pain on athletic performance, many of the medications used to treat headache can produce somnolence or decreased exercise tolerance.

PATHOPHYSIOLOGY OF HEADACHE

The pathophysiology of headache is complex and differs among headache types. Among the various types of headache, the mechanisms involved in migraine headache have been the most widely investigated. The migraine process involves vasodilation of the intracranial and extracranial vasculature, neurogenic inflammation of perivascular structures, and activation of the trigeminal system. These changes are mediated through complex neurotransmitter systems primarily involving serotonin, norepinephrine, dopamine, and gamma-aminobutyric acid (GABA).

The factors that precipitate this cascade of pathologic changes are equally complex. As previously discussed, genetics clearly play a role in many patients. Additionally, migraine headaches are often associated with specific endogenous or exogenous triggers. Women with migraine headache often report an association between their menstrual cycle and headache frequency and/or severity. A hormonal influence is

TABLE 23–1. COMMON HEADACHE TRIGGERS

Diet:	Alcohol
	Nitrites/nitrates
	Monosodium glutamate
	Caffeine
	Chocolate
	Tyramine-containing foods
Hormonal:	Oral contraceptive pills
	Menses
	Hormone replacement therapy
	Pregnancy
Sleep:	Excessive sleep
	Sleep deprivation
Environmental:	Barometric changes
	Strong odors
	Bright light
Medications:	Nitroglycerin
	Hydralazine
	Histamine
Miscellaneous:	Fatigue
	Tobacco
	Hunger
	Stress

also suggested by the commonly observed increase in migraine headaches among women on oral contraceptives and in postmenopausal women on hormone replacement therapy. A list of common headache triggers is provided in Table 23–1.

The mechanisms involved in exercise-induced headaches are not as clearly understood. This is most likely true because exercise-induced headaches are a heterogeneous group. Exercise-induced headaches include migraine headache with and without aura, tension-type headache, benign exertional headaches, and headaches due to specific intracranial or systemic disease.

Cerebral oxygenation, and possibly perfusion, may be involved in exercise-induced headaches. This is supported by the observation that some athletes competing at high altitudes develop migrainous headaches that do not occur when they compete at sea level.[9] In such cases, the lower partial pressure of oxygen at higher elevations may produce a relative cerebral hypoxia. Exercise-related headaches have also been associated with cerebral infarction and myocardial ischemia.[10,11]

Although most exercise-induced headaches are benign, they can be an indicator of serious pathology. Up to 10% of patients with exertional headaches have an intracranial structural lesion as do as many as 25% of patients with cough- or Valsalva-induced headache.[12,13] These structural lesions include vascular malformations, benign and malignant neoplasms, prior cerebral contusions or infarctions, cerebral arterial dissections, or other structural abnormalities such as Chiari malformations. Other conditions that may be associated with exercise-induced headaches include severe hypertension, hypoglycemia, pheochromocytoma, cardiac ischemia or dysrhythmias, dehydration, and sinus disease. Many of the performance-enhancing drugs such as thermogenic aids and androgenic steroids can also produce headache.

COMMON HEADACHE TYPES

Migraine Headache

Migraine headache will likely be the most commonly encountered headache in athletes. Although migraine headaches are usually of moderate to severe intensity, migraine is defined by a set of characteristics that distinguish it from other headache types. A summary of characteristics that distinguish the most common types of headache encountered in the athlete is provided in Table 23–2.

Migraine headaches are generally unilateral and retro-orbital. However, patients often describe their headaches as they are at maximum intensity. Patients who describe their headaches as diffuse may actually have a unilateral onset. Even so, a diffuse headache does not exclude the diagnosis of migraine. Migraine headaches may vary in which side they occur in the same patient, but generally one side is predominant. Headaches that occur exclusively in one area should be explored for an underlying structural abnormality.

Migraine headaches reach maximum intensity from 20 minutes to a couple of hours. Rarely, migraines will be at maximum intensity at the onset or within a few minutes. These headaches have been termed *crash migraines*,[14] and may be mistaken for the headache of subarachnoid hemorrhage. Migraine headaches generally last between 4 and 72 hours.

The quality of migraine headache pain is usually dull and throbbing. This is due to the intracranial and extracranial vasodilation of neurogenic inflammation. A throbbing quality is not pathognomonic of migraine and may be seen in headaches associated with fever or intracranial neoplasms.

Because of the nausea and vomiting often associated with migraines, they are sometimes described as *sick headaches*. This phenomenon is likely secondary to associated meningeal irritation, brain stem activation, or possibly elevated intracranial pressure. Factors that normally increase intracranial pressure such as coughing, Valsalva's maneuver, or bending over generally increase the pain of migraine headache.

During migraine headaches patients often experience increased sensory perception which manifests as photophobia and phonophobia. Aversion to certain odors and especially to movement also occur. Generally, the patient with a migraine headache prefers to lie still in a dark, quiet location and tries to go to sleep. Sleep will often alleviate, or at least lessen, the headache. Clearly, the athlete with a migraine headache will not be able to perform at his or her expected level, if at all.

As mentioned previously, a minority of migraine headache patients will experience an aura. The aura is a neurologic symptom or sign generated by a focal area of neuronal dysfunction, and it manifests as a visual, motor, or sensory abnormality. The most common auras are visual such as scotomas, photopsias (brightly colored dots of light), or visual distortions. Visual

TABLE 23–2. SUMMARY OF HEADACHE CLASSIFICATION

Feature	Migraine Headache	Tension-Type Headache	Cluster Headache	Benign Exertional Headache
Location	Unilateral	Bilateral	Unilateral	Bilateral, often posterior
Duration	4–72 hr	30 min–7 days	15–180 min	5 min–24 hr
Quality	Dull, throbbing	Pressing, tightening	Constant, boring	Variable
Intensity	Moderate to severe	Mild to moderate	Severe	Variable
Nausea/vomiting	Usually present	No	May be present	No
Phonophobia and/or photophobia	Usually present	No	No	No
Aura	Sometimes	No	No	No
Unilateral lacrimation, nasal congestion, and scleral injection	No	No	Yes	No
Precipitated by exercise	Possible	Possible	No	Yes

Source: Adapted from International Headache Society.[1]

auras generally occur in a hemianoptic distribution. Other manifestations of aura include focal weakness or hemiparesis, paresthesias, numbness, or even brain stem dysfunction. The aura will either precede the headache or occur concurrently with it. The aura usually does not last longer than 60 minutes.

Tension-Type Headache

Overall, tension-type headache may be the most common headache; however, the intensity is generally less than that of other types of headache. Therefore, many patients treat these headaches with over-the-counter medications and never seek medical advice. It is probably the rare person that has never experienced a tension-type headache at some time.

Tension-type headaches tend to be diffuse. The pain may begin posteriorly around the suboccipital and high cervical regions or over the vertex. The headache will generally become bilateral and may be described as a band-like pressure around the head. The headache tends to be constant rather than throbbing, although a throbbing quality may be present when the headache is at its peak intensity.

The associated features of migraine headache are notably absent with tension-type headaches. There will be no prodrome or aura, and the patient does not complain of nausea or vomiting. Mild-to-moderate phonophobia or photophobia may be present, but not both. Strenuous activity may need to be limited but rarely stopped altogether.

The onset of tension-type headaches is usually insidious with gradual progression over hours. A pattern of progression over the course of the day is typical. Tension-type headaches are quite variable in frequency. Tension-type headaches are considered episodic if they occur less than 15 days per month and chronic if they occur 15 or more days per month.

Chronic tension-type headaches may occur daily, or near daily, and be present during all waking hours. This pattern of headache is often associated with chronic, excessive use of analgesic medications and has been termed *rebound headache* or *analgesic withdrawal headache*. Rebound headaches are not considered tension-type headaches by the International Headache Society classification, but rather "Headache associated with substances or their withdrawal."

Headaches due to excessive analgesic use may occur with any analgesic medication, but especially with medications containing caffeine or butalbital. These headaches tend to increase in frequency with escalating use of the medication, thus creating a vicious cycle. The effectiveness of the abused analgesic medication generally decreases over time and patients frequently need to switch medications. Additionally,

analgesic abuse headaches do not respond as well to prophylactic medications. The cornerstone of treatment is withdrawal of the offending analgesic medication.

Cluster Headache

Cluster headaches are relatively uncommon but particularly disabling. Cluster headaches cause a severe, often excruciating, pain that is described as "sharp" or "boring." The pain is nonthrobbing in nature and generally located behind one eye or temporal area. Cluster headaches are always unilateral.

Cluster headaches occur more often in men and usually begin in the third decade of life. These headaches are generally spontaneous but may be provoked by vasodilating substances such as alcohol or nitrates. Cluster headaches often begin approximately 1 to 2 hours after the onset of sleep and promptly wake the patient. During a cluster headache it is difficult for the patient to sit still and he or she will often pace or rock back and forth in severe pain.

Cluster headaches generally last 45 minutes to 1 hour with a range of 15 minutes to 3 hours. Patients may experience up to eight or more headaches in a day. Cluster headaches derive their name from their tendency to occur in clusters. Cluster headache periods usually last between 1 and 3 months but occasionally occur on a chronic basis. Each cluster headache period may be separated by headache-free periods lasting months to years. The onset of cluster headache periods is often in the late fall and/or late spring seasons.

Cluster headaches are associated with distinctive clinical signs. These associated signs are unilateral and must occur on the same side as the headache pain. The most common associated signs are conjunctival injection and/or lacrimation, nasal congestion and/or rhinorrhea, and facial flushing and/or sweating. The location and character of the pain and the associated signs of cluster headache tend to be highly stereotypic for an individual patient. It is rare for the headache to switch sides during a cluster period; however, the headache may switch sides from cycle to cycle.

Benign Exertional Headache

Headaches specifically induced by exercise have been described using varying terminology by different authors. The term *effort headache* has been used to define headaches precipitated by sustained aerobic activity, whereas *exertional headache* has been used when short bursts of anaerobic activity such as weightlifting precipitated the headache. This author believes that adherence to the International Headache Society classification simplifies diagnosis and provides a common nomenclature for all physicians to use.

Benign exertional headaches are headaches precipitated by any form of exercise. Since different activities may induce headaches of differing characteristics, subvarieties such as *weightlifter's headache* are recognized. As previously mentioned, up to 10% of patients with exertional headaches will have an intracranial structural lesion. Therefore, benign exertional headache should only be diagnosed when the cause of the headache is proved to be benign.

By definition, benign exertional headaches are precipitated by exercise. In like fashion, avoiding the inciting activity prevents the headache. Although all forms of exercise may induce the headache, aerobic activities such as running, swimming, cycling, or skiing are most often implicated. Benign exertional headaches are more common in men than women.

Benign exertional headaches can begin at any time during the exercise period. Typically, the headache will not begin immediately; instead it starts after the exercise is well underway. The intensity of the headache generally builds as exercise continues. Benign exertional headaches tend to be diffuse and have a throbbing quality. The headache may last for 4 to 6 hours after cessation of exercise.

A common variant of benign exertional headache, weightlifter's headache, occurs with anaerobic activities involving straining or with Valsalva's maneuver. This headache tends to begin abruptly during or immediately following the activity. The headache is predominantly posterior and has a throbbing quality. Weightlifter's headache generally lasts seconds to minutes but may be followed by a diffuse, dull headache lasting hours.

IDENTIFICATION AND EVALUATION OF DANGEROUS HEADACHES

The identification of potentially dangerous headaches is primarily dependent on taking a detailed history. The physical examination may be entirely normal despite the presence of an underlying medical condition or intracranial structural lesion. A summary of worrisome headache features is provided in Table 23–3. A directed laboratory and/or neuroimaging evaluation can complement the clinical evaluation, and if results are normal they assure the patient of the benign nature of the headache. Clinically useful testing modalities are provided in Table 23–4.

Headaches that begin suddenly or at maximum intensity are suggestive of an acute neurologic event. These headaches are often described as the worst

TABLE 23–3. WORRISOME HEADACHE CHARACTERISTICS

Abrupt, severe onset ("thunderclap" onset)
Change in previously existing headache character
Onset of headache after age 50 years
Headache associated with head and/or neck trauma
Associated neurologic deficits or papilledema
Nocturnal onset
Headache increases in severity after lying down
Headache that is constant, or near constant, and progressive
Headache that occurs exclusively over one region
History of cancer or infection with human immunodeficiency virus
Associated loss of consciousness or confusional state

headache of the patient's life. The most urgent example of such a headache is an intracranial hemorrhage, such as subarachnoid hemorrhage. Other possible etiologies of a sudden, severe headache include arterial dissections, central nervous system infections, and vasculitis. Although migraine headache and other benign forms of headache can present in this fashion, these would be diagnosed by exclusion. An algorithm for the evaluation of the acute, severe headache is provided in Fig. 23–1.

Intracranial mass lesions may present with headache. Initially, the headache will often be mild to moderate in severity and will progressively worsen over time. Intracranial mass lesions will generally be associated with a neurologic deficit elicited on history or neurologic examination. However, the deficit may be subtle and difficult to identify, especially early in the course. Headaches in patients over the age of 50 years should be investigated for intracranial neoplasms or temporal arteritis. Similarly, headache in patients with a history of cancer or human immunodeficiency virus infection should be investigated.

Conditions that raise the intracranial pressure, such as mass lesions, central nervous system infections, vasculitis, and pseudotumor cerebri often produce a bilateral or posterior headache. The headache is often constant in severity, but may be aggravated by lying flat or during sleep. Although papilledema is a

TABLE 23–4. EVALUATION OF WORRISOME HEADACHE

Laboratory:	Complete blood cell count (CBC)
	Basic chemistry panel with blood urea nitrogen (BUN) and creatinine
	Erythrocyte sedimentation rate (ESR)
Neuroimaging:	Computed tomography (CT scan) with and without contrast *or* magnetic resonance imaging of the brain (MRI), magnetic resonance angiography (MRA) of the intracranial vasculature
Cerebrospinal fluid:	Useful to evaluate for subarachnoid blood, infection, inflammation, and opening pressure

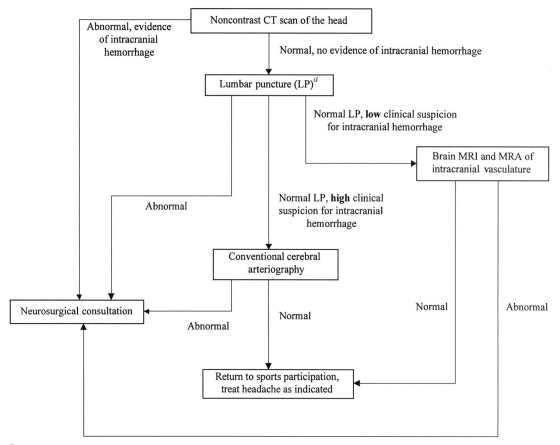

^aLumbar puncture used to evaluate cerebrospinal fluid for blood and/or xanthochromia, protein content, pleocytosis, and measurement of intracranial pressure.

CT = computed tomography; MRI = magnetic resonance imaging; MRA = magnetic resonance angiography.

Figure 23–1. Algorithm for the evaluation of the acute, severe headache.

sign of elevated intracranial pressure, it may take weeks to develop and cannot be relied upon to exclude these conditions or rule out an intracranial abnormality.

Headaches associated with head and/or neck trauma should be investigated for subdural hematoma, arterial dissection, or cerebral contusion. Headache is a common manifestation of postconcussion syndrome.

Benign headaches tend to be episodic in nature and rather stereotypic. A history of headaches that vary in location is reassuring of a benign nature. Any patient that presents with a significant change in a previously existing headache or a strictly one-sided headache deserves further investigation.

TREATMENT OF HEADACHE

Establishing an accurate diagnosis is the foundation of an effective treatment plan. The next step is formulating a regimen that adequately controls the patient's

headaches while producing little or no negative impact on athletic performance. Complete resolution of all headaches may not be a realistic goal for many patients. Instead, reducing the headache frequency and/or severity and providing adequate abortive therapy to the patient's satisfaction will define success. This occurs when the headache burden and medication side effects are acceptable to the patient and allow participation in the activities he or she enjoys.

There are multiple approaches to headache treatment, including the avoidance of triggering factors, use of abortive and prophylactic medications, and various nonpharmacologic modalities. Patients often respond best when these options are used together. The value of patient education cannot be stressed enough. Education regarding common headache triggers and beneficial lifestyle modifications empowers the patient to take a more active role in his or her treatment.

There are two general approaches to the pharmacologic treatment of headache: abortive and prophylactic. Abortive therapy is used to stop, or at least lessen, a headache that has already begun. The goal of prophylactic therapy is to reduce the frequency and/or severity of future headaches. Prophylactic treatment generally requires adherence to a daily medication regimen. However, some patients are able to prevent their headaches by using an abortive agent prior to engaging in an activity that would normally induce a headache. This approach is often effective in the athlete. The most common abortive and prophylactic medications and recommendations for their use are provided in Tables 23–5 and 23–6, respectively.

There are no strict guidelines as to when prophylactic treatment is indicated. However, prophylactic therapy should be strongly considered in the following situations: (1) when headaches occur with such frequency that abortive treatment is no longer safe or desirable, (2) the headaches do not adequately respond to abortive treatment, or (3) the headaches are of such severity or duration that significant disability results. In general, I begin prophylactic treatment when abortive medications are required more often than once or twice a week.

Since many of the medications used to treat headache are associated with side effects that may interfere with athletic performance, athletes may be motivated to try nonpharmacologic modalities. Such interventions often help reduce the frequency and severity of headaches but rarely stop them altogether. As previously mentioned, identifying and avoiding headache triggers is effective and should be a part of every headache treatment plan. Regularity in sleep and meal times should be encouraged. Biofeedback may be helpful in those patients motivated to learn the necessary principles and techniques. Athletes are less likely to develop benign exertional headaches if they adequately warm up prior to strenuous exercise.

Treatment of Migraine Headache

There are numerous options for the abortive treatment of migraine headaches. As a general rule, abortive therapy is most successful when used early in the course of the headache. Some patients, especially those with mild or moderate symptoms, will respond to acetaminophen (Tylenol) or a nonsteroidal anti-inflammatory drug (NSAID). These agents rarely produce sedation or impact athletic performance.

The majority of patients will require a medication more specific for migraine. A medication containing isometheptine (Midrin) is often effective if used soon after headache onset. Alternatively, medications containing caffeine and butalbital (Fiorinal, Fioricet) may be used. Although effective, these medications often

produce sedation which may make exercise difficult or impossible.

The ergotamine preparations act as nonspecific 5-HT$_1$ agonists. These agents can be administered orally, sublingually, or rectally. Dihydroergotamine mesylate is available as a subcutaneous injection or nasal spray. Nausea is a common side effect of the ergots and concomitant use of an antiemetic may be necessary. Sublingual ergot use is convenient and has a rapid onset of action, generally less than 30 minutes.

Some authors, myself included, believe the triptan medications are the agents of choice in exercise-induced migraines.[15] There are currently three triptans suitable to rapidly abort a migraine headache: sumatriptan (Imitrex), rizatriptan (Maxalt), and zolmitriptan (Zomig). A fourth triptan, naratriptan (Amerge), is also used for the abortive treatment of migraine headache. However, its half-life is longer than that of the other triptans, thus making it an ideal medication for patients who tend to have recurrent migraine headaches within a relatively short time or those that require multiple doses of a shorter-acting triptan. Each of these medications act as selective 5-HT$_1$ agonists. Sumatriptan can be administered orally, nasally, or subcutaneously. Rizatriptan and zolmitriptan are oral agents. When given orally, these medications have an onset of action of approximately 30 minutes. Repeat dosing after 2 hours is often necessary for sustained benefit.

The most common side effects of the triptans are somnolence, atypical pain sensations, and dizziness. Sedation is less of a problem with the triptans than with the other migraine agents. As with the ergot preparations, athletic participation is generally possible after treatment with triptans if the headache has been effectively treated. The triptans should not be used in patients with evidence of coronary artery disease, Prinzmetal's angina, or uncontrolled hypertension. The triptans and ergot preparations should not be used within 24 hours of each other.

Prophylactic therapy can significantly improve the patient's quality of life by decreasing headache frequency and thus decreasing the need for abortive medications. Many of the medications used for migraine prophylaxis cause sedation or reduce exercise tolerance. For this reason, prophylactic medications should be started at a low dose and increased slowly. Patients need to be educated that the benefits of prophylactic therapy may not be realized for a number of weeks following their initiation or upward titration. Once initiated, a prophylactic agent should be continued for at least 6 months before changing to a different agent.

The tricyclic antidepressant medications are often used effectively for migraine prophylaxis. The two

TABLE 23–5. COMMONLY USED ABORTIVE MEDICATIONS FOR HEADACHE

Category and Agent	Trade Name	Route	Suggested Dose	Potential Impact on Exercise Performance
Analgesic				
Acetaminophen	Tylenol	Oral	325–1000 mg given orally every 4–6 hr as needed	None
Nonsteroidal Anti-inflammatory Drugs				
Aspirin	Ecotrin	Oral	325–650 mg given orally every 4–6 hr as needed	None
Ibuprofen	Motrin, Advil, Nuprin	Oral	200–800 mg given orally every 8 hr as needed	None
Indomethacin	Indocin	Oral	25–50 mg given orally every 8 hr as needed	None
Naproxen	Naprosyn, Anaprox, Aleve	Oral	220–500 mg given orally twice daily as needed	None
Muscle Relaxants				
Cyclobezaprine HCl	Flexeril	Oral	10 mg given orally twice daily as needed	Sedation
Methocarbamol	Robaxin	Oral	500–1500 mg given orally up to four times daily as needed	Sedation
Carisoprodol	Soma	Oral	350 mg given orally up to three times daily as needed	Sedation, habit forming
Orphenadrine citrate	Norflex, Norgesic	Oral	50–100 mg given orally twice daily as needed	Sedation, impaired sweating, dry mouth
Antimigraine Sedatives				
Butalbital, acetaminophen, caffeine	Fioricet, Esgic	Oral	One tablet given orally four times daily as needed	Sedation, habit forming
Butalbital, aspirin, caffeine	Fiorinal	Oral	One tablet given orally four times daily as needed	Sedation, habit forming
Isometheptine, dichloralphenazone, acetaminophen	Midrin	Oral	Two capsules given orally at onset of headache, then one every hour until headache is gone. Maximum of 5 capsules per 24 hr and 10/week	Sedation
Ergotamines				
Ergotamine tartrate, caffeine	Cafergot, Ercaf	Oral	Two capsules given orally at onset of headache, then one every hour until headache is gone. Maximum of 5 capsules per 24 hr and 10/week	None
Ergotamine tartrate	Ergomar	Sublingual	One 2-mg tablet sublingually at onset of headache, may repeat every 30–60 min to maximum of 3 per 24 hours and 6/week	None
Dihydroergotamine mesylate, caffeine	Migranol nasal spray	Nasal	One spray in each nostril, repeat spray in each nostril in 15 min	None
Triptans				
Sumatriptan	Imitrex	Oral	50-mg tablet given orally at onset of headache, may repeat at 2 hr intervals to maximum dose of 200 mg	None
Sumatriptan	Imitrex	Nasal	One 20-mg spray in one nostril at onset of headache; may repeat one time after 2 hr	None
Sumatriptan	Imitrex	Subcutaneous	6-mg injection at onset of headache; may repeat once after 1 hour	None
Rizatriptan	Maxalt, Maxalt MLT[a]	Oral	10 mg given orally at onset of headache, may repeat at 2-hr intervals to a maximum of 30 mg[b]	None
Zolmitriptan	Zomig	Oral	2.5 mg given orally at onset of headache; may repeat at 2-hr intervals to maximum of 10 mg	None

(Continued)

TABLE 23–5. CONTINUED.

Category and Agent	Trade Name	Route	Suggested Dose	Potential Impact on Exercise Performance
Naratriptan	Amerge	Oral	2.5 mg given orally at onset of headache; may repeat once after 4 hours. Maximum dose of 5 mg per 24 hr	None

[a]The Maxalt MLT formulation is an orally-disintegrating tablet and is easily administered without water.
[b]Patients concurrently using propranolol should use half the standard dose of rizatriptan (5 mg given orally at onset of headache, may repeat at 2-hr intervals to maximum of 15 mg).

most common tricyclic antidepressants are amitriptyline (Elavil) and nortriptyline (Pamelor). Nortriptyline produces less sedation and anticholinergic side effects than amitriptyline and is better tolerated by young, active adults. As with other prophylactic medications, the tricyclic antidepressants should be started at a low dose and gradually increased until a clinical benefit is realized. I prefer to begin nortriptyline at 10 mg given orally at bedtime with an increase to 20 to 25 mg after 2 weeks if the medication is well tolerated. I then reevaluate the patient 6 to 8 weeks later and titrate the medication as needed. Sedation, dry mouth, and dizziness are the most common side effects. Medications with anticholinergic properties, including the tricyclic antidepressants, can inhibit sweating and thus increase the risk of heat-related injury or illness.

Perhaps the most commonly used prophylactic agents are the beta blockers. Propranolol (Inderal) is the beta blocker of choice in migraine prophylaxis. Propranolol is available in short- and long-acting formulations. I prefer to start patients on regular propranolol 20 mg given orally 3 times daily. If the patient tolerates this dosage, I change to the longer-acting Inderal LA 80 mg after 1 to 2 weeks. Further increases can be made based on response and side effects. Propranolol can produce sedation, hypotension, and sexual dysfunction. Additionally, propranolol can reduce exercise tolerance by blunting the normal physiologic heart rate response during exercise.

Other medications that have been used for migraine prophylaxis include verapamil (Calan), the selective serotonin reuptake inhibitors (Prozac, Zoloft, Paxil), and the antiepileptic drugs. Verapamil and the selective serotonin reuptake inhibitors are often used for migraine prophylaxis, but with limited benefit. Sodium valproate (Depakote) is an effective prophylactic agent, but is often poorly tolerated by athletes due to sedation and weight gain. Gabapentin (Neurontin) is less sedating and better tolerated than sodium valproate and has been used with reasonable success.

Treatment of Tension-Type Headache

The treatment of tension-type headache is often more difficult than the treatment of migraine headache. This is most likely due to the fact that tension-type headache is a more heterogeneous entity often with complex psychosocial influences. The etiology and pathophysiology of tension-type headache is less clearly understood than that of migraine and there are likely subgroups of tension-type headache mediated by different mechanisms.

There is often a component of stress, anxiety, and/or depression with tension-type headache. It may be for this reason that tension-type headaches tend to be more chronic and frequent than migraine headaches. It is not unusual for a patient with tension-type headaches to complain of daily, or near-daily, headaches.

Given the chronic nature of tension-type headaches, addressing contributing factors and emphasizing prophylactic therapy generally produces better results. The frequent use of analgesic medications should be avoided because this may lead to analgesic withdrawal headaches, often referred to as rebound headaches, which further complicate treatment. This is especially true for medications that tend to be habit forming, such as narcotics, benzodiazepines, or medications containing butalbital.

Simple analgesics and NSAIDs are the agents of choice for episodic tension-type headaches, those involving fewer than 15 headache days per month. The NSAIDs are effective for most patients. In fact, the majority of patients with tension-type headaches self-medicate with over-the-counter NSAIDs and never seek medical attention. My first choice of NSAID is naproxen (Naprosyn) 500 mg given orally twice daily as needed. Orally administered muscle relaxants may be used where muscle tension is a feature. Muscle relaxants may be used alone or in combination with NSAIDs.

In the patient with episodic tension-type headaches that are refractory to analgesics, NSAIDs, and muscle relaxants, an agent containing isomethleptine may be effective. Isometheptine is most likely effective in this setting due to shared pathophysiologic

TABLE 23–6. COMMONLY USED PROPHYLACTIC MEDICATIONS FOR HEADACHE

Category and Agent	Trade Name	Suggested Dose	Potential Impact on Exercise Performance
Tricyclic Antidepressants			
Amitriptyline	Elavil	Begin with 10–25 mg given orally at bedtime. Increase every 3–4 weeks by 10–25 mg based on response and side effects. Dosage range 10–150 mg/day.	Sedation, dry mouth, impaired sweating, weight gain
Nortriptyline	Pamelor	Begin with 10–25 mg given orally at bedtime. Increase every 3–4 weeks by 10–25 mg based on response and side effects. Dosage range 10–100 mg/day.	Sedation, dry mouth, impaired sweating, weight gain
Beta Blockers			
Atenolol	Tenormin	Begin with 25 mg given orally once daily. Increase every 3–4 weeks based on response and side effects. Dosage range 25–100 mg/day, given once daily or divided twice daily.	Sedation, reduced exercise tolerance
Propranolol	Inderal, Inderal LA	Begin with 20 mg given orally three times daily. Change to 80 mg LA after 2 weeks. Increase every 3–4 weeks based on response and side effects. Dosage range 60–240 mg/day.	Sedation, reduced exercise tolerance
Selective Serotonin Reuptake Inhibitors			
Fluoxetine	Prozac	Begin with 20 mg given orally once daily, generally in the morning. Increase every 3–4 weeks based on response and side effects. Dosage range 20–80 mg/day, given once daily or divided twice daily.	Weight loss, insomnia
Paroxetine	Paxil	Begin with 20 mg given orally once daily, generally in the morning. Increase every 3–4 weeks based on response and side effects. Dosage range 20–50 mg/day.	Weight loss, insomnia
Sertraline	Zoloft	Begin with 50 mg given orally once daily, generally in the morning. Increase in 3–4 weeks based on response and side effects. Dosage range 50–100 mg/day.	Weight loss, insomnia
Other Antidepressants			
Bupropion	Wellbutrin, Wellbutrin SR	Begin with 100 mg given orally twice daily, increase to three times daily after 1 week. The sustained-release formulation is dosed 150 mg once daily, increase to twice daily after 1 week.	Anxiety, weight loss
Nefazodone	Serzone	Begin with 50 mg given orally twice daily. Increase at weekly intervals by 100 mg (total daily dose) based on response and side effects until a dosage of 150 mg twice daily is reached. Dosage range 300–600 mg/day, divided twice daily.	Sedation
Anticonvulsants			
Gabapentin	Neurontin	Begin with 100–300 mg given orally at bedtime. Increase weekly by 100–300 mg based on response and side effects until a dosage of 900 mg given three times daily is reached. Dosage range 300–3700 mg/day, divided three times daily.	Sedation
Valproate sodium	Depakote	Begin with 125 mg given orally at bedtime. Increase by 125 mg every week based on response and side effects until a dosage of 500 mg twice daily is reached. Dosage range 1000–2000 mg/day, divided twice daily.	Sedation, tremor, weight gain
Other Medications			
Cyproheptadine	Periactin	Begin with 2 mg given orally at bedtime, increase to 4 mg after 2 weeks. Increase every 3–4 weeks based on response and side effects to 4 mg three times per day. Dosage range 2–12 mg/day, divided three times daily.	Sedation, dry mouth, impaired sweating, weight gain
Verapamil	Calan SR	Begin with 120 mg sustained-release formulation given orally once daily. Increase every 3–4 weeks based on response and side effects. Dosage range 120–480 mg/day.	Reduced exercise tolerance

mechanisms between some tension-type headaches and migraine. When using isometheptine for tension-type headache, it may be dosed the same as for the treatment of migraine headache.

The treatment of chronic tension-type headache occurring 15 or more days per month should rely more heavily on prophylactic medications and nonpharmacologic therapies. The use of abortive medications should be reserved only for the more intense headaches so as to avoid an analgesic withdrawal (rebound) reaction. Initiation of an antidepressant medication and gradual upward titration based on response and side effects is appropriate. I prefer to begin nortriptyline at 10 mg given orally at bedtime with an increase to 20 to 25 mg after 2 weeks. If the patient does not tolerate this, generally due to sedation, I switch to a selective serotonin reuptake inhibitor such as paroxetine (Paxil) or fluoxetine (Prozac), or to bupropion (Wellbutrin).

Nonpharmacologic therapies should be utilized in athletes with chronic tension-type headaches. I generally refer these patients to physical therapy for cervical stretching and strengthening exercises. This form of therapy encourages the patient to take a more active role in his or her headache management and acts as a stepping-stone to further instruction in relaxation techniques. In patients who are motivated to learn the necessary techniques, biofeedback may be a powerful tool to aid in stress reduction.

Treatment of Cluster Headache

The treatment of cluster headache is often complex with three overlapping goals: abortive treatment of acute cluster headaches, abortive management of episodic cluster periods, and long-term prophylactic treatment of chronic cluster headaches or frequent episodic cluster headaches. Given the disability from cluster headaches due to their severity and frequency, complexity of management, and unique toxicities of medications useful for their treatment, it is recommended that neurologic consultation be obtained.

In general, the acute cluster headache is severe and of relatively short duration, around 45 minutes. For this reason, effective abortive treatment must be readily available and have rapid onset of action. High-flow oxygen delivered by face mask early in the headache is highly effective. However, due to obvious accessibility limitations it is most effective when utilized in the home setting where rapid access is possible. The ergotamine-related medications remain the standard treatment. Dihydroergotamine mesylate administered subcutaneously or intranasally often provides rapid relief. Sublingually administered ergotamine tartrate is also effective; however, orally administered ergotamine preparations are not, due to

poor gastrointestinal absorption. Sumatriptan used subcutaneously or intranasally is a good alternative to the ergotamine-related agents but these should not be used with 24 hours of each other.

Episodic cluster headache is characterized by cluster periods lasting weeks to months. The two primary forms of treatment used to abort the cluster period, or lessen the frequency and/or severity of acute cluster headaches, are oral corticosteroids and ergotamine-related medications. Prednisone (prednisolone) given orally 60 to 80 mg per day generally produces clinical improvement within a few days. This is followed by a 10- to 14-day taper of the drug. It is not unusual for the headaches to return or worsen as the prednisone taper progresses. Orally administered ergotamine tartrate or methysergide (Sansert) is often begun concurrently with oral corticosteroids and continued past the corticosteroid taper. These agents are tapered once the expected duration of the cluster has passed. Methysergide can cause fibrosis of the retroperitoneum, lung, or heart valves. For this reason, methysergide should not be used for longer than 5 months without a drug holiday, and appropriate monitoring is necessary.

Chronic cluster headaches and frequently occurring episodic cluster headaches often require long-term prophylaxis. Verapamil is a safe, generally well-tolerated, and effective medication for this purpose. Other medications useful for cluster headache prophylaxis are valproic acid, lithium carbonate (Eskalith), and methysergide. Due to potential toxicities, lithium carbonate and methysergide require regular monitoring and should be prescribed only by those familiar with their use.

Treatment of Benign Exertional Headache

The first step in the treatment of benign exertional headache should be reconsideration of the benign nature of the headache. As previously described, up to 25% of patients presenting with headaches precipitated by exercise or straining will have an intracranial structural lesion. If such a lesion is identified the athlete should cease strenuous activity, and neurologic or neurosurgical consultation should be obtained.

Headache precipitated by exercise may represent migraine headache, tension-type headache, or true benign exertional headache. In the case of migraine and tension-type headaches, treatment is the same regardless of whether or not exercise is a precipitating factor. An algorithm for the systematic treatment of exercise-induced headache is provided in Fig. 23–2.

Benign exertional headaches are often effectively treated with a NSAID. The NSAIDs may be used alone or in combination with acetaminophen. These agents are not expected to adversely impact athletic performance.

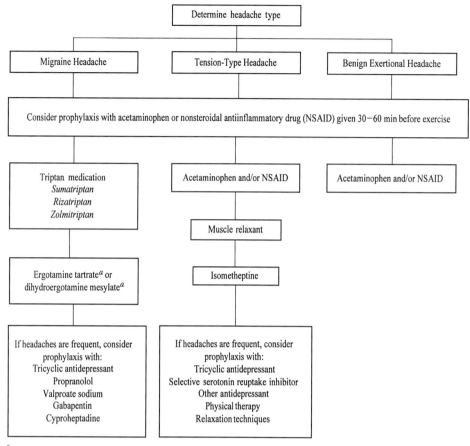

^aErgot-containing medications should not be used within 24 hours of a triptan agent.

Figure 23–2. Algorithm for the management of exercise-induced headache.

The most commonly used medication is indomethacin (Indocin) 25 to 50 mg given orally up to 3 times daily. A 25- to 50-mg dose of indomethacin (Indocin) given 30 to 60 minutes before exercise is often effective in preventing the headache. Although indomethacin (Indocin) is generally effective, I have had good results with naproxen 250 to 500 mg used in the same fashion before exercise.

REFERENCES

1. International Headache Society: Classification and diagnostic criteria for headache disorders, cranial neuralgias, and facial pain. *Cephalalgia* 1988:8, 1.
2. Lipton RB, Stewart WF: Migraine in the United States: Epidemiology and health care use. *Neurology* 1993:43, 6.
3. Rasmussen BK, Jensen R, Schroll M, et al.: Epidemiology of headache in a general population—a prevalence study. *J Clin Epidemiol* 1991:44, 1147.
4. Stewart WF, Lipton RB, Liberman J: Variation in migraine prevalence by race. *Neurology* 1996:16, 231.
5. Mathew NT: Diagnosis and modern treatment of migraine. *Prog Neurol* 1999:1, 3.
6. Swain R, Rosencrance G: Headache occurrence and classification among distance runners. *West Virginia Med J* 1999:95, 76.
7. Williams SJ, Nukada H: Sport and exercise headache: Part 1. Prevalence among university students. *Br J Sports Med* 1994:28, 90.
8. Williams SJ, Nukada H: Sport and exercise headache: Part 2. Diagnosis and classification. *Br J Sports Med* 1994:28, 96.
9. Jokl E: Olympic medicine and sports cardiology. *Ann Sports Med* 1984:1, 127.
10. Seelinger DF, Coin GC, Carlow TJ: Effort headache with cerebral infarction. *Headache* 1975:15, 142.
11. Lance JW, Lambros J: Unilateral exertional headache as a symptom of cardiac ischemia. *Headache* 1998:38, 315.
12. Rooke ED: Benign exertional headache. *Med Clin North Am* 1968:52, 801.
13. Raskin NH: Migraine and other headaches, in Rowland LP (ed.), *Merritt's Textbook of Neurology*, 9th ed., Baltimore, Williams & Wilkins, 1995:837.
14. Fisher CM: Painful states: A neurological commentary. *Clin Neurosurg* 1984:31, 32.
15. Diamond S: Managing migraines in active people. *Phys Sports Med* 1996:24, 41.

Chapter 24

GASTROINTESTINAL PROBLEMS
IN RUNNERS

Janus D. Butcher and David Brown

INTRODUCTION AND EPIDEMIOLOGY

Nearly every runner has experienced gastrointestinal (GI) symptoms during a workout at some point in their running career. While exercise-induced GI complaints are typically quite distressing for the athlete, fortunately they tend to be episodic and self-limited.[1] The GI symptoms that are most often reported by runners include gastroesophageal (GE) reflux, abdominal pain, diarrhea, and nausea with the incidence reported to be greater than 80% in certain groups of running athletes.[2] These symptoms are not restricted to runners, however. Other athletes, including rowers, cross-country skiers, swimmers, and cyclists report similar problems. Peters and colleagues[3] noted several interesting patterns of GI symptoms in a recent study conducted on runners, cyclists, and triathletes. Runners had a higher incidence of lower GI symptoms vs. upper GI symptoms (71% vs. 36%), while cyclists had a fairly even split between upper and lower GI symptoms (67% vs. 64%).

Because these symptoms are so common, there is a tendency to attribute all GI symptoms in the athlete strictly to their exercise behaviors. The clinician must keep in mind, however, that athletes are at risk for the same disease processes as nonathletes and the differential diagnosis of their symptoms should include those diseases found in the nonrunning population. For instance, chronic dyspepsia in a runner should lead one to consider *Helicobacter pylori* infection. Similarly, the workup for bloody diarrhea should include consideration of inflammatory bowel disease. Additionally, non-GI processes such as cardiovascular disease should be considered in certain athletes complaining of upper GI complaints.

UPPER GI SYMPTOMS

Common upper GI symptoms include belching, nausea, vomiting, and epigastric pain. These are usually experienced during maximal exertion and can cause a great deal of concern for the athlete because they may mimic symptoms of cardiac disease. Although these symptoms are reported in a variety of sports, they are most frequently encountered in running.[4] These symptoms are generally worse with increasing intensity or prolonged duration of exercise and are more severe with immediate postprandial exercise (within 3 hours of eating).[5]

Several possible causes of GE reflux have been suggested. Transient relaxation of the lower esophageal sphincter (LES) due to air swallowing is a likely contributor.[6] Other factors that can decrease LES tone

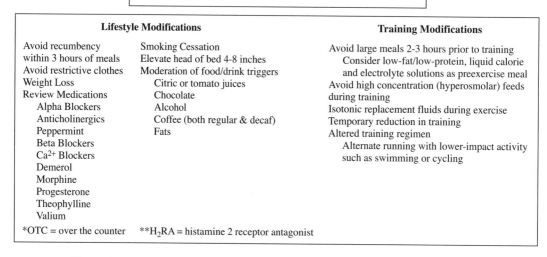

Figure 24–1. Therapeutic pyramid for exercise-related gastroesophageal reflux disease.

include alcohol, caffeine, high-fat foods, smoking, and many drugs (Fig. 24–1).

An increase in acid production has also been suggested as a cause of GE reflux; however, recent studies indicate that decreased gastric mucosal secretion resulting from reduced splanchnic blood flow is a more likely cause. This reduction in the protective stomach lining lowers the resistance to gastric acid secretion.[7] This effect may be accentuated by NSAID use, emotional stress, or any factor that increases acid production. The delayed gastric emptying seen with strenuous exercise may also contribute to upper GI symptoms.[8]

H pylori infection has in recent years taken center stage as a cause of peptic ulcer disease and chronic gastritis. This very common infection should be considered in cases of chronic or recurrent upper GI symptoms. Screening can be done with urea breath testing. Serologic testing to measure the *H pylori* IgG level can be used if urea breath testing is unavailable. Mucosal biopsy is reserved for patients who have other symptoms or findings requiring upper endoscopy. Once an infection has been diagnosed, several efficacious eradication regimens are available (Table 24–1). A negative follow-up breath test or a 50% drop in the antibody titer is diagnostic of successful eradication.

TABLE 24–1. REGIMENS FOR TREATMENT OF *HELICOBACTER PYLORI* INFECTION

Regimen	Eradication Rate[a]
Omeprazole 20 mg BID Bismuth subsalicylate 525 mg QID Tetracycline 500 mg QID Metronidazole 250 mg QID	85–90%
Omeprazole 20 mg BID Amoxicillin 1000 mg BID Clarithromycin 500 mg BID	96.4%
Omeprazole 20 mg BID Metronidazole 500 mg BID Clarithromycin 500 mg BID	89.8%
Omeprazole 20 mg BID Amoxicillin 1000 mg BID Metronidazole 500 mg BID	79.0%

[a]All eradication rates based on a 7-day regimen. European data suggest 7 days are adequate; however, this has not been confirmed by U.S. studies. Thus, a full 14-day treatment course is recommended.
Source: Adapted from Lind T, Veldhuyzen van Zanten S J O, Unge P, et al.: Eradication of Helicobacter pylori *using one week triple therapies combing omeprazole with two antimicrobials—The MACH 1 study.* Helicobacter *1996:1, 138.*

Evaluation (Figure 24–2)

The evaluation of upper GI symptoms in athletes should begin with careful documentation of training habits, nonsteroidal anti-inflammatory drugs (NSAIDs)

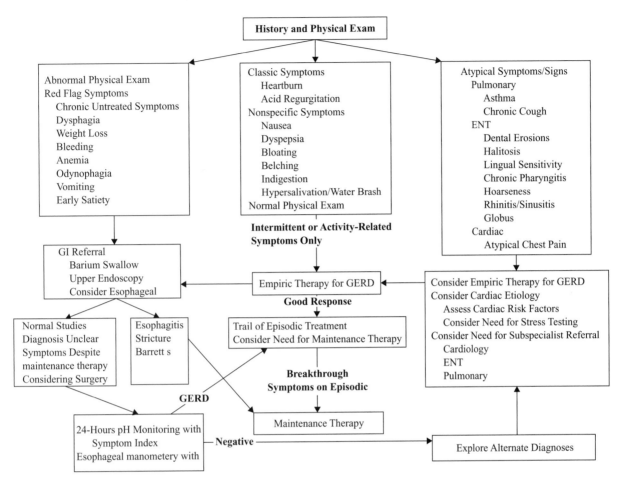

Figure 24–2. Evaluation of gastroesophageal symptoms.

use, diet, and prior history (and family history) of gastritis, peptic ulcer disease, inflammatory bowel disease, or other GI problems. Care must be taken to rule out more serious causes of epigastric pain, most importantly those of a cardiac etiology. An electrocardiogram (ECG) or electrocardiographic stress test should be obtained in athletes presenting with epigastric pain and associated cardiac risk factors (age over 40, smoking history, family history, hyperlipidemia, or comorbid disease state) or if associated symptoms suggest cardiac origin (shortness of breath, diaphoresis, radiating pain). Laboratory evaluation should include a complete blood cell count to assess hemoglobin and hematocrit to ensure that there is no significant blood loss. Liver function testing with transaminases, bilirubin, and amylase are relatively inexpensive and will help to exclude other causes of upper GI symptoms, such as hepatitis, pancreatitis, and biliary tract disease. As mentioned above, serologic testing or urea breath testing for *H pylori* is indicated in the runner with chronic dyspepsia. Endoscopy should be performed in patients with recurrent or persistent symptoms despite treatment. Ambulatory pH monitoring and LES manometry have also been advocated to evaluate patients with refractory symptoms following an otherwise normal evaluation.[9]

Treatment

Treatment options for GE reflux are many and should be approached stepwise in association with the evaluation outlined in Fig. 24–2. Most often, simple changes in diet, meal timing, and training habits will alleviate these symptoms. Avoiding large meals 2 to 3 hours prior to training and high concentration (hyperosmolar) feeds while training may prevent symptoms. The use of low-fat, low-protein, liquid calorie and electrolyte solutions is an effective means of supplying immediate preexercise calories while minimizing GE reflux. Isotonic fluids tend to cause fewer upper GI symptoms and are the best source for calorie replacement while exercising.[10] Athletes may also reduce these symptoms by temporarily decreasing training or by alternating running with a lower-impact workout, such as cycling or swimming.[5]

Medical therapy of GE reflux disease is a multibillion dollar industry in the United States. There are a multitude of options for therapy, most of which are effective. In general, a stepwise approach incorporating dietary changes, training modifications, and medications is the most practical treatment regimen (Fig. 24–1). It is best to start simply and inexpensively and progress as needed.

Antacids such as aluminum hydroxide and magnesium salts are useful in the treatment of mild symptoms. These should be taken immediately before beginning exercise and can be repeated during the workout as needed. H_2 receptor blockers (ranitidine, 150 mg twice a day; famotidine, 20 mg a day; and cimetidine, 400 mg twice a day) have been shown to be effective in decreasing upper GI symptoms in runners.[6,11,12] These medications have the advantage of being available without prescription and are considerably cheaper than newer medications. Initially, GE reflux can be treated empirically with these H_2 blocking agents. If symptoms persist, further evaluation as outlined in Fig. 24–2 is indicated. The gastric proton pump inhibitors (omeprazole, 20 mg once a day; lansoprazole, 15 mg once a day) are very effective in the treatment of gastritis; however, these require a prescription and are considerably more expensive than H_2 blockers. Discontinuation of NSAIDs or the substitution of COX-2 selective anti-inflammatory agents (celecoxib, 200 mg once a day; rofecoxib, 25 mg once a day) is usually prudent.

LOWER GI SYMPTOMS

Lower GI symptoms including fecal urgency, loose stools, and frank diarrhea are very common in runners. Studies have found that 37% to 54% of runners experience bowel urgency either during or immediately following a strenuous workout.[2,13] These symptoms are usually precipitated by increasing training mileage or particularly intensive workouts.[14] Frequently the athlete is forced to interrupt the workout as a result of these symptoms.[13] In severe cases, runner's diarrhea may result in significant dehydration and has been implicated in the development of rhabdomyolysis and acute tubular necrosis.[14] Bloody diarrhea has also been suggested as a cause of runner's anemia.[15]

The precise physiology of runner's diarrhea is not well understood, although a number of etiologies have been suggested. One theory proposes that a rapid shift in intestinal fluid and electrolytes with strenuous exercise results in colonic irritability and cramping.[13,16] Another possible mechanism involves the autonomic nervous system. The increased parasympathetic tone seen with moderate exercise causes increased peristalsis, leading to rapid bowel transit and cramping. In more strenuous exercise, sympathetic nervous system stimulation increases the release of gastroenteropancreatic hormones (gastrin, motilin, and endogenous opioids), which may account for increased bowel activity.[8,17] Ischemic enteropathy and GI bleeding may also cause runner's diarrhea.[18] Infectious etiologies should also be considered in acute diarrheal illnesses in runners. This is particularly true in the setting of recent international or wilderness travel or in focal outbreaks among team or family members.

GI Bleeding

In recent years a great deal of interest has arisen regarding GI bleeding in runners. Although this phenomenon is rarely clinically significant, the incidence is quite remarkable in some studies. In one such study, McCabe and colleagues[19] demonstrated a 20% incidence of occult blood in the stools of runners completing a marathon. Of their respondents, 6% reported frank hematochezia following that race, while 17% reported at least one previous episode of running-associated bloody diarrhea. More dramatic is the report of an 87% positive conversion rate on stool occult blood testing in runners following an ultradistance running event.[11] Review of these studies suggests that the GI bleeding may be distance- or effort-related (dose-dependent).

Several possible mechanisms for GI bleeding in runners have been suggested. A running-induced ischemic enteropathy has been proposed by several authors.[4,12–15,19,20] Splanchnic blood flow is reduced to approximately 70% to 80% of normal with strenuous cardiovascular exercise.[21] When this low blood flow is maintained for a long period, as in a long-distance run, it can lead to local tissue ischemia, necrosis, and superficial mucosal erosions resulting in intraluminal bleeding.[20] By a similar mechanism, reduced GI blood flow also contributes to the development of hemorrhagic gastritis, which is associated with GI blood loss in long-distance runners.[11,22]

Another theory involves mechanical trauma to the bowel similar to that described in other hollow viscera such as the bladder and ureters.[16,23] The repetitive, high-impact characteristics of running cause jarring of the intestines, which may result in serosal and mucosal injury.[14,19] Hemorrhagic gastritis may result from mechanical stress via traction forces of the diaphragm and gastrophrenic ligaments on the gastric fundus.[11] This mechanical trauma theory is refuted somewhat by the report of GI bleeding associated with competitive bicycling.[24,25]

The relationship between NSAID use and GI blood loss is not clear. NSAIDs have been associated with the development of gastritis and peptic ulcer disease;

TABLE 24–2. EVALUATION OF LOWER GI SYMPTOMS

Historical Data/Test	Diagnostic Utility
Training diary	Lower GI symptoms often develop with increased intensity or frequency of training
Bloody diarrhea/hematochezia	Associated with ischemic enteropathy, inflammatory bowel disease, and infectious diseases
NSAID use	Gastritis/ulcer as potential cause for bleeding or occult blood
Travel history	Heightened suspicion for infectious diarrhea
Family history	Inflammatory bowel disease Irritable bowel disease
Stool occult blood testing	Assessment for GI blood loss
Fecal leukocytes, ova/parasites, culture	Evaluate for infectious etiologies
Barium enema	Rule out mechanical, structural, or inflammatory conditions
Endoscopy	Rule out inflammatory, ischemic, neoplastic, and infectious processes

however, the studies on GI blood loss in the athlete have not shown any direct correlation.[11] Perianal disease, including hemorrhoids, fissures, and perianal chafing, is another possible cause of GI blood loss in athletes.

Evaluation of Lower GI Symptoms (Table 24–2)

The approach to lower GI symptoms in the runner begins with a careful history of symptom character and severity. Specifically, inquire about the presence of diarrhea, melena, hematochezia, or hematemesis and their association with exercise, meals, or other stressors. Any recent changes in training intensity, duration, or distance should be quantified. NSAID use, the athlete's history of recent travel, and preexisting illness are also important etiologic factors. A past history or family history of inflammatory bowel disease, gastritis, peptic ulcer disease, and other causes of GI bleeding should be undertaken if indicated by the patient's presenting circumstances. Laboratory assessment should include stool evaluation for fecal heme content, leukocytes, ova and parasites, and stool cultures, to determine the presence of inflammatory or infectious etiologies. A complete blood cell count should be done to evaluate for possible anemia. In persons with evidence of bloody diarrhea, further evaluation with a barium enema, flexible sigmoidoscopy, colonoscopy, and esophagogastroduodenoscopy (EGD) may be warranted to determine the focus of blood loss.

Treatment: Nonbloody Diarrhea

Treatment of runner's diarrhea begins with a reduction in training intensity or distance for 1 to 2 weeks with a gradual return to the previous high-intensity workouts. In most cases this will be effective in stopping the symptoms without recurrence.[14] Exercise substitution and cross-training with low-impact (nonrunning) activities also help to reduce the symptoms while allowing the athlete to maintain cardiovascular fitness.

Dietary manipulations may be of some use in the prevention of lower GI symptoms. A complete liquid diet on the day prior to a long-distance competition or planned strenuous workout may decrease symptoms during the event. This is obviously of limited value in the treatment of long-term running-induced diarrhea; however, a low-residue (low-fiber) diet may be helpful in some athletes.[10]

Antidiarrhea medications should be used with caution due to potential side effects. Antispasmodics such as loperamide (4 mg initially then 2 mg as needed, up to 16 mg/day) are usually safe. Anticholinergic medications such as diphenoxylate or modafinil should be avoided because they can affect sweating and increase risk of heat injury.

Treatment: Bloody Diarrhea

The treatment of bloody diarrhea in the athlete includes a short-term reduction in training along with exercise substitution as discussed above.[20] In cases related to hemorrhagic gastritis, the use of H_2 antagonists (ranitidine, 150 mg twice a day; famotidine, 20 mg once a day; or cimetidine, 400 mg twice a day) is very effective over the course of several days.[11,20] In endurance athletes predisposed to upper GI blood loss (ultra runners, or those with a previous history of upper GI blood loss), prerace treatment with H_2 antagonists is effective in preventing blood loss.[11] Discontinuation of NSAIDs or substitution of a COX-2 selective medication (celecoxib, 200 mg once a day; rofecoxib 25 mg once a day) should be advised in most cases of bloody diarrhea.

Traveler's Diarrhea

Traveler's diarrhea (TD) is a common health risk among travelers to developing countries. With the large number of international competitions and growing numbers of adventure travelers visiting remote locations, TD is a great concern for these athletes. Of the 8 million Americans who will travel to a third-world country this year, approximately one third will develop diarrhea during the trip. The risk varies depending on the destination, but infection rates range from 20% to 59%.[26–28]

The infection is transmitted through the fecal/oral route, generally in food or water. Many pathogens have been described in traveler's diarrhea, although in most cases the specific etiology is not determined. In up to 50% of cases studied, the infection was found to be due to enterotoxigenic *Escherichia coli* species.[27] *Shigella*, *Salmonella*, and *Campylobacter* species are other possible bacterial causes. Viral and amoebic sources are less commonly implicated in outbreaks. TD usually strikes in the first week of travel with symptoms lasting for 3 to 7 days. Occasionally symptoms may persist for 1 month or more. Diarrhea, vomiting, and abdominal pain are the most common symptoms. Fever, bloody diarrhea, and malaise occur less often but can be quite debilitating. Dehydration is common and is the major concern in the treatment of TD. While the duration of TD is usually brief, the impact that even a short illness may have in the running athlete increases the need for early recognition and treatment.

Prevention

Avoidance of TD is clearly the most effective treatment. Minimizing the risk of exposure to the agents by following a few simple rules has been shown to decrease the incidence of disease. Travelers should be advised to avoid the following sources of infection when traveling: unpeeled fruits, uncooked vegetables, dairy products, ice, and untreated water. Bottled or treated water should be used for drinking and brushing teeth.[28] In addition, bottled soft drinks and beer are generally considered to be safe. These recommendations are often difficult to follow when traveling, and as a result individuals often ask about prophylactic antimicrobial medications.

The use of bismuth subsalicylate has been shown to reduce the incidence of TD by up to 65%.[29] Although it is effective, the relatively high dose required for maximal protection, two 262 mg tablets four times a day, has been associated with several side effects including salicylate-induced tinnitus and a blackened tongue. Prophylactic use of trimethoprim-sulfamethoxazole (one double-strength tablet each day) and doxycycline (100 mg once a day) have previously been shown to reduce the incidence of TD by approximately 50% to 85%.[30] However, due to growing bacterial resistance to these medications and the risk of potentially serious drug reactions, their usefulness is limited. Prophylaxis may be considered in patients with underlying GI illnesses or in other particularly high-risk situations.[31] An argument can easily be made to use prophylactic antibiotics in athletes on short trips to compete in highly endemic regions. This must be weighed against the potential for side effects and adverse reactions for the chosen antibiotic. Currently the fluoroquinolone antibiotics (ofloxacin 400 mg, ciprofloxacin 500 mg, norfloxacin 400 mg) taken in a single dose once a day have the lowest resistance profiles and are the drugs of choice when prophylaxis is indicated.[28]

Treatment

The most important consideration in the treatment of TD is the replacement of fluid losses. Most cases can be satisfactorily managed by the use of noncaffeinated, nonalcoholic oral fluid replacements. More severe illnesses may require intravenous fluids (normal saline or lactated Ringer's solution) in volumes adequate to replace estimated losses.

The course of TD can be significantly shortened by initiating antibiotic therapy early in the infection.[32] Ideally, the antibiotics should be started with the first loose stool, but may still shorten the illness if taken up to 48 hours after symptoms begin. The most commonly used medications are trimethoprim-sulfamethoxazole, one double-strength tablet twice a day, or doxycycline, 100 mg twice a day for 3 days. Unfortunately, growing resistance worldwide has significantly limited the usefulness of both of these medications. Fluoroquinolone antibiotics are currently the antibiotics of choice.[32] Ofloxacin 400 mg, ciprofloxacin 500 mg, or norfloxacin 400 mg, each taken twice a day for 3 to 5 days are all very effective.

Antidiarrheal agents such as loperamide, two capsules (4 mg) initially, and then one capsule (2 mg) following each loose stool, or diphenoxylate, two tablets four times a day, are useful in reducing symptoms in uncomplicated TD. In the presence of fever or bloody diarrhea, however, these agents may actually prolong the course of illness and are contraindicated. These medications are not useful for prophylaxis against TD. The current recommendation is for combined therapy with both a fluoroquinolone antibiotic and loperamide at the first loose stool, then continuing the antibiotic for 3 to 5 days.[32]

HEPATIC INJURY

Abnormal Liver Function Tests (LFTs)

Liver enzyme elevations have been described in many types of exercise but are most affected by long-distance running. Exercise-induced hepatic injury probably results from ischemic insult due to decreased oxygen tension in the hepatic blood supply. The damage to the liver is readily reversible when exercise is stopped, with enzyme levels usually returning to normal within 1 week.[33] While there is no evidence that these exercise-related enzyme elevations lead to long-term sequelae, it would seem prudent to limit exercise until LFTs normalize.

Increased serum glutamate oxaloacetate transaminase (SGOT), alanine aminotransferase (ALT), creatine kinase, aspartate aminotransferase (AST), bilirubin, alkaline phosphatase, creatinine phosphatase, and lactic dehydrogenase (LDH), have all been described in runners.[34,35] While these can indicate liver injury, they may also be related to musculoskeletal trauma. More specific indicators of hepatocellular injury, glutamic dehydrogenase (GLDH) and gamma-glutamyl transferase (GGT) have been found to be elevated in long-distance runners.[36] The gradual serum reductions of albumin seen in ultradistance runners further support the possibility of hepatic injury in these athletes.[36]

Hepatitis

In the athlete with acute viral hepatitis, no specific exercise restrictions are indicated. However, the symptoms commonly associated with the acute phase of infection, including fever, malaise, nausea, vomiting, and abdominal pain, will often limit the athlete's ability to train. The continuation of low-intensity exercise in the acute phase may actually allow the athlete to return to preillness levels of performance more quickly in the recovery phase of the illness.[37] No specific exercise restrictions are necessary in chronic liver disease; however, the patient's overall condition as a result of the illness must be considered when developing an exercise program.

Immunization against hepatitis B is currently recommended for all adults.[38] Two preparations are currently available (Recombivax HB and Engerix-B). Each is administered as three inoculations at 0, 1 month, and 6 months. Immunization against hepatitis A is recommended for persons living in or traveling to areas of high incidence of hepatitis A infection. Low-incidence areas include the United States, Canada, western Europe, New Zealand, Australia, and Japan. With the increasing interest in international competition and adventure travel, the importance of hepatitis A vaccination is growing. Two immunization preparations are available (Havrix or Vaqta), and both are administered in two doses at 0 and between 6 and 12 months. Intramuscular immunoglobulin (0.02 mg/kg) administration is also effective for up to 3 months of protection.

ABDOMINAL PAIN

Exertion-related abdominal pain is quite common. Although many etiologies have been described, most often this is a benign symptom. The "side stitch" is the most common form of this complaint in runners. Typically it is described as an aching sensation in the right upper abdominal quadrant, affecting athletes as they significantly increase their mileage and untrained persons initiating an exercise program. Although the precise etiology is not known, the most likely cause is diaphragmatic muscle spasm related to hypoxia.[39] Other possible explanations include hepatic capsule irritation, pleural irritation, abdominal adhesions, and right colonic gas pains.[40] These pains are often worse with postprandial exercise.

The athlete may get some relief by stretching the right arm over the head or by forced expiration against pursed lips.[41] Stopping exercise nearly always results in immediate cessation of symptoms. The frequency and severity of side stitches usually decrease as the overall fitness of the athlete improves.

More serious causes of abdominal pain in runners have been described, including omental infarction, bowel infarction, and hepatic vein thrombosis.[42] These are fortunately very rare events and are generally accompanied by unremitting pain, severe systemic illness, collapse, and multisystem failure. These are typically reported after long-distance competition and require emergent surgical intervention.

CONCLUSION

GI symptoms are very common in the running population. These entities include both upper and lower tract problems including running-specific illnesses as well as those also seen in the general population. Accurate diagnosis and prompt therapy will limit the impact of these symptoms on training and competition.

REFERENCES

1. Sullivan SN, Wong C: Does running cause gastrointestinal symptoms? A survey of 93 randomly selected runners compared with controls. *N Z Med J* 1994:107, 328.
2. Worobetz LJ, Gerrard DF: Gastrointestinal symptoms during exercise in endurance athletes. *N Z Med J* 1985:98, 644.
3. Peters HPF, Bos M, Seebrgts L, Akkermans LMA, et al.: Gastrointestinal symptoms in long-distance runners, cyclists, and triathletes: Prevalence, medication, and etiology. *Am J Gastroenterol* 1999:94, 1570.
4. Shawdon YE, Beasley I, Evans DF: The effects of different types of exercise on gastroesophageal reflux. *Aust J Sci Med Sport* 1996:28, 93.
5. Clark S, Kraus B, Sinclair J, et al.: Gastroesophageal reflux induced by exercise in healthy volunteers. *JAMA* 1989:261, 3599.

6. Krause BS, Sinclair JW, Castell DO: Gastroesophageal reflux in runners. *Ann Intern Med* 1990:112, 429.

7. Gaudin C, Zerath E, Guezennec C: Gastric lesions secondary to long-distance running. *Dig Dis Sci* 1990:35, 1239.

8. Read N, Houghton L: Physiology of gastric emptying and pathophysiology of gastroparesis. *Gastroenterol Clin North Am* 1989:18, 359.

9. Shawdon A: Gastro-oesophageal reflux and exercise. *Sports Med* 1995:20, 109.

10. Brouns F, Saris W, Reher N: Abdominal complaints and gastrointestinal function during long-lasting exercise. *Int J Sports Med* 1987:8, 175.

11. Baska R, Moses F, Deuster P: Cimetidine reduces running-associated gastrointestinal bleeding. *Dig Dis Sci* 1990:35, 956.

12. Cooper BT, Douglas SA, Firth LA, et al.: Erosive gastritis and gastrointestinal bleeding in a female runner. *Gastroenterology* 1987:92, 2019.

13. Keeffe EB, Lowe DK, Goss JR, et al.: Gastrointestinal symptoms of marathon runners. *West J Med* 1984:141, 481.

14. Fogoros R. Runner's trots. *JAMA* 1980:243, 1743.

15. Stewart J, Ahlquist D, McGill D, et al.: Gastrointestinal blood loss and anemia in runners. *Ann Intern Med* 1984:100, 843.

16. Rehrer N, Janssen G, Brouns F, et al.: Fluid intake and gastrointestinal problems in runners competing in a 25-km marathon. *Int J Sports Med* 1989:10, s22.

17. Cammack J, Read N, Cann PA, et al.: Effect of prolonged exercise on the passage of a solid meal through the stomach and small intestine. *Gut* 1982:23, 957.

18. Bounous G, McArdle AH: Marathon runners: The intestinal handicap. *Med Hypothesis* 1990:33, 261.

19. McCabe M, Peura D, Kadakia S, et al.: Gastrointestinal blood loss associated with running a marathon. *Dig Dis Sci* 1986:31, 1229.

20. Heer M, Repond F, et al.: Acute ischemic colitis in a female long distance runner. *Gut* 1987:28, 896.

21. Clausen JP: Effect of physical training on cardiovascular adjustments to exercise in man. *Physiol Rev* 1977:57, 779.

22. Rudzki SJ, Hazard H, Collinson D: Gastrointestinal blood loss in triathletes. *Aust J Sci Med Sports* 1995:27, 3.

23. Blaklock NJ: Bladder trauma in the long distance runner: 10,000 metres haematuria. *Br J Urol* 1977:49, 129.

24. Rubin RB, Saltzman JR, Zawacki JK: Bicycle racing, Raynaud's phenomenon, and gastrointestinal bleeding. *Am J Gastro* 1994:89, 291.

25. Wilhite J, Mellion M: Occult gastrointestinal bleeding in endurance cyclists. *Phys Sportsmed* 1990:18, 75.

26. Bruins J, Bwire R, Slootman EJH, et al.: Diarrhea morbidity among Dutch military service men in Goma, Zaire. *Military Med* 1995:160, 446.

27. Wolfe M: Acute diarrhea associated with travel. *Am J Med* 1990:88, 34s.

28. Statement on traveller's diarrhea. *Can Med Assoc J* 1995:152, 205.

29. Dupont H, Ericsson C, et al.: Prevention of traveler's diarrhea by the tablet form of bismuth subsalicylate. *JAMA* 1987:257, 1347.

30. Consensus conference. Traveler's diarrhea. *JAMA* 1985:253, 2699.

31. Ferenchick G, Havlichek D: Primary prevention and international travel. *J Gen Intern Med* 1989:4, 247.

32. Dupont HL, Erickson CD: Prevention and treatment of travelers diarrhea. *N Engl J Med* 1993:328, 1821.

33. Lijnen P, Hespel P, Fagard R, et al.: Indicators of cell breakdown in plasma in men during and after a marathon race. *Int J Sports Med* 1988:9, 108.

34. Bunch T: Blood test abnormalities in runners. *Mayo Clin Proc* 1980:55, 113.

35. De Paz JA, Villa JG, Lopez P, Gonzalez-Gallego J: Effects of long-distance running on serum bilirubin. *Med Sci Sports Exerc* 1995:27, 1590.

36. Nagel D, Seiler D, Franz H, et al.: Ultra-long-distance running and the liver. *Int J Sports Med* 1990:11, 441.

37. Ritland S: Exercise and liver disease. *Sports Med* 1988:6, 121.

38. Dick L: Travel medicine: Helping patients prepare for trips abroad. *Am Fam Phys* 1998:58, 383.

39. Pate R: Principles of training, in Kulund D, (ed.), *The Injured Athlete*, Philadelphia, Lippincott, 1988.

40. Lauder TD, Moses FM: Recurrent abdominal pain from abdominal adhesions in an endurance triathlete. *Med Sci Sports Exerc* 1995:27, 623.

41. Stamford B: A "stitch" in the side. *Phys Sportsmed* 1985:13, 187.

42. Scobie BA: Gastrointestinal emergencies with marathon type running: Omental infarction with pancreatitis and liver failure with portal vein thrombosis. *N Z Med J* 1998:111, 211.

Chapter 25

GENITOURINARY DISORDERS

Michael W. Johnson

INTRODUCTION

Running is one of the most visible expressions of the fitness boom that began in the 1970s. Running is an efficient, effective, and enjoyable activity that improves cardiovascular and musculoskeletal fitness. It is inexpensive and readily available. Strenuous exercise, such as running, places great demands on all organ systems. The musculoskeletal system adapts to the increased demands by becoming stronger, and the cardiovascular system becomes more efficient. During exercise, blood is shunted from the kidneys to the working muscles. This decreased renal blood flow is a major contributor to disorders of the genitourinary system seen in the runner. Subjects covered in this chapter include exercise-induced hematuria and proteinuria, acute renal failure, rhabdomyolysis, genitourinary infection, and genital pain.

EPIDEMIOLOGY

Hematuria and proteinuria are the most common urinary findings in runners. In fact, a study of 383 runners noted that 17% developed hematuria and 30% developed proteinuria following the completion of a marathon. Interestingly, there was no difference in incidence based on gender.[1] Acute renal failure in runners

is a rare event and is usually associated with volume depletion, rhabdomyolysis, or the nephrotoxic effects of nonsteroidal anti-inflammatory drugs (NSAIDs). The prevalence of sexually transmitted diseases (STDs) in runners is similar to that of the general population, although a study of college athletes showed that they tend to be at higher risk for certain lifestyle behaviors. These maladaptive behaviors include less safe sex, greater number of sexual partners, and less contraceptive use when compared with their nonathlete peers.[2]

GENITOURINARY ANATOMY AND PHYSIOLOGY

Anatomy

The genitourinary system, located in the lower abdomen and pelvis, is composed of the kidneys, ureters, bladder, urethra, and genital organs. The kidneys can be found high in the retroperitoneum bilaterally and are well protected. A solitary or malpositioned kidney is prone to injury. The urinary bladder is located in the anterior pelvis and is rarely acutely injured. The male genitalia, owing to its external location, is often subject to injury and infection. The scrotal skin, with its hair follicles and sweat glands, is frequently the site of local infection or irritation.

Physiology

Renal Physiology at Rest

Renal blood flow at rest is approximately 1200 ml/min, which is 20% of cardiac output. In fact, the kidneys receive more blood flow per unit weight than any other organ in the body. Renal plasma flow is 700 ml/min, of which 15% is filtered through the glomeruli. Renal blood travels to the glomerulus via the afferent arteriole and exits through the efferent arteriole. It is important to understand the physiologic effect arteriole vasoconstriction has on glomerular pressure. When the afferent arteriole constricts, a pressure drop occurs within the glomerulus, and the filtration fraction decreases. When efferent arteriole vasoconstriction occurs, pressure increases within the glomerulus, thereby increasing the filtration fraction. Plasma is filtered at the glomerulus, and the ultrafiltrate is modified by a variety of secretive and absorptive processes in its course through the renal tubules.

Glomerular filtration rate (GFR) and renal plasma flow are well maintained until the fifth decade, when a steady, slow decline occurs. This decline is greater in diabetic and hypertensive patients. As elderly patients are more prone to dehydration, they should be adequately hydrated prior to and throughout exercise.[3]

Renal Physiology With Exercise

The simple act of running causes acute changes in a variety of organ systems, as exercising muscle requires a significantly larger proportion of the cardiac output. Blood flow is shunted away from the kidney to meet the demands of working muscle. Studies have noted a drop in renal blood flow from 1000 ml/min to as little as 200 ml/min.[4]

Increased cardiac output and peripheral vasodilation are mediated through amplified sympathetic nervous system output. Increased sympathetic drive causes both afferent and efferent renal arteriole vasoconstriction. In an attempt to maintain GFR, the efferent arteriole constricts to a greater degree than the afferent arteriole. This creates an increased "pressure-head" at the glomerulus that increases the kidney's filtration fraction, accounting for many of the renal changes seen with exercise. The increase in filtration fraction is proportional to the intensity of exercise and is attenuated by increasing the runner's hydration status. Poorly hydrated individuals have a significantly larger decrease in renal blood flow compared with normally hydrated individuals. With moderate exercise (50% $\dot{V}O_2$max), renal plasma flow decreases by 30%; with heavy exercise (65% $\dot{V}O_2$max), renal plasma flow decreases by 75%. Fortunately, these changes are temporary, as renal blood flow typically returns to preexercise levels within 60 minutes of exercise cessation.[5]

Exercise-induced renal changes are also due to increases in a variety of hormones such as antidiuretic hormone, aldosterone, and endothelin. Antidiuretic hormone levels increase with running to help protect against free-water loss. Additionally, water and sodium are preserved through increased aldosterone release. Endothelin is a potent vasoconstrictor.

HEMATURIA

Exercise-induced hematuria is known by a variety of names: sports hematuria, stress hematuria, and 10,000-meter hematuria. It was described as early as 1793, when Bernadini Ramazziani, an Italian physician, described the passage of bloody urine by runners and attributed it to a ruptured vein in the kidney. Barach first noted hematuria in runners in 1910, and Gardner described the entity nearly a half century ago, terming it "athletic pseudonephritis." Sports hematuria, as exercise-induced hematuria is currently known, is defined as hematuria, gross or microscopic, that occurs following vigorous exercise and resolves promptly with rest.

Hematuria occurs in a variety of contact and noncontact sports and is related to the duration and intensity of the event. The longer and more strenuous the event, the more prominent the hematuria. Sports hematuria is most common in swimmers and distance runners. The incidence of hematuria in runners ranges from 20% of marathoners to 50% of ultramarathoners. One study reported an incidence of 18% in marathoners who were known to be free of renal disease and had negative urinalysis prior to the marathon[6]; another found bloody urine in 69% of 48 runners who ran 9 to 14 km.[7] Sports hematuria does not appear to be gender specific, as a study of 383 marathoners revealed hematuria in 17% of the runners, regardless of gender.[1]

Patient History

A thorough history should be obtained in runners who present with gross hematuria. One should inquire about the presence of urinary urgency, dysuria, frequency, and the presence of clots, as well as trauma, penile discharge, or a history of nephrolithiasis. General historical questions should include the presence of bleeding disorders, ongoing menses, recent streptococcal infection, generalized swelling, or risk factors for urologic cancer such as tobacco use, age greater than 40, and pelvic irradiation. Other important historical questions include prescription and over-the-counter drug use, dietary supplement use, family history, and diet history. In addition, a complete exercise history should be obtained when microscopic hematuria is discovered incidentally.

An important historical feature is the timing of gross hematuria. Presence of blood upon initiating urination is probably urethral in origin. Hematuria upon termination of urination originates from the bladder or posterior urethra. Continuous hematuria probably originates from the upper urinary tract.

Physical Examination

A thorough and meticulous physical examination should be completed. Vital signs, especially blood pressure, should always be obtained. The back, flank, abdomen, and genitalia are examined, paying particular attention to signs of trauma or infection.

Laboratory Findings

The crucial step in the evaluation of sports hematuria is the urinalysis, which consists of dipstick and microscopic evaluation. Chemical detection of blood by dipstick is based on the peroxidase-like activity of hemoglobin. The degree of color change is directly related to the amount of hemoglobin present. The sensitivity of urinary dipsticks is over 90%, although the specificity is somewhat lower when compared with microscopy. False-positive dipstick readings are usually associated with menstrual blood. Other confounding factors include the intake of large amounts of ascorbic acid (vitamin C), which inhibits the peroxidase activity and ingestion of foodstuffs with high concentrations of oxidants.

Microscopy should always accompany dipstick analysis. Normal urine contains fewer than three red blood cells per high power field. Microscopic hematuria is common in the general population, with a prevalence ranging from 4% in children to 13% in men older than 35 years of age and postmenopausal women. Erythrocytes, leukocytes, and the presence of bacteria point toward an infectious etiology. Dysmorphic red blood cells, erythrocyte casts, and marked proteinuria indicate a glomerular process. The evaluation of pediatric hematuria should include a spot calcium-to-creatinine ratio to look for benign hypercalcuria. African-American athletes should be tested for the presence of sickle cell trait or disease.[8]

A positive dipstick for blood with an absence of red blood cells on microscopy indicates the presence of hemoglobinuria or myoglobinuria. Hemoglobinuria may be due to *foot strike hemolysis*, which usually appears 1 to 3 hours after vigorous exercise. The etiology is felt to be hemolysis of the erythrocytes as they pass through the heel. Eventually the body's ability to bind hemoglobin is surpassed, and hemoglobin is passed in the urine. Myoglobinuria is much rarer and is indicative of significant muscle breakdown. It is felt that poorly trained runners or those with preexisting muscle disease are at higher risk for myoglobinuria.

Etiology

The etiology of sports hematuria is multifactorial and includes hypoxic damage to the nephron and direct or indirect trauma to the bladder, prostate, or urethra. The lower urinary tract is the most common source of exercise-induced hematuria.

Renal vasoconstriction leads to decreased afferent blood flow but an increased pressure head due to a relatively greater efferent vasoconstriction. Hypoxic damage occurs as well, which is proportional to the intensity and duration of exercise. The cumulative effect is increased glomerular permeability and excretion of erythrocytes into the urine.

In 1977, Blacklock[9] described contusions of the urinary bladder as a source of sports hematuria. He performed cystoscopy on 18 British servicemen who presented with hematuria after a 10,000-meter run and described predictable contusions on the anterior wall of the bladder with corresponding mirror images on the posterior wall. Most distinctive was a posterior-wall contusion that arose from "bladder wall slap" onto the internal meatus located at the fixed bladder base. Repeat cystoscopy performed 1 week later revealed complete healing of the contusions. Blacklock theorized that this minor trauma repeated thousands of times over the course of a long run accounted for the contusions and subsequent hematuria. For this mechanism of injury to occur, the bladder must be empty or nearly empty. Variable urine volumes within the bladder would account for the seemingly random nature of the hematuria observed.[9]

Repetitive "bladder slap" and hypoxic damage can both contribute to sports hematuria in runners. Bloody urine can also arise from prostatic contusion associated with bicycle seat use, which is an important consideration in runners who compete in triathlons.

Additionally, hematuria may not be related to running at all. Of most concern is hematuria in a runner older than 40 years of age that fails to clear after a rest from running for 48 to 72 hours. This gross hematuria is worrisome for neoplasm. A broad differential diagnosis including urinary tract infection, nephrolithiasis, urethritis, prostatitis, glomerulonephritis, and medications should be entertained. Exercise-induced hematuria may be the first sign of IgA nephropathy.

Evaluation

In suspected sports hematuria, a urinalysis should be repeated after 24 to 72 hours of rest. With a negative history and physical examination, the absence of red blood cells clinches the diagnosis of sports hematuria. Men over the age of 40 years, a large segment of the running population, require a thorough evaluation to exclude cancer of the urinary tract as the etiology of their hematuria. Further workup is needed if the hematuria is persistent or is not associated with exercise.

An appropriate workup could include urine culture, serum markers of renal function, sickle cell preparation, and imaging (intravenous pyelogram, sonogram, or magnetic resonance imaging) based on presenting symptoms and physical examination findings. In patients over the age of 40 years, bladder lesions should be excluded through intravenous pyelography, cystoscopy, and bladder cytology (Fig. 25–1). New-onset hypertension associated with proteinuria and hematuria is consistent with glomerulonephritis and requires a thorough evaluation, possibly including renal biopsy. With a negative evaluation, repeat episodes of exercise-induced

hematuria do not require repeated evaluation. If the runner exhibits new symptoms or if the hematuria is not exercise related, further evaluation in needed.[10]

Treatment

Sports hematuria is treated with rest from the offending activity and repeat urinalysis to confirm resolution. If another medical condition is found to be responsible for the hematuria, it should be treated appropriately. Athletes may return to running after an episode of sports hematuria without risk of long-term sequelae. Runners should be encouraged to drink adequate amounts of fluids and avoid urinating before running, to decrease the incidence of bladder contusions. If heel strike hemolysis is suspected, a change to running shoes with better cushioning or a softer running surface is recommended. Recurrent cases of proven exercise-induced hematuria need not

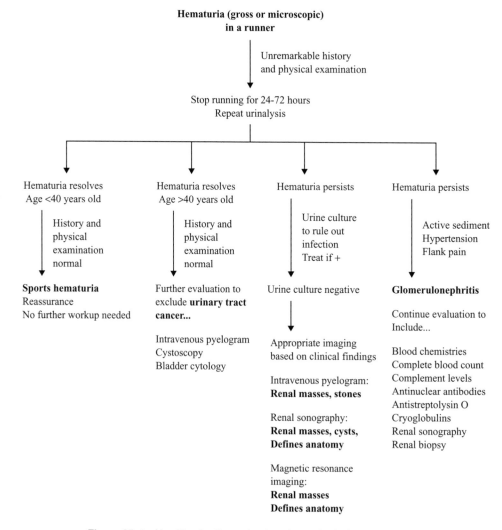

Figure 25–1. Algorithm for the evaluation of exercise-induced hematuria.

be evaluated and activity need not be stopped, although modification of intensity and/or duration is suggested.

PROTEINURIA

Normal urine protein is composed of 30% albumin, 30% serum globulins, and 40% tissue proteins. This composition is altered by conditions that change glomerular filtration, tubular reabsorption, or excretion of urine protein. Proteinuria of glomerular origin is typically in the 1- to 3-g a day range and is predominantly albumin. Conversely, proteinuria of tubular origin is of low molecular weight (immunoglobulins) and seldom exceeds 2 to 3 g a day.

Postexercise proteinuria is relatively common and has been described for well over 120 years. Leube described postexertional proteinuria in soldiers in 1878. In a study of 383 marathoners, the incidence of proteinuria was 30% in both men and women.[1] It has been described in a variety of sports, both contact and noncontact. Proteinuria is associated with more strenuous activity, such as maximal short-term effort, rather than prolonged activity.

Patient History

As with the sports hematuria, a thorough yet focused history should be obtained. Important historical questions include exposure to nephrotoxic drugs, IV drug use, and chronic conditions such as diabetes, systemic lupus erythematosus, or chronic active hepatitis. A family history of hereditary nephritis or polycystic kidney disease is important. More often than not, the proteinuria is an incidental finding, and the patient should be questioned about prior exercise, its duration, and, more importantly, its intensity.

Physical Examination

A meticulous physical examination should be completed. Vital signs, especially blood pressure, should always be obtained. The back, flank, abdomen, skin, and genitalia are examined in routine fashion. The extremities are evaluated for any signs of edema. The crucial step in the evaluation of sports proteinuria, as in hematuria, is the urinalysis.

Laboratory Findings

Proteinuria is defined as more than 150 mg of protein excreted in a 24-hour period. Proteinuria is measured on a urine dipstick by a pH shift when urine proteins, mainly albumin, come in contact with tetrabromophenol blue dye. False-negative readings can occur with alkaline or dilute urine, or when the primary protein is not albumin. False positives may occur with highly concentrated urine, gross hematuria, highly alkaline urine, and phenazopyridine HCl. Confirmatory tests for proteinuria include the sulfosalicylic acid test, a more sensitive test for low molecular weight proteins, and urine protein electrophoresis.[8]

Dipstick measurement of exercise-induced proteinuria is usually in the 2+ to 3+ range and is maximal within the first 20 to 30 minutes following exercise. A urine dipstick reading of 2+ is equivalent to 100 to 299 mg/dl of protein; 3+ readings are in the 300- to 999-mg/dl range. The specific gravity should be taken into account when proteinuria is present. If 1+ proteinuria is present and the urine is highly concentrated, a repeat sample should be analyzed after adequate hydration. Specific gravity is less important with 2+ to 3+ readings, as this level of proteinuria is always abnormal and requires evaluation.

As an aside, urinalysis has been a routine component of the preparticipation examination for youth activities. Rest proteinuria is a common finding in children, and exercise-induced proteinuria is as common as in adults, if not more so. A study of 170 children revealed that postexercise proteinuria was present throughout childhood and adolescence and was directly related to running intensity.[11] Rest proteinuria in this age group is benign in all but 0.1% of cases, and the monetary and emotional costs involved in further evaluation are large; therefore, routine urinalysis screening in this population is no longer recommended.[5]

Etiology

In postexercise proteinuria, the proteins are from plasma, and their composition is different from those found in physiologic proteinuria. The composition of proteinuria was analyzed in 12 runners following an agonistic mountain footrace. This study revealed significantly increased levels of albumin and beta$_2$-microglobulin that are of glomerular and tubular origin, respectively.[12] A study of 10 professional cyclists before and after a vigorous training session confirmed that the proteinuria was of both glomerular and tubular origin.[13]

As mentioned in the physiology section, the relative difference in decreased renal blood flow and GFR results in an increased filtration fraction, allowing macromolecules to diffuse into the tubular lumen. Brief intense running yields proteins of glomerular origin while more prolonged running yields mixed glomerular and tubular proteins. A study of 13 men who ran at maximal exertion revealed short distances primarily affected glomerular permeability while longer distances affected both glomerular and tubular sites.[14] Severe exercise overloads the renal tubule's ability to reabsorb plasma proteins.

Evaluation

Exercise-induced proteinuria is expected to clear within 24 to 48 hours after exercise cessation. Repeat resting urinalysis with microscopic examination must be performed in all cases of exercise-induced proteinuria. Exercise-induced proteinuria carries a benign prognosis, but other causes of proteinuria must not be overlooked. If urinalysis after 24 to 48 hours of rest still reveals proteinuria, a thorough evaluation for its etiology should be undertaken (Fig. 25–2). Causes include benign orthostatic proteinuria, recent streptococcal infections, collagen vascular disease, polycystic kidneys, nephritis, renal disease, and multiple myeloma. An appropriate workup should include serum tests for renal function and a 24-hour urine collection for protein, creatinine, and creatinine clearance. Other tests may include a complete blood count, serum chemistry profile, and a fasting glucose level. The kidneys may be imaged utilizing intravenous pyelography, sonography, or magnetic resonance imaging.

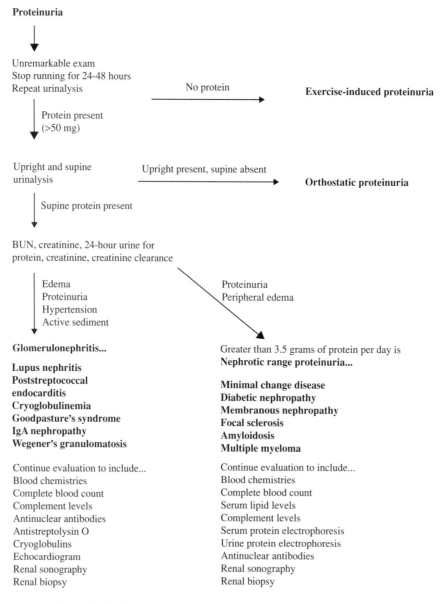

Figure 25–2. Algorithm for the evaluation of exercise-induced proteinuria.

Treatment

Exercise-induced proteinuria has a benign prognosis, and the runner is not at any higher risk for chronic renal disease. The runner may exhibit proteinuria in the future, depending on the level of exertion. If a renal disorder is uncovered, referral to a nephrologist for further evaluation and treatment is appropriate.

ACUTE RENAL FAILURE

Acute renal failure in runners is typically due to complications associated with strenuous exercise such as rhabdomyolysis, dehydration, or hyperpyrexia. The magnitude and duration of dehydration can lead to acute tubular necrosis. Hemolysis due to hyperpyrexia or heel strike contributes to the acute tubular necrosis and renal failure. NSAIDs inhibit prostaglandins (thereby decreasing renal blood flow) and contribute to acute renal failure in runners who "premedicate" in the hopes of decreasing postrun muscle soreness. NSAIDs as a group are also known to decrease glomerular filtration, with consequent salt and water retention, and are responsible for 2% of all cases of chronic renal failure. Experienced runners are at a much lower risk of developing acute renal failure than are untrained athletes.

In most cases, acute renal failure occurs in a setting of "run to exhaustion," dehydration, hyperpyrexia, and rhabdomyolysis. The runner in acute renal failure often presents with nonspecific complaints such as malaise, weakness, loss of appetite, nausea, anuria or oliguria, and symptoms of dehydration. If the cause of acute renal failure is volume depletion, vigorous intravenous fluid (IVF) therapy is required. Appropriate dietary changes, avoidance of nephrotoxic drugs, and adjustment of medication dosing are all important. If acute tubular necrosis is the cause, treatment includes appropriate IVF hydration, electrolyte management, and removal of the offending nephrotoxic agent. Note that diuretics are only indicated in fluid overload states, as evidenced by pulmonary edema, peripheral edema, or anasarca. Indications for dialysis include the need for ultrafiltration of a volume-overloaded patient or the need for solute clearance.

Rhabdomyolysis

Rhabdomyolysis has been implicated as one cause of acute renal failure. Myoglobin from damaged muscle precipitates in the renal tubules, obstructing urine flow and causing further damage to the hypoxemic renal tubular cell. In the past, rhabdomyolysis alone has been blamed for acute renal failure. A recent study of 35 runners with exercise-induced rhabdomyolysis revealed that none developed acute renal failure in the absence of other nephrotoxic cofactors such as hypovolemia or aciduria.[15] All runners should avoid nephrotoxic drugs and ensure adequate hydration to prevent acute renal failure.

EXERCISE IN CHRONIC RENAL FAILURE

Exercise is difficult in patients with chronic renal failure or end-stage renal disease. Uremia is felt to be the cause of reduced exercise capability, as those who undergo renal transplantation return to near-normal aerobic capacity. The decreased erythropoietin levels found in those with end-stage renal disease contribute to a decreased oxygen-carrying capacity, although peripheral oxygen extraction is maintained. Those with impaired renal function do not respond to exercise in a normal fashion, as there is a significant fall in GFR and inability to conserve free water when compared with those who have normal kidney function.[16] However, patients with chronic renal failure can still benefit from exercise. Exercise capacity can be increased, blood pressure reduced, and lipid profiles improved with moderate activity.

TESTICULAR FUNCTION

Short bouts of intense exercise increase testosterone levels, whereas sustained submaximal exercise has been shown to decrease serum testosterone levels. It is unclear whether long-term intense exercise decreases testosterone levels chronically. Theories as to the etiology of the decreased testosterone levels include decreased production, decreased protein binding, or increased clearance. The most likely cause is decreased production due to repetitive microtrauma to the testes and elevated testicular temperature.[17] A study of eight male runners who trained at increasing distances revealed no change in sperm characteristics or testosterone levels compared with age-matched sedentary controls. Twenty-five percent of the runners' sperm counts fell to oligospermatic levels by the end of the intense exercise period but promptly returned to normal levels with decreased workload.[18] It is not felt that running causes long-term reproductive or endocrine problems, but more research in this area is needed.

GENITOURINARY INFECTIONS

Sexually Transmitted Diseases

STDs are common in athletes, nongonococcal urethritis being the most common. Patients present with dysuria and a urethral discharge. As with all STDs, a thorough evaluation for concomitant STDs should be undertaken. A sexual history should be obtained and sexual contacts appropriately treated. Gonococcal infections involve a history of dysuria, penile or vaginal discharge, and positive gonococcal culture. *Chlamydia* coinfection is common, and all patients with a gonococcal infection should also be treated for this condition. Other common STDs include genital warts (condyloma acuminatum) and herpes simplex infection.

Superficial Skin Infections

Tinea cruris, or "jock itch," is a superficial fungal infection located in the groin and inner thighs; it often occurs in runners. It is a result of poor hygiene, inadequate drying, or local skin breakdown due to chafing. The most common organisms include *Trichophyton rubrum, T. mentagrophytes,* and *Candida* species. The runner often complains of itching, burning, and pain. The rash is often quite erythematous, with well-demarcated borders sparing the penis and scrotum. Treatment includes effective drying methods with the application of cornstarch or talcum powder along with topical antifungal medications and low-potency topical corticosteroids.

GENITAL PAIN

Owing to their external location, the male genital organs are more likely to be subject to trauma and extremes of temperature. Injury to the female external genitalia has been reported but much less commonly than in men.

Testicular Torsion

Acute scrotal pain is typically caused by one of three disorders: testicular torsion, testicular appendage torsion, and epididymitis. Of the three, testicular torsion is by far the most common accounting for 90% of cases. Testicular torsion typically occurs between the ages of 12 and 18, although incidence at all ages has been reported. It can occur with exercise or at rest. Testicular torsion typically presents with abrupt onset of severe testicular pain and associated abdominal or groin pain, nausea, vomiting, or anorexia. Physical examination reveals a tender, enlarged testis that is often elevated or in an abnormal lie. The cremasteric reflex is absent.

The importance of prompt recognition and treatment cannot be understated. Salvage of the testis requires relief of the vascular obstruction. Manual derotation may be attempted while awaiting surgery. At surgery, derotation in an attempt to salvage the affected testis and contralateral orchiopexy to prevent future torsion is the current procedure of choice.[19]

Frostbite

Runners in cold climates should be aware of the risk of frostbite. Many recognize the importance of face, hand, and foot protection yet forget that any minimally protected area is at risk. Runners know that they generate heat as they exercise and can be lulled into a false sense of security. Abrupt changes in weather, fatigue, and injury can leave a runner at risk for frostbite.

Frostbite involves crystallization of fluids in the skin or subcutaneous tissue and can occur within seconds to hours depending on air temperature, wind speed, and amount of insulating clothing. Runners prefer freedom of movement and often wear insufficient running gear. Penile or scrotal frostbite presents like that of any other body part. Initially the affected area will have a burning sensation followed by numbness. Frostbitten skin ranges from white to purple in color and is hard, waxy, and insensate to touch. Treatment involves prompt rewarming, at which time the skin becomes red, swollen, and intensely painful. Blister formation is indicative of more severe tissue damage. Loss of tissue is a possibility with prolonged exposure. As always, prevention of frostbite through education and appropriate attire is the best treatment.[20]

CONCLUSIONS

Running offers many advantages over a sedentary lifestyle. Unfortunately, the genitourinary system does not benefit from aerobic training as do the cardiovascular and musculoskeletal systems. In fact, blood flow is shunted away from the urinary system during running to provide for the increased demand of exercising muscle. This can lead to a variety of disorders such as hematuria, proteinuria, and genital pain. Adequate hydration, avoidance of nephrotoxic drugs, and appropriate runner education give the genitourinary system a fighting chance in the body's natural response to exercise.

REFERENCES

1. Boileau M, Fuchs E, Barry JM, et al.: Stress hematuria: athletic pseudonephritis in marathoners. *Urology* 1980:15; 471.
2. Nattiv A, Puffer JC, Green GA: Lifestyle and health risks of collegiate athletes: a multi-center study. *Clin J Sport Med* 1997:7, 262.
3. Lowenthal DT, Kirschner DA, Scarpace NT, et al.: Effects of exercise on age and disease. *South Med J* 1994:87, S5.
4. Jones GR, Newhouse I: Sports-related hematuria: A review. *Clin J Sports Med* 1997:7, 119.

5. Cianflocco AJ: Renal complications of exercise. *Clin Sports Med* 1992:11, 437.

6. Siegel AJ, Hennekens CH, Solomon HS, et al.: Exercise-related hematuria. Findings in a group of marathon runners. *JAMA* 1979:241, 391.

7. Fassett RG, Owen JE, Fairley J, et al.: Urinary red-cell morphology during exercise. *BMJ* 1982:285, 1455.

8. Brendler CB: Evaluation of the urologic patient, in Campbell MF (ed.), *Campbell's Urology*, 7th ed., Philadelphia, WB Saunders, 1998:139.

9. Blacklock, NJ. Bladder trauma in the long-distance runner: "10,000 Metres Haematuria." *Br J Urol* 1977:49, 129.

10. Gambrell RC, Blount BW: Exercise-induced hematuria. *Am Fam Physician* 1996:53, 905.

11. Poortmans JR, Geudvert C, Schorokoff K: Postexercise proteinuria in childhood and adolescence. *Int J Sports Med* 1996:17, 448.

12. Estevi P, Urbino R, Tetta C, et al.: Urinary protein excretion induced by exercise: Effect of a mountain agonistic footrace in healthy subjects. Renal function and mountain footrace. *J Sports Med Phys Fitness* 1992:32, 196.

13. Clerico A: Exercise-induced proteinuria in well-trained athletes. *Clin Chem* 1990:36, 562.

14. Poortmans JR, Mathieu N, De Plaen P: Influence of running different distances on renal glomerular and tubular impairment in humans. *Eur J Appl Physiol* 1996:72, 552.

15. Sinert R, Kohl L, Rainone T, et al.: Exercise-induced rhabdomyolysis. *Ann Emerg Med* 1994:23, 1301.

16. Tavener D, Craig K, Mackay I, et al.: Effects of exercise on renal function in patients with moderate impairment of renal function compared to normal men. *Nephron* 1991:57, 288.

17. Brukner P, Fricker PA: Endocrinologic conditions, in Fields KB, Fricker PA (eds.), *Medical Problems in Athletes*, Malden, MA, Blackwell Science, Publishers, 1997:225.

18. Hall HL: Effects of intensified training and detraining on testicular function. *Clin J Sports Med* 1999:9, 203.

19. Burgher SW: Acute scrotal pain. *Emerg Med Clin North Am* 1998:16, 781.

20. Armstrong LE: American College of Sports Medicine position stand. Heat and cold illnesses during distance running. *Med Sci Sports Exerc* 1996:28, i.

Chapter 26

HEMATOLOGIC CONCERNS IN THE RUNNER

William B. Adams

INTRODUCTION

This chapter reviews the effects of running on hematologic parameters and manifestations of certain hematologic disturbances in runners. This includes a review of the interplay between exercise and alterations of hematologic cell lines, as well as the evaluation of various hematologic disorders in athletes. Also included is a discussion of exertional rhabdomyolysis.

HEMATOLOGY IN THE RUNNER

Running and other forms of exercise generally do not predispose athletes to hematologic disease states. Although runners typically are healthier, they are susceptible to the same hematologic diseases as nonathletes. Hematologic disturbances, however, may cause symptoms earlier and at lower severity, often initially presenting as impaired physical performance.[1]

Maximal or prolonged exertion often causes transient perturbations of several hematologic values. Endurance and altitude training typically result in more sustained alterations of hematologic parameters.[2] Dietary inadequacies often encountered in athletes may also cause hematologic problems due to a deficit of calories or critical nutrients.[3]

EFFECTS OF RUNNING ON HEMATOLOGIC PARAMETERS

Acute and chronic effects of running on hematologic parameters are influenced by several factors. These include the individual's level of conditioning, the intensity and duration of the exercise event, hydration status, environmental conditions in which the exercise is performed, and frequency of endurance-level training.[2,4] Brief anaerobic-type exercise typically causes little change in hematologic values in either the short or long term. However, prolonged exertional activity (i.e., longer than 1 hour) frequently causes short-term alterations in hematologic parameters. Sustained effects are seen when endurance-type training is performed with regularity.[5]

Acute Effects

RBC Parameters
Sustained aerobic exercise typically causes a transient increase in hemoglobin (Hgb) and hematocrit (Hct). These acute changes in red blood cell (RBC) parameters (particularly Hct) result exclusively from intravascular fluid shifts because there are no major reservoirs for mobilization of RBCs.[5] Plasma volume often decreases as much as 5% to 20%. This is caused

by sweat losses plus mobilization of fluids into muscle tissues as capillary hydrostatic pressure and intracellular oncotic pressure increase.[1,2]

WBC Parameters

Vigorous exertion causes marked but transient increases in total white cell (WBC) count with increases in several leukocyte lines. The magnitude of this leukocytosis depends primarily on the intensity of the exercise activity, whereas the duration of leukocytosis correlates more with the length of time high-intensity exertion is sustained.[6,7] WBC count may double for 10 to 15 minutes after exercise, even with brief exertion.[5,7] Neutrophil numbers can increase to two to three times normal levels, with lesser increases seen in lymphocytes.[6] The neutrophil increase arises primarily from acceleration of cardiac output that causes movement of neutrophils from the marginal circulatory pool into the main circulation (demargination). The increase in lymphocytes appears to be primarily mediated by catecholamine action.[7] If exercise is brief, neutrophil levels typically return to normal within 1 hour.[6] With more sustained or higher-intensity exertion, these elevations persist longer due to cortisol stimulation.[7] Following the increase during exercise, lymphocytes often manifest a rebound drop below preexercise levels. This drop persists for 30 minutes to several hours after moderate to heavy exertion. Monocyte numbers may show a mild transient rise with exercise as well. This results either from demargination or catecholamine-mediated alteration of monocyte-endothelial interaction, or both.[8]

In prolonged high-intensity exertion, such as marathon running or similar endurance events, the total leukocyte count may triple and remain there for several hours. This arises from mobilization of white cells from bone marrow due to cortisol-mediated stress response.[5–7]

Platelets and Coagulation System Parameters

With strenuous exertion, platelet counts increase significantly. This is thought to arise from mobilization of platelets from pulmonary and splenic pools. There is also a slight increase in mean platelet size, presumably due to mobilization of larger, more immature platelets from these sites.[5,9] This increase tends to resolve within 1 hour.[9]

Studies of acute effects of exercise on platelet action are conflicting, but most evidence suggests no modification of platelet activity unless exercise produces endothelial injury.[9] Strenuous exertion tends to increase both fibrinolytic and coagulation potential in a balanced fashion during exercise. However, after exercise the balance may favor coagulation due to the shorter half-life

of fibrinolytic factors. In unconditioned exercisers, there is thought to be a slight tendency toward enhanced thrombosis following strenuous exertion. However, this seems to reverse with regular exercise because conditioned athletes demonstrate enhanced fibrinolytic activity.[9]

Sustained Effects

RBC Parameters

Regular, sustained aerobic exercise stimulates an increase in RBC mass (up to 18%). During exercise, increased capillary hydrostatic pressure and intracellular oncotic pressure in exercising muscle couple with fluid losses from sweating to decrease plasma volume 5% to 20%. This plasma volume contraction is more pronounced in trained athletes; however, this fluid loss is offset by resting state or preexercise volume expansion.[1,2] Dehydration during exercise activates the renin-angiotensin-aldosterone hormonal axis, promoting increases in albumin and intravascular volume expansion (typically 20%).[2] While this plasma expansion decreases Hgb and Hct values, total RBC mass is actually increased. The net effect of increased RBC mass with greater expansion of plasma volume allows greater delivery of oxygen and substrates to exercising muscles and more effective removal of metabolites. It also offsets potential hyperviscosity from fluid shifts during exercise (see discussion of athletic pseudoanemia below).[1,2] Deformability of RBCs may also be enhanced by regular exercise.[2] The cumulative effect of these physiologic changes are adaptations that optimize perfusion of exercising muscles.

WBC Parameters

Running and similar aerobic activity appear to have little sustained effect on WBC populations.[7,8] There is some suggestion that regular moderate-level training increases neutrophil counts whereas prolonged high-intensity exertion appears to lower neutrophil counts. This, coupled with a reduction in immunoglobulin A levels, is thought to have some correlation with the increase in upper respiratory illness seen in overtraining.[7,8,10]

Platelets and Coagulation System Parameters

Regular aerobic training or conditioning decreases resting platelet counts slightly and blunts the rise in platelet count seen in response to vigorous exercise. This appears to be primarily due to the expansion of plasma volume as physiologic adaptation to training occurs. Findings of studies regarding platelet function in conditioned athletes are contradictory, but most indicate that regular exercise slightly reduces clotting activity.[9] As one first begins regular exercise training, there appears to be a slight tendency toward enhanced thrombosis following strenuous exertion. With regular training, however, the balance reverses toward enhanced fibrinolysis, particularly as conditioning is achieved.[9]

HEMATOLOGIC DISORDERS IN THE RUNNER

RBC Abnormalities

Anemia

Anemia is the reduction of total RBC volume (Hct) or Hgb concentration below normal values. It is a common clinical condition with a multitude of causes.[11] The prevalence of anemia for males in the United States ranges from 6/1000 for those below age 45 to 18.5/1000 males aged 75 and above. For females the prevalence is 30/1000 for all ages.[12] Though runners and other athletes tend to be healthier, they are susceptible to the same conditions that cause anemia as nonathletes.[1] There may, however, be a tendency toward anemia from nutritional deficiencies, particularly in athletes trying to restrict weight or those following special diets that are deficient in iron, vitamins, or calories.[2,4]

Anemia arises either from excessive loss or inadequate production of RBCs, or a combination of both. Symptoms and physical manifestations depend on the decrement of oxygen delivery capacity to tissues, change in blood volume, the rate at which these changes occur, cardiopulmonary compensatory capacity, and direct manifestations of the illness causing the anemia.[11,13] The following sections describe manifestations of some of the more common anemias seen in runners and details an approach for evaluation of anemia.

ATHLETIC PSEUDOANEMIA (SPORTS ANEMIA). As noted above, sweat losses and intravascular fluid shifts during sustained aerobic exercise may decrease plasma volume 5% to 20%. Trained endurance runners tend to have a greater reduction in plasma volume during exercise due to greater sweat losses. This reduction, however, is offset by a physiologic plasma volume expansion in the resting or preexercise state. While RBC production is increased with regular endurance training, the increase in RBC mass is offset by a greater expansion of plasma volume. This results in a slight reduction in Hgb and Hct levels in the resting state. This is not a true anemia, but rather a physiologic adaptation that promotes increased cardiac output, enhanced oxygen delivery to tissues, and protects against hyperviscosity. Hence it is termed "athletic pseudoanemia," or sports anemia.[2,14,15] Typically the Hgb values run 0.5 g/dl lower for runners pursuing moderate-intensity training and 1.0 g/dl lower for elite level athletes.[15] This hemodilution from conditioning is temporary, however, and may resolve within days of terminating endurance-level training.[2] Diagnosis may be confirmed by testing the runner after several days' rest from training, or inferred from clinical blood count (CBC) testing revealing normal RBC indices and RBC distribution width (RDW) with a normal reticulocyte count and normal serum ferritin level. Beware that serum ferritin levels tend to run lower with moderate- to high-intensity training, particularly in the initial weeks of training. For athletes, a ferritin level $\geq 12 \, \mu g/L$ is considered normal.[4] If iron deficiency anemia is in question, a trial of oral iron supplementation (325 mg TID) with a repeat reticulocyte count at 1 to 2 weeks may resolve the question. A rise in the reticulocyte count confirms iron deficiency as the etiology of the anemia.[16] One should be cautious about giving routine iron supplementation simply for an isolated low serum ferritin due to potential of producing an iron overload state.[4]

IRON DEFICIENCY ANEMIA. Iron deficiency anemia is the most common cause of true anemia in the runner as it is in the nonathlete.[14,15] It is more often seen in female athletes, typically due to inadequate dietary consumption coupled with ongoing menstrual losses. Reduction in meat consumption without compensatory increases in other iron sources may diminish intestinal iron absorption as heme iron is more efficiently assimilated.[4,14] Laboratory testing reveals low Hgb and Hct levels with low mean corpuscular volume (MCV) and mean corpuscular Hgb (MCH) and increased RDW (unless iron deficiency is very prolonged). Peripheral smear reveals hypochromic microcytic cells. The reticulocyte count is low to normal and serum ferritin levels are low. Due to considerable variation, serum iron levels are not reliable for assessment of iron status. Total iron-binding capacity (TIBC) and transferrin saturation (serum iron × 100/TIBC) more accurately reflect iron status. In isolated iron deficiency, TIBC tends to be elevated, while transferrin saturation tends to be low (particularly <16%). Serum ferritin provides an indirect assessment of iron stores with levels $<12 \, \mu g/L$ indicative of iron deficiency.[11,13] However, isolated low ferritin levels (i.e., 12 to 20 $\mu g/L$) without anemia is not unusual in runners and does not indicate iron deficiency.[4,13]

In evaluation of iron deficiency anemia it is imperative to determine the cause of the deficiency state in order to best effect therapy and avoid overlooking potentially serious conditions. Iron replacement should continue until 6 to 12 months after anemia has resolved.[16]

BLOOD LOSS. Acute heavy bleeding may cause anemia before the onset of iron deficiency. Typically the diagnosis is obvious from history or examination findings of gross blood, melena, or signs of hypovolemia. Bleeding contained within tissues or the body cavity may be less obvious, particularly in the retroperitoneal space. Initially the Hgb and Hct are normal. Platelet counts transiently drop but become elevated within an hour if no ongoing hemorrhage is present. Without intravenous fluid administration, the decline in Hgb and Hct may require a few days to manifest as slower endogenous plasma expansion restores intravascular volume. At this point Hgb and Hct decline but RBC indices may still be normal. After 3 to 5 days, a reticulocytosis develops that increases MCV and RDW. Bilirubin levels are normal unless internal bleeding is present. Internal bleeding mimics hemolysis with a rise in unconjugated bilirubin and lactate dehydrogenase (LDH), but indicators of hemolysis on peripheral smear are absent.[11,17]

If blood loss is slow and insidious, anemia may not manifest until iron stores are depleted. Often this occurs with gastrointestinal (GI) bleeding and with menstrual blood loss in women. However, prior to iron depletion, a reticulocytosis with increase in RDW still manifests.

GI LOSSES. GI bleeding is a very common and often serious cause of anemia. Accordingly, a stool occult blood test is indicated in initial assessment of any anemia workup.[12] GI bleeding may arise from the mucosa due to peptic ulcer disease or medication use (e.g., NSAID use), vascular anomalies, inflammatory bowel diseases, ischemic syndromes, infection, diverticuli, or tumors. In prolonged endurance events, low-grade GI bleeding is very common. The source of this bleeding is seldom detectable and is theorized to arise from acute transient ischemia or mechanical contusion (e.g., cecal slap syndrome).[2–4,16] Athletes frequently participating in long-distance running and those using nonsteroidal anti-inflammatory drugs (NSAIDs) may accrue enough cumulative blood loss to impact RBC mass.[2,15,16] In the absence of this or other pathology, however, GI bleeding from running alone is seldom significant enough to cause anemia.[1] Regardless, any GI bleeding warrants thorough investigation to rule out serious conditions. The reader is referred to Chapter 24 for a more detailed review of etiologies and evaluation of GI bleeding in the runner.

MENSTRUAL LOSSES. Blood loss from menstruation may be significant, particularly if a woman is prone to heavy or frequent menses or her diet is inadequate to compensate for cumulative menstrual losses. Characteristics of excessive flow are requirement for 12 or more pads per menstrual period, passage of clots after the first day, or duration of flow greater than 7 days.[11] Quantitation of menstrual flow and assessment of adequacy of iron replacement for chronic menstrual losses should be considered in the evaluation of all women runners with anemia. Treatment is geared toward measures to reduce menstrual flow if excessive, along with iron replacement.

HEMATURIA/HEMOGLOBINURIA. Bleeding from the urologic system is not typically of high enough volume to produce anemia. Some runners experience hematuria that is thought to arise either from increased filtration of RBCs into the urine (as a result of vascular shunting) or from bladder wall contusion during prolonged running. However, any gross or microscopic hematuria requires evaluation, particularly to rule out urologic tumors.[2] Hemoglobinuria secondary to hemolysis is occasionally seen in long-distance running. It has been attributed to foot-strike hemolysis and typically is a not a significant source of blood or iron loss.[4,16] For a more detailed review of etiologies and evaluation of genitourinary bleeding in the runner see Chapter 25.

HEMOLYSIS

HEMOLYTIC CONDITIONS. Hemolytic anemia is a condition in which accelerated RBC destruction exceeds the erythropoietic capacity of normal bone marrow. States in which erythropoiesis compensates for hemolysis without anemia developing are termed *compensated hemolytic disease.*[18] There are numerous and varied etiologies of hemolysis. They range from infections, drug- or toxin-induced, autoimmune-mediated and inherited defects in the erythrocyte cell membrane, cellular enzymes, and globulin synthesis. Manifestations of hemolysis and development of anemia depend on the intensity and duration of erythrocyte destruction vs. RBC production capacity. If the hemolysis is low grade, as in many chronic forms, there may be few or no manifestations other than incidental findings on a CBC and peripheral smear. With slightly more aggressive hemolysis, symptoms are often those of a viral illness, with fatigue, myalgias, arthralgias, fever, and chills. Massive acute hemolysis typically manifests as shock, but most cases develop insidiously, presenting as weakness, tachycardia, or fatigue.[18] Physical examination may reveal mild scleral icterus or jaundice as well as abdominal tenderness and splenic enlargement.

Characteristically, fragmented or unusual RBC morphologies are seen on peripheral smear. Reticulocytes increase and, accordingly, RDW and MCV become elevated. However, with long-standing hemolysis MCV and MCH may be low due to iron deficiency and inability to sustain erythropoiesis. Serum bilirubin (primarily unconjugated or indirect) is typically elevated, though normal values do not exclude hemolysis. LDH is elevated and haptoglobin is reduced. Urinalysis may reveal elevated urobilinogen and positive hemoglobin reaction on urine dipstick test.[18]

EXERTIONAL HEMOLYSIS (E.G., FOOT-STRIKE HEMOLYSIS). Exertional hemolysis is a condition of intravascular destruction of RBCs in association with various exertional activities. Originally described as "march hemoglobinuria" in foot soldiers in the late 1800s, it was thought to arise from the foot strike, causing compression of capillaries and rupturing RBCs. However it is also seen in swimmers, rowers, and weightlifters, though typically to a much lesser degree.[2,14,16] It is now hypothesized that intravascular turbulence, acidosis, and elevated temperatures in muscle tissues may be causative factors as well.[15] In either situation, hemolysis typically is not significant enough to affect CBC parameters. However, if enough hemolysis occurs, the reticulocyte count, RDW, and MCV may be elevated with reduction in haptoglobin levels. Transient hemoglobinuria may occur if hemolysis exceeds the capacity of serum haptoglobin to bind released hemoglobin (approximately 20 cc of blood).[2,14,15] Generally no treatment is necessary. Reducing impact forces to the feet (e.g., improved shoe cushioning, softer running terrain) may benefit some, particularly elite level runners.[15]

Vitamin Deficiency: Cyanocobalamin (Vitamin B_{12}) Deficiency and Folate Deficiency

Vitamin B_{12} and folate deficiencies produce a macrocytic anemia with impaired erythropoiesis. With these deficiencies DNA synthesis is impaired and RNA synthesis is uninhibited. Accordingly, the RBC precursor continues to grow without appropriate cell division. This produces an enlarged cell with excessive cytoplasmic components, hence these anemias are classified as megaloblastic anemias.[11,13] Vitamin B_{12} and folate deficiencies are uncommon in the United States. The typical western diet provides ample amounts of these vitamins and many athletes supplement their intake of these vitamins.[2] However, runners on special diets deficient in these vitamins (e.g., vitamin B_{12} in vegans), or individuals on drugs that inhibit folate activity or DNA synthesis may be at risk for deficiency and require supplementation. In the absence of dietary insufficiency and drug interference, deficiencies of vitamin B_{12} or folate should prompt investigation for conditions that interfere with intestinal absorption and metabolism.[11,13]

Anemia from vitamin B_{12} or folate deficiency tends to develop gradually and symptoms may be mild in comparison to the degree of anemia present. MCV values may persist in the normal range for months, and then initially show only mild elevation.[11,13] Also, if the deficiency is associated with concomitant iron deficiency, the tendency toward macrocytosis may be masked.[2,11,13] The RDW typically becomes elevated very early on with a lack of reticulocytes on peripheral smear. Hypersegmented neutrophils and oval macrocytic erythrocytes also appear early on the peripheral smear, often weeks to months before MCV is affected. When enlarged RBCs are seen, they often appear hyperchromic due to loss of central pallor, but the mean corpuscular hemoglobin concentration (MCHC) is actually normal. Diagnosis can be confirmed with serum B_{12} and folate levels. Treatment is directed toward correction of dietary inadequacies or problems of vitamin assimilation and utilization.[11,13]

Hemoglobinopathies

Thalassemia

Thalassemia is a genetic condition involving defective synthesis of the α or β globulin chains that make up hemoglobin. Anemia arises from both ineffective erythropoiesis and accelerated loss due to shortened life span of affected erythrocytes. The thalassemias are classified according to which globulin subunit is affected (α- or β-thalassemia) and whether impact on RBC populations is mild (thalassemia minor) or severe (thalassemia major). The thalassemias are very prevalent, particularly in certain regions and populations. Prevalence of α-thalassemia is higher in blacks, American Indians, and Asians, whereas β-thalassemia is more common in individuals of Italian and Greek descent.[1,19]

Because genes for α-thalassemia are present at two loci (four alleles), it is less likely to manifest significant deficiency. β-thalassemia, however, is coded for at one locus (two alleles), therefore the defect is more likely to manifest hematologic abnormality. β-thalassemia major typically becomes apparent in childhood, with marked anemia, growth disturbance, and jaundice. β-thalassemia minor, however, is often unrecognized until adulthood. Both β-thalassemia minor and α-thalassemia manifest minimal to mild hypochromic microcytic anemia, frequently asymptomatic. The patient may relate a family history of anemia, and physical examination may reveal mild splenomegaly. Laboratory studies reveal decreased Hgb and Hct with markedly low MCV. RDW, however, is normal and peripheral smear reveals microcytic RBCs with many RBCs having various abnormal morphologies. In contrast to iron deficiency anemia, ferritin and TIBC are normal. Diagnosis of β-thalassemia can be confirmed by hemoglobin electrophoresis yielding elevated hemoglobin A_2 and hemoglobin F. Treatment typically is unnecessary. If anemia is significant, assess for concomitant iron deficiency and treat as indicated. Otherwise, RBC mass can be increased by using transfusions or erythropoietin (problematic due to prohibitions in competitive athletics).[1,19]

Sickle Cell Trait

Sickle cell trait (SCT) is a common condition present in 8% of blacks in the United States. It typically does not cause anemia and seems to have little effect on athletic performance.[1,20] However, SCT may confer heightened risk of complications with exercise at altitude, heat stress environments, settings of rapid conditioning, or sustained maximal exertion. Individuals with SCT may also manifest mild microscopic hematuria which appears to occur independent of physical exertion.[20] This hematuria is rarely significant, but should be diagnosed as hematuria from SCT only after other etiologies are ruled out.[20,21]

Hypoxic environments, particularly altitudes above 10,000 feet, may stimulate sickling and cause a clinical picture similar to sickle cell anemia. Exertion at altitudes of 5000 feet or more may produce enough hypoxic and metabolic stress to induce sickling and its sequelae.[20,21]

Individuals with sickle cell trait may be at higher risk of exertion-related rhabdomyolysis, particularly in heat stress conditions. Retrospective studies of military recruit populations indicate that SCT may confer increased risk of sudden death and exertional rhabdomyolysis. Though total incidence is low, the occurrence of sudden death and exertional rhabdomyolysis in blacks with SCT were 30 times higher than those without, and 100 times higher than nonblack recruits without SCT.[21] While causative factors are difficult to discern, it is suggested that risk is heightened with overly rapid conditioning and events involving sustained maximal exertion efforts (e.g., >10 mets for 5 or more minutes).[20,21]

In light of exertion-related risks, it may be prudent to screen individuals for SCT who are in higher prevalence groups or those with a family history of sickle cell disease or SCT. With known SCT, avoidance of hypoxic environments and strict adherence to heat illness prevention is crucial. Also, avoidance of accelerated training and maximal sustained exertion in unconditioned individuals with SCT may be warranted.

Hemoglobin SC

Hemoglobin C is present in 2% of the blacks in the United States. Typically the heterozygous state (Hgb AC) presents no problems. Homozygous (Hgb CC) states or coupling with sickle hemoglobin (Hgb SC) may manifest hemolysis and splenic infarctions at altitude.[1,21]

Other Disorders Causing Anemia

Several other conditions may cause anemia as part of the disease process, often through impaired erythropoiesis. Hypothyroidism and liver and myelodysplastic diseases typically manifest a macrocytic anemia with enlarged RBCs having thin walls. Alcoholism may produce a mild macrocytosis with or without anemia, even in absence of liver disease. Renal disease (acute and chronic) typically produces a normocytic anemia, though microcytosis can develop. This arises from inadequate erythropoietin production.[11,13,19] Sideroblastic anemia presents as a microcytic anemia in its hereditary form and macrocytic anemia in acquired forms. Diagnosis is best confirmed by findings of excess ringed sideroblasts on bone marrow study because detection of siderocytes in circulation is inconsistent.[13]

In myelodysplastic syndrome, maturation of several cell lines may be impaired. There is hyperproliferative response in the marrow, but maturation and delivery of cells to the circulation is impaired. It manifests as a persistent normocytic anemia, often with deficiencies in other cell lines. Myelodysplasia may occur in isolation, as a consequence of radiation or chemotherapy treatment, or as a prelude to the development of leukemia. Anemia of chronic disease manifests as a persistent anemia with elevated ferritin levels and low TIBC. Initially anemia is normocytic and normochromic, but it may subsequently become microcytic. It is characterized by inadequate transport of iron from storage sites, but the exact defect causing impaired erythropoiesis is unclear.[13,19]

EVALUATION OF HEMATOLOGIC DISORDERS IN THE RUNNER

In the absence of pathologic indicators, it may be prudent to initially repeat the CBC after the runner has rested for several days to eliminate acute transient hematologic perturbations as cited above. Ideally, blood drawn for hematologic study should be collected when the patient is normally hydrated and in a calm, well-rested state. There should be no recent food intake or use of caffeine, nicotine, or other stimulants. Stress, emotional disturbance, and stimulants may artificially increase the WBC and platelet counts. Dehydration and overhydration may alter all parameters through hemoconcentration or dilutional effects. The possible influence of these factors should be considered in analyzing results of blood collected under these conditions.[5,11]

Evaluation of Anemia

History

The evaluation of anemia in the runner should start with a search for historical clues, symptoms, and physical signs that point toward a specific etiology. Historical factors to solicit include character and duration of symptoms and whether onset was abrupt or insidious. Prior history of hematologic problems, malignancy, chronic diseases, or any family history of blood disorders is important as well. Assessment of caloric intake versus expenditure, endeavors at weight control, and use of exclusionary diets may reveal problems of caloric inadequacy or deficiency of critical nutrients. Use of nutritional aids, supplements, ergogenic agents, medications (particularly NSAIDs, inhibitors of DNA synthesis and folic acid), tobacco, or alcohol may be contributory as well.[5,11]

Anemia classically presents with fatigue or malaise, but athletes often complain of a decline in performance or endurance, or elevated heart rate.[1] Reports of petechiae, bruising or bleeding problems, abdominal discomfort, jaundice, alteration of bowel patterns, dyspnea, fever, or pica may suggest particular etiologies. It is important to seek out indicators of GI bleeding because this is a common and often serious cause of anemia. In women, menstrual blood loss commonly contributes to anemia and should be quantified. Chemical exposure through work or hobbies may have hemolytic or hematopoietic effects as well.[11]

Examination

The physical examination should assess overall health and nutrition as well as hemodynamic status, particularly orthostasis. Pallor and relative or absolute resting tachycardia indicate significant anemia. Findings of scleral icterus, jaundice, and splenomegaly suggest a hemolytic process. Bruising and petechiae may indicate a coagulation or platelet disorder. Certain integumentary changes may characterize dietary deficiencies or hypothyroidism. Findings of adenopathy, foci of skeletal tenderness in limbs or sternum, and abdominal or pelvic masses may suggest underlying malignancy. Signs of chronic diseases (particularly renal and hepatic), infection, endocrinopathies, and malignancies in particular should be sought out and stool should be tested for occult blood.[11]

Studies

Evidence of heavy bleeding, severe hemolysis, malignancy, or profound deficiency in one or more hematologic cell lines may necessitate specialized testing and specialist referral early on. Otherwise, if the history, physical examination, and testing for occult bleeding do not point toward a specific etiology, a systematic laboratory evaluation should ensue.[11]

In approaching laboratory studies, verify conditions under which the blood was collected, assessing for factors that spuriously alter hematologic parameters as noted above. Repeating studies after several days of rest may preclude much unnecessary workup and anxiety.[5,11] Stool occult blood testing is indicated early because GI bleeding is a common cause of anemia.[19] Otherwise, initial laboratory testing should start with a CBC, differential count, peripheral smear review, and reticulocyte count. These studies allow classification of anemia according to conditions of excessive loss (bleeding or hemolysis) or inadequate production (ineffective erythropoiesis). Using this scheme with subsequent subcategorization according to RBC size (MCV) and hemoglobin content (MCH) allows for a more focused approach in determining the etiology of the anemia. If initial assessment reveals gross or occult bleeding, the evaluation is directed toward identification of the source and implementation of corrective measures (to include iron and blood replacement as indicated).

The first step in assessing hematologic parameters is to determine if the condition is one of excessive blood loss or inadequate RBC production. This requires review of the reticulocyte count with determination of the reticulocyte production index (RPI). The RPI accounts for expected variance in reticulocyte percentage for different hematocrit values, thus it tends to be a more reliable parameter. The formula for determination of RPI is as follows:

Reticulocyte Production Index

$$RPI = \frac{\text{Reticulocyte percentage}}{\text{Reticulocyte maturation time (days)}} \times \frac{\text{Hct}}{0.45}$$

Reticulocyte maturation time

= 1.0 for Hct of 0.45
= 1.5 for Hct of 0.35
= 2.0 for Hct of 0.25
= 2.5 for Hct of 0.15

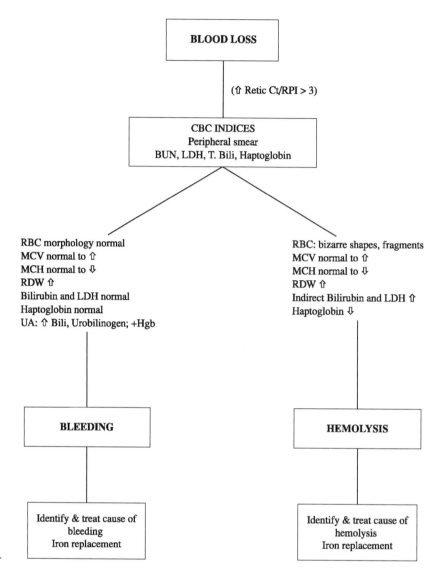

Figure 26–1. Initial evaluation of anemia.

RPI values of 3 or more indicate increased erythrocyte production as is seen with blood loss (Fig. 26–1).[11] Elevations of serum bilirubin (particularly unconjugated), LDH, and urobilinogen, with decreased haptoglobin indicate hemolysis.[11] In this setting, determine the cause of hemolysis and implement corrective measures.[13] Normal values for these tests indicate bleeding and should be followed with investigations to identify and treat the source. However, internal bleeding may mimic hemolysis, yielding the same chemistry disturbances as RBCs are broken down and reabsorbed. The difference is distinguished by history, examination findings, and paucity of fragmented cells on peripheral smear.[11,13,17,18]

Anemia with RPI values less than 2 indicates impaired erythropoiesis (Fig. 26–2). In this setting the next step involves using CBC results to subcategorize anemia according to erythrocyte indices of MCV and MCH. The MCV allows classification of the anemia as normocytic (normal MCV), microcytic (low MCV), or macrocytic (elevated MCV). Decreased MCH indicates hypochromia as seen in prolonged iron deficiency. It is important to realize that these parameters are averages and may not adequately reflect the clinical state early on when morphologic variation within the RBC population is averaged out. This situation, however, is revealed by an increase in the RDW. The RDW reflects size variance in the RBC population and can identify acute alterations in RBC morphology long before MCV is affected (e.g., early iron-deficiency anemia). The peripheral smear may also reveal morphologic characteristics in RBCs or other cell lines indicative of certain pathologic processes (e.g., hematologic malignancies, hemolysis, hemoglobinopathies, etc.).[5,11,13]

Another useful study at this stage, particularly in evaluating microcytic anemia, is the serum ferritin

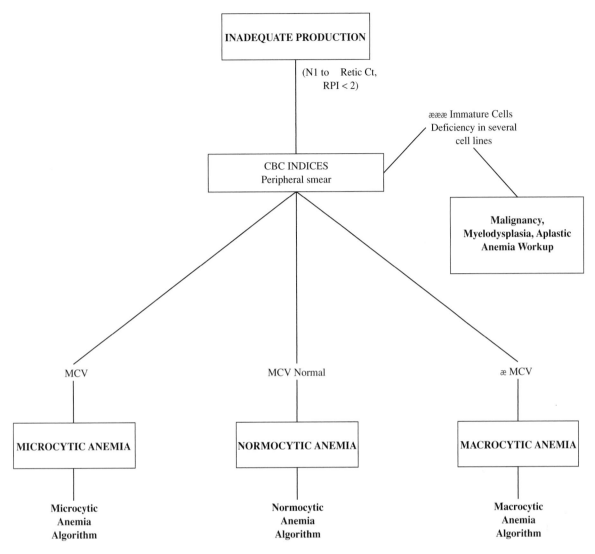

Figure 26–2. Evaluation of anemia secondary to impaired production.

level (Fig. 26–3). In the absence of concomitant disease processes, serum ferritin reflects total body iron stores. Serum ferritin tends to be low in iron deficiency (typically <12 μg/L). However, inflammatory disease processes may elevate ferritin levels into the normal range, masking the presence of iron deficiency.[13] Ferritin levels tend to be elevated in thalassemia, anemia of chronic disease, liver disease, and various malignancies. Determination of TIBC and transferrin saturation (serum iron $\times$ 100/TIBC) may further aid in determination of etiology. TIBC tends to be elevated in iron deficiency and decreased in anemia of chronic disease. Transferrin saturation tends to be lower in iron deficiency than anemia of chronic disease, particularly for values <16%.[13] Various etiologies of microcytic anemia are listed in Table 26–1.

Macrocytic anemia may be either a megaloblastic or nonmegaloblastic anemia (Fig. 26–4). The former typically results from a deficiency of vitamin B_{12} or folate, though drugs that inhibit folate or DNA synthesis, as well as defects in DNA synthesis, may be at fault. Nonmegaloblastic anemias typically result from alcoholism, liver disease, or hemolytic anemia. Megaloblastic anemia tends to manifest higher MCV values and is often associated with pancytopenia, hypersegmentation of neutrophils, and oval macrocytes on peripheral smear. LDH is significantly elevated as well. Serum or erythrocyte B_{12} or folate assays help differentiate between these etiologies. In unclear situations a bone marrow examination may be necessary.[13] Table 26–2 lists many etiologies of macrocytic anemia.

A normocytic anemia may be a mild manifestation of systemic disease, an anemia in transition to becoming macrocytic or microcytic, or a state in which concomitant conditions yield mixed microcytic

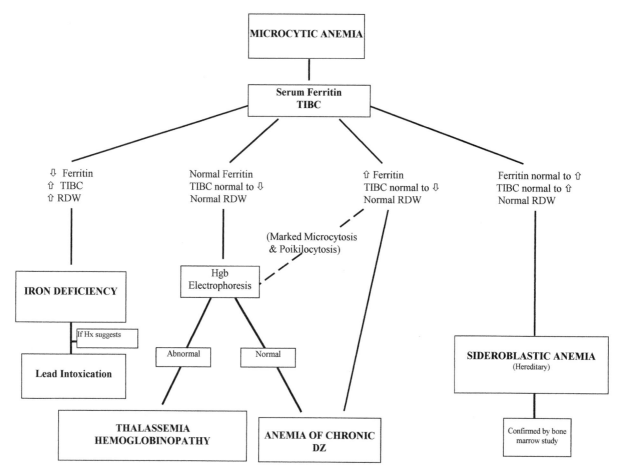

Figure 26–3. Evaluation of macrocytic anemia.

and macrocytic erythrocyte populations with normal indices due to averaging. The latter situations would be apparent from elevation of RDW and review of the peripheral smear. Normocytic anemia may represent early acute hemolysis or bleeding. These states should be distinguishable from clinical examination findings and laboratory results as detailed above (Fig. 26–1). Otherwise, the remainder of etiologies fall into the category of impaired erythropoiesis. This may arise from impaired marrow activity (hypoplastic or aplastic anemia, leukemia, and similar marrow infiltrative diseases) or decreased

erythropoietin activity as seen in renal and liver disease, endocrinopathies, and severe malnutrition. Also anemia of chronic disease often manifests a normocytic anemia. This condition is characterized by elevated ferritin levels. Intrinsic marrow diseases are typically characterized by pancytopenia and immature or bizarre morphologies on peripheral smear. These are confirmed by bone marrow biopsy.[13] Renal, liver, and endocrine diseases should be identified through clinical evaluation, but may be missed if symptoms are mild or more insidious in development. Figure 26–5 outlines an approach to evaluating normocytic anemia and Table 26–3 lists common etiologies.

Erythrocythemia (Polycythemia) and Erythropoietin

RBC mass may be increased as a physiologic response to hypoxic stress or disease processes or induced by drug use. Smoking, carbon monoxide exposure (e.g., ice rinks), and training at altitude may also increase RBC mass in athletes. A spurious erythrocytosis may

TABLE 26–1. CAUSES OF MICROCYTIC ANEMIA

Iron Deficiency Anemia
Anemia of Chronic Disease
Disorders of Iron Metabolism
Disorders of Globulin Synthesis (Thalassemias)
Disorders of Porphyrin and Heme Synthesis
Sideroblastic Anemia
Lead Intoxication

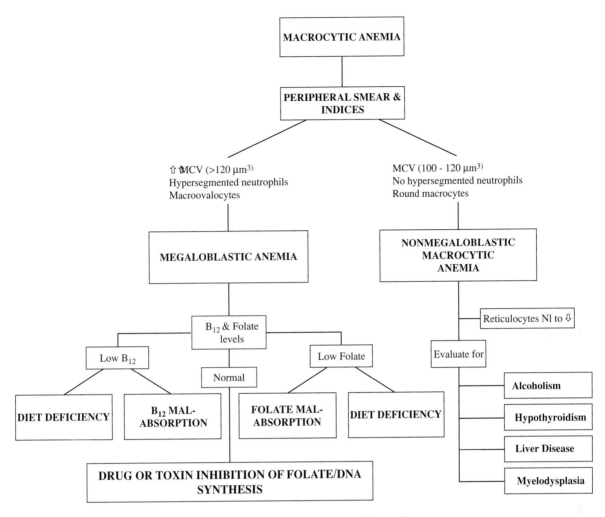

Figure 26–4. Evaluation of macrocytic anemia.

also arise from transient plasma volume contraction (e.g., exercise, dehydrated status).[22] True polycythemia arises from conditions of excess RBC production, either as part of a hyperplastic marrow response

TABLE 26–2. CAUSES OF MACROCYTIC ANEMIA

Vitamin B_{12} Deficiency
Folate Deficiency
Combined B_{12} and Folate Deficiency
Disorders of DNA Synthesis (Inherited)
Alcoholism
Drug or toxin inhibition of DNA Synthesis
Erythroleukemia
Blood Loss (Hemolysis or Hemorrhage)
Liver Disease
Hypothyroidism
COPD
Myelodysplastic Anemia
Myeloophthisic Anemia
Aquired Sideroblastic Anemia

(polycythemia vera), or a secondary response to excess erythropoietin production (secondary polycythemia). Polycythemia vera is a myeloproliferative disorder involving trilineage marrow hyperplasia. Thus the elevations of RBC mass often occur with concomitant leukocytosis and thrombocytosis. It is typically characterized by low erythropoietin levels in the presence of markedly elevated hematocrit. These patients require regular phlebotomy to prevent a hyperviscosity state.[23]

Secondary polycythemia is a response to elevated erythropoietin. This arises either as a physiologic response to hypoxia or from reduced oxygen delivery to tissues due to hemoglobin variants with excessively high oxygen affinity. These conditions typically manifest no associated elevations of WBC or platelet counts but erythropoietin levels are elevated. Use of exogenous erythropoietin technically falls into this category but is discussed in the next section under induced errthrocythemia.

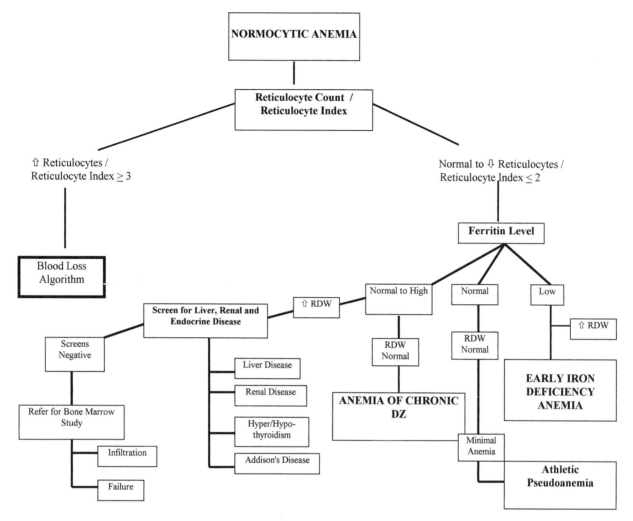

Figure 26–5. Evaluation of normocytic anemia.

Induced Erythrocythemia and Blood Doping

Much focus in recent years has been focused on boosting hematocrit with the goal of enhancing athletic performance. Increased RBC mass improves athletic performance primarily through improvements in oxygen-carrying capacity of blood and enhanced oxygen delivery to tissues. Additional but less dramatic enhancements include increased cardiac output and heat dissipation though intravascular volume (RBC and plasma) expansion and enhanced buffering capacity of blood against lactic acid accumulation.[24] Enhancement of endurance is difficult to quantify, though laboratory measurements of performance gains are greatest in moderately fit individuals.[2] To achieve optimal performance benefit from increased RBC mass, the increase in total RBCs must be balanced against detrimental increases in blood viscosity. Most studies indicate an ideal peak Hgb of 17 mg/dl or Hct of 50%. Higher levels (particularly Hct >55%) are detrimental because viscosity becomes excessive, causing impairment of blood flow and oxygen delivery.[24]

For years athletes have attempted to boost their Hct through training at altitude, phlebotomy with

---

TABLE 26–3. CAUSES OF NORMOCYTIC ANEMIA

Blood Loss (early)
Hemolysis (early)
Anemia with Impaired Marrow Response
Aplastic/Hypoplastic Anemia
Leukemia
Multiple Myeloma
Myelodysplastic Anemia
Early Iron Deficiency
Renal Disease
Mixed Anemia (Iron Deficiency/Thalassemia and Megaloblastic Anemia)
Anemia of Chronic Disease
Malnutrition

subsequent blood transfusion, and by pharmacologic stimulation of erythropoiesis with androgenic steroids and exogenous erythropoietin. Training at altitude (or in similar low-oxygen environments) stimulates erythropoietin production, resulting in increased RBC numbers (and thus total Hgb), expansion of blood volume and the tissue capillary network, plus enhancement of the oxidative capacity of muscle tissues. Phlebotomy with subsequent autologous transfusion (after a period of re-equilibration) has given way to boosting Hct with recombinant erythropoietin (rEpo) in recent years. Erythropoietin was purified in 1977 and recent recombinant DNA technology has allowed production in large quantities for clinical use and athletic abuse.[2,14,24,25] This has sparked a proliferation of regulatory prohibitions against blood doping in competitive athletics. Aside from the ethical considerations, induction of erythrocytosis is hazardous. Excessive elevations of Hct, particularly when coupled with intravascular plasma contraction (exercise-associated fluid shifts, fluid losses with sweating) may create a hyperviscosity state with consequent CNS disturbances and death.[2] Unfortunately, discriminating endogenous erythropoietin from rEpo is difficult, making detection of rEpo use problematic. However, new methods which show promise are actively being pursued.[14,24–26]

WBC Line Abnormalities

Strenuous or prolonged vigorous exercise may produce acute profound perturbations of WBC populations. This effect, however, resolves with rest and is not typically associated with persistent abnormalities of WBC lines. Various drugs may either elevate or depress WBC production, as may infection. Persistent leukopenia may be indicative of human immunodeficiency virus infection or marrow disorders. Some populations (e.g., black males) may manifest a mild neutropenia that is nonpathologic.[5]

If blood work indicates a pathologic alteration of the WBC population, examination should include a thorough assessment of lymphatic and hematologic systems with investigation for infectious, toxic, or oncologic causes.

Readily treatable etiologies such as infection are addressed as indicated. Otherwise, early referral to a hematologist for bone marrow assessment may be necessary, particularly if the etiology is unclear or there is profound leukopenia, leukocytosis, or disturbances of other cell lines suggestive of hematologic malignancy.[27]

Abnormalities of Platelets and Coagulation

Exercise, particularly high-endurance activities, seems to have a net neutral effect on platelets and coagulation.

Certain drugs, toxins, autoimmune disorders, infections, malignancies, and other conditions that trigger disseminated intravascular coagulation (DIC) may produce thrombocytopenia ranging from mild to severe.[27]

Acute development of petechiae, bruising, and bleeding problems should prompt investigation for etiologies in these areas. Longstanding history of mild bleeding or bruising problems may indicate von Willebrand's disease or mild factor VIII or IX deficiency. Also, diets deficient in green vegetables may manifest coagulopathy due to impairment of vitamin K-dependent factors.[27]

Evaluation of platelet and coagulation disorders focuses on identification of causative conditions as listed above. Laboratory assessment should start with a CBC with peripheral smear looking for abnormalities in all hematologic cell lines. Coagulation studies [prothrombin time (PT), partial thromboplastin time (PTT), and international normalized ratio (INR)] should be conducted as well. If the clinical picture suggests DIC (low platelets, fragmented RBCs, prolonged coagulation times), confirmatory testing to include fibrinogen, fibrin split products, and D-dimer should be added.[27]

Thrombocytosis is often a transient condition, typically a manifestation of an acute response to physiologic stress. Transient isolated thrombocytosis is rarely of significance. Persistent thrombocytosis should prompt investigation for infection, inflammatory disorders, malignancies, or other hyperproliferative disorders (e.g., polycythemia vera, myeloproliferative diseases).[23]

Special Considerations

Runners on Anticoagulants

There has been little written about running while on anticoagulant therapy, but issues of mechanical trauma inducing bleeding raise concern. Jarring from the impact of running may cause bruising and subcutaneous or intramuscular hematomas in susceptible individuals. Also, the risk of GI bleeding associated with vigorous or prolonged running may be increased, though there is no formal study of these issues to quantify risk. Outside of prolonged endurance events and strenuous exertion, running carries a relatively low risk for inducing bleeding. Emphasis must be placed on cushioning of foot strike and avoidance of shear stress through use of proper footwear and running on softer surfaces. Also close regular monitoring of coagulation studies becomes even more critical with curtailment of running as excessive anticoagulation may manifest.

Often, limitations for individuals on anticoagulants are more to control the condition requiring anticoagulation (atrial fibrillation, peripheral vascular disease, stroke) than the risk from the anticoagulation itself. Patients with artificial heart valves manifest more hemolysis in hyperdynamic states, but this is not an effect of the anticoagulant.

Exertional Rhabdomyolysis

Rhabdomyolysis is the breakdown of skeletal muscle with release of myocyte contents into the circulation. Biochemically, muscle injury causes a release of myoglobin and muscle enzymes (creatine phosphokinase, LDH, transaminases). Severe conditions that promote breakdown of a large amount of muscle tissue typically cause electrolyte disturbances (potassium, phosphate, and calcium), and acidosis plus extracellular fluid shifts into injured tissues.[28] Rhabdomyolysis may arise from a variety of insults to muscle tissue. These include drug or toxin exposure, infection, ischemia, direct trauma from crush injury or electrical shock, and heatstroke.[28] Excessive overload as in weightlifting can produce rhabdomyolysis of an isolated muscle or muscle group. Typically this is self-limited and rarely manifests systemic effects beyond the involved muscle. *Exertional rhabdomyolysis* is the term applied to rhabdomyolysis associated with vigorous exercise. It is most frequently seen in running activity and is often associated with exertional heat illness (heat exhaustion and heat-stroke).[21,29] Certain individuals have higher susceptibility to exertional rhabdomyolysis, particularly those with underlying muscle enzyme deficiencies or metabolic diseases such as diabetes or thyroid disease.[28] There is an increased risk of severe rhabdomyolysis associated with SCT as well. This typically occurs in conjunction with exertional heat illness (particularly heatstroke) but occasionally manifests in settings of rapidly accelerated physical training and events involving sustained maximal exertion (see SCT section, above).[20,21,29] Alcohol consumption, infection, dehydration, preexisting electrolyte disturbances, and chronic acidosis also enhance susceptibility to exertional rhabdomyolysis.[28]

The spectrum of exertional rhabdomyolysis ranges from mild muscle injury with negligible symptoms or systemic effects, to fulminant cases with large muscle mass injury, severe metabolic derangements, DIC, and death.[21,28,29] Many cases fall between these extremes with symptoms and laboratory studies indicative of mild to moderate injury. While not at imminent risk, these individuals may incur renal injury from myoglobin release and be susceptible to severe rhabdomyolysis if injured muscles are overtaxed prior to completion of healing. The renal toxicity from myoglobin may correlate with both total myoglobin load and duration of renal tubule exposure.[28]

Therefore patients with myoglobinuria or myoglobinemia must be treated with aggressive hydration to maintain high urine output until the myoglobin has cleared.

Management of rhabdomyolysis focuses on recognizing the occurrence of significant myocyte injury, determining the magnitude of injury, and initiating the appropriate interventions. Clinical red flags are marked muscle pain or weakness, particularly if more severe than expected for the activity performed. Of note, symptoms may be mild initially but can progress in intensity in subsequent hours. Concomitant onset of darkened urine indicates myoglobinuria. Initial laboratory studies should include basic electrolyte panel ("Chem 7"), CPK, transaminases, LDH, uric acid, CBC, and urinalysis with microscopy. In more severe cases, calcium, phosphate, PT, PTT, fibrinogen, and fibrin-split products should be added.[28,29] It is important to note that muscle enzyme abnormalities often peak 1 to 2 days after the injury.[29] Finding on urinalysis of positive hemoglobin with no RBCs is used as an indicator of myoglobinuria because myoglobin studies are not quickly available in most settings.[30] Muddy casts indicate a heavy myoglobin load and likely renal toxicity.[28]

Severity of rhabdomyolysis is gauged initially by magnitude of symptoms and perturbations of blood chemistries. Extreme pain, collapse during exertion, and early electrolyte shifts with acidosis are ominous indicators. In the presence of heatstroke, mental status alterations are typical with multisystem toxicity manifesting early.[26] Assessment for the presence and resolution of myoglobinuria is important because myoglobin-associated renal failure may occur even with mild symptoms.[28]

Initial treatment in all cases of rhabdomyolysis is hydration. Mild cases manifest minimal symptoms that quickly resolve and stable CPK levels (typically ≤1000 IU/L) with no other laboratory abnormality. If these individuals remain asymptomatic they may be treated with oral rehydration and rest with return to activity the next day. With more prominent symptoms, rapid intravenous hydration with 2 L isotonic fluids is indicated. If heat illness is present, rapid cooling measures must be implemented. The patient should be reassessed as fluid bolus is completed and laboratory studies become available. The patient with near or complete resolution of symptoms, modest muscle enzyme elevations (e.g., CPK < 5000, transaminases less than twice normal) and otherwise normal studies, may be released with continued oral hydration and restricted activity. The patient must be reevaluated within 12 to 24 hours to assess for lack of symptom resolution or significant rise in muscle enzymes (e.g., CPK rise >1000 mg/dl or transaminase values more than three times normal). Serial evaluations should continue until all parameters return to normal. Any case with severe or inadequately improving symptoms, continually rising muscle enzymes, early metabolic derangement, or myoglobinuria requires more aggressive fluid treatment that is optimally done in a hospital setting.[30] Additionally, hospitalization may be warranted if the clinical picture is unclear, other concerning features are present, or compliance with rest is suspect.

Occasionally patients present with fulminant rhabdomyolysis with massive muscle necrosis. These individuals manifest early severe metabolic derangements with acidosis often accompanied by shock. Many cases of noncardiac exertional sudden death are believed to arise from this because of electrolyte-induced dysrhythmias.[21] These cases require treatment according to advanced life support protocols for the dysrhythmias and transfer to an intensive care facility for management of the metabolic derangements. Muscle necrosis in these cases is often perpetuated by increased compartment pressures, even small increases, and improves with early fasciotomy of involved muscle areas.[31]

Experience with Marine recruits has shown that healthy individuals with uncomplicated mild to moderate rhabdomyolysis may return to activity after all enzymes have returned to normal. It may be prudent, though, to resume exercise in a graduated manner, particularly if activity restriction is required for more than a few days. Recurrent bouts of rhabdomyolysis or any severe episodes warrant investigation for an underlying disease process or muscle enzyme deficiency.[21,28]

CONCLUSION

With the exception of athletic pseudoanemia, it is uncommon to encounter significant persistent hematologic alterations caused by running. While high-intensity and prolonged endurance training may result in alterations of several hematologic parameters, and occasionally lysis of RBCs, rarely are these of pathologic significance. However, signs and symptoms of hematologic disease may manifest at an earlier stage in runners due to physiologic demands that require maximal hematologic system performance.

The condition of exertional rhabdomyolysis may occasionally manifest in runners that advance their training too rapidly, it but may also appear in a conditioned runner in association with underlying disease states or as a consequence of exertional heat illness.

Identification and early treatment of runners with myoglobin release or severe myocyte injury is crucial to preclude serious complications.

REFERENCES

1. Fields KB: The athlete with anemia, in Fields KB, Fricker PA, (eds.), *Medical Problems in Athletes*, Malden, Mass, Blackwell Science, 1997:259.
2. Selby GB, Eichner ER: Hematocrit and performance: The effect of endurance training on blood volume. *Semin Hematol* 1994:31, 122.
3. Harris SS: Helping active women avoid anemia. *Physician Sportsmed* 1995:23, 35.
4. Cook JD: The effect of endurance training on iron metabolism. *Semin Hematol* 1994:31, 146.
5. Jandl JH: Blood cell formation, in Jandl JH, *Blood Textbook of Hematology*, New York, Little Brown, 1996:53.
6. Lee GR: Granulocytes—neutrophils, in Lee GR, Bithell TC, Foerster J, et al., (eds.), *Wintrobe's Clinical Hematology*, 9th ed., Philadelphia, Lea & Febiger 1993:247.
7. Nieman DC, Nehlsen-Cannarella SL: The immune response to exercise. *Semin Hematol* 1994:31, 166.
8. Woods JA, Davis M, Smith JA, et al.: Exercise and cellular innate immune function. *Med Sci Sports Exerc* 1999:31, 57.
9. Streiff M, Bell WR: Exercise and hemostasis in humans. *Semin Hematol* 1994:31, 155.
10. Eichner ER: Infection, immunity, and exercise: What to tell patients. *Physician Sportsmed* 1993:21, 125.
11. Lee GR: Anemia: General aspects, in *Wintrobe's Clinical Hematology*, 10th ed., Lippincott Williams & Wilkins, Philadelphia, 1999:897.
12. Little DR: Ambulatory management of common forms of anemia. *Am Fam Physician* 1999:59, 1598 1999.
13. Lee GR: Anemia: A diagnostic strategy, in *Wintrobe's Clinical Hematology*, 10th ed, Lippincott Williams & Wilkins, Philadelphia, 1999:908.
14. Eichner ER: Sports anemia, iron supplements and blood doping. *Med Sci Sports Exerc* 1992:24(suppl.), 315.
15. Eichner ER: Anemia and blood doping, in Sallis RE, Massimino F (eds.), *Essentials of Sports Medicine*, Mosby, St. Louis, MO 1997:35 (Chap. 6).
16. Selby G: When does an athlete need iron? *Physician Sportsmed* 1991:19, 96.
17. Lee GR: Acute posthemorrhagic anemia, in *Wintrobe's Clinical Hematology*, 10th ed, Lippincott Williams & Wilkins, Philadelphia, 1999:1485.
18. Lee GR: Hemolytic disorders: General considerations, in *Wintrobe's Clinical Hematology*, 10th ed, Lippincott Williams & Wilkins, Philadelphia, 1999:1109 (Chap. 7).
19. Abramson SD, Aramson N: "Common" uncommon anemias. *Am Fam Physician* 1999:59, 851.
20. Eichner ER: Sickle cell trait, heroic exercise and fatal collapse. *Physician Sportsmed* 1993:21, 51.
21. Kark JA, Ward FT: Exercise and hemoglobin S. *Semin Hematol* 1994:31, 181.

22. Means RT: Polycythemia: Erythrocytosis, in *Wintrobe's Clinical Hematology*, 10th ed, Lippincott Williams & Wilkins, Philadelphia, 1999:1538.

23. Levine SP: Thrombocytosis, in *Wintrobe's Clinical Hematology*, 10th ed, Lippincott Williams & Wilkins, Philadelphia, 1999:89, 1109, 1485, 1648.

24. Simon TL: Induced erythrocythemia and athletic performance. *Semin Hematol* 1994:31, 128.

25. Porter DL, Goldberg MA: Physiology of erythropoietin production. *Semin Hematol* 1994:31, 112.

26. Bressolle F, Audran M, Guidicelli C, et al.: Population pharmacodynamics for monitoring epoetin in athletes. *Clin Drug Invest* 1997:14, 233.

27. Tenglin R: Hematologic abnormalities, in Lillegard WA, Butcher JD, Rucker, KS (eds.), *Handbook of Sports Medicine: A Symptom-Oriented Approach*, 2nd ed, Boston, Butterworth-Heinemann, 1999:331.

28. Vivweswaran P, Guntupalli J: Environmental emergencies: Rhabdomyolysis. *Crit Care Clin* 1999:15, 415.

29. Gardner JW, Kark JA: Clinical diagnosis , management, and surveillance of exertional heat illness, in *Textbook of Military Medicine, Medical Aspects of Deployment to Harsh Environments* (in press).

30. Gardner JW, Kark JA: Heat-associated illness, in Srickland GT, (ed.), *Hunter's Tropical Medicine*, 8th ed., Philadelphia, Saunders, 2000:140.

31. Wise JJ, Fortin PT: Bilateral exercise induced thigh compartment syndrome diagnosed as exertional rhabdomyolysis. A case report and review of the literature. *Am J Sports Med* 1997:25, 126.

Chapter 27

CARDIOVASCULAR CONSIDERATIONS IN THE RUNNER

John P. Kugler, Francis G. O'Connor, and Ralph G. Oriscello

INTRODUCTION

Both the cardiovascular benefits and risks associated with aerobic activity are highly relevant to medical providers caring for both the serious and casual runner. Indeed, as a unique physical activity running seems to attract both the most cardiovascular fit as well as those at considerable cardiovascular risk. While there are abundant data that aerobic exercise clearly modifies risk, there is also a small but definable increased risk of sudden death. It is imperative that primary care providers be both proponents of safe and regular exercise for the general population, as well as careful screeners for those at unique risk for sudden death.

This chapter will discuss specific cardiovascular considerations for the runner, including a discussion of the benefits of exercise; an epidemiologic summary of exercise-associated sudden death and its etiologies; preparticipation risk assessment and screening; syncope and exercise-associated collapse; and finally the role of running as a form of exercise in patients with hypertension and coronary artery disease.

CARDIOVASCULAR BENEFITS OF RUNNING

It is widely accepted that there are risk factors that increase the likelihood of an individual developing atherosclerotic heart disease (coronary artery disease), coronary artery obstruction, or partial obstruction due to lesions related to cholesterol deposition. While they may be weighted differently from individual to individual, the usual culprits include gender, genetics, age, blood pressure, smoking, cholesterol level, obesity, diabetes mellitus, personality type (how stress is handled), and inactivity. Recently, serum levels of homocysteine, an amino acid that disrupts the integrity of the endothelium of the coronary arteries and leads to cholesterol deposition, has been listed as a risk factor in those being evaluated for premature coronary artery disease.[1]

While ways to increase the life expectancy of the physically active individuals have been sought, no factor seems to do so with certainty. It has been difficult to discern whether preexisting disease causes inactivity or inactivity causes coronary artery disease.[2] There is a body of literature that states that substantial health benefits accrue from increasing increments of physical activity, partially reflected by increasing levels of high density lipoprotein (HDL) cholesterol, diminished obesity, improved glucose handling, lowering of blood pressure, and altered total cholesterol/HDL ratios. All of these factors potentially lower the estimated risk of developing coronary artery disease.[3]

In a large survey of 8283 male recreational runners, it was concluded that exercise exceeding minimum

341

guidelines led to substantial health benefits.[4] There did not appear to be a point of diminishing returns of the health benefits of running up to 50 miles per week. Higher levels of HDL cholesterol were a major effect of longer weekly running distances. There were no other factors (e.g., alcohol intake or diet alteration) that seemed to correlate with the increased HDL levels.

The Centers for Disease Control and Prevention and the American College of Sports Medicine indicate that the greatest reduction in mortality risk is achieved by moving from a sedentary to a moderately active lifestyle.[5] It is thought that the amount of improvement in risk diminishes at higher levels of exercise. This is confirmed by the Cooper Institute's Aerobic Center Longitudinal Study that showed that initially unfit men who improved to at least a moderately fit level had a 44% reduction in risk of death in comparison to those who remained unfit.[6] The moderately fit men who improved to the highly fit category had only a 15% reduction in the age-adjusted all-cause death rate. Data from the Harvard Alumni study[7] show a 17% reduction in mortality in men who increased their weekly energy expenditure from inactive to moderate activity in accordance with current public health recommendations. A further reduction in mortality rate of 7% was seen in those who increased their level of activity further. In this review Paffenbarger supports public health officials' recommendation for moderate exercise.

The Cooper group emphasizes the need to carefully evaluate the benefit-risk ratio at various activity levels. There is a major concern that excessive mileage may increase the incidence of musculoskeletal injuries, chronic fatigue, menstrual disorders, and altered immune function, and lead to other overuse problems and possibly even increased incidence of disease. They agree that "some activity is better than none and more is better than a little."[6]

If the disease is already established, does exercise in the form of running lead to its reversal? In this case there is an acute cardiac risk associated with moderate to strenuous activity. The most important risk is that of sudden cardiac death due to exercise-induced ventricular fibrillation. Most recommendations are more geared to the primary prevention of coronary artery disease. Few would disagree that favorably altering risk factors, allowing for uncertainties, could favorably alter the course of patients with known coronary artery disease. Without other treatment (angioplasty, coronary artery bypass grafting, diet alterations, statin drugs, aspirin, etc.), exercise has not shown demonstrable benefits in lessening the extent of the disease or likelihood of reinfarction, or to reduce the rates of complex arrhythmias or mortality.

THE RISK AND ETIOLOGIES OF SUDDEN DEATH WITH EXERCISE

While sudden death is a relatively common cause of death in western societies, accounting for 50% of coronary heart disease mortality, sudden death during exercise is an uncommon event. In a Seattle retrospective study,[8] 6% of sudden cardiac deaths occurred during an acute episode of moderate exercise and 9% of cases occurred during less intense exercise. Incidence rates have ranged from estimates of 1 death per 15,240 joggers per year in Rhode Island[9] to 1 cardiac arrest per 20,000 exercisers in Seattle/King County.[8] Thompson and colleagues[9] reported the incidence of cardiac arrest related to running or jogging and found that during a 6-year period in Rhode Island, 12 deaths were reported, representing 13 deaths per 100,000 joggers per year, or 1 death per 396,000 hours of jogging. The total death rate for nonvigorous activity, including both expected and unexpected deaths, was 1 death per 3,000,000 person hours, a 10-fold difference, pointing to a causal relation between physical exertion and sudden death.

In younger populations the incidence is extremely low, with a recent estimate in the U.S. of approximately 1 to 5 cases per million competitive athletes annually.[10] In younger athletes the highest incidence is in the late teens. Maron and coworkers[11] estimate the incidence of sudden death in high school athletes to be between 1 in 100,000 and 1 in 300,000. In high school and college athletes, Van Camp and colleagues[12] estimated a rate of 7.47 per 1,000,000 per year for male athletes and a rate of 1.33 per 1,000,000 in female athletes.

Several case series studies in the past 20 years have clearly demonstrated that the etiology of sudden death during exercise is strongly related to age. The rare sudden death in the young athlete (younger than age 35) is most often associated with a congenital cardiovascular structural abnormality. In the United States hypertrophic cardiomyopathy has consistently led the list of congenital abnormalities since one of the earliest studies was published in 1980.[13–15] Interestingly, a study in northern Italy[16] in 1990 identified right ventricular dysplasia as the leading likely etiology of sudden death in young athletes, suggesting that in certain population groups there may be some variance in etiology. Table 27–1 is a summary of the possible causes of sudden exercise-related cardiac deaths in younger athletes, organized in estimated descending order of frequency.[17] For older athletes, atherosclerosis is clearly the predominant cause of sudden death, and it predictably increases in frequency with age, reflecting its role as one of the cardiovascular risk factors for both men and women.

TABLE 27–1. THE MOST COMMON ETIOLOGIES FOR SUDDEN CARDIAC DEATH IN YOUNG ATHLETES[a]

Hypertrophic cardiomyopathy
Coronary artery anomalies
Atherosclerotic coronary artery disease
Myocarditis (including Kawasaki's)
Other etiologies (less common)
    Arrhythmogenic right ventricular dysplasia
    Marfan's syndrome
    Conduction system abnormalities
    Idiopathic concentric left ventricular hypertrophy
    Substance abuse (e.g., cocaine, steroids)
    Aortic stenosis
    Mitral valve prolapse
    Commotio cordis
    Exertion-induced rhabdomyolysis with sickle cell trait

[a]In order of descending frequency.
Source: Adapted and updated from O'Connor et al.[17]

Identifying asymptomatic or early symptomatic cardiac conditions, which increase the risk of sudden death for the runner, is a challenging but critical task for the primary care provider. It requires an appreciation for very subtle historical and physical examination cues that some athletes would prefer not be revealed for fear of disqualification or restrictions on activity. Key to the detection of these conditions is a basic knowledge of their clinical presentation and clinical course. What follows is a brief discussion of the most common conditions.

While coronary artery disease is primarily a disease of the older athlete, it can appear in younger age groups and should always be considered in the differential diagnosis of exercise-related symptoms. Early fatigue or dyspnea, exercise-related syncope, or angina-type pain, especially in a setting with coexisting risk factors, mandates a complete workup, regardless of age. Many individuals with known risk factors for coronary artery disease start vigorous exercise programs without proper screening and may deny prodromal symptoms. The clinician should rigorously pursue classic ischemic symptoms regardless of risk factors and be highly cautious in the screening of individuals with known risk factors.

Hypertrophic cardiomyopathy is a congenital disorder that has an autosomal dominant inheritance pattern and is characterized by a disarray of ventricular muscle fibers and asymmetric septal hypertrophy resulting in left ventricular outflow obstruction. The condition is thought to predispose to malignant ventricular arrhythmias that can result in syncope or sudden cardiac death. Its prevalence is estimated at 2 per 1000 young adults.[18] Most often the condition is clinically silent before presenting with sudden cardiac death. There may be a personal or family history of syncope

with exertion or of sudden death. Patients may have a systolic murmur that increases with Valsalva and standing and decreases with squatting and handgrip. While a chest x-ray or electrocardiogram may show evidence of left ventricular hypertrophy, these studies may be normal, and a two-dimensional echocardiogram is the best confirmatory test. Unfortunately the routine screening history and physical examination is notoriously insensitive for diagnosing this disorder.[19]

Anomalous coronary arteries have multiple manifestations, but the two most frequent anomalies associated with exercise-related sudden death involve the origins of both the left and right coronary arteries arising from the left or right sinus of Valsalva.[20] It is postulated that the acute angle of the anomalous coronary artery at the takeoff point creates a narrowing of the coronary ostium. With exercise, there is aortic dilatation which further narrows the orifice and compromises coronary blood flow. Unfortunately, most patients are asymptomatic[21] prior to the terminal event, although effort-related syncope, early fatigue, or angina may be prodromal symptoms and should prompt an evaluation with a cross-sectional two-dimensional echocardiogram and/or cardiac magnetic resonance imaging (MRI) study. Diagnosis can be confirmed with coronary angiography and surgical correction can be attempted.

While acute myocarditis is rare, its clinical manifestations can be extremely subtle and outcome can be devastating. It is usually secondary to a virus, most often coxsackie B.[22] Early indications may include congestive heart failure symptoms such as dyspnea, cough, and orthopnea, or merely early fatigue and symptoms of exercise intolerance. Subtle clinical signs may include sinus tachycardia without other explanation, pulsus alternans, or the classical clinical signs of congestive heart failure. Unfortunately, most patients have few if any prodromal signs or symptoms and may abruptly present with sudden death secondary to a ventricular arrhythmia.

Several other conditions have been less frequently associated with sudden death during exercise. Marfan's syndrome is associated with ruptured aortic aneurysms and may be detectable by a careful history and physical examination that is sensitive to phenotypic cues.[23] Arrhythmogenic right ventricular dysplasia, the most common etiology for sudden cardiac death in young athletes in northern Italy, is very rare in the United States. It frequently presents with right ventricular tachycardia precipitated by exercise. There may be subtle baseline ECG changes (e.g., persistent precordial T wave inversion) and an elaborate workup may be needed to confirm the diagnosis. Other congenital conditions include conduction system abnormalities, aortic stenosis, mitral valve prolapse, and idiopathic concentric left ventricular hypertrophy. Preventable conditions induced by substance abuse, especially cocaine, amphetamines, and anabolic steroids, should also be carefully considered. Other events related to exercise have also been identified as rare causes of sudden death.[20] These include commotio cordis (cardiac concussion), sudden cardiac death induced by a nonpenetrating precordial blow to a person with a structurally normal heart. Another cause is exertion-induced rhabdomyolysis with sickle cell trait, a condition that may rarely occur in certain predisposed individuals, in which exertion triggers hypoxia, lactic acidosis, and red blood cell sickling.

SCREENING

What is the primary care physician's role in screening athletes of all ages that may be at risk for sudden death? The primary goal of the cardiovascular portion of the preparticipation medical examination should be to identify individuals with conditions that put them at high risk of sudden death. The American Heart Association (AHA) Science and Advisory Committee published consensus recommendations for preparticipation cardiovascular screening for high school and college athletes in 1996.[24] The AHA recommended that a complete and careful personal and family history and physical examination be conducted for athletes of all ages. This evaluation should be designed to identify cardiovascular conditions known to cause sudden death. The screening should be done every 2 years, with interim histories obtained in the intervening years. The 26th Bethesda Conference gives guidelines on conditions for which exercise is contraindicated or activity level should be limited,[25] and these conditions are summarized in Table 27–2. It is the physician's primary responsibility to conduct a thorough history and physical examination to evaluate for these conditions. The cardiology consultant should provide expert assistance in definitive diagnosis and severity assessment, as well as assistance in formulating specific recommendations for exercise limitations when indicated.[26]

The patient's history should be assessed for risk factors, including a family history of premature coronary heart disease, diabetes mellitus, sudden death, syncope, hypertension, or significant disability from cardiovascular disease in close relatives younger than age 50. It should include an assessment for a past personal history of a heart murmur, diabetes mellitus, hypertension, hyperlipidemia, and smoking; and a recent personal history of syncope, near syncope, profound

TABLE 27–2. GUIDELINES ON RESTRICTION OF EXERCISE FOR PATIENTS WITH CARDIOVASCULAR DISEASE

Contraindications to vigorous exercise
Hypertrophic cardiomyopathy
Idiopathic concentric left ventricular hypertrophy
Marfan's syndrome
Coronary heart disease
Uncontrolled ventricular arrhythmias
Severe valvular heart disease (especially aortic stenosis and pulmonic stenosis)
Coarctation of the aorta
Acute myocarditis
Dilated cardiomyopathy
Congestive heart failure
Congenital anomalies of the coronary arteries
Cyanotic congenital heart disease
Pulmonary hypertension
Right ventricular cardiomyopathy
Ebstein's anomaly of the tricuspid valve
Idiopathic long QT syndrome

Require close monitoring and possible restriction
Uncontrolled hypertension
Uncontrolled atrial arrhythmias
Hemodynamic significant valvular heart disease (aortic insufficiency, mitral stenosis, mitral regurgitation)

Source: Adapted from 26th Bethesda Conference.[25]

exercise intolerance, and exertional chest discomfort, dyspnea, or excessive fatigue. It should also address specific knowledge of a personal or family history of certain cardiovascular conditions, including hypertrophic cardiomyopathy (HCM), dilated cardiomyopathy, Marfan's syndrome, long QT syndrome, or significant arrhythmias.[24,26–27]

The physical examination should particularly focus on the detection of hypertension, the cardiac rhythm, the presence of a heart murmur, and any findings of unusual facies or body habitus characteristic of syndromes with associated cardiovascular defects, especially Marfan's syndrome. The specific features of Marfan's syndrome that the clinician should be alert for include[26,28] 1) various skeletal features, such as tall stature; relatively long arms, legs, and fingers; highly arched palate; joint hyperextensibility; anterior chest deformity; loss of thoracic kyphosis; scoliosis; and congenital contractures; 2) ocular features such as flat cornea, myopia, lens subluxation, and retinal detachment; and 3) cardiovascular conditions such as dilatation of the ascending aorta, mitral valve prolapse, mitral regurgitation, aortic regurgitation, aortic dissection, and dysrhythmia. The cardiac examination begins with palpation in an attempt to identify the point of maximal impulse, as well as any thrills or heaves that may indicate pathologic conditions. Auscultation should be done in the supine, seated, and standing positions. Murmurs, gallops, and pathologic splitting should all be noted. Echocardiography should be considered for the evaluation of murmurs that are diastolic, continuous, holosystolic or of intensity grade 3 or greater. Listening while squatting, standing, and during a Valsalva maneuver should be performed to rule out dynamic outflow obstruction. A systolic murmur that gets louder with standing or Valsalva suggests the obstruction of hypertrophic cardiomyopathy.

The patient's history, physical examination, and age should guide specific laboratory and procedural testing. Lipid profiles for total cholesterol and HDL should be checked in the older athlete and may be useful at any age. Exercise stress testing is not routinely recommended as a screening procedure for the early detection of coronary artery disease because of its low predictive value and high rate of false-positive and false-negative results. Van Camp does recommend, however, that serious consideration of stress test screening be given to the following categories of patients before starting an exercise program: 1) males older than age 45 years; 2) females older than age 55 years; 3) all individuals with total cholesterol higher than 250 or HDL less than 30, hypertensives, smokers, diabetics, or those with a family history of premature coronary heart disease; 4) all individuals with symptoms (e.g., exertional chest discomfort, profound exercise intolerance, syncope, and frequent premature ventricular contractions).[27]

The American College of Sports Medicine (ACSM) has also published guidelines for recommending exercise stress testing prior to beginning an exercise program.[29] The ACSM recommends treadmill stress testing in the following individuals: those with suggestive symptoms of heart disease; those individuals with two or more cardiac risk factors; those individuals with known cardiac, pulmonary, or metabolic disease; and apparently healthy older (male >40, women >50) adults who wish to engage in vigorous activity. The ACSM defines moderate activity as exercise that maintains a level of less than 60% of $\dot{V}o_2$max, or an activity that is at an intensity well within an individual's exercise capacity, and which can comfortably be sustained for a prolonged period of time.

Many patients and physicians express concern about stress testing and the risk of death during the procedure. There is a small but measurable incidence of death during and shortly after testing. In a multicenter survey, a combined morbidity and mortality rate of 4 per 10,000 tests was found.[30] There was no single protocol and the patient group was heterogeneous. In a similar large group (10,751 patients), symptom-limited exercise tests were followed by 5 cases of cardiac arrest, all within the first 4 minutes of recovery and all recovering with defibrillation or cardioversion. The rate stands at 1 arrest per 2000 tests. The risk may be substantially lower in a group in which coronary artery disease is not predominant.

Chest x-rays and echocardiograms are not currently routinely recommended for screening and should be reserved for direct assessments of suspected underlying conditions. In particular, echocardiography is not only costly, but the low prevalence of disease has potential to create a high rate of false positive results. One study did demonstrate that a limited screening echocardiogram can be incorporated into a preparticipation program; however, the validation of the limited echocardiogram as a screening tool remains to be established.[31] It should only be used for individuals with a family history or symptoms and signs of hypertrophic cardiomyopathy or aortic stenosis, pulmonic stenosis, Marfan's syndrome, or nonfunctional cardiac murmurs that have not been previously assessed.[26]

Even though there is a lack of solid data to support the cost-effectiveness of widespread preparticipation cardiovascular evaluations, it still seems clinically prudent. When given in the setting of an overall health maintenance visit, the thorough preparticipation evaluation can certainly yield benefits far beyond the prevention of the rare exercise-related sudden death. A strong endorsement of sensible lifestyle modifications by the primary care physician is a valuable goal of the preparticipation evaluation, and the astute clinician takes full advantage of every opportunity to urge the patient to exercise good health habits.[26]

SYNCOPE AND EXERCISE-ASSOCIATED COLLAPSE

Definition

Syncope is best defined as a sudden and temporary loss of consciousness in the absence of head trauma, that is associated with a loss of postural tone, from which the individual recovers spontaneously without electrical or chemical cardioversion.[32] Consciousness is dependent on proper functioning of the reticular activating system and both cerebral hemispheres. Dysfunction leading to syncope, while multifactorial and complex, is most commonly thought to be secondary to insufficient cerebral cellular perfusion and/or metabolism.

Exercise-related syncope occurs when the above events take place either during or immediately after a period of exercise. The sports medicine literature additionally recognizes the term *exercise-associated collapse* (EAC) to describe athletes who are unable to stand or walk unaided as a result of lightheadedness, faintness, dizziness, or syncope.[33,34] EAC specifically excludes orthopedic injuries (e.g., sprained ankle, leg cramps) that would preclude completing an event.

Epidemiology

While the literature on exercise-related syncope is limited, several consistent themes are clear. Studies at centers that have evaluated young adults presenting with syncope found that exertion is associated with a minority of these events, representing only 3% to 20% of clinical cases.[35,36] The second observation in the literature is that while the great majority of cases are benign and have a favorable outcome, young and otherwise healthy adults who present with exertional as opposed to nonexertional syncope have a greater probability of an organic etiology (e.g., hypertrophic cardiomyopathy, arrhythmogenic right ventricular dysplasia).[32,35,37] Accordingly, most authors conclude that exertional syncope warrants a higher index of suspicion and a thorough investigative evaluation for a pathologic etiology.[32,35-40]

Finally, one study evaluated the characteristics of collapsed ultramarathoners.[33] The researchers found that 85% of exercise-associated collapse occurred after crossing the finish line, and tended to be associated with individuals nearing cutoff times for medals and race closure times. The 15% of runners collapsing during the event were much more likely to have a readily identifiable medical condition (e.g., heatstroke, hyponatremia). This study confirmed long-standing anecdotal observations by sports medicine professionals that collapse before crossing the finish line is a much more ominous event than collapse after crossing it.

Differential Diagnosis

While syncope has an extensive differential diagnosis, with nearly as many classification systems as authors on the topic, exercise-related syncope in the young athlete presents a more limited diagnostic profile. Table 27–3 summarizes common etiologies, with clinical clues and suggested diagnostic testing.

Evaluation

Exercise-related syncope, while generally a benign event, may be a precursor to sudden death and requires a thorough investigation. However, at this time the literature has not clearly identified a diagnostic gold standard or a consensus algorithm to replace clinical judgment.[41]

History

The patient who presents with "passing out with exercise" requires a careful history to discern pathologic from benign etiology. The evaluating physician must first distinguish between true syncope involving a loss of consciousness and presumably hemodynamic compromise, and the exercise-associated collapse associated with exhaustive effort. In true syncope from hemodynamic causes, the athlete typically recovers quickly, with restoration of arterial pressure unless resuscitation is required. After collapse associated with an exhaustive effort, athletes usually will have prolonged periods of "being out of it," even in the supine position, with normal heart rate and blood pressure. This picture is in contrast to patients with syncope due to heat stress who are universally hypotensive and tachycardic. Athletes who describe being "unconscious" but are able to assist in their own evacuation are unlikely to be in the throes of a life-threatening arrhythmia, though other metabolic abnormalities are possible (e.g., hyponatremia). It is in the postevent state that important clues to the etiology, such as seizures, incontinence, and immediate vital signs (including body temperature) should be sought. It must be emphasized, however, that seizures commonly occur as a result of hypotension and reduced cerebral perfusion and therefore do not necessarily imply epilepsy as the underlying cause of syncope.[42]

The second critical distinction that must be made is whether the syncopal event occurred during or immediately after exercise. Orthostatic hypotension occurring after exercise, and usually associated with sudden cessation of activity, is much less ominous than the sudden loss of consciousness that occurs during exercise, which suggests an arrhythmic etiology. Prodromal symptoms, occurring during exercise or other precipitating events, such as palpitations (suggesting arrhythmia), chest pain (ischemia, aortic dissection), nausea (ischemia or high levels of vagal activity), or wheezing and pruritus (anaphylaxis) are also significant. As in the evaluation of syncope in nonathletes, it is also important to identify whether syncope or dizziness occurs only in the upright position (orthostatic hypotension) or also sitting or supine (arrhythmia or nonhemodynamic cause).[42]

The practice of high-risk behaviors such as recreational drug use, or the presence of eating disorders should be carefully investigated, though athletes may not always acknowledge such activity. A comprehensive medication list, including over-the-counter medications and ergogenic aids, is necessary. Finally, a family history of sudden death is critical to obtain, and if present, may identify very high-risk subgroups with hypertrophic cardiomyopathy, long QT syndrome, or arrhythmogenic right ventricular dysplasia.[42]

Physical Examination

The physical examination is adjunctive to the history in assisting the physician in arriving at a differential diagnosis. Vital signs, including orthostatics, are taken

TABLE 27–3. CLINICAL CLUES TO COMMON ETIOLOGIES PRESENTING WITH EXERCISE-RELATED SYNCOPE

Clinical Clues	Suspected Diagnosis	Electrocardiogram	Suggested Diagnostic Testing
Noxious stimulus, prolonged upright position	Neurocardiogenic syncope	Normal	Exercise testing
Palpitations, response to carotid sinus pressure	Supraventricular tachyarrhythmias	Preexcitation	Electrophysiologic study and definitive therapy
Grade III/VI systolic murmur, louder with Valsalva, when present; family history of sudden death	Hypertrophic cardiomyopathy	Normal; pseudoinfarction pattern; left ventricular hypertrophy with strain	Echocardiography with Doppler
Prior upper respiratory tract infection, pneumonia, shortness of breath, recreational drug use	Myocarditis	Simulating a myocardial infarction with ectopy	Viral studies, echocardiogram, drug screening
Exertional syncope, grade III/VI harsh systolic crescendo-decrescendo murmur	Aortic stenosis	Left ventricular hypertrophy	Echocardiography with Doppler
"Thumping heart," midsystolic click with or without a murmur	Mitral valve prolapse	QT interval may be prolonged	Echocardiography with Doppler
Recurrent syncope with family history of sudden death	Prolonged QT syndrome	Prolonged corrected QT interval (>.44)	Family history; exercise stress test with ECG after exercise
Usually asymptomatic, sudden death event, family history of sudden death	Coronary anomalies	Normal rest electrocardiogram	Coronary angiography, cardiac MRI
Chest pain syndrome, family history of sudden death	Acquired coronary artery diseases	Ischemia; may be normal	Exercise testing with or without perfusion or contractile imaging, lipid studies
Asymptomatic until syncope, tachyarrhythmias, family history of sudden death	Right ventricular dysplasia	T wave inversion v1–v3 premature ventricular contractions with left bundle branch block configuration	Echo/Doppler study, electrocardiography
Prolonged endurance event, altered consciousness with normal temperature	Exertional hyponatremia	Nonspecific changes; may be normal	Serum electrolytes, urine and serum osmolality
Prolonged endurance event, altered consciousness with elevated temperature	Hyperthermia, heat stroke	Nonspecific changes; may be normal	Rectal temperature, electrolytes, CPK, LFTs, CBC, urine myoglobin, sickle cell screen
Incontinence, prolonged post-ictal state	Seizure	Nonspecific changes, may be normal	Electroencephalogram, cranial MRI

before the examination. Blood pressure should be measured in both the arms and legs as well as after at least 5 minutes of standing to induce orthostatic hypotension. The body habitus should be screened for features of Marfan's syndrome. Careful evaluation of the carotid or radial pulse may demonstrate the bifid (two systolic peaks) pulse of hypertrophic cardiomyopathy or the slow rising pulse (pulsus parvus et tardus) of aortic stenosis. The cardiac examination should be performed as previously described in the section on screening.

Electrocardiogram

The electrocardiogram (ECG) offers useful information to the physician evaluating the athlete with syncope.

The ECG should be carefully evaluated for rate, rhythm, and repolarization abnormalities, specifically the long QT syndrome, preexcitation, left or right ventricular hypertrophy, and the complications of ischemic heart disease. Electrocardiographic evidence of left ventricular hypertrophy or ventricular extrasystoles, while not uncommon in athletes, may represent subtle clues to hypertrophic cardiomyopathy or arrythmogenic right ventricular dysplasia, respectively. Conversely, a completely normal electrocardiogram is rare in patients with hypertrophic cardiomyopathy. Electrocardiographic clues to common pathologic conditions that present with syncope are found in Table 27–3.

Special Tests and Referral

Numerous special tests are potentially warranted in the evaluation of the young athlete with exercise-induced syncope. The two tests that are pivotal to the diagnostic evaluation are the echocardiogram and the exercise stress test. Echocardiography should precede exercise stress testing, and allows the clinician to assess ventricular size and function, estimate pulmonary pressures, and rule out valvular dysfunction. In the young athlete, echocardiography can specifically assist in making the diagnosis of hypertrophic cardiomyopathy, aortic stenosis, and pulmonary hypertension. The echocardiogram should be closely examined for the presence of the left coronary ostium, which should arise from the left sinus of Valsalva. If present, it excludes an important congenital coronary anomaly often reported to cause sudden cardiac death. If it is not clearly identified, further testing could be required.[42]

The exercise stress test should be performed after the echocardiogram. Rather than a standard Bruce protocol, a test should be designed to reproduce the conditions that provoked the specific syncopal event. For example, a stuttering start-stop test for a basketball or soccer player or a prolonged high-intensity test for a runner might be performed. The exercise electrocardiogram should also be examined for appropriate shortening of the QT interval.[42]

Videotape analysis and discussions with witnesses can be useful because differentiating specific features of the syncopal event can be difficult even in the most experienced of hands. Upright tilt-table testing, frequently used in the evaluation of patients with syncope of undetermined etiology, is *not* useful in well-trained athletes, because many athletes with no clinical history of syncope will have it provoked with orthostatic stress.[40,43] In fact, reliance on tilt-table testing to make a diagnosis of neurocardiogenic syncope in an athlete may provide a false sense of security with potentially catastrophic consequences.

A complete review of all the advanced cardiac diagnostic tests available for the evaluation of exertional syncope is beyond the scope of this chapter. The exact sequencing of these studies, as well as a decision as to whether an athlete can return to full activity during ongoing evaluation, requires individualization as well as consideration for consultation.

The clinician should bear in mind that not all syncope is cardiogenic. Athletes whose history suggests seizure activity may require an electroencephalogram and magnetic resonance resonance imaging study of the brain to exclude a structural lesion of the brain. Hematologic and metabolic abnormalities require testing as indicated. Diabetics on insulin, and athletes with eating disorders or patients on beta blockers should be assessed for hypoglycemia. African-American athletes with a history of collapse associated with high altitude training, dehydration, or hyperthermia should be screened for sickle cell trait.[42]

Putting It All Together

We present an algorithm (Fig. 27–1) to provide a framework for primary care providers in evaluating young athletes presenting with a history of exercise-related syncope. After a careful history, physical, ECG, and selected lab tests, the clinician categorizes the patient's syncopal etiology as diagnostic, suggestive, or unexplained. The diagnostic/suggestive categories include those diagnoses in which the clinician clearly has identified or suspects an etiology based on careful review, and appropriate management follows, which may include reassurance, restriction, and/or referral.

In cases where the provider clearly suspects the young athlete had a postrace exercise-associated collapse secondary to an exhaustive effort, a suggestive diagnosis of a non–life-threatening neurocardiogenic syncopal event may be made and appropriate management prescribed. The clinician is reminded that this diagnosis is the result of a carefully performed history and physical, with electrocardiographic analysis. The history of the event is critical in establishing the diagnosis as previously discussed. Mandatory diagnostic features for benign syncope include postexertional nonrecurrent nature, unremarkable family history, and normal cardiac examination and electrocardiogram. Any doubt in the clinician's mind should prompt a diagnosis of the athlete's syncopal event as unexplained and warrants further diagnostic evaluation.

Unexplained exercise-related syncope, in the authors' opinion, warrants restriction and evaluation, beginning with echocardiography and then exercise stress testing. A diagnosis made with these tests should be managed as is appropriate, while negative testing may warrant either careful observation or referral to a cardiologist and consideration for more advanced testing.[42]

In the patient with an unremarkable echocardiogram and exercise stress test, a presumptive diagnosis of neurocardiogenic syncope can be made. Again, if the event was clearly postexertional by history, nonrecurrent, associated with a normal physical examination with no family history of early sudden death or recurrent syncope, and the patient has a normal ECG, we believe these athletes may safely return to vigorous activity with careful observation. Athletes whose clinical pictures do not meet these criteria, on the other hand, warrant further evaluation by a cardiologist.[42]

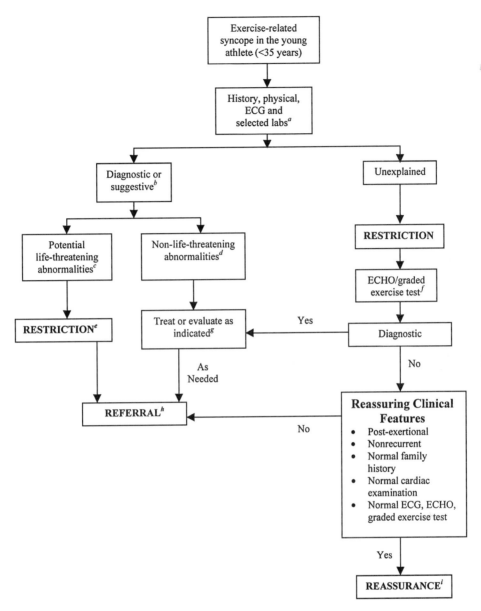

Figure 27–1. Algorithm for the primary care evaluation of exertional syncope in the athlete less than 35 years of age.

[a]After a thorough history, physical examination, and electrocardiogram, lab tests should be ordered only as clinically indicated (e.g., CBC in suspected anemia, glucose in hypoglycemia, sickle cell screening as appropriate).

[b]Diagnostic or suggestive: The history, physical examination, and electrocardiographic analysis result in a definitive or presumptive diagnosis (e.g., hypertrophic cardiomyopathy, exertional hyponatremia).

[c]Potentially life-threatening diagnoses may include hypertrophic cardiomyopathy, arrhythmogenic right ventricular dysplasia, prolonged QT syndrome, and heatstroke.

[d]Non–life-threatening diagnoses may include hypoglycemia, mild hyponatremia, neurocardiogenic syncope, and mild heat exhaustion.

[e]Restriction: This individual should be restricted from strenuous/vigorous exercise pending completion of the syncope evaluation.

[f]An echocardiogram and exercise stress test is warranted in all cases of unexplained exertional syncope, including postexertional syncope. Echocardiography should precede exercise stress testing.

[g]The diagnostic evaluation should be ordered as indicated according to the diagnosis being entertained; this may be in consultation with a cardiologist, neurologist, and/or psychiatrist. Temporary restriction from vigorous activity should be considered on an individual basis.

[h]Referral: Consultation is warranted and may include Holter or event monitoring, tilt-table testing, electrophysiologic studies, coronary angiography, electrophysiologic studies, cardiac and/or brain MRI, electroencephalography, and/or psychiatric testing.

[i]Reassurance: The athlete may return to vigorous activity with an appropriate follow-up plan.

HYPERTENSION

Systemic hypertension affects athletes of all ages and is one of the most common life-threatening disorders in the United States. Clearly, patients benefit from early diagnosis and management. Care should be taken, however, not to overdiagnose this condition in young people, and an accurate diagnosis is especially important.[25] Blood pressures should be compared with norms for the appropriate age, height, and weight categories. Blood pressure cuffs of proper size should be used, and at least three different blood pressures should be measured on three different days before the diagnosis of hypertension is confirmed.

The evaluation of hypertension should not differ between the athlete and nonathlete, and was well described in the JNC-VI recommendations in 1997.[44] It should be initially categorized by stage of severity as delineated by the JNC-VI guidelines (Table 27–4). Specifically, it should include a search for secondary causes as well as a thorough assessment of potential target organ damage, coexistent cardiovascular disease, and other cardiovascular risk factors. The evaluation requires a full history (including inquiries about the use of performance-enhancing substances such as anabolic steroids), a physical examination, ECG, urinalysis, CBC, electrolytes, fasting glucose, lipid profile, BUN and creatinine, and uric acid. It may include a chest x-ray, an echocardiogram to evaluate for left ventricular hypertrophy, and possibly an exercise stress test to assist in determining level of allowable sports participation.[25,45] Additional studies may be indicated if the initial screening uncovers abnormalities.

Hypertensive patients are at particular risk for target organ damage to the brain, eyes, kidneys, and heart. The untreated or poorly controlled are at greatest risk. Because of the asymptomatic nature of early hypertensive disease, detection requires vigilance, and difficulty with follow-up and compliance should be anticipated, particularly in younger athletes.

TABLE 27–4. JNC VI CATEGORIES OF ADULT BLOOD PRESSURE LEVELS

Category	Systolic		Diastolic
Optimal	<120	and	<80
Normal	<130	and	<85
High-normal	130–139	or	85–89
Hypertension			
Stage 1	140–159	or	90–99
Stage 2	160–179	or	100–109
Stage 3	>179	or	>109

Source: Adapted from Grubb et al.[43]

Treatment

JNC-VI recommendations for treatment[44] stress the prompt initiation of lifestyle modifications as initial therapy. Both aerobic and resistance exercise have been documented to have a useful role in the therapy of mild to borderline hypertension. Weight reduction, limitation of salt and alcohol intake, adequate dietary potassium, calcium, and magnesium intake, smoking cessation, and reduced intake of saturated fat and cholesterol are all useful in the motivated patient in both improving blood pressure control (with or without medication) and in improving general cardiovascular health. If lifestyle modifications are insufficient or if there are indications for immediate pharmacologic intervention, JNC-VI recommends several choices for initial drug therapy. The choice of drug depends on the presence of comorbid conditions and complications.

For the uncomplicated hypertensive, JNC-VI strongly encourages the use of either a diuretic or a beta blocker. However, this presents a dilemma for the active athlete and requires tailoring the medication to the individual. Drug therapy is not a contraindication to participation in vigorous athletics, but it does merit close monitoring for potential drug-exercise interactions, especially hypokalemia with diuretics, hyperkalemia with potassium-sparing diuretics and angiotensin-converting enzyme (ACE) inhibitors, bradycardia and bronchospasm with beta blockers, and fatigue and postexercise blood pressure elevation with adrenergic inhibitors. Usually, ACE inhibitors, calcium channel blockers, and prazosin are tolerated best by competitive athletes. Diuretics should generally be avoided in competitive athletes because of potassium balance issues and the risk of arrhythmias and dehydration. Beta blockers will have an adverse impact on the cardiovascular training effect of exercise. Fatigue is more common and oxygen consumption and work capacity can be impaired. As a result of these concerns, it is generally preferable to avoid diuretics and beta blockers as first-line therapy in young competitive athletes.[46] The reader is encouraged to consult a reference on NCAA and USOC restrictions.[47] Several antihypertensives, including diuretics and beta blockers, are on the banned drug list for both organizations. For the average runner, the physician should carefully balance the comorbidities of the patient with the potential drug-exercise interactions and design an intervention plan that maximizes the benefits of exercise and directed pharmacology.

Limitations

It is unclear whether hypertensive individuals are at any increased overall risk of developing target organ

TABLE 27–5. THE 26TH BETHESDA CONFERENCE CLASSIFICATION OF SPORTS

	A. Low Dynamic	B. Moderate	C. High Dynamic
I. Low Static	Billiards Bowling Cricket Curling Golf Riflery	Baseball Softball Table tennis Tennis (doubles) Volleyball	Badminton Cross-country skiing (classic technique) Field hockey Orienteering Race walking Racquetball Running (long distance) Soccer Squash Tennis (singles)
II. Moderate Static	Archery Auto racing Diving Equestrian Motorcycling	Fencing Field events (jumping) Figure skating Football (American) Rodeo Rugby Running (sprint) Surfing Synchronized swimming	Basketball Ice hockey Cross-country skiing (skating technique) Football (Australian rules) Lacrosse Running (middle-distance) Swimming Team handball
III. High Static	Bobsledding Field events (throwing) Gymnastics Karate/judo Luge Sailing Rock climbing Water skiing Weightlifting Wind surfing	Bodybuilding Downhill skiing Wrestling	Boxing Canoeing/kayaking Cycling Decathlon Rowing Speed skating

complications if they participate in competitive sports.[45] Generally, athletic participation depends on target organ involvement and overall blood pressure control. Most patients who have controlled (BP <140/90 at rest for adults) mild to moderate hypertension, with no target organ involvement, can participate in all competitive sports.[25] Patients with uncontrolled hypertension therapy should be limited to low-intensity sports. Patients with severe but controlled hypertension, with no target organ damage, may participate in low-intensity sports. Some patients may selectively participate in high to moderate dynamic and low static sports. In young athletes, the exercise stress test may be useful in stratifying risk and selecting which patients might safely compete.[45] Patients whose blood pressure is controlled but who have target organ damage should be limited to low-intensity sports.[25,46] See Table 27–5 for the 26th Bethesda Conference classification of sports for specific guidance. Note that running is considered a high dynamic exercise, with long distance being low static and middle distance being moderate static.

THE RUNNER WITH CORONARY ARTERY DISEASE

Over a quarter of a century ago there were those who believed that running to the extreme by completing a marathon was associated with immunity from sudden death (then considered death during ventricular fibrillation).[48] The "Bassler Hypothesis," as it was subsequently known, suggested that running that exceeded a predetermined threshold intensity protected against coronary artery disease. The hypothesis stated that if it did not completely protect one from coronary artery disease (CAD), marathon training in some way altered the threshold for life-threatening ventricular fibrillation. Shortly thereafter articles appeared documenting death from occluded coronary arteries while participating in marathons in super-trained individuals who had proven coronary artery disease.[49] But the event that absolutely disproved the hypotheses was the death of James F. Fixx, the man who more than anyone else started the running craze through his bestselling books and zeal as a preacher of the gospel that active people live longer. He died of a coronary artery disease-related event while jogging.[50]

It is evident from the literature that the most frequent cause of exercise-related cardiac events and sudden death in adults is atherosclerotic heart disease.[9,25] Studies have also demonstrated that exercise transiently increases the risk of cardiac events, including myocardial infarction, cardiac arrest, and sudden cardiac death.[8] Accordingly, Thompson and colleagues, in the report on CAD in the 26th Bethesda Conference Report, postulate that it is likely that the risk of exercise-related cardiac events for patients with previously diagnosed coronary artery disease is higher than that for apparently healthy individuals.[25] Despite these risks, runners are anxious to return to physical activity and require prudent recommendations from knowledgeable clinicians. This section on coronary artery disease will discuss issues important to returning the runner with CAD to competition/training, including diagnosis of CAD, postmyocardial infarction evaluation, risk assessment for athletic participation, and recommendations for returning to competition.

Diagnosis of CAD

Coronary artery disease is the leading case of death in the United States, accounting for over 500,000 deaths each year. The principal manifestations of this disorder include angina pectoris, myocardial infarction (MI), and sudden death. Unfortunately, sudden death is the first and only manifestation of CAD in approximately 18% of all CAD patients and occurs at a rate of 0.8 per 10,000 every 2 years in healthy men aged 45 and younger and 6.0 per 10,000 in men aged 65 to 74 years, according to data from the Framingham Heart Study.[51] Well-described risk factors for CAD include hyperlipidemia, hypertension, tobacco use, diabetes mellitus, family history of CAD, and sedentary lifestyle.

Coronary artery disease may be confidently diagnosed if any of the following criteria are met: 1) coronary angiography demonstrates coronary artery atherosclerotic luminal narrowing of at least one major coronary artery; or 2) a history of MI can be confirmed by conventional ECG or enzyme criteria; or 3) a history suggestive of angina pectoris is supported by objective data such as an ischemic ST segment or abnormal myocardial perfusion response to exercise.[25]

Postmyocardial Infarction Evaluation

Since 1996, primary coronary artery angioplasty has been added to thrombolysis for initial management of MI. Patients receiving angioplasty have the earliest warning of disease involvement in coronary arteries other than the culprit vessel. Those receiving thrombolysis are currently evaluated after MI by submaximal exercise and myocardial perfusion imaging or angiography with early intervention (angioplasty, stenting, bypass grafting). In the early period after an MI, the use of dobutamine infusion with echocardiographic scanning is not recommended, because of the effect of increased heart rate on myocardial oxygen demands. Intravenous dipyridamole-99mTc-sestamibi imaging is the early test of choice for risk stratification after acute infarction in the absence of primary angioplasty.[52] This early evaluation is intended to reduce the incidence of recurrent events during the index hospital stay or in the early recovery period, the time the majority of reinfarctions occur.

It is presumed that by the time an MI patient seeks advice regarding returning to full physical activity, he or she has fully recovered, is on infarction-limiting medications (beta blocker therapy, aspirin, with or without ACE inhibitors), and has had early postinfarction testing to determine the timing, type, and appropriateness of mechanical intervention. After the initial evaluation as described above, and an appropriate period of supervised cardiac rehabilitation, further imaging should be unnecessary to determine when an individual may return to running. In the absence of significant ventricular ectopic activity, a stress test without nuclear imaging is all that is required. In the absence of ST/T changes in regions remote from the original infarction, significant ventricular ecotpy, hypotension, and typical angina pain, and in the presence of normal blood pressure response, the patient can return to regular activity with a risk factor profile similar to that of a normal individual.

In the presence of left ventricular hypertrophy, new or old left bundle branch block, the requirement for medications that affect repolarization (e.g., digitalis), the presence of Wolff-Parkinson-White syndrome, or female gender, stress testing with a radionuclide is recommended. If a fixed lesion corresponding to the area identified by ECG as the site of infarction is all that is found, the person can return to full activity.

The American College of Sports Medicine offers guidelines for the patient with CAD who participates in a home exercise program, as opposed to a supervised cardiac rehabilitation program (Table 27–6).[29] These guidelines require careful assessment of a graded exercise stress test and the patient's ability to ascertain a pulse and self-assess symptoms. These guidelines are geared toward exercising at an intensity well below the "anginal threshold." Clinicians should keep in mind that all programs for these patients should be carefully individualized.

Risk Assessment for Athletic Participation

Runners returning to competitive athletics with a diagnosis of CAD warrant a careful risk assessment. While there are no data that clearly correlate the risk of participation in competitive athletics with the severity of CAD, most authors recommend careful risk stratification

TABLE 27–6. PRESCRIPTION GUIDELINES FOR HOME EXERCISE

Angina Patients	Recommended Intensity
• 0 to 1.5 mm ST segment depression and no angina on discharge GXT	70% to 85% peak HR
• ST-segment depression >2 mm at HR >135	70% to 85% of HR associated with onset of 1 mm ST-segment depression
• ST-segment depression >2 mm at HR <135	High-risk: suggest consultation
• Angina with or without ST-segment depression	70% to 85% of HR at onset of angina
Other Considerations	
• Deconditioned patients (4–5 METs)	60% to 75% of peak HR
• Noncardiac limitations	60% to 85% of peak HR
• Initiation of beta-blockade (in the absence of graded exercise test)	RPE-based intensity

prior to participation. The risk stratification process attempts to identify those athletes with severe disease, left ventricular dysfunction, inducible ischemia, and electrical instability. The 26th Bethesda Conference Report recommends that the evaluation process include the following: left ventricular assessment by two-dimensional echocardiography, radionuclide angiography, or left ventricular angiography; maximal treadmill testing to determine functional capacity; and finally, testing for inducible ischemia by exercise electrocardiography, radionuclide perfusion imaging, or exercise echocardiography. Clinicians are reminded that patients should be tested on their medications, because athletes will undoubtedly be participating on medications. Following testing, patients may be stratified into one of two categories: those at mildly increased risk and those at substantially increased risk, as described below.[25]

Mildly increased risk:

- Normal or near normal resting left ventricular systolic function (i.e., ejection fraction >50%);
- Normal exercise tolerance for age (>10 METs if aged <50; >9 METs for ages 50 to 59; >8 METs for ages 60 to 69; and >7 METs if aged >70);
- Absence of exercise-induced ischemia by exercise testing;
- Absence of exercise-induced complex ventricular arrhythmias; absence of hemodynamically significant stenosis in all major coronary arteries if coronary angiography is performed; or successful myocardial revascularization by surgical or percutaneous techniques.

Substantially increased risk:

- Impaired left ventricular systolic function at rest (i.e., ejection fraction <50%);
- Evidence of exercise-induced myocardial ischemia;
- Evidence of exercise-induced complex ventricular arrhythmias;

- Hemodynamically significant stenosis of a major coronary artery (>50%) if angiography was performed.

Current Recommendations

While there are no data specific to participation of athletes with underlying CAD, all authors agree that these participants are at a higher risk than normal.[25] Both the clinician and the patient need to acknowledge this increased risk with activity, and then carefully individualize the treatment and exercise regimen. All patients with underlying CAD should optimize risk factor modification and be carefully screened and instructed as to warning signs and symptoms.

The 26th Bethesda Conference Report offers recommendations for patients with CAD who wish to participate in competitive sports (Table 27–7).[25] However, the recommendations are clearly for those participants who are involved in competitive athletics. For example, long-distance running is classified by the Bethesda Conference

TABLE 27–7. SUMMARY OF 26TH BETHESDA CONFERENCE RECOMMENDATIONS FOR PATIENTS WITH CORONARY ARTERY DISEASE

General:
1. All athletes should understand that the risk of a cardiac event with exertion is probably increased once coronary artery disease is present.
2. Athletes should be informed of the nature of prodromal symptoms and should be instructed to promptly cease their sports activity and contact their physician if symptoms appear.

Specific:
1. **Mildly increased risk.** May participate in low and moderate static and low dynamic competitive sports (IA and IIA) and avoid intensely competitive situations.
2. **Substantially increased risk.** May participate in low-intensity competitive sports (IA) after careful assessment and individualization. These patients should be reevaluated every 6 months and should undergo repeat exercise testing at least yearly.

as a high dynamic, low static activity (Table 27–5), which would be contraindicated for a patient with CAD.[25] Jogging as a recreational activity or running in races as a participant as opposed to a competitor is not specifically addressed. Again, each patient's treatment and exercise should be carefully individualized. Athletes with CAD who do participate in competitive sports should be reevaluated for risk stratification at least annually.

REFERENCES

1. Fallest-Strobl PC, Koch DD, Stein JH, et al.: Homocysteine: A new risk factor for atherosclerosis. *Am Fam Physician* 1997:56, 1607.
2. Williams PT: Relationships of heart disease risk factors to exercise quantity and intensity. *Arch Intern Med* 1998:158, 237.
3. Pate RR, Pratt M, Blair SN, et al.: Physical activity and public health. *JAMA* 1995:273, 402.
4. Williams PT: Relationship of distance run per week to coronary heart disease risk factors in 8283 male runners. *Arch Intern Med* 1997:157, 191.
5. Centers for Disease Control and Prevention and American College of Sports Medicine, in cooperation with the President's Council on Physical Fitness and Sports: Summary Statement: Workshop on Physical Activity and Public Health. American College of Sports Medicine, July 29, 1993.
6. Blair SN: Dose of exercise and health benefits. *Arch Intern Med* 1997:157, 153.
7. Paffenbarger RS Jr, Kampert JB, Lee IM, et al.: Changes in physical activity and other lifeway patterns influencing longevity. *Med Sci Sports Exerc* 1994:26, 857.
8. Siscovick DS, Weiss NS, Fletcher RH, et al.: The incidence of primary cardiac arrest during vigorous exercise. *N Engl J Med* 1984:311, 874.
9. Thompson PD, Funk EJ, Carleton RA, et al.: Incidence of death during jogging in Rhode Island from 1975 through 1980. *JAMA* 1982:247, 2535.
10. Rich BS: Sudden death screening. *Med Clin North Am* 1994:78, 267.
11. Maron BJ, Thompson PD, Puffer JC, et al.: Cardiovascular pre-participation screening of competitive athletes. *Circulation* 1996:94, 850.
12. Van Camp SP, Bloor CM, Mueller FO, et al.: Nontraumatic sports death in high school and college athletes. *Med Sci Sports Exerc* 1995:27, 641.
13. Maron BJ, Roberts WC, McAllister HA, et al.: Sudden death in young athletes. *Circulation* 1980:62, 218.
14. McCaffrey FM, Braden DS, Strong WB: Sudden cardiac death in young athletes. *Am J Dis Child* 1991:145, 177.
15. Burke AP, Farb A, Virmani R, et al.: Sports-related and non-sports-related sudden cardiac death in young adults. *Am Heart J* 1991:121, 568.
16. Corrado D, Thiene G, Nava A, et al.: Sudden death in young competitive athletes: Clinicopathologic correlations in 22 cases. *Am J Med* 1990:89, 588.
17. O'Connor FG, Kugler JP, Oriscello RG: Sudden death in young athletes: Screening for the needle in the haystack. *Am Fam Physician* 1998:57, 2763.
18. Maron BJ, Gardin JM, Flack JM, et al.: Prevalence of hypertrophic cardiomyopathy in a general population of young adults. Echocardiographic analysis of 4111 subjects in the CARDIA Study. Coronary Artery Risk Development in (Young) Adults. *Circulation* 1995:92, 785.
19. Maron BJ, Shirani J, Poliac LC, et al.: Sudden death in young competitive athletes. Clinical, demographic, and pathological profiles. *JAMA* 1996:276, 199.
20. Futterman LG, Myerburg R: Sudden death in athletes: An update. *Sports Med* 1998:26, 335.
21. Taylor AJ, Rogan KM, Virmani R: Sudden cardiac death associated with isolated congenital coronary artery anomalies. *J Am Coll Cardiol* 1992:20, 640.
22. Bresler MJ: Acute pericarditis and myocarditis. *Emerg Med* 1992:24, 35.
23. McKeag DB: Preparticipation screening of the potential athlete. *Clin Sports Med* 1989:8, 373.
24. Maron BJ, Thompson PD, Puffer JC, et al.: Cardiovascular Preparticipation Screening of Competitive Athletes: A statement for health professionals from the Sudden Death Committee (Clinical Cardiology) and Congenital Cardiac Defects Committee (Cardiovascular Disease in the Young), American Heart Association. *Circulation* 1996:94, 850.
25. 26th Bethesda Conference: Recommendations for determining eligibility for competition in athletes with cardiovascular abnormalities. *Am J Cardiol* 1994:24, 845.
26. Kugler JP, O'Connor FG: Cardiovascular problems, in Lillegard WA, Butcher JD, Rucker KS, (eds.), *Handbook of Sports Medicine,* 2nd ed., Butterworth/Heinemann, Boston, 1999:339.
27. Van Camp SP: Exercise-related sudden death: Cardiovascular evaluation of exercisers (part 2 of 2). *Phys Sportsmed* 1988:16, 47.
28. Pyeritz RE: The Marfan syndrome. *Fam Physician* 1986: 34, 83.
29. American College of Sports Medicine: *ACSM's Guidelines for Exercise Testing and Prescription,* 5th ed., Philadelphia, Williams & Wilkins, 1995:188.
30. Rochmis P, Blackburn H: Exercise tests: A survey of procedures, safety and litigation experience in approximately 170,000 tests. *JAMA* 1971:217, 1061.
31. Lembo NJ, Dell-Italia LJ, Crawford MH, O'Rourke RA: Bedside diagnosis of systolic murmurs. *N Engl J Med* 1988:318, 1572.
32. Kapoor WN: Approach to the patient with syncope, in Goldman L, Braunwald E, (eds.), *Primary Cardiology,* Philadelphia, Saunders, 1998:144.
33. Holtzhausen L, Noakes TD, Kroning B, et al.: Clinical and biochemical characteristics of collapsed ultramarathon runners. *Med Sci Sports Exerc* 1994:26, 1095.
34. Roberts WO: Exercise-associated collapse in endurance events. A classification system. *Physician Sportsmed* 1989:17, 49.
35. Driscoll DJ, Jacobsen SJ, Porter CJ, et al.: Syncope in children and adolescents. *J Am Coll Cardiol* 1997:29, 1039.

36. Kapoor W: Evaluation and outcome of patients with syncope. *Medicine* 1990:69, 160.
37. Maron BJ, Shirani J, Poliac LC, et al.: Sudden death in young competitive athletes. *JAMA* 1996:276, 199.
38. Corrado D, Basso C, Schiavon M et al.: Screening for hypertrophic cardiomyopathy in young athletes. *N Engl J Med* 1998:339, 364.
39. Corrado D, et al.: Sudden arrhythmic death in young people: Warning symptoms and pathologic substrates. Presented at the annual meeting of the North American Society of Pacing and Electrophysiology, San Diego, 1998. Unpublished.
40. When does fainting represent a deadly condition? *Sports Med Digest* 1998:20, 118.
41. Linzer M, Yang EH, Estes M, et al.: Diagnosing syncope. Part 1: Value of history, physical examination, and electrocardiography. *Ann Intern Med* 1997:126, 989.
42. O'Connor FG, Oriscello RG, Levine BD: Exercise-related syncope in the young athlete: Reassurance, restriction or referral? *Am Fam Physician* 1999:60, 2001.
43. Grubb BP, Temsey-Armos PN, Samoil D, et al.: Tilt table testing in the evaluation of athletes with recurrent exercise-induced syncope. *Med Sci Sports Exerc* 1993:25, 24.
44. Joint National Committee on Prevention, Detection, Evaluation, and Treatment of High Blood Pressure. The sixth report of the Joint National Committee on Prevention, Detection, Evaluation, and Treatment of High Blood Pressure. *Arch Intern Med* 1997:157, 2413.
45. Strong WB, Steed D: Cardiovascular evaluation of the young athlete. *Pediatr Clin North Am* 1982:29, 1325.
46. Kugler JP, O'Connor FG: Cardiovascular problems, in Lillegard WA, Butcher JD, Rucker KS, (eds.), *Handbook of Sports Medicine*, 2nd ed., Butterworth/Heinemann, Boston, 1999:341.
47. Fuentes RJ, Rosenberg JM, Davis A, (eds.): *Athletic Drug Reference '96*, Durham, NC, Clean Data Inc., 1996.
48. Bassler TJ: Athletic activity and longevity. *Lancet* 1972:2, 712.
49. Noakes TD, Opie LH, Rose AG: Marathon running and immunity to coronary heart disease: Fact versus fiction. *Clin Sports Med* 1984:3, 527.
50. Gross J: James F. Fixx Dies Jogging. *New York Times*, July 22, 1984.
51. Anderson KM, Wilson PWF, Odell PM, et al.: An updated coronary risk profile: A statement for health professionals. *Circulation* 1991:83, 356.
52. Wackers FT, Zaret BL: Risk stratification after acute infarction. *Circulation* 1999:100, 2040.

Chapter 28

INFECTIOUS DISEASE IN THE RUNNER

John P. Metz, W. Scott Deitche, and Thomas M. Howard

INTRODUCTION

Most people would agree that exercise helps maintain overall health and decreases one's vulnerability to common infections. In a survey of nonelite athletes who engaged in regular, moderate exercise, 90% reported that they rarely got sick.[1-3] Elite athletes, however, feel that intense training lowers their immunity and makes them more susceptible to illness.[2,3] Many studies show that exercise influences the immune system in both elite and recreational athletes. The current opinion is that moderate exercise, such as recreational running, is an immune stimulant. Intense exercise, such as training for and running a marathon, however, may suppress immune system function. Some authors submit that this relationship between exercise and immune function supports the proposed J-shaped model[1-7] (Fig. 28–1).

This chapter will detail how exercise affects the immune system, highlight common symptoms and illnesses which often affect runners, review some common immune modulators that may serve a treatment and preventive role, and discuss how a runner should return to training after illness. We hope to provide health care providers of athletes, especially runners, some insights into the prevention, diagnosis, and treatment of these common infectious illnesses.

IMMUNOLOGY AND EXERCISE

To better understand the effects of exercise on the immune system, a brief review of the body's immune system is needed. The immune system can be considered as two parts, the innate and the acquired, that work together to prevent illness.

The innate portion is rather nonspecific when it comes to host defense. Its components include the skin, mucous membranes, phagocytes, natural killer (NK) cells, tumor necrosis factor (TNF), cytokines, and complement factors. Both complement and cytokines are soluble factors that control and mediate immune function and play a key role in activating T and B lymphocytes of the acquired immune system.[8]

The body's first lines of defense against many pathogens are physical barriers, namely the skin and mucous membranes. At the skin, physical factors such as temperature, wind, sun, humidity, and trauma can impair its barrier function.[6] Similarly, the structures and cells lining the mucous membranes of the upper respiratory system add to our body's front-line defenses. Many viruses and other pathogens are airborne and are therefore affected by airflow patterns, mechanical barriers, and ciliary action in the respiratory tract.

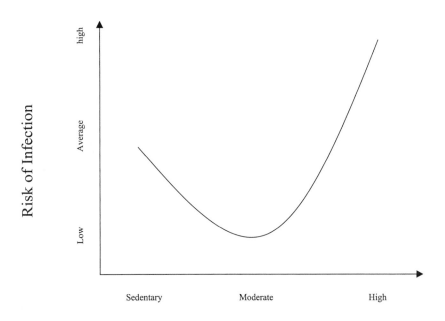

Figure 28–1. J curve of exercise and immune function.

At rest, turbulent flow through the nasal turbinates of the nose precipitates large particles in the nasal mucosa. Smaller particles such as viruses remain suspended until they reach the bronchi and bronchioles. The physical mucous barrier in the respiratory tract then impedes invasion of the underlying respiratory mucosa.[4] Within the mucous barrier are IgA-rich secretions produced by glandular cells of the mucosa that reduce viral load by opsonizing viral particles to facilitate their removal by phagocytosis.[3,4,7,9] Finally, the ciliary action of the mucosa, augmented by coughing, helps clear harmful organisms by moving mucus to the throat where it is cleared either through expectoration or swallowing.[4]

During exercise, the body changes from predominantly nasal breathing to predominantly mouth breathing, leading to increased deposition of harmful particles in the lower respiratory tract. It also causes increased cooling and drying of the respiratory mucosa which slows ciliary movement and increases mucus viscosity.[4] Depressed secretory IgA levels and increased occurrence of upper respiratory infections have also been noted in cross-country skiers, cyclists, and swimmers.[2–4,7,9] This ultimately leads to decreased clearance of microorganisms and other harmful particles from the bronchial tree and possibly an increased risk of infection.[3,4]

As mentioned above, the nonbarrier components of the innate immune system are complement factors, cytokines, TNF, phagocytes, and NK cells. Exercise has little effect on complement factors.[9] Of all the

immune functioning cells, NK cells appear to be the most sensitive to exercise. Several studies have documented elevations in NK cell counts in athletes in response to brief bouts of exercise.[1–7] Woods and colleagues[10] reported an increase of 150% to 300% in the number of NK cells found in peripheral smears after acute exercise (i.e., lasting <1 hour). Some authors suggest that the acute rise in NK cell counts is due to stimulation of the NK cell β_2-adrenergic sites by high concentrations of epinephrine present during the early phases of exercise.[3,7,10] However, this elevation of the NK cell count is only temporary. After longer periods of exercise (lasting >1 hour), NK counts fall below preexercise levels[10] and NK cell activity is decreased by 40% to 60% for at least 6 hours. This drop in NK cell activity is thought to be due to cortisol-induced redistribution of NK cells from the circulation to the tissues.[3]

Macrophages phagocytose foreign particles in response to complement and cytokines. They also play a role in presenting antigens to lymphocytes of the acquired immune system, as well as producing lymphocyte-stimulating cytokines. Moderate exercise increases macrophage count and activity. These values return to normal after several hours of rest. Intense exercise, however, reduces macrophage function acutely, and long-term intense training reduces macrophage response to inflammation. This may be in response to increased production of prostaglandin E_2 (PGE$_2$), which is produced by overuse muscular trauma.[4]

Similarly, the cytokine interleukin-1 (IL-1) appears to increase in response to the stress of exercise. IL-1 plays an important role in increasing the levels of T- and B-lymphocytes, a finding consistent with other studies that link leukocytosis to periods of exercise. In one study, IL-1 levels in the serum were elevated after test subjects exercised at 60% of maximum aerobic capacity.[11]

Proinflammatory cytokines like IL-1, TNF-α, and IL-6[3] are also responsible for the symptoms that we experience with illness and severe exercise.[1–5,7,11] Elevated cytokine levels produce fever, arthralgias, and myalgias with illness as well as the classic muscle pain felt after intense, eccentric exercise with muscle breakdown. In this setting, the cytokines aid in the complex events associated with muscle repair at the cellular level by communicating that damage has occurred and rest is needed to prevent further damage and allow healing. When muscle breakdown occurs, an inflammatory response attracts monocytes and neutrophils to the area to phagocytose debris. This correlates with the known increase in blood granulocyte and monocyte phagocytic activity with exercise. However, phagocytic activity is depressed in the nasal mucosa after periods of prolonged, intense exercise.[3]

The acquired portion of the immune system has the ability to form a memory and attack specific foreign particles that have invaded the body previously. The main components of this part of the system are T and B lymphocytes and plasma cell–secreted antibodies.[8] As mentioned above, factors from the innate immune system trigger proliferation of T and B lymphocytes through the stress of both exercise and infection. In both elite and nonelite athletes, serum T lymphocyte counts have been found to be elevated shortly after a brief period of moderate exercise.[1–7] Additionally, if the level of exercise is intense and lasts longer than 30 minutes, the lymphocyte count increases even more.[1–5,7,11] Two to 4 hours after longer (>1 hour) periods of intense eccentric exercise lymphocyte counts fall below preexercise levels.[1–5,7,11] The time it takes for the counts to return to baseline varies, but in most cases is 24 hours or more.[1–4,7]

Antibody production is affected by intense, prolonged exercise. Cross-country skiers and cyclists have been found to have low baseline salivary IgA levels, which further declined after racing.[2–7,9] Similar findings have been found in other athletes at rest and after stressful exercise. IgG does not seem to be affected as much by intense training, though some elite athletes show a small decrease during the peak of their training period.[4]

Among T lymphocytes are the CD4+ (T helper) and CD8+ (T suppressor) cells, which contribute to cell-mediated immunity. A ratio of CD4+/CD8+ cells of 1.5 is considered necessary for proper immune function. Heavy exercise and training can cause a decrease in this ratio via a decrease in CD4+ cells and an increase in CD8+ cells. A decreased CD4+ count also leads to diminished production of cytokines that activate NK cells and macrophages, and cause B cell stimulation and proliferation.[4] In one study[12] of cell-mediated immunity and antibody response, male triathletes showed diminished skin test measures of cellular immunity 48 hours after competing in a half ironman triathlon compared with noncompeting triathletes and recreational athletes. These changes in the T lymphocyte population contribute to immune system suppression with heavy exercise.[4] The clinical significance of these data remains to be seen.

Researchers have identified and named the period of brief immunosuppression, when ciliary action, IgA levels, NK cell count, macrophage number and activity, T lymphocyte count, and CD4+/CD8+ ratio are decreased after intense exercise, as the immunologic "open window."[3–5,7]

INFECTION AND TRAINING

Fever

Fever and the accompanying fatigue and malaise that occur with some acute illnesses can limit or even completely prevent a runner from training or competing. Fever is defined as an oral or rectal temperature of 100.4°F or higher. Fever is one of the most common presenting complaints, accounting for roughly 15% of visits to a health care provider.[13] It is commonly associated with acute or chronic infections, as well as muscle trauma, prolonged exercise (such as marathons), heat-related illness, medications, and neoplasms.

The body's temperature is controlled through a neurobiochemical process at the periphery and at the hypothalamus. Peripherally, the body employs vasodilation, sweating, and the shunting of blood flow to help maintain an euthermic state. At the level of the hypothalamus, local production of interleukin 1B (IL-1B) causes an increase in local PGE_2 levels, thereby causing an elevation of cyclic adenosine monophosphate (cAMP). In the case of fever, the ultimate rise in cAMP induces an elevation in body temperature by raising the temperature set point.[13]

Fever has been shown to reduce the rate of viral replication during viral infections. Fever, therefore, may be a sign of pathology or a function of normal physiology. Fever impairs concentric muscle strength, mental cognition, and pulmonary perfusion. In addition, fever increases overall systemic metabolism and insensible fluid loss resulting in increased caloric, oxygen, and fluid requirements. All of these factors can greatly impair the athlete's performance and increase the risk of injury.[7]

To best treat fever, the provider should consider the actual source, as in the case of infection, and concentrate on treating the infection rather than the fever. Treatment of fever should not be based purely on the degree of temperature elevation, but rather on the level of patient discomfort. The treatment of fever should start with oral antipyretics. These drugs work centrally by limiting the synthesis of PGE_2, which in turn interrupts the signal for temperature elevation at the hypothalamus. Both acetaminophen and nonsteroidal anti-inflammatory drugs (NSAIDs) work in this way. NSAIDs tend to be more effective inhibitors of prostaglandin and are effective both centrally and peripherally. Acetaminophen tends to be more effective in inhibiting prostaglandin synthesis centrally at the hypothalamus. This difference may explain why NSAIDs are often more effective at reducing myalgias associated with infection and muscle breakdown.[13] One should caution runners that in the setting of dehydration, the use of NSAIDs may reduce renal blood flow to the point of renal failure. Also, during an upper respiratory infection, acetaminophen increases nasal symptoms and signs and the duration of viral shedding when compared with ibuprofen.[14] Typical doses are acetaminophen 650 to 1000 mg every 4 to 6 hours (maximum dose, 4000 mg in a 24-hour period) and ibuprofen 400 mg every 4 hours, 600 mg every 6 hours, or 800 mg every 8 hours.

Runny Nose and Congestion

Probably the most common complaints related to infectious diseases among runners are rhinorrhea and nasal congestion. Common causes of acute nasal symptoms include upper respiratory infections (URIs), acute sinusitis, and allergic and nonallergic rhinitis. Though allergic and nonallergic rhinitis are not infectious diseases, their symptoms overlap with the other two conditions and will be described here to aid the provider in diagnosis and treatment.

Upper Respiratory Infections

URIs are quite common, with adolescents and adults getting an average of 2 to 4 colds per year. The symptoms usually include rhinorrhea with nasal congestion (80% to 100%) and sneezing (70%), and may also include sore throat (50%), cough (40%), hoarseness (30%), malaise (20 to 25%), and headache (30%). Temperature greater than 100°F (37.7°C) occurs less than 1% of the time and should prompt a search for other causes. Physical examination findings typically include nasal mucosa edema and erythema with clear to cloudy rhinorrhea, oropharyngeal erythema, and occasionally cervical lymphadenopathy.[15]

Treatment is relatively straightforward and is aimed primarily at symptom relief until the infection resolves, usually within 7 to 10 days. Rest and maintenance of adequate hydration are paramount. Oral or nasal decongestants can help relieve nasal stuffiness, but side effects can include nervousness, insomnia, tachycardia, and increased blood pressure. If rhinorrhea and sneezing are dominant symptoms, nonsedating antihistamines are good choices. Their anticholinergic action causes drying of the nasal mucosa and increased mucus viscosity. The main side effects of these medications are sedation, dry mouth, and constipation, which some people are unable to tolerate.[15] Runners in warm climates should use these medications with caution since they impair sweat production and increase the risk of heat exhaustion or heatstroke.[16] Nasal ipratropium will provide the anticholinergic effect of the nonsedating antihistamines without the systemic side effects.[17] See Table 28–1 for details on names and doses of specific medications.

Acute Sinusitis

In the United States acute sinusitis accounts for over 16 million office visits to a physician a year and is the fifth most common reason that doctors prescribe antibiotics. There is no single sign or symptom that is pathognomonic for acute sinusitis. A constellation of signs and symptoms must be combined into a single impression. Common clinical indicators are unilateral sinus pain and tenderness, purulent rhinorrhea by history and examination, lack of response to standard URI therapy, sinus pain increased with leaning forward, maxillary toothache, and "double sickening." Double sickening refers to a patient who has a cold that starts to improve, but then gets acutely worse. Fever and other constitutional symptoms may or may not be present. Transillumination of the sinuses is not always reliable to diagnose sinusitis. Radiographs of the sinuses are generally not useful when the clinical picture suggests sinusitis.[18]

Treatment of acute sinusitis is the same as that for URIs, at least with regard to symptomatic relief with analgesics and decongestants. Nasal saline rinses, available as over-the-counter mixtures or by mixing $1/4$ teaspoon of table salt in 8 ounces of warm water, can give short-term relief and aid in the removal of mucous. Placing a warm washcloth over the affected sinus and its corresponding nostril may also decrease sinus pain and pressure. Sedating antihistamines are not recommended for the treatment of sinusitis since the increased mucus viscosity may impede drainage from the sinuses and

TABLE 28–1. COMMON MEDICATIONS AND DOSES

Medication Type	Medication Name	Dose
Decongestant, oral	Pseudoephedrine	30–60 mg qid
Decongestant, nasal	Phenylephrine 0.5%, 1.0%	2–3 sprays q4hr prn, max 3 days
	Oxymetazoline 0.05%	1–2 sprays bid, max 3 days
Antihistamine, sedating	Chlorpheniramine	4 mg q4–6hr
	Brompheniramine	4 mg q4–6hr
	Diphenhydramine	25–50 mg q4–6hr
	Clemastine	0.5–1.0 mg bid
Antihistamine, nasal	Azelastine	2 sprays bid
Antihistamine, low sedating	Cetirizine	5–10 mg qd
Antihistamine, nonsedating	Loratidine	10 mg qd
	Fexofenadine	60 mg qd–bid
Anticholinergic, nasal	Ipratropium 0.03%[a]	2 sprays bid–tid
	Ipratropium 0.06%[b]	2 sprays tid–qid
Corticosteroid, nasal	Beclomethasone	1 spray bid–qid
	Budesonide	4 sprays qd or 2 sprays bid
	Flunisolide	2 sprays bid or 1 spray tid
	Fluticasone	2 sprays qd
	Mometasone	2 sprays qd
	Triamcinilone	2 sprays qd
Cromolyn, nasal	Cromolyn sodium	1 spray q4–6hr

[a]for allergic and nonallergic rhinitis.
[b]for rhinitis associated with upper respiratory infection.

prolong symptoms or prevent cure. Antibiotics should cover the common causative pathogens, *Streptococcus pneumoniae*, *Haemophilus influenzae*, and *Moraxella catarrhalis*. Appropriate first-line choices include a 10- to 14-day regimen of amoxicillin (500 mg three times a day), and trimethoprim-sulfamethoxazole (double strength; 1 pill twice a day). Second-line choices include cefuroxime (250 to 500 mg twice a day), amoxicillin-clavulanate (500 mg three times a day or 875 mg twice a day), doxycycline (100 mg twice a day), and clarithromycin (500 mg twice a day).[18]

Allergic and Nonallergic Rhinitis

When evaluating the athlete with nasal symptoms, allergic and nonallergic rhinitis must be kept in the differential diagnosis since their symptoms can and do often overlap. Allergic rhinitis is an IgE-mediated phenomenon in which mast cells in the respiratory mucosa release histamine in response to certain allergens such as pollen, mold, animal dander, and dust mites. Common symptoms of allergic rhinitis are nasal congestion and rhinorrhea, sneezing, nasal and palatal itching, and itchy or watery eyes. The diagnosis of allergic rhinitis is important since it often goes undiagnosed and is strongly associated with asthma exacerbations and sinusitis.[19] Nonallergic rhinitis, also sometimes called vasomotor rhinitis, can cause similar symptoms but is not IgE-mediated. The pathophysiology is not understood at this time, but it is thought to

be a type of inflammatory response to nonallergen airway irritants such as smoke, odors, chemicals, pollution, and changes in temperature or humidity.[20] In the absence of constitutional or other symptoms of URI and sinusitis, rhinorrhea is often due to allergic rhinitis, especially when symptoms last for more than 2 hours a day for 9 months of the year.[19] The patient's history will often yield a parent or sibling with similar symptoms because genetic factors contribute greatly to allergic rhinitis. A history of other atopic disease such as eczema or asthma may also be present.[20]

Physical findings are often nonspecific. Bluish-colored, edematous nasal mucosa is present in only 60% of allergic rhinitis patients. In nonallergic rhinitis patients the nasal mucosa usually has a more erythematous appearance. Faint ecchymosis under the eyes (allergic shiners) can also be seen, but are found in other nasal conditions as well.[20]

Allergy skin testing, while not necessary for the diagnosis of allergic rhinitis, can be useful to inform patients as to what allergic stimulants to avoid or reduce their exposure to (e.g., dust mites, cockroaches, molds), or to initiate immunotherapy if the patient chooses that treatment option.[20]

The treatment goal for allergic rhinitis is to dry and shrink the inflamed nasal mucosa and block the histamine-induced nasal symptoms. Nonallergic rhinitis is treated in a similar fashion though therapy is directed primarily at reducing and blocking nasal mucosal inflammation since histamine does not play a predominant role. An important aspect of achieving this goal is to avoid the triggers that cause the symptoms, if possible. Pharmacologic treatment offers several options. The sedating antihistamines are an effective and inexpensive choice. The anticholinergic action, however, may cause intolerable side effects, and these agents must be used with caution in warm climates, as noted above. The newer, low-sedating and nonsedating antihistamines are very effective in the setting of allergic rhinitis and have few if any irritating side effects.[20] A potential downside to these medications is their cost. Inhaled nasal corticosteroids have been found to reduce nasal inflammation and have minimal side effects.[19] Fluticasone probably has a more rapid onset of action, but beclomethasone also comes in an aqueous form to reduce nasal drying and irritation. When congestion is a prominent symptom or is not controlled with other medications, decongestants may be used. A final option for allergic, but not nonallergic, rhinitis is nasally inhaled cromolyn sodium. It has virtually no side effects, but may take a few weeks to take full effect. All of these medications may be used alone or in combination to optimize symptom reduction.[17]

Cough

Acute Cough

Cough is among the top five reasons that patients see physicians, resulting in approximately 30 million office visits per year. The American public spends roughly $600 million dollars a year on cough medications.[21] Acute cough, defined as cough lasting less than 3 weeks, accounts for about 50% of office visits for cough. Acute cough may be due to infectious or noninfectious etiologies. The most common infections that cause acute cough are URIs, sinusitis, bronchitis, and pneumonia.[22] The signs and symptoms of common causes of cough are displayed in Table 28–2.

The diagnostic indicators of URI and sinusitis are discussed above in the nasal symptom section. Acute bronchitis is another diagnosis that is quite common in the primary care setting. The symptoms can include any of the symptoms that are associated with URI, but the cough is the most predominant and troubling feature. The cough may be productive or nonproductive. Fever may or may not be present. Predisposing factors include smoke exposure, asthma, chronic obstructive pulmonary disease (COPD), alcohol use, and IgA deficiency.[15] Most cases of acute bronchitis, in the absence of any predisposing factors, are viral in etiology. Certain bacteria such as *Mycoplasma pneumoniae* and *Chlamydia trachomatis* may also cause bronchitis in a small percentage of cases. Pulmonary findings on physical examination are variable and can range from normal to diffuse rhonchi, and wheezing. Chest x-rays are usually normal and are more useful to exclude other diseases such as pneumonia.[22]

The treatment of cough associated with URI and acute sinusitis must first focus on treating not the cough, but the underlying cause, as outlined above.[23] Second, if the patient is a smoker, he or she should be advised to quit. Third, adequate hydration helps reduce the viscosity of mucous and makes it easier to expectorate. Often these measures may provide significant relief without taking additional cough medicines.[23] If cough is especially irritating, however, it may be treated symptomatically. Not only may this provide the patient some comfort, but it may decrease the risk of complications of repetitive coughing: pneumothorax, chest wall muscle strains, rib fractures, and posttussive syncope. The most effective cough suppressant is a narcotic cough medicine such as codeine (10 to 30 mg every 3 to 4 hours) in syrup or tablet form. In addition to cough suppression, it will provide sedation to help the patient sleep. For patients who cannot take narcotics, there are several nonnarcotic options. First is the cough suppressant dextromethorphan, available

TABLE 28–2. DIFFERENTIAL DIAGNOSIS AND SYMPTOMS OF COMMON CAUSES OF ACUTE COUGH

	Fever	Shortness of Breath	Mucus Production	Reflux Symptoms	Nasal Symptoms	Symptom Duration
URI	−	−	+/−	−	+	<2 weeks
Postnasal drip	−	−	+[a]	−	+	Variable
Sinusitis	+/−	−	+	−	+	>2 weeks
Bronchitis	+/−	+/−	+/−	−	−	Variable
Pneumonia	+	+	+[b]	−	−	<2 weeks
Asthma	−	+	+/−	+/−	−	>2 weeks
GERD	−	−	−	+/−	−	>2 weeks

+ = usually present. +/− = variably present. − = not commonly present. URI = upper respiratory infection. GERD = gastroesophageal reflux disease.
[a]usually greater upon awakening than any other part of the day.
[b]for typical pneumonia. A typical pneumonia typically has a severe dry cough.

in a number of different cough and cold combination medicines. Benzonatate (100 mg three times a day) is another choice that comes in pill form. Some cough medicines are expectorants and in theory work by decreasing mucus viscosity, thus making it easier to expectorate. The most commonly used of these medications is guaifenesin (600 to 1200 mg twice a day); it is commonly found in combination cold and cough medicines. Alone, though, it has never proven to be effective in the treatment of cough. Since many of these cough medicines are available in combination with other cold medicines (decongestants, antihistamines, analgesics, etc.), the provider must be vigilant to ensure that the patient is not receiving a potential overdose of other cold medicines.[23]

The treatment of cough due to bronchitis follows the same strategy as for cough associated with URIs and acute sinusitis with rest and hydration again being paramount. Bronchodilators such as albuterol (1 to 2 puffs every 4 to 6 hours) may be useful as well, especially in patients with wheezing on examination. Antibiotics are often not indicated because most cases in patients with normal pulmonary function are due to viruses. The clinician must provide the patient with a lot of reassurance because a course of acute bronchitis may last as long as 4 to 5 weeks.[22] The decision to prescribe antibiotics, however, may involve some nonmedical factors and must be individualized to the athlete. For instance, one may prescribe more quickly to an elite runner with an upcoming major competition rather than wait several days and risk deconditioning or poor perfomance.[14] In recreational runners, however, watchful waiting and withholding antibiotic treatment until it is clearly indicated is a reasonable approach. Antibiotic treatment should target *Mycoplasma* and *Chlamydia* species.[24] Reasonable first-line choices include erythromycin (250 mg four times a day or 500 mg twice a day) or doxycycline (100 mg twice a day). Second-line choices include clarithromycin (250 to 500 mg twice a day) or azithromycin (500 mg a day for one day, then 250 mg a day for 4 days).

In the patient returning to running after acute bronchitis, keep in mind that the inflamed bronchi are more prone to spasm. Also, with exercise comes increased minute ventilation and inhalation of antigens and irritants, as well as drying and cooling of inspired air, all of which can cause bronchospastic symptoms. Bronchodilators may also reduce bronchospastic symptoms during this period.[14]

Acute cough with a history of fever with or without rigors, sputum production, myalgias, pleuritic chest pain, and shortness of breath, and physical findings which may include hypoxia, tachypnea, and localized pulmonary rales or rhonchi suggests the diagnosis of community-acquired pneumonia. Pneumonia is the sixth leading cause of death in the United States and the leading cause of death among infectious diseases. Community-acquired pneumonia affects about 3 million persons in the United States per year, and about one sixth of this group requires hospitalization.[25]

Chest x-rays often show infiltrates which can be localized or diffuse. Early in the course of the illness the chest x-ray may be normal because radiologic findings may lag behind clinical findings. Sputum examination and culture may provide clues as to the causative organism provided that the sample is adequate [less than 10 epithelial cells and greater than 25 white blood cells per high-power field (HPF)].[25]

In otherwise healthy subjects, treatment can usually be done on an outpatient basis.[15] Proper rest, hydration, and nutrition are critical to success. Antibiotics should cover the most common bacterial pathogens (*Streptococcus pneumoniae, Mycoplasma pneumoniae, Legionella pneumoniae, Chlamydia pneumoniae, Haemophilus influenzae*). First-line therapy includes erythromycin (500 mg four times a day for 7 to 10 days), doxycycline (100 mg twice a day for 7 to 10 days), azithromycin (500 mg for 1 day then 250 mg a day for 4 days), or clarithromycin (500 mg twice a day for 7 to 10 days).[24]

Due to the damaged pulmonary parenchyma, the pneumonia patient will require more time to recover and return to full training than a patient with sinusitis or bronchitis. Absolute rest while the patient is symptomatic is critical to avoid prolonged illness, pulmonary abscess, and empyema. The period of absolute rest is usually at least several days but may be for as long as several weeks. Chest x-rays should not be used to guide return to activity since findings of pneumonia may persist for up to 6 weeks after the initial diagnosis.[14]

Chronic Cough

The dilemma in diagnosing and treating cough comes when it is of a chronic nature, lasting more than 3 weeks. In a nonsmoker, 65% to 95% of the time chronic cough is due to one or more of four causes: postnasal drip (PND), asthma, gastroesophageal reflux disease (GERD), and postinfectious bronchial inflammation.[21] Other less common causes to consider are listed in Table 28–2.

Postnasal drip is a common clinical entity and can be due to several causes. It causes a nagging, nocturnal cough with some sputum production, mostly in the morning upon awakening. Daytime symptoms are usually less severe than nighttime symptoms. The cough may accompany URI symptoms or symptoms of allergic rhinitis. Other possible causes include acute or chronic sinusitis. Treatment can be tailored to the individual. Nighttime doses of a decongestant (Table 28–1) may help decrease mucus production and relieve nasal congestion. They may, however, cause insomnia. Further treatment is similar to that of URI, sinusitis, or rhinitis.

Asthma is a clinical syndrome characterized by episodes of reversible airway obstruction and hyperresponsive airways. About 5% of the population of the United States have symptoms consistent with asthma.[26] In the athlete it often presents as a cough that occurs shortly into or just after a run. There may also be a history of nocturnal coughing, cough induced by cold, dry weather, or cough triggered by airway irritants (smoke, dust, pollution) or allergens (animal dander, pollen). Dyspnea and chest tightness may be associated with the cough.[14] There may also be a history of childhood asthma that the patient supposedly "grew out of." Physical examination while the patient is acutely symptomatic often reveals tachypnea, use of accessory respiratory muscles, increased expiration:inspiration ratio, decreased breath sounds, audible wheezing, and decreased peak flow rate.[26] Differentiation of asthma from exercise-induced bronchospasm may be difficult at first, but patients with exercise-induced bronchospasm usually do not have symptoms other than when they exercise.[14] Chest radiographs are often normal, but may show hyperinflation in severe cases. Pulmonary function testing may be necessary in some cases to make the diagnosis.[26] Treatment of asthma is beyond the scope of this chapter, but is discussed more fully in Chapter 22.

GERD affects an estimated 25% to 35% of Americans. Cough may be the sole presenting symptom in as many as 40% of patients with GERD.[21] For further diagnostic and management strategies see Chapter 24.

Postinfective bronchoirritation may last 4 to 6 weeks after other symptoms of URI or bronchitis have resolved. It often manifests as an irritating or nighttime cough that produces little to no sputum and is exacerbated by exercise. Diagnosis relies on excluding other causes such as atypical pneumonia, bronchitis, GERD, asthma, and PND. Management relies on

avoiding irritant stimuli such as smoke, fumes, dust, and molds. Bronchodilators such as albuterol (2 puffs every 4 to 6 hours) may relieve symptoms as well. Finally, inhaled corticosteroids such as fluticasone (88 to 440 μg twice a day), beclomethasone (2 to 4 puffs 4 times a day), flunisolide (2 to 4 puffs twice a day), or triamcinolone (2 to 4 puffs two to four times a day) may be useful until the condition resolves.

Sore Throat

Sore throat is another common complaint that prompts the patient to seek medical attention to reduce pain and/or to rule out strep throat. The differential diagnosis of the sore throat (Table 28–3) includes PND and significant illnesses as group A beta-hemolytic streptococcal (GABS) pharyngitis and infectious mononucleosis (IM), and enterovirus infections like coxsackievirus, which have been linked to infectious myocarditis.[27,28]

History should target questions such as time of onset, ill contacts, time when the pain is the worst, presentation of cough, whether or not fever is present, difficulty swallowing, and difficulty in speaking. The provider should also look for tonsillar exudates, asymmetric tonsillar swelling, ulcerations, palatal petechiae, fever, cervical adenopathy, and splenomegaly. The presence of a sore throat, fever, cervical adenopathy, and tonsillar exudates with the absence of cough and nasal symptoms, in a patient with known contact to someone with strep throat indicates empiric antibiotic treatment and a greater than 50% likelihood that the etiology is GABS.[29]

The most common cause of adult pharyngitis is adenovirus, followed closely by PND.[27] Therefore the treatment of choice in a majority of the cases is supportive care. Saltwater gargles, humidified air, throat lozenges, and acetaminophen 650 to 1000 mg or ibuprofen 400 mg given every 4 to 6 hours for mild sore throat pain are often effective means in addressing this complaint.

When the diagnosis of strep throat is unclear, then any one of a number of rapid strep tests (which have

---

TABLE 28–3. SYMPTOMS AND SIGNS SEEN WITH COMMON FORMS OF ACUTE PHARYNGITIS

	Fever	Adenopathy	Splenomegaly	Rhinorrhea	Ulcerations	Exudate	Fatigue
URI	−	+/−	−	+	−	+/−	+/−
GABS	+	+[a]	−	−	−	+	+/−
IM	+	+[b]	+/−	−	−	+	+
Enterovirus	+/−	+/−	−	−	+	−	+/−

+ = usually present. +/− = variably present. − = not commonly present. URI = upper respiratory infection. GABS = group A beta-hemolytic streptococcus. IM = infectious mononucleosis.
[a]more typically in the anterior cervical chains.
[b]more typically in posterior cervical chains.

an 86% positive predictive value) may be done. If positive the patient should be treated. If negative, then a throat culture should be done and the patient treated based on the results. Treatment with penicillin 500 mg twice a day for 10 days remains the drug of choice. A suitable second-line antibiotic is either azithromycin 500 mg once a day for 1 day and then 250 mg a day for 4 days or erythromycin 250 mg four times a day for 10 days.[27] Treatment with antibiotics not only hastens recovery, but also renders the patient noninfectious after 24 hours and protects him or her from the rare complication of rheumatic fever.[14] Failure to respond to antibiotic therapy may indicate poor compliance or other infectious sources such as viruses or other bacteria (i.e., gonococcus, mycoplasma). A patient who gets considerably worse despite treatment must also be checked for peritonsillar or retropharyngeal abscess, because these demand urgent referral to an otolaryngologist.

Another common cause of pharyngitis in the high school and college age patient is infectious mononucleosis (IM) caused by Epstein-Barr virus (EBV). It is a ubiquitous infection with >90% of the population demonstrating antibody titers by age 30.[29] In most cases, it is self-limiting, with sore throat, fever, lymphadenopathy, and fatigue as the classic presentation. Anorexia and nausea are often present and may complicate recovery. The typical course involves a 5-day prodromal period of headache, anorexia, and malaise, followed by 1 to 4 weeks of the above symptoms. Fatigue and malaise may occasionally persist beyond 4 weeks. This feature alone can limit an athlete's return to training.

Findings include fever, diffuse posterior lymphadenopathy, and dense tonsillar exudates. A morbilliform rash may occur, particularly in cases in whom the individual is prescribed ampicillin or amoxicillin to treat a presumed strep throat. This does not represent drug allergy, but rather an atypical reaction with the viral infection which can aid in the diagnosis of IM. Laboratory studies that can aid in the diagnosis include lymphocytosis (>50%; >10% atypical lymphocytes on the peripheral smear), and a positive heterophil antibody (monospot) test. Keep in mind that 10% of IM sufferers will have a negative monospot.[29] In such a case EBV serology might be considered. One quarter of affected individuals will have concomitant GABS pharyngitis, so a rapid strep test and/or throat culture should be performed and the patient treated if positive.[29]

Supportive care should be instituted, with bed rest in the early acute stages, as well as oral hydration, saline gargles, and pain and fever relief with acetaminophen or ibuprofen. Aspirin should not be used because of the possibility of inducing Reye's syndrome. Treatment with antibiotics is not recommended nor is the routine use of antivirals like acyclovir.[29]

Fortunately, in most cases of IM the disease course is self-limited. Complications can occur and include splenomegaly, airway obstruction, thrombocytopenia, hemolytic anemia, agranulocytosis, hepatitis, myocarditis, Guillain-Barré syndrome, Bell's palsy, and pneumonia.[14] Splenic enlargement is reported in 40% to 70% of cases of IM and peaks in the second to third week of the illness. Splenic rupture occurs in about 0.3% to 0.5% of cases and can occur during normal daily activities such as lifting, bending, or straining at stool. Patients must be made aware that any development of left upper quadrant pain that radiates to the left shoulder (Kehr's sign) demands immediate medical attention to rule out splenic rupture.[14,30] Tonsillar swelling is common and can rarely lead to airway obstruction. This condition, if caught early, may respond to a short course of oral corticosteroids such as prednisone 40 to 60 mg once a day for 7 to 10 days.[29]

Runners should avoid any exercise for the first 21 days of the illness. After that, light exercise may be initiated if the athlete feels ready to exercise and does not have symptomatic splenomegaly. Significant splenic enlargement with left upper quadrant pain may necessitate restriction from running until it resolves, although generally this is not the case.[16] If in doubt, ultrasound measurement of the spleen and left kidney every 2 weeks can be used to track splenomegaly. When the spleen to kidney ratio reaches 1.25 or less, then splenomegaly is considered to have resolved.[31] The recovery period and time to return to full activity is highly variable, but can be as long as 2 to 3 months.[14]

Acute Diarrhea

Diarrhea is defined as three or more loose stools a day for up to 7 days.[32] Acute diarrhea is most often due to infections—most being viral infections in the United States—but other causes to consider include endocrine disorders (such as hyperthyroidism), inflammatory bowel disease, and antibiotic-induced colitis.[32] Diarrheal diseases due to infection in the runner are often best managed by supportive measures and time. In most cases, it is an inconvenience to the runner and has a benign course. This does not mean that this disease process should be taken lightly because roughly 10,000 deaths a year occur secondary to diarrhea in the United States.[32]

Through a detailed history, the cause of diarrhea can often be narrowed down to one of the above categories. In the history, keys that are often helpful in identifying an etiology include travel history, hobbies, animal contacts, antibiotic usage, dietary habits, and ill contacts. The review of systems should cover items as the stool appearance (mucous, bloody, or watery), presence or absence of fever, weight loss (both acutely and chronically), and presence or absence of abdominal pain. Often, the overall presentation of the diarrheal disease may aid in identifying where in the gastrointestinal tract an infection has occurred.

In most cases the morbidity from diarrhea is related to fluid losses and subsequent dehydration and electrolyte imbalances. Anecdotal findings indicate that runners tend to live in a relatively dehydrated state due to fluid losses from running. Further dehydration through enteric losses can increase the risk of suffering morbidity related to diarrhea.

Stool examination for fecal leukocytes and occult blood, as well as stool culture and *C. difficile* toxin assay in the patient with antecedent antibiotic use, are helpful in identifying the infectious cause. The presence of fecal leukocytes, especially >5/HPF, strongly suggests the presence of a bacterial infection and warrants antibiotic treatment. Some clues to differentiating among the different types of acute diarrhea are shown in Table 28–4.

As mentioned earlier, treatment in most cases of diarrheal disease focuses on rehydration. In severe cases, intravenous (IV) rehydration with isotonic crystalloid may be indicated. However, oral intake of glucose and electrolyte solutions to recover fluid and electrolyte losses remains a safer, often more effective, and cheaper form of therapy than IV rehydration. Beyond rehydration and rest, antibiotics play a treatment role when diarrhea is caused by a proven or strongly suspected bacterial or protozoan organism.[32] Ultimately, the decision to use antibiotics empirically in the treatment of diarrhea remains in the hands of the provider.

When bacterial colitis (*Salmonella, Shigella, E. coli, Campylobacter*) is suspected, either ciprofloxacin 500 mg twice a day for 3 to 5 days or trimethoprim-sulfamethoxazole, one DS pill twice a day for 3 to 5 days may be given. *Salmonella* should not be treated unless the illness is severe or the patient immunocompromised, because antibiotic treatment may prolong the carrier state. If there is a suspicion that the diarrhea may be due to *C. difficile,* one should add metronidazole 250 to 500 mg three times a day for 7 to 14 days or vancomycin 125 mg orally four times a day for 7 to 14 days. Giardiasis can be treated with metronidazole 250 mg three times a day for 5 days.[24]

Antimotility agents should generally be avoided. If absolutely necessary use loperamide (4 mg after the first loose stool, then 2 mg after each subsequent loose stool, to a maximum of 16 mg a day) instead of lomotil (2 tabs four times a day) because lomotil contains atropine and may have unwanted anticholinergic side effects.

Viral Myocarditis

Establishing guidelines for the runner to return to training after an illness is not an easy endeavor. Exercising when one is systemically ill (i.e., with fever, myalgias, and other systemic symptoms) theoretically increases one's risk of viral myocarditis. This finding has been borne out in animal studies but has not been replicated in humans.[14] Infectious myocarditis is an inflammatory disorder of the myocardium. Most of these infections are due to viruses, especially those in the enterovirus family, but can also be due to bacteria, fungi, *Rickettsia* spp., *Mycobacteria* spp., and protozoa. Myocarditis carries potential morbidity related to congestive heart failure, arrhythmias, and sudden death. Unfortunately, there are no good indicators of who will and will not develop viral myocarditis.[33] Therefore, physicians who treat runners must be able to recognize the nonspecific signs and symptoms of myocarditis.

Symptoms that should alert the physician to the diagnosis of myocarditis include lower extremity edema, fatigue, dyspnea, decreased exercise tolerance, chest pain, palpitations, and presyncope/syncope that occurs during exertion in the postinfection period. Some cases of myocarditis may clinically mimic a myocardial infarction. Symptoms of congestive heart failure (CHF) usually do not occur unless the case is severe. An almost universal sign is tachycardia. In severe cases one may notice pulmonary rales, jugular venous distension, lower extremity edema, an audible S$_3$,

TABLE 28–4. SYMPTOMS AND SIGNS SEEN WITH COMMON FORMS OF ACUTE DIARRHEA

	Fever	Abdominal Cramps	Weight Loss	Foreign Travel	Ill Contacts	Antibiotic Use	Blood/Mucus in Stools
Viral	−	+/−	−	−	+	−	−
Bacterial	+	+	+/−	+	−	−	−
IBD	+	+	+	−	−	−	+
Endocrine	−	−	+	−	−	−	+
C. difficile	+	+	−	−	−	+	+

+ = usually present. +/− = variably present. − = not commonly present. IBD = inflammatory bowel disease.

and other signs of CHF. The symptoms of myocarditis often do not occur for up to several weeks after the inciting illness, so a high index of suspicion is needed to make the diagnosis.[33]

Initial workup should include a CBC, erythrocyte sedimentation rate (ESR), cardiac enzymes, ECG, and echocardiogram. CBC may show a leukocytosis and the ESR is often elevated. Cardiac enzymes would be elevated, and the degree of elevation correlates with the degree of myocardial necrosis.[14] ECG findings include nonspecific ST-T wave changes, injury pattern, atrial and ventricular arrhythmias, and AV conduction blocks.[33] Echocardiogram is a crucial test to demonstrate diminished cardiac function and wall motion abnormalities. Other tests to consider include acute and convalescent titers to identify the pathogen, but this would not change treatment in any way in the case of viral myocarditis.[14] Medical treatment is aimed at reducing cardiac afterload with diuretics and angiotensin-converting enzyme (ACE) inhibitors. Cardiology consultation should be considered for management and guidance for return to running.[28]

For individuals diagnosed with myocarditis, the 26th Bethesda Conference[34] recommends a 6-month convalescent period after the onset of symptoms. During this time, the runner should not participate in any kind of exercise or training. Before returning to training, the runner should have a full cardiac evaluation to include Holter monitoring, echocardiogram, and treadmill testing. The runner may return to training when cardiac dimensions and resting and exertional ventricular function have returned to normal and there are no clinically relevant arrhythmias on ambulatory monitoring.

Immune Modulators

While intense, prolonged exercise may increase one's susceptibility to infection, it is also absolutely necessary to allow the elite athlete to compete successfully. Since an elite runner may be unable or unwilling to reduce his or her training load, he or she may turn instead to a number of different medications and substances to counteract exercise-induced immunosuppression and/or prevent common infections. Among these substances are vitamin C, echinacea, glutamine, and carbohydrate supplementation.

VITAMIN C. Researchers in South Africa found in double-blind placebo-controlled studies that 3 weeks of vitamin C supplementation, 600 mg/day in ultramarathoners led to fewer reports of URIs. Other teams did not replicate this finding, however. In fact, another study showed no benefit from vitamin C supplementation.[3] More studies must be done before vitamin C

supplementation can be recommended to ward off illness in the elite athlete.

ECHINACEA. Extracts from plants of the genus *Echinacea* are widely used in Europe and North America for the treatment and prevention of URIs. Surveys have indicated that echinacea is one of the biggest selling herbal preparations in the United States, accounting for 10% of the total herbal medicine market.

Echinacea is thought to have an immunostimulating effect and has been found in studies to enhance phagocytosis, increase secretion of complement factors and cytokines, and enhance leukocytosis. Anti-inflammatory and antimicrobial properties have been reported also. Echinacea does seem to decrease the severity and duration of URIs, especially when started early in the course of the illness and taken in sufficient doses. More studies of higher quality are needed because past studies suffer from errors in design. The evidence supporting the use of echinacea to prevent URIs is less convincing. These studies also have methodological shortcomings and do not report statistically significant results (though they do report trends in favor of echinacea). Echinacea does not seem to have any significant toxicity other than occasionally reported severe allergic reactions and anaphylaxis. Therefore its use for the treatment of URIs can be cautiously recommended, but not for the prevention of them.[35]

GLUTAMINE. Glutamine, a precursor for nucleoside biosynthesis, is a vital fuel for immune cell proliferation. It is found in the diet in meats and greens, but the vast majority is produced by skeletal muscle, lung tissue, and the GI mucosa. Glutamine utilization increases during times of physiologic stress, such as infection, after trauma or surgery, and with prolonged physical exertion.

Within the immune system, T and B lymphocyte proliferation, and synthesis of antibodies and interleukin-2 are all glutamine-dependent. While short (<1 hour) bouts of high-intensity exercise can raise glutamine levels, prolonged exercise leads to depressed glutamine levels and decreased lymphocyte proliferation. This decrease in glutamine is thought to be multifactorial. Prolonged exercise causes a rise in cortisol, which increases protein catabolism as well as gluconeogenesis, for which glutamine is a prime fuel source. The kidney uses glutamine as a buffer during periods of metabolic acidosis. Glutamine release from muscle tissues during catabolic states may fall as well.

From a clinical standpoint, plasma glutamine levels have been found to be lower in overtrained athletes vs. well-trained athletes and sedentary individuals. There have also been reports of increased rates of URIs in athletes with depressed glutamine levels, though some reports in swimmers do not show this. Whether glutamine supplementation decreases the risk of infection is unclear at this time. One study of marathon and ultramarathon runners found that those who had glutamine drinks immediately and 2 hours after a race had a 49% incidence of self-reported URI within a week, while a placebo group had an 81% rate. There is good evidence that glutamine is vital to immune function and that prolonged exercise decreases glutamine levels. How much this contributes to one's risk of infection and whether glutamine supplementation can decrease that risk remains to be proven.[36]

CARBOHYDRATES. Carbohydrate consumption is postulated to decrease immunosuppression by maintaining higher levels of blood glucose, thus leading to decreased excretion of cortisol and other stress hormones. Several studies, summarized in two articles by Nieman,[3,37] do in fact show an attenuation of stress hormone levels, decreased changes in immune cell counts, and attenuation of the cytokine response when endurance athletes consume carbohydrates before, during, and after exercise. Carbohydrates therefore seem to reduce the physiological stress that prolonged exercise puts on the immune system.[3,37] One could postulate that carbohydrate supplementation, by reducing the need for gluconeogenesis, could have a glutamine-sparing effect. Human and animal studies of this theory have so far provided conflicting results and no clear conclusions.[36] In general, there has been no clinical research, however, to determine if carbohydrate consumption among athletes actually leads to a decreased incidence of infections.[3,37]

RETURN TO RUNNING

When a runner can return to a full running schedule after an acute illness can be a vague and frustrating topic for both the runner and physician. The habitual runner is concerned about deconditioning during illness and recovery periods. Unlike the runner who is recovering from IM or viral myocarditis, there are no absolute guidelines for runners to resume training after an acute illness.

One method for establishing a return plan for the runner is the "neck check" as described by Eichner[2] and Primos.[39] If symptoms are above the neck (i.e., runny nose, nasal congestion, sore throat, or sneezing) and not associated with below-the-neck symptoms (i.e., fever, myalgias, arthralgias, severe cough, GI symptoms), then the runner may run at half speed for 10 minutes. If the symptoms do not worsen or

improve, then the workout may be continued at full pace. If, however, the symptoms worsen in the initial half-speed 10-minute period, the workout should end and the runner should rest until symptoms improve. Exercise should be delayed until all below-the-neck symptoms have resolved.[2] When resuming training after recovering from an illness, the runner should start at a moderate pace and gradually increase his or her training intensity to preillness level over 1 to 2 days for every training day missed.[39]

The training delay outlined above serves three purposes. First, training with any below-the-neck symptoms hampers the workout and limits the runner's desired training effects. Second, without a medical evaluation a runner may not know if his or her illness is a benign URI or the beginnings of an infection that could be made worse with exercise, such as pneumonia or a viral infection that may predispose to viral myocarditis.[2] Third, not training may prevent the spread of disease to fellow training partners.[39]

Once the athlete has rested for an appropriate period the next question is how quickly to return to full activity. Runners should start at about 50% intensity, and should pay attention to overall energy status and sense of well-being as they advance.[39] Recovery from a significant illness such as pneumonia may take as long as 8 weeks before return to preillness levels of performance.[14]

As alluded to earlier in the chapter, the physician may find that his or her advice presented to the casual runner is often well received. However, runners with a more competitive drive may be somewhat more resistant to limitation of training efforts during recovery periods. For these patients, knowledge of the runner's short- and long-term running goals may be of benefit. For example, a runner may be trying to improve on a 10-K time in an upcoming race. In this case, the runner might appreciate hearing that these goals may be better served by competing in a race at a later date. Persistent training during an illness may lead to injury or overtraining effects, creating further delay in recovery. This approach links potential outcomes unique to runners and their training with the long-term consequences.

This brings up an additional tip for physicians who frequently treat runners. Make an effort to be knowledgeable of the races within your region. Awareness to regional races could prove helpful in advising the patient to consider training for an alternate race at a later date when full recovery is more likely to have occurred. This type of approach further personalizes the patient's treatment plan.

For the runner who is assessed at a clinical level where some reduction of training is indicated, cross-training utilizing stationary bicycles or treadmills may

TABLE 28–5. DIFFERENTIAL DIAGNOSIS IN THE RUNNER WHO FAILS TO RECOVER

Overtraining
Thyroid disorders
HIV (acute or chronic)
Hepatic disease
Depression
Eating disorders
Diabetes
Cancer
Pregnancy
Malnutrition/malabsorption disease
Anemia
Autoimmune disorders
Alcohol/drug abuse
Parasitic/spirochete infections
Myocarditis
Asthma

be considered. These devices are often found in local gyms and can make it easy for the runner to quantify his or her efforts, with the added benefit of adding a measure of intensity to the workout through the recovery period. Working out in the gym while recovering from an illness will also allow the runner to exercise indoors, away from potentially inclement or extreme weather that can weaken the innate immune system.

Finally, the physician should be wary of the athlete that does not recover from illness. The differential diagnosis (Table 28–5) of these athletes is complicated and should be quickly undertaken in cases in which the athlete does not recover in a reasonable period of time.

CONCLUSION

It is widely believed that moderate-intensity exercise is an immune stimulant and that intense exercise may cause immune suppression. When, despite their best efforts runners become ill, it is important to properly care for them to minimize lost training time. Correct diagnosis, treatment, and slowing or suspending training according to Eichner's "neck check" protocol are critical to a speedy return to full training. With a sensible, balanced training program, and proper sleep, nutrition, and training load, runners can accomplish their goals without sacrificing their health.

REFERENCES

1. Pedersen B, Bruunsgaard H: How exercise influences the establishment of infections. *Sports Med* 1995:19, 393.
2. Eichner R: Infection, immunity, and exercise: What to tell patients. *Phys Sportsmed* 1993:21, 125.
3. Nieman D: Nutrition, exercise, and immune system function. *Clin Sports Med* 1999:18, 537.
4. Shephard R, Shek P: Exercise, immunity, and susceptibility to infection. *Phys Sportsmed* 1999:27, 47.
5. Pedersen B, Rohde T, Zacho M: Immunity in athletes. *J Sports Med Phys Fitness* 1996:36, 36.
6. Simon H: Exercise and infection. *Phys Sportsmed* 1987:15, 135.
7. Brenner I, Shek P, Shephard R: Infection in athletes. *Sports Med* 1994:17, 86.
8. Goodman J: The immune response, in Stites D, Terr A, (eds.), *Basic Clinical Immunology*, 7th ed., Appleton & Lange, 1991:34.
9. Gleeson M, McDonald WA, Pyne DB, et al.: Salivary IgA levels and infection risks in elite swimmers. *Med Sci Sports Exerc* 1999:31, 67.
10. Woods J, Davis J, Smith J, Niemann D: Exercise and cellular innate immune function. *Med Sci Sports Exerc* 1999:31, 57.
11. Cannon J, Kluger M: Endogenous pyrogen activity in human plasma after exercise. *Science* 1983:220, 617.
12. Bruunsgaard H, Hartkopp A, Mohr T, et al.: In vivo cell-mediated immunity and vaccination response following prolonged, intense exercise. *Med Sci Sports Exerc* 1997:29, 1176.
13. Kauffman R: Fever, in Rakel RE, (ed.), *Conn's Current Therapy*, 51st ed., Philadelphia, Saunders, 1999:23.
14. McDonald W: Upper respiratory tract infections, in Fields KB, Fricker PA, (eds.), *Medical Problems in Athletes*, Malden, Mass, Blackwell Scientific, 1997:9.
15. Levy BT, Kelly MW: Common cold, in *Griffith's 5 Minute Clinical Consult*, Baltimore, Lippincott Williams & Wilkins, 1999:246.
16. Lillegard WA, Butcher JD, Rucker KS: *Handbook of Sports Medicine: A Symptoms Oriented Approach*, 2nd ed., Stoneham, Butterworth-Heinemann, 1999:353.
17. Middleton: *Allergy: Principles and Practice*, 5th ed., St. Louis, Mosby-Yearbook, 1998, p 674.
18. Fagnan LL: Acute sinusitis: A cost effective approach to diagnosis and treatment. *Am Fam Physician* 1998:58, 1795.
19. Naclerio R, Solomon W: Rhinitis and inhalant allergens. *JAMA* 1997:278, 1842.
20. Middleton: *Allergy: Principles and Practice*, 5th ed., St. Louis, Mosby-Yearbook, 1998:1005.
21. Lawler W: An office approach to the diagnosis of chronic cough. *Am Fam Physician* 1998:58, 2015.
22. Williamson HA: Acute bronchitis, in Rakel RE, (ed.), *Conn's Current Therapy*, 51st ed., Philadelphia, Saunders, 1999:210.
23. Simon HB: Management of the common cold, in *Primary Care Medicine*, 3rd ed., Philadelphia, Lippincott-Raven, 1995:277.
24. Gilbert DN, Moellering RC, Sande MA: *The Sanford Guide to Antimicrobial Therapy*, 28th ed., Antimicrobial Therapy Inc., 1998.
25. Masters PA, Weitekemp MR: Community-acquired pneumonia, in *Pulmonary and Critical Care Medicine*, St. Louis, Mosby-Yearbook, 1998:J1–16.

26. Drazen JM: Asthma, in *Cecil's Textbook of Medicine,* 20th ed., Philadelphia, Saunders, 1996:376.

27. Perkins A: An approach to diagnosing the acute sore throat. *Am Fam Physician* 1997:55, 131.

28. Francis G: Viral myocarditis detection and management. *Phys Sportsmed* 1995:23, 63.

29. Bailey R: Diagnosis and treatment of infectious mononucleosis. *Am Fam Physician* 1994:49, 879.

30. Asgari M, Begos D: Spontaneous splenic rupture in infectious mononucleosis: A review. *Yale J Biol Med* 1997:70, 175.

31. Loftus W, Metreweli C: Ultrasound assessment of mild splenomegaly: Spleen/kidney ratio. *Pediatr Radiol* 1998:28, 98.

32. Mayer M, Wanke C: Acute infectious diarrhea, in Rakel RE (ed.), *Conn's Current Therapy,* 51st ed., Philadelphia, Saunders, 1999:13.

33. Braunwald E: Myocarditis, in *Heart Disease: A Textbook of Cardiovascular Medicine,* 5th ed., Philadelphia, Saunders, 1997:1435.

34. Maron BJ, Isner JM, McKenna WJ: Hypertrophic cardiomyopathy, myocarditis, and other myopericardial diseases and mitral valve prolapse. *Med Sci Sport Exerc* 1994:26(suppl), S261.

35. Barrett B, Vohamnn M, Calabrese C: Echinacea for upper respiratory infection. *J Fam Pract* 1999:48, 1999.

36. Walsh NP, Blannin AK, Robson PJ, et al.: Glutamine, exercise, and immune function: Links and possible mechanisms. *Sports Med* 1998:26, 177.

37. Niemann D, Pedersen B: Exercise and immune function. Recent developments. *Sport Med* 27:73, 1999.

38. Primos WA: Sports and exercise during acute illness. Recommending the right course for patients. *Phys Sports Med* 1996:24, 44.

Chapter 29

THE RUNNER WITH DIABETES

Russell D. White

INTRODUCTION

Diabetes mellitus is a group of metabolic diseases characterized by hyperglycemia resulting from defects in insulin secretion, insulin action, or both. This hyperglycemia produces long-term microvascular and macrovascular complications.[1] Diabetes mellitus is the most common endocrine disease. Diabetes is increasing in incidence in the western world and is estimated to affect 216 million individuals worldwide by the year 2010.[2,3] In the U.S. there are currently 16 million diabetic patients. Of these, 90% have type 2 diabetes and the remainder have type 1 disease.[4]

Type 1 diabetes is caused by loss of insulin secretion due to progressive destruction of the pancreatic beta cells.[5] Type 1A is an autoimmune disease characterized by cellular antibodies that may form against islet cells (islet cell antibodies, ICA), insulin (insulin autoantibodies, IAA), and glutamic acid decarboxylase (GAD_{65}). These antibodies destroy endogenous insulin production and the patient becomes metabolically unstable. Type 1B is an idiopathic, nonautoimmune disease state with loss of beta cell function.[6] Type 1 patients demonstrate hyperglycemia, experience weight loss, and are prone to ketoacidosis. Death may occur if exogenous insulin is not administered and the acidotic state is reversed. Typical onset is before age 30 with peak incidence during adolescence.

Type 2 diabetes is characterized by defects in both insulin secretion and insulin action. The pathogenesis involves impaired insulin secretion, increased hepatic glucose production, and decreased muscle glucose uptake. These latter phenomena are due to hepatic and peripheral resistance to the physiological action of insulin. Due to both genetic (family history, familial hyperlipidemia) and environmental (sedentary lifestyle, inappropriate diet with increased caloric intake) factors, insulin resistance is associated with obesity, hypertension, hyperlipidemia, and type 2 diabetes. This constellation of diseases has been defined as syndrome X. These individuals exhibit a defect in the timing and amount of insulin secretion. As postprandial blood glucose increases followed by elevated fasting glucose levels, serum insulin levels gradually rise. As the insulin receptors "downregulate," peripheral tissues and the liver develop "insulin resistance" and fail to respond to insulin.[7] In long-term studies insulin resistance may precede the onset of diagnosed diabetes by 10 to 20 years.[8] There are many variations of the above clinical scenario, but most patients are older than age 40 years when diabetes develops.

There is an alarming increase in the number of adolescents developing type 2 diabetes. These patients are typically overweight, maintain an inappropriate calorie-laden diet, and participate in no physical activity. A few individuals may develop maturity-onset diabetes of the young (MODY).[9] MODY is a specific autosomal dominant subtype of type 2 diabetes with a genetic predisposition for development in adolescence or early adulthood. They do not demonstrate autosomal antibodies and are treated similarly to those with classical type 2 diabetes. Criteria for the diagnosis of MODY include 1) elevated blood glucose level for diagnosis of diabetes, 2) absence of ketosis, 3) correction of fasting hyperglycemia without insulin use for at least 2 years, and 4) age of onset under age 25 years in at least one family member.[9,10]

The treatment triad for diabetes mellitus includes medication, medical nutritional therapy, and exercise.[11] Diabetic patients may either participate in running as adjunctive treatment of their disease or as a recreational or competitive sport. Ironically, type 1 patients often *want* to exercise as runners but sometimes should not, while type 2 patients should exercise or run but often *will not*. Proper diabetic management before, during, and after running is crucial.

PHYSIOLOGICAL EFFECTS OF EXERCISE ON DISEASE STATES

Effects of Exercise on Glucose Metabolism

Exercise has been utilized as a treatment for diabetes mellitus since the time of Hippocrates. In 1926 Lawrence first published the effect of insulin alone and in combination with exercise in diabetic patients[12] (Fig. 29–1). Since then clinicians have known that both type 1 and type 2 patients may benefit from regular exercise.[13–16]

Exercise augments the effect of insulin, facilitating glucose transport across the cell membrane, and may increase muscle glucose uptake 20-fold.[17,18] The main facilitator is glucose transporter 4 (GLUT-4), a transmembrane protein encoded by specific genes. Obesity and diabetes impair this protein. The activity of this transporter is enhanced not only by insulin-like growth factors, thyroid hormone, bradykinins, nitric oxide, biguanides, and thiazolidinediones, but also exercise.[19] A single exercise session (45 minutes) may increase insulin sensitivity by 40% and continue for the subsequent 48 hours.[20] This glucose-lowering effect via exercise helps normal persons, as well as type 1 and type 2 diabetic patients.[21] However, type 2 diabetic patients benefit the most.

Long-term exercise does not enhance glucose control (based on HbA$_{1C}$ determinations) in type 1 patients. Unfortunately, many type 1 athletes experience hypoglycemia with exercise. Consequently, these athletes compensate with extra food either during or following exercise. With excess this calorie ingestion, the benefit of exercise is offset by the supplemental

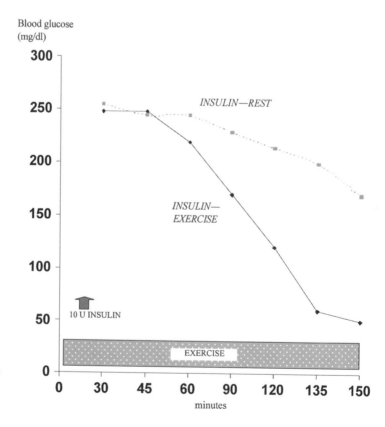

Figure 29–1. Effect of exercise on action of insulin. *(Source: Adapted with permission from Lawrence.[12])*

calories and long-term diabetic control is not improved.

Other Effects of Exercise in Diabetic Patients[22-24]

Hyperlipidemia

Exercise in diabetic patients improves the lipid profile by both direct and indirect effects. Exercise stimulates lipoprotein lipase activity and facilitates a negative energy balance. Exercise lowers the levels of very low-density lipoprotein (VLDL), triglycerides, and low-density lipoprotein (LDL) cholesterol. Exercise also increases levels of high-density lipoprotein (HDL) cholesterol.[25]

Hypertension

Regular aerobic exercise decreases both systolic (average, 11 mm Hg) and diastolic (average, 9 mm Hg) blood pressure components.[26] With exercise and weight loss, insulin levels decrease, the expanded plasma volume contracts, and there is less hypertrophy in the tunica media of smooth muscle vasculature. The overall prognosis in diabetic patients is improved via a combination of decreased blood pressure, decreased weight, and improved serum glucose levels.

Obesity

This major cardiovascular risk factor is a pathologic component of the type 2 patient. Aerobic exercise such as running is crucial to the management and treatment of weight loss. A minimal weight loss of 15 to 20 pounds has been found to decrease the fasting insulin levels by 30% to 50% and improve glycemic control.

Fibrinolysis

Many type 2 diabetic patients have elevated levels of plasminogen activator inhibitor-1 (PAI-1). This factor inhibits naturally occurring tissue plasminogen activator and places type 2 patients at risk for increased thrombotic activity. Regular aerobic activity decreases PAI-1 levels, improves fibrinolysis, and reverses this tendency for thrombosis.

Psychological Benefits

While running may be an individual sport, this activity may improve peer interaction of the adolescent type 1 diabetic athlete and promote socialization as the athlete grows older. Likewise, type 2 patients may enjoy jogging or running with groups or clubs. This social interaction contributes to the overall psychological well-being of the diabetic runner.

To promote these beneficial effects in both type 1 and type 2 patients, aerobic exercise such as running

should be performed 30 to 40 minutes, 3 to 4 times per week at a minimum of 30% to 40% of the individual's $\dot{V}o_2$max. Intensity at 50% to 80% of $\dot{V}o_2$max is necessary for marked improvement in glucose tolerance.[11,25] Recent data indicate that *accumulation* of several short bouts, rather than a single episode of 30 minutes of daily activity, is beneficial for cardiovascular health. The benefit of accumulated activity in diabetic patients is unclear.

RISKS OF EXERCISE IN DIABETIC PATIENTS

Hypoglycemia and Coronary Artery Disease

Potential risks in diabetic athletes must be evaluated prior to starting a running program. Hypoglycemia is the major risk in type 1 athletes. In addition, the risk of exacerbation of hyperglycemia or ketoacidosis in insulinopenic type 1 runners may occur. Additional risks from running in older type 1 patients include asymptomatic coronary heart disease. Coronary artery disease is also the major risk for type 2 patients. More than 20% of type 2 patients have coronary artery disease when diagnosed with diabetes. Associated peripheral vascular disease must also be evaluated. An exercise stress test is indicated for diabetic runners if criteria in Table 29–1 are met.[14]

Other Risks

Other risks include exacerbation of retinopathy, injury from neuropathy, or autonomic dysfunction. Running is prohibited with active proliferative retinopathy. Once treated and stabilized, the ophthalmologist may clear the patient for running activity. Likewise, foot and ankle injuries commonly occur in diabetic runners with neuropathy. The inability to perceive ill-fitting

---

TABLE 29–1. INDICATIONS FOR GRADED EXERCISE TESTING IN DIABETES MELLITUS

A graded exercise test *may* be helpful if a patient is about to embark on a moderate- to high-intensity exercise program and meets any of the following criteria:

- Age >35 years
- Type 1 diabetes of >15 years' duration
- Type 2 diabetes of >10 years' duration
- Presence of any additional risk factor for coronary artery disease
- Presence of microvascular disease
  Retinopathy
  Nephropathy, including microalbuminuria
  Neuropathy, including autonomic neuropathy
- Presence of macrovascular disease
  Cerebrovascular disease
  Coronary artery disease
  Peripheral vascular disease

Source: Adapted with permission from American Diabetes Association.[14]

shoes, tissue injury, or simple blisters places the diabetic runner at increased risk of further complications. Finally, autonomic dysfunction exposes diabetic runners to specific risks: 1) abnormal sweating mechanisms may affect efficient heat dissipation, 2) runners with asymptomatic heart disease may not experience anginal symptoms until serious disease occurs, and 3) symptoms of hypoglycemia may not occur until the runner experiences central nervous system dysfunction. Finally, patients with autonomic dysfunction may lack the normal heart rate response to exercise. These runners cannot rely on target heart rate to gauge exercise intensity. Instead, they must rely on the Borg scale (rate of perceived exertion) when monitoring exercise activity.

NORMAL PHYSIOLOGY OF EXERCISE

Energy Sources

The normal exercise physiology of running involves an intricate interaction of the energy sources via hormonal control. The type of energy utilized depends on the running intensity and duration[27] (Table 29–2). The

TABLE 29–2. TYPES OF EXERCISE AND ENERGY SOURCES

Duration of Exercise	Intensity of Exercise	Energy Source
Short	Strenuous	Glucose
Medium	Vigorous	Glucose/FFA[a]
Long	Mild	FFA[a]

[a]FFA, free fatty acids.

initial immediate source of energy is intramuscular adenosine triphosphate (ATP), creatine phosphate, and mobilization of muscle glycogen. As the vascular reservoir of circulating glucose is utilized, hepatic glycogen is reconverted to glucose (glycogenolysis), and glucose is formed from lactate, glycerol, and amino acids (gluconeogenesis). Finally, adipose tissue supplies free fatty acids (FFA) and glycerol from the breakdown of triglycerides (lipolysis). This steady-state of energy sources and peripheral muscle utilization maintains the blood glucose within a narrow range during exercise (Fig. 29–2). Intact hormonal systems provide homeostatic control of the blood glucose in the normal person without diabetes.[28] This homeostatic control in

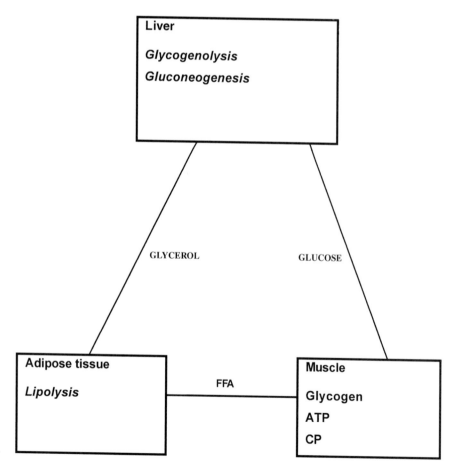

Figure 29–2. Energy sources for exercise.

TABLE 29–3. REGULATORY HORMONES AND ACTIONS

Hormone	Physiologic Action
Insulin	Facilitates glucose transfer into cells and promotes glycogen synthesis. Inhibits glucagon secretion. Inhibits gluconeogenesis. Converts glucose to triglycerides in lipid tissue.
Glucagon	Stimulates hepatic glycogenolysis and gluconeogenesis.
Catecholamines Epinephrine Norepinephrine	Promote hepatic glycogenolysis and gluconeogenesis. Suppress insulin secretion. Limit peripheral glucose utilization.
Growth hormone	Inhibits carbohydrate metabolism. Neutralizes free fatty acids.
Cortisol	Inhibits peripheral glucose utilization. Promotes gluconeogenesis.

aerobic exercise, such as running, involves the interaction of insulin, glucagon, catecholamines, growth hormone, and cortisol (Table 29–3).

Hormonal Control

Insulin facilitates glucose transfer into the cell and conversion to glycogen, inhibits gluconeogenesis to spare proteins, and functions as an anabolic hormone in converting glucose to triglycerides in lipid tissue. Basal insulin levels normally decrease by 50% with exercise.[29] In addition, insulin promotes glycogen synthesis in the liver and inhibits glucagon secretion. The net effect of the above mechanisms is to *lower* the circulating blood glucose level.

Glucagon is a counterregulatory hormone, which stimulates hepatic glycogenolysis and gluconeogenesis. The net effect of glucagon is to *raise* the circulating blood glucose level. *Catecholamines* (epinephrine and norepinephrine) also function as counterregulatory hormones and promote hepatic glycogenolysis and gluconeogenesis while suppressing insulin secretion. These hormones limit peripheral glucose utilization, thus maintaining a ready source of immediate glucose for energy requirements where needed in the body. The net effect of the catecholamines is to *raise* circulating blood glucose levels. *Growth hormone* inhibits carbohydrate metabolism and mobilizes FFA for energy. Exercise itself may be a stimulus for growth hormone release.[30] The net effect of growth hormone is to *raise* circulating blood glucose levels. Finally, *cortisol* initially inhibits peripheral glucose utilization. The late effect of cortisol mobilizes amino acids and glycerol for gluconeogenesis. The net effect of cortisol is to *raise* circulating blood glucose levels.

Normal Hormonal Changes With Exercise

The normal runner experiences the following hormonal changes with aerobic exercise: 1) catecholamine and glucagon levels rise, 2) insulin levels fall, 3) glycogen stores are mobilized for fuel and gradually become exhausted, 4) growth hormone and cortisol may increase, and 5) energy becomes available from either ingested glucose, gluconeogenesis, or free fatty acids. Sutton has represented this graphically[31] (Fig. 29–3).

In summary, the other counterregulatory hormones balance the action of insulin when the athlete is running. In the normal nondiabetic runner the blood glucose level is maintained in a narrow range of 70 to 85 mg/dl. When the actions of insulin, glucagon, and the catecholamines do not occur as expected in the diabetic runner, problems may occur.

PHYSIOLOGY OF EXERCISE IN DIABETIC RUNNERS

Competitive diabetic runners report optimal performance when they maintain blood glucose levels between 70 and 150 mg/dl. Described below are the expected hormonal changes in the diabetic runner.[32,33]

Type 1 Diabetic Runners[34]

First, the expected physiological *decline* in insulin levels is not reproduced by exogenous insulin administration. In fact, circulating insulin levels may increase with exercise due to enhanced absorption from injection sites. Excessive insulin levels may also attenuate mobilization of glycogen for energy. Second, after 10 years of diabetes, dysregulation often occurs and desensitization to the counterregulatory hormone system ensues. As blood glucose levels decrease, the release of glucagon and catecholamines is delayed and hypoglycemia may occur.[35] Thus, the diabetic runner with type 1 diabetes is exercising without a normal functioning hormonal control system. As glycogen stores become exhausted from endurance running, this athlete must rely on an *exogenous* energy source. If this is not available, immediate hypoglycemia may occur.

In contrast, if the type 1 diabetic runner is insulin-deficient and the blood sugar is excessive, endurance running may exacerbate the diabetic state. First, osmotic diuresis with relative dehydration affects performance. Next, as the blood glucose rises, the risk of causing higher blood glucose levels increases.[36,37] Further strenuous exercise may either precipitate or exacerbate existing ketoacidosis (Table 29–4). Instead of exercise, this athlete requires rest, fluid replacement, and insulin to correct the insulinopenic state.

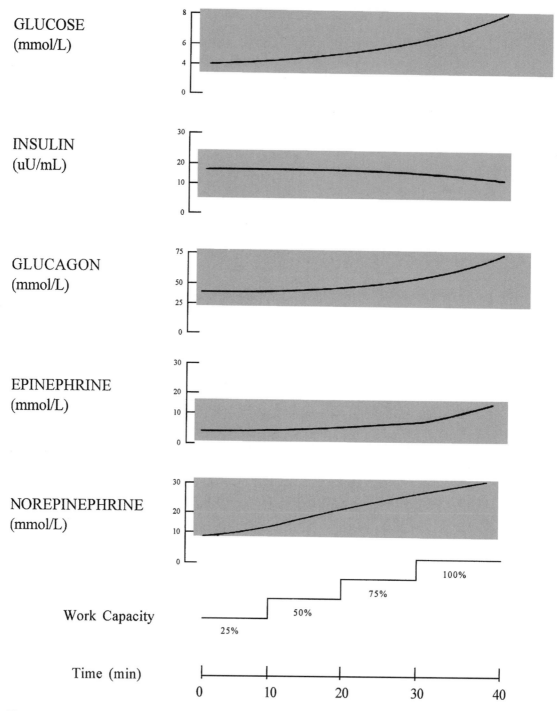

Figure 29–3. Hormonal changes with exercise in normal subjects. *(Source: Adapted with permission from Sutton.[31])*

Wahren and colleagues[38] compared the levels of blood glucose in normal, nonketotic diabetic, and ketotic diabetic athletes. Stimulation of the counterregulatory hormones in the insulinopenic, ketotic state only serves to worsen this condition (Fig. 29–4). Berger and coworkers[37] also studied athletes subjected to 3 hours of exercise. A similar effect was found when compared with normal controls (Fig. 29–5).

Type 2 Diabetic Runners

In type 2 diabetes, exercise improves insulin sensitivity and decreases insulin resistance.[39,40] Hepatic insulin sensitivity is also improved with decreased

TABLE 29–4. METABOLIC EFFECTS OF SERUM INSULIN LEVELS

Serum Insulin Level	Effect on Counterregulatory Hormones	Effect on Energy Sources	Effect on Blood Glucose Level	Athlete Performance
Low	Increased stimulation	Decreased transfer of glucose into the exercising muscles; increased free fatty acids and gluconeogenesis	Hyperglycemia, possible ketoacidosis	Osmotic diuresis, dehydration, increased fatigue, decreased performance
Optimal	Normal stimulation	Normal glucose transfer into cells of exercising muscle; normal glycogenolysis, gluconeogenesis and release of free fatty acids	Euglycemia	Optimal athletic performance
High	Decreased stimulation	Increased glucose transfer into exercising muscle; inhibits gluconeogenesis	Hypoglycemia	Decreased performance

gluconeogenesis. Many of the studies in type 2 patients have focused on aerobic exercise at high metabolic levels. Holloszy and colleagues[41] noted dramatic improvement with subjects running 25 to 35 kilometers per week at 70% to 80% $\dot{V}O_2$max. However, this activity level is not appropriate for many type 2 individuals. In addition, insulin resistance tends to increase with age due to a progressive loss of lean muscle mass. This change may correlate with decreased GLUT-4 production seen with aging.[19] Scientific evidence does support the use of resistance training in type 2 diabetes to increase the lean body mass and improve insulin sensitivity.[42] In turn, this improved insulin sensitivity

due to resistance training increases the aerobic performance in type 2 athletes.[43]

Specific Application to Running

Short-Distance (Sprint)

Short-distance, intense (anaerobic) running events should not pose significant metabolic problems for the type 1 athlete. Maintaining the ideal preexercise glucose level between 120 and 180 mg/dl and proper hydration will maximize performance. The individual blood glucose levels should be reviewed during the training periods to predict the response during

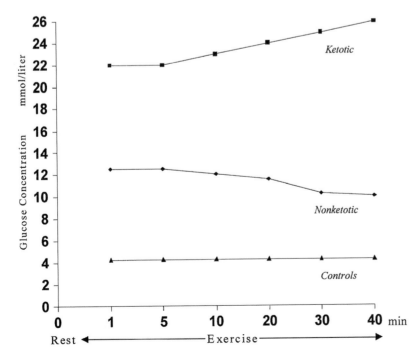

Figure 29–4. Comparison of normal, ketotic, and nonketotic diabetic athletes. *(Source: Adapted with permission from Wahren et al.[38])*

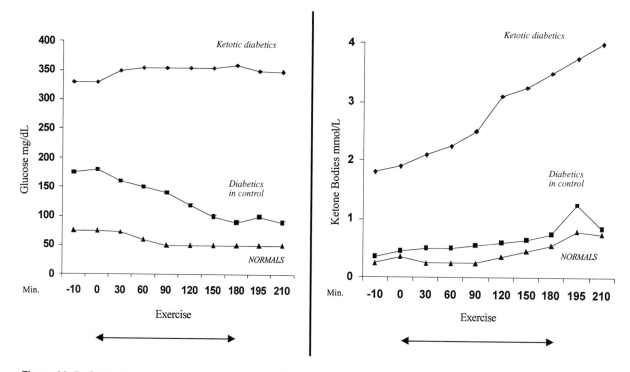

Figure 29–5. Comparison of normal, ketotic, and controlled diabetic athletes. *(Source: Adapted with permission from Berger.[37])*

competition. Serial warm-up sprinting will utilize some energy and this can be monitored. Mitchell and coworkers[44] demonstrated that hyperglycemia may occur in some athletes who exercise at high intensity for short periods of time. The competitive event itself may result in an increase in blood glucose levels secondary to acute catecholamine release. One would not expect delayed hypoglycemia to occur.

The predictable response for sprinting in the type 2 athlete is a reduction in the serum glucose levels without causing hypoglycemia. Over time improved insulin sensitivity may dictate a reduction in dosage of antidiabetic medication (sulfonylureas or insulin). Delayed hypoglycemia is uncommon in these runners.

Long-Distance (Endurance)[45]

Long-distance (aerobic) running requires careful management of fuel sources and insulin management for the type 1 diabetic runner.[46] With prolonged exercise, the body's fuel stores may become exhausted. Individual glucose utilization rates can be calculated. Many endurance runners strive for an optimal prerun blood glucose, take minimal insulin, and estimate a glucose decrease of 10 to 15 mg/dl per mile. When running for periods of 30 to 60 minutes, self-monitoring of blood glucose (SMBG) during the training period will delineate the individual's predicted response. The insulin is adjusted to achieve a prerun glucose of 120 to 180 mg/dl. When the measurement

is closer to 100 mg/dl, 15 to 30 grams of carbohydrates will need to be ingested prior to the exercise. With subcutaneous intermittent insulin injection, *some* insulin is required and it cannot be totally eliminated. When the runner is utilizing NPH (or Lente) combined with insulin lispro or regular, the intermediate-acting insulin is often decreased by 50% and the short-acting insulin is decreased by 25% to 75%, depending on the distance, time of exercise, and the individual's recorded response during training.[47] If a type 1 endurance runner experiences difficulty in maintaining satisfactory blood glucose levels, changing to more frequent insulin injections (3 to 4 per day) may improve control.

When exercising with continuous subcutaneous insulin infusion (CSII) or insulin-pump therapy, the runner may either remove the pump or continue the infusion with modified dosing. The pump may be removed for exercise periods shorter than 1 hour. With careful SMBG the runner can determine whether to abruptly cease infusion or to administer a bolus (usually no more than 50% of the planned infusion for the time exercised) before ceasing infusion.

If CSII is continued during the run, the infusion rate is modified. When running in the basal state (before breakfast or more than 4 hours since the last meal), the basal infusion rate is initially reduced by 50% during the exercise period. Subsequently, this infusion rate is adjusted according to SMBG. For example, if a runner with a basal rate of 1.4 units per hour jogs for 1 hour in the early morning before breakfast, this rate is reduced to 0.7 units per hour. Following individual SMBG, this temporary basal infusion rate can be adjusted to the specific runner. Some athletes elect to decrease the infusion rate 30 minutes before exercise or during the postexercise period due to increased insulin sensitivity. In addition, the subsequent mealtime bolus is often reduced by 30% to 50% due to persistent insulin sensitivity. When use of the insulin pump is continued during any running exercise, the athlete should monitor for hyperglycemia secondary to malfunction or dislodgment of the infusion needle. Special belts, cases, and protective covers are available for use during running and other sports activity.[48]

When running greater distances, external fuel sources become more important. The risk of hypoglycemia is increased since insulin levels do not wane in the type 1 diabetic runner as in the runner with normal hormonal control[31](Fig. 29–3). Carbohydrate-containing fluids and exogenous fuel sources will be required as exercise progresses. In addition, these endurance runners will need to ingest adequate carbohydrates (1.5 grams of carbohydrate per kg body weight) in the "golden recovery period" at the finish line.[49] If glycogen stores are not adequately replenished, the risk of delayed hypoglycemia is high. Table 29–5 outlines a management plan for type 1 runners competing in marathons and utilizing CSII.

Type 2 diabetic runners may participate in endurance running, but these persons are less likely to compete because they are frequently obese. However, some may have achieved weight loss, improved their cardiovascular fitness, and will participate. Unless these persons are taking insulin or sulfonylureas for treatment, one would not expect either immediate or delayed hypoglycemia. The period of increased insulin sensitivity should persist for 12 to 48 hours without clinical hypoglycemia.[20,50] Those treated with sulfonylureas or insulin may require reduction in dosage as they train, improve physical fitness, reduce body fat, and improve insulin resistance.

NUTRITIONAL REQUIREMENTS FOR DIABETIC RUNNERS (TABLE 29–6)[51]

General Requirements
The runner requires protein, fat, carbohydrates, and adequate fluids for proper performance. For each kilogram of body weight per day the endurance runner should consume at least 1.2 grams of protein, less than 1.4 grams of fat, along with 8 to 10 grams of carbohydrate, depending on the intensity and duration of training. The calories derived from this diet average 55% to 60% carbohydrate, 30% fat, and 10% to 15% protein. Total carbohydrate fuel stores in the runner average 1600 calories in muscle and 300 calories in the liver. Fat stores are almost unlimited and may approach one million calories in obese individuals.

Carbohydrate-Loading
Carbohydrate-loading is done cautiously in the type 1 runner. In the fit type 1 runner, insulin can be adjusted to balance carbohydrate-loading in the precompetition period. Meticulous glucose control with adequate exogenous insulin will promote adequate glycogen stores. Likewise, the well-trained type 2

TABLE 29–5. MARATHON MANAGEMENT PLAN FOR TYPE 1 RUNNER WITH CSII[a]

1. Bolus with insulin and eat 3 to 4 hours prior to event, if possible.
2. Check glucose prior to event and strive for level of 120 to 180 mg/dl prior to event. (Some elite runners ingest carbohydrate if glucose is less than 150 mg/dl at starting time.)
3. Reduce temporary basal rate to 40% to 50% of usual basal rate (or predetermined historical basal rate) during event and for 1 hour after event. (Some elite runners set temporary basal rate at 0.1 to 0.2 units per hour during event and for 1 hour afterward.)
4. During marathon event measure blood glucose at these points:
   Starting line
   6 mile marker
   12 mile marker
   18 mile marker
   22 mile marker
   Finish line
5. Carry quick forms of glucose (e.g., Quick Surge).
6. Ingest water and fuel sources depending on level of measured glucose and runner's response to exercise.
7. Replenish depleted glycogen stores following event!
8. During shorter events (<1 hour) or for the swimming portion of triathlons, one may discontinue CSII therapy.
9. The best guidelines are derived from the individual runner's historical response to endurance exercise or running.

[a]CSII, continuous subcutaneous insulin infusion.

TABLE 29–6. SUMMARY OF NUTRITIONAL STRATEGIES

Phase of Training	Recreational Athlete	Endurance Athlete
Baseline recommended total calories per day		>50 kcal (men). 45–50 kcal (women).
Daily training	Ingest <30% total daily energy from fat; 10%–12% from protein; balance from CHO.	Ingest <1.4 g fat/kg body wt/day; 0.8–1.2 g protein; 8–10 g CHO.
CHO loading (week before event)	Not applicable.	*CAUTION:* For type 1 runners: Do 90, 40, 40, 20, 20, 0 min of moderate-intensity exercise per day; consume 5 g CHO/kg BW/day during first 3 days; consume 8–10 g CHO/kg BW during next 3 days.
Hours before event	Exercise need not be taken on empty stomach; work-enhancing effect of preexercise CHO meal is doubtful; consume adequate fluids.	Consume 4–5 g liquid CHO/kg 3–4 hr preevent and/or consume 1–2 g liquid CHO kg 1 hr preevent. Solids may be substituted.
During event	Consume 250 ml of fluid every 20 minutes or at rate equal to sweat loss; fluids may be CHO/electrolyte beverages, water, or other preferred fluids.	Consume 250 ml of fluid every 20 minutes or at rate equal to sweat loss; preferred fluids are CHO/electrolyte (6%–10% wt/vol) beverages at a rate to provide 40–65 g CHO/hr. If CHO consumption is delayed, consume 200 g of liquid CHO before completing 2 hr of exercise and then consume 40–65 g CHO/hr.
4–6 Hours postevent	Not applicable.	Consume 0.7–3.0 g CHO/kg *immediately* postevent and every 2 hr for 4 hr; if tolerated, 0.4 g CHO/kg every 15 min postevent for 4 hr.
24 Hours postevent	Follow daily training schedule.	Consume 8–10 g CHO/kg/day; mixed CHO foods can be consumed; high-glycemic index foods promote glycogen synthesis.

CHO, carbohydrate; BW, body weight.
Individual response patterns may vary. The specific response to exercise can be monitored with self-monitoring of blood glucose.
Source: Adapted with permission from Sherman et al.[51]

athlete with enhanced insulin sensitivity should also have adequate glycogen stores. Studies have confirmed normal muscle glycogen synthesis during endurance exercise in well-controlled diabetic patients.

Ideally, the diabetic runner should ingest liquid or solid foods containing carbohydrate 3 to 4 hours prior to the event. Intake of additional liquid carbohydrate 1 hour prior to the event is optional. Adequate fluid intake is crucial to promote optimal performance.

Endurance Running Requirements

With endurance running, hypoglycemia is the major risk in type 1 athletes and in type 2 athletes receiving certain medications. These runners must adjust medications and maintain an intake of exogenous carbohydrates, especially with activities lasting more than 1 hour. Carbohydrate-containing fluids (e.g., 8% weight/volume) are acceptable for ingestion by the diabetic runner. However, one must calculate the grams of carbohydrate consumed carefully because an excessive intake may elevate glucose levels and decrease performance. Runners may either monitor glucose levels and adjust carbohydrate intake or follow predetermined energy requirements based on training experience. Immediately following the event, the runner must consume adequate carbohydrates to prevent delayed hypoglycemia. These recommendations are summarized in Table 29–6.

Finally, adequate fluid ingestion in the diabetic runner is critical for optimal metabolic performance. These requirements are similar to those of the nondiabetic runner.

SPECIAL PRECAUTIONS/HAZARDS

Exercise-Induced Hypoglycemia

Immediate Hypoglycemia

Hypoglycemia in the diabetic runner is either immediate or delayed. Immediate hypoglycemia occurs during or shortly after exercise. This condition is most common in the type 1 patient and usually occurs due to caloric intake inadequate to meet metabolic demands. Other causes include excessive exogenous insulin administration or injection of insulin into exercising muscle or overlying subcutaneous tissue, resulting in increased absorption.

To prevent immediate hypoglycemia one should avoid injection of insulin into an area of exercising muscles (e.g., use of anterior thigh in a runner).[52] Instead, injection into the abdominal area is recommended. Then one should continuously replace calories during a period of prolonged activity. For example, a runner might require 800 to 1000 calories per hour to maintain a constant energy source while exercising. Athletes can refer to published tables to obtain a range for energy requirements when performing different activities[53] (Table 29–7). With careful SMBG during such activities, the athlete can then determine individual caloric requirements and make necessary adjustments. To avoid weight gain, the runner may emphasize insulin adjustment rather than supplemental calories. In general, with improved fitness level and favorable environmental conditions, fewer calories are necessary. In contrast, exercising at a lower fitness level in cold weather may consume more calories (Table 29–8). In a hot environment some diabetic runners experience hypoglycemia due to poor appetite and decreased caloric intake.

Delayed Hypoglycemia

Delayed hypoglycemia usually occurs 6 to 12 hours after exercise and has been reported up to 28 hours postexercise.[54] Also called nocturnal hypoglycemia, this

TABLE 29–8. PHYSIOLOGIC FACTORS WHICH PREDISPOSE TO HYPOGLYCEMIA

- Longer exercise time
- Greater exercise intensity
- Inadequate caloric intake
- Poor fitness level
- Excessive insulin dose
- Colder environmental temperatures
- Insulin injection site and typical absorption rate
    Abdomen above umbilicus > below umbilicus
    Abdomen > arm
    Arm > thigh/hip
- Insulin injection into exercising muscle
- Insulin injection over area of exercising muscle
- Massage or heat application to area of insulin injection

phenomenon often occurs at nighttime, when the athlete is least likely to perceive and recognize this condition. The pathophysiology involves vigorous exercise, which severely depletes body glycogen stores. Then, in the postexercise ("golden replenishment period") interval, the athlete fails to adequately replace these glycogen stores. (Glycogen-depleting activity may require up to 550 grams of carbohydrate for repletion.) Instead, the athlete either underestimates caloric requirements or ingests limited calories and defers eating until later. Over the ensuing hours, liver and muscle tissues extract circulating blood glucose to replenish depleted glycogen stores and glycogen synthetase is activated.[55] In addition, the peripheral muscle tissues are more sensitive to any available insulin postexercise.[56] The subsequent severe and persistent delayed hypoglycemia often requires continuous caloric intake over several hours to correct.

Effects of Medications

Some medications are prone to cause hypoglycemia with exercise (Table 29–9). Foremost is insulin therapy as discussed above. Intermediate- and long-acting types are more likely to produce late hypoglycemia. Conversely, lispro insulin (Humalog), with its more rapid absorption and shorter duration of action, is less likely to produce these effects. Insulin injection site and environmental factors, as well as the insulin type used, may affect the absorption and subsequent effect on blood glucose (Table 29–10).

Sulfonylureas and meglitinides, which stimulate endogenous insulin secretion, may cause hypoglycemia and require dosage adjustment. Meglitinides have a more immediate effect, are more predictable, and are less likely to cause late effects. Agents such as metformin, oligosaccharidases, and the thiazoladinediones rarely produce hypoglycemia with exercise. Concomitant drugs given with these medications are

TABLE 29–7. ENERGY EXPENDITURE FOR RUNNING ACTIVITIES

Activity	Estimated Kilocalories per Hour[a]
Walking at 2 mph	185
Walking at 4 mph	335
Running at 5 mph	560
Running at 6 mph	660
Running at 10 mph	1120

[a]Based on body weight of 70 kg.
Source: Derived from Passmore et al.[53]

TABLE 29–9. ANTIDIABETIC AGENTS AND HYPOGLYCEMIA

Agent	Hypoglycemia With Exercise	Mechanism of Action	Treatment
Insulin			
Rapid acting Lispro	Yes	Increased absorption from injection site; suppression of gluconeogenesis; promotes glucose transfer into cells.	Administer oral carbohydrates; consider insulin reduction (25%–75%) with moderate to prolonged exercise.
Short acting Regular	Yes		
Intermediate NPH Lente	Yes		Administer oral carbohydrates; consider insulin dose reduction by 30%–60% prior to exercise.
Long acting Ultralente	Yes		Administer oral carbohydrates; consider holding or reducing prior to prolonged exercise.
Sulfonylurea	Yes	Increased insulin levels and subsequent physiologic response of insulin.	Administer oral carbohydrates, adjust dose with exercise.
Meglitinide	Yes		
Metformin[a]	No	NA	NA
Oligosaccharidase[a]	Rare, only in combination	NA	Must administer glucose or dextrose.
Thiazoldinedione[a]	No	NA	NA

NA, not applicable.

[a]If hypoglycemia occurs when these agents are used in combination, the other responsible agents must be adjusted. These agents do not cause hypoglycemia with exercise.

TABLE 29–10. TIME COURSE OF ACTION FOR INSULIN PREPARATIONS[a]

Insulin Preparation	Onset of Action (hr)	Peak Action (hr)	Duration of Action (hr)
Rapid onset			
Insulin lispro (analogue)	0.1–0.5	1–2	3–5
Short acting			
Regular (crystalline, soluble)	0.5–1.0	2–4	6–8
Intermediate acting			
NPH (isophane suspension)	1–4	6–8	12–18
Lente (insulin zinc suspension)	1–3	4–8	12–20
Long acting			
Ultralente (extended insulin zinc suspension)	2–4	8–14	18–24
Combinations of insulin			
70/30 (70% NPH; 30% regular)	0.5–1.0	Dual	12–18
50/50 (50% NPH; 50% regular)	0.5–1.0	Dual	12–18

[a]Based on human insulin injected into abdomen.

usually the offending agents. If an athlete treated with oligosaccharidases becomes hypoglycemic, treatment will require a monosaccharide or simple sugar, such as glucose or fructose. The absorption of sucrose (table sugar) is inhibited.

TEAM APPROACH TO THE DIABETIC RUNNER

The team approach to the management of the diabetic runner includes the physician, coach, athletic trainer, teammates, and family, as well as the athlete. The physician should offer guidelines and enforce principles of training for the runner with special metabolic needs. Ideally, this physician should be competent in diabetes management, sports medicine training, and exercise physiology. The coach outlines a training program that includes the frequency, duration, time of day, and training goals with the athlete. The diurnal timing will be important when coordinating meals and medications with the training schedule. The athletic trainer works one on one with the athlete and monitors performance. The trainer is often the person who maintains appropriate glucose monitoring equipment, initially diagnoses hypoglycemia, and then treats the athlete following a predetermined protocol.[57] This protocol should include both immediate-acting glucose and injectable glucagon. Family members and teammates should be aware of hypoglycemic signs, symptoms, and appropriate treatment. Finally, the athlete must be an active participant in the management team. Adolescent diabetic runners may be uncooperative, fail to eat properly, or administer insulin incorrectly. Type 1 runners of any age must not only possess a glucose self-monitoring device but also use it diligently while exercising. While type 2 runners should rarely encounter hypoglycemia, a treatment plan must be in place.

Many type 1 distance runners wear a fanny pack and develop skill at SMBG and determining appropriate fuel ingestion at distance markers. Alternatively, the runner may train and compete with a supporting "pit team." The runner passes off an impregnated test strip to a team member along the side of the course. The team member measures the capillary glucose, and radios ahead to a second team member who tells the runner the result. Together the runner and team then decide whether the athlete must ingest more calories or only water at the next station. These team members often leapfrog along the course as the runner advances. Special permission from race officials may be necessary for this sort of arrangement.

SUMMARY

The diabetic runner faces specific metabolic challenges. The type 1 runner must control the preexercise glucose level, monitor the intraexercise blood glucose level, and adjust insulin and carbohydrate fuel intake carefully to maximize performance. Immediate and delayed hypoglycemia are always risks in this athlete. The type 2 runner faces fewer adjustments of medications and fuel intake and the risk of hypoglycemia is lower. Individual metabolic responses to running are determined by historical SMBG data collected during training sessions. Cooperation by all members of the athlete's team ensures successful participation. By following established principles and guidelines, diabetic athletes can participate, compete, and enjoy the benefits of running.

A DOZEN TIPS FOR THE DIABETIC RUNNER

1. Have a preexercise evaluation and exercise stress test, if indicated.
2. *ALWAYS* run with a partner.
3. Diabetic runners must wear identification (e.g., Medic-Alert jewelry) and have a strategy for treating hypoglycemia experienced while running.
4. Diabetic runners must not only possess but also *USE* a glucose-monitoring device.
5. Well-controlled type 1 diabetic runners of less than 10 years' experience usually have few complications.
6. Type 1 diabetics of greater than 10 years' experience often have dysregulation.
7. Sites of insulin injection in type 1 runners *MAY* affect absorption rate with exercise; certain medications may cause hypoglycemia in type 2 runners.
8. Meals should be eaten 3 to 4 hours before running.
9. Avoid exercising during times of peak insulin activity (consider using Humalog insulin).
10. Check blood sugar before exercise. Ideal range for a type 1 runner is 120 to 180 mg/dl.
    a. If <100 mg/dl snack before exercise
    b. If 100 to 250 mg/dl, exercise
    c. If >250 mg/dl, delay exercise, check ketones, treat blood sugar/dehydration
    d. Supplement with glucose-containing fluids every 30 minutes during periods of strenuous exercise
11. Be aware of *DELAYED HYPOGLYCEMIA*. After exercise, replenish glycogen stores based on duration and intensity of exercise.

12. Each diabetic runner must be aware of his or her personal pattern of blood glucose response to exercise.

REFERENCES

1. American Diabetes Association: Report of the expert committee on the diagnosis and classification of diabetes mellitus. *Diabetes Care* 1997:20, 1183.
2. Valle T, Tuomilehto J, Eriksson J: Epidemiology of NIDDM in Europoids, in Alberti KGMM, Simmet P, DeFronzo RA, et al. (eds.), *International Textbook of Diabetes Mellitus,* Chichester, UK, John Wiley & Sons, 1997: 125.
3. McCarthy D, Simmet P: Diabetes 1994 to 2010: Global estimates and projections. Melbourne, International Diabetes Institute, 1994.
4. Harris MI, Zimmet P: Classification of diabetes mellitus and other categories of glucose intolerance, in Alberti KGMN, Zimmet P DeFronzo RA (eds.), *International Textbook of Diabetes Mellitus,* 2nd ed., London, John Wiley and Sons, 1998:15.
5. Atkinson MA, Maclaren NK: The pathogenesis of insulin-dependent diabetes mellitus. *N Engl J Med* 1994:331, 1428.
6. Imagawa A, Hanafusa T, Miyagawa J, et al.: A novel subtype of type 1 diabetes mellitus characterized by a rapid onset and an absence of diabetes-related antibodies. *N Engl J Med* 2000:342, 301.
7. Kahn CR: Insulin receptors and insulin signaling in normal and disease states, in Alberti KGMN, Zimmet P, DeFronzo RA (eds.), *International Textbook of Diabetes Mellitus,* 2nd ed., London, John Wiley and Sons, 1998: 446.
8. Warram JH, Martin BC, Krolewaski AS, et al.: Slow glucose removal rate and hyperinsulinemia precede the development of type II diabetes in the offspring of diabetic parents. *Ann Intern Med* 1990:113, 909.
9. Fajans SS: Maturity-onset diabetes of the young (MODY). *Diabetes Metab Rev* 1989:5, 579.
10. Scheuner MT, Raffel LJ, Rotter JI: Genetics of diabetes, in Alberti KGMN, Zimmet P, DeFronzo RA (eds.), *International Textbook of Diabetes Mellitus,* 2nd ed. London, John Wiley and Sons, 1998:58.
11. American Diabetes Association: Standards of medical care for patients with diabetes mellitus. *Diabetes Care* 2001:24(suppl 1), S33.
12. Lawrence RD: The effect of exercise on insulin action in diabetes. *British Med J* 1926:1, 648.
13. American College of Sports Medicine and American Diabetes Association: Joint Position Statement: Diabetes mellitus and exercise. *Med Sci Sports Exerc* 1997:29, i.
14. American Diabetes Association: Diabetes mellitus and exercise. *Diabetes Care* 2001:24(suppl 1), S51.
15. White RD, Sherman C: Exercise in diabetes management: Maximizing benefits, controlling risks. *Phys Sportsmed* 1999:27, 63.
16. Jarett RJ, Shipley MJ, Hunt R: Physical activity, glucose tolerance, and diabetes mellitus: The Whitehall Study. *Diabetic Med* 1987:3, 549.
17. DeFronzo RA, Ferrannini E, Sato Y, et al.: Synergistic interaction between exercise and insulin on peripheral glucose uptake. *J Clin Invest* 1981:68, 1468.
18. Eriksson JG: Exercise and the treatment of type 2 diabetes mellitus: An update. *Sports Med* 1999:27, 381.
19. Shepherd PR, Kahn BB: Glucose transporters and insulin action. *N Engl J Med* 1999:341, 248.
20. Petrseghin G, Price TB, Peterson KF, et al.: Increased glucose transport-phosphorylation and muscle glycogen synthesis after exercise training in insulin-resistant subjects. *N Engl J Med* 1996:335, 1357.
21. Koivisto VA, DeFronzo RA: Physical training and insulin sensitivity. *Diabetes Metab Rev* 1986:1, 445.
22. Lehmann R, Kaplan V, Bingisser R, et al.: Impact of physical activity on cardiovascular risk factors in IDDM. *Diabetes Care* 1997:20, 1603.
23. Lehmann R, Vokac A, Niedermann K, et al.: Loss of abdominal fat and improvement of the cardiovascular risk profile by regular moderate exercise in patients with NIDDM. *Diabetologia* 1995:38, 1313.
24. Beaser RS, White RD: Strategies for the prevention and treatment of macrovascular complications of Type 2 diabetes. Monograph of the American Academy of Family Physicians and American Diabetes Association. Kansas City, Mo, September 1998.
25. Schneider SH, Morgado A: Exercise in the management of Type 2 diabetes mellitus, in DeFronzo RA (ed.), *Current Therapy of Diabetes Mellitus,* St. Louis, Mosby-Year Book, 1998:90.
26. American College of Sports Medicine Position Stand: Physical activity, physical fitness, and hypertension. *Med Sci Sports Exerc* 1993:25, i.
27. Powers SK: Fundamentals of exercise metabolism, in Durstine JL, King AC, Painter PL, et al. (eds.), *Resource Manual for Guidelines for Exercise Testing and Prescription,* 2nd ed., Philadelphia, Lea and Febiger, 1993:59.
28. Felig P, Wahren J: Fuel homeostasis in exercise. *N Engl J Med* 1975:293, 1078.
29. Zinman B: Adjusting the treatment regimen for exercise in Type I diabetes. *Practical Diabetology* 1993:12, 17.
30. McCardle WD, Katch FI, Katch VL: *Exercise Physiology,* 4th ed, Baltimore, Williams & Wilkins, 1996:361.
31. Sutton JR: Diabetes and exercise, in Strauss RH (ed.), *Sports Medicine,* 2nd ed., Philadelphia, Saunders, 1991:221.
32. Horton ES: Role and management of exercise in diabetes mellitus. *Diabetes Care* 1988:11, 210.
33. Vranic M, Berger M: Exercise and diabetes mellitus. *Diabetes* 1979:28, 147.
34. Devlin JT: Exercise in the management of Type 1 diabetes mellitus, in DeFronzo RA (ed.), *Current Therapy of Diabetes Mellitus,* St. Louis, Mosby-Year Book, 1998:62.
35. Hirsch IB, Marker JC, Smith LJ, et al.: Insulin and glucagon in prevention of hypoglycemia during exercise in humans. *Am J Physiol* 1991:260 (*Endocrinol Metab* 23), E695.

36. Marble A, Smith RM: Exercise in diabetes mellitus. *Arch Intern Med* 1938:58, 577.

37. Berger M, Berchtold P, Cuppers H-J, et al.: Metabolic and hormonal effects of muscular exercise in juvenile type diabetics. *Diabetologia* 1977:13, 355.

38. Wahren J, Hagenfeldt L, Felig P: Splanchnic and leg exchange of glucose, amino acids, and free fatty acids during exercise in diabetes. *J Clin Invest* 1975:55, 1303.

39. Mayer-Davis EJ, D'Agostino R, Karter AJ, et al.: Intensity and amount of physical activity in relation to insulin sensitivity. *JAMA* 1998:279, 669.

40. Hughes VA, Fiatarone MA, Fielding RA, et al.: Exercise increases muscle GLUT-4 levels and insulin action in subjects with impaired glucose tolerance. *Am J Physiol* 1993:264, E855.

41. Holloszy JO, Schultz J, Kusnierkiewicz J, et al.: Effects of exercise on glucose tolerance and insulin resistance. *Acta Med Scand Suppl* 1986:711, 55.

42. Miller WJ, Sherman WM, Ivy JL: Effect of strength training on glucose tolerance and post-glucose insulin response. *Med Sci Sports Exercise* 1984:16, 539.

43. Schneider SH, Ruderman NV: Exercise and NIDDM. *Diabetes Care* 1990:13, 785.

44. Mitchell TH, Abraham G, Schiffrin A, et al.: Hyperglycemia after intense exercise in IDDM subjects during continuous subcutaneous insulin infusion. *Diabetes Care* 1988:11, 311.

45. Richter EA, Turcotte L, Hespel P, et al.: Metabolic responses to exercise: Effects of endurance training and implications for diabetes. *Diabetes Care* 1992:15, 1767.

46. Sane T, Helve E, Pelkonen R, et al.: The adjustment of diet and insulin dose during long term endurance exercise on Type I (insulin-dependent) diabetic men. *Diabetologia* 1988:31, 35.

47. Berger M: Adjustment of insulin therapy, in Ruderman N, Devlin JT (eds.), *The Health Professional's Guide to Diabetes and Exercise*, Alexandria, Va, American Diabetes Association, 1995:117.

48. Walsh J, Roberts R: *Pumping Insulin,* San Diego, Torrey Pines, 1994.

49. Ivy JL: Muscle glycogen synthesis before and after exercise. *Sports Medicine* 1991:11, 6.

50. Maynard T: Exercise. Part I Physiological response to exercise in diabetes mellitus. *Diabetes Educator* 1991:17, 196.

51. Sherman WM, Ferrara C, Schneider B: Nutritional strategies to optimize athletic performance, in Ruderman N, Devlin JT (eds.), *The Health Professional's Guide to Diabetes and Exercise*, Alexandria, Va, American Diabetes Association, 1995:94.

52. Frid A, Ostman J, Linde B: Hypoglycemia risk during exercise after intramuscular injection of insulin in the thigh in IDDM. *Diabetes Care* 1990:11, 410.

53. Passmore R, Durnin JVGA: Human energy expenditure. *Physiol Rev* 1955:35, 801.

54. MacDonald J: Postexercise late-onset hypoglycemia in insulin-dependent diabetic patients. *Diabetes Care* 1978:10, 584.

55. Mikines KJ, Sonne B: Insulin sensitivity and responsiveness after acute exercise in man. *Clin Physiol* 5(suppl 4), A67.

56. Hough DO: Diabetes mellitus in sports. *Med Clin North Am* 1994:78, 423.

57. Jimenez CC: Diabetes and exercise: The role of the athletic trainer. *J Athletic Training* 1997:32, 339.

Chapter 30

RUNNING AND OSTEOARTHRITIS

Stuart E. Willick

INTRODUCTION

Running has many benefits. It can be personally and socially rewarding. Running has been shown to improve cardiovascular endurance and help control blood pressure, lipids, and cholesterol.[1] Running is a useful form of weight management and can improve strength, endurance, and mood.[1,2]

Yet running is not without risk. As outlined in Part III of this book, running overload injuries to muscle, tendon, and bone are common. Less well understood, however, is the relationship between running and joint injury. The sports medicine practitioner will frequently hear runners ask if they can do permanent damage to their joints if they continue running. This is a logical question because all mechanical devices eventually break down with repetitive loading. Biological joints differ from nonbiological mechanical constructions in that they possess intrinsic healing mechanisms designed to combat the inevitable breakdown process. Repetitive loading of joints during running may favor the breakdown process. It is also possible, however, that running might stimulate joint healing and joint health.

This chapter reviews the available literature on the association between running and the development of osteoarthritis. Serving as background, the first part of the chapter briefly reviews the clinical, histologic, and radiologic findings of osteoarthritis. The second part summarizes in vitro and human epidemiologic studies that offer theoretical considerations regarding the relationship between running and osteoarthritis. The third section covers in vivo animal studies. The final, most clinically relevant section examines in vivo human studies that explore the association between running and the development of osteoarthritis.

Osteoarthritis

Osteoarthritis is the most common form of joint disease. It is characterized by degeneration of the articular cartilage with eburnation of subchondral bone and hypertrophy of bone at the articular margins resulting in osteophyte formation.[3] Osteoarthritis may be classified as primary (idiopathic) or secondary. Secondary osteoarthritis has many causes, including trauma, damage from other inflammatory diseases, and developmental anomalies such as hip dysplasia. Osteoarthritis usually has an insidious onset and follows a slow progressive course. The clinical findings include joint stiffness, variable pain that is worsened by use and weightbearing, deformity, limitation of motion, crepitus, and synovitis or other signs of local inflammation without systemic manifestations. Radiologic findings of osteoarthritis include joint space narrowing, osteophyte formation, intraarticular osseous bodies, subchondral sclerosis, and subchondral cysts.[4] The physical findings often do not correlate with the radiographic findings. Sometimes people have marked degenerative joint changes on x-ray with minimal or no symptoms. Radiographically, 86% of women and 78% of men over 65 years of age show evidence of osteoarthritis, but 40% to 70% of people with radiographic changes of osteoarthritis are symptom free.[5–7] Therefore, the diagnosis of osteoarthritis should be based on a combination of clinical and radiographic findings.

THEORETICAL CONSIDERATIONS

Theoretical evidence regarding a proposed association between running and degenerative joint disease can be broadly classified into two categories: human epidemiologic evidence and in vitro laboratory evidence.

An association between running and the development of osteoarthritis is theoretically supported by abundant epidemiologic evidence supporting the concept that osteoarthritis is more common in joints that sustain greater loads over extended periods of time.[8–14] Additionally, in vitro laboratory studies have provided evidence suggesting that the stresses of joint loading can be associated with changes in articular cartilage.[15–19] In light of this evidence indicating that loading of joints in at least some form is associated with osteoarthritis, it is reasonable to entertain the idea that repetitive loading of joints during years of running might also lead to greater wear and tear in those joints.

Human Epidemiologic Studies
Numerous epidemiologic studies suggest a relationship between repetitive exposure to increased mechanical stress and the development of degenerative joint changes. Buckwalter and Mankin[10] suggested that high-impact and torsional loads might increase the risk of degeneration of normal joints, and individuals that have abnormal anatomy, joint instability, disturbances of joint or muscle innervation, or inadequate muscle strength have a greater risk of degenerative joint disease.

Lindberg and Montgomery[11] investigated the prevalence of primary osteoarthrosis in men who performed heavy labor for at least 30 years. Their data show a significantly higher prevalence of primary osteoarthrosis among subjects who performed heavy labor versus age-matched controls who did not, as demonstrated by symptomatic complaints and knee roentgenography. The reported association between degenerative joint changes and heavy labor in the Lindberg study concurs with findings from other studies that have suggested that performing heavy labor for many years has been shown to be an independent predictor for the development of osteoarthritis in load-bearing joints.[8]

In a study by Felson and colleagues[12] members of the Framingham Heart Study cohort were followed longitudinally to assess occupational joint use and osteoarthritis. The findings of this study suggest that men whose jobs required repetitive knee bending and at least moderate physical demands had higher rates of radiographic knee osteoarthritis than men whose jobs required neither.

In a related study, the same researchers used cohort analysis of the Framingham Heart Study group to evaluate the effect of weight loss in preventing symptomatic osteoarthritis in women.[13] The results suggest that a decrease in body mass index of 2 units or more over the 10 years prior to the study period decreased the odds for developing osteoarthritis by over 50%. The investigators concluded that weight loss significantly reduces the risk for symptomatic knee osteoarthritis in women.

Findings from the Felson[13] weight loss study as well as other studies demonstrating an association between obesity[9] and osteoarthritis provide important information regarding the possible destructive effects of loading on joints. This information combined with the observed association between heavy labor and osteoarthritis[12] seems to support a proposed relationship between repetitive exposure to increased mechanical stress and the development of degenerative joint changes. Whether or not the results from these populations are applicable to runners warrants closer attention.

In Vitro Studies
The ability of joints to withstand destructive forces is dependent on intrinsic and extrinsic factors. Intrinsic factors include water content, proteoglycan content and matrix integrity of the articular cartilage, thickness of the articular cartilage, subchondral bone integrity, the ability of periarticular ligaments and muscles to support the joint, and the body's inherent healing mechanisms. Extrinsic factors include the magnitude, frequency, rate, and direction of forces applied to the joint.

A number of in vitro laboratory studies have provided information suggesting that joint use in the normal physiologic range does not lead to degenerative changes. In a study of articular surface pressures, Adams and Swanson[15] used direct pressure measurements in cadaveric hip joints during simulated activity to examine the effects of physical activity on joint surfaces. The findings of this study suggest that physical activities under normal conditions result in articular surface pressures ranging between 4.93 and

9.57 MN/m^2. These pressures were not observed to cause fibrillation in joint cartilage, and the authors concluded that physiologic stresses do not cause apparent injury to normal joints.

A related study by Repo and Finlay[20] examined survival of articular cartilage after controlled impact. Autoradiography and light and scanning electron microscopy revealed no evidence of chondrocyte death or structural damage until stress levels of 25 MN/m^2 or greater were reached. These levels of stress correlated with loads sufficient to fracture a femoral shaft and are therefore greater than those sustained during normal physical activity.[20] The findings of this study, combined with the aforementioned findings of Adams and Swanson,[15] suggest that activities such as running and jumping are not likely to result in maximal joint stresses great enough to cause disruption of normal articular cartilage.

In contrast to the above referenced studies suggesting that joint use within the normal physiologic range does not cause damage to articular cartilage, several in vitro studies have suggested that certain types of applied loads and repetitive motion can produce degenerative changes in joints.[21–27]

In one study examining the behavior of articular cartilage subjected to an applied load, Newton and coworkers[21] suggested that the ability of articular cartilage to distribute forces is dependent on the rate at which the force is applied. When a load is applied to the surface of normal articular cartilage, movement of fluid within the matrix of the cartilage occurs to optimally distribute forces throughout the cartilage and to the subchondral bone.[22] When the load is applied slowly, there is time for the fluid within the matrix to redistribute, thus allowing the cartilage to undergo the necessary deformation and absorb the impulse sustained by the macromolecular cartilaginous framework. If a force is applied too quickly for this fluid redistribution within the cartilage to occur, such as with sudden torsional joint loading or sudden axial joint impact during sports, a greater stress is applied to the macromolecular framework of the matrix.[22]

Examining the effects of applied loads and repetitive motion on joints, Weightman and colleagues[23] cyclically loaded in vitro samples of human cartilage to the point at which fibrillation of the cartilage surface was induced. Extrapolation of the results of this study suggests that tensile fatigue failure of articular cartilage may occur at physiologic stress levels if the loads are applied at high enough frequency.

In a related study, Radin and Paul[24] demonstrated articular cartilage degeneration of in vitro bovine metacarpophalangeal joints subjected to repetitive motion combined with impact loading. Their data suggested that degenerative changes may occur when in vitro articular cartilage is subjected to physiologic stress levels if the joint is simultaneously subjected to repetitive rotation and axial loading.

Deckel and Weissman[25] used rabbit knee joints to investigate the effects of repetitive joint rotation and rotation combined with axial peak overloading. The investigators in this study, as in the studies by Weightman et al.[23] and Radin and Paul,[24] reported physical and biochemical changes in the articular cartilage surface with these types of joint stress. Additionally, Deckel and Weissman[25] attempted to separate the two types of stress to which weightbearing joints are subjected. One type is a shear stress produced by reciprocal friction of articulating surfaces, and axial loading produces the other type. Interestingly, these researchers observed degenerative changes in knees subjected to simultaneous shear stress and axial overloading, but not in those subjected to repetitive shear overuse alone. This distinction suggests that it is the added peak axial overloading that is responsible for degenerative physical and biochemical changes in joints.

Zimmerman and coworkers[26] used in vitro cartilage plugs to show that repetitive loading can be a cause of cartilage disruption. They found the extent of damage increased as the load increased and as the number of loading cycles increased. When the investigators used 1000 pounds per square inch ($1000 \text{ psi/inch}^2 = 7 \times 10^6 \text{ N/m}^2$) they found surface abrasions after 250 cycles. These observers noted primary fissures that penetrated to the calcified cartilage after 500 cycles. Secondary fissures coming from the primary fissures formed after 1000 cycles, and after 8000 cycles fissures coalesced and undercut cartilage fragments. With higher loads, similar changes were seen after fewer cycles. The findings of this study indicate that repetitive loads can cause progression of cartilage damage from surface abrasions to vertical fissures and can ultimately extend the damage to create free fragments and cartilage flaps. It must be noted, however, that the forces applied in this study are several orders of magnitude greater than those encountered under normal physiologic conditions.

An investigation of the proposed threshold of stress for joint injury by Newberry and colleagues[27] involved the impaction of rabbit patellofemoral joints at varying intensities. Their data suggest that low-intensity impacts produced acute tissue stresses below the injury threshold, while high-intensity impacts produced stresses that exceeded the threshold for disease pathogenesis.

In a general sense, these studies begin to identify "safe" and "unsafe" ranges of tissue stress, which may have future utility in the design of safe training programs for humans.[27] To date the extrapolation of these designated low- and high-intensity stresses from in vitro laboratory studies to human terms remains ill defined. The clinical question remains, however, whether the act of running generates mechanical stress sufficient to cause disruption of normal articular cartilage.

In Vivo Animal Studies

Several studies have examined joint responses to running in animal models.[28–38]

A series of animal studies from Germany have shown that the histologic joint effects from running are dependent on the distance run. Dogs that ran moderate distances (4 km/day, 5 days/week for 40 weeks) showed increased cartilage thickness, proteoglycan content, and indentation stiffness.[28,29] Higher-volume running (20 km/day, 5 days/week for 15 weeks) resulted in decreased proteoglycan content and cartilage thickness. During longer-term, very high-volume running (40 km/day for up to 1 year), a decrease in indentation stiffness and cartilage proteoglycan concentration was seen along with stimulation of subchondral bone remodeling.[30,31] However, the clinical relevance of the changes in the articular cartilage and subchondral bone seen in these studies is unclear. They may be the result of healthy joint adaptation to repetitive motion and loading instead of true joint degeneration with production of symptomatic osteoarthritis.

Newton and coworkers[21] examined the effects of moderate lifelong running with added weight in beagles. In this study the animals ran 4 km per day, 5 days per week for 550 weeks. While running, the animals wore jackets that weighed 130% of their body weight. At the end of the study the synovial joints of the exercised animals were compared with the synovial joints of control animals (beagles with cage activity for 550 weeks). No difference in the synovial joints was seen between the two groups macroscopically, microscopically, or mechanically. This study suggests that moderate running with greater than normal body weight does not increase the risk of joint degeneration.

Videman[32] investigated the effect of running on the osteoarthritic joint in rabbits. This researcher experimentally induced osteoarthritis-type changes in rabbits by immobilization, which is known to produce joint changes similar to those seen in osteoarthritis. After a period of immobilization the rabbits ran at near maximal levels for 14 weeks. The control group included rabbits that also had joints immobilized but were not exercised. The joints were then examined clinically, histologically, and radiologically. No difference was found in joint range of motion, histology, or radiographic appearance. In this experimental model,

running did not accelerate osteoarthritis in animals that already had degenerative joint changes.

Kaiki and colleagues[33] studied experimental osteoarthritis and running in rats. They found that running led to worse osteoarthritis in rats whose joints had been injected with 2% hydrogen peroxide, which is also known to produce degenerative changes. Two control groups included rats whose joints were injected with saline and then exercised and rats whose joints were injected with 2% peroxide but were not exercised.

Palmoski and Brandt[34] investigated the effect of running on the reversal of atrophic changes in canine knee cartilage. The animals' knees were immobilized in casts for 6 weeks. The investigators found that immobilization resulted in an increase in cartilage water content and a decrease in cartilage thickness, proteoglycan synthesis, and proteoglycan aggregation. While ad lib activities appeared to slowly reverse these changes, running 6 miles per day not only prevented the reversal of the proteoglycan aggregation changes, it also caused a further decrease in cartilage thickness. In a related study, Palmoski and Brandt[35] showed that immobilization of the knee after an anterior cruciate ligament resection may help prevent joint degeneration, whereas forced activity can cause joint degeneration. These two studies taken together suggest that rest or limited activity of a joint immediately after a joint injury may result in a better outcome than excessive repetitive motion and loading.

Taken together, the findings of these in vivo animal studies clearly indicate that running can affect the composition and mechanical properties of articular cartilage. Moderate-volume running seems to have a beneficial effect on articular cartilage.[21,28,29] High-volume running can lead to subchondral bone changes and decreased cartilage indentation stiffness and proteoglycan concentration, but it remains unclear from these animal studies if this is equivalent to symptomatic osteoarthritis.[30,31] The experimental models designed to assess the effect of running in the setting of preexisting osteoarthritis show mixed results. The immobilization study[32] suggested no worsening of osteoarthritis, but the hydrogen peroxide study[33] indicated that running does worsen osteoarthritis. Finally, running may lead to worse outcomes than rest after acute joint injury.[34,35]

HUMAN STUDIES

Studies Suggesting a Link Between Running and Osteoarthritis

There are two clinical reports in the human literature that suggest a link between running and osteoarthritis.

The first is of dubious value due to methodological problems. The second found an association between high-volume running and the development of osteoarthritis.

McDermott and Freyne[14] published a report on the incidence of osteoarthritis in runners with knee pain. They evaluated 20 distance runners who complained of knee pain and found that 6 out of the 20 had radiographic signs of osteoarthritis. Because 30% of the subjects had radiographic evidence of knee arthritis, the authors suggested that distance running is a risk factor for degenerative joint disease. They appropriately caution, however, that there were several confounding factors. For example, the 6 runners who had radiographic evidence of knee osteoarthritis also had a higher incidence of traumatic knee injuries and greater genu varum than the 14 runners without radiographic evidence of osteoarthritis. Methodological flaws that further detract from the value of this case series include the lack of nonrunning controls and the omission of the cause of knee pain in most of the subjects.

Marti and Knobloch[39] investigated the relationship between distance running and hip osteoarthritis. They obtained histories and performed physical examinations on 27 elite distance runners, 9 bobsledders, and 23 sedentary controls. The runners had significantly more radiographic evidence of hip osteoarthritis than the bobsledders or nonrunning controls, as judged by blinded radiologists. They found age, mileage run, and running pace to be independent predictors of hip osteoarthritis. This latter finding provides clinical correlation to basic science research[21–23] that suggested that higher rates of applied load are associated with cartilage breakdown. There were significantly more degenerative changes seen in the hips of those who ran an average of more than 65 miles per week compared with those who ran less. Running pace was a stronger predictor of the development of hip osteoarthritis than running mileage. Interestingly, $\dot{V}O_2$max was inversely correlated with radiographic findings of osteoarthritis.

Studies Refuting a Link Between Running and Osteoarthritis

In contrast to the small volume of literature cited in the previous section, there are several published reports in the human literature that provide evidence against a causal effect of running on the development of osteoarthritis.

Panush and colleagues[40] compared runners with nonrunners to investigate a possible link between running and degenerative joint disease. They examined 17 male runners and 18 male nonrunners, with a mean age of 56 years. The runners ran an average of 28 miles per week for 12 years. The study and control groups reported no differences in pain, swelling, or other musculoskeletal complaints. There were no differences between the two groups in terms of musculoskeletal examinations or radiographic findings. Although the study numbers were small, the authors concluded that their data did not support an association between running and osteoarthritis.

In a similar but larger study, Sohn and Micheli[41] retrospectively studied the effect of running on osteoarthritis of the hips and knees. They administered questionnaires to 504 former collegiate cross-country runners and 287 former collegiate swimmers. The subjects ranged from 23 to 77 years of age with a mean age of 57. They were between 2 and 55 years postgraduation with a mean of 25 years postgraduation. The investigators found the incidence of severe hip or knee pain to be 2% in the runners and 2.4% in the swimmers. The incidence of any knee pain was 15.5% in the runners and 19.5% in the swimmers. The incidence of surgery for osteoarthritis was 0.8% in runners and 2.1% in swimmers. No difference in joint pain was found between high mileage (40 to 140 miles/week) and low mileage (25 miles/week) runners. Based on these findings, Sohn's group concluded that collegiate level running was not associated with the development of osteoarthritis of the knees or hips, when compared with collegiate level swimming.

Lane and coworkers[42] investigated long-distance running and its effect on bone density and osteoarthritis. They examined 41 runners between 50 and 72 years of age, and 41 age-matched controls. Unfortunately, running distance was not recorded. They administered an extensive questionnaire, performed musculoskeletal examinations, and obtained knee x-rays. Quantitative computed tomography (CT) of the first lumbar vertebra was performed to assess bone density. The examiners were blinded to subject status. They found the runners had a 40% greater bone density in the first lumbar vertebra in comparison to the nonrunners. There were no differences between the two groups with respect to abnormal radiographs, crepitus, joint stability, or symptomatic osteoarthritis. These data suggest that running is not associated with osteoarthritis, but does promote greater bone density.

Lane's group continued their investigation of the relationship between running, osteoarthritis, and bone mineral density in a subsequent study.[43] They did a 9-year follow-up of 28 runners from 60 to 70 years of age and 27 age-matched nonrunners. They compared joint examinations, knee and hip x-rays, and quantitative CT of the first lumbar vertebra. They found that the radiographic findings of osteoarthritis had progressed in both groups, but there was no significant difference in the rate of progression between the two groups. The runners, however, maintained a greater bone mineral density. These results strengthened their conclusions from the previous study.

Konradsen and colleagues[44] also looked at the association between long-term running and osteoarthritis. They examined 27 former competitive runners who ran 12 to 24 miles/week for an average of 40 years and 27 age-matched sedentary controls. The mean age of both groups was 58 years. The researchers found no difference in joint alignment, range of motion, or pain. There was also no difference in radiographic appearance of the subjects' hips, knees, or ankles. The authors concluded that their data did not support an association between long-term running and osteoarthritis.

In a broader study Kohatsu and Schurman[45] examined several risk factors for the development of knee osteoarthritis using a different perspective. Rather than comparing runners and nonrunners, these investigators performed histories, x-rays, and physical examinations on 46 subjects with severe knee osteoarthritis and 46 age-matched controls without knee osteoarthritis. They found that knee osteoarthritis was associated with higher body mass index, prior knee injury, and heavy manual labor. They found no association, however, between knee osteoarthritis and the subjects' participation in athletic activities. Notably, there were twice as many runners in the control group as in the osteoarthritis group. These data also suggest that running is not associated with the development of osteoarthritis, unlike obesity, prior knee injury, and heavy manual labor.

Kujala and coworkers[46] investigated knee osteoarthritis in former runners, soccer players, weightlifters, and shooters. These researchers performed a history, physical examination, and knee radiographs on 117 former world-class athletes. The examiners and radiologists were both blinded to subject status. Confirming the data of Kohatsu and Schurman, they found that knee osteoarthritis was significantly associated with prior knee injury (OR 4.73) and greater body mass index (OR 1.76). Radiographic evidence of osteoarthritis was seen in 31% of the weightlifters, 29% of the soccer players, 14% of the runners, and 3% of the shooters. When compared with weightlifting and soccer, running seemed to cause less osteoarthritis, although it appears to be harder on the knees than shooting.

In a cross-sectional population study, Lane and colleagues[47] looked at running and the development of musculoskeletal disability in general. The investigators compared 498 runners between 50 and 72 years of age and 365 age-matched controls. They found runners had less physical disability, greater functional capacity, sought medical care less, and weighed less than their nonrunning counterparts. The authors concluded that running protected against musculoskeletal disability, although they could not comment specifically on osteoarthritis.

Ward and associates[48] also surveyed physical disability in runners by sending yearly questionnaires to 454 older runners (mean age, 58 years; average distance ran, 25 miles/week) and nonrunners (mean age, 62 years) over a period of 5 to 7 years. They collected sociodemographic, clinical, lifestyle, and disability data. They found that 49% of the runners and 77% of the nonrunners reported some physical disability. Age, greater body mass index, strenuous work-related activity, and the use of more medications were associated with a greater likelihood of disability. In agreement with Lane's research, their data indicate that running is not associated with physical disability, and may even be protective against physical disability.

LIMITATIONS OF EXISTING LITERATURE

The inherent limitations of the existing literature warrant discussion. One limitation is that the studies available focus on the hips and knees. There is no research on whether running might be associated with (or protective against) degenerative changes in the ankle or lumbar spine. The existing literature is also lacking more comprehensive controls. For example, the influences of running surface, athletic footwear, running gait, presence of biomechanical deficits, gender, and cross-training have not been studied. Furthermore, the studies cited are primarily retrospective. Prospective studies require time, patience, and careful planning because osteoarthritis usually develops over many years. Another limitation is that there are scant data on the effect of running on joints that are already osteoarthritic, although experience tells us that athletes with symptomatic disease of weightbearing joints tend to participate in lower-impact sports. Finally, and perhaps most importantly, the effect of selection bias on the existing data is unclear. For example, if a study finds that older runners have less osteoarthritis than older nonrunners, perhaps it is because individuals who previously were runners but subsequently developed osteoarthritis have already been "selected" into the nonrunning group.

CONCLUSIONS

There is strong evidence that age, prior joint injury, greater body mass index, and heavy manual labor are associated with the development of osteoarthritis. The existing literature *does not* support a causal relationship between low- or moderate-distance running and osteoarthritis. The literature is inconclusive regarding a causal relationship between very-high-volume running and osteoarthritis. The study by Marti and colleagues[39] found an association between running pace and high-volume running and osteoarthritis, while the study by Sohn and Micheli[41] found no difference in joint pathology between high- and low-volume runners. In general, older runners tend to be healthier than their nonrunning counterparts.

Further research is needed to investigate the following areas:

- the relationship between running and the development of osteoarthritis of the ankle and lumbar spine;
- the relationship between high-volume running and the development of osteoarthritis;
- the influences of running pace, running surface, shoes, and gait; and
- the effect of selection bias on the studies performed to date.

RECOMMENDATIONS

Patients do not generally ask: "What does the literature say?" More likely, a runner will ask: "Am I doing permanent damage to my joints? Is there anything I can do to lessen the chance of developing arthritis?" Based on the data presented, the sports medicine practitioner can feel comfortable telling the patient that low- and moderate-volume running do not predispose to knee or hip osteoarthritis. The clinician might also consider making some common-sense recommendations, including

- Wear appropriate running shoes
- Acquire new running shoes every 200 to 300 miles
- Run on soft surfaces
- Cross-train
- Correct running gait abnormalities
- Treat injuries appropriately
- Maintain optimal body mass index and nutritional status
- Correct biomechanical deficits and maximize flexibility, strength, endurance, and motor control along the kinetic chain

Those athletes who require more aggressive measures for symptom control (intraarticular steroid injections, Synvisc injections, or arthroscopic debridement for chronic osteoarthritis) should be counseled

regarding appropriate activity level. Although in some cases a certain level of running may be permitted, recommendations for lower-impact forms of cross-training are generally indicated.

REFERENCES

1. Powell KE, Paffenbarger RS: Workshop on epidemiologic and public health aspects of physical activity and exercise: A summary. *Public Health Rep* 1985:100, 118.
2. Sherwood DE, Selder DJ: Cardiorespiratory health, reaction time, and aging. *Med Sci Sports* 1979:11, 186.
3. Buckwalter JA: Osteoarthritis and articular cartilage use, disuse, and abuse: Experimental studies. *J Rheumatol Suppl* 1995:43, 13.
4. Lane NE, Buckwalter JA: Exercise: A cause of osteoarthritis? *Rheum Dis Clin North Am* 1993:19, 617.
5. Alexander CJ: Osteoarthritis: A review of old myths and current concepts. *Skeletal Radiol* 1990:19, 327.
6. Lane NE, Michel B, Bjorkengren A, et al.: The risk of osteoarthritis with running and aging. *J Rheumatol* 1993:20, 661.
7. Panush RS, Lane NE: Exercise and the musculoskeletal system. *Baillieres Clin Rheumatol* 1994:8, 79.
8. Paty JG: Running injuries. *Curr Opin Rheumatol* 1994:6, 203.
9. Davis MA, Ettinger WH, Neuhaus JM, et al.: The association of knee injury and obesity with bilateral osteoarthritis of the knee. *Am J Epidemiol* 1989:130, 278.
10. Buckwalter JA, Mankin HJ: Articular cartilage: Degeneration and osteoarthritis, repair, regeneration, and transplantation. *Instr Course Lect* 1998:47, 487.
11. Lindberg H, Montgomery F: Heavy labor and the occurrence of arthrosis. *Clin Orthop* 1987:214, 235.
12. Felson DT, Hannan MT, Naimark A, et al.: Occupational physical demands, knee bending, and knee osteoarthritis: Results from the Framingham study. *J Rheumatol* 1991:18, 1587.
13. Felson DT, Zhang Y, Anthony JM, et al.: Weight loss reduces the risk for symptomatic knee osteoarthritis in women: The Framingham study. *Ann Intern Med* 1992:116, 535.
14. McDermott M, Freyne P: Osteoarthritis in runners with knee pain. *Br J Sports Med* 1983:17, 84.
15. Adams D, Swanson SAV: Direct measurement of local pressures in the cadaveric human hip joint during simulated level walking. *Ann Rheum Dis* 1985:44, 658.
16. Brown TD, Anderson DD, Nepola JV, et al.: Contact stress aberrations following imprecise reduction of simple tibial plateau fractures. *J Orthop Res* 1988:6, 851.
17. Brown TD, Pope DF, Hale JE, et al.: Effects of osteochondral defect size on cartilage contact stress. *J Orthop Res* 1991:9, 559.
18. Brown TD, Shaw DT: In vitro contact stress distributions in the natural human hip. *J Biomech* 1983:16, 373.
19. Miyanaga Y, Fukubayashi T, Kurosawa H: Contact study of the hip joint: Load deformation pattern, contact

area and contact pressure. *Arch Orthop Trauma Surg* 1984: 103, 13.

20. Repo RU, Finlay JB: Survival of articular cartilage after controlled impact. *Bone Joint Surg* 1977:59A, 1068.

21. Newton PM, Mow VC, Gardner TR, et al.: The effect of lifelong exercise on canine articular cartilage. *Am J Sports Med* 1997:25, 282.

22. Mow V, Rosenwasser M: Articular cartilage: Biomechanics, in Woo SL-Y, Buckwalter JA, (eds.), *Injury and Repair of the Musculoskeletal Soft Tissues,* Park Ridge, Ill, American Academy of Orthopedic Surgeons, 1988:427.

23. Weightman B, Chappell DJ, Jenkins EA: A second study of tensile fatigue properties of human cartilage. *Ann Rheum Dis* 1978:37, 58.

24. Radin EL, Paul IL: Response of joints to impact loading: In vitro wear. *Arthritis Rheum* 1971:14, 356.

25. Dekel S, Weissman SL: Joint changes after overuse and peak overloading of rabbit knees in vivo. *Acta Orthop Scand* 1978:49, 519.

26. Zimmerman NB, Smith DG, Pottenger LA, et al.: Mechanical disruption of human patellar cartilage by repetitive loading in vitro. *Clin Orthop* 1988:229, 302.

27. Newberry WN, Garcia JJ, Mackenzie CD, et al.: Analysis of acute mechanical stress in an animal model of post-traumatic osteoarthritis. *J Biomech Eng* 1998:120, 704.

28. Kiviranta I, Tammi M, Jurvelin J, et al: Articular cartilage thickness and glycosaminoglycan distribution in the canine knee joint after strenuous running exercise. *Clin Orthop* 1992:283, 302.

29. Kiviranta I, Tammi M, Jurvelin J, et al.: Moderate running exercise augments glycosaminoglycans and thickness of articular cartilage in the knee joint of young beagle dogs. *J Orthop Res* 1988:16, 188.

30. Arokoski J, Kiviranta I, Jurvelin J, et al.: Long-distance running causes site-dependent decrease of cartilage glycosaminoglycan content in the knee joints of beagle dogs. *Arthritis Rheum* 1993:36, 1451.

31. Oettmeier R, Arokoski J, Roth AJ, et al.: Subchondral bone and articular cartilage response to long distance running training (40 km per day) in the beagle knee joint. *Eur J Exp Musculoskel Res* 1992:1, 145.

32. Videman T: The effect of running on the osteoarthritic joint: An experimental matched-pair study with rabbits. *Rheumatol Rehabil* 1982:21, 1.

33. Kaiki G, Suji H, Yonesawa T, et al.: Osteoarthritis induced by intra-articular hydrogen peroxide injection and running load. *J Orthop Res* 1990:8, 730.

34. Palmoski MJ, Brandt KD: Running inhibits the reversal of atrophic changes in canine knee cartilage after removal of a leg cast. *Arthritis Rheum* 1981:24, 1329.

35. Palmoski MJ, Brandt KD: Immobilization of the knee prevents osteoarthritis after anterior cruciate ligament resection. *Arthritis Rheum* 1982:25, 1201.

36. Radin EL, Ehrlich MG, Chemack R, et al.: Effect of repetitive impulse loading on the knee joint of rabbits. *Clin Orthop* 1978:131, 288.

37. Radin EL, Martin RB, Burr DB, et al.: Effects of mechanical loading on the tissues of rabbit knee. *J Orthop Res* 1984:2, 221.

38. Lukoschek M, Boyd RD, Schaffler MB, et al.: Comparison of joint degeneration models. Surgical instability and repetitive impulse loading. *Acta Orthop Scand* 1986:57, 349.

39. Marti B, Knobloch M, Tschopp A, et al.: Is excessive running predictive of degenerative hip disease? *Br Med J* 1989:299, 91.

40. Panush RS, Schmidt C, Caldwell JR, et al.: Is running associated with degenerative joint disease? *JAMA* 1986:255, 1152.

41. Sohn RS, Micheli LJ: The effect of running on the pathogenesis of osteoarthritis of the hips and knees. *Clin Orthop Rel Res* 1985:198, 106.

42. Lane NE, Bloch DA, Jones HH, et al: Long-distance running, bone density, and osteoarthritis. *JAMA* 1986:255, 1141.

43. Lane NE, Oehlert JW, Bloch DA, et al.: The relationship of running to osteoarthritis of the knee and hip and bone mineral density of the lumbar spine: A 9 year longitudinal study. *J Rheumatol* 1998:25, 334.

44. Konradsen L, Hansen EMB, Songard L: Long distance running and osteoarthritis. *Am J Sports Med* 1990:18, 379.

45. Kohatsu ND, Schurman DJ: Risk factors for the development of osteoarthritis of the knee. *Clin Orthop Rel Res* 1990:261, 242.

46. Kujala UM, Kettunen J, Paananen H, et al.: Knee osteoarthritis in former runners, soccer players, weight lifters, and shooters. *Arthritis Rheum* 1995:38, 539.

47. Lane NE, Bloch DA, Wood PD, et al.: Aging, long-distance running, and the development of musculoskeletal disability. *Am J Med* 1987:82, 772.

48. Ward MM, Hubert HB, Shi H, et al.: Physical disability in older runners: Prevalence, risk factors, and progression with age. *J Gerontol* 1995:50A, M70.

Chapter 31

OVERTRAINING

Joseph Kosinski and
Thomas M. Howard

INTRODUCTION

In the competitive world of athletics in the new millennium, athletes train harder and risk injury in order to achieve small gains in performance that could mean the difference between victory and fame, defeat and anonymity. One need only watch a championship sporting event where the difference between winning a gold medal and a silver medal is just a few fractions of a second. Increasing amounts of training time are required for incremental gains in performance. Unfortunately, this increased training time increases exposure of the athlete to injury.

Although training methods have become more sophisticated, science has lagged behind, and much of the physiology of training still remains a mystery. This chapter will review the subject of overtraining, with a review of definitions, current theories, evaluation techniques, and treatment and preventive strategies.

TRAINING PHYSIOLOGY

A thorough discussion of exercise physiology is beyond the scope of this chapter, but a rudimentary knowledge is necessary to understand overtraining syndrome (see Chapters 11 and 48). Training alters the body's homeostasis, causing muscular fatigue and a decrease in performance. During the recovery period, the body regenerates in order to reestablish homeostasis. However, this regeneration does not stop at homeostasis. Some overcompensation occurs in which the stress placed on the body during training causes the body to adapt, so that by the next training period, performance capability has actually increased. This is known as the *training response* or *overload principle*.[1-6] Ideally, to maximize the benefits of training the next training period should not occur until this overcompensation phase has been completed, but it is not known exactly when this occurs (Fig. 31–1). Training intensity imposes a high stress level to gain the desired training effect, but also has the highest potential to create overload. It should also be noted that the total stress on the athlete in training is the sum of physiological, psychological, and social stressors.

Recovery from overload training can be divided into four major categories: hydration and nutrition, sleep and rest, relaxation and emotional support, and stretching and active rest.[7] Failing to replenish fluid and metabolic losses after intense training or get adequate sleep and rest will result in excessive fatigue at the beginning of the next session. Stretching and active rest (cross-training) aid in muscle recovery and accelerate the recovery process. Mental training for relaxation as well as emotional and social support allows athletes to train more effectively.

Although training schedules vary, all training encompasses gradually increasing stressors as the body fights to adapt to this increased training load.

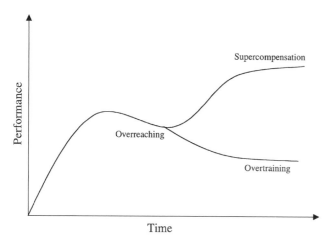

Figure 31–1. Overload Principle of Training.

Occasionally coaches and athletes incorporate into their training schedule a sequence of planned short periods of greatly increased load with little time for regeneration. It is thought that when the athlete resumes a less-rigorous training schedule, there will ultimately be a larger gain in performance.

Typical Case Presentation of Overtraining (Case 1)

A 16-year-old high school runner presented with his mother to a sports medicine specialist with a complaint of fatigue and declining performance over the past 2 to 3 months. He had recently quit the high school cross-country team because of disagreement with his coach about training schedules and was currently training on his own. He was running 60+ miles per week, was a full-time high school student maintaining an "A" average, and working 20 hours a week in a local bookstore. He was an only child and his father was the CEO of a medium-sized company. He complained of fatigue and lack of energy, and had chronic upper respiratory symptoms of rhinorrhea, sore throat, and an intermittent cough. He did not smoke or drink alcohol and denied recreational drug use. His past medical history was unremarkable and he was on no medications or supplements. On examination he was found to be a fit, thin male (height, 5' 10"; weight, 145 lb). His head, ears, eyes, nose, and throat (HEENT) examination was normal, neck supple, and cardiovascular, pulmonary, and abdominal examinations were unremarkable. His skin and genitourinary (GU) examinations were normal. Standard laboratory tests were also normal.

DEFINITIONS

Overreaching is defined as a short-term decrement in performance after a period of overload. This period is usually 1 to 2 weeks. Some authors even consider overreaching to represent normal physiologic fatigue in response to overload training.

Overtraining syndrome, also known as staleness, is defined as prolonged decreased sport-specific performance, usually lasting greater than 2 weeks. It is also manifested by premature fatigability, emotional and mood changes, lack of motivation, and overuse injuries, as well as various sorts of infections. Recovery is markedly longer and variable among affected runners, sometimes taking months before the athlete returns to baseline performance.

Periodization is the process of varying intensity of training, alternating periods of lower intensity or cross-training with more intense training periods to allow adequate recovery.

Epidemiology and Importance

Overtraining is not a new problem. Indeed, this condition was recognized as far back as the beginning of the century. In 1923, in an early article on training, D. C. Parmenter warned, "Overtraining or staleness is the bug-a-boo of every experienced trainer."[3] Overtraining is also not a rare problem. Morgan and colleagues[8] reported that 65% of elite runners had at some time in their career experienced staleness. The issue facing coaches and athletes is to find the optimum amount and intensity of training. If athletes train too little or too much they will not compete at their full potential. This results in poor performance in key events, injury, and/or early retirement.

Some say that overtraining is not limited to elite athletes, but this is controversial.[9] Recreational athletes may not exercise as hard as elite athletes, but they do suffer from different stressors, such as scheduling conflicts with their jobs and a lack of coaching. Recreational athletes also overexercise, and suffer from the many injuries associated with overuse. Indeed, 45% to 70% of all runners will suffer an injury in a given year.[10] Therefore, for a weekend warrior, overreaching or overtraining syndrome is a very real possibility.

Classification

Overtraining is not a diagnosis with one particular set of signs and symptoms. Numerous psychological and physical complaints can be seen. Historically, there are 2 clinical forms of overtraining syndrome recognized: sympathetic or Basedowian type, and parasympathetic or Addisonian type. Current thinking is that they represent different points on the overtraining continuum.[7,11–13]

Sympathetic overtraining is characterized by an increase in sympathetic tone in the resting state. The term "Basedowian" refers to *morbus Basedow* (hyperthyroidism), and although it is not likely that a thyroid dysfunction exists, the symptoms associated with the sympathetic form are reminiscent of the symptoms of hyperthyroidism. In addition to decreased athletic performance and fatigue, symptoms of the sympathetic type are jitteriness, increase in baseline heart rate and blood pressure, weight loss, and insomnia. Sympathetic overtraining probably represents an intermediate stage on the overtraining continuum, on the way to parasympathetic, or more chronic or severe, overtraining.[7]

Parasympathetic overtraining is also known as Addisonoid-type overtraining. The term "Addisonoid" refers to adrenal dysfunction, although again, no adrenal pathology has been reported. Symptoms of this more chronic and severe form of overtraining consist of depression, hypersomnia, low baseline heart rate and blood pressure, and decreased libido.[7,14]

CURRENT THEORIES

There currently is no unified theory to explain overtraining syndrome. Commonly described theories are the autonomic imbalance hypothesis, the glycogen depletion hypothesis, the branched-chain amino acid hypothesis, the neuroendocrine dysfunction hypothesis, and the cytokine hypothesis. Further research into all theories is still ongoing. Research on overtraining is difficult. Small populations, problems with standardization, and confounding variables hamper studies. Overtraining syndrome is likely multifactorial, incorporating aspects of all these theories.

Autonomic Imbalance Hypothesis

This theory proposes that an underlying imbalance in the autonomic system is responsible for the symptoms of overtraining. From a clinical standpoint, many distinguish between the sympathetic and parasympathetic types of overtraining discussed above. Currently, this theory only accounts for the parasympathetic form of overtraining. It is hypothesized that an autonomic imbalance results from an altered sympathetic nervous system, resulting in the parasympathetic form of overtraining. This theory supports the concept of a decrease in the intrinsic activity of the sympathetic nervous system. Basal urinary catecholamine release is thought to reflect the baseline "tone" of the sympathetic nervous system, as this is the time when arousal and stimulus are lowest. This has consistently been shown to be decreased in overtrained athletes. This decrease might not be the result of fatigue, but rather the result of inhibitory effects on the sympathetic nervous system.

Lehmann and associates[14] hypothesize that the decrease in this resting tone of the sympathetic nervous system is the result of three conditions:

- First, there is a negative feedback mechanism, which occurs as a result of the surge of catecholamines released during periods of heavy training. This causes a downregulation of baseline catecholamine secretion.
- Second, an increase in metabolism during exercise causes two major changes: (1) A plasma amino acid imbalance and altered brain neurotransmitter metabolism occur, with an increase in the levels of aromatic amino acids (phenylalanine, tryptophan, and tyrosine), causing increased hypothalamic tryptophan and dopamine concentrations in the brain. This causes metabolic "error signals" with inhibitory effects on the sympathetic nervous system. (2) There is an increase in the body's core temperature, which causes an inhibitory effect on the hypothalamic sympathetic centers during prolonged training.
- Third, there is an afferent neuronal negative feedback system of the receptive centers of overloaded muscles (nociception, proprioception) resulting in receptor downregulation. This implies that prolonged stimulation of these receptive centers causes less sympathetic activity with time.

There is also evidence of decreased responsiveness of target organs to catecholamines.[14] Evidence for this includes studies that show increased plasma resting norepinephrine and increased submaximal plasma catecholamine responses to exercise, decreased β-adrenergic receptor density, and decreased β-adrenergic receptor responses.

In summary, this theory states that the parasympathetic form of overtraining can be explained by imbalances in the autonomic nervous system. As a result of sustained stimulus from exercise, a negative feedback response occurs which decreases the resting tone of the sympathetic system.

Glycogen Depletion Hypothesis

Essentially, this hypothesis states that extensive periods of heavy training lead to glycogen depletion in muscles. Because muscle glycogen is the prime source of energy for moderate to intense exercise,[15] low levels can result in muscular fatigue and a decrease in performance leading to the symptoms of overtraining syndrome. Also, low levels of glycogen can lead to increased oxidation of the branched-chain amino acids (BCAA) to glucose, in an attempt to use alternative energy supplies. This lowers the body's total pool of the

BCAA, and can also lead to central fatigue[16] (see section on central fatigue theory).

Costill and associates,[15] in a study of 12 swimmers, found that a lack of response (those with difficulty completing an increase in training load) resulted in those athletes with low levels of muscle glycogen and an inadequate dietary intake of carbohydrates. This lends support to the hypothesis, but it seems that this is not the complete picture. In a contrasting study by Synder,[16] cyclists who increased their training load and also increased their dietary carbohydrate intake (thus hoping to avoid glycogen depletion), were still able to meet the defined criteria for overreaching, and it is assumed that they would have progressed to overtraining syndrome had the study continued long enough. Thus, although low muscle glycogen is associated with muscle fatigue and central fatigue, it is likely only a contributing factor, given that overreaching can also occur with normal muscle glycogen levels.

Branched-Chain Amino Acid Hypothesis (Central Fatigue Theory)

According to the branched-chain amino acid (BCAA) hypothesis, overtraining syndrome is caused by an increase in the synthesis of 5-hydroxytryptamine (5-HT) in the central nervous system. With extensive exercise, glycogen levels become depleted in muscles, leading to the use of secondary energy sources by the muscles. The BCAAs (leucine, isoleucine, and valine) are oxidized to glucose. A concurrent increase in the level of fatty acids also occurs. The fatty acids compete with tryptophan for albumin binding sites, leading to an increase in plasma tryptophan. As both the BCAA and tryptophan use the same neutral carrier to pass through the blood-brain barrier, a decrease in plasma BCAA and an increase in plasma tryptophan lead to an increase in tryptophan passing through the blood-brain barrier.

In the brain, tryptophan is converted into the neurotransmitter 5-HT. 5-HT is well known to play a role in various neuroendocrine and emotional functions, all of which can be seen with overtraining syndrome. Given this, it is this connection between overtraining syndrome and an increase in the free tryptophan:BCAA ratio that forms the basis for the BCAA hypothesis.[1,5,17,18]

In animal studies done by Chaouloff and associates,[19,20] it was shown that an increase in exercise intensity did in fact lead to an increase in plasma levels of free tryptophan (f-TRP), 5-HT, and 5-hydroxyindoleacetic acid (5-HIAA), and in the cerebrospinal fluid (CSF) an increase in tryptophan and 5-HIAA.

In humans, the results are not as clear-cut. In a study by Lehmann and associates,[14] it was found that deteriorating performance was seen with an increase in the f-TRP:BCAA ratio. However, an even larger increase in the f-TRP:BCAA ratio was seen with an improvement in performance. These results are contradictory, but conclusions cannot be inferred from them because the methodology between the two was not standardized, and there were confounding variables. More research still needs to be done.

Neuroendocrine Imbalance Hypothesis

This theory points to an interruption of the neuroendocrine axis during periods of increased training as the cause of overtraining syndrome. Specifically, there are alterations that occur between the hypothalamic-pituitary-adrenal (HPA) and the hypothalamic-pituitary-gonadal (HPG) axes, as well growth hormone (GH) and thyrotropin-releasing hormone/thyroid-stimulating hormone (TRH/TSH) secretion as a result of physical exertion.[9,11]

Barron and associates[21] noted a decrease in response in GH, adrenocorticotropic hormone (ACTH), and cortisol to insulin-induced hypoglycemia. Response to TRH and luteinizing hormone-releasing hormone (LHRH) did not show a change, and from this it was inferred that the level of dysfunction was at the hypothalamus, with intact pituitary function. Other studies[22] have shown pituitary dysfunction with a decrease in β-endorphin released from the pituitary, but data here are also contradictory.

Cytokine Hypothesis

The basis of this hypothesis is the adaptive response to overload in tissues. Tissue injury from overload results in a mild local inflammatory response with resultant adaptation of the tissue in the recovery period. When local recovery does not occur, this local acute inflammatory response becomes chronic, leading to a systemic immune and inflammatory response. Much of this local and systemic response is mediated by cytokines. Cytokines are soluble hormone-like proteins that function as chemical communicators, and are produced by immune cells and endothelial cells. They include interleukins (IL), interferons (INF), tumor necrosis factors (TNF), growth factors, and chemokines. The most active proinflammatory cytokines involved in overtraining are IL-1β, TNF-α, and IL-6. Elevated cytokines act on the CNS to induce the "sick behavior" that manifests as fatigue, anorexia, and depression, as well activate the HPA axis and inhibit the HPG axis. Additionally, these elevated cytokines induce hepatic gluconeogenesis and production of acute phase reactants. Finally, systemic immune activation as well the inadequate recovery of the peripheral tissues increases glutamine consumption and decreases production.[23]

CLINICAL PRESENTATION OF OVERTRAINING

Fry and colleagues[24] defined four major categories of symptoms associated with overtraining: physiological, psychological, biochemical, and immunologic. Runners may present anywhere along the continuum from physiologic fatigue to staleness. Common presenting symptoms are listed in Table 31–1. It is important for the care provider to realize that the total stress on an athlete is the sum of physiologic, social, and psychological stressors during any particular period in the runner's life. Therefore, presentations may take the form of medical visits for infection or injury or visits for mood disorders, stress, or fatigue. There are many subjective complaints, such as fatigue, lack of motivation or competitive spirit, hypersomnolence, depression, irritability, lack of cooperation with teammates or coaching staff, and difficulty concentrating. There are also physical findings, including chronic overuse injuries refractory to treatment, change in heart rate or blood pressure, weight loss, and increased incidence of infection (see Chapter 28).

DIAGNOSIS AND DIFFERENTIAL DIAGNOSIS

There are no specific guidelines to establish the diagnosis, partly because the spectrum of symptoms is so large. There are sport-specific parameters of dysfunc-

tion, such as increased running times for an event. There are not yet any useful laboratory parameters to diagnose overtraining syndrome, although there are many hematologic and hormonal changes associated with overtraining.

Overtraining is a diagnosis of exclusion and the differential diagnosis is similar to that of fatigue (see Table 31–2), including various infectious etiologies, collagen vascular disorders, cancer, metabolic dysfunction, substance abuse, and psychiatric disorders.[2,25–28]

To establish the diagnosis, as always one must first perform a thorough history and physical examination. Questions about symptoms of congestion, rhinorrhea, myalgias, nausea/vomiting, and diarrhea may rule out a postviral syndrome as a cause of the patient's symptoms. Sore throat, exposure to someone with mononucleosis, or splenomegaly on physical examination would be good indications to consider infectious mononucleosis as the cause. A history of tick exposure or a characteristic rash may indicate Lyme or other rickettsial diseases. Other infectious etiologies that could mimic overtraining syndrome include viral hepatitis and myocarditis.

TABLE 31–1. COMMON SYMPTOMS OF OVERTRAINING

Sport-specific performance complaints
    Inability to meet prior performance standards
    Prolonged recovery time
    Decreased coordination
    Decreased muscular strength
Physiologic findings
    Blood pressure changes
    Increased resting heart rate
    Weight loss
    Increased incidence of injuries
    Increased incidence of infections
    Amenorrhea
Subjective complaints
    Fatigue
    Feelings of depression
    Anorexia
    Hypersomnia/disturbed sleep
    Myalgias
    Gastrointestinal disturbances
    Headaches
    Increased irritability
    Concentration difficulties
    Apathy

Source: Compiled from references 3, 11, 22, 39–41.

TABLE 31–2. DIFFERENTIAL DIAGNOSIS OF OVERTRAINING

Infectious etiologies
    Postviral syndrome
    Infectious mononucleosis
    Lyme disease
    Viral hepatitis
    Myocarditis
Collagen vascular disorders
    Polymyalgia rheumatica
    Systemic lupus erythematosus
    Fibromyalgia
    Chronic fatigue syndrome
Metabolic
    Hypothyroidism or hyperthyroidism
    Anemia
    Electrolyte disorders
Pharmacological
    Alcohol
    Caffeine
    Illegal or performance-enhancing drugs
Psychiatric
    Depression
    Physical abuse
    Sexual abuse
    Emotional abuse
    Posttraumatic stress disorder
    Malingering
Other
    Cancer
    Acquired nutritional problems
    Pregnancy
    Sleep deprivation

Fibromyalgia and chronic fatigue syndrome may present similarly with fatigue, sleep disturbance, and tender or trigger points. Endocrine disorders should also be considered, in particular hypothyroidism and hyperthyroidism, hypoglycemia, and anemia.

Another important and often overlooked problem is the subject of substance abuse. This problem is present throughout society and is sometimes seen in athletes. In fact, the elite athlete may be at high risk, suffering from many lifestyle stressors such as excessive exercise, poor nutrition, lack of sleep, jet lag, and anxiety over upcoming competitions. It is also important to ask questions about excessive alcohol or caffeine intake, as well as about the use of illicit or performance-enhancing drugs. Keep in mind that more than one drug may be at work.

Finally, the last element to consider in the differential, but certainly not the least important, are psychiatric issues. The athlete may suffer from depression, physical, emotional, or sexual abuse, or posttraumatic stress disorder. It should be remembered that a psychiatric condition can often coexist with substance abuse, as the patient makes attempts at self-medication.

After working through the differential diagnosis, the physician needs to assess the patient's baseline level of fitness. This should not only be done quantitatively (miles per week) and documented in the records, but also subjectively, as an assessment of how the patient perceives his or her training schedule. Also important is any history of a recent increase in duration or intensity of exercise prior to onset of symptoms. In many cases an athlete may have increased his or her training schedule in preparation for an upcoming event. A suggested initial evaluation and laboratory workup is outlined in Fig. 31–2.[9]

TREATMENT

Just as the etiology of overtraining is not yet fully understood, the treatment strategy is based more on intuition than science. The first line of treatment should

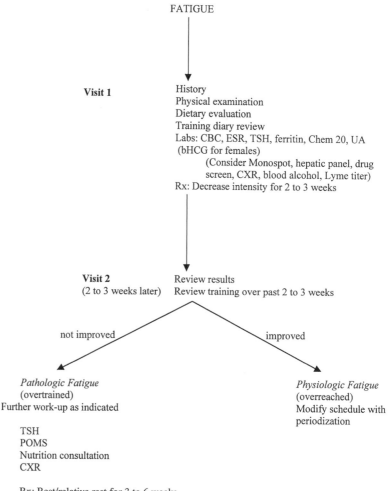

Figure 31–2. Evaluation Algorithm for Overtraining.[25]

be prevention. A review of the athlete's training schedule, exploration of the concepts of cross-training and periodization, as well as adequate rest and minimization of coexisting lifestyle stressors should all be used in an effort to prevent overtraining syndrome.

When prevention fails, what the athlete needs most is rest. It is important to realize that there is no quick fix for overtraining syndrome. Ultimately, rest is curative, but several key points need to be made. First, early detection is most helpful. If caught in the early stages of overreaching, overtraining may be prevented. It cannot be stressed enough that prevention is the best and most effective treatment.

A proposed treatment and evaluation protocol is seen in Fig. 31–2. If an athlete presents early with signs of fatigue and declining performance, merely decreasing the training intensity by 50% to 75% for 1 or 2 weeks may be enough to result in improved performance in competition. If the symptoms are more severe, of longer duration, or have failed to respond to decreased intensity, then more significant restrictions should be considered. An initial rest period of 2 to 4 weeks should be considered. Both the relative rest and total rest periods will be very hard to enforce in runners. During this rest period, education is essential in order to ensure better compliance with the training break and to prevent future occurrences. Life stressors should be reviewed in depth. A review of the athlete's diet and sleep schedule is just as important in reducing stress, as is a review of the training and competition schedules. Consultation with a nutritionist and sports psychologist can be beneficial. Additionally, continuous surveillance for signs of other conditions in the differential diagnosis of fatigue should be considered. Anecdotal reports of the use of selective serotonin reuptake inhibitors (SSRIs) such as fluoxetine in the successful management of such cases probably reflect the management of primary or secondary depression while physical recovery is occurring.

Upon return to practice and competition the athlete should pay careful attention to sleep, nutrition, school and work load, and competition stress, and slowly advance the pace of training. The sequence of advancing activity should focus on frequency, then duration, and finally the intensity of the sessions.

MONITORING AND PREVENTION

There has been extensive research in an attempt to find a reliable blood marker or test to predict when an athlete is suffering from or approaching overtraining syndrome, but to date there is no such indicator for this disorder. Coaches and trainers have had to use their experience and instinct to predict the optimal training intensity and duration for each individual athlete, taking into account individual stressors and recovery time. Identification of markers of overtraining would allow coaches and trainers to maximize training duration and intensity without fear of compromising performance, and allow the athlete to train as intensively as possible, stopping short of the onset of overtraining.

It was once believed that creatinine kinase (CK) was a good indicator of overtraining.[29] High CK levels indicate increased permeability from muscle cell membrane damage as a result of intense exercise. However, this has been shown to be a normal finding in athletes without performance impairment, and has been absent in athletes with overtraining syndrome. Similarly unfortunate findings have been seen after attempts to use hematocrit, red blood cell count, cortisol, testosterone, serum ferritin, lactate, and growth hormones as markers for overtraining.[11,13,24,30,31]

Recently, glutamine has been investigated as a possible marker of overtraining. Glutamine is an amino acid that is depleted during catabolic states such as in infection, surgery or trauma, and acidosis. If recovery between training sessions is inadequate, then the effects of depleted glutamine become cumulative. It has been shown that athletes with overtraining syndrome have low glutamine levels.[4,32–34] It is difficult to perform reliable studies, since confounding factors (diurnal variation, diet, and infection, to name but a few) that may alter glutamine metabolism must be accounted for. Early research is promising, but more research needs to be done.

Physiological markers have also been investigated. Resting and postexercise heart rate and resting and exercising oxygen consumption ($\dot{V}_{O_2}$) are two examples.[30,35] The resting heart rate has too many confounding factors (fever or illness, stimulant use) to make this a reliable marker of overtraining. However, this is still a frequently utilized monitoring tool, with a >10 BPM increase indicating poor recovery and a need to modify the training load.

Some of the earliest changes seen in overtraining syndrome are psychiatric. There are numerous questionnaires that have been used in an attempt to detect overtraining. The Profile of Mood States (POMS) is one such test.[36] The POMS consists of 65 items and yields a global measurement of affect or mood by examining tension/anxiety, depression/dejection, anger/hostility, vigor/activity, fatigue/inertia, and confusion/bewilderment. The patient responds on a five-point scale to 65 adjectives that describe the feelings and moods that he or she experienced in the previous week. A global score calculates the sum of the negative mood states (tension, depression, anger, and fatigue), and subtracts the positive mood state (vigor). The "Iceberg Profile" has been used to define the normal profile with high vigor and low negative mood states. It has been shown that mood disturbances increase with increased training loads and return to baseline after reduction in training load.[8,30] Athletes who experience overtraining syndrome have higher POMS total mood disturbance scores than athletes without it. It has also been shown to predict which athletes are prone to overtraining.[30] It is still not clear if POMS will predict overtraining in all athletes, and it does appear that some athletes experience alterations in mood states without having decrements in their performance.[8,37] The results of POMS testing in overtrained athletes are promising, but its use may not be practical for athletes and coaches.

A more useful monitoring tool recently described is the Total Quality Recovery (TQR) score studied by Kentta and Hassmen.[7] TQR can be subdivided into the TQR perceived (TQRper) and TQR action (TQRact). The action score is self reported by assessing the athlete's recovery in the four major areas of recovery mentioned earlier using the following scoring scheme: nutrition and hydration (10 points), sleep and rest (3 points), relaxation and emotional support (4 points), and stretching and active rest (3 points). The maximum total score is 20 points. The perceived score utilizes a scale similar to the Borg Relative Perceived Exertion Scale, in which the athlete self reports his or her overall perception of recovery. This scale can be adjusted according to individual differences among subjects (Table 31–3). This combination of TQRact and TQRper allows the coach or athlete to continually assess adequacy of recovery and readiness for continued high-intensity training.

Because of the uncertainty of psychological and physiological markers of overtraining, many believe that analyzing a combination of both with self-monitoring is best. Many athletes use daily training logs[38,39] such as the Daily Analyses of Life Demands for Athletes (used by Australian Olympic teams) and the Psycho-Behavioral Overtraining Scale (used by some British athletes). Both these diaries include training details (type of training, time, distance, and intensity), in addition to a combination of well-being and life stressors and potential causes, along with symptoms of stress (fatigue, depression, and irritability). Also included are physiological parameters (resting heart rate, muscle soreness) and any injuries or illnesses. These self-rating schemes may prove to be valuable predictors of overtraining syndrome in some athletes.

EVALUATION AND TREATMENT OF CASE 1

After initial evaluation the attending physician, suspecting overtraining, prescribed a 2-week rest period with no running and referred the athlete to a nutritionist and psychologist for evaluation. The patient and his mother were initially reluctant, thinking there must be an overlooked disorder or chronic infection, and they requested a course of antibiotic treatment prior to further evaluation. A 5-day course of azithromycin failed to improve symptoms and eventually the patient complied with the recommended plan.

Further history taken by the psychologist noted increased stress levels over performance on the upcoming SATs and the admission process for a service academy. The nutritionist noted substandard caloric and fluid intake and suggestions were made to the athlete and his parents.

He stopped running for a period of 3 weeks and changed his sleep, study, and work schedules to allow 7 to 8 hours of sleep each night and limiting work to weekends. He and his parents were offered individual and group counseling with the psychologist, but only the athlete attended 4 sessions. He resumed running 3 weeks later, running 2 miles per day at a slow 8 min/ mile pace 5 days a week. The length and pace were advanced over the next 3 weeks until he was running 25 miles per week with 2 sessions of interval training per week.

At this point in his training he was continuing to feel well. Much of his stress dissipated after successful performance on the SATs and an interview for appointment to the service academy. He joined the winter track team and had a successful season, running

TABLE 31–3. TQR PERCEIVED (TQRper) SCALE

Rating of Perceived Exertion (RPE)	Total Quality Recover (TQR)
6	6
7 very, very light	7 very, very poor recovery
8	8
9 very light	9 very poor recovery
10	10
11 faintly light	11 poor recovery
12	12
13 somewhat hard	13 reasonable recovery
14	14
15 hard	15 good recovery
16	16
17 very hard	17 very good recovery
18	18
19 very, very hard	19 very, very good recovery
20	20

Source: From Kentta et al.[7]

the 1000 M and 3000 M, and qualifying for the regional and state meets.

CONCLUSION

The most difficult aspect of training and competition is finding the right program that will allow an athlete to improve his or her performance without falling prey to overtraining. Overtraining syndrome is a poorly understood disorder manifested by systemic symptoms and declining performance that probably has a multifactorial etiology.

Prevention is the best strategy, and coaches, athletes, trainers, and physicians should pay close attention to every athlete. Runners who supervise their own training programs need to pay attention to their own symptoms.

Adequate recovery during training and rest, whether it is absolute or relative, is the most important aspect of treatment. With careful attention to diet, sleep, hydration, social stressors, and training and competition schedules, runners can avoid this condition and perform at their peak at all times.

REFERENCES

1. Dishman RK: Brain monoamines, exercise, and behavioral stress: Animal models. *Med Sci Sports Exerc* 1996:29, 63.
2. Hendrickson CD, Verde TJ: Inadequate recovery from vigorous exercise: Recognizing overtraining. *Phys Sportsmed* 1994:22, 56.
3. Parmenter DC: Some medical aspects of the training of college athletes. *Br Med Surg J* 1923:189, 45.
4. Rowbottom DG, Keast D, Morton AR, et al.: The emerging role of glutamine as an indicator of stress and overtraining. *Sports Med* 1996:21, 80.
5. Sharpe M, Hawton K, Clements A, Cowen PJ: Increased brain serotonin function in men with chronic fatigue syndrome. *BMJ* 1997:315, 164.
6. Steinacker JM, Lormes W, Lehmann M, Altenberg D: Training of rowers before world championships. *Med Sci Sports Exerc* 1998:30, 1158.
7. Kentta G, Hassmen P: Overtraining and recovery. A conceptual model. *Sports Med* 1998:26, 1.
8. Morgan WP, Brown DR, Raglin JS, et al.: Psychological monitoring of overtraining and staleness. *J Sportsmed* 1987:21, 107.
9. Lehmann M, Mann H, Gastmann U, et al.: Influence of unaccustomed high mileage vs. intensity training related changes in performance and serum amino acid levels. *Int J Sports Med* 1996:17, 187.
10. Ballas MT, Tytko J, Cookson D: Common overuse running injuries: Diagnosis and management. *Am Fam Physician* 1997:15, 2473.
11. Fry AC, Kraemer WJ: Resistance exercise overtraining and overreaching: Neuroendocrine responses. *Sports Med* 1997:23, 106.
12. Israel S: Zur problematik das ubertrainings aus intemistiseher und Ieistungsphysiolgishtr siclit. *Med Sport* 1976:16, 51.
13. Kuipers H, Keizer HA: Overtraining in elite athletes. *Sports Med* 1988:6, 79.
14. Lehmann M, Foster C, Dickhuth HH, Gastmann U: Autonomic imbalance hypothesis and overtraining syndrome. *Med Sci Sports Exerc* 1998:30, 1140.
15. Costill DC, Flynn MG, Kirwan JP, et al.: Effects of repeated days of intensified training on muscle glycogen and swimming performance. *Med Sci Sports Exerc* 1988:20, 249.
16. Synder AC: Overtraining and glycogen depletion hypothesis. *Med Sci Sports Exerc* 1998:30, 1146.
17. Gastmann U, Lehmann M: Overtraining and the BCAA hypothesis. *Med Sci Sports Exerc* 1998:30, 1173.
18. Mittleman KD, Ricci MR, Bailey SP: Branched-chain amino acids prolong exercise during heat stress in men and women. *Med Sci Sports Exerc* 1998:30, 83.
19. Chaouloff F, Elghozi JL, Guezeïnnec Y, Laude D, et al.: Effects of conditioned running on plasma, liver, and brain tryptophan, and on brain 5-hydroxytryptophan metabolism of the rat. *Br J Pharmacol* 1985:86, 33.
20. Chaouloff F, Kennett GA, Serrurier B, et al.: Amino acid analysis demonstrates that increased plasma free tryptophan causes the increase of brain tryptophan during exercise in rats. *J Neurochem* 1986:46, 1647.
21. Barron JL, Noakes TD, Levy W, et al.: Hypothalamic dysfunction in overtrained athletes. *J Endocrin Metab* 1985:60, 803.
22. Russell JB, Mitchell DE, Musey PI, Collins DC: The role of beta-endorphins and catechol estrogen on the pituitary axis in female athletes. *Fertil Steril* 1984:42, 690.
23. Smith LL: Cytokine hypothesis of overtraining: A physiologic adaptation to excessive stress? *Med Sci Sports Exerc* 2000:32, 317.
24. Fry RW, Morton AR, Keast D, et al.: Overtraining in athletes: An update. *Sports Med* 1991:12, 32.
25. Derman W, Schwellnus MP, Lambert MI, et al: The "Worn-out athlete": A clinical approach to chronic fatigue in athletes. *J Sports Sci* 1997:15, 341.
26. Dyment PG: Frustrated by chronic fatigue? Try this systematic approach. *Phys Sportsmed* 1993:21, 47.
27. Levin S: Overtraining causes Olympic sized problems. *Phys Sportsmed* 1991:19, 112.
28. Miller TW, Vaughan MP, Miller JM: Clinical issues and treatment strategies in stress-oriented athletes. *Sports Med* 1990:9, 370.
29. Ryan AJ, Brown RL, Frederick EC, et al.: Overtraining and athletes. *Phys Sportsmed* 1983:11, 92.
30. Hooper SL, Mackinnon LT: Monitoring overtraining in athletes. *Sports Med* 1995:30, 321.
31. Kuipers H: Training and overtraining: An introduction. *Med Sci Sports Exerc* 1998:30, 1137.
32. Hiscock N, Mackinnon LT: A comparison of plasma glutamine concentration in athletes from different sports. *Med Sci Sports Exerc* 1998:30, 1693.

33. Mackinnon LT, Hooper SL: Plasma glutamine and upper respiratory tract infection during intensified training in swimmers. *Med Sci Sports Exerc* 1996:28, 285.

34. Mackinnon LT, Hooper SL, Jones S, et al.: Hormonal, immunological, and hematological responses to intensified training in elite swimmers. *Med Sci Sports Exerc* 1997:29, 1637.

35. Gilmann MB: The use of heart rate to monitor the intensity of endurance training. *Sports Med* 1996:21, 73.

36. McNair DM, Lorr M, Droppleman L: Profile of mood states (POMS), Educational & Industrial Testing Service, San Diego, Calif, 1990.

37. Mondin GW, Morgan WP, Piering PN, et al.: Psychological consequences of exercise deprivation in habitual exercisers. *Med Sci Sports Exerc* 1996:28, 1199.

38. Rushall BS: A tool for measuring stress tolerance in elite athletes. *Appl Sport Psych* 1990:2, 51.

39. Collins D: Early detection of overtraining problems in athletes. *Coaching Focus* 1995:28, 17.

40. Foster C: Monitoring overtraining in athletes with reference to overtraining syndrome. *Med Sci Sports Exerc* 1998:30, 164.

41. Fry RW, Morton AR, Garcia-Webb D, et al.: Biological - responses to overload training in endurance sports. *Eur J Appl Physiol* 1992:64, 335.

Chapter 32

ENVIRONMENTAL INJURIES

Jonathan S. Halperin and
Karim Khan

*This chapter is dedicated in fond
memory of John Sutton, M.D.
John Sutton was a medical pioneer.
He made significant contributions to
the fields of sports medicine and
pulmonary physiology. He was a dear
friend, a wonderful colleague, and an
inspiring teacher. He assisted the
climbing elite in pursuit of the world's
highest peaks and stimulated those of
us in the medical profession to ascend
to both personal and professional
milestones. His spirit, friendship,
guidance, and companionship will be
sorely missed.*
Jonathan S. Halperin and Karim Khan

INTRODUCTION

The pursuit of physical fitness and the desire to challenge ourselves in athletic competition are accepted behaviors as we commence the 21st century. The most devoted will travel to the highest peaks, to the most inhospitable deserts, or to the Alaskan tundra to train or compete. There are marathons that take place near the Arctic circle. The Ironman™ triathlon takes place in heat and humidity that can be oppressive. Many running races and triathlons take place in an alpine environment.

Our physiological responses to exercise will vary depending on the environment in which the exercise is performed. These responses are intended to allow the human body to maintain a constant internal temperature and oxygen homeostasis.[1] If this exposure is gradual and prolonged, adaptations will occur that improve the human body's ability to exercise in extreme environments.

It is important to emphasize, however, that the most important factors that allow one to exercise under varied environmental conditions are behavioral and not physiologic.[1] We can choose to wear appropriate clothing in the heat or cold. We can seek shelter when conditions become inhospitable. We can drink fluids, even though we are not thirsty.

This chapter will outline the physiological adaptations and possible medical complications that occur when one exercises or races in an adverse environment.

THERMOREGULATION

The human body is able to maintain a relatively constant internal temperature over a wide range of environmental conditions. We can walk briskly on a warm, humid summer night or ice skate outdoors on a cold winter day. The physiological responses to an exercise demand will vary with the environmental conditions. The goal of these adaptations is to maintain thermal homeostasis. Outside of a narrow range of internal core temperature (±2°C), essential body functions break down. At 45°C there is denaturation of many body proteins. Below 32°C there is significant impairment of cardiovascular and neurologic function.

Cellular metabolism produces heat as a by-product. Work or exercise above resting levels increases heat production dramatically. In addition, the body can be heated by or lose heat to the environment. The body has a finite ability to either dissipate a heat load or to metabolically produce heat to offset a loss of heat to the environment.

Normal Thermal Exchange (Table 32–1)

The body can either gain or lose heat when it interacts with the environment. Heat is either retained or lost via conduction, convection, or radiation. Heat is also lost through cooling from evaporation of sweat into the environment. This relationship is expressed in the heat storage equation of Winslow[2]:

$$S = M \pm R \pm Cv \pm Cd - E$$

where S is heat storage, M is metabolic heat production, R is heat gained or lost by radiation, Cv is heat gained or lost by convection, Cd is heat gained or lost by conduction, and E is heat lost by evaporation. Body core temperature increases during exercise. The mean body temperature is the result of a dynamic balance between those processes that produce heat and those responsible for heat loss.

Mechanisms of Heat Production and Heat Gain

The body can generate heat in a number of ways. A certain amount of heat is generated from the body's basic metabolic processes. Heat will be gained from the environment when the ambient temperature is greater than the skin temperature. Solar radiation on a clear, bright day can be a significant source of heat gain. During exercise, however, the most important source of heat production is muscular work. A runner working at 80% $\dot{V}O_2$max may increase his or her heat production by three- to fourfold.[3]

From an energy standpoint, the body is inefficient when it comes to muscular work. Seventy-five percent of the energy used to produce muscle activity is dissipated as heat. Thus it is easy to surmise that if metabolic heat production is not compensated for by an equivalent heat loss, the body's core temperature will rapidly rise and symptoms of heat illness will develop.

Mechanisms of Heat Loss

At rest, the body is able to dissipate an internal or external thermal load through radiation and convection. Heat loss via radiation involves a simple physical transfer of heat from the body to the cooler outside environment. Obviously this transfer is more efficient if the ambient temperature is lower than body temperature. Movement of cool air over the body surface causes heat loss via convection. During exercise, the body will shunt blood from the core to the extremities and body surface where additional heat is lost by conduction and convection. If the thermal load is great enough, sweat glands will be activated. As sweat is produced, evaporative heat loss occurs and the body is cooled. In most cases, the combination of direct heat loss to the environment and the evaporative loss of sweating is usually sufficient to prevent a substantial rise in body temperature.

EXERCISE IN THE HEAT

The human body has an inherent ability to adapt to a thermal load. Excessive heat and humidity, lack of conditioning, poor acclimatization, and dehydration are factors that will overwhelm the human thermoregulatory system. When the rate of heat elimination is exceeded by the rate of heat gain, body temperature rises and heat illness will ensue.

Heat Illness

Heat illness is a dynamic continuum. It may present clinically as mild discomfort, but if unrecognized or untreated, it may quickly progress and become life threatening. Heat illness may be classified as mild, moderate, or severe (Table 32–2).

Mild heat illness can present as generalized fatigue, muscular cramping, or syncope. In moderate or severe illness, the human thermoregulatory system is

---

TABLE 32–1. NORMAL THERMAL EXCHANGE

Conduction:	Heat exchange that occurs when two objects are in contact with one another. Heat will flow to the cooler object.
Convection:	Heat loss or heat gain that is secondary to air moving across a warmer or cooler object.
Radiation:	Heat exchange that occurs between two objects that are not in contact with one another.
Evaporation:	Heat loss that occurs when water (sweat) is converted to water vapor.

TABLE 32–2. CLASSIFICATION OF HEAT-RELATED ILLNESS

Classification	Mild	Moderate	Severe
Type	Heat cramps Heat syncope	Heat exhaustion	Heatstroke
Symptoms	Muscle cramps Light-headedness	Headache, exhaustion, weakness, nausea, vomiting, confusion, ataxia	Impaired consciousness
Signs	Muscle tightness or spasm Postural hypotension Increased pulse	Increased sweating Decreased blood pressure Increased heart rate	Decreased blood pressure Increased heart rate Hot, dry skin or cold, clammy skin
Treatment	Rest, ice, massage Oral glucose-electrolyte Remove from sun Lie down Elevate legs and pelvis Cool with ice bath	Rest, ice, massage May need intravenous fluids (other treatment per mild)	Medical emergency: Hospital transport for rapid cooling, intravenous fluids, assisted respiration

Adapted with permission: Brukner et al.[31]

overwhelmed. Significant cardiovascular, neurologic, and renal impairment can rapidly ensue if progressive heat injury is not diagnosed and treated.

Predisposing Factors

Some individuals are at greater risk than others for heat injury. These include the overweight, the unfit, the elderly, and the very young. Lack of sleep, coexisting febrile illness, and lack of heat acclimatization will put the athlete at risk. It appears that trained individuals have a greater heat dissipating capacity than do the untrained.[1] Training in a hot, humid environment (acclimatization) has been shown to lower the sweating threshold and increase the efficiency of the sweat response.[4,5] If dehydration is present, or lost water (via sweat and respiration) is not adequately replenished, the risk of heat injury is markedly increased.[6]

Use of drugs that impair sweating (major tranquilizers and antihistamines), drugs that interfere with cardiovascular performance (diuretics, antihypertensives, and beta blockers), and drugs that contribute to endogenous heat production (amphetamines, cocaine, neuroleptics, and tricyclic antidepressants) may predispose an individual to develop heat illness.[7]

Mild Heat Illness

The athlete with mild heat illness may present clinically in a number of ways. The most common presentation is that of fatigue, weakness, and headache. This has been called *heat fatigue,* and it responds to cessation of activity, moving out of direct sunlight, and oral fluids. Heat cramps are commonly seen with mild heat illness. They are seen in the calf, thigh, and periscapular region. The etiology of muscular cramping and pain postexercise is unclear, although an alteration of salt:water balance has been suggested.[7] Treatment involves rest and gentle ice massage to the affected muscles. Oral rehydration with a cool beverage that contains glucose and electrolytes will assist in recovery.

Heat syncope presents as a fainting episode that usually occurs immediately postexercise in hot and humid conditions. It can be mistaken for a more serious problem such as heatstroke or heat exhaustion. During exercise in a warm environment, blood is shunted from the core to the periphery. When exercise ceases, blood tends to pool in the venous circulation, causing weakness or dizziness that may progress to a syncopal episode. The athlete usually responds to elevation of the legs and pelvis, rest, and oral fluids. Heat syncope needs to be differentiated from the more serious forms of heat illness such as heat exhaustion or heatstroke.

Moderate Heat Illness: Heat Exhaustion

Heat exhaustion is a clinical condition that results from exercise in a hot and humid environment. Loss of total body water from sweat loss during these conditions can be significant. It tends to occur in individuals who are poorly acclimatized to exercise in the heat, are unfit, and are extracellular fluid (ECF) volume–contracted.[8] Exercise-induced ECF volume contraction (dehydration) produces a decrease in circulating blood volume, blood pressure, and sweat production.[9] If the athlete continues to exercise while in this state, the ability to offset the resultant increase in body core temperature will be significantly impaired and severe heat illness (exertional heatstroke) will occur.

Heat exhaustion represents the inability of the cardiovascular system to further respond adequately to an ongoing workload in a hot and humid environment.[9] Symptoms include headache, weakness, nausea, vomiting, and confusion. The athlete is usually mildly hypotensive with an increased heart rate. Syncopal episodes may occur. Mild to moderate elevation of rectal temperature may be observed.

Treatment consists of rehydration, rest, and removal from the hot environment. If the athlete cannot tolerate oral fluids, intravenous fluid administration may be needed. In those athletes that cannot be rapidly transported to a medical facility, it is best to use an isotonic solution such as Ringer's lactate or 0.9% sodium chloride. Ideally, serum and urine electrolytes should be known prior to giving intravenous fluids.

Severe Heat Illness: Heatstroke

Exertional heatstroke occurs when the athlete's thermoregulatory system is no longer able to cope with the thermal load that is being generated by ongoing muscular work. The body temperature becomes significantly elevated to the point that tissue and organ damage occurs (Table 32–3).

The athlete with exertional heatstroke typically presents with central nervous system dysfunction. The athlete may display inappropriate behavior and frank psychosis before lapsing into a coma. Rectal temperature is significantly elevated (usually >40°C), and the skin may be hot and dry or cool and sweaty. Hypotension, tachycardia, and tachypnea are seen. Electrolyte disturbances such as hypokalemia, hypocalcemia, and hyponatremia are commonly observed.[10]

TABLE 32–3. COMPLICATIONS OF SEVERE HEAT ILLNESS

System	Abnormality
Cardiovascular	Arrhythmias
	Myocardial infarction
	Hypotension
Pulmonary	Dyspnea
	Pulmonary edema
Neurological	Delirium
	Coma
	Convulsion
	Stroke
Gastrointestinal	Hepatic damage
	GI bleeding
Hematological	Disseminated intravascular coagulation
Muscular	Rhabdomyolysis
Renal	Acute nephropathy
	Interstitial nephritis

Adapted with permission: Sutton.[1]

Severe heat illness or exertional heatstroke is a true medical emergency. It may be fatal if not immediately diagnosed and properly treated. The factors that determine successful treatment of this condition are anticipation, prompt recognition, and rapid cooling.[7] Delay in treatment may lead to rhabdomyolysis and acute renal failure.[11] Morbidity and mortality from this condition are directly related to the intensity and duration of hyperthermia.[8]

Many whole-body cooling techniques have been used to treat exertional heatstroke (cold water immersion; application of cool damp towels; ice packs placed on the groin, neck, and axilla; cool moist air driven by fans). Although there is disagreement as to which method is most effective, rapid cooling is the mainstay of initial treatment.[10]

Intravenous fluid replacement is usually needed. The rate of infusion and type of infusion solution used should be guided by serum and urine electrolyte levels. Ideally, an athlete with exertional heatstroke would best be managed in a tertiary care center that can provide laboratory analysis and cardiovascular monitoring.

Heat-Related Illness: Management on the Run

The foundation of management of heat-related illness is early recognition and prompt treatment. The medical staff at a running race or triathlon should be keenly aware of environmental conditions, have adequate supplies of ice and fluids, and have a working triage system to facilitate rapid transport to a hospital or emergency room.

On the race course, trained medical personnel should be able to recognize early signs of heat injury. These may include impaired performance, excessive fatigue, poor coordination, and confusion. Alert race officials should intervene early and remove the athlete from the hot environment and place him or her in a shaded area where further assessment can be made and treatment administered. One of the most important steps in initial assessment is to measure body temperature. Unfortunately, oral and axillary temperature measurements are unreliable in these situations. Rectal temperature should be measured because it gives the best indication of body core temperature. A significantly elevated rectal temperature will help confirm the diagnosis of heat-related illness, and in conjunction with the patient's clinical condition help dictate appropriate initial management and triage.[7]

If the rectal temperature is elevated, immediate steps should be taken to cool down the athlete. Cooling should continue until the rectal temperature starts to decline (some recommend cooling until the rectal temperature declines to 102°F). If the rectal temperature remains significantly elevated despite aggressive cooling in the field, rapid transport to a medical facility is warranted.

In most cases of hyperthermia, some degree of ECF volume contraction will be present. Evidence of hypovolemia (hypotension, tachycardia) is an indication for fluid replacement. If the patient is alert, rehydration may be begun with cool oral fluids, preferably a glucose-electrolyte solution. If the patient has impaired consciousness or is unable to tolerate oral fluids, intravenous fluids may be needed.

Heat Acclimatization

Athletes are better able to cope with exercise in hot and humid conditions if they are acclimatized.[4,12,13] Lack of acclimatization is a particular problem for athletes who have to train or compete in warm, humid climates. In addition, athletes may be at risk for heat injury in their own locales if conditions change rapidly, such as the first hot spell of summer that comes after a particularly cool spring.

After prolonged exposure the human body will adjust to hot and humid conditions by increasing blood volume and venous tone. Of particular importance are alterations of the sweating mechanism. It has been observed that athletes who train in hot and humid conditions sweat more profusely, sweat earlier in response to a thermal load, and produce sweat with a higher water content.[3,6] These changes produce an increased rate of heat loss for a given set of environmental conditions and a smaller rise in body temperature.

Guidelines for Prevention of Heat Illness— ACSM Position Statement

In most cases, heat illness resulting from exercising in a warm environment can be prevented if both the athlete and race organizers are aware of the inherent risks and take steps to prevent it. The following guidelines were developed by experts in the fields of sports medicine and exercise science[9]:

1. Athletes should be adequately trained and conditioned to compete at their desired level.
2. If an athlete is preparing to compete in hot, humid conditions to which he or she is unaccustomed, the necessary level of acclimatization must be undertaken.
3. Event organizers should ensure that their events are not scheduled when high humidity and temperature are most likely to occur. If possible, events should be held in the early morning or late afternoon to avoid the midday sun.

TABLE 32–4. RISK OF HEAT INJURY DUE TO ENVIRONMENTAL STRESS
Wet bulb globe temperature (WBGT) index[a]

WBGT Index	Risk of Heat Injury	Flag Color
>28°C	Very high risk	Black
23°C–28°C	High risk	Red
18°C–23°C	Moderate risk	Yellow
<18°C	Low risk	Green

[a]WBGT = (0.7 Twb) + (0.2 Tg) + (0.1 Tdb)
Twb: wet bulb temperature
Tg: black globe temperature
Tdb: dry bulb temperature
Source: Adapted from Armstrong et al.[9]

4. Event organizers and competitors should be aware of the wet bulb globe temperature (WBGT) index (Table 32–4). The WBGT index should be posted at the race starting point and at other points along the race course. If the WBGT index is greater than 28°C, consideration should given to canceling the race or rescheduling it.
5. Athletes should wear appropriate clothing while training and racing. Loose fitting, light colored clothing with a mesh weave is ideal.
6. Athletes should be well hydrated before, during, and after exercise. It is recommended that participants drink plenty of fluids for 24 to 48 hours prior to competing in a warm, humid environment. At least 500 ml of fluid should be ingested $\frac{1}{2}$ hour prior to exercise or competition.

   During exercise, athletes should drink fluids at regular intervals. Ideally, 150 to 200 ml of fluid should be consumed every 15 minutes in hot conditions. If the training session or event is shorter than 1 hour in duration, plain water is adequate. In events lasting longer than 1 hour, a dilute glucose-electrolyte solution should be used.[14]
7. Race organizers should ensure that adequate medical support is available. A well-equipped and well-trained medical team should be present at all endurance events taking place in hot and humid conditions. Race-site medical facilities should have equipment and personnel to provide necessary resuscitation if needed.

Exercise-Associated Collapse

Heat illness is the most likely cause of distress or collapse while exercising in hot weather. It is important to consider other possible causes of distress or collapse that may also occur in these conditions.[15] A list of these possible clinical scenarios is shown in Table 32–5.

TABLE 32–5. EXERCISE-ASSOCIATED COLLAPSE

Condition	Possible Causes
Hypoglycemia	Excess medication by diabetic athlete
	Poor carbohydrate loading and intake
Hyponatremia	Endurance event greater than 3 hours
	Ingestion of large amounts of plain water
	Inadequate sodium intake
Hypothermia	Slower athlete in an endurance event
	Change in weather (cool wind)
Drug toxicity	Cocaine, amphetamines, tricyclic
	antidepressants
Ischemic heart disease	Arrhythmias
	Myocardial infarction
Cerebrovascular disease	Stroke
	Transient ischemic attack
Convulsion/coma	Epilepsy
	Hyponatremia

Adapted with permission: Brukner et al.[31]

The importance of obtaining a rectal temperature cannot be overemphasized as one of the key steps in the assessment of a collapsed athlete in hot weather. A rectal temperature greater than 40ºC to 41°C indicates that heat illness is the most likely cause of collapse. A rectal temperature of less than 40°C should compel the medical staff to consider other causes of collapse.

Another important cause of distress or collapse while exercising in hot weather is hyponatremia.[16] Although the pathophysiology of this condition is not yet entirely clear, athletes in endurance events of longer than 3 to 4 hours' duration sometimes display significant hyponatremia. Ongoing sodium replacement with dilute glucose and electrolyte solutions as well as salty foods such a pretzels are recommended. When symptomatic, athletes may show signs of central nervous system (CNS) dysfunction. In severe cases seizures may occur. Treatment consists of early recognition and electrolyte replacement. (Exercise-associated collapse is discussed in more detail in Chapter 27.)

EXERCISE IN THE COLD: HYPOTHERMIA

Exercise in a cool environment puts athletes at risk of developing hypothermia. The ability to exercise in cold weather is temperature dependent. At some point, the body will lose more heat than it can generate, there will be a lowering of the body's core temperature, and hypothermia will result.

Body Heat Production in Cold Weather

In normal conditions, the body relies on basal metabolism to maintain core temperature. In cold weather the body uses thermogenesis (shivering) to produce heat, and peripheral vasoconstriction to minimize heat loss.

Shivering—involuntary muscular contraction—is under control of the hypothalamus and occurs in response to a decrease in body core temperature. The metabolic rate can be increased up to three times over the resting state by shivering thermogenesis.[17] However, this type of muscular contraction is dependent on glycogen stores and thus has a limited ability to generate heat in a cold environment. Shivering results in decreased muscular coordination and is therefore a disadvantage in sporting activity.

Peripheral vasoconstriction allows the body to shunt blood from the skin surface to the body core and minimize heat loss by conduction and convection. Because this mechanism is not active in the skin of the hands and scalp, hats and gloves are essential to minimize heat loss in cool environments.[18]

Heat Loss in Cold Weather

Heat loss in a cool environment occurs mainly from the skin and can be regulated somewhat by vasoconstriction. Heat loss via conduction is not a significant problem because air is a poor conductor of heat, but it can become a major factor if the athlete becomes wet from snow, rain, or excessive perspiration. Heat loss from convection is normally low when wearing adequate clothing. It can become important in windy conditions when the air temperature drops below 20°C. Evaporative heat loss can be an issue, often unrecognized by the athlete, in cold, dry conditions.

Factors Minimizing Heat Loss

The human body adapts to racing or training in cold weather by shunting blood from the periphery to the core. This response is mediated by sensors at the skin surface and in the hypothalamus. Peripheral vasoconstriction thus acts to reduce external heat loss through the skin. It establishes a countercurrent heat exchange between the cold periphery and the warmer body core.[19]

Appropriate clothing is essential to minimize heat loss in a cold, windy, and sometimes wet environment. The head and scalp must be covered because significant heat loss occurs in these areas. Wearing multiple, thin layers of clothing and a water-resistant outer shell allows comfortable exercise and minimizes heat loss. Clothing should be made of an effective insulating material (wool, wool blends, or polypropylene). It is always better to overdress and shed clothing during a run or race than to risk developing hypothermia.

Physiological Consequences of Hypothermia

When exercising in cold weather, the body attempts to maintain thermal balance by generating heat and

TABLE 32–6. SYMPTOMS AND SIGNS OF HYPOTHERMIA

Core temperature (°C)	Symptoms and Signs
36	Goose pimples
35	Shivering
	Dysarthria
	Impaired mentation
34	Numbness
	Loss of coordination
	Muscular fatigue
32	Disorientation
	Ataxia
31	Semicoma
	Bradycardia
	Muscle rigidity
28	Ventricular fibrillation
	Cardiovascular death

Adapted with permission: Sutton.[1]

minimizing heat loss. Over time, there are likely to be adaptations that allow the body to perform more efficiently in this environment. However, the athlete who is unprepared or unacclimatized risks serious and possibly fatal complications (Table 32–6).

Cardiovascular Consequences

Vasoconstriction may eventually lead to fluid shifts by increasing the central blood volume. This can stimulate increased renal output (cold diuresis), which combined with fluid loss from respiration and sweating may result in a reduction of the total circulating blood volume. Upon cessation of exercise and rewarming, there is a resultant shift of blood volume to the periphery and further reduction of cardiac output. When combined with a cold myocardium, circulatory collapse may occur.[19]

Decreased cardiac output may also occur as a result of impaired electrical conductance. Electrocardiographic changes observed in hypothermia include bradycardia and prolongation of all segments of the QRS waveform. The presence of a J wave in the ST segment is indicative of hypothermia. Both atrial and ventricular fibrillation may occur. Cardiac arrhythmias can be refractory to treatment at low body core temperatures.[20]

Respiratory Consequences

Cold exposure stimulates hyperventilation. Over time, this will result in heat and water loss via the respiratory tract. The athlete may experience bronchospasm and in some cases dyspnea. These effects can be magnified and lead to hypoxia and decreased pulmonary function when the athlete is exercising at altitude in a cold environment.[18] There is no direct damage to the lungs from exposure to cold air because the upper airways provide effective warming and humidification of inspired air.

Neuromuscular Consequences

Nerve conduction and neuromuscular function are adversely affected by hypothermia. Impaired coordination and ataxia may be early signs of hypothermia. As hypothermia progresses, cognition and consciousness are impaired. In severe cases the patient may appear comatose.[19]

A reduction in muscle strength and flexibility is seen with a decrease in ambient temperature. The athlete is at risk for muscle strain or frank tears in a cool environment. If the core temperature falls below 34°C, increased tissue viscosity and impaired oxidative coupling will significantly diminish muscular activity.[17]

A proper warm-up consisting of gentle stretching and a low-intensity activity such as jogging or walking is recommended to prevent injury in a cold environment.

Clinical Features of Hypothermia

The clinical features of hypothermia will vary depending on the degree of reduction in core temperature. It is important to stress that rectal temperature is the only reliable indirect measure of body core temperature. Oral and axillary temperatures are affected by wind, rain, and ambient temperature. Tympanic membrane temperature measurements can be used if a rectal temperature cannot be practically obtained.[20]

Mild hypothermia is seen when the body core temperature is 35°C or greater. Shivering, tachycardia, tachypnea, and cool extremities are usual symptoms. There may be urinary urgency and slight incoordination.

Moderate hypothermia is seen when the body core temperature drops below 34°C. At this stage, there will be signs of CNS depression. The athlete is confused and displays gross incoordination, slurred speech, and drowsiness; he or she may become dehydrated. Shivering is diminished or may not be present at all.

In severe hypothermia, the body core temperature is less than 32°C. At this stage the athlete displays marked cognitive impairment and may be comatose. The body is rigid and cool and there is no shivering. The athlete is hypotensive with bradycardia. At this point cardiac arrhythmias are commonly seen and refractory ventricular fibrillation is a real concern.

Treatment of Hypothermia: General Principles

Management of the hypothermic athlete requires early recognition and prompt treatment. The athlete should be removed immediately from cold, wet, or windy conditions. Once stable, a rectal or auricular temperature should be obtained. The athlete should initially be passively rewarmed with warm blankets and ingestion of warm fluids. Cold, wet clothing should be removed. The extremities should be examined to rule out frostbite. If the athlete's condition does not improve, transportation to a medical facility should be arranged.

Treatment of Mild and Moderate Hypothermia

An athlete with mild hypothermia should be removed from the cold, insulated, and given warm fluids containing glucose and electrolytes. Although the application of external heat will make the athlete more comfortable, it is probably not needed. Mild activity may be performed provided the rectal temperature remains above 35°C.

The athlete with moderate hypothermia needs more aggressive treatment. He or she should be removed from the cold and insulated. In the field, the patient should be rewarmed by passive means until the rectal temperature has reached 34°C.[20] If possible, the athlete should be continually monitored for the presence of cardiovascular instability and arrhythmias. When stable, the patient can be rewarmed by more aggressive techniques in a hospital setting that provides continuous monitoring, intravenous hydration, and resuscitation equipment. Moderate hypothermia is a serious condition that may progress to severe hypothermia, which carries significant risk of mortality.

Treatment of Severe Hypothermia

The athlete with severe hypothermia is at risk for ventricular fibrillation, so the patient should be handled as gently as possible to minimize this risk. Appropriate medical facilities are necessary to effectively treat severe hypothermia. If the athlete can be transported quickly and safely with minimal handling to a hospital equipped with an intensive care unit, the chances of survival are greatly improved. In the hospital setting more invasive rewarming techniques and close cardiovascular monitoring will be available.[20]

The athlete with severe hypothermia often appears gravely ill or dead. On closer observation, there may be slow respirations and a slow, weak carotid pulse. This condition must not be mistaken for cardiac asystole, because cardiopulmonary resuscitation may precipitate ventricular fibrillation. The axiom "The patient is not clinically dead until he or she is warm and dead" is important to bear in mind when treating the hypothermic patient. Aggressive treatment and rewarming in a hospital setting may prove fruitful.

Rewarming Techniques in Hypothermia

The question of whether to actively or passively rewarm the athlete with moderate or severe hypothermia is controversial. The medical staff is faced with the dilemma of rewarming in the field or waiting to transfer the athlete to a medical facility where more aggressive rewarming techniques can take place. Delaying treatment can lead to more severe hypothermia. Rewarming in the field may provoke ventricular fibrillation.

Passive Rewarming

Passive rewarming involves adequately insulating the athlete to allow for thermogenesis to heat the body from within. If possible, the athlete should be placed in a warm environment. Wet clothing should be gently removed and the athlete should be covered with dry, warm blankets. If evacuation from the cold is impossible, the athlete may be covered with a plastic bag from the neck down and then covered with blankets until transfer is possible. "Space" or mylar blankets provide little added protection and are easily torn by sharp twigs and rocks in the field.

Active Rewarming

Active rewarming can performed by both internal and external methods. External active rewarming is used in cases of mild hypothermia. The athlete can be gently immersed in a tub of hot water or have hot packs applied to the torso. Surface rewarming can cause an increase in peripheral blood flow and relative central hypovolemia. Surface rewarming also results in a subjective feeling of warmth that reduces the rate of shivering.

Internal active rewarming is used in severe cases of hypothermia and is only possible in a hospital setting. Numerous techniques have been used, including cardiopulmonary bypass, hemodialysis, warm intravenous infusions, and peritoneal lavage. This type of treatment requires an experienced medical staff and close monitoring in an intensive care unit.[20]

Frostbite

Frostbite is the actual freezing of tissues secondary to exposure to the extreme cold. It most commonly occurs in the peripheral limbs and on the exposed areas of the face (cheeks, ears, and tip of the nose). It can involve the superficial skin and subcutaneous tissue, or in more severe cases involve the full skin thickness and deeper structures.

Male runners need to provide adequate insulation in the genital areas in cold, windy conditions. Frostbite of the penis is one of the most painful injuries a runner will endure. Learn from our experience, otherwise you will only let it happen once!

Clinical Features and Treatment

Patients with superficial frostbite complain of burning local pain with paresthesia. On examination, the skin is initially pale and grey, and it becomes red and edematous after thawing. Superficial blisters may be present.

Superficial frostbite can be treated by local thawing. The most reliable method is direct contact with body heat. The injured part should not be rubbed because skin sloughing may occur. No attempt should be made to thaw the injured area unless it is possible to prevent refreezing. Subsequent freezing and rethawing can produce a more serious injury.[21]

Deep frostbite is initially very painful and then tissues becomes numb. The affected area appears as a frozen block of hard, white tissue. Areas of gangrene and deep hemoserous blisters can occur in severe cases.

The affected area should be rapidly rewarmed in a hot water bath. A whirlpool with antiseptic added is ideal. The rewarming process is often acutely painful and adequate analgesia should be administered. Radiant heat from a fire or radiator should not be used because skin burns may occur. The tissue should continue to be rewarmed until it becomes soft and pliable and normal sensation returns. Intravenous infusion of low molecular weight dextran may help reduce swelling and maintain vasodilatation. Antibiotics may be needed if signs of infection develop.[21]

EXERCISE AT ALTITUDE

The allure of traveling to high-altitude locations for recreation and pleasure has increased over the past few decades. The increased popularity of the mountain lifestyle has brought more athletes to live, train, and race at altitude. In addition, there has been an unhealthy pursuit of some of the world's highest peaks by novice climbers.

The enjoyment of alpine travel needs to be balanced with the physiologic stress of adapting to hypoxia and decreased barometric pressure. At extreme altitudes, or with rapid ascent to moderate altitude, the athlete or climber can face the significant risk of morbidity or mortality from altitude-related illness.

Physiological Adaptations to Altitude

As one ascends to higher altitudes, the barometric pressure and partial pressure of oxygen decrease (Table 32–7). Physical activity, which is critically dependent on oxygen transport and delivery, will be adversely affected. In addition, there will likely be cold temperatures in an alpine environment, increasing the risk of hypothermia.

TABLE 32–7. RELATIVE HYPOXEMIA AT ALTITUDE

Altitude	Pao_2
Sea level	80–100 mm Hg
3000 meters	60 mm hg
6000 meters	30 mm hg
8848 meters (Everest summit)	28 mm hg

Source: Adapted from Foulke.[25]

There are many physiological adaptations that occur with increasing altitude (Table 32–8). Initially there is an increase in the ventilation rate. This produces a fall in alveolar carbon dioxide concentration ($Paco_2$) and an increase in alveolar oxygen concentration (Pao_2). This effect is immediate and continues while the athlete or climber remains at altitude. This ultimately leads to a rise in arterial oxygen concentration (Pao_2). Over the next 7 to 10 days, erythropoiesis is stimulated causing an increase in hemoglobin (Hgb) and hematocrit (Hct). This combined with the rise in Pao_2 results in increased oxygen-carrying capacity in the bloodstream. There is a resultant shift in the oxygen/Hgb dissociation curve that facilitates oxygen loading in the lungs and unloading in the tissues. Over the next few weeks changes occur in the tissues. These include increased capillary density, increased mitochondrial density, mild muscle atrophy, and an apparent optimization of muscle oxidative enzymes.[22]

An ascent to altitude that has been sufficiently gradual will allow an athlete to make appropriate physiological adjustments and enable the athlete to exercise in an alpine environment. However, if the rate of ascent or the altitude reached are greater than the capacity of the body to adapt, potentially life-threatening problems may ensue.

TABLE 32–8. PHYSIOLOGICAL ADAPTATIONS AND RESPONSES TO ALTITUDE

Observed Physiological Change	Exposure Needed to Produce Changes	Exposure Time to Maximum Change
Increased ventilation	Immediate	Weeks
Increased heart rate	Immediate	Weeks
Increased hemoglobin	Days to weeks	Weeks
Increased capillary density	Weeks	Months to years
Increased aerobic enzyme activity in muscle	Weeks	Months
Increased mitochondrial density in muscle	Weeks	Months

Source: Adapted from Sutton.[30]

TABLE 32–9. CLINICAL FEATURES OF ALTITUDE-RELATED ILLNESS

Clinical Syndrome	Features
Acute mountain sickness (AMS)	Headache, insomnia, nausea, vomiting, ataxia, and impaired mentation Affects those who ascend too high and too fast Symptoms are accentuated by physical exercise Descent brings dramatic relief Prophylaxis and acute treatment with acetazolamide
High-altitude pulmonary edema (HAPE)	Initially dyspnea with dry cough. Can progress to severe respiratory distress with pink, frothy sputum, hypoxemia, and cyanosis Serious; rapid descent mandatory Oxygen administration can relieve symptoms Dexamethasone routinely given but effects not proven May need emergency evacuation and hospitalization
High-altitude cerebral edema (HACE)	Severe headache, mental confusion, hallucinations, ataxia, weakness, and eventually coma Rare, but very serious Descent to lower altitude mandatory Dexamethasone routinely given by intramuscular or intravenous routes
High-altitude retinal hemorrhage (HARH)	Common above 5000 meters Usually asymptomatic; resolves without treatment Descent recommended if visual defects occur
Miscellaneous conditions	Edema of face and periphery Weight loss Increased risk of thrombophlebitis and embolism Sickle cell crisis (can occur at moderate altitude in those with sickle cell trait)

Reproduced with permission: Sutton.[1]

Altitude-Related Illness (Table 32–9)

Altitude-related illness is a spectrum of conditions that may have overlapping clinical presentations. The common feature seen in all cases is hypobaric hypoxia.[23] Athletes present with varying degrees of weakness, malaise, nausea, and headache. There are signs of increasing pulmonary work (hyperventilation, dyspnea, and tachycardia), progressing in severe cases to pulmonary distress and central nervous system dysfunction.

This is a condition of the young and fit. A wanton disregard for personal safety combined with the wide range of individual rates of acclimatization to altitude is a prescription for possible tragedy. While healthy people do not usually develop symptoms below 2500 meters, a rapid ascent to levels of 3500 meters and above will likely precipitate severe forms of altitude-related illness.[24–26]

Acute Mountain Sickness (AMS)

AMS is the most common manifestation of altitude-related illness. The symptoms are somewhat variable and nonspecific. It usually occurs within the first 12 to 36 hours after arrival at an altitude greater than 2500 meters.[22] Symptoms include headache, malaise, nausea, anorexia, and insomnia. The athlete or climber may have difficulty concentrating and poor judgment.

There may be associated hypothermia, hypovolemia, and physical exhaustion that can potentiate symptoms.

It has been proposed that there is an imbalance between cerebral vasodilation (mediated by hypoxia) and cerebral vasoconstriction (mediated by hypocarbia). This can produce alterations in cerebral circulation and relative cerebral hypoxia.[27]

AMS is best prevented by a gradual ascent to altitude. This allows for appropriate acclimatization. Many strategies have been employed. In general, one should not climb more than 500 meters/day and should sleep at a lower altitude than the maximum attained that day.[25] The athlete or climber should avoid alcohol and sedatives. Once symptoms develop, a rapid descent is imperative. Oxygen administration will provide some relief but is not a substitute for transport to lower altitude.

The use of acetazolamide has been proposed as both a treatment for and prophylaxis against altitude-related illness. It appears to work by enhancing bicarbonate excretion and stimulating ventilation. It has not been shown, however, to prevent high-altitude pulmonary edema (HAPE) or high-altitude cerebral edema (HACE).[27] The recommended dosage of acetazolamide is 125 to 250 mg orally twice daily commencing the day before ascent and continuing for 3 days thereafter.[22,27] If the climber or athlete is allergic to sulfa-based drugs, dexamethasone (4 mg twice or four times a day) can be used instead.

High-Altitude Cerebral Edema (HACE)

The climber or athlete who presents with evidence of cognitive impairment and gait ataxia should be suspected of having developed HACE. It can come on rapidly and can be fatal. It tends to occur at altitudes greater than 3500 meters or with rapid ascent. Fortunately, it is less common than other forms of altitude-related illness.[22]

In contrast to AMS, with HACE there is a severe headache that may not be relieved by analgesics. In addition, there are definite changes in mental status and evidence of neurologic dysfunction.[22] The pathophysiology of HACE is unclear. It has been proposed that alterations in cerebrovascular tone lead to increased membrane permeability and progressive cerebral edema.[28]

The signs and symptoms of HACE must be recognized quickly. Rapid descent is imperative and should occur as quickly as conditions allow. High-flow oxygen administration may be helpful. Dexamethasone given intramuscularly (10 mg) or orally (4 mg four times a day) is commonly used, yet there is no definitive proof of its effectiveness. There is no prophylactic drug regimen.[27]

High-Altitude Pulmonary Edema (HAPE)

The young, active climber or athlete who rapidly ascends to altitudes greater than 2500 meters is at risk of developing HAPE.[29] Symptoms may develop at a slower rate than with AMS and HACE. The athlete or climber will complain of a nonproductive cough, dyspnea, and headache. There may be signs of pulmonary distress, including tachypnea, tachycardia, rales, and cyanosis. In severe cases, severe hypoxia and pulmonary hypertension can induce pulmonary edema.[25]

Supplemental oxygen and rapid descent are the mainstays of treatment. Descents of only 500 to 1000 meters are often very helpful. Subsequent exercise may worsen hypoxemia and exacerbate pulmonary hypertension, therefore a period of bed rest is often recommended. If the patient presents with marked pulmonary edema and respiratory distress, morphine and diuretics may be needed.[22]

High-Altitude Retinal Hemorrhage (HARH)

This form of retinopathy is commonly seen with physical exertion above 4000 meters. It has been observed in up to 50% of climbers who ascend to levels greater than 5000 meters.[25] Alterations of vasoregulation and membrane permeability are thought to be responsible.

These small retinal hemorrhages are usually asymptomatic and require no treatment. However, rapid descent is recommended if visual defects are present.

Altitude Training

While most athletes are not at risk of developing severe altitude-related illness, there has been recent interest in the effects of altitude on exercise performance. As was described earlier, there are physiological changes that occur when one enters a high-altitude environment. These include enhanced erythropoiesis—an increase in red cell mass—that may prove advantageous when an athlete competes after a return to sea level.

An analysis of the results at the Mexico City Olympics demonstrated that to perform well in events lasting longer than 2 minutes at high altitude one needs to be adequately acclimatized or to have been born and raised at altitude. The suggestion that training at altitude will benefit performance at sea level, while theoretically plausible, has not yet been scientifically proven or refuted. Most studies to date have serious deficiencies in experimental design (lack of control groups, numerous uncontrolled variables) that make an accurate determination of the benefits of training at altitude difficult at best.[30]

The presumed effect of training at altitude is enhancement of the transport and utilization of oxygen (as measured by $\dot{V}O_2max$). However, it is well documented that oxygen uptake decreases progressively with increasing altitude.[28] Hence, an athlete training at altitude cannot achieve the same level of training intensity that he or she can achieve at sea level. In addition, training in a cool alpine environment will prove a distinct disadvantage when the athlete returns to a warm or humid climate to train or compete. Finally, any individual who is foolish enough to exercise at altitude before his or her body has physiologically adapted is at significant risk of developing altitude-related illness.[31] More recent data suggest that living at altitude but training at sea level may provide the greatest enhancement in performance at sea level.[32]

Guidelines for the Prevention of Altitude-Related Illness (Table 32–10)

The athlete who trains or competes in an alpine environment must be aware of the inherent risks that occur with an ascent to altitude. Common sense and caution are the foundations of prevention and treatment. There are physiological changes that occur as one gradually climbs to higher altitudes. Some are beneficial, but others, if ignored, can lead to serious health consequences. Impulsive and reckless behavior,

TABLE 32–10. STRATEGIES TO PREVENT ALTITUDE-RELATED ILLNESS

1. Commence ascent below 2500 to 3000 meters.
2. Avoid significant exertion for the first 24 hours.
3. Avoid or minimize alcohol consumption.
4. Keep daily rate of ascent below 300 meters.
5. Sleep at a lower altitude than maximum altitude achieved that day.
6. Keep well hydrated and avoid sedatives.

Source: Adapted from Sutton.[1]

while perhaps tolerable at sea level, can be fatal at altitude.

CONCLUSIONS

The thrill of competing may take the avid athlete to many wonderful and exotic locales. The desire to compete and train year round will expose the fitness enthusiast to different environmental conditions.

As this chapter has elucidated, there are potential dangers and risk of serious injury or illness if common sense is not used and appropriate precautions are not taken. Athletic competition and physical training are the foundation of a healthy, active lifestyle. The human body has an amazing ability to adapt to a wide range of environmental conditions. Lack of preparation combined with a callous disregard for the risks of exercise in hot, cold, or high-altitude environments can lead to potentially serious consequences.

REFERENCES

1. Sutton JR: Exercise and the environment, in Bouchard C, Shepard RJ (eds.), *Exercise, Fitness and Health*, Champaign, Ill, Human Kinetics, 1989:165.
2. Winslow CEA, Herrington LP, Gagge AP: Physiological reactions of the human body to various atmospheric humidities. *Am J Physiol* 1937:120, 288.
3. Gisolfi CV, Wenger CB: Temperature regulation during exercise: Old concepts, new ideas. *Exerc Sport Sci Rev* 1984:12, 339.
4. Nadel ER, Pandolf KP, Roberts MF, et al.: Mechanisms of thermal acclimatization to exercise and heat. *J App Physiol* 1974:37, 515.
5. Maughan RJ, Shirreffs SM: Preparing athletes for competition in the heat: Developing an effective acclimatization strategy. *Sports Sci Exch (Gatorade Sports Sci Inst)* 1997:10, 2.
6. Nadel ER: Limits imposed on exercise in a hot environment. *Sports Sci Exch (Gatorade Sports Sci Inst)* 1990:3, 7.
7. Knochel JP: Heat illness, in Callaham ML (ed.), *Current Practice of Emergency Medicine*, Toronto, BC Decker, 1991:1098.
8. Armstrong LE, De Luca JP, Hubbard RW: Time course of recovery and heat acclimation ability of prior exertional heat stroke patients. *Med Sci Sports Exerc* 1990: 22, 36.
9. Armstrong LE, Epstein Y, Greenleaf JE, et al.: American College of Sports Medicine position stand: Heat and cold illness during distance running. *Med Sci Sports Exerc* 1996:28, i.
10. Callaham ML: Heat illness, in Rosen P (ed.), *Emergency Medicine: Concepts and Clinical Practice*, St. Louis, Mosby, 1988:693.
11. Clarkson P: Worst case scenarios: Exertional rhabdomyolysis and acute renal failure. *Sports Sci Exch (Gatorade Sports Sci Inst)* 1993:6, 1.
12. Armstrong LE, Maresh CM: The exertional heat illness: A risk of athletic participation. *Med Exerc Nutr Health* 1993:2, 125.
13. Shapiro YD, Moran D, Epstein Y: Acclimatization strategies: Preparing for exercise in the heat. *Int J Sports Med* 1998:19, 161.
14. Convertino VA, Armstrong LE, Coyle EF, et al.: American College of Sports Medicine position stand: Exercise and fluid replacement. *Med Sci Sports Exerc* 1996:28, i.
15. Roberts WO: Exercise associated collapse in endurance events: A classification system. *Phys Sportsmed* 1989: 19, 67.
16. Maughan RJ: Fluid requirements and exercise in the heat, in Maughan RJ (ed.), *Basic and Applied Sciences for Sports Medicine*, Oxford, Butterworth-Heinemann, 1999:170.
17. Pate R: Special considerations for exercise in cold weather. *Sports Sci Exch (Gatorade Sports Sci Inst)* 1988:1–10.
18. Shepard RJ: Adaptation to exercise in the cold. *Sports Med* 1985:2, 59.
19. Doubt TJ: Physiology of exercise in the cold. *Sports Med* 1991:11, 367.
20. Scott SK, Marx JA: Hypothermia, in Callaham ML (ed.), *Current Practice of Emergency Medicine*, Toronto, BC Decker, 1991:1090.
21. Phillips LG, Heggers JP, Robson MC: Frostbite and local cold injury, in Callaham ML (ed.), *Current Practice of Emergency Medicine*, Toronto, BC Decker, 1991:1096.
22. Schoene RB: High altitude, in Safran MR, McKeag DB, Van Camp SP (eds.), *Manual of Sports Medicine*, Philadelphia, Lippincott-Raven, 1998:110.
23. Sutton JR, Lassen N: Pathophysiology of acute mountain sickness and high altitude pulmonary oedema. *Bull Eur Physiopath Respir* 1979:15, 1045.
24. Sutton JR, Jones NL, Houston CS: *Hypoxia: Man at Altitude*, New York, Thieme-Stratton, 1982.
25. Foulke GE: Altitude related illness. *Am J Emerg Med* 1985:3, 217.
26. Hackett PH, Roach RC: Medical therapy of altitude illness. *Ann Emerg Med* 1987:16, 980.
27. Foulke G: Emergencies of high altitude travel, in Callaham ML (ed.), *Current Practice of Emergency Medicine*, Toronto, BC Decker, 1991:1104.

28. Sutton JR, Reeves JT, Wagner PD, et al.: Operation Everest II: Oxygen transport during exercise at extreme simulated altitude. *J Appl Physiol* 1988:64, 1309.

29. Schoene RB: High altitude pulmonary edema: Pathophysiology and clinical review. *Ann Emerg Med* 1987:16, 987.

30. Sutton JR: Exercise training at high altitude: Does it improve endurance performance at sea level? *Sports Sci Exch (Gatorade Sports Sci Inst)* 1993:6, 4.

31. Brukner P, Kahn K: *Clinical Sports Medicine,* Sydney, McGraw-Hill, 1993.

32. Levine BD, Stray Gunderson J: "Living high-training low": Effect of moderate altitude acclimatization with low-altitude training on performance. *J App Physiol* 1997:83, 102.

Part V

SPECIAL CONSIDERATIONS

Chapter 33

SPECIAL CONSIDERATIONS FOR THE PEDIATRIC RUNNING POPULATION

Wade A. Lillegard

INTRODUCTION

Health-related physical fitness includes cardiorespiratory endurance, muscular strength and endurance, body composition, and flexibility.[1] Physical activity is a behavior or attribute that is a significant determinate of physical fitness.[2] Both physical activity and physical fitness are encouraged among our youth. One of the Healthy People 2000 goals is to have 75% of children under the age of 18 participate in vigorous physical activity for more than 20 minutes, three times a week.[3] Unfortunately, only 71% of boys and 66% of girls at age 12 meet this goal, and by 21 years of age the percentages are 42% and 30%, respectively.[4]

Running is an excellent mode of exercise because it is inexpensive, convenient, and safe. It fulfills most of the above-mentioned criteria by being vigorous and improving cardiorespiratory endurance, strength, and body composition. Increased fitness also leads to improvements in classroom behavior, self-control, self-esteem, alertness, enthusiasm, creativity, and maturity and less destructive behavior.[5] As with any sport, the potential for adverse consequences of training and possible injuries inherent in running must be considered. Knowledge of these risks allows the physician to help prevent injury or illness and to intervene when necessary in an effort to return the athlete to running

in the least amount of time. This chapter reviews pediatric exercise physiology as well as common orthopedic and medical problems that are relevant to the care of the young runner.

PHYSIOLOGY

Aerobic Capacity Related to Growth

Absolute maximal aerobic capacity increases curvilinearly with age, from 1 L/min at age 6 to 3 L/min at age 15. This translates to an annual increase of approximately 200 ml/min, which seems to parallel skeletal maturation and development of $\dot{V}_{O_2}$-dependent organs (heart, lungs, and blood volume).[4] This rate continues in boys until 18 years of age but plateaus in girls between 12 and 14 years (Fig. 33–1). $\dot{V}_{O_2}$max relative to body weight (ml/kg/min) averages in the high 40s to low 50s in children and changes little during growth in males but decreases in females after puberty.[4,6] These gender differences are largely due to different postpubescent morphologic changes. The amount of metabolically active muscle is similar in prepubescent boys and girls comprising 25% to 30% of their body weight. After puberty, this increases to 40% to 45% in boys, but only 35% to 38% in girls.[7] If this difference (in percent body fat) is factored out, aerobic capacity relative to

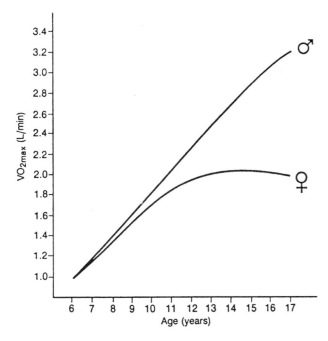

Figure 33–1. Aerobic capacity related to body weight linearly increases in boys into young adulthood, whereas girls plateau in their peripubertal years. (*Source Bale P: The functional performance of children in relation to growth, maturation and exercise.* Sports Med *1992:13, 152.*)

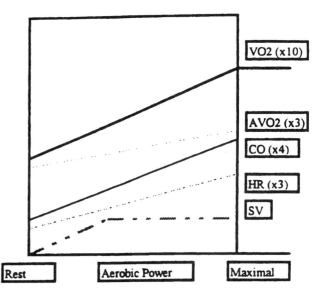

Figure 33–2. Summary of cardiovascular changes related to intensity of exercise in healthy adults. (*Source: From Braden and Carroll JF.*[4])

lean body mass becomes similar in boys and girls.[8] Furthermore, the weight-adjusted female heart size and stroke volume is 85% that of males, and females have slightly lower hemoglobin levels after puberty.[7]

Physiologic Response to Exercise

The normal physiologic response to exercise is different in children and adults. Regardless of age, oxygen consumption ($\dot{V}_{O_2}$) is a product of cardiac output (CO) and oxygen extraction ($A\dot{V}_{O_2}$ difference), and cardiac output is determined by both heart rate (HR) and stroke volume (SV). This is summarized in the basic formula

$$\dot{V}_{O_2} = HR \times SV \times A\dot{V}_{O_2} \text{ diff}$$

Adults exercising at a mild intensity (30% to 40% $\dot{V}_{O_2}$max) increase oxygen delivery by increasing their stroke volume 1.3 to 1.5 times resting values with a slight increase in HR.[4] At moderate intensities (40% to 60% $\dot{V}_{O_2}$max), the stroke volume increases to a lesser degree (1.5 to 2 times resting), but cardiac output is maintained by increasing the heart rate, and more oxygen is extracted by the working muscle ($A\dot{V}_{O_2}$ difference increases). At maximal effort the stroke volume is 1.5 times resting values, HR is 2.5 to 3 times resting, and the $A\dot{V}_{O_2}$ difference is three times resting values.[4] Figure 33–2 summarizes these cardiovascular responses to exercise in adults.

Children's stroke volume and cardiac output are lower than those of adults, yet their $\dot{V}_{O_2}$max (ml/kg/mm) is generally higher. The higher oxygen consumption then must come from either an increased delivery (via heart rate) or increased extraction of oxygen ($A\dot{V}_{O_2}$ difference). The maximal heart rate of children is higher than in adults, and their resting heart rate is lower, the net yield being a higher heart rate reserve (HR max − HR rest) and heart rate scope (HR max/HR rest). The maximal $A\dot{V}_{O_2}$ difference with exercise is not significantly different in children than in adults. Children, however, have a higher $A\dot{V}_{O_2}$ difference at submaximal levels of exercise so that at a given submaximal $\dot{V}_{O_2}$ (L/min) their $A\dot{V}_{O_2}$ difference is nearer their maximal values.[4] Indeed, the $A\dot{V}_{O_2}$ difference nearly doubles in early exercise in children and then slowly increases to 2.5 to 3 times resting values as the intensity increases to maximal exertion.[9]

Both the heart rate and oxygen extraction differences are probably attributable to the children's smaller muscle mass. For a child to perform the same rate of work ($\dot{V}_{O_2}$) as an adult, children must use a smaller absolute muscle mass. This smaller muscle mass is then stressed to a greater degree, resulting in increased metabolite formation, which provides feedback to the medulla to increase the heart rate.[10] Furthermore, the $A\dot{V}_{O_2}$ difference would be enhanced because the increased heat generated per unit of muscle would decrease the O_2 affinity for hemoglobin and increase the vasodilation of the arteries entering the working muscle.[6]

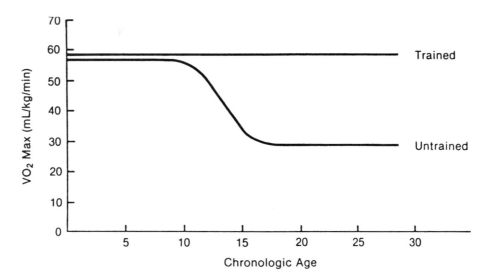

Figure 33–3. Continued aerobic training maintains aerobic capacity after puberty. Cessation of training leads to a rapid decline through puberty. (*Source: McKeag DB: The role of exercise in children and adolescents.* Clin Sports Med *1991:10, 124.*)

Aerobic Trainability of Children

The ability of children to increase their aerobic capacity with training is somewhat less than that of adults, who typically will improve by 25% to 30%. $\dot{V}O_2$max improvements in aerobically trained children younger than 14 years average 11% or less, and older children improve 20% to 25%.[4] One reason for this blunted training response may be an inadequate training stimulus secondary to an immature anaerobic metabolism system (and hence a higher anaerobic threshold). Younger children demonstrate lower lactate accumulation and lactate/pyruvate ratios during intense exercise than older children or adults.[11] This implies a relatively underdeveloped glycolytic pathway in younger children, possibly due to lower phosphofructokinase activity and/or lower sympathetic activity. The latter relatively increases splanchnic blood flow, which enhances hepatic metabolism of lactate. Younger children, therefore, must train at a higher intensity to meet their anaerobic threshold. Prepubescents reach their anaerobic threshold at an intensity of 165 to 170 beats/min, which is equivalent to 85% of their maximal heart rate.[12,13] This is generally a higher threshold than for adults and may indicate that prepubescent children need to exercise at higher intensities if they are to improve aerobic capacity.[14] Regardless, it appears that endurance and submaximal heart rates at a given exercise intensity may improve with training. As children become more economical in their gait, they utilize less oxygen. As they get older, or through neuromuscular training, this translates into a larger metabolic reserve and allows them to compete more successfully over long distances. For prepubescents then, neuromuscular skill proficiency may be the only substantial physiologic enhancement derived from run training. Older children (14 to 18 years) have more trainability and show aerobic capacity improvements similar to those of adults if they train with the appropriate intensity, frequency, and duration.[15] Their improvement is due less to neuromuscular efficiency and more to increased stroke volume and cardiac output.

The healthy prepubescent child is at near maximal aerobic capacity due to normal growth and development, and this is marginally effected by exercise training. After puberty, aerobic capacity will decline unless it is actively maintained through aerobic exercise training (Fig. 33–3).

COMMON INJURIES IN THE YOUNG RUNNER

Hip and Pelvis Injuries
Apophysitis and Apophyseal Avulsions
The apophyseal attachments of tendons are the weak link in the kinetic chain. Repetitive stresses frequently cause microinjury to these attachments, resulting in apophysitis.[16] A sudden, forceful contraction of the attached muscle can avulse the apophysis and cause acute pain. A number of pelvic areas are at risk in the running child including the iliac crest, anterior superior iliac spine (ASIS), anterior inferior iliac spine (AIIS), and ischial tuberosity (IT) (Fig. 33–4).[17]

ISCHIAL TUBEROSITY APOPHYSIS. Avulsion injuries of the IT result from a violent hamstring muscle contraction while the hamstrings are taut (e.g., sprinting) and are the most frequent avulsion injuries to the pelvis.[16,18]

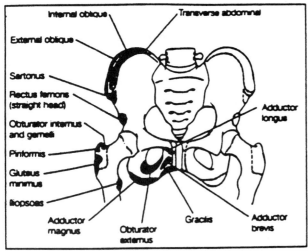

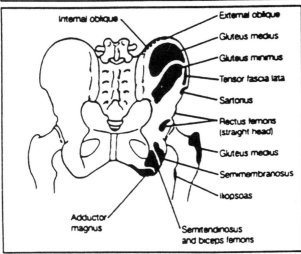

Figure 33–4. Origins of muscles attached to the pelvis illustrating sites of avulsion fractures. (*Source: From Combs.*[17])

Tendon repture without a bone fragment is uncommon in the growing child. Apophysitis may result from repetitive microtrauma due to tight hamstrings, speed work, hill running, or any combination of these factors. Both types of injury are characterized by pain in the buttock region at the origin of the hamstrings and adductor magnus.

Physical examination reveals point tenderness at the IT; the pain is aggravated by resisted knee flexion or a passive hamstring stretch. Plain radiographs may demonstrate an avulsed fragment; bone scans may be helpful in equivocal cases by demonstrating increased uptake at the tuberosity in apophyseal injury.[18]

Treatment for IT apophysitis consists of relative rest, ice, nonsteroidal anti-inflammatory agents (NSAIDs), and stretching of the hamstrings and adductors. Most avulsions are initially treated with crutch walking until pain ceases. Stretching and strengthening are instituted when they can be performed without pain. Surgical treatment may be considered for high-demand athletes with avulsion fractures, as up to two-thirds of conservatively treated avulsions will not unite. Urgent surgical intervention is recommended for those patients with total or near total proximal hamstring rupture or an avulsion fragment displaced more than 2 cm.[18]

Chronic pain may develop secondarily to enlargement of the tuberosity, chronic bursitis, or a tight or soft tissue "cord" impinging on the proximal hamstring. These chronic problems require aggressive physical therapy and possible steroid injections.[18] Surgical intervention is warranted in resistant cases.

ANTERIOR INFERIOR ILIAC SPINE APOPHYSIS. Avulsion of the AIIS apophysis is the second most common avulsion fracture of pelvis.[16] This avulsion is due to a sudden contraction of the rectus femoris muscle while the hip is extended and the knee is flexed.[19] Repetitive microtrauma from traction by the rectus femoris can cause apophysitis and is characterized by an insidious onset of anterior hip pain.

The affected runner has pain with weightbearing, and there is tenderness to palpation over the AIIS. Active flexion or passive hyperextension of the hip aggravates the pain. The diagnosis is clinical, but pelvic radiographs may be used if an avulsion is suspected.

Treatment of avulsions is usually conservative and depends on the severity of symptoms. Severe pain may require a short period of bed rest followed by crutch walking with progressive weightbearing. Quadriceps stretching and progressive resistance exercises are added when the athlete can ambulate without pain. Progressive running may resume as symptoms resolve. Complications are rare but may require surgical resection.[19]

ANTERIOR SUPERIOR ILIAC SPINE APOPHYSIS. A sudden contraction of the sartorius muscle can avulse the ASIS apophysis from its attachment to the ilium.[20] This is the third most common avulsion fracture in the pelvis and accounts for 1.4% of hip and pelvis injuries.[16]

The patient with an ASIS avulsion usually describes a sudden, sharp pain following a forced extension of the hip. On examination the ASIS is swollen and tender, and hip extension is painful. Displacement of an avulsed fragment may be seen on plain radiographs. Severe pain may require a period of bed rest followed by a Brown splint, keeping the hip in 60 degrees of flexion, and crutch walking for up to 5 weeks. Patients with less severe pain may require only protected weightbearing with crutches until they can ambulate without pain. This is followed by a program of progressive stretching and strengthening.

The avulsion usually heals with a deformity but with good function. Surgery is considered for large avulsions, severe displacement, or rotation. In athletes, surgery may allow a more rapid return to training and competition.[20]

ASIS apophysitis presents with a gradual onset of pain and possibly swelling after running. Treatment is relative rest, ice, NSAIDs, and stretching of the quadriceps and hip flexors, with a gradual return to running as pain abates.

ILIAC CREST APOPHYSIS. The long iliac crest is the attachment site for the transverse, the internal oblique, and external oblique abdominal muscles. Injuries to the iliac crest apophysis can come from direct trauma, sudden forceful traction, or repetitive microtrauma. Sudden forceful contraction of the abdominal muscle, such as those experienced by runners while abruptly changing direction, can result in avulsions of the apophysis with a sudden onset of symptoms.[17] Apophysitis is the result of repetitive traction microtrauma found usually in distance runners and has a gradual onset.

Symptoms consist of localized pain at the iliac crest with running and, at times, even with walking. The "gluteus medius lurch" is characterized by leaning into the affected side while stepping with the ipsilateral foot. Iliac apophysitis is a clinical diagnosis, and radiographs are only necessary if a fracture or avulsion is considered. A bone scan will generally be positive but is rarely necessary.

Initial treatment consists of ice, NSAIDs, and stretching of the abdominal musculature. If a fracture is present or pain is severe, crutch walking with a gradual return to activity is recommended. Symptoms usually subside in about 4 weeks.[17]

Legg-Calvé-Perthes Syndrome

Legg-Calvé-Perthes syndrome is an idiopathic avascular necrosis of the proximal femoral epiphysis. It occurs in children between the ages of 3 and 12 years but most commonly presents between 5 and 7 years. Boys are affected three to five times more frequently than girls, and both hips are involved in 10% to 20% of cases.[21]

The affected young runner presents with a limp and vague pain in the groin, hip, thigh, or knee. (When a child has vague knee pain, the examiner should evaluate the hip.) Physical examination reveals variable shortening of the involved leg, which may accentuate a limp. Almost all affected children will have limited hip abduction and internal rotation when tested in both hip flexion and extension, even in early stages of the disease. Anteroposterior and frog leg radiographs

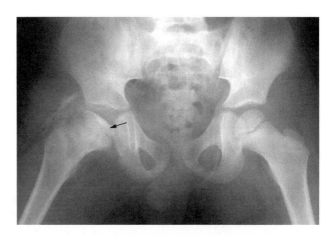

Figure 33–5. Radiograph demonstrating the dense, collapsed epiphysis (arrow) consistent with advanced avascular necrosis.

should be carefully scrutinized in suspected cases. Early disease is characterized by a dense epiphysis, which is patchy, more distal, and uneven at the margins. Later stages show more involvement of the femoral head with cystic changes and fragmentation (Fig. 33–5). Magnetic resonance imaging (MRI) should be performed if plain radiographs are normal but clinical suspicion is high.

Treatment is sufficiently controversial to warrant referral of all cases to an orthopedic surgeon for management.[21] Nonoperative treatment consists of range-of-motion exercises, bracing, and varying degrees of weightbearing. In general, children diagnosed before 5 years of age have a more favorable prognosis, and those diagnosed after 8 years old have a less favorable outcome.

Slipped Capital Femoral Epiphysis

Both acute and chronic slips result in displacement of the capital femoral epiphysis. Posterior medial slips are the most common, and they are bilateral in approximately 60% of cases.[22] The high-risk period for developing a slip is during periods of peak height velocity (10 to 13 years old for girls and 12 to 15 years old for boys).[23] Children large for age or maturity are also at higher risk.

Runners with a chronic slip or preslip (the growth plate is damaged but no slip has occurred) may have a mild limp and complain of vague groin, hip, or knee pain. Medial knee pain, referred from the hip via the obturator nerve, may be the only complaint. As the slip progresses, the affected child develops progressive out-toeing and a worsening limp. Acute slips result in severe pain and are more likely to be identified early. Physical examination reveals a decreased range of motion, especially in flexion, internal rotation, and

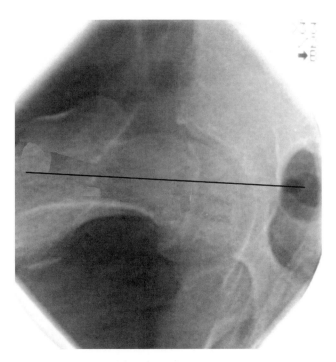

Figure 33–6. Frog leg lateral view of a slipped capital femoral epiphysis (SCFE). The epiphysis is slipped medial (inferior) relative to the femoral neck. In a normal hip, a line through the middle of the femoral neck should bisect the epiphysis on both the anteroposterior and frog leg views.

abduction. The classic finding is a hip that rotates externally as it is passively flexed.

In normal hips, a line drawn through the center of the femoral neck should bisect the epiphysis on both the anteroposterior and frog leg lateral radiographs.[23] (Fig. 33–6). Comparison views are of questionable help as most slips are bilateral. Suspected preslips with normal radiographs should be evaluated further using a bone scan with pin-hole colimetry or an MRI (urgently).

Slips are considered a relative orthopedic emergency once the diagnosis is made or suspected. Even minimally displaced chronic slips are prone to sudden progression with a misstep or twist of the leg. Patients should be placed on nonweightbearing crutches or bed rest pending transportation to a surgeon for definitive treatment.

Knee Pain

Osgood-Schlatter Disease
Osgood-Schlatter disease is a traction apophysitis of the tibial tuberosity that most commonly affects the growing adolescent. It represents a painful healing response to a chronic avulsion injury from the pull of the patellar tendon on the developing tibial tuberosity.[24] This leads to cartilage and bone proliferation and frequently

inflammation. It affects girls and boys equally and is more likely in siblings of affected individuals.[25]

Physical examination reveals a tender, swollen, and prominent tibial tuberosity. There may be a mild extensor lag, and pain is aggravated by resisted knee extension or partial squats. Quadriceps and hamstring muscle tightness are common findings and are predisposing factors. Routine radiographs are not necessary unless some other condition such as tumor or infection is suspected.

Treatment depends on the severity of symptoms. Athletes should be cautioned against jumping or cutting activities as the inherent violent quadriceps contractions predispose these individuals to an acute avulsion injury. Immobilization for 2 to 3 weeks is only indicated for severe symptoms or in patients who may be unreliable or noncompliant. Most require relative rest, ice massage, and analgesics until pain abates. A general guideline is to prohibit any activity that causes limping. Quadriceps and hamstring flexibility exercises are begun immediately, and a strength program is instituted when pain no longer occurs with activities of daily living. The strengthening program consists of straight leg raises, 3 sets of 10 repetitions. The athlete starts with 3 to 5 lb and progresses to 12 lb of resistance.[26] Neoprene knee braces and infrapatellar straps may offer symptomatic relief. Running can begin when there is no pain with walking or rehabilitation exercises and is progressed as long as there is no pain.

Sinding-Larsen-Johansson Syndrome
This syndrome refers to a partial ligamentous avulsion and soft-tissue calcification, or stress fracture, at the inferior pole of the patella.[25] The etiology is probably chronic stress from repetitive use of the knee extensor mechanism during running. Children may present with an acute exacerbation of a chronic condition.

Physical examination reveals tenderness localized to the inferior pole of the patella. The pain is aggravated by resisted knee extension and partial squats. Tight quadriceps and hamstrings are frequently present. An extensor lag indicates a possible inferior pole sleeve avulsion fracture.

Radiographs may reveal calcification at the inferior pole or an avulsion fracture. Partial ligamentous tears cause pain but normal radiographs are seen.

Patients with an extensor lag and a sleeve avulsion fracture should be referred for possible surgical treatment. Acute trauma superimposed on a chornic Sinding-Larsen-Johansson syndrome, with no sleeve avulsion, requires 4 to 6 weeks of immobilization to rest the area and allow healing.[25] Subacute and chronic pain is treated in the same manner as Osgood-Schlatter disease.

Foot and Ankle Pain

Freiberg's Infraction

Freiberg's infraction is an osteochondrosis of the distal metatarsal epiphysis, more prevalent in girls, and most commonly affecting the second metatarsal and occasionally the third or fourth metatarsal. The etiology is unclear, but the disease results in articular surface flattening and subchondral bone collapse. Athletes generally become symptomatic between 12 and 15 years old but can present as early as 8 years.[27]

Affected runners complain of an insidious onset of pain in the metatarsophalangeal joint or vague forefoot pain that worsens with running and improves with rest. Physical examination reveals tenderness with or without soft tissue thickening over the metatarsal head. Pain may be aggravated by axial compression of the proximal phalanx. Motion is limited by pain and soft-tissue thickening.

Radiographs demonstrate squaring off of the metatarsal head in early disease. More progressive disease results in joint space narrowing, hypertrophy of the metatarsal head, irregular base of the proximal phalanx, collapse, and fragmentation.[28] A bone scan or MRI will be positive prior to plain radiographic changes and can be helpful in diagnosing early cases.

Treatment revolves around relieving stress on the involved joint. Mild cases can be treated with a metatarsal pad proximal to the joint and an orthosis to correct for overpronation if present. A semirigid full-length foot plate (spring steel or carbon fiber) can be used under a corrective orthosis to decrease stress on the metatarsal head further. More significant pain should be treated with cast immobilization until symptoms obate, followed by a staged return to full activity using a metatarsal pad and orthosis.[28] Athletes who have advanced disease or persistent pain in spite of conservative therapy should be referred for possible surgical treatment.

Köhler's Disease

Köhler's disease is an osteochondroses of the tarsal navicular that results in medial foot and arch pain. It is characterized by an insidious onset of navicular pain in children 2 to 9 years of age.[29] Physical findings are limited to tenderness of the tarsal navicular with minimal swelling. Plain radiographs reveal narrowing and increased density of the tarsal navicular.

Treatment is to support the navicular area with medial longitudinal arch supports and relative rest. Short-term casting may be indicated in young runners with significant pain. This is generally a completely reversible condition.[29]

Accessory Navicular Syndrome

Pain over the medial prominence of the tarsal navicular may be due to a symptomatic accessory navicular bone. There may be erythema and tenderness over the medial prominence due to bursal irritation. With apophysitis, there is tenderness to palpation, and pain is elicited with resisted foot inversion and plantarflexion (due to traction from the pull of the posterior tibialis tendon). Radiographs reveal the characteristic prominence and smooth margins of the accessory navicular but are otherwise normal (Fig. 33–7).

The superficial bursitis is treated by modifying the footwear to accommodate the medial prominence and/or placing an orthopedic felt donut pad over the area. Accessory navicular apophysitis is treated with a longitudinal arch support, ice, NSAIDs, and decreased

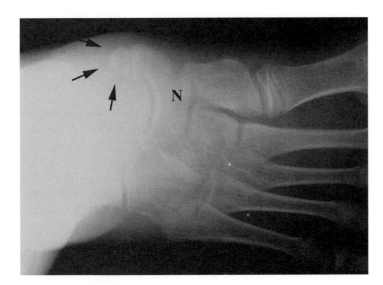

Figure 33–7. The accessory navicular bone (arrows) is best seen on the anteroposterior view. N, navicular bone.

activities. More severe cases can initially be treated with a range of motion walker or short-leg walking cast for 3 to 4 weeks followed by arch supports. Surgical excision can be considered if conservative measures fail.[30]

Sever's Disease (Calcaneal Apophysitis)

This is the most common cause of heel pain in the 9- to 11-year-old runner and is caused by repetitive trauma to the calcaneal apophysis. There is a history of insidious onset of heel pain aggravated by walking barefoot on hard surfaces or with running. Affected children may have an antalgic gait or even walk on tiptoe to avoid direct trauma. On physical examination there is minimal to no swelling around the heel, but it is tender to palpation, especially with a mediolateral squeeze. Heel cord tightness and/or calcaneal eversion can both predispose to and aggravate this condition. Radiographs are generally not helpful or necessary unless other conditions are being ruled out.

Treatment depends on the severity of symptoms. Minimally symptomatic children can be treated with a cushioned heel lift, orthosis (with planovalgus feet), heel cord stretching, and running as tolerated. More severe cases should be treated with a short leg walking cast for 10 to 14 days to rest the heel completely.[29] This is followed by a heel cup, corrective orthosis if indicated, heel cord stretching, and a gradual return to running.

Osteochondral Lesions of the Talar Dome

Osteochondral lesions of the talar dome can cause deep ankle pain and variable swelling. There may be mechanical symptoms of locking or catching, and symptoms are aggravated by running. Posteromedial lesions (55% of cases) are not typically associated with trauma, whereas anterolateral lesions (45% of cases) are.[31]

Physical examination findings may be absent or limited to a reactive synovitis around the ankle. There may be focal tenderness over the anterolateral talus when examined with the foot plantarflexed and inverted.

Posteroanterior, lateral, and mortice views will identify 70% to 100% of the lesions, and they are staged as follows based on their radiographic appearance (Fig. 33–8)[32]:

    Stage 1 small area of compression of subchondral bone
    Stage 2 partially attached osteochondral fragment
    Stage 3 completely detached, nondisplaced fragment
    Stage 4 completely detached, displaced fragment

An MRI or computed tomography (CT) scan can readily identify lesions not detected by plain radiographs.

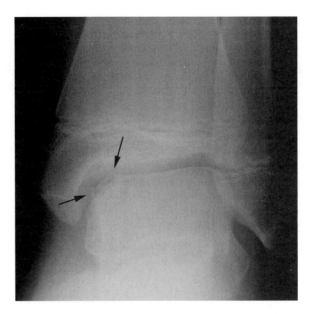

Figure 33–8. Stage 3 osteochondral lesion of the medial talus (arrows).

Asymptomatic stage 1, 2, and 3 lesions do not require treatment.[31] Symptomatic stage 1 lesions can be treated with restricted activity and limited motion until symptoms resolve. Treatment of symptomatic stage 2 lesions with a short-leg walking cast for at least 6 weeks is effective in 90% of cases.[33] Patients with symptomatic stage 3 or 4 lesions, or stage 2 lesions that have failed up to 4 to 6 months of casting, should be referred to an orthopedic surgeon.

Rigid (Peroneal Spastic) Flatfoot or Tarsal Coalition

Rigid flatfoot is a congenital deformity caused by a developmental failure of the tarsal bones to separate, leaving a bony, cartilaginous, or fibrous bridge between two or more of the tarsal bones (Fig. 33–9). This limits normal subtalar and midfoot motion, leading to inflammation of the involved joints. The peroneal tendon crosses over the subtalar joint and often goes into spasm secondary to subtalar inflammation, hence the term "peroneal spastic flatfoot." Tarsal coalition is present in approximately 1% of the population and is bilateral in 50% to 60% of patients.[34] Talocalcaneal coalitions comprise 48% of all coalitions and generally become symptomatic between 8 and 12 years of age.[34] Calcaneonavicular coalitions occur in 43% of the patients and become symptomatic between 12 and 16 years of age.[34]

Patients with tarsal coalition develop insidious, or occasionally acute, onset of arch, ankle, midfoot, or hindfoot pain. Patients may have a history of frequent ankle sprains due to the limited subtalar motion. On

(a)

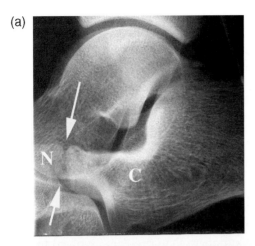

(b)

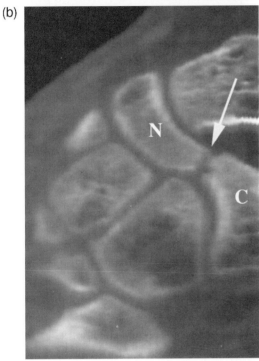

Figure 33–9. (*a*) Lateral ankle radiograph demonstrating a square appearance of the anterior calcaneal process contiguous with the navicula. The narrow gap between (arrows) is consistent with a cartilaginous but not bony calcaneaonavicular coalition. N, navicular bone; C, calcaneus. (*b*) Computed tomogram (CT) of a cartilaginous calcaneonavicular coalition. Note the narrow pseudo-articulation (arrow) and the crenulated surfaces of the calcaneous (C) and navicular bone (N).

physical examination the patient will have a slightly flat or flattened arch. While standing in neutral, the calcaneus will be everted and will minimally invert upon standing tiptoe. There is little to no motion in the subtalar and transverse tarsal joints, and stress on these joints frequently causes pain. Standard roentgenographic evaluation includes anteroposterior, lateral, 45-degree oblique, and Broden's (subtalar) views. Bony

calcaneonavicular bars are best visualized with the 45-degree oblique view, and the Broden's view best demonstrates talocalcaneal bars. A fine-cut CT is often necessary to demonstrate a tarsal coalition as it better visualizes small bony bridges and changes consistent with cartilaginous coalitions (crenulation and eburnation) (Fig. 33–9b). Technitium bone scans generally show increased uptake in the involved joints.

A child with a symptomatic tarsal coalition should be treated initially with a short-leg walking cast for 4 to 6 weeks to allow the inflamed joints to rest. This is followed by an ankle-foot orthosis (AFO) or prescription foot orthosis to minimize the subtalar and transverse tarsal motion. Orthopedic referral should be considered in individuals who fail to respond to conservative treatment or are involved in competitive athletics.

NONMUSCULOSKELETAL CONSIDERATIONS

Heat Intolerance

A hot environment imposes two separate but additive physiologic stressors to the exercising individual. Environmental heat stress alone, in a euhydrated athlete, can decrease maximal aerobic power by up to 7%.[35] Mild dehydration (1% to 2% body weight) in a temperate climate can result in a decrease in physical work capacity,[36,37] and dehydration of 3% will decrease maximal aerobic power.[38,39] In hot climates, smaller fluid losses (2%) can result in a large decrement in both aerobic power and physical work capacity.[39] Adults commonly dehydrate by 2% to 8% of their body weight during exercise in the heat,[38] and children appear to demonstrate a similar degree of hypohydration.[40] There is a direct relationship between increases in water deficits and increases in core temperatures in both children and adults.[41] Children, however, manifest a higher core temperature for any degree of hypohydration than do adults (Fig. 33–10).

Children absorb more heat than adults due to their higher body surface area-to-mass ratio. They have a less-efficient sweating mechanism and therefore rely more on nonevaporative mechanisms for heat dissipation than do adults.[41] Although the potential for heat storage is greater in children, they are able to thermoregulate as well as adults when exercising in an environment up to 5°C to 7°C above skin temperature and less than 50% relative humidity.[41] In climates 10°C greater than skin temperature, children have decreased heat tolerance manifested by higher core temperatures and lower sweating rates than adults.[41]

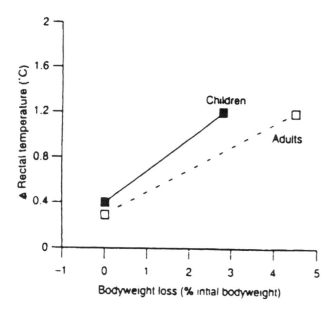

Figure 33–10. Children manifest a higher core temperature at any level of dehydration than do adults. (*Source: Bar-Or O: Voluntary hypohydration in 10- to 12-year-old boys.* J Appl Physiol *1980:48, 106.*)

Fluids and Electrolytes

It is apparent from the above discussion that euhydration is critical in minimizing heat stress in exercising children. In adults, thirst is stimulated by increased plasma osmolality consequent to sodium losses in sweat. Thirst, unfortunately, is not perceived in adults until they have lost 2% of body weight in fluid.[39] Children, in spite of lower sweat sodium losses, have an increased thirst intensity even with losses of body water as low as 100 g.[42] Neither children nor adults will voluntarily fully replenish fluids when allowed to drink plain water during exercise in hot climates.[43] Children drinking flavored glycogen replacement drinks will, however, maintain adequate hydration during prolonged exercise in the heat. Wilk and Bar-Or[43,44] investigated the drinking behavior of prepubescent children offered three different drink types while exercising in the heat. Subjects were allowed to drink either plain water, grape-flavored water, or grape-flavored water with a 6% carbohydrate solution. Children drinking either plain water or grape-flavored water failed to maintain adequate hydration, whereas those given grape-flavored water with carbohydrates consistently maintained adequate hydration.

The primary purpose of a sport drink is to maintain hydration. A secondary purpose is to supply extra energy (glucose) for the working muscle. Sodium is included in most sports drinks becuase it (1) replaces sodium losses from sweating; (2) facilitates glucose transport across the gut lumen; and (3) enhances water absorption secondary to the increased plasma osmolality from the glucose and sodium in the plasma. The sodium concentration of commercial sports drinks is 20 to 25 mmol/L, which is slightly below the concentration of children's sweat. This relatively low concentration prevents sodium overload. For moderate exercise in dry heat, children should ingest 7 ml/kg/hr of a sport drink to prevent dehydration.[40] The amount should be increased with higher temperatures, exercise at higher intensities, and in acclimatized children. (Acclimatization results in higher sweat rates.)

PSYCHOLOGICAL CONCERNS

A large number of children are involved in sports, yet only a small percentage train and compete intensively. Competition has less psychological impact on the young athlete than the rigors of training. Competitive 8- to 12-year-olds will frequently train 10 to 15 hours a week, and adolescents may train up to 28 hours a week. The effects of training are compounded by other factors such as family/peer relationships, education demands, and other life events. Unrealistic expectations can lead to adverse effects on emotional growth and interpersonal development.[45,46] A runner's self-concept may become tied to athletic success, with loss in competition producing a decreased feeling of self-worth. Promising child athletes who drop out of competition in adolescence may require special support.[47]

Successful athletes usually enjoy improved group status, but long hours of training may prevent the making and retaining of lasting friendships. Training and competing behaviors lessen helping and sharing behaviors, which may lead to impaired social behavior.

Psychological stresses from sports may lead to an increased risk of injury or illness. Interestingly, elite runners have been shown to be more somatically focused and hypochondriacal than age-matched peers and are more likely to deny the impact of stresses on their lives.[48] Extremely motivated athletes, however, may ignore injuries, feeling that this signifies mental toughness or courage. The treating physician must also be aware that injuries may serve as an acceptable "out" for an athlete who no longer desires to compete but feels compelled to continue by the expectations of others. Desire to achieve a lean, competitive body may encourage anorexia, bulimia, or excessive exercise, leading to amenorrhea, with a poor self-image and sense of self-worth.[47]

Goal Setting

Goal setting can be useful in helping a young runner improve performance. The goals one sets can be based on a personal best time, time for an individual race, or finishing position. It is recommended that most young runners (not necessarily the elite) base their goal on a time for each race rather than position of finish.[49] This goal should be challenging yet attainable based on course conditions and the individual's training. The process of setting this specific goal for each race raises the runner's self-awareness of current ability, which helps in planning effort and strategy. Goal setting based on finishing position is not recommended because the athlete has no control over how competitors will run. Failure to meet this type of goal may then reduce the athlete's future motivation.[50]

AMENORRHEA

Primary amenorrhea is the absence of menstruation by age 16, and secondary amenorrhea is the absence of at least three contiguous menstrual cycles after menarche. Either form is of particular concern in young runners due to the potential metabolic consequnces. Peak bone mass is accrued between 16 and 30 years, with 48% accrued in the adolescent years. Adequate estrogen is essential for this to occur, and amenorrhea is frequently a sign of hypoestrogenemia. These young girls then, may be losing bone when they should be building bone—placing them at risk for osteoporosis in later years.

The American Academy of Pediatrics recommends the following actions for prevention and treatment of athletic amenorrhea[51]:

1. Investigation of menstrual history and diet as part of the preparticipation physical
2. Diet and nutrition education for athletes, parents, and coaches
3. Monitoring of menses, growth velocity, diet, weight, and skin folds while training and competing
4. Consideration of anorexia nervosa as a diagnosis
5. Calcium supplementation if the diet has less than 1200 mg/day
6. Decreased intensity of exercise if amenorrhea occurs within 3 years of onset of menses
7. Consideration of pregnancy as a cause!
8. Estrogen supplementation in adult women (16 years old or more than 3 years past menarche) if amenorrhea occurs and the patient is hypoestrogenemic

Please refer to the next chapter on "The Female Runner"for a detailed discussion of the diagnosis and treatment of this disorder.

GUIDELINES FOR THE YOUNG RUNNER

Organized exercises in children should have three main goals: (1) to improve general fitness and coordination, (2) to minimize injuries, and (3) to enhance social development through group activities.[52] Adult supervision is essential for a successful organized sport. The focus of this supervision is to ensure broad participation in a wide variety of activities. This seems to prevent "burnout," provide enhancement of sport-specific and general skills, prevent injury, and prevent training and competition from dominating the child's life.[53]

Running as aerobic conditioning is integral to sports such as soccer and basketball and is recommended for others such as football and baseball.[54] Aerobic conditioning or endurance is a function of intensity, duration, and frequency of training. General recommendations are a minimum frequency of three times a week, at 75% of the maximum heart rate or 50% of the $\dot{V}O_2$max, and a duration 30 to 60 minutes a session.[55]

Training should be preceded by a warm-up and followed by a cool-down, which includes adequate time for stretching. Training should start at a low intensity for 3 to 4 weeks and then progress at a rate of no more than 10% a week.

Recommended Distances for Children

The American Academy of Pediatrics takes a very simple and straightforward approach in its running guidelines: if the child enjoys the sport and is asymptomatic, there are no restrictions on distance.[46]

The Australian Sports Medicine Federation recommends the following distance guidelines:

Competition Distance

Age (Yr)	Distance (km)
<9	3
9–11	5
12–14	10
15–16	21.1 (half marathon)
17	30
18+	42.2 (full marathon)

Competition Frequency

Ten kilometers or less can be done weekly; longer than 10 km requires a longer recovery and must be tailored to the athlete. Sprinters have greater risk of muscle-tendon unit tears, strains, and avulsions and should train and compete with this concern in mind.[52]

Training Frequency and Duration

Training should be three times a week for those under 14 years and five times a week for athletes older than

14 years. Training sessions should not last longer than 90 minutes including warm-up and cool-down.[52]

CONCLUSIONS

Running sports for the pediatric population are a beneficial investment in time and effort. Children and adolescents are not just small adults and require special consideration. Although a number of specific risks are inherent in running children, these can be avoided with proper anticipation and guidance. All adults involved with children's sport must be educated to avoid or recognize problems before they have a significant impact on the athlete. With appropriate cooperation among coaches, teachers, family, peers, and the athlete, participation in running sports can be a rewarding experience.

REFERENCES

1. Raunicar AR, Strong WB: The status of adolescent physical fitness. *Adoles Med State Art Rev* 1991:2, 65.
2. Blair SN, Kohl HW, Paffenbarger RS, et al.: Physical fitness and all cause mortality: A prospective study of healthy men and women. *JAMA* 1989:262, 2395.
3. U.S. Public Health Service: *Healthy People 2000: National Health Promotion and Disease Prevention Objectives*, Washington, DC, U.S. Department of Health and Human Services, 1991.
4. Braden DS, Carroll JF: Normative cardiovascular responses to exercise in children. *Pediatr Cardiol* 1999:20, 4.
5. Tuckman B, Hinkle J: An experimental study of the physical and psychological effects of aerobic exercise on schoolchildren. *Health Psychol* 1986:5, 197.
6. Turley KR, Wilmore JH: Cardiovascular responses to treadmill and cycle ergometer exercise in children and adults. *J Appl Physiol* 1997:83, 948.
7. Wells C: The limits of female performance, in Clark DH, Eckert HM (eds.), *American Academy of Physical Education Papers 18*. Champaign, IL, Human Kinetic Publishers, 1985:68.
8. Bar-Or O: *Pediatric Sports Medicine for the Practitioner*, New York Springer-Verlag, 1983.
9. Rosenthal M, Bush A: Haemodynamics in children during rest and exercise: Methods and normal values. *Eur Respir J* 1998:11, 854.
10. Coyle EF: Cardiovascular function during exercise: Neural control factors. *Gatorade Sports Sci Inst* 1991:4, 1.
11. Pianosi P, Seargeant L, Hawarth JC: Blood lactate and pyruvate concentrations, and their ratio during exercise in healthy children: Developmental perspective. *Eur J Appl Physiol* 1995:71, 518.
12. Rowland TW, Green GM: Anaerobic threshold and the determination of target training heart rates in premenarcheal girls. *Pediatr Cardiol* 1989:10, 75.
13. Washington RL, Gundy JC van, Cohen C, et al.: Normal aerobic and anaerobic exercise data for North American school-age children. *J Pediatr* 1988:112, 223.
14. Rowland TW: Trainability of the cardiorespiratory system during childhood. *Can J Sports Sci* 1992:17, 259.
15. Payne VG, Morrow JR: Exercise and $\dot{V}o_2$max in children: A meta-analysis. *Res Q Exerc Sport* 1993:64, 305.
16. Draper D, Dustman A: Avulsion fracture of the anterior superior iliac spine in a collegiate distance runner. *Arch Phys Med Rehabilit* 1992:73, 881.
17. Combs J: Hip and pelvis avulsion fractures in adolescents. *Physician Sportsmed* 1994:22, 41.
18. Kujala U, Orava S: Ischial apophysis injuries in athletes. *Sports Med* 1993:16, 290.
19. Mader T: Avulsion of the rectus femoris tendon: An unusual type of pelvic fracture. *Pediatrc Emerg Care* 1990:6, 198.
20. Veselko M, Smrkolj V: Avulsion of the anterior-superior iliac spine in athletes: Case reports. *J Trauma* 1994:36, 444.
21. Wenger DR, Ward WT, Herring JA: Current concepts review: Legg-Calvé-Perthes disease. *J Bone Joint Surg Am* 1991:73A, 778.
22. Hagglund G, Hansson LI, Ordeberg G, et al.: Bilaterality in slipped upper femoral epiphysis. *J Bone Joint Surg Br* 1988:70-B, 179.
23. Kendig RJ, Field L, Fischer LC: Slipped capital femoral epiphysis, a problem of diagnosis. *J Miss State Med Assoc* 1993:34, 147.
24. Ogden JA, Southwick W: Osgood-Schlatter's disease and tibial tuberosity development. *Clin Orthop* 1976:116, 180.
25. Thabit G, Micheli LJ: Patellofemoral pain in the pediatric patient. *Orthop Clin North Am* 1992:23, 567.
26. Micheli LJ: The traction apophysitises. *Clin Sports Med* 1987:6, 389.
27. Smillie I: Freiberg's infarction (Kohler's second disease). *J Bone Joint Surg Br* 1957:39B, 580.
28. Katcherian DA: Treatment of Freiberg's disease. *Orthop Clin North Am* 1994:25, 69.
29. Griffin LY: Common sports injuries of the foot and ankle seen in children and adolescent. *Orthop Clin North Am* 1994:25, 83.
30. Bennett GL, Weiner DS, Leighley B: Surgical treatment of symptomatic accesory tarsal navicular. *J Pediatr Orthop* 1990:10, 445.
31. Shea MP, Manoli A: Osteochondral lesions of the talar dome. *Foot Ankle* 1993:14, 48.
32. Berndt AL, Harty M: Transchondral fractures (osteochondritis dissecans) of the talus. *J Bone Joint Surg Am* 1959:41A, 988.
33. Pettine KA, Morrey BF: Osteochondral fractures of the talus—a long term follow-up. *J Bone Joint Surg Br* 1987:69B, 89.
34. Bordelon RL: Flatfoot in children and young adults, in Mann RA, Coughlin MJ (eds.); *Surgery of the Foot and Ankle*, vol 1, St. Louis, MO, CV Mosby, 1993:717.
35. Sawka MN, Young AJ, Caderette BS, et al.: Influence of heat stress and acclimation on maximal aerobic power. *Eur J Appl Physiol* 1985:53, 294.

36. Armstrong LE, Costill DL, Fink WJ: Influence of diuretic-induced dehydration on competitive running performance. *Med Sci Sports Exerc* 1985:17, 456.

37. Caldwell JE, Ahonen E, Nousiainen U: Differential effects of sauna diuretic, and exercise-induced hypohydration. *J Appl Physiol* 1984:57, 1018.

38. Sawka MW: Physiological consequeness of hypohydration: Exercise performance and thermoregulation. *Med Sci Sports Exerc* 1992:24, 657.

39. Sawka MN, Latzka WA, Matott RP, et al.: Hydration effects on temperature regulation. *Int J Sports Med* 1998:19, S108.

40. Meyer F, Bar-Or O: Fluid and electrolyte loss during exercise: The paediatric angle. *Sports Med* 1994:18, 4.

41. Falk B, Bar-Or O, MacDougall JD: Thermoregulatory responses of pre-, mid, and late-pubertal boys to exercise in dry heat. *Med Sci Sports Exerc* 1992:24, 688.

42. Meyer F, Bar-Or O, Passe D, et al.: Hypohydration in children during exercise in the heat: Effect on thirst, drink preferences and rehydration. *Int J Sport Nutr* 1994:4, 22.

43. Wilk B, Kriemler S, Keller H, et al.: Consistency in preventing voluntary dehydration in boys who drink a flavored carbohydrate-NaCl beverage during exercise in the heat. *Int J Sport Nutr* 1998:8, 1.

44. Wilk B, Bar-Or O: Effect of drink flavor and NaCl on voluntary drinking and hydration in boys exercising in the heat. *J Appl Physiol* 1996:80, 1112.

45. Maffulli N: The growing child in sport. *Br Med Bull* 1992:48, 561.

46. Committee on Sports Medicine: Risks in distance running for children. *Pediatrics* 1990:86, 799.

47. Rowley S: Psychological effects of intensive training in young athletes. *J Child Psychol Psychiatry (England)* 1987:28, 371.

48. Currie A, Potts SG, Donovan W, et al.: Illness behaviour in elite middle and long distance runners. *Br J Sports Med* 1999:33, 19.

49. Lane AM, Karageorghis CI: Goal confidence and difficulty as predictors of goal attainment in junior high school cross-country runners. *Percept Mot Skills* 1997:84, 747.

50. Burton D: Winning isn't everything: Examining the impact of performance goals on collegiate swimmers' cognitions and performance. *Sports Psychol* 1989:3, 105.

51. Committee on Sports Medicine: Amenorrhea in adolescent athletes. *Pediatrics* 1989:84, 394.

52. Australian Sports Medicine Federation: *Track and Field. Guidelines for Safety in Children's Sport.*

53. The prevention of sports injuries of children and adolescents. *Sidelines* 1993:3, 3.

54. Westcott W: *Guidelines. National Youth Sports Foundation for the Prevention of Athletic Injuries,* 1991.

55. American Alliance for Health, Physical Education, Recreation, and Dance: *Health Related Physical Fitness Test Manual,* 1980.

Chapter 34

THE FEMALE RUNNER

Catherine M. Fieseler

During the past 2 to 3 decades there has been tremendous growth in the amount of information available regarding female athletes, as increasing numbers of women become active in sports and exercise. Since running is a simple sport to master, requiring no special equipment or skill, it has attracted a large number of women. In 1978, 769 women ran the New York City Marathon; in 1998, 8952 women finished the race.[1] The female runner presents the clinician with several unique medical concerns. This chapter will review anatomic and physiologic differences between men and women and the medical, musculoskeletal, and reproductive concerns of caring for female runners.

ANATOMY AND PHYSIOLOGY

Prior to puberty there are no significant differences between males and females in aerobic capacity or strength. The production of gonadotropins at puberty results in the major male-female differences (see Table 34–1). Puberty begins earlier in girls, causing the growth spurt at a younger age and closure of bony growth plates an average of 2 years earlier than in boys. The average female is 10% shorter than her male counterpart and weighs 30 to 40 pounds less.[2–6]

Due to the effect of androgens, the average 20- to 24-year-old male has greater lean body mass than a comparably aged female. Females have a higher percentage of body fat due to the effects of estrogen. The average female has approximately 20% to 26% body fat, whereas the body fat of the average male is 12% to 16%. The greater percentage of body fat translates into the extra pounds of fat carried by female runners, which increases the amount of energy needed for running with no increase in energy production.[2–6]

Body fat distribution is influenced by gonadotropins. Women tend to have a greater concentration of fat in the hips and thighs (gynoidal distribution), whereas males accumulate fat in the abdominal area (androidal distribution). Androidal obesity, which is associated with a higher prevalence of cardiovascular disease, hypertension, blood lipid abnormalities, and glucose intolerance, can be reduced through exercise. These adipose cells have greater lipolytic activity than the gynoidal adipocytes, thus gynoidal obesity is much more resistant to reduction by exercise.[4,5]

Bone density is lower in the postpubescent female as compared with the male.[5,7] It is unknown if there is a clinical correlation between this lower bone density and the higher incidence of stress fractures in female athletes.[8–12]

In addition to size, there are other anatomic differences between men and women that can affect performance. Although the male pelvis is generally larger, the female pelvis is wider. This wider pelvis produces a decreased femoral angle (<125 degrees)

TABLE 34–1. DIFFERENCES BETWEEN POSTPUBERTAL MALES AND FEMALES

The female has shorter stature
The female has less lean body mass
The female has a greater percentage of body fat
The female has lower bone density
The female has a wider pelvis
The female has a greater Q angle
The female has fewer and smaller muscle fibers
The female has fewer RBCs
The female has a lower hematocrit and hemoglobin concentration
The female has a smaller heart and therefore a smaller stroke volume
The female has a smaller vital capacity and residual lung volume
The female has a lower $\dot{V}O_2$max

and is often associated with increased femoral anteversion. These factors result in greater valgus at the knee and an increased Q angle[4,5] which may play a role in patellofemoral disorders.[13–16]

The muscular system differs quantitatively, with males having larger and a greater number of muscle fibers. Prior to puberty, there is little difference in the cross-sectional area (CSA) of muscle in males and females. The difference increases significantly after puberty, reaching a 30% to 50% difference in the CSA of muscle between men and women by 20 years of age. This difference is greater in the upper extremities compared with the lower extremities; females have 50% of male muscle CSA in the upper extremities and 70% in the lower extremities.[6] The percentages of fast twitch and slow twitch fibers are similar between males and females, though a few studies have reported a greater percentage of type I (slow twitch) fibers in the vastus lateralis of women and a greater percentage of type II fibers in men.[6] The greater muscle mass results in greater strength in men, predominantly in the upper body. Differences in absolute strength are less significant when expressed relative to fat-free weight (lean body mass).[2,5,6]

Differences also exist in the hematopoietic system. Women have approximately 6% fewer red blood cells than men; hemoglobin concentration and hematocrit average 10% to 15% less in women than average male levels. As a result of the lower hemoglobin concentration, oxygen-carrying capacity is lower.[2,4,5,17]

Finally, there are significant differences in cardiopulmonary function that affect performance. A woman's heart is smaller, therefore stroke volume is reduced.[17] At an equal workload a woman must achieve a higher heart rate than a man; the maximal heart rate is similar in both genders.[5,17] Due to her smaller size, the thorax and therefore the vital capacity and residual volume are less in a postpubertal woman.[2,4,5,17] Due to the combination of all of these factors, a female at the same weight and level of conditioning as a male counterpart has a lower baseline maximal oxygen uptake ($\dot{V}O_2$max).[5,17]

MUSCULOSKELETAL INJURIES IN THE FEMALE RUNNER

An excellent review article on running injuries by van Mechelen[18] examined multiple factors and how they were related to injuries in the runner. A history of previous injury, lack of running experience, competitive running, and excessive weekly mileage were factors significantly related to running injuries. Interestingly, gender did not prove to be a significant risk factor for injuries.

Patellofemoral Pain Syndrome

Despite van Mechelen's findings, a number of authors feel that there is an increased incidence of patellofemoral stress syndrome in female athletes, due to anatomic factors that result in lateral tracking of the patella.[12–16,19] These factors include a wide pelvis, increased valgus of the knee, and increased femoral anteversion. Lack of development of the vastus medialis obliquus, thought to be more common in women, also results in lateral tracking of the patella. Other predisposing factors, such as pes planus and overpronation, occur with similar frequency in males and females. Treatment involves activity modification, correction of foot malalignments, and quadriceps strengthening exercises (especially the vastus medialis obliquus).

Iliotibial Band Friction Syndrome

The wider female pelvis and more prominent greater trochanter may also predispose women to a slightly increased incidence of iliotibial band inflammation.[12,14] These anatomic features increase the span of the iliotibial band, potentially making it tighter. This may produce a friction syndrome and pain at the level of the greater trochanter, the lateral femoral condyle, or at its insertion on Gerdy's tubercle. The most important factor in the treatment of this disorder is flexibility exercises.

Foot Disorders

There is an increased incidence of several foot disorders in women, which in part is due to inappropriate footwear. There is a genetic basis for the development of prominent first and fifth metatarsal heads. Wearing narrow shoes creates pressure on the overlying bursa, resulting in pain and swelling there; eventually, continued pressure may result in thickening of the metatarsal head. Inappropriate shoes may cause corns and calluses, and exacerbate bunions and bunionettes.[13–16,18] Treatment of these disorders includes proper shoes, padding, and good foot care.

Stress Fractures

An increased incidence of stress fractures has been reported in female runners, especially in association with menstrual irregularities.[7–11] Several reviews on this subject[8,20] suggest that a lack of conditioning as opposed to female gender is a major predisposing factor to stress fractures. To some degree, this problem is related to decreased bone density, poor nutrition, and low estrogen levels; training errors are a major factor in the development of stress fractures in both men and women. Stress fractures in runners occur most commonly in weightbearing bones—tibia, metatarsals, tarsals, fibula, and occasionally femur and pelvis.[11,14,15,21,22] Treatment primarily consists of rest. Preventive measures, such as adequate intake of calcium and hormone replacement supplementation, along with proper training, may be helpful in decreasing the incidence of stress fractures.

MEDICAL CONCERNS IN THE FEMALE RUNNER

The Female Athlete Triad

The female athlete triad is an entity described in 1992 referring to the interrelatedness of disordered eating, amenorrhea, and osteoporosis in athletic women.[23–27] As separate entities, each of these disorders is of significant concern; in combination, there is potential for serious morbidity and mortality. Compared with other athletes, women runners have a higher incidence of both amenorrhea and disordered eating, increasing the likelihood that the triad will be present in these athletes. The presence of one of these disorders in a high-risk athlete should prompt the physician to evaluate for the other disorders of the triad. The evaluation and treatment of each of these disorders are reviewed in this chapter.

Nutrition

Disordered Eating

Eating disorders are fairly common among female runners, ranging from mild abnormalities in nutrition to the severe disorders of anorexia nervosa and bulimia nervosa. In some cases, this is a misguided attempt to lose the extra body fat that is part of normal female anatomy, often with the encouragement of the coach. The misconception that "thinner is faster" is still prevalent. Often, this may involve missing meals and avoidance of certain foods.[28]

Although this state of disordered eating often results in inadequate intake of carbohydrates, protein, vitamins, and minerals (especially calcium, iron, and zinc),[29] a more pressing concern is the possible progression to a more severe form of eating disorder.[15,27,30]

Anorexia nervosa is a disorder in perception of body image, no matter how underweight the athlete may be. A body weight less than 85% of the expected weight, an intense fear of gaining weight, and amenorrhea are the other major features of this disorder.[27,30–32] The prevalence of anorexia nervosa in adolescent and young adult females is estimated to be 1%.

The *Diagnostic and Statistical Manual of Mental Disorders*, Fourth Edition (DSM-IV) describes two subtypes of anorexia nervosa. The restrictive type involves a drastic reduction in food intake and/or excessive exercise. The binge eating/purging type involves regular binge eating or purging behavior (self-induced vomiting, use of laxatives and diuretics).[31,32]

The more common disorder, bulimia nervosa, is characterized by recurrent episodes of binge eating, with an associated sense of lack of control and inappropriate behavior to avoid weight gain after binging. Episodes that occur at least twice a week for at least 3 months qualify for the diagnosis.[30,33] DSM-IV describes two subtypes of bulimia nervosa. The purging type involves the regular misuse of laxatives, diuretics, or enemas or self-induced vomiting. The nonpurging type involves compensatory behavior, such as fasting or excessive exercise. Prevalence is estimated to be 1% to 3% of adolescent and young adult females.

Eating disorder not otherwise specified (EDNOS) is a diagnostic category for patients who do not meet all of the diagnostic criteria for anorexia nervosa or bulimia nervosa.[33] Prevalence is estimated to be 3% to 5%.

A complex interaction of biologic, psychological, and sociocultural factors contribute to the development of eating disorders. Eating disorders are ten times more common in females than males. In western culture, thinness is emphasized as the ideal, a factor contributing to disordered eating in athletes and nonathletes alike. Difficulty coping with stress may manifest as disordered eating. Low self esteem is common in these women. A woman's identity as an athlete is strongly linked to her appearance; if she has no other sense of identity, "ideal" body image may become an obsession. A personal history of abuse is common.[30–32]

A high level of suspicion is necessary to diagnose eating disorders (Tables 34–2 and 34–3). It is difficult to differentiate the athlete who runs extra miles to improve performance from the one who does so to lose weight. Menstrual abnormalities are common in athletes and in women with disordered eating. Low body weight and bradycardia are also common to both groups.[5,30,31]

TABLE 34–2. SIMILARITIES BETWEEN ATHLETES AND ANORECTICS

Low body weight
Controlled caloric consumption
Dietary faddism
Increased physical activity
Resting bradycardia and hypotension
Anemia
Oligomenorrhea/amenorrhea

Factors that distinguish disordered eating are aimless physical activity, decreasing exercise performance, poor muscular development, cardiac dysrhythmias, cold intolerance, and distorted body image. Lanugo may be present in anorectics. Dental erosions, parotid gland enlargement, and calluses on the dorsum of the hand may be seen with bulimia.[30,31]

Making the diagnosis of an eating disorder is difficult but critical. Potential consequences include severe electrolyte disturbance, cardiac dysrhythmias, and death. The prognosis for recovery from anorexia nervosa is not good; the mortality rate is 5% to 18%. Treatment involves a multidisciplinary team, including a primary care physician, nutritionist, and mental health professional. Family members and coaches are often involved in the treatment.[28,30–32]

Educating coaches, athletes, and families about eating disorders and proper nutrition is essential. If a coach feels that an athlete needs to lose weight, proper nutritional guidance should be available. Teammates should be encouraged to express their concerns about a colleague's eating habits. The preparticipation physical should include menstrual history and a nutrition screen. The athlete should be asked about any food restrictions, her heaviest and lowest competitive weights, and general dietary habits. She should be asked about use of vomiting, diuretics, and laxatives to control weight, and about her perception of body image.[30,31] Eating disorders are serious, life-threatening conditions; the earlier the diagnosis is made, the better the prognosis.

General Nutritional Guidelines

The basal metabolic rate is lower in women; therefore, caloric expenditure for a given activity is less. To avoid

TABLE 34–3. FEATURES DISTINGUISHING ATHLETES AND ANORECTICS

Athletes		Anorectics
purposeful	TRAINING	aimless
increasing	EXERCISE TOLERANCE	poor/decreasing
good	MUSCLE DEVELOPMENT	poor
accurate	BODY IMAGE	inaccurate

weight gain female athletes typically consume fewer calories than their male counterparts, and in the process often have diets deficient in carbohydrates, protein, vitamins, and minerals. Without proper dietary guidelines, female athletes often have inadequate intake of calcium, zinc, magnesium, iron, and B complex vitamins, with a resultant decrease in bone density, suboptimal healing and immune function, and anemia.[5,29] Estrogen alters the metabolism of vitamin C, resulting in a greater daily requirement. Exercise also increases the requirement for vitamin C. Nutritional instruction should be given and supplementation recommended.[2,3,29]

Iron Deficiency

Iron deficiency anemia is present in 20% to 25% of female athletes. It is very common in female distance runners due to gastrointestinal losses, in addition to lower iron stores, monthly loss through menses, and inadequate dietary intake. Ferritin levels are lower in competitive distance runners than in the normal population. Because iron deficiency with or without anemia is common in female distance runners and may impair performance, screening for this with a serum ferritin and hemoglobin level is advisable. If ferritin levels are low, treatment with supplemental ferrous iron is recommended.[3,5,29] The recommended daily dosage is 150 to 300 mg of ferrous iron in cases of anemia and 50 to 100 mg of ferrous iron for low ferritin levels in the absence of anemia.[34]

Breast Complaints

Breast soreness due to excessive movement of the breasts during exercise has been described in women runners. This complaint is more common in larger-breasted women (bra cup sizes C and D). A sports bra may alleviate this discomfort. An appropriate bra for athletic participation should have a complete cup to prevent motion of the breasts relative to the body, straps which are wide and nonelastic, and fasteners (if present) which are covered on both sides.[5,35]

Another complaint, which is also common in male runners, is jogger's nipple—a raw nipple due to prolonged friction from the bra or shirt. This may be treated and prevented by the application of bandages or petroleum jelly prior to running.[5]

REPRODUCTIVE CONCERNS IN THE FEMALE RUNNER

The normal menstrual cycle is dependent on a coordinated feedback system of gonadal hormones. Gonadotropin-releasing hormone (GnRH) is released by the hypothalamus and stimulates the release of follicle-stimulating hormone (FSH) and luteinizing hormone (LH) by the pituitary. During the follicular phase, FSH acts on the ovarian follicle, resulting in estrogen production. During the luteal phase, the increasing level of estrogen causes the pituitary to release a large burst of LH; this acts on the maturing follicle resulting in ovulation. The corpus luteum responds to LH by producing progesterone.[36,37]

The Effect of the Menstrual Cycle on Exercise

A number of studies have evaluated the effect of various phases of the menstrual cycle on athletic performance; no significant effect has been noted for most athletes.[5,38–40] De Souza and colleagues[38] compared exercise performance during the early follicular and the midluteal phases of eumenorrheic runners with the performance of amenorrheic runners. Not only was there no difference in performance during the different menstrual phases, the results were comparable to those of the amenorrheic runners. Lebrun and co-workers[40] found the absolute and relative $\dot{V}O_2$max slightly lower in the luteal phase of the menstrual cycle, but the differences were not statistically significant. Another study reported an increase in $\dot{V}O_2$ (less economical oxygen consumption) at 80% $\dot{V}O_2$max during the midluteal phase compared with the early follicular phase, but no difference in $\dot{V}O_2$ at 55% $\dot{V}O_2$max.[41]

Menstrual Disorders

Women runners have a high incidence of menstrual irregularities. These menstrual changes may be classified as luteal phase deficiency, anovulation, and exercise-associated amenorrhea, which represent various stages in the spectrum of menstrual disorders. Delayed menarche and primary amenorrhea may occur in younger runners.[5,27,37,42–45]

Luteal Phase Deficiency

Luteal phase deficiency occurs when the luteal phase of the menstrual cycle (ovulation to menses) is decreased in length and progesterone production is inadequate. Many women are unaware of this problem because the total length of the menstrual cycle is often normal. A number of studies have shown a decrease in length of the luteal cycle with training, in addition to a negative energy balance.[46,47] This causes suppression of GnRH production. Infertility is usually the presenting complaint for this disorder. Luteal phase deficiency may be evaluated using basal body temperatures, detection of urine LH level, or midluteal phase serum progesterone levels. This diagnosis is likely if menses occurs less than 10 days after a rise in basal body temperature or a surge in urinary LH levels. A midluteal progesterone level less than 10 ng/ml suggests luteal phase deficiency, which can be confirmed by endometrial biopsy.[37,42–44,48,49]

Hyperprolactinemia can also result in a luteal phase deficiency, so a serum prolactin level should be checked. Other hormone levels should be obtained if the history or physical examination suggests an abnormality [i.e., hirsutism—dehydroepiandrosterone sulfate (DHEAS)]. If the results of this workup are normal, an extensive evaluation is probably not warranted unless the athlete is concerned about fertility.[37,42–44,48,49]

Infertility and recurrent spontaneous abortions are sequelae of luteal phase deficiency. Although it has not been reported, a potential risk of inadequate progesterone levels is inadequate endometrial protection and its attendant risks of endometrial hyperplasia and adenocarcinoma.[37,42–44] A decrease in lumbar spine bone mineral density (BMD) has been reported in cyclically menstruating runners. These women were found to have lower estrogen levels than their moderately active counterparts, but had a higher intake of calcium.[50]

Although this study raises concerns about BMD, there are currently no treatment recommendations for luteal phase deficiency other than an adequate diet. Supplemental training such as weightlifting or rowing may help improve lumbar spine BMD.[51,52] When fertility is desired, treatment may include decreased exercise intensity or hormonal treatment such as clomiphene citrate and progesterone suppositories.[37,43,44]

Anovulation

When anovulation occurs, estrogen is produced but progesterone levels are extremely low. There is no rise in basal body temperature. Several different patterns of irregular bleeding may occur, ranging from short cycles (less than 21 days) to long cycles and oligomenorrhea (35 to 150 days). The secretion of unopposed estrogen results in proliferative growth of endometrial tissue. Bleeding is not cyclic and unpredictable. Menorrhagia often occurs, which may lead to anemia. Because ovulation has not occurred, the athlete is infertile. The previously mentioned risks associated with unopposed and low levels of estrogen may occur with anovulation.[37,42–44] A study by Micklesfield and associates[53] found decreased BMD of the lumbar spine in mature female runners (ages 25 to 39 years) with a history of oligomenorrhea but not amenorrhea, even if they had resumed a normal menstrual cycle. Oligomenorrhea was defined as 9 or fewer menstrual periods per year.

Exercise-Associated Amenorrhea

The absence of menstrual bleeding is called amenorrhea. In the case of a woman who has never menstruated, it is known as primary amenorrhea, whereas secondary amenorrhea refers to the cessation of menses once it has become established. There are no precise criteria defining the length of time that menstrual bleeding must be absent to make this diagnosis (different studies have used anywhere from 3 to 12 months without menstrual bleeding to define amenorrhea). This has resulted in wide variability in the reported incidence of this disorder.[37,42–44,48,49]

Primary amenorrhea refers to the absence of menses by the age of 16 years. This has been associated with an increased incidence of stress fractures in ballet dancers.[37,43,45]

Exercise-associated amenorrhea is a diagnosis of exclusion; other causes of this disorder, including pregnancy, must be excluded. Exercise-associated amenorrhea is a type of hypothalamic amenorrhea. Although a single cause of this disorder has not been identified, a number of factors have been associated with its development: delayed menarche, previous menstrual dysfunction, nulliparity, young age, psychological stress, intensive exercise, caloric restriction, weight loss, and eating disorders.[37,42–45,48,49]

Two popular hypotheses for the cause of exercise-associated amenorrhea are hypothalamic suppression and an energy drain.[54] There may be inhibition of the hypothalamic GnRH pulse generator in response to activation of the adrenal axis. Amenorrheic athletes have mildly elevated levels of cortisol.

An energy deficit occurs when caloric intake is insufficient to meet the demands of energy expended during exercise. Studies have shown a reduction in resting metabolic rate in amenorrheic runners compared with eumenorrheic runners and sedentary controls,[55] in addition to lower levels of thyroid hormone (triiodothyronine).[9,55] This may be an adaptive response, conserving energy at the expense of ovulation and menses.

Until the early 1980s, it was thought that athletes did not have to worry about the effects of amenorrhea on BMD because of the positive effects of exercise on bone. Unfortunately, the most significant sequela of amenorrhea is the loss of bone density that is sometimes associated with this disorder.[9,52,53,56–58] Several studies have reported that female runners with a history of stress fracture were more likely to have a history of oligomenorrhea and amenorrhea.[9–11,50]

Tomten and colleagues[58] evaluated the BMD at multiple sites in eumenorrheic and oligomenorrheic/amenorrheic runners and a control group. Lumbar spine BMD was significantly lower in the runners with menstrual irregularities than in the eumenorrheic runners and controls. The eumenorrheic runners had significantly greater BMD of the femoral neck compared with the control group. The oligomenorrheic/amenorrheic group had similar femoral neck BMD compared with controls.

Another study compared gymnasts, runners, and a control group. The rate of menstrual irregularities was similar in the gymnasts and runners as was the percentage of body fat and calcium intake. Menarche was later in the gymnasts than the other two groups and the gymnasts started training at a much younger age than the runners. The gymnasts had significantly greater BMD of the lumbar spine and femoral neck than the controls, who in turn had greater BMD at these sites than the runners.[59] The greater BMD at all measured sites in gymnasts was confirmed by Kirchner and coworkers.[60]

The follow-up study by Drinkwater and associates[61] in 1986 on 9 of the original amenorrheic runners and 9 controls reported resumption of menses in 7 women. Lumbar spine BMD had increased in this group, whereas the amenorrheic runners experienced further loss of BMD. The BMD in both groups remained lower than the control group. In 1990, Drinkwater and colleagues[62] compared BMD with menstrual history. The greatest BMD was found in women with normal cycles, and the lowest BMD was found in amenorrheic women with a history of chronic menstrual irregularities. This raised concerns about the possibility of irreversible loss of BMD. Low vertebral BMD in women with a history of previous menstrual irregularities was reported in the previously mentioned study by Micklesfield and associates.[53] Keay and co-workers[63] reported decreased vertebral BMD in dancers who had stopped training and resumed normal cycles; femoral neck BMD was normal. The concern generated by these studies is for the development of early osteoporosis.

Evaluation of oligomenorrhea and amenorrhea begins with a thorough history and physical examination. The past medical history should note any fractures, endocrine abnormalities, chronic diseases, medications, and congenital anomalies. A thorough menstrual history should be taken, including age of menarche, past menstrual irregularities, last menstrual period, duration and frequency of menses, premenstrual symptoms, obstetric history, gynecologic surgery and infections, sexual activity, use of contraception, and family history of age of menarche/menopause. The athlete should be questioned about her training, including the age at which she started, frequency and intensity of training, participation in competition, and any correlation she has noted between training intensity and her menstrual cycles. The review of systems should address signs of androgen excess (male hair distribution, stria, acne), vision changes, headaches, and galactorrhea. A dietary history should address caloric intake; calcium, iron, and protein intake; eating disorders; body image; and the athlete's heaviest and lowest weight in the past few years and any correlation of weight with menstrual cycle.[37,42–45,48,49]

A complete physical examination should be performed with special attention paid to the following: vital signs, especially height and weight; and body composition if available. Funduscopic examination and visual fields by confrontation should be performed. Look for signs of androgen excess. Lanugo and carotenemia may be present in anorectic women. The thyroid should be evaluated for enlargement and masses; look for signs of hyper- or hypothyroidism. Examine the breasts for galactorrhea.[36,37,42–45,48]

A pelvic examination should be performed, including a Pap smear and cultures. In cases of primary amenorrhea, evaluate for the presence of a uterus (to rule out testicular feminization) and perform Tanner staging. If a uterus is not palpable, ultrasound evaluation should be performed.[36,37,42–45,48]

In cases of secondary amenorrhea, rule out ovarian enlargement (polycystic ovarian syndrome) with a bimanual pelvic examination. A pelvic ultrasound may confirm any abnormal findings. Evaluate the cervical mucus; if estrogen is present, ferning will occur.[37,43]

Recommendations regarding laboratory evaluation (Fig. 34–1) differ slightly between various authors. Initially, a pregnancy test and TSH and prolactin levels should be obtained. Measurement of FSH and possibly LH may also be done at this time. Marshall[37] states that checking LH levels is not necessary in most cases, although it is helpful in diagnosing polycystic ovarian syndrome. If signs of androgen excess are present, testosterone and DHEAS levels should be checked. (Shangold and associates[44] feel that these levels should be measured in all patients.[36,37,42–44,48])

Some authors feel that a progestin challenge (following a negative pregnancy test) provides useful

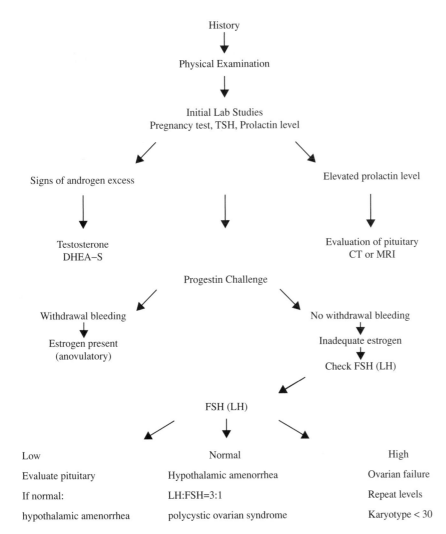

Figure 34–1. Evaluation of oligomenorrhea and amenorrhea.

information. If withdrawal bleeding occurs following the administration of progestin (10 mg of medroxyprogesterone acetate) for 5 to 10 days, endometrial tissue is present and has been prepared by endogenous estrogens. It also confirms that the genital outflow tract is intact and unobstructed. If bleeding does not occur, severe hypoestrogenemia, an obstructed genital outflow tract, pregnancy, or excessive androgen effect may be present.[36,37,42]

If FSH and LH are elevated, the levels should be repeated prior to making the diagnosis of ovarian failure. In women younger than 30 years of age, a karyotype should be performed in cases of elevated FSH and amenorrhea or if the uterus is absent.[37,43]

If FSH and LH are low and the progestin challenge is negative, the sella turcica should be evaluated, even in the presence of normal prolactin levels. Traditionally this has been done with a lateral coned-down view of the sella, but due to the low sensitivity of this study many institutions now use computed tomography (CT) scan or magnetic resonance imaging (MRI) to evaluate the sella.[36,37,43,44]

In polycystic ovarian syndrome the LH:FSH ratio is 3:1 or greater. These women usually have normal or high levels of estrogen plus anovulation. If an amenorrheic patient is 30 years of age or older and has an elevated LH:FSH ratio, an endometrial biopsy should be performed to evaluate for endometrial hyperplasia or carcinoma.[37]

When the evaluation has led to the diagnosis of exercise-associated amenorrhea, several factors need to be taken into consideration, including the athlete's current desire for fertility and her willingness to make lifestyle changes.[37,42–45]

If the athlete does not desire conception, hormone replacement therapy should be considered, in conjunction with optimizing her weight, exercise intensity, and nutrition. No studies have shown that the use of exogenous estrogen causes an increase in BMD of young women with hypoestrogenic oligomenorrhea/amenorrhea.[7,21,60,63] Several studies have reported a decreased incidence of stress fractures in runners on oral contraceptive pills (OCP)[9–11]; this may be due to an improved quality of bone. Recommendations should be made to decrease exercise intensity by 10% to 20% or increase weight by 2% to 3%; many athletes are very reluctant to make these changes. She should receive dietary counseling and increase her calcium intake to 1500 mg per day.[7,37,42–44,48,49,52]

Significant bone loss probably occurs early in the course of amenorrhea, so treatment should be initiated promptly following the diagnosis.[57] Oral contraceptives are a good choice for the sexually active athlete who does not have any contraindication for the use of hormone therapy. If contraception is not a concern, cyclic estrogen and progestin therapy may be used. The most widely used protocols for hormone replacement are similar to those used for postmenopausal women (i.e., conjugated equine estrogen 0.625 mg once a day for days 1 to 25 and medroxyprogesterone acetate 10 mg once a day for days 16 to 25); currently there are no available long-term data on hormone dosage for young women with amenorrhea.[7,37,42–44]

If the athlete desires fertility, she should be strongly encouraged to decrease her exercise intensity and to gain weight. After evaluation for other causes of infertility, ovulation may be induced.[37,43,44]

There is even less knowledge about the adolescent athlete with amenorrhea. A decrease in exercise intensity should be encouraged and proper nutrition stressed. The American Academy of Pediatrics[64] recommends these measures for younger amenorrheic athletes (within 3 years of menarche and less than 16 years of age). In cases involving older amenorrheic adolescent athletes estrogen supplementation is recommended. Estrogen therapy is also recommended for the amenorrheic adolescent athlete who has had stress fractures.[37,43–45,64]

As more data are collected on the long-term effects of amenorrhea on BMD, these treatment recommendations may change.

Osteoporosis

The skeleton is composed of trabecular and cortical bone, the proportions of which vary in different bones. The axial skeleton is predominantly trabecular bone; the appendicular skeleton is predominantly cortical bone. Trabecular bone is porous and has a high turnover rate. Cortical bone is dense and has a slow turnover rate.[21]

Osteoporosis is characterized by the loss of bone mass and deterioration of the microarchitecture of the bone tissue.[65] The World Health Organization defines osteoporosis as BMD greater than 2.5 standard deviations below the mean normal value in young adults. Osteopenia is defined as 1 to 2.5 standard deviations below this mean.[65–67]

As discussed earlier in the chapter, estrogen deficiency is a major risk factor for osteoporosis (Table 34–4); this may be due to late menarche, early menopause, and/or menstrual irregularities. Loss of bone density is greatest in the first 5 to 7 years following the cessation of menses. Other risk factors include white race, family history, medications (glucocorticoids, excess thyroid hormone, phenytoin), sedentary lifestyle, poor nutrition, and use of tobacco or alcohol abuse.[66,68]

TABLE 34–4. RISK FACTORS FOR OSTEOPOROSIS

Female gender	Medications
White race	Tobacco use
Early menopause	Alcohol abuse
Late menarche	Sedentary lifestyle
Family history	Poor nutrition

Bone density can be evaluated by several different methods: dual energy x-ray absorptiometry (DEXA), dual photon absorptiometry (DPA), and quantitative computed tomography (QCT). DEXA delivers the lowest dose of radiation, is the least expensive, and is accurate and reproducible.[65,67]

Treatment of osteoporosis should include modification of as many risk factors as possible. Calcium is recommended for everyone; if women are on hormone replacement therapy (HRT), 1000 mg per day is recommended. For women not on HRT, 1500 mg per day is the recommended dosage. Vitamin D, 600 to 800 IU per day should also be recommended.[66,68,69]

Exercise has been shown to maintain BMD in postmenopausal women.[70] As discussed in the section on amenorrhea, exercise can increase BMD.

Estrogen has been shown to decrease loss or increase BMD in postmenopausal women.[21,69,71,72] This may be given orally (daily or cyclically) or transdermally. The primary concern for many women is the potential of an increased risk of breast cancer. Contraindications to HRT include unexplained vaginal bleeding, history of breast or endometrial carcinoma, active liver disease, and recent vascular thrombosis (Table 34–5).[72]

Postmenopausal osteoporotic women who cannot or will not take HRT may be placed on alendronate. This oral bisphosphonate has been shown to increase BMD. The major side effects involve the gastrointestinal tract. Alendronate has a very long half-life and has not been adequately studied in premenopausal women. It is not recommended in women desiring future childbearing.[7,66,69]

Calcitonin may be given subcutaneously or intranasally. It has not proven to be as effective as HRT or alendronate.[7,66,69]

TABLE 34–5. CONTRAINDICATIONS TO HORMONE REPLACEMENT THERAPY

Unexplained vaginal bleeding
History of breast carcinoma
History of endometrial carcinoma
Active liver disease
Recent vascular thrombosis

Pregnancy

Multiple concerns exist regarding exercise during pregnancy—the effect of increased body temperature on the fetus, the effect of increased blood flow to muscles diverted from the placenta, the effect of exercise on the nutrients available to the fetus, the effect of exercise on the mother's health, and the effects of exercise on birthweight and Apgar scores. A number of adaptive changes protect the fetus during exercise. An increase in maternal hematocrit and cardiac output, along with improved oxygen extraction as uteroplacental blood flow decreases, help prevent impairment of fetal oxygenation. Maternal temperature decreases and fetal temperature is slightly higher than maternal temperature. This gradient facilitates the dissipation of heat from the fetus to the mother. An increase in minute ventilation and increased blood flow to the skin augment maternal dissipation of heat. As pregnancy progresses, alterations in glucose metabolism enhance maternal fat mobilization, sparing glucose for fetal nutrition.[73–78]

A number of musculoskeletal changes occur during pregnancy. Despite these changes, no significant problems associated with exercise have been reported during healthy pregnancies. Pregnant women who exercise report fewer symptoms related to pregnancy—nausea, fatigue, back pain, etc.—than their inactive counterparts.[76,79,80] Exercise has not been shown to adversely affect the growth and development of the fetus.[76,79–81]

In 1985, the American College of Obstetrics and Gynecology (ACOG) made recommendations regarding exercise during pregnancy and the postpartum period. These were fairly restrictive, limiting exercise to 15 minutes and maternal heart rate to 140 beats per minute.[82] As more data on the effects of exercise on pregnancy became available, ACOG amended their recommendations in 1994.[83] General recommendations are made for healthy women with uncomplicated pregnancies. The pregnancy and the exercise program should be carefully monitored and the following general guidelines reviewed with the pregnant athlete:

- Most women can exercise safely during pregnancy.
- Regular exercise is encouraged instead of intermittent activity.
- The pregnant runner should be advised to stop running and seek evaluation if she experiences any problems.
- After the first trimester exercise in the supine position should be avoided.
- Exercise intensity should be modified by any symptoms that are experienced. She should not exercise to exhaustion.

- Adequate caloric and fluid intake should be ensured. This is extremely important to avoid dehydration and hypoglycemia.
- She should dress appropriately to augment heat dissipation and should avoid extremes in environmental conditions.

There are a number of medical conditions that are contraindications to exercise during pregnancy: pregnancy-induced hypertension, premature rupture of membranes, preterm labor during any pregnancy, incompetent cervix (even with a cerclage in place), persistent bleeding after the first trimester, and intrauterine growth retardation. Several other conditions mandate careful evaluation of the risks and benefits of exercise during pregnancy, including chronic hypertension, and active thyroid, pulmonary, cardiac, or vascular disease.[83]

Many women continue running during pregnancy until it becomes too uncomfortable to do so. At that point, encouragement may be given to switch to nonweightbearing exercises, such as pool running or swimming.

During the postpartum period there is a gradual return to the prepregnant condition, with many of the physiologic changes of pregnancy persisting for up to 6 weeks. Resumption of exercise should be gradual and the recommendations for exercise during pregnancy should be extended to the postpartum period. Special concerns during this time are adequate hydration (especially if she is breastfeeding—it is best if the runner breastfeeds prior to her workout); a supportive bra; and urinary incontinence (use of Kegel exercises should be encouraged).[5,83,84]

Menopause

Women should be encouraged to continue running throughout their menopausal years. Two of the major health concerns in postmenopausal women are osteoporosis and coronary artery disease. Weightbearing exercise and supplemental calcium slow the loss of bone density. Aerobic exercise may help decrease the risk of cardiovascular disease in postmenopausal women.[5,85,86]

Around the time of menopause, hormone replacement therapy should be discussed with all women without contraindications for it, and the decision to proceed with HRT should be made on an individual basis.[5,85,86]

Stress urinary incontinence is a common problem for the adult female athlete. There is a positive correlation between incontinence and the number of vaginal deliveries a woman has had.[87,89] Episodes of incontinence are more common during high-impact

---

TABLE 34–6. KEGEL EXERCISES

Goals: Increase tone and strength of levator ani.

Instruct the patient to tighten (lift) the anal sphincter and perivaginal muscles; avoid the Valsalva maneuver. The accuracy of the exercise can be confirmed by digital vaginal examination in the office. The patient may be advised to insert her finger in her vagina to feel the muscle contraction when she is initially learning the exercises. Weighted vaginal cones may be used to increase strength.

Source: From Wallace.[88]

---

activities such as running. The incidence is greater in postmenopausal women, but it also occurs in young nulliparous women. Thus the potential for stress urinary incontinence is great in the multiparous postmenopausal runner.

This problem should be addressed with all female runners, especially those who are postmenopausal. Evaluation includes a careful history and physical examination. A simple test is to ask the woman to stop urinating approximately 5 seconds after she begins to void (the functional stop test). This test assesses the pelvic floor musculature. Inability to stop the flow of urine requires further evaluation; the reader is referred to the articles by Wallace and Elia for further details.[88,89]

Prior to seeking evaluation, measures taken by women with this complaint include stopping or changing exercises, urinating immediately prior to exercising and exercising with access to a bathroom, performing Kegel exercises (Table 34–6), and wearing a protective pad during exercise. Medical management may include biofeedback, pharmacologic measures, intravaginal and barrier devices, and surgery.[87–89] Pseudoephedrine 15 to 30 mg orally twice a day is sometimes used in the treatment of stress urinary incontinence.[88,89]

SUMMARY

Female runners are subject to all of the overuse injuries seen in male runners. There may be a greater incidence of several of these injuries in women due to anatomic differences. Major areas of concern when caring for these athletes include eating disorders and amenorrhea, both of which may produce significant consequences. Screening for these disorders should be a routine part of preparticipation examinations. Early detection and treatment improve the overall prognosis for both conditions.

Special consideration should be given to pregnant and postmenopausal runners. Continued activity with close supervision should be encouraged for both groups.

REFERENCES

1. *Runner's World* 1999:34, 91.
2. Hale RW: Differences and similarities between the sexes, in Hale RW (ed.), *Caring for the Exercising Female*, New York, Elsevier, 1991:31.
3. Hale RW: Factors important to women engaged in vigorous physical activity, in Strauss RH (ed.), *Sports Medicine*, 2nd ed., Philadelphia, Saunders, 1991:487.
4. Sanborn CF, Jankowski CM: Physiologic considerations for women in sport. *Clin Sports Med* 1994:13, 315.
5. Wells CL: *Women, Sport & Performance*, 2nd ed., Champaign, Ill, Human Kinetics Books, 1991.
6. Sale D, Spriet L: Skeletal muscle function and energy metabolism, in Bar-Or O, Lamb D, Clarkson P (eds.), *Perspectives in Exercise Science and Sports Medicine*, Vol. 9, *Exercise and the Female*, Carmel, Ind, Cooper, 1996:289.
7. Nattiv A, Armsey T: Stress injury to the bone in the female athlete. *Clin Sports Med* 1997:16, 197.
8. Goldberg B, Pecora C: Stress fractures: A risk of increased training in freshmen. *Phys Sports Med* 1994:22, 68.
9. Marcus R, Cann C, Madvig P, et al.: Menstrual function and bone mass in elite women distance runners. *Ann Intern Med* 1985:102, 158.
10. Barrow G, Saha S: Menstrual irregularity and stress fractures in collegiate female distance runners. *Am J Sports Med* 1988:16, 209.
11. Bennell K, Malcolm S, Thomas S, et al.: Risk factors for stress fractures in female track-and-field athletes: A retrospective analysis. *Clin J Sport Med* 1995:5, 229.
12. O'Toole M: Prevention and treatment of injuries to runners. *Med Sci Sports Exerc* 1992:24, S360.
13. Griffin LY: The female athlete, in DeLee JC, Drez D (eds.), *Orthopaedic Sports Medicine: Principles and Practice*, Philadelphia, Saunders, 1994:356.
14. Hunter-Griffin LY: Aspects of injuries to the lower extremity unique to the female athlete, in Nicholas JA, Hershman EB (eds.), *The Lower Extremity and Spine in Sports Medicine*, 2nd ed., St. Louis, Mosby, 1995:141.
15. Ireland ML: Special concerns of the female athlete, in Fu FH, Stone DA (eds.), *Sports Injuries: Mechanisms, Prevention and Treatment*, Baltimore, Williams & Wilkins, 1994:153.
16. Arendt E: Common musculoskeletal injuries in women. *Phys Sportsmed* 1996:24, 39.
17. Perrault H: Cardiorespiratory function, in Bar-Or O, Lamb D, Clarkson P (eds.), *Perspectives in Exercise Science and Sports Medicine*, Vol. 9, *Exercise and the Female*, Carmel, Ind, Cooper, 1996:215.
18. Van Mechelen W: Running injuries: A review of the epidemiological literature. *Sports Med* 1992:14, 320.
19. Arendt EA: Orthopaedic issues for active and athletic women. *Clin Sports Med* 1994:13, 483.
20. Welch MJ: Women in the military academies: US Army. *Phys Sports Med* 1989:17, 89.
21. Snow-Harter CM: Bone health and prevention of osteoporosis in active and athletic women. *Clin Sports Med* 1994:13, 389.
22. Brukner P, Bradshaw C, Khan K, et al.: Stress fractures: A review of 180 cases. *Clin J Sport Med* 1996:6, 85.
23. Nattiv A, Agostini R, Drinkwater B, et al.: The female athlete triad: The inter-relatedness of disordered eating, amenorrhea, and osteoporosis. *Clin Sports Med* 1994:13, 405.
24. Nattiv A, Lynch L: The female athlete triad: Managing an acute risk to long-term health. *Phys Sports Med* 1994:22, 60.
25. Yeager KK, Agostini R, Nattiv A, et al.: The female athlete triad: Disordered eating, amenorrhea, osteoporosis. *Med Sci Sports Exerc* 1993:25, 775.
26. Smith A: The female athlete triad. *Phys Sportsmed* 1996:24, 67.
27. ACSM position stand on the female athlete triad. *Med Sci Sports Exerc* 1997:29, i.
28. Noden M: Dying to win. *Sports Illustrated*, Aug 1994:52.
29. Manore M: Nutritional needs of the female athlete. *Clin Sports Med* 1999:18, 549.
30. Johnson MD: Disordered eating in active and athletic women. *Clin Sports Med* 1994:13, 355.
31. Hobbs W, Johnson C: Anorexia nervosa: An overview. *Am Fam Physician* 1996:54, 1273.
32. Vollmer S: To eat or not to eat: The question of anorexia nervosa. *Family Practice Recertification* 1999:21, 37.
33. McGilley B, Pryor T: Assessment and treatment of bulimia nervosa. *Am Fam Physician* 1998:57, 2743.
34. Risser WL, Risser JM: Iron deficiency in adolescents and young adults. *Phys Sports Med* 1990:18, 87.
35. Hindle WH: The breast and exercise, in Hale RW (ed.), *Caring for the Exercising Female*, New York, Elsevier, 1991:83.
36. Speroff L, Glass RR, Kase NG: Amenorrhea, in Speroff L, Glass RR, Kase NG (eds.), *Clinical Endocrinology and Infertility*, 3rd ed., Baltimore, Williams & Wilkins, 1982:141.
37. Marshall LA: Clinical evaluation of amenorrhea in active and athletic women. *Clin Sports Med* 1994:13, 371.
38. De Souza MJ, Maquire MS, Rubin KR, et al.: Effects of menstrual phase and amenorrhea on exercise performance in runners. *Med Sci Sports Exerc* 1990:22, 575.
39. Lebrun CM: The effect of the phase of the menstrual cycle and the birth control pill on athletic performance. *Clin Sports Med* 1994:13, 419.
40. Lebrun C, McKenzie D, Prior J, et al.: Effects of menstrual cycle phase on athletic performance. *Med Sci Sports Exerc* 1995:27, 437.
41. Williams T, Krahenbuhl G: Menstrual cycle phase and running economy. *Med Sci Sports Exerc* 1997:29, 1609.
42. Otis CL: Exercise-associated amenorrhea. *Clin Sports Med* 1992:11, 351.
43. Shangold M: Menstruation, in Shangold M, Mirkin G (eds.), *Women and Exercise*, Philadelphia, FA Davis, 1988:129.
44. Shangold M, Rebar RW, Wentz AC, et al.: Evaluation and management of menstrual dysfunction in athletes. *JAMA* 1990:63, 1665.
45. White CM, Hergenroeder AC: Amenorrhea, osteopenia and the female athlete. *Pediatr Clin North Am* 1990:37, 1125.
46. Kaiserauer A, Snyder A, Sleeper M, et al.: Nutritional, physiological, and menstrual status of distance runners. *Med Sci Sports Exerc* 1989:21, 120.

47. Williams N, Young J, McArthur J, et al.: Strenuous exercise with caloric restriction: Effect on luteinizing hormone secretion. *Med Sci Sports Exerc* 1995:27, 1390.

48. Kiningham R, Apgar B, Schwenk T: Evaluation of amenorrhea. *Am Fam Physician* 1996:53, 1185.

49. McIver B, Romanski S, Nippoldt T: Evaluation and management of amenorrhea. *Mayo Clin Proc* 1997:72, 1161.

50. Winters K, Adams W, Meredith C, et al.: Bone density and cyclic ovarian function in trained runners and active controls. *Med Sci Sports Exerc* 1996:28, 776.

51. Lee E, Long K, Risser W, et al.: Variations in bone status of contralateral and regional sites in young athletic women. *Med Sci Sports Exerc* 1995:27, 1354.

52. Wolman R, Clark P, McNally E, et al.: Menstrual state and exercise as determinants of spinal trabecular bone density in female athletes. *Br Med J* 1990:301, 516.

53. Micklesfield L, Lambert E, Fataar A, et al.: Bone mineral density in mature, premenopausal ultramarathon runners. *Med Sci Sports Exerc* 1995:27, 688.

54. Loucks A, Vaitukaitis J, Cameron J, et al.: The reproductive system and exercise in women. *Med Sci Sports Exerc* 1992:24, S288.

55. Myerson M, Gutin B, Warren M, et al.: Resting metabolic rate and energy balance in amenorrheic and eumenorrheic runners. *Med Sci Sports Exerc* 1991:23, 15.

56. Drinkwater BL, Nilson K, Chestnut III CH, et al.: Bone mineral content of amenorrheic and eumenorrheic athletes. *N Engl J Med* 1984:311, 277.

57. Myburgh K, Bachrach L, Lewis B, et al.: Low bone mineral density at axial and appendicular sites in amenorrheic athletes. *Med Sci Sports Exerc* 1993:25, 1197.

58. Tomten S, Falch J, Birkeland K, et al.: Bone mineral density and menstrual irregularities. A comparative study on cortical and trabecular bone structures in runners with alleged normal eating behavior. *Int J Sports Med* 1998:19, 92.

59. Robinson T, Snow-Harter C, Gillis D, et al.: Bone mineral density and menstrual cycle status in competitive female runners and gymnasts (abstract). *Med Sci Sports Exerc* 1993:25, S49.

60. Kirchner E, Lewis R, O'Connor P: Bone mineral density and dietary intake of female college gymnasts. *Med Sci Sports Exerc* 1995:27, 543.

61. Drinkwater B, Nilson K, Ott S, et al.: Bone mineral density after resumption of menses in amenorrheic athletes. *JAMA* 1986:256, 380.

62. Drinkwater B, Bruemner B, Chestnut C: Menstrual history as a determinant of current bone density in young athletes. *JAMA* 1990:263, 545.

63. Keay N, Fogelman I, Blake G: Bone mineral density in professional female dancers. *Br J Sports Med* 1997:31, 143.

64. American Academy of Pediatrics, Committee on Sports Medicine: Amenorrhea in adolescent athletes. *Pediatrics* 1989:84, 394.

65. Dalsky G: Guidelines for diagnosing osteoporosis. *Phys Sportsmed* 1996:24, 96.

66. Goodman T, Simon L: Osteoporosis: Current issues in diagnosis and management. *J Musculoskel Med* 1997:14, 10.

67. Staud R: Osteoporosis: Guidelines for measuring bone mineral density. *J Musculoskel Med* 1998:15, 25.

68. Bowman M, Spangler J: Osteoporosis in women. *Primary Care Clin Office Pract* 1997:24, 27.

69. Moussa J, Elias Y, Libanati C: Osteoporosis: Prevention and treatment in the primary care setting. *Primary Care Rep* 1997:3, 1.

70. Grove K, Londeree B: Bone density in postmenopausal women: High impact vs. low impact exercise. *Med Sci Sports Exerc* 1992:24, 1190.

71. Metka M, Holzer G, Heytmanek G, et al.: Hypergonadotropic hypogonadic amenorrhea (WHO III) and osteoporosis. *Fertil Steril* 1992:57, 37.

72. American College of Obstetricians and Gynecologists: Hormone replacement therapy. *ACOG Tech Bull* 166, 1992.

73. Wolfe L, Brenner I, Mottola MF: Maternal exercise, fetal well-being and pregnancy outcome, in Holloszy J (ed.): *Exercise and Sport Science Reviews*, Vol. 22, Baltimore, Williams & Wilkins, 1994:145.

74. Artal R: Exercise during pregnancy. *Phys Sports Med* 1999:27, 51.

75. Wang T, Apgar B: Exercise during pregnancy. *Am Fam Physician* 1998:57, 1846.

76. Sternfeld B: Physical activity and pregnancy outcome: Review and recommendations. *Sports Med* 1997:23, 33.

77. Artal R: Exercise and fetal responses during pregnancy, in Hale RW (ed.), *Caring for the Exercising Woman*, New York, Elsevier, 1991:103.

78. Artal R: Exercise during pregnancy, in Strauss RH (ed.), *Sports Medicine*, 2nd ed., Philadelphia, Saunders, 1991:503.

79. Sternfeld B, Quesenberry C, Eskenazi B, et al.: Exercise during pregnancy and pregnancy outcome. *Med Sci Sports Exerc* 1995:27, 634.

80. Clapp J: The effect of continuing regular endurance exercise on the physiologic adaptations to pregnancy and pregnancy outcome. *Am J Sports Med* 1996:24, S28.

81. Clapp J, Little K: Effect of recreational exercise on pregnancy weight gain and subcutaneous fat deposition. *Med Sci Sports Exerc* 1995:27, 170.

82. American College of Obstetricians & Gynecologists: Exercise during pregnancy and the postnatal period. *ACOG Tech Bull*, 1985.

83. American College of Obstetricians & Gynecologists: Exercise during pregnancy and the postpartum period. *ACOG Tech Bull* 189, 1994.

84. Clapp III JF: A clinical approach to exercise during pregnancy. *Clin Sports Med* 1994:13, 443.

85. Blanchette PL, Hale RW: Exercise and aging, in Hale RW (ed.), *Caring for the Exercising Woman*, New York, Elsevier, 1991:93.

86. Shangold M: An active menopause: Using exercise to combat symptoms. *Phys Sportsmed* 1996:24, 30.

87. Kulpa P: Conservative treatment of urinary stress incontinence. *Phys Sportsmed* 1996:24, 51.

88. Wallace K: Female pelvic floor functions, dysfunctions, and behavioral approaches to treatment. *Clin Sports Med* 1994:13, 459.

89. Elia G: Stress urinary incontinence in women: Removing the barriers to exercise. *Phys Sportsmed* 1999:27, 39.

Chapter 35

THE GERIATRIC RUNNER

William Micheo, David A. Soto-Quijano,
Carlos Rivera-Tavarez, Eduardo Amy,
Robert P. Wilder, and George Fuller

INTRODUCTION

With improvement in medical care there has been a significant increase in the aging population. In 1990 approximately 12.5% of the population of the United States was over the age of 65, and by 2030 will that number will swell to approximately 20%.[1] By definition, the elderly can be divided into three categories: the young old (ages 65 to 74); the old (ages 75 to 85); and the old old (age >85).[2] Between 1960 and 1990, the population of the very old increased by 140%. It is anticipated that the number of old old in the United States will grow from 4 million to 13 million by 2040.[3]

In the past, the aging paradigm has been that increasing age invariably leads to progressive loss of function, chronic illness, use of medications, and finally disability. The aging process appears to be multifactorial with a genetic component contributing to some of the physiologic changes we see in elderly individuals; however, lack of physical activity also plays a role in the loss of function and disability typically associated with aging.[4] Structured physical activity in the form of regular exercise appears to have a significant role in reversing some of the physiologic changes typically associated with aging.[5] Regular exercise benefits older adults through improved overall health and physical fitness, increased opportunities for social contacts, gain in cerebral function,

lower rates of mortality, and fewer years of disability later in life.[3] Running is a form of regular exercise that can be performed throughout the lifetime and results in physiologic as well as functional benefits, which may in turn improve the quality of life of the elderly.

The older runner, however, is at a higher risk of injury because of age-related changes including prior joint injuries, loss of flexibility, and strength deficits. Thus it is important for the practitioner treating the geriatric runner to be knowledgeable about the demands of the sport, the physiologic changes seen in the elderly, their response to an appropriate training program, and the treatment of injuries in this patient population.

PHYSIOLOGIC EFFECTS OF AGING

Several physiologic changes are associated with normal aging. Alterations have been noted in virtually all body systems. Many of these changes, however, are influenced by chronic inactivity. Aging and inactivity-related changes can be attenuated by regular exercise (Table 35–1). Commonly recognized benefits from regular exercise include improvement in aerobic capacity, strength, and flexibility. Additional benefits include improved postural stability, which reduces the risk of falling and associated injuries, psychological

TABLE 35–1. PHYSIOLOGIC CHANGES ASSOCIATED WITH TYPICAL AGING AND EXERCISE

Physiological Variables	Aging	Exercise
Cardiovascular		
$\dot{V}O_2$max	↓	↑
Max HR	↓	No changes
Max stroke volume	↓	↑
A-$\dot{V}O_2$ difference	↓	↑
Neuromuscular Changes		
Muscle strength	↓	↑
Type II fibers	↓	↑
Type I fibers	↑	↑
Number of fibers	↓	No changes
Fiber size	↓	↑
Muscle fiber area	↓	↑
Muscle oxidative capacity	↓	↑
Motor unit function	↓	↑
Bone and Connective		
Tissue Changes		
Tensile strength	↓	↑
Bone resorption	↑	↓
Bone mass	↓	↑
Stiffness	↑	↓

Source: Modified from Pu CT, Nelson ME.[1]

benefits, including improved cognitive function and alleviation of depression, and reduction in risk factors associated with disease states, including heart disease, diabetes, and osteoporosis.[6–8]

Cardiovascular Changes

Maximal oxygen consumption ($\dot{V}O_2$max) decreases 5% to 15% per decade after age 25[7–9] as a result of decreases in both maximal cardiac output and maximal arteriovenous oxygen (a-v O_2) difference.[7,10–13] The age-associated decrease in maximal cardiac output is largely due to an age-associated decrease in maximal heart rate of 6 to 10 beats per minute per decade, as well as a smaller stroke volume during exercise in the older adult.[7,11–14] Red blood cell count and plasma and total blood volumes are also lower in older adults.[15] Older adults have reduced early diastolic filling during rest and exercise due to reduced left ventricular compliance.[16,17] End-diastolic volumes during maximal exercise are larger in older adults and result in reduced ejection fractions.[10,12,13] Left ventricular contractility is reduced, and blood pressure and systemic vascular resistance are higher during maximal exercise.

Skeletal Muscle Changes

Loss of muscle mass and strength is a component of normal aging. After age 30, there is a decrease in the cross-sectional area of the thigh, decreased muscle density, and an increase in intramuscular fat. These changes are more pronounced in women than in men.[7,18] This decrease in mass is largely due to fiber atrophy. After age 70, there is loss of muscle fibers associated with loss of strength and power.[19–22] Fiber loss appears to be equally distributed between fast and slow twitch types. The loss in type II fiber cross-sectional area is associated with preferential atrophy.[21,23–25] Other effects associated with aging include a deterioration of the excitation coupling process and a loss in the number of functioning motor units, with the remaining ones becoming larger. With normal aging, this contributes to a reduction in muscle strength of 15% per decade from age 50 to 70, and 30% per decade thereafter.[7,26–29] In addition to its effects on athletic performance, the decline in strength with age carries with it implications related to functional ability, including walking; a significant correlation between muscle strength and walking speed and ability has been reported.[7,30] The extent to which strength loss is related to aging itself vs. inactivity is unclear. Aniansson and associates reported isometric quadriceps strength losses of up to 4% per year after age 70. However, Greig and associates identified no loss of quadriceps strength between the ages of 74 and 82 in regularly active persons.[23,31–33] Also seen is a decrease in basal metabolic rate. On the cellular level, ultrastructural changes occur in muscle and are difficult to distinguish from changes of inactivity superimposed on aging. Muscle biopsies from elderly, inactive subjects demonstrate lower IIa-IIb fiber ratios, lower capillary-to-fiber ratios, and poorer oxidative capacity when compared with muscle tissue from younger persons.[20,21,23] These differences are not apparent, however, in habitually active elderly men. Active elderly men seem to have similar oxidative enzyme to those of younger men, and differences seem to appear only when younger athletes train harder.[23,34–37] Glycolytic enzymes and high-energy phosphagen levels appear to be maintained even beyond age 65.[23,31,32] Regular endurance training induces increases in type I fibers, shifting of type II fibers from IIb to IIa, increased muscle capillarization, increased mitochondrial protein, and increased ability to use free fatty acid metabolism during exercise.

Respiratory Changes

Between the ages of 30 and 70 years, maximum lung capacity diminishes by up to 50%, residual volume (RV) increases 30% to 50%, and vital capacity (VC) decreases 40% to 50%.[3] Forced expiratory volume in one second (FEV_1) decreases linearly with age starting at 20 to 30 years of age. Total lung capacity (TLC) does not change with age, creating an increased residual volume/TLC ratio that results in decreased air exchange capabilities.

These changes are probably the result of loss of elasticity in lung tissue and the chest wall which ultimately results in an increase in the work of breathing and reduction in maximal ventilation. Additionally, there is a decrease in activity of the cilia within the bronchi that allows secretions to accumulate.

Cartilage, Ligament, and Tendon Changes

Elasticity of connective tissue declines with age, commencing in the late to mid 20s for both males and females.[6] This decline is thought to be related largely to age-associated changes in collagen and elastin. Collagen is the primary component of fibrous connective tissue that forms ligaments and tendons. It provides high tensile strength and stiffness and protects against overextension. The amount of collagen in ligaments and tendons decreases with aging.[8,38] Increases in density and stability also occur in collagen as a result of increased cross-linkage and diminished action by collagenase.[39] Consequently, aging is associated with increased stiffness of tendons, an increase in the time required to regain original dimensions after stretching, and a more limited range of stretching beyond which full recovery is possible.[40] In later states of senescence, there may actually be increased collagenase activity, resulting in weakening of the tendons.[39] Therefore, aging collagen is less extensible and more subject to overload failure. Elastin, on the other hand, is roughly 15 times as extensible as collagen. It confers elasticity, whereas collagen protects against overextension. As a person ages, the elastic fibers lose water, fray, undergo fragmentation, and gradually disappear.[41] Cross-linkages are increased.[42] Also noted is a reduction in size of proteoglycan subunits; a decrease in connective tissue, glycosaminoglycan, and water content; disruption of cartilage matrix; and a decline in the rate of new collagen synthesis.

The loss of resilience in collagen makes strains, sprains, and tendon ruptures more frequent complications of overly vigorous or unusual activity in the elderly. Capillary blood supply to the tendons also decreases with age, so local ischemia may contribute to rupture. Aging also modifies insertion of tendons onto bone. The cortex of the bones becomes thinner, and the marrow extends into the tendon through small fissures, allowing bone formation to occur in proximal parts of the tendons. Joint mobility and flexibility are also influenced by factors that affect joint kinematics (i.e., degenerative joint disease or internal injury) and the neurophysiology of motor control (i.e., neural inhibition, spasticity, movement disorders, and shortening of muscles due to chronic nerve irritation). These problems, however, can be alleviated by an extended warm-up, proper flexibility, a gradually progressive exercise program, and an emphasis on activities in which tendon strain is minimized, such as walking on a smooth surface.

Bone Changes

Aging is associated with a reduction in bone mass, and consequently bone strength, rendering the skeletal system more vulnerable to fracture. Bone density peaks by the end of the third decade and is higher in men than in women. Genetic factors also influence bone density. African Americans tend to have higher bone density than whites or Asians.[8,43] Bone density remains stable through the mid to late 40s. In women, bone density starts to decline at or before menopause at a rate of 2% to 5% per year for 5 to 8 years, after which the rate slows to 0.5% to 1.0% per year. In men, bone density may remain stable up to age 65, after which density declines 0.5% to 1.0% per year.[8]

PHYSIOLOGIC EFFECTS OF TRAINING

Aerobic Exercise

At least 50% of the reduction in $\dot{V}O_2max$ associated with aging and inactivity can be countered with vigorous aerobic exercise training, at least through age 70.[7,19,23,44,45] Older adults elicit the same 10% to 30% increases in $\dot{V}O_2max$ with prolonged endurance exercise training as do young adults. The magnitude of the increase in $\dot{V}O_2max$ in older adults is a function of training intensity.[7] Active elderly men seem to have similar oxidative enzyme levels as younger men, and differences seem to appear only when younger athletes train harder.[23,34–37] The decline in $\dot{V}O_2max$ for endurance-trained athletes over age 70 appears to be similar to that of sedentary adults and is probably a result of their inability to maintain the same training stimulus they had when they were younger.[7,14]

In addition to the relative preservation of $\dot{V}O_2max$, other factors may contribute to an endurance-trained athlete's ability to maintain a high level of athletic performance, including the ability to use a higher relative fraction of the maximal aerobic power during exercise.[23,46,47] Thus, a fall in $\dot{V}O_2max$ of 5% to 10% with age may not affect performance. Furthermore, if an athlete develops greater mechanical efficiency, the energy cost for any given workload is reduced, thereby allowing maintenance of performance.

Resistance Exercise

Strength training can help offset the loss of muscle mass and strength associated with normal aging. Muscle strength has been shown to increase in response to training between 60% and 100% of the "one repetition maximum" (1RM).[7,48] A number of studies have demonstrated that older men and women can achieve strength gains similar to those of younger persons as a result of resistance training when given an adequate stimulus.[49,50] Increases in muscle cross-section area, however, have been smaller and less consistent. This suggests that strength gains in the elderly following resistance exercise programs are affected by neural adaptations, motor learning, coordination of voluntary motor unit firing, and body coordination in general.[19,21,25,49,51–57]

As with aerobic activity, strength training is also thought to increase metabolic rate, decrease body fat, improve insulin action, lessen the decline in bone mineral density, and improve dynamic balance and level of physical activity.[8]

Flexibility

Research regarding flexibility in the elderly is limited. It is generally accepted, however, that flexibility training can optimize joint range of motion and musculoskeletal function, and thus reduce injury potential (i.e., risk of muscle strains, ligament strains, and low back problems) and enhance functional capability.[6,7]

TRAINING RECOMMENDATIONS

Exercise prescriptions must be individualized to a particular runner's chosen event (long distance vs. short distance) and goals (recreation vs. fitness vs. competition). Following are minimum guidelines for exercise prescription based on recommendations of the American College of Sports Medicine.[6]

Preparticipation Screening

Prior to commencing an exercise program, any athlete can benefit from preparticipation health screening. Medical examination and a clinical exercise stress test are specifically recommended for the following groups[6]:

1. Men >40 years old and women >50 years old pursuing vigorous (>60% $\dot{V}_{O_2}$max) exercise programs
2. Persons with known cardiac, pulmonary, or metabolic disease, or symptoms suggestive of these
3. Persons with or one or more major signs or symptoms suggestive of cardiopulmonary disease (Table 35–2), or two or more coronary artery disease risk factors (Table 35–3)

TABLE 35–2. MAJOR SYMPTOMS OR SIGNS SUGGESTIVE OF CARDIOPULMONARY DISEASE

1. Pain, discomfort (or other anginal equivalent) in the chest
2. Shortness of breath at rest or with mild exertion
3. Dizziness or syncope
4. Orthopnea or paroxysmal nocturnal dyspnea
5. Ankle edema
6. Palpitations or tachycardia
7. Intermittent claudication
8. Known heart murmur
9. Unusual fatigue or shortness of breath with usual activities

These symptoms must be interpreted in the clinical context in which they appear, since they are not all specific for cardiopulmonary or metabolic disease. *Source: From Mahler DA.[6]*

Aerobic Exercise

The exercise prescription for cardiovascular training of the older adult follows the general guidelines for exercise prescription, with some additional recommendations.[6] Exercise should be performed at an intensity of 60% to 90% of one's maximal heart rate, or 50% to 85% of $\dot{V}_{O_2}$max or heart rate reserve. Exercise should be performed for 20 to 60 continuous minutes, 3 to 5 times per week. The exercise modality should be one that does not induce excessive joint or soft-tissue damage in the individual athlete. Because there is a wide range in maximal heart rate in persons over age 65, it is better to use a measured maximal heart rate when possible, rather than an age-predicted heart rate. For similar reasons, the heart-rate reserve method is recommended for establishing a training heart rate in older persons, rather than using a percentage of the maximal predicted heart rate (Table 35–4). Because some older persons may be unable to sustain aerobic exercise for 20 continuous minutes, one viable alternative is to perform exercise in several 10-minute intervals throughout the day.

Strength Training

Strength training should include exercises that train all the major muscle groups: gluteals, quadriceps, hamstrings, pectorals, latissimus dorsi, deltoids, biceps, triceps, scapular stabilizers, and abdominals. One to three sets of 8 to 12 repetitions at a Borg Perceived Exertion Rating of 12 to 13 (somewhat hard), or 60% to 80% 1RM, should be performed 2 to 3 times per week with at least 48 hours between sessions. Because sessions lasting longer than 60 minutes may have a detrimental effect on adherence to exercise, resistance training sessions should be designed to be completed in 20 to 30 minutes.[6,7]

Furthermore, aging and inactivity appears to affect recovery from hard exercise. Following eccentric

TABLE 35–3. CORONARY ARTERY RISK DISEASE FACTORS

	Defining Criteria
Positive risk factors	
1. Age	Men >45 years; women >55 years or premature menopause without estrogen replacement
2. Family history	Myocardial infarction or sudden death before 55 years of age in father or other male first-degree relative, or before 65 years of age in mother or other female first-degree relative
3. Current cigarette smoking	
4. Hypertension	Blood pressure ≥140/90 mm Hg, confirmed by measurements on at least two separate occasions, or on antihypertensive medication
5. Hypercholesterolemia	Total serum cholesterol >200 mg/dL (5.2 mmol/L) (if lipoprotein profile is unavailable) or HDL <35 mg/dL (0.9 mmol/L)
6. Diabetes mellitus	Persons with insulin-dependent diabetes mellitus (IDDM) who are >30 years of age, or have had IDDM for >15 years, and persons with non-insulin-dependent diabetes mellitus (NIDDM) who are >35 years of age should be classified as patients with known disease
7. Sedentary lifestyle/ physical inactivity	Persons comprising the least active 25% of the population, as defined by the combination of sedentary jobs involving sitting for a large part of the day and no regular exercise or active recreational pursuits
Negative risk factors	
1. High serum HDL cholesterol	>60 mg/dL (1.6 mmol/L)

Notes: It is common to sum risk factors in making clinical judgements. If HDL is high, subtract one risk factor from the sum of positive risk factors, since high HDL decreases coronary artery disease risk. Obesity is not listed as an independent positive risk factor because its effects are exerted through other risk factors (e.g., hypertension, hyperlipidemia, diabetes). Obesity should be considered as an independent target for intervention.
Adapted in part from Expert Panel *JAMA* 1993:269, 3015.
Source: Reproduced with permission from Mahler DA.[6]

TABLE 35–4. KARVONEN FORMULA

Subtract standing resting heart rate (HR_{rest}) from maximal heart rate (HR_{max}) to obtain heart rate reserve.

Calculate 50% and 85% of the heart rate reserve.

Add each of these values to resting heart rate to obtain the target heart rate, e.g.,

Target heart rate range = $[(HR_{max} - HR_{rest}) \times 0.50 \text{ and } 0.85] + HR_{rest}$

Source: From Mahler DA.[6]

exercise.[25] This finding reinforces the importance of adequate rest between training sessions for the aging athlete.

Flexibility

Although no one specific protocol for stretching has been established, the American College of Sports Medicine offers a number of recommendations. Flexibility exercises should be prescribed for every muscle group (pectorals, latissimus dorsi, hip abductors and adductors, hip flexors, gluteals, hamstrings, quadriceps, gastrocsoleus). Stretching should be preceded by warm-up activity to increase circulation and internal body temperature. Three to five repetitions of each stretch should be performed. Exercise should incorporate slow movement followed by a static stretch of 10 to 30 seconds. The degree of stretch should not cause pain, but rather mild discomfort. Stretching should be performed at least three times per week, preferably daily, and should be included as an integral part of warm-up and cool-down exercises.

Regular flexibility, strength, and aerobic conditioning that follows the previously described guidelines will enhance athletic performance and minimize risk for injury. Event-specific functional activities, including anaerobic sprints, plyometric drills, and start training should be incorporated into training as indicated.

Before training, a warm-up period of light running should be followed by stretching. Training should commence slowly, with a gradual increase to peak intensity. A cool-down period and stretching should follow training and competition.

SPECIAL CONSIDERATIONS

Osteoarthritis and Running (See Chapter 30)

Osteoarthritis (OA) is the most common form of arthritis. It is characterized by chemical changes within affected articular cartilage, including a decrease in

exercise, 90% of muscle fibers of older men (age 60) exhibit signs of injury, compared with only 5% to 50% of muscle fibers of younger men (age 20 to 30).[58] Older muscle also demonstrates a slower return to resting contractile function following endurance content as well as an aggregation of proteoglycans. These abnormalities have been attributed to stimulation followed by failure of chondrocytes and by associated enzyme (cathepsin, hyaluronidase, collagenase) activity. Exostoses of bone develop at sites of cartilage damage. Potential contributors include repetitive trauma and autoimmune disorders, although their role remains controversial.[59,60] Up to 80% of 60-year-olds have radiographic evidence of osteoarthritis, but findings are poorly correlated with symptoms. Thus, treatment is based primarily on clinical presentation as opposed to radiographic findings alone.

Additionally, the role of exercise in preventing OA has been recognized more widely in the public health community than by medical practitioners.[61] Exercise plays a role in primary (weight loss), secondary [strengthening and range-of-motion (ROM) exercises] and tertiary (reducing risk of inactivity-related diseases) prevention of OA. It is an effective, malleable, and inexpensive modality used to achieve optimal outcomes in patients with the disease.[62] Information available about the effects of sports activity on the synovial joint and in the development of OA is not conclusive and sometimes contradictory. A systematic review of randomized clinical trials published by Van Baar and colleagues in 1999[63] found exercise therapy improves pain control, self-reported disability, walking performance, and the patient's global assessment. There was no difference in the effect of any particular type of exercise when comparing hospital-based vs. home-based programs.

Although a definitive link between sports activity and OA has not been established, reports have suggested a predisposition to certain injuries: spine, knees, and elbows in wrestlers; patella in cyclists; fingers in cricket players; shoulders, elbows, and wrists in gymnasts; hips, knees, and ankles in soccer players; and knees and ankles in football players.[8] Various occupational stresses may also be associated with the development of OA: hands in garment, textile, cotton, and diamond workers; shoulders and elbows in pneumatic drillers; and knees in occupations that require bending, such as mining.[64]

A number of investigations have focused on long-distance running, and in general conclude that running does not necessarily contribute to OA in otherwise normal joints.[65–67] The variability of exercise patterns and the predisposition to develop joint injuries make studies of the relationship of running and sports participation to OA in humans difficult to perform and evaluate. Controlled studies[68–71] in dogs showed an increase in cartilage thickness, proteoglycan content, and indentation stiffness with moderate running after 40 weeks. With more strenuous running, the cartilage and

proteoglycan content decreased, but the animals did not develop joint degeneration. Another study[72] followed dogs for 550 weeks and concluded that there is no increase in the probability of degenerative joint disease (DJD) with lifelong moderate exercise. Buckwalter and Lane[73] reviewed some of the clinical studies in humans and concluded that lifelong jogging or moderate low-impact running does not appear to increase the risk for development of OA in people with normal strength and joints, but appears to lead to an increased risk of developing marginal osteophytes not associated with articular cartilage degeneration. On the other hand, Sutter and Herzog[74] suggest that muscle inhibition secondary to incompletely rehabilitated knee injuries can be a predisposing factor for knee OA.

Although a direct link between sports activity and OA has not been confirmed, it remains prudent to avoid power sports in which excessive forces are applied to affected joints.[75]

It appears that much of the disability associated with OA is secondary to deconditioning and weakness.[76] There is, however, very little objective evidence regarding the value of physical therapy or exercise programs in reducing disability.[77,78] Current approaches include the use of analgesics to control pain and inflammation, as well as active exercises to increase ROM and to strengthen muscles about the joint and thus maximize functional ability.[8,79] Athletes with OA may benefit from alternative forms of exercise that place less stress on the joints, including water exercise. Patients with advanced symptomatic OA who have failed to respond to conservative measures may benefit from surgical remediation, including arthroscopic debridement and even arthroplasty to improve function and decrease symptoms. With increasing emphasis being placed on the health benefits of exercise, more patients want to be active in sports after joint arthroplasty. Different reports in the literature found 29% to 56% of subjects were able to return to sports after hip replacements.[80,81]

Visuri and Honkanen[82] found an increase in recreational exercise after total hip replacement (walking increased from 2% to 55% and cycling from 7% to 29%). Bradbury and colleagues[83] found that 65% of patients who participated in sports before total knee replacement returned to exercise. The majority of patients return to low-impact sports like golf and bowling. Patients who did not participate in sports preoperatively are less likely to begin sports after surgery. There is still debate about the long-term effect of sports activity on the rate of wear of prostheses and loosening and revision rates. Ritter and Medding concluded that light exercise has no deleterious effects on replaced hips.[81] Other studies have found the risk of loosening to be lower in patients with total hip replacement who returned to sports.[80,82] Bradbury and colleagues[83] advise against high-impact activity, but allow low-impact sports and recreation after total knee replacement. Potential complications of returning to sports should be balanced by the beneficial effects of exercise on the cardiovascular system. It is generally accepted, however, that running should be avoided in patients following hip or knee arthroplasty. Walking, cycling, and deep water running are safe fitness alternatives.

Osteoporosis and Running

Health care costs related to osteoporosis are estimated to be $3.8 million per day or $14 billion per year, so prevention of this problem is a major public health concern.[84] Osteoporosis is defined as a bone mass loss of 2.5 standard deviations below that of a young adult woman.[85] Its consequences include decreased quality of life and independence, and increased morbidity and mortality.[86] In runners it can also contribute to stress fractures.

Risk factors for developing osteoporosis as described by the World Health Organization[85] include sedentary lifestyle as one of the modifiable elements. Exercise is an important part of the prevention and treatment of the disease. Among persons who exercise, those who do strenuous or moderate exercise have higher bone mass density at the hip than those who do mild exercise. A similar association was found between lifelong regular exercise and higher hip bone mass density.[87] Postmenopausal women who exercised and took calcium supplementation had less bone loss than those who received calcium supplementation alone.[88]

Type I osteoporosis is seen primarily in postmenopausal women, is associated with estrogen deficiency, and primarily affects spongy (trabecular) bone, predisposing to fractures of the thoracic and upper lumbar vertebrae and the wrist (Colles' fracture). Type II osteoporosis affects older persons (age >75) of both genders. It mainly affects cortical bone and is associated with fractures of the hip and femoral neck.[8]

Osteoporosis is also classified as primary (due to aging) or secondary (due to an identifiable cause). Aging may be related to any number of factors that result in bone mass loss. An age-related decrease in renal mass and a deterioration in renal function reduce blood levels of vitamin D, but increase serum levels of parathyroid hormone (PTH). Aging also reduces the ability of PTH to stimulate formation of 1,25-dihydroxyvitamin D.[8,89] In women, estrogen loss further accelerates bone mineral loss after menopause. Other suggested contributors of bone mass loss include a decrease in calcitonin,[90] prolactin,[91] and testos-

terone.[8,92–94] Contributors to secondary osteoporosis are numerous (Table 35–5). The prophylaxis and treatment of osteoporosis are multifaceted. In secondary osteoporosis, correction of the underlying causes is paramount. High-intensity strength training is effective in maintaining femoral neck bone mass density as well as improving muscle mass, strength, and balance in postmenopausal women compared with unexercised controls.[95] Thus, weightbearing exercises such as walking and running are recommended in older adults for prevention of osteoporosis. Runners with established osteoporosis, particularly those who have experienced stress fractures, should consider minimizing running activity. Cross-training can supplement a modified running program, and can incorporate lower-impact forms of modified weightbearing exercises such as

---

TABLE 35–5. SECONDARY OSTEOPOROSIS*

1. Hyperparathyroidism
2. Cushing's disease
3. Multiple myeloma
4. Hyperthyroidism (endogenous and iatrogenic)
5. Idiopathic hypercalciuria
   a. Due to renal calcium leak
   b. Due to renal phosphate leak
6. Malabsorption (including partial gastrectomy)
7. 25-OH vitamin D deficiency
   a. Due to chronic liver disease
   b. Due to chronic anticonvulsant therapy (phenytoin, barbiturates)
8. 1,25 (OH) 2 vitamin D deficiency due to lack of renal synthesis
   a. Due to chronic renal failure
9. Adult hypophosphatasia
10. Osteogenesis imperfecta tarda
11. Male hypogonadism (Klinefelter's syndrome)
12. Female hypogonadism (Turner's syndrome)
13. Conditions consistent with hypoestrogenism secondary to anorexia and/or exercise
    a. Anorexia nervosa
    b. Exercise-induced amenorrhea
14. Conditions associated with disuse
    a. Paraplegia/hemiplegia
    b. Immobilization
    c. Prolonged bed rest
15. Alcoholism
16. Diabetes mellitus
17. Rheumatoid arthritis
18. Chronic obstructive pulmonary disease
19. Systemic mastocytosis
20. Conditions associated with the use of medications
    a. Corticosteroids
    b. Heparin
    c. Anticonvulsants
    d. Excess thyroid hormone
21. Malignancy

*Secondary to inherited or acquired abnormalities or diseases or to physiological aberrations.
Source: From Chestnut CH: Osteoporosis, in DeLisa JA, (ed.), *Rehabilitation Medicine Principles and Practice,* Philadelphia, Lippincott, 1988:866.

power walking and fitness machines, as well as deep water running for cardiovascular training. Exercise, lifestyle, nutrition, and medications are also important. Young adults who participate in regular, weightbearing exercise develop higher bone mineral content than sedentary persons. The ability to augment bone mineral content through physical activity continues at least into late middle age (up to age 65).[96,97] The capacity of exercise to curtail bone density loss in more elderly subjects is less clear, although subjects who engage in regular physical activity appear to have a continuing advantage over sedentary controls.[8,98–101] The type of exercise performed appears important, as not all exercise programs lead to increased mechanical loading of the bones. In particular, pool exercises and swimming lack the capacity to increase mechanical loading of the skeleton.[8] Lifestyle habits, such as cigarette smoking and excessive alcohol and caffeine use, can adversely affect bone mineral content and should be discouraged.[102] Adequate intake of calcium (1000 to 1500 mg per day) and vitamin D (400 IU per day) is important, especially in postmenopausal women. Postmenopausal women may benefit from estrogen replacement, which limits bone resorption.[8,103] In patients with established osteoporosis, administration of calcitonin also helps to decrease bone resorption, and reduce the risk of fracture.[104] Alendronate is the first drug to receive FDA approval for restoring previously lost bone in postmenopausal women with osteoporosis, and it may be indicated for postmenopausal women who have osteoporosis as defined by the FDA (i.e., lumbar spine bone mineral density of at least 2 standard deviations below the premenopausal mean).

Thermoregulation in Older Adults

Epidemiologic data suggest that individuals over 60 years old are less tolerant to heat than younger patients, but controlled research has not supported this conclusion. Laboratory studies have demonstrated that older individuals respond to heat challenges with higher core temperature and heart rate, lower sweating rates, and higher loss of body fluids than younger individuals, but it is not clear if there is a direct decrease in heat tolerance with age or if this is an indirect consequence of other variables affected during aging. For example, decreased $\dot{V}O_2max$, sedentary lifestyle, altered body composition (decreased body mass), chronic hypohydration, increased prevalence of chronic diseases, and increased use of medications are common phenomena in older adults that may induce heat tolerance independently of age. These variables should also be considered in studies that compare older and younger populations since there are no comprehensive longitudinal studies of aging and thermoregulation.[105]

The two basic mechanisms to eliminate excess heat generated by muscle activity are increasing skin blood flow and producing and evaporating sweat. Studies by Kenney[106,107] have shown significantly lower skin blood flow in older athletes that appears to be secondary to structural changes in cutaneous vessels. It appears that heat-acclimated older athletes activate the same number of sweat glands as young adults for a given skin area, but sweat production is lower. Heat acclimation has a beneficial effect on heat tolerance and athletic performance: lower core temperature and heart rate, higher sweating rates, increased blood volume, and production of more dilute sweat. Studies have demonstrated heat acclimation in older athletes similar to that of younger individuals.[106,107] However, older patients may present in a state of hyperosmolar hypohydration secondary to reduced thirst and increased water excretion, so older athletes should pay close attention to proper hydration.

Advancing age seems to be associated with attenuated vasoconstrictor response during cold exposure. This, added to sarcopenia and a lower basal metabolic rate, has an impact on thermoregulation during exercise in a cold environment, again underscoring the importance of caution when exercising in temperature extremes.

RUNNING INJURIES

Although greater detail for each injury is provided elsewhere in the text, common running injuries in older athletes are reviewed here.

Running injuries occur due to overload of the muscles, tendons, bones, or joints. The knee, foot, and ankle are the most common sites of injury. The causes of injury can be divided into intrinsic factors (i.e., poor flexibility, malalignment) and extrinsic factors (i.e., training errors, worn shoes, irregular running surface).

Training errors account for 60% of running injuries and include increasing weekly mileage to more than 40 to 45 miles per week, running on hilly terrain, and doing interval training.[108] Thorough diagnosis of the running injury should be done using the musculoskeletal injury model described by Kibler.[109] This model identifies the anatomic site of injuries, the clinical symptoms, and functional deficits (Table 35–6).

Achilles' Tendinitis

The triceps surae includes the medial and lateral heads of the gastrocnemius and soleus muscles. The Achilles'

TABLE 35–6. OVERVIEW OF MUSCULOSKELETAL INJURIES

Clinical alterations
  Symptoms

Anatomic alterations
  Tissue injuries
  Tissue overload

Functional alterations
  Biomechanical deficits
  Subclinical adaptations

Source: Modified from Kibler WB.[109]

tendon is the largest and strongest tendon in the body. During running it can receive tensile loads of over eight times body weight and it is not covered by a synovial sheath. The area just proximal to the insertion on the calcaneus is at highest risk of injury due to relative avascularity.[110] Constant repetitive stress eventually leads to degenerative changes at the tissue level, initially peritendinitis and subsequently intrasubstance tendinosis degeneration.

Achilles' tendinitis is one of the most common sports injuries, frequently occurring in mature male athletes who are active in running and jumping activities. It can be elicited by use of inadequate footwear with a soft heel counter, tibia vara, a tight or underdeveloped hamstring, and cavus foot. Male to female ratios vary from 2:1 to 12:1.[110] The diagnosis is mostly clinical, with patients complaining of localized pain of the Achilles' tendon associated with decreased motion and swelling and weakness during activity. Occasionally, a nodule can be palpated on the tendon 2 to 6 cm from its insertion.

Inflexibility of dorsiflexor muscles or weakness of plantarflexors are associated with Achilles' tendinitis. This puts an extra load on the Achilles' tendon that worsens the condition. To compensate, patients suffering from Achilles' tendinitis may run with a shortened stride, landing on the heel with a tendency to jump off the opposite leg.[111] Conservative treatment for Achilles' tendinitis includes rest, physical modalities, and exercises to resolve the biomechanical deficits (i.e., stretching of the dorsiflexors and plantarflexors and strengthening of the plantarflexors and ankle invertors and evertors). A heel lift used in the initial stages of treatment can relieve pain by reducing tensile loading, but long-term use can perpetuate the inflexibility.

Degenerative changes may lead to Achilles' tendon rupture, with 75% of cases occurring in athletes. A high level of suspicion is required to make the diagnosis. Patients may report feeling a pop after rapid eccentric loading when the ankle and foot are in dorsiflexion. Pain is not necessarily severe, but edema and ecchymosis develop, and the patient is unable to continue athletic activity. On physical examination there is a palpable defect proximal to tendon insertion. The patient is able to plantarflex the foot, but cannot perform a toe raise. The Thompson's test can be performed by squeezing the posterior calf in the prone position and observing passive plantarflexion in an intact tendon.

In the case of a complete tear, nonsurgical management carries a higher risk of rerupture and should be reserved for patients who are not interested in high levels of activity. Surgical procedures restore the anatomy, but should be followed by a ROM, flexibility, and strengthening program.

Plantar Fasciitis

The plantar fascia is a tough, fibrous, aponeurotic structure arising from the medial calcaneal tubercle and inserting into the plantar plates of the metatarsophalangeal joints, the bases of the proximal phalanges of the toes, and the flexor tendon sheaths.[112] It provides shape and support to the longitudinal arch and acts as a shock absorber on foot impact. During walking and running it is repeatedly stretching and relaxing.

Plantar fasciitis is a common cause of heel pain, affecting as many as 15% to 20% of runners.[113] It is a microtrauma overload injury usually associated with biomechanical abnormalities. Tight plantarflexors, short flexor muscles, and weakness of the posterior calf create a biomechanical pronation that causes increased load on the plantar fascia insertion to the calcaneus bone and eventually inflammation and pain.[113] Other biomechanical abnormalities of the lower extremity including hip abductor weakness, externally rotated leg, and supinated foot posture may also be present. Patients usually complain of heel pain in the morning that decreases during the day and then worsens with increased activity. Commonly this is not associated with trauma and presents with an insidious onset. It may be diffuse or migratory, but with time it localizes to the medial calcaneus. The patient may relate the onset of symptoms to a rapid increase in distance, speed, intensity, or frequency of running, or to a change to a more flexible shoe.

The diagnosis is based mainly on history and physical examination. The patient will present with tenderness to palpation over the medial calcaneal tubercle and in more advanced cases, over the proximal medial longitudinal arch. Slight swelling in the area may be found. Achilles' tendon tightness is found in most patients. Other associated findings include pronated and everted foot, supinated foot, and tightness of hamstrings.

Initial treatment is directed at relieving pain and includes anti-inflammatory medications (NSAIDs) and icing the affected area. Heel pads and arch supports to maintain longitudinal arch support during ambulation minimize biomechanical abnormalities.

Advice on proper footwear is also helpful, and exercise programs to correct muscular imbalances (i.e., stretching and strengthening of plantar flexors, stretching of hamstring, short foot flexors, and the plantar fascia) are the definitive treatment. Correction of other inflexibilities and weaknesses in the kinetic chain are also addressed. Localized steroid and anesthetic injection can provide pain relief, but physicians should be careful to avoid the interior surface that can cause fat pad atrophy, osteomyelitis of the calcaneus, or iatrogenic rupture of fascia. The use of night splints or in severe cases casting, can reduce pain. Surgery should be considered only if the pain has not responded to conservative treatment after 12 months. The athlete may return to play when full ROM in the ankle is present, heel pain is minimal, and strength is equal to that of the other side.

Stress Fractures

Stress fractures occur at the origin of powerful extremity muscles (the area of greatest local stress), most commonly in the tibia (12 to 15 cm proximal to the medial malleolus), followed by the pelvis, femoral neck, metatarsals, and fibula.[111] Clinically, this injury presents with a gradual increase in activity-related pain that is aggravated by repetitive, forceful loading and improved by rest; and pain and tenderness in a discrete, localized region with minimal soft-tissue swelling. Runners may have recently increased their mileage or intensity, changed their terrain, or switched to a different running shoe.[114] During the first 4 weeks, postinjury bone scan, CT, or MRI can help with diagnosis, while radiographs show reactive sclerosis 2 to 4 weeks' postinjury.

Stress fractures are seen most commonly when the ability of the bone to repair the microtrauma of repetitive overloading is overcome. Factors that increase ground reactive forces tend to aggravate this condition. In addition, poor lower-extremity alignment, inadequate footwear, an improper training surface, decreased flexibility, and accelerated training programs contribute to the development of stress fractures.[115]

This injury is increasingly encountered in elderly athletes. In many cases, they have never previously engaged in regular physical activity, and the skeletal system thus is not prepared to withstand mechanical stress. It is thought that rather than being stress fractures, the injuries suffered are really insufficiency fractures, because they are caused by repeated microtrauma of a bone with lowered resistance.[108]

Treatment during the acute phase consists of rest, ice, and NSAIDs. To maintain cardiovascular fitness, cross-training is recommended. When the patient is asymptomatic, there should be a progressive return to running with decreased intensity. Initially, pain-free runs are allowed on an even, soft surface with new shoes and orthotics if needed.[112]

Medial Tibial Stress Syndrome (MTSS)

MTSS, commonly known as shin splints, is a common example of a runner's overuse injury. The diagnosis is based on the finding of diffuse tenderness over the posteromedial aspect of the distal third of the tibia that is associated with a history of running, with pain improving with rest. The clinical diagnosis can be confirmed with the aid of a three-phase bone scan (the third phase usually being positive as severity increases), and in chronic cases there will be periosteal thickening on plain radiographs. Although the exact anatomic changes that cause MTSS have been debated, most experts agree that there is an inflammatory process of the periosteum caused by overuse and biomechanical abnormalities. Several predisposing factors have been identified in the etiology of MTSS. Among them are mechanical problems that increase valgus forces on the rear foot, such as running courses with tight corners; increased external rotation of the hip; genu varum; large Q angle; excessive pronation; pes planus; pes cavus; and lower extremity length and muscle imbalances.[111] Training errors such as inadequate footwear, inadequate warm-up, uneven terrain, hard surfaces, and cold weather may also contribute.

The best treatment for this condition is prevention, but once the athlete becomes symptomatic, relative rest, ice, NSAIDs, and gentle stretching activities are part of the initial intervention. Strengthening of the lower leg and foot intrinsic muscles is then begun. As symptoms begin to subside, a gradual return to activities is recommended with a decrease in training intensity, and running on soft, flat surfaces. This should be accompanied by flexibility exercises for the lower extremities and cross-training activities to maintain cardiovascular conditioning. New shoes and orthotic equipment may also be necessary. Shin sleeves may alleviate discomfort via a counterforce effect.

Meniscal Tears

The menisci serve as shock absorbers, decrease load concentrations, and help to guide normal knee kinematics.[115] As much as 50% of the compressive load across the knee is transmitted through the menisci (this load increases with flexion). Any injury to the menisci reduces the weight contact area of the knee, placing the articular cartilage at risk for failure or degenerative changes. Common causes of injury include acute microtrauma following hyperflexion or twisting, and chronic microtrauma due to running or jumping. Meniscal cartilage deteriorates with aging, therefore it can tear by shear failure in the older runner without acute trauma. Symptoms include pain with activity, or mechanical symptoms of catching, grinding, locking, and slight swelling. Clinical findings include joint line tenderness and pain upon hyperflexion or hyperextension.

Many patients improve with a rehabilitative regimen of 4 to 6 weeks that includes ice, NSAIDs, and protective strengthening. Surgical consultation is recommended in refractory cases.

Patellofemoral Pain Syndrome

Anterior knee pain is very common among runners and may be secondary to more than one pathologic process with a common clinical manifestation. Patellofemoral pain syndrome can be caused by chronic repetitive overload, particularly with activities that increase joint loading such as running on hilly terrain.

Biomechanical abnormalities associated with anterior knee pain include increased femoral internal rotation, tight hip flexors, hamstrings, iliotibial band, and Achilles' tendon, and increased foot pronation. In addition muscle imbalances, particularly quadriceps weakness, may be associated with patellar pain.[116]

The pain generators include the subchondral bone, synovial capsular and retinacular soft tissues, and the tendon's insertion on the patella. Symptoms include dull, aching retropatellar or peripatellar pain of insidious onset that increases with activities involving knee flexion, such as squatting, sitting for prolonged periods (theatre sign), descending stairs, or running on hilly terrain. On physical examination, the patient may present with patella crepitus, pain with patella compression or quadriceps contraction, and quadriceps muscle atrophy. The previously mentioned biomechanical abnormalities such as hip flexor, iliotibial band, and hamstring and quadriceps tightness may also be found. Gluteal weakness is also a common finding.

Treatment is similar to that of the other conditions discussed above, and includes rest, ice, and NSAIDs during the acute phase. Stretching the tight structures and a strengthening program that avoids excessive knee flexion should be instituted early, in combination with cross-training strategies. Other interventions may include a patella tendon strap or knee sleeves to promote proper patellar tracking, and foot orthotics to correct hyperpronation.[112]

In summary, injuries in the older athlete often result from the combined effects of training and the natural changes aging brings to tendons, cartilage, and bones. Attention to proper training, with a gradual increase in the amount and intensity of exercise, is especially important in avoiding injury in this older population of athletes.[117]

REFERENCES

1. Pu CT, Nelson ME: Aging, function, and exercise, in Frontera WR (ed.), *Exercise in Rehabilitation Medicine,* 1st ed., Champaign, Ill, Human Kinetics, 1999:39.
2. Ting AJ: Running and the older athlete. *Clin Sports Med* 1991:10, 319.
3. Daley MJ, Spinks WL: Exercise, mobility, and aging. *Clin Sports Med* 2000:29, 1.
4. Crespo CJ: Exercise and the prevention of chronic disabling illness, in Frontera WR (ed.), *Exercise in Rehabilitation Medicine,* 1st ed., Champaign, Ill, Human Kinetics, 1999:151.
5. Rogers MA, Evans WJ: Changes in skeletal muscles with aging: Effects of exercise training. *Exerc Sport Sci Rev* 1993:21, 65.
6. Mahler DA: *American College of Sports Medicine's Guidelines for Exercise Testing and Prescription,* 5th ed., Baltimore, Williams & Wilkins, 1997.
7. American College of Sports Medicine Position Stand. Exercise and physical activity for older adults. *Med Sci Sports Exerc* 1998:30, 992.
8. Shephard JR: *Aging, Physical Activity, and Health,* Champaign, Ill, Human Kinetics, 1997.
9. Heath GW, Hagberg JM, Ehsani AA, et al.: A physiological comparison of young and older endurance athletes. *J Appl Physiol* 1981:51, 634.
10. Fleg JL, O'Connor F, Gerstenblith G, et al.: Impact of age on the cardiovascular response to dynamic upright exercise in healthy men and women. *J Appl Physiol* 1995: 78, 890.
11. Ogawa T, Spina RJ, Martin WH III, et al.: Effects of aging, sex and physical training on cardiovascular responses to exercise. *Circulation* 1992:86, 494.
12. Rodeheffer RG, Gerstenblith G, Becker LC, et al.: Exercise cardiac output is maintained with advancing age in healthy human subjects: Cardiac dilation and increased stroke volume compensate for a diminished heart rate. *Circulation* 1984:69, 203.
13. Stratton JR, Levy WC, Cerqueira MD, et al.: Cardiovascular responses to exercise: Effects of aging and exercise training in healthy men. *Circulation* 1994:89, 1648.
14. Pollock ML, Mengelkock LJ, Graves JE, et al.: Twenty-year follow-up of aerobic power and body composition of older track athletes. *J Appl Physiol* 1997:82, 1508.
15. Davy KP, Seals DR: Total blood volume in healthy young and older men. *J Appl Physiol* 1994:76, 2059.
16. Levy WC, Cerqueira MD, Abrass IB, et al.: Endurance exercise training augments diastolic filling at rest and during exercise in healthy young and older men. *Circulation* 1993:88, 116.

17. Miller TR, Grossman SJ, Schectman KB, et al.: Left ventricular diastolic filling and its association with age. *Am J Cardiol* 1986:58, 531.

18. Imamura K, Ashida H, Ishikawa T, et al.: Human major psoas muscle and sacrospinalis muscle in relation to age: A study by computed tomography. *J Gerontology* 1983:38, 678.

19. Frontera WR, Hughes VA, Lutz KJ, et al.: A cross-sectional study of muscle strength and mass in 45- to 78-yr-old men and women. *J Appl Physiol* 1991:71, 644.

20. Aoyagi Y, Katsuta S: Relationship between the starting age of training and physical fitness in old age. *Can J Sports Sci* 1990:15, 65.

21. Cartee GD: Aging skeletal muscle: Response to exercise. *Exerc Sport Sci Rev* 1994:22, 91.

22. Larson L, Grimby G, Karlsson J: Muscle strength and speed of movement in relation to age and muscle morphology. *J Appl Physiol* 1979:46, 451.

23. Young JL, Press JM: Athletic performance—must it decline with age? *J Back Musculoskel Rehabil* 1995:5, 7.

24. Lexell J, Taylor CC, Sjostrom M: What is the cause of ageing atrophy? Total number, size and proportion of different fiber types studied in whole vastus lateralis muscle from 15- to 83-year-old men. *J Neurol Sci* 1988:84, 275.

25. Rogers MA, Evans WJ: Changes in skeletal muscle with aging: Effects of exercise training. *Exerc Sports Sci Rev* 1993:21, 65.

26. Dannekiold-Samsøe B, Kofod V, Munter J, et al.: Muscle strength and functional capacity in 78–81-year-old men and women. *Eur J Appl Physiol* 1984:52, 310.

27. Harries UJ, Bassey EJ: Torque-velocity relationships for the knee extensors in women in their 3rd and 7th decades. *Eur J Appl Physiol* 1990:60, 187.

28. Larsson L: Morphological and functional characteristics of the ageing skeletal muscle in man: A cross-sectional study. *Acta Physiol Scand* 1978:457(suppl), 1.

29. Murray MP, Duthie EH Jr, Gambert SR, et al.: Age related differences in knee muscle strength in normal women. *J Gerontol* 1985:40, 275.

30. Bassey EJ, Bendel MJ, Pearson M: Muscle strength in the triceps surae and objectively measured customary walking activity in men and women over 65 years of age. *Clin Sci* 1988:74, 85.

31. Aniansson A, Grimby G, Hedberg M, et al.: Muscle morphology, enzyme activity and muscle strength in elderly men and women. *Clin Physiol* 1981:1, 73.

32. Aniansson A, Hedberg M, Henning GB, et al.: Muscle morphology, enzymatic activity, and muscle strength in elderly men: A follow-up study. *Muscle Nerve* 1986:9, 585.

33. Greig CA, Botella J, Young A: The quadriceps strength of healthy elderly people re-measured after eight years. *Muscle Nerve* 1993:16, 6.

34. Coggan AR, Spina RJ, Rogers MA, et al.: Histochemical and enzymatic characteristics of skeletal muscle in master athletes. *J Appl Physiol* 1990:72, 1896.

35. Coggan AR, Spina RJ, Rogers MA, et al.: Skeletal muscle adaptations to endurance training in 60- to 70-year-old men and women. *J Appl Physiol* 1992:72, 1780.

36. Minor MA, Hewett JE, Webel RR, et al.: Efficacy of physical conditioning exercise in patients with rheumatoid arthritis and osteoarthritis. *Arthritis Rheum* 1989:32, 1396.

37. Minor MA, Hewett JE, Webel RR, et al.: Exercise tolerance and disease related measures in patient rheumatoid arthritis and osteoarthritis. *J Rheumatol* 1988:15, 905.

38. Haut RC, Lancaster RL, DeCamp CE: Mechanical properties of the canine patellar tendon: Some correlations with age and the content of collagen. *J Biomech* 1992:25, 163.

39. Bloomfield SA: Bone, ligament, and tendon, in Lamb DR, Gisolfi CV, Nadel E (eds.), *Exercise in Older Athletes*, Carmel, Ind, Cooper, 1995:175.

40. Viidik A: Adaptability of connective tissue, in Saltin B (ed.), *Biochemistry of Exercise VI*, Champaign, Ill, Human Kinetics, 1986:545.

41. Maurel E, Bouissou H, Pieraggi MT, et al.: Age dependent biochemical changes in dermal connective tissue: Relationship to histological and ultrastructural observations. *Connect Tissue Res* 1980:8, 33.

42. Spina M, Volpin D, Giro MG: Age related changes in the content of cross-links and their precursors in elastin of human thoracic aortae, in Robert AM, Robert L (eds.), *Biochemie des tissus conjunctifs normaux et pathologiques* (Biochemistry of normal and pathological connective tissues), Paris, CNRS, 1980:125.

43. Favus MJ: Osteoporosis and the aging athlete. *J Back Musculoskel Rehabil* 1994:5, 19.

44. Åstrand I: Aerobic work capacity in men and women with special reference to age. *Acta Physiol Scand* 1960:169(suppl), 45.

45. Siegel AJ, Warhol MJ, Lang G: Muscle injury and repair in ultra long distance runners, in Sutton JR, Brock RM (eds.), *Sports Medicine for the Mature Athlete*, Indianapolis, Benchmark Press, 1986:35.

46. Costill DL, Thomason H, Roberts E: Fractional utilization of the aerobic capacity during distance running. *Med Sci Sports Exerc* 1973:5, 248.

47. Young JL, Press JM: The physiologic basis of sports rehabilitation. *Phys Med Rehabil Clin North Am* 1994:5, 9.

48. MacDougall JD: Adapatability of muscle to strength training—a cellular approach, in, Saltin B (ed.), *Biochemistry of Exercise*, Vol. 5, Champaign, Ill, Human Kinetics, 1986:501.

49. Frontera WR, Merideth CN, O'Reilly KP, et al.: Strength conditioning in older men: Skeletal muscle and hypertrophy and improved function. *J Appl Physiol* 1988:64, 1038.

50. Fontera WR, Meredith CN, O'Reilly KP, et al.: Strength training and determinants of $\dot{V}O_2$max in older men. *J Appl Physiol* 1990:68, 329.

51. Cress ME, Thomas DP, Johnson J, et al.: Effect of training on $\dot{V}O_2$max, thigh strength, and muscle morphology in septuagenarian women. *Med Sci Sports Exerc* 1991:23, 752.

52. Fiatarone MA, Marks EC, Ryan ND, et al.: High-intensity strength training in nonagenarians: Effects on skeletal muscles. *JAMA* 1990:263, 3029.

53. Fiatarone MA, O'Neill EF, Ryan ND, et al.: Exercise training and nutritional supplementation for physical frailty in very elderly people. *N Engl J Med* 1994:330, 1769.

54. Heislein DM, Harris BA, Jette AM: A strength training program for post-menopausal women: A pilot study. *Arch Phys Med Rehabil* 1994:75, 198.

55. McMurdo MET, Rennie L: A controlled trial of exercise by resident's of old people's homes. *Age Ageing* 1993:22, 11.

56. Moritani T: Training adaptations in the muscles of older men, in Smith EL, Serfass RC (eds.), *Exercise and Aging: The Scientific Basis*, Hillside, NJ, Enslow Publishers, 1981.

57. Pyka G, Lindenberger E, Charette S, et al.: Muscle strength and fiber adaptations to a year-long resistance training program in elderly men and women. *J Gerontol* 1994:49, M22.

58. Manifredi TG, Feilding RA, O'Reilly KP, et al.: Plasma creatine kinase activity and exercise-induced muscle damage in older men. *Med Sci Sports Exerc* 1991:23, 1028.

59. Lane NE, Bloch DA, Jones HH, et al.: Long-distance running, bone density, and osteoarthritis. *JAMA* 1986:255, 1147.

60. Panush RS: Physical activity, fitness and osteoarthritis, in Bouchard C, Shephard RJ, Stephens T (eds.), *Physical Activity, Fitness and Health*, Champaign, Ill, Human Kinetics, 1994:712.

61. Pate RR: Physical activity and public health: Recommendations by CDC and ACSM. *JAMA* 1995:273, 402.

62. Minor MA: Exercise in the treatment of osteoarthritis. *Rheum Dis Clin North Am* 1999:25, 397.

63. Van Baar MA, Assendelft WJJ, Dekker J, et al.: Effectiveness of exercise therapy in the patients with osteoarthritis of the hip and knee. *Arthritis Rheum* 1999:42, 1361.

64. Panush RS, Brown DG: Exercise and arthritis. *Sports Med* 1987:4, 54.

65. Lane NE, Bloch DA, Wood PD, et al.: Aging, long-distance running, and the development of musculoskeletal disability. A controlled study. *Am J Med* 1987:82, 772.

66. Lane NE, Michael B, Bjorkengren A, et al.: The risk of osteoarthritis with running and aging: A 5-year longitudinal study. *J Rheumatol* 1993:20, 461.

67. Sohn RS, Micheli LJ: The effect of running on the pathogenesis of osteoarthritis of the hips and knees. *Clin Orthop* 1985:198, 106.

68. Kiviranti I: Articular cartilage thickness and glycosaminoglycan distribution in the canine knee joint after strenuous exercise. *Clin Orthop* 1992:283, 302.

69. Kiviranti I: Moderate running exercises augment glycosaminoglycans and thickness of articular cartilage in the knee joint of young beagle dogs. *J Orthop Res* 1988:6, 188.

70. Oettmeier R: Subchondral bone and articular cartilage responses to long distance running training in the beagle knee joint. *Euro J Exp Musculoskel Res* 1992:1, 145.

71. Arokoski J: Long-distance running causes size dependent decrease of cartilage glycosaminoglycan content in the knee joint of beagle dogs. *Arthritis Rheum* 1993:36, 1451.

72. Newton PM: The effects of lifelong exercise on canine articular cartilage. *Am J Sports Med* 1997:25, 282.

73. Buckwalter JA, Lane NE: Athletics and osteoporosis. *Am J Sports Med* 1997:25, 873.

74. Suter E, Herzog W: Does muscle inhibition after knee injury increase the risk of osteoarthritis? *Exerc Sports Sci Rev* 2000:28, 15.

75. Kujala UM, Kapiro J, Sarna S: Osteoarthritis of weight bearing joints of lower limbs in former élite male athletes. *Br Med J* 1994:308, 231.

76. Ettinger WH, Fried LP: Aerobic exercise as therapy to prevent functional decline in patients with osteoarthritis, in Ory M, Weindruch R (eds.), *Preventing Frailty and Falls in the Elderly*, Springfield, Ill, Thomas, 1991:210.

77. Basmajian JV: Therapeutic exercise in the management of rheumatic diseases. *J Rheumatol* 1987:14(suppl), 22.

78. Fisher NM, Pendergast DR: Effects of a muscle exercise program on exercise capacity in subjects with osteoarthritis. *Arch Phys Med Rehabil* 1994:75, 792.

79. Kovar PA, Allegrante JP, MacKenzie CR, et al.: Supervised fitness walking in patients with osteoarthritis of the knee: A randomized controlled trial. *Ann Intern Med* 1992:116, 529.

80. Dubs L, Schwend N, Munzinger E: Sports after total hip arthroplasty. *Arch Orthop Trauma Surg* 1983:101, 161.

81. Ritter MA, Medding JB: Total hip replacement: Can the patient play sports again? *Orthopedics* 1987:10, 1447.

82. Visuri T, Honkanen R: Total hip replacement: Its influence on spontaneous recreation exercise habits. *Arch Phys Med Rehabil* 1980:61, 325.

83. Bradbury N, Borton D, Spoo T, et al: Participation in sports after total knee replacement. *Am J Sports Med* 1998:26, 530.

84. Cummings SR, Kelsey JI, Velvitt MC: Epidemiology of osteoporosis and osteoporotic fractures. *Epidemiol Rev* 1985:7, 178.

85. World Health Organization Technical Report Series #843: Assessment of fracture risks and its applications to screening for post-menopausal osteoporosis, Geneva, 1994.

86. Prestwood KM, Kenny AM: Osteoporosis: Pathogenesis, diagnosis and treatment in older adults. *Clin Geriatr Med* 1998:14, 577.

87. Greendale GA, Barett-Connor E, Eldstein S: Lifetime leisure exercise and osteoporosis; The Rancho Bernardo Study. *Am J Epidemiol* 1995:141, 951.

88. Prince R, Devine A, Dick I: The effects of calcium supplementation (milk powder, or tablets) and exercise in bone density in post-menopausal women. *J Bone Min Res* 1995:10, 1068.

89. Armbrecht HJ, Perry HM, Martin KJ: Changes in mineral and bone metabolism with age, in Perry HM, Morley JE, Coe RM (eds.), *Aging and Musculoskeletal Disorders*, New York, Springer, 1993:68.

90. MacIntyre I, Stevenson JC, Whitehead MI, et al.: Calcitonin for prevention of postmenopausal bone loss. *Lancet* 1988:1, 900.

91. Chestnut CH: Osteoporosis, in Hazzard WH, Bierman EL, Blass JP, et al. (eds.), *Principles of Geriatric Medicine and Gerontology*, New York, McGraw-Hill, 1994:897.

92. Baylick DJ, Jennings JC: Calcium and bone homeostasis and changes with aging, in Hazzard WH, Bierman EL, Blass JP, et al. (eds.), *Principles of Geriatric Medicine and Gerontology*, New York, McGraw-Hill, 1994:879.

93. Kasperk CH, Wergedal JE, Farley JR, et al.: Androgens directly stimulate proliferation of bone cells in vitro. *Endocrinology* 1989:124, 1576.

94. Slemenda CW, Hui SL, Longcope C, et al.: Sex steroids and bone mass. A study of changes about the time of menopause. *J Clin Invest* 1987:80, 1261.

95. Nelson ME, Fiatarone MA, Morganti CM: Effects of high-intensity strength training on multiple risk factors for osteoporotic fractures: A randomized, controlled trial. *JAMA* 1994:272, 1909.

96. Chow R, Harrison JE, Notarius C: Effect of two randomized exercise programmes on bone mass of healthy postmenopausal women. *Br Med J (Clin Res Ed)* 1987:295, 1441.

97. Sidney KH, Shephard RJ, Harrison JE: Endurance training and body composition of the elderly. *Am J Clin Nutr* 1977:30, 326.

98. Cheng S, Suominen H, Era P, et al.: Bone density of the calcaneus and fractures in 75- and 80-year-old men. *Osteoporosis Int* 1994:4, 48.

99. Krall EA, Dawson-Highes B: Walking is related to bone density and rates of bone loss. *Am J Med* 1994:96, 20.

100. Suominen H, Rahkila P: Bone mineral density of the calcaneus in 70- to 81-year-old male athletes and a population sample. *Med Sci Sports Exerc* 1991:23, 1227.

101. Suominen H: Bone mineral density and long term exercise. An overview of cross-sectional athlete studies. *Sports Med* 1993:16, 316.

102. Cummings SR, Kelsey JL, Mevitt MC, et al.: Epidemiology of osteoporosis and osteoporotic features. *Epidemiol Rev* 1985:7, 178.

103. Drinkwater B: Physical activity, fitness, and osteoporosis, in Bouchard C, Shephard RJ, Stephens T (eds.), *Physical Activity, Fitness, and Health*, Champaign, Ill, Human Kinetics, 1994:724.

104. Kanis JA, Johnell O, Gullberg B, et al.: Evidence for efficacy of drugs affecting bone metabolism in preventing hip fracture. *Br Med J* 1992:305, 1124.

105. Buono MJ, McKenzie BK, Kasch FW: Effects of aging and physical training on the peripheral sweat production of the human eccrine sweat gland. *Age Ageing* 1991:20, 439.

106. Kenney WL: Thermoregulation at rest and during exercise in healthy older adults. *Exerc Sports Sci Rev* 1997:25, 41.

107. Kenney WL: The older athlete: Exercise in hot environments. *Sports Sci Exch* 1993:6, 44.

108. Carpintero P, Berral F, Baena P, et al.: Delayed diagnosis of fatigue fractures in the elderly. *Am J Sports Med* 1997:25, 659.

109. Kibler WB: A framework for sports medicine. *Phys Med Rehab Clin North Am* 1994:5, 1.

110. Soma CA, Mandelbaum BR: Achilles tendon disorders. *Clin Sports Med* 1994:3, 811.

111. Windsor RE, Chambers K: Overuse injuries of the leg, in Press J (ed.), *Functional Rehabilitation of Sports and Musculoskeletal Injuries*, 1st ed., Gaithersburg, Md, Aspen Publishers, 1998:265.

112. Fredericson M: Common injuries in runners. *Sports Med* 1996:21, 49.

113. Kibler WB: *ACSM Handbook for the Team Physician*, Baltimore, Williams & Wilkins, 1996:380.

114. Maitra RS, Johnson DL: Stress fractures: Clinical history and physical examination. *Clin Sports Med* 1997:16, 259.

115. Kibler WB: *ACSM Handbook for the Team Physician*, Baltimore, Williams & Wilkins, 1996:312.

116. Press J, Young J: Rehabilitation of patellofemoral pain syndrome, in Press J (ed.), *Functional Rehabilitation of Sports and Musculoskeletal Injuries*, 1st ed., Gaithersburg, Md, Aspen, 1998:254.

117. Maharam LG, Bauman PA, Kalman D: Master athletes: Factors affecting performance. *Sports Med* 1999:28, 273.

Chapter 36

THE DISABLED RUNNER

Paul F. Pasquina

INTRODUCTION

Pioneering efforts of disabled individuals, especially World War II veterans, and their eagerness to engage in competitive sports have led to a worldwide movement in the area of disabled sports.[1] Today, opportunities to compete exist in both the national and international arena in virtually all sports and recreational activities ranging from wheelchair basketball to bungee jumping. This chapter pays special attention to track athletes.

In the not so distant past, individuals with disabilities were viewed as *spectators* rather than as *participants*. In fact, only 10 to 20 years ago, psychologists were advocating that such individuals should participate in "sanitized" games in order to ensure "success" of all participants. It was believed that individuals with disabilities should be protected from participating in sports where winning or losing was a possibility, as these individuals had already "lost" enough. We now know, however, that these artificial situations do not correlate well with real life, nor do they reflect the true desires of the participants to compete. In addition, it would be a tragedy if such individuals were not afforded all the other benefits that sport and recreation have to offer. Today, despite the efforts of many pioneers and international organizations, the two greatest limiting factors to participation include access and awareness.

Two highly publicized athletic events available for individuals with disabilities include the Special Olympics and the Paralympics. Both involve national and international competition. The Special Olympics are for people with mental retardation, and the Paralympics are for athletes with physical or visual impairment. The goals of the two events are different. Participation is the goal of the Special Olympics, whereas elite athletic competition is the goal of the Paralympics.

Health care practitioners are encouraged to become involved with disabled sporting events in their communities. Not only will you find the experience rewarding, but the athletic competition is often as exciting if not more so than some able-body athletic events. Finally, if you or someone you know has a disability, you can help by making him or her aware of the opportunities in sport and recreation that exist for him or her.

LEGAL IMPLICATIONS

All individuals, especially those who practice sports medicine, should be aware of the legal implications of the Federal Rehabilitation Act of 1973 and the Americans with Disabilities Act of 1990 (ADA). The Federal Rehabilitation Act prohibits the exclusion of otherwise qualified individuals from participating in federally funded programs. The ADA was later passed, which extended these rights to include the public and private sector. The ADA specifies that a disabled individual must be "qualified for participation" and that "with or without reasonable accommodations, he or she can perform the essential functions of the position that he or she holds or desires." Similar to NCAA regulations, which are described later in this chapter, the ADA allows participation in athletic competition, provided that the participant does not present a direct threat or harm to the health and safety of others. It does not expressly state that such participation cannot pose a direct threat to the participant's own health. Therefore, sports medicine professionals must be cognizant of the potential conflict between medical safety recommendations and the expanded legal rights of disabled individuals.[2]

In addition to those laws designed to protect the rights of adults, section 504 of the Federal Rehabilitation Act of 1973 has recognized the physical, cognitive, and affective benefits of athletic participation in childhood development and education. It states that public schools are prohibited from discriminating against students with disabilities and are required to develop an individualized education plan (IEP) for these individuals. IEPs routinely include physical, occupational, and cognitive therapy.

TERMS AND DEFINITIONS

It is essential that individuals who work with disabled athletes first understand some basic terminology. The terms *disease, impairment, functional limitation, handicap,* and *disability* are often used interchangeably; however, they each have distinct meanings and implications.

Disease
Disease refers to the interruption or interference of normal bodily processes or structure. Most health care practitioners are familiar with such disease processes as Duchenne's muscular dystrophy, amytrophic lateral sclerosis, multiple sclerosis, spina bifida, etc. A denervated muscle after trauma is also an example.

Impairment
Impairment refers to the loss or abnormality of mental, emotional, physiologic, or anatomic structure or function. Examples may include atrophy or paralysis of a certain muscle or muscle group.

Functional Limitation
Functional limitation refers to a restriction or lack of ability to perform an action or activity in the manner or within the range of what society considers normal. This typically involves activities of daily living such as dressing, ambulating, toileting, etc.

Handicap
Handicap refers to the social and environmental consequences to an individual, which may include architectural, economic, or attitudinal barriers. Handicaps exist not from a particular impairment but primarily from barriers created by nondisabled persons.[3] An example would be the inability of a person in a wheelchair to negotiate a staircase at home or at work. If, for example, an elevator were installed, this particular handicap would not exist.

Disability
Disability refers to the expression of the physical or mental limitation in a social context. A classic example is a concert pianist who loses a finger and has minimal impairment and functional limitation but may be completely "disabled" because he/she can no longer earn a livelihood. This term, however, should not be limited to vocational activities, as sports and recreation also have a place in society.

Despite these definitions, the term "disability" remains confusing, partly because many persons who consider themselves experts in the field as well as those who have disabilities themselves cannot always come to agreement. Therefore, the ADA and NCAA have published their own definitions.

The ADA defines "disability" as having one of the following: (1) an impairment that limits a major life activity; (2) a record of an impairment, such as that which may appear in a preparticipation examination form or a physician's notes or charts; or (3) a perception by the public that an impairment limits a major life activity.

The NCAA has chosen the term "impairment" in their regulations and recognizes the right of impaired individuals to participate in intercollegiate programs, provided such individuals qualify for a team without lowering the standards and they do not put others at risk. An "impairment," as defined by the NCAA, exists when individuals are confined to a wheelchair; are deaf, blind, or missing a limb; and have only one of a paired set of organs.

Types of Disabilities
A variety of diseases and pathologic conditions may lead to disability. These include both acquired and congenital conditions (Table 36–1). Disabled athletes are susceptible to many of the same sports-related injuries that occur in able-bodied athletes. Their disease or pathologic state, however, makes them particularly vulnerable to other conditions, of which the sports medicine practitioner must be aware. For example, an individual who acquires an amputation secondary to an infected diabetic limb ulcer will most likely also suffer from a peripheral neuropathy that may alter proprioception and balance

TABLE 36–1. ACQUIRED AND CONGENITAL DISABILITIES

Congenital	Acquired
Limb deficiencies	Amputation
Spina bifida	Spinal cord injury (SCI)
Cerebral palsy	Traumatic brain injury (TBI)
Erbs palsy	Traumatic plexopathy
Muscular dystrophy	Myopathies
MS/ALS	Polio/post polio
Visual/hearing	Visual/hearing

putting the athlete at risk for injury to the intact limb. Other examples include individuals with spinal cord injuries, who are at an increased risk of temperature-related injuries, bladder infections, and pressure ulcers. Therefore, knowing the specific disease process affecting athletes will help not only in guiding treatment but also in the prevention of injury.

ROLE OF THE SPORTS MEDICINE TEAM

Members of the sports medicine team must be aware of special considerations when caring for disabled athletes. By understanding the requirements of a specific sport, the medical team will be able to provide more appropriate recommendations to the athlete in terms of preparticipation conditioning, appropriate clothing, and padding, so as to help prevent injury. Although the team may be called on to treat these individuals for many of the same conditions affecting able-bodied athletes (gastrointestinal disorders, dehydration, infection, sprains, strains, or fracture), they must also consider a much broader differential diagnosis and may be more limited in terms of treatment options. For example, a wheelchair athlete complaining of leg swelling or pain may not have a simple strain or contusion but a deep venous thrombosis (DVT) or possibly a fracture, as these individuals are at higher risk for such conditions secondary to their immobility status and disuse osteoporosis. Another example is that of a wheelchair athlete who sustains a strain to the shoulder. Although the treatment of choice may be rest, this may be difficult to achieve, as the athlete depends on the use of the upper extremity for mobility.

As in treating able-bodied athletes, when prescribing medications or modalities to disabled athletes, one must consider other collateral medical problems or concurrent medications that may interfere with the prescribed treatment or increase the risk of harm to the patient. For example, athletes taking anticholinergic medications such as ditropan for bladder control may be more susceptible to the combined affects of prescribing antihistamines. In addition, the use of heat or cold modalities on sensory-impaired tissues should be avoided or performed with extreme caution.

Aside from these more obvious roles of the medical team, members should also be aware of the possible barriers to access to sporting arenas faced by disabled athletes. During the 1996 Paralympic Games in Atlanta, the athletes used the same facilities as the able-bodied athletes. Before these facilities were accessible to wheelchair athletes, however, modifications such as widening over 350 bathroom doors, installing 750 hand-held shower heads, supplying 700 transfer benches, and changing all door handles had to be performed. Therefore, medical care providers must be sensitive to these issues and be advocates for the athletes.

Finally, medical team members may be asked to participate in classification of athletes, which is discussed in the following section.

MEDICAL CLASSIFICATION

As with most sports, creating an equal playing ground fosters a competitive spirit and the joy of participation. Disabled sports are no different. Just as different weight classifications exist in boxing or different divisions exist in college football, athletes with disabilities compete against athletes with similar abilities. This is primarily achieved through the medical classification process. This system is somewhat complex and exists for the visually and mentally impaired, as well as for amputees, wheelchair athletes, and individuals with cerebral palsy. Each classification typically includes a letter followed by a number. The letter represents the event (T for track, F for field, S for swimming, etc.), and the number describes a specific functional activity or strength level that the athlete is able to perform or a specific level in the case of an amputee (Table 36–2).[4] The Wheelchair Road Racing Classification used at the

TABLE 36–2. CLASSIFICATION SYSTEM FOR AMPUTEES

Class A1	Double AK—Both legs amputated above the knee
Class A2	Single AK—One leg amputated above the knee
Class A3	Double BK—Both legs amputated below the knee
Class A4	Single BK—One leg amputated below the knee
Class A5	Double AE—Both arms amputated above or through the elbow joint
Class A6	Single AE—One arm amputated above or through the elbow joint
Class A7	Double BE—Both arms amputated below the elbow, but through or above the wrist joint
Class A8	Single BE—One arm amputated below the elbow, but through or above the wrist joint
Class A9	Combinations of amputations of the upper and lower extremities

TABLE 36–3. WHEELCHAIR ROAD RACING CLASSIFICATIONS AT THE BOSTON MARATHON

Class T1*	Have functional elbow flexors and wrist dorsi-flexors. No functional elbow extensors or wrist palmar-flexors. May have shoulder weakness.
Class T2*	Have functional elbow flexors and extensors, wrist dorsi-flexors, and palmar-flexors. Have functional pectoral muscles. May have finger flexors and extensors.
Class T3**	Have normal or nearly normal upper-limb function. Have no abdominal muscle function . . . May have weak upper-spinal extension.
Class T4**	Have back extension, usually including both upper and lower extensors. Usually have trunk rotation (i.e., abdominal muscles.

*Quad Class is composed of Classes 1 and 2
**Open Division is composed of Classes 3 and 4

Boston Marathon (Table 36–3) and International Stoke Mandeville Wheelchair Sports Federation (ISMWSF) classifications (Table 36–4) have been listed for reference. In addition to these classification systems, most sports have their own variations of classifications based on the athlete's ability to perform functions specific to that particular sport. One example is the National Wheelchair Basketball Association (NWBA) classification system, which has been standardized for national and international competition. For more information regarding this process, the reader is encouraged to contact these specific organizations or refer to the references provided.[5,6]

WHEELCHAIR ATHLETIC INJURIES

Although there are numerous publications examining the injury patterns in able-bodied athletics, a relative paucity exists for wheelchair and disabled athletes. It appears, however, that the risk of injury/illness for disabled athletes is not significantly different from that of able-bodied athletes.[7] This is especially true in skiers.[8] In addition, it also appears there is no relationship between disability type, classification, or sex and the number of injuries reported except for the fact that temperature regulation problems and pressure sores are much more prevalent in spinal cord–injured athletes.

As with most athletics, risk of injury increases with increased participation. Most wheelchair athletic injuries are associated with track, basketball, and road racing.[9] Strains and muscular injuries account for most injuries, followed by blisters and abrasions. Injuries usually involve the upper extremities, especially the shoulders, wrists, and fingers. Further investigation by health care practitioners typically reveals a relationship between the injury and a recent change in the athlete's level of training intensity or technique, for example, "increasing mileage in preparation for an upcoming race," "altering seat position in the wheelchair," or "learning a new propulsion technique." Therefore, athletes should be encouraged to follow good training practices.

TABLE 36–4. ISMWSF CLASSIFICATION

Class 1A	Lower cervical lesions between C4 and C6 with involvement of all four extremities. Nonfunctional triceps muscles (test = 0 to 3)
Class 1B	Lower cervical lesions (up to C7) with involvement of all four extremities. Triceps good or normal (test = 4 or 5). Poor flexion and extension of the wrist (test = 0 to 3).
Class 1C	Lower cervical lesions (up to C8) with involvement of all four extremities. Triceps good or normal (test = 4 to 5). Good or normal function of wrist extensors and flexors (test = 4 or 5). Poor functioning of the interossei and lumbricals of the hand (test = 0 to 3).
Class 2	Thoracic lesions from T1 to T5. Involvement of the trunk and lower extremities. No use of abdominal muscles. No sitting balance.
Class 3	Thoracic lesions from T6 to T10. Involvement of the abdomen and lower extremities. Good upper abdominal muscles. No use of lower abdominal muscles. No use of lower trunk extensors. Slight capacity to maintain sitting balance.
Class 4	Thoracic and lumbar lesions from T6 to T10. Involvement of the lower extremities. Good abdominal and dorsal spinal muscles. Fair hip flexors and abductors. Good sitting balance. Lower Extremity Test*: traumatics from 1 to 20 points, nontraumatics from 1 to 15 points.
Class 5	Lumbar lesion at or above L5. Involvement of the lower extremities. Good sitting balance. Good abdominal muscles. Lower Extremity Test*: traumatics from 21 to 40 points, nontraumatics from 16 to 35 points.
Class 6	Sacral lesions from S1 to S3, involvement of one lower extremity or slight involvement of both lower extremities. Lower Extremity Test*: traumatics from 41 to 60 points, nontraumatics from 36 to 50 points.

*Lower Extremity Tests include testing of muscles involved in: Hip flexion, extension, abduction and adduction; Knee flexion and extension; Ankle plantar and dorsi flexion. Points are based on a 0 to 5 manual muscle strength scale.

This includes gradually increasing their intensity or distance, as well as slowly introducing new techniques, so that their bodies may adjust to the new demands.

Rotator Cuff Dysfunction

Wheelchair athletes are particularly susceptible to rotator cuff injuries. Injuries may be prevented by adequate warm-up as well as an appropriate shoulder strengthening program prior to participation in sporting activities. It is essential that these athletes strengthen not only their rotator cuff muscles, but also their scapula stabilizers (trapezius, levator, pectoralis, latissimus, serratus, and rhomboids). Rotator cuff injuries can typically be managed conservatively, although treatment should be aggressive as the shoulder joint is a weight-bearing joint for wheelchair athletes and critical to mobility. Therefore, further imaging and orthopedic consultation should not be delayed, if so indicated.

Skin Injuries

Blisters and abrasions commonly occur on the hands and fingers. These typically are caused by traction or irritation from contact with the wheelchair rim, tire, or locking mechanism. In addition to callus formation, proper padding can often prevent such injuries. Wearing gloves, taping fingers, placing plastic spoke protectors, or proper placement of brakes can all help prevent hand or finger injuries. Wheelchair athletes are also susceptible to skin injuries to the inner upper arm, which can come into contact with the wheel. Many athletes use their inner arms as a means of braking. Pads or even cut-out tube socks can be worn to cover the upper arms to help prevent such injuries. Another prevention technique is to change the angle of the wheel (camber), so that the wheels tilt in. This allows more clearance through the axilla region and also increases the base of support for the chair.

Pressure sores are another major concern for wheelchair athletes. Although as a general rule active wheelchair users are less likely to develop pressure sores than nonactive users, the size and shape of today's modern sports chairs, coupled with the athlete's altered sensory perception as well as perspiration, predispose the athlete to such injuries. Wheelchair racers often find themselves in a knees-up, forward leaning position for extended periods; this position causes excessive skin pressures, which impair circulation and can lead to ulcer formation. Preventing such conditions requires diligent skin observation and care. In addition, wheelchair athletes should wear absorbent clothing, maintain proper hygiene and nutrition, and also perform pressure relief techniques regularly. This can be achieved by arm pushups to relieve pressure on the buttocks, particularly the areas of the ischial tuberosities.

Temperature Regulation Injuries

Heat and cold injuries are of special concern for wheelchair athletes, especially individuals with spinal cord injuries in whom the ability to maintain thermal regulation has been disrupted. In excessive heat environments, athletes rely on the dissipation of heat by means of evaporation from perspiration. Some spinal cord injuries do not allow an athlete to perspire below the level of the lesion, thus impairing the ability to dissipate heat generated during athletic activities. In addition, increased skin surface contact with the chair also impairs the dissipation of heat. Early signs of heat injury might include clumsiness, erratic wheelchair propulsion, and complaints of headache, nausea, and dizziness, as well as apathy and evidence of confusion or mental status change.[10] Athletes at risk must be advised on the appropriate use of clothing and hydration. In hotter climates, training schedules and competitions should be performed in the cooler early morning hours, and rest/finish stations should be placed in shaded areas. In addition, care should be taken when cooling heat-injured patients too aggressively, especially in areas of altered sensation. Axilla, neck, and head areas are typically appropriate areas to apply ice packs in such conditions. In addition, as with able-bodied athletes, acclimatization is an important consideration for wheelchair athletes who may be scheduled to compete in national and international competitions in foreign climates. This usually takes approximately 2 weeks, although benefits have been reported within 1 week.

Hypothermia is also a critical problem in wheelchair athletics. In cold environments, able-bodied athletes with an intact autonomic nervous system are able to shunt blood flow appropriately as well as shiver to generate heat as needed. These protective mechanisms, however, are altered in many spinal cord injured individuals. Wheelchair athletes may also have significant atrophy of paralyzed musculature, which not only decreases the effectiveness of shivering in generating significant heat but also decreases soft-tissue insulation. One must be aware that in extreme cold-weather conditions, insensate extremities, especially the toes, may be particularly susceptible to frostbite. As with cooling heat-injured athletes, great care must be taken when heating cold-injured athletes, especially in insensate areas. Proper clothing is therefore paramount in extreme climate situations, especially alpine skiers.

Nerve Entrapments

Upper-extremity nerve entrapments are common in individuals who rely on manual wheelchairs for mobility. The most common sites are the median nerve at the carpal tunnel, the ulnar nerve at the wrist and across the elbow, and the distal radial sensory nerve.

Clinical evidence of nerve injury involves numbness of the hand and fingers in the classic nerve distribution. Symptoms, however, are often nondescript. Localizing findings may include a positive Tinel's sign at the wrist and atrophy/weakness of the thenar muscles (median) or a positive Tinel's sign along the ulnar groove at the elbow or Guyon's canal at the wrist and atrophy/weakness of the hypothenar or interossei muscles (ulnar). Although clinical symptoms occur in approximately 23% of wheelchair athletes, electromyographic diagnostic studies have demonstrated abnormalities in 64% of these athletes.[11] These rates are much higher than in able-bodied athletes; however, they are comparable to nonathletic wheelchair users.

Boninger et al.[12] recently studied the prevalence of upper-limb nerve entrapments in elite wheelchair racers and discovered that "despite the amount of time spent training, these wheelchair athletes have a similar or even lower prevalence of median mononeuropathy than reported for the general wheelchair-using population." The authors attribute this finding to several possible hypotheses. First, wheelchair athletes are generally in better physical condition, which eases general activities of daily living as well as transfers in and out of the wheelchair. Second, it is possible that wheelchair athletes pay more attention to the size and proper fit of their wheelchair, which may alter the forces expressed across the carpal tunnel during their daily activities.

The importance of this finding is that individuals who rely on manual wheelchairs for mobility should not be discouraged from participating in athletics because of presumed increased risk of nerve injury. In fact, the opposite may be true. Even so, medical practitioners should be aware of the high prevalence of such injuries and act accordingly. When a peripheral nerve entrapment is suspected, it is recommended that electrodiagnostic studies be obtained to help localize and give some indication of the severity of the injury. Although conservative treatment is the recommended first step, including wrist splints, nonsteroidal antiinflamatory agents, and possibly steroid injections, a low threshold for surgical referral is suggested as the upper extremities serve as weightbearing limbs for these individuals, and critical for mobility.

Autonomic Dysreflexia

Individuals with spinal cord injuries at or above T-6 are at risk for developing autonomic dysreflexia. Typical symptoms include headache, facial flushing, severe hypertension, and tachycardia or bradycardia. Recognition and immediate treatment of this condition is critical as it may lead to seizure, stroke, or even death. The condition occurs because of the injured individual's inability to control his/her sympathetic

nervous system. This phenomenon is believed to be the result of a massive sympathetic discharge initiated by a spinal reflex mechanism from a noxious stimulus below the level of the spinal cord lesion. The most common stimuli are usually produced by a distended bowel or bladder, but other causes may include urinary tract infections, venous thrombosis, or extremity injuries. Initial treatment should include head elevation, followed by identification and removal of the noxious stimulus. This usually involves disimpacting the colon or draining the bladder, especially in the event of an occluded/kinked catheter, which may require irrigation. If this is not successful, a thorough physical examination will often reveal the source. In the presence of persistent hypertension, one should have a low threshold for administering a fast-acting blood pressure-lowering agent. Some athletes may attempt to induce a level of autonomic dysreflexia, such as by clamping an indwelling catheter during competition, in order to enhance performance. This practice should be discouraged, and the health care provider should consider it in the differential diagnosis of the athlete with autonomic dysreflexia.

SPORT/RACING WHEELCHAIRS

Many types of wheelchairs exist for individuals with disabilities. The type and specific features of the chair should be tailored to the individual's needs. Sport wheelchairs have a rigid frame as opposed to a folding or collapsible frame. A rigid frame provides more stability to the athlete and also requires fewer chair components, thereby reducing weight and improving energy efficiency. One disadvantage to a rigid frame, however, is the difficulty in transporting it. Unlike a folding chair, which can be easily stored in the trunk or back seat of a car, a rigid frame chair often needs to be disassembled prior to transport.

Sport chairs (Fig. 36–1) can be expensive and are generally not the primary chair of the user. They are

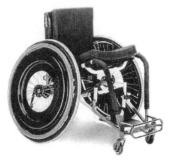

Figure 36-1. Sports wheelchair.

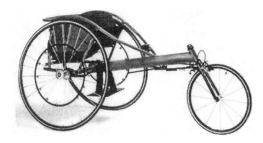

Figure 36-2. Racing wheelchair.

typically used for such sports as basketball, rugby, and tennis. They have thin indoor-type wheels with little tread and small front casters, which allow for more maneuverability. In addition, sports chairs have a large camber. Camber is the angle of the wheel. The farther the bottom of the wheel is moved outward, the larger the camber. A larger camber provides more stability, tightens the turning radius of the chair, and allows the user to propel the wheelchair at higher speeds.

Racing chairs (Fig. 36–2) are highly specialized and are also not the primary chair of the user. They are made of lightweight material, such as titanium, and have seats designed to hold the body in a very compact shape. They have small-diameter hand rims to help maximize distance from each arm stroke and, like other sports chairs, have a large camber.

AMPUTEES

Today's modern prosthetics enable individuals with amputations to participate in nearly all athletic and recreational activities. Prosthetics exist for sprinting as well as long-distance running. It is not uncommon to see individuals with amputations competing against able-bodied athletes in marathons and ironman triathlons. Different prosthetic devices and components are necessary depending on the type of activity and level of amputation. Modifications can be made to prosthetics to accommodate participation in activities ranging from swimming to skydiving.

When evaluating an athlete with a limb deficiency, it is important to obtain a good history. Not all problems should be attributed to the prosthesis itself. It is not uncommon for an individual with a below-knee (transtibial) amputation to develop knee, hip, or back injuries similar to those of an able-bodied athlete. Special attention should be paid to any recent change in intensity, mileage, running surfaces, hills, etc. In addition, one should consider the age and fit of the prosthesis. The typical life of a prosthesis is approximately 5 years, although in active individuals components can become worn much sooner. It is rare for an athlete to use the same prosthesis during athletics as that used for daily activities.

When prescribing a prosthesis one should follow a standard approach to minimize the possibility of omission of an important component. One method is to start proximally and work distally. This includes first choosing an appropriate socket (usually total contact), followed by the type of knee (if above-knee or transfemoral amputation), the type of shank (lower-leg component), the type of ankle (rare in most prosthetics, especially those used for running), the type of foot (typically energy storing), and finally the type of suspension (usually suction, suprapatellar cuff, or Neopryn sleeve). Modern lightweight durable materials such as titanium, carbon fibers, and Kevlar have allowed manufacturers to develop prosthetics better suited not only for a more active lifestyle but also for rigorous sports participation. Hydraulic components and shock absorbers added to knees and shanks give a more natural and fluid gait and running form.

Athletes complaining of residual limb pain should also be examined closely. Possible etiologies include skin breakdown from poorly fitting sockets, causing pressure points or abnormal shear forces, inappropriate blood and lymphatic drainage, or even development of a neuroma. The athlete should next be examined with the prosthesis on to check for static and dynamic alignment as well as altered gait. This process can often become complicated, and therefore consultation with a rehabilitation specialist and/or prosthetist is recommended.

SPECIAL OLYMPICS

The Special Olympics offers worldwide participation in summer and winter sports to over 1 million people, both children and adults with mental retardation. All participants are required to complete a preparticipation questionnaire and obtain a physical examination from a qualified health care practitioner. Physicians should pay special attention to the cervical spine when examining individuals with Down's syndrome (trisomy 21). Up to 15% of individuals with Down's syndrome have laxity of the transverse ligament of C-1 (atlas), which stabilizes the articulation between it and the odontoid process of C-2 (axis). If excessive laxity exists, this may cause C-1 to sublux on C-2, resulting in spinal cord compression. It is therefore important for physicians to perform a complete neurologic examination and also obtain preparticipation x-rays of the cervical spine including lateral views in neutral, flexion, and extension positions. Individuals with evidence of instability or any symptoms or signs of upper motor neuron disease suggestive of spinal cord injury warrant an immediate neurosurgical consultation.

Cardiac defects are also common in individuals with Down's syndrome as well as other causes of mental retardation. All diastolic or systolic murmurs (grade 3/6 or louder) require further evaluation. Individuals with seizure disorders must be evaluated closely for seizure control and therapeutic drug levels. Those with poorly controlled seizure disorders should be prohibited from participating in events such as swimming, diving, gymnastics, skiing, speed skating, and equestrian events. When in doubt, a neurology consultation should be obtained.

REFERENCES

1. Botvin Modorsky JG, Curtis KA: Wheelchair sports medicine. *Am J Sports Med* 1984:12, 128.
2. Nichols AW: Sports medicine and the Americans with Disabilities Act. *Clin J Sport Med* 1996:6, 190.
3. Messner DG, Benedick JR: The disabled athlete, in Nicholson, Hershman (eds.), *The Lower Extremity & Spine,* 2nd ed., St. Louis, Mosby, 1995:159.
4. van Eijsden-Besseling MDF: The (non)sense of the present-day classification system of sports for the disabled, regarding paralyzed and amputee athletes. *Paraplegia* 1985:23, 288.
5. National Wheelchair Basketball Association: *NWBA Physical Classification Handbook,* Lexington, KY, University of Kentucky, 1979.
6. National Wheelchair Athletic Association, 2107 Templeton Gap Road, Suite C, Colorado Springs, CO 80907. (303) 632-0698.
7. Reynolds J, Stirk A, Thomas A, et al.: Paralympics–Barcelona 1992. *Br J Sports Med* 1994:28, 14.
8. Ferrara MS, Buckley WE, Messner DG, et al.: The injury experience and training history of the competitive skier with a disability. *Am J Sport Med* 1992:20, 55.
9. Curtis KA, Dillon DA: Survey of wheelchair athletic injuries: Common patterns and prevention. *Paraplegia* 1985:23, 170.
10. Burnham RS, Steadward RD: Upper Extremity Peripheral Nerve Entrapments Among Wheelchair Athletes: Prevalence, Location, and Risk Factors. *Arch Phys Med Rehabil* 1994:75, 519.
11. Boninger ML, Robertson RN, Wolff, M, et al.: Upper Limb Nerve Entrapments In Elite Wheelchair Racers. *Am J Phys Med Rehabil* 1996:75, 170.
12. Pasquina PF, Houston, Belandres: Beta Blockade in the Treatment of Autonomic Dysreflexia: A Case Report and Review. *Arch of Phys Med and Rehab,* May 1998.

Chapter 37

THE ULTRAMARATHONER

Catherine M. Fieseler

The challenge of running long distances has prompted tens of thousands of people to train for and complete marathons. Some runners have taken this challenge to the next level—ultramarathons. Training for and racing distances longer than a marathon creates unique stresses on the runner, which may cause a number of medical and orthopedic problems. Proper training and nutrition are also extremely important for ultramarathoners. These issues will be presented in this chapter.

An ultramarathon is a race longer than the traditional marathon distance of 26.2 miles. Races may be run over a specified distance or may be run for a specified amount of time. Common distance events include 50K, 50 miles, 100K, and 100 miles; there are specific cut-off times for these races. A runner will be pulled out of the race if aid stations are not reached within a specified time. These races may be run on trails or roads. Timed events include: 6 hour, 12 hour, 24 hour, 48 hour, and multiday events. These races are run on a measured course. The runner attempts to cover as much distance as possible within the specified time. In multiday events, runners typically take sleeping breaks.

Trail races present a variety of challenges for participants. Most of these races involve a wide variety of terrain; hills and mountains, tree roots, rocks, and streams are a few of the obstacles. There may be major changes in elevation or altitude. There are often significant temperature changes during the race because many participants are running for 24 hours or longer. Wildlife may be encountered, in addition to poison ivy and other troublesome plant life. Courses are marked in a variety of ways, but it is not unusual for runners to wander off the trail, especially if they are running at night (typically using a flashlight to navigate). Races have aid stations at a number of points along the course. The distance between stations can be quite variable, ranging from a few miles to more than 10 miles apart. A variety of fluids and food are usually available. Most runners wear a pack to carry fluids, food, and other supplies between aid stations. Many races allow runners to have a crew meet them at various points during the race. The crew may provide clothing, shoes, and supplies for their runner. Drop bags with supplies may be prepared by a runner without a crew; these are sent to designated sites along the course.

Timed events allow frequent access to supplies and it is much easier to keep track of the participants. One problem is the number of repetitive turns a runner must make. Runners in many of the timed events held on a 400-meter track will reverse their running direction on a regular basis.

MEDICAL CONCERNS IN ULTRAMARATHONERS

Cardiac

A number of studies have reported an elevated level of serum creatine kinase (CK) and the proportion of CK myocardial bands (CK-MB) in runners who have completed an ultramarathon.[1,2] This has raised the concern of possible subclinical myocardial damage during prolonged exertion. Laslett and Eisenbud[1] performed CK-MB and cardiac troponin T levels on runners at the Western States 100 Mile Endurance Run. Levels were taken pre- and postrace. CK-MB levels were elevated and cardiac troponin T levels were normal in all subjects.

Davila-Roman and colleagues[2] studied 14 runners who completed the 1994 Hardrock 100, one of the most difficult races in the country as indicated by the 48-hour cutoff time and high altitude course. Prior to the race, a physical examination and an echocardiogram were performed, and serum cardiac troponin I and CK-MB levels were drawn. Baseline studies were normal in all cases. Immediately upon completion of the race, vital signs were taken, a physical examination and echocardiogram performed, and more lab work was done. Postrace heart rates were elevated and diastolic blood pressure was decreased; systolic blood pressure was unchanged. CK-MB levels were elevated in all runners, but cardiac troponin I levels were undetectable in all but one of the subjects. All echocardiograms showed an augmentation of left ventricular function, as manifested by a decrease in left ventricular end-systolic and end-diastolic areas and volumes, without a change in the ejection fraction. The right ventricle was normal in nine subjects, but in five subjects there was marked right ventricular dilation and global right ventricular hypokinesia. Paradoxical septal motion was noted and estimated right atrial pressure was elevated in each of these cases. Each of these five subjects experienced wheezing during and upon completion of the race. The subject with an elevated cardiac troponin I level had marked right ventricular dysfunction. Repeat studies performed 18 to 24 hours after the race showed normal CK-MB levels. The isolated elevated cardiac troponin I level was still detectable, but within normal limits. All echocardiograms were normal. The pulmonary hypertension that developed in 5 subjects may have been due to the high-altitude site of this race. The incidence of right ventricular dysfunction in ultraendurance competitors who race at lower altitudes is unknown. None of the subjects required significant medical intervention and all recovered without sequelae.

Rhabdomyolysis

Lind and colleagues[3] measured CK levels in 161 of the finishers (of a total of 198) of the 1995 Western States 100 Mile Endurance Run. CK levels were greater than 20,000 IU/L in 31 subjects (Table 37–1). The highest measured level was 101,000 IU/L. This runner maintained the same weight at the start and finish of the race, and he experienced what appeared to be blood in the urine during the race. He did not require medical treatment. None of the subjects with significantly elevated CK levels sought medical attention.

The previous year, a finisher began to feel ill the day after completing the race. After a 24-hour period of nausea and vomiting, he was hospitalized with acute renal failure. He required dialysis several times. One other runner in 1994 developed renal failure, but responded to supportive therapy without dialysis.

The highest CK level measured at the Western States 100 race was 221,200 IU/L in 1999.[4] This male runner did not lose any weight during the race and ingested approximately 45 liters of fluid. Immediately postrace, his blood urea nitrogen (BUN) was 56 mg/dl, creatinine was 1.7 mg/dl, and sodium was 133 mmol/L; he noted that his urine was dark in color. Two days later, he felt as if he had a fever and his quadriceps were sore. Repeat lab work at that time revealed a CK of 49,120 IU/L, BUN of 49 mg/dl, and creatinine of 2.1 mg/dl. He was hospitalized for 36 hours of intravenous hydration and his symptoms resolved and lab studies improved: CK was 16,076 IU/L, BUN was 29 mg/dl, and creatinine was 1.4 mg/dl. He has resumed running without any problems.

Although a number of ultramarathoners use aspirin or nonsteroidal anti-inflammatory drugs (NSAIDs) during a race, Lind and associates did not note any correlation of medication use with elevated CK levels or the development of acute renal failure.[3]

Laboratory Studies

Elevated bilirubin levels have been reported in distance runners.[5] This was thought to be secondary to the breakdown of red blood cells. DePaz and coworkers[6] evaluated 13 runners before and following completion

TABLE 37–1. CREATINE KINASE LEVELS IN COMPETITORS IN THE 1995 WESTERN STATES 100 MILE ENDURANCE RUN

No. of Subjects	CK (IU/L)
31	>20,000
38	10,000–20,000
37	5000–10,000
55	1000–5000

Source: From Lind et al.[3]

of a 100K race. Laboratory studies showed a 66% decrease in haptoglobin (indicating the presence of hemolysis). Additionally, there was an increase in alanine aminotransferase (ALT; 42%), aspartate aminotransferase (AST; 193%), gamma-glutamyl transferase (GGT; 56%), total bilirubin (106%), unconjugated bilirubin (96%), and conjugated bilirubin (283%). Although hemolysis was present in these subjects, findings were also consistent with a hepatic disturbance.

Low serum ferritin has been reported frequently in long-distance runners, but not in other endurance athletes.[7,8] Dickson and colleagues[7] noted marked elevation of serum ferritin levels following two ultramarathons. During one of these races, levels were checked prior to and 48 hours after completion of the event. During the second race, laboratory studies were performed prior to, immediately following, and 2 and 6 days after the event. In this latter study, ferritin levels returned to baseline by 6 days following the race. Immediate postrace white blood cell counts were markedly elevated, with a significant increase in neutrophils. Results were normal 48 hours after the race.

One of the concerns raised by these studies is that a falsely elevated ferritin level in an endurance runner may result in missing the diagnosis of iron deficiency.

Dehydration

Many 100-mile trail races in the United States have mandatory weight checks prior to and at specific points during the race. The goal of weight checks is to minimize the possibility that a dehydrated runner might collapse miles away from any medical care. Typical guidelines for weight loss include the medical disqualification of a runner with a 7% or greater loss in weight. Significant weight gain may also result in removal of the runner from competition.

The main concern about dehydration is the potential collapse of the runner. The majority of runners who collapse at a race do so after finishing.[9] If dehydration is the cause of collapse, the runner should collapse during the race, when stroke volume is greatest and would be most affected by a decrease in circulating blood volume.[10] All of the runners who collapsed during the race had a known medical condition, compared with only 34% of those who collapsed after finishing.[9]

Asymptomatic postrace postural hypotension was found to be common following an ultramarathon.[11] Thirty-one runners were evaluated prior to and following an 80K race. The average weight loss was 3.5 kg, representing 4.6% dehydration. Following the race, there was a significant decrease in supine and erect blood pressure and an increase in heart rate. With postural change (supine to erect), 68% of the subjects had asymptomatic postural hypotension (systolic blood pressure decrease of 20 mm Hg or greater), compared with 7% prior to the race. There were no significant differences in total weight loss, change in plasma volume, or heart rate between runners with and without postural hypotension.

Hyponatremia

A decreased level of sodium has been reported in athletes following a marathon,[12] ultramarathons,[9,13] ultradistance multisport triathlon,[14] and ultradistance triathlons.[15–17] Many of these athletes were found to be asymptomatic. Mild symptoms of hyponatremia are nonspecific and include malaise, confusion, fatigue, and nausea. More severe symptoms include hyperreflexia, seizures, coma, and death.[16]

In a study of runners who suffered exercise-associated collapse following an ultramarathon, 9% were found to have sodium levels lower than 130 mmol/L.[13] Each of these runners consumed a significant amount of fluid during the 90K race, typically water or cola and water. The average rate of ingestion was 1.3 L/hr. The authors calculated that 0.29% of race finishers were likely to develop symptomatic hyponatremia.

A number of studies have shown that hyponatremia is more likely to develop in runners who did not lose, and in some cases gained, weight during the race.[14–17] An inverse relationship between postrace sodium levels and percent change in body weight was noted in each of these studies. Barr and colleagues[18] studied the effects of ingesting water, saline, and no fluids during prolonged exercise. Serum sodium concentration decreased in both groups ingesting fluids (average weight loss, <1 kg) and increased in the no-fluid group (average weight loss, 4.5 kg).

O'Toole and associates[15] performed neuromuscular excitability tests on triathletes prior to and following an ultraendurance event, looking for clinical tests indicating electrolyte abnormalities. This testing included deep tendon reflexes at three sites, evaluation of hand tremor, evaluation of weight, Trousseau's sign, and Chvostek's sign. During the race, most athletes lost weight, many had electrolyte abnormalities, and many had altered neuromuscular excitability. The changes in neuromuscular excitability tests were unrelated to significant fluid loss or electrolyte abnormalities.

Speedy and co-workers[17] evaluated 540 athletes who completed an ultradistance triathlon. Twenty-three percent of the athletes who sought medical attention were hyponatremic, and 15% of those who did not seek treatment were hyponatremic, with 1.5% having a sodium level <130 mmol/L. All of the athletes with sodium concentration below 125 mmol/L were symptomatic; the majority with a sodium concentration >130 mmol/L were asymptomatic. Female athletes were noted to have significantly lower postrace sodium concentrations than their male counterparts, and 45% of female finishers were hyponatremic, compared with 14% of the male finishers.

The etiology of hyponatremia in ultraendurance athletes is uncertain. Researchers reporting an inverse relationship between postrace sodium concentration and percentage change in body weight suggest fluid overload as the cause. It is not known why normal renal mechanisms do not cope with this fluid overload.[17]

Noakes[19] recommends fluid intake at a rate of 500 ml/hr for slower runners in an ultramarathon. Available data led to his conclusion that this much fluid is sufficient to prevent significant dehydration, and is much lower than the ingestion rates calculated in cases of hyponatremia. Rate of fluid ingestion is quite variable among different runners in different running environments. Competing on a hot, humid day requires a greater rate of ingestion than running on a cold day. The ideal rate of fluid ingestion that will avoid both dehydration and hyponatremia has not been determined.

Gastrointestinal Problems

Nausea and gastrointestinal (GI) bleeding are two common problems for ultrarunners. Nausea may occur for a number of reasons. Hyponatremia, dehydration, and a diet consisting only of carbohydrates during a race are controllable factors contributing to the development of nausea and vomiting.[20] Running for hours causes a rise in stress hormones, and this can cause nausea. Proper attention to hydration, diet, electrolyte replacement, and training will reduce the risk of developing nausea.[20]

Occult GI bleeding has been reported in 8% to 30% of marathon runners.[21] In a study by Baska and colleagues,[22] 35 runners performed three hemoccult stool tests prior to a 100-mile race and on the first three stools following the race. Of the runners with negative hemoccults prior to the race, 85% converted to positive following the race. The runners with occult blood in the stool had a greater incidence of lower GI symptoms (i.e., bloating, diarrhea, and abdominal cramping) than the runners with negative postrace hemoccult tests.

Cimetidine was administered to 9 of 25 runners in another study by Baska and coworkers.[23] Only one of the nine runners receiving cimetidine had postrace hemoccult-positive stools, while 14 of 16 runners in the control group had positive tests.

Blisters

Blisters are a very common problem for ultramarathoners. A blister is the result of shear stress acting on the stratum corneum, resulting in separation of the skin into two layers. Hemodynamic forces cause this newly developed space to fill with fluid.[24]

Factors predisposing a runner to the development of blisters include new or poorly fitted shoes, prolonged running, increased speed or intensity, and moisture and debris (dirt or rocks) in the shoes.[25] Many runners use preventive measures to avoid blister formation.[25,26] These include taping sites prone to blister formation, modifying shoes and laces to alleviate pressure points, using skin tougheners (benzoin, Betadine soaks), using lubricants, wearing synthetic socks, ankle-length nylons, or double-layer socks, wearing properly fitted shoes, wearing gaiters (sleeves that fit over the ankles and into the shoes to keep dirt and rocks out), and changing shoes and socks during the race.

If a blister develops during a race, it should be cleaned, drained, and treated with a blister care product, such as moleskin, adhesive felt, Spenco secondskin dressing, or Compeed.[26]

Subungual Hematoma

A subungual hematoma is the collection of blood under the toenail. This is caused by trauma to the nail and can be quite painful. Steep downhill running, especially on loose gravel, increases the risk of getting a subungual hematoma. Ensuring that there is adequate room in the toebox of the shoes lowers the risk of a subungual hematoma. Kicking rocks on trails is another hazard. Trail shoes have extra protection around the toebox to prevent this type of trauma.

If a painful subungual hematoma develops during a race, the pressure can be relieved by draining the hematoma. The nail should be cleaned with alcohol and a needle or pin (such as the safety pin on the race number) that has been heated in a flame should be pressed against the involved nail. As soon as the blood begins to flow, needle or pin should be removed. Pressure should be maintained on the nail until most of the blood is released. The runner should then be able to continue running.[26]

MUSCULOSKELETAL CONCERNS IN ULTRAMARATHONERS

Very few studies have evaluated the musculoskeletal injuries that occur during an ultramarathon. During trail races, acute injuries (i.e., sprains and fractures) are not uncommon. Overuse injuries are much more common in ultramarathoners.[27–29] Hutson[27] reviewed the medical records after a 6-day race in 1982. The race was run on a 400-meter track and the running direction was changed every 12 hours. Sixty percent of the runners developed injuries severe enough to affect performance. One runner had to drop out due to severe bilateral Achilles' tendinitis. Injuries occurred with equal frequency in either leg. The most common injury was tendinitis of the muscles of the anterior compartment of the lower leg. Anterior knee pain (patellar tendinitis and patellofemoral pain syndrome) was also common, with Achilles tendinitis occurring with slightly less frequency.

Fallon[28] reported on injuries suffered during the 1990 Westfield Sydney to Melbourne Run. This is a 1005K race run on public roads (left-hand side), that must be completed within 8.5 days. The 32 starters suffered 64 injuries, and the majority of these (90%) involved the lower extremity with only one acute injury. The most common diagnoses were tendinitis of the muscles of the anterior compartment of the lower leg and anterior knee pain. Bishop and Fallon[29] reported on injuries during a 6-day track race in which the running direction was reversed every 2 hours. Sixty-five percent of the runners sustained injuries significant enough to affect their performance. Achilles' tendinitis was the most common injury, followed by extensor digitorum longus tendinitis, retropatellar pain syndrome, and anterior compartment syndrome.

Tendinitis of the muscles of the anterior compartment of the lower leg, also known as ultramarathoner's ankle, is an injury fairly specific to ultramarathoners. The site of inflammation noted in two of the studies[28,29] was at the extensor retinaculum at the anterior aspect of the ankle. While footwear and biomechanics play a role in developing this injury, the shuffling gait adopted by most ultramarathoners while racing is probably the major culprit.[28,29] The limited dorsiflexion and plantarflexion at the ankle restricts the length of the tendons which pass under the retinaculum with each step, producing increased friction at this site.

TRAINING FOR ULTRAMARATHONS

The single most important factor in training for an ultramarathon is the long run. The length of the race should determine training strategies. Preparing for a 50K race should be similar to preparation for a marathon, with the addition of training on trails if the race is run on a trail. Trail races are typically slower than road races due to rougher terrain and obstacles (downed trees, streams, tree roots, etc.). Running on trails demands close attention to foot placement to avoid falling. Many runners will walk on difficult

sections of trail, especially in longer races. The energy expended running up a very steep hill will usually cost the runner dearly later in the race. Energy conservation is key. For longer races, there are a number of different approaches to training. The long run is still the most important factor, but most runners cannot do 60-mile training runs due to the time commitment required and risk of injury. Other than races themselves, many runners limit the long run to 35 to 40 miles, and one race is often used as training for the next event. A common training regimen is a run of 25 to 30 miles on one day (typically Saturday), followed by a 10- to 15-mile run the following day. The pace for the long run is slow and easy, perhaps 7 minutes per mile for an elite runner or 13 minutes per mile for a slower runner. The long run may include walking if the runner anticipates walking in the race. Practice walking quickly; slow runners are often passed by fast walkers in an ultramarathon. Access to fluids and carbohydrates is important during these runs because they will last about 3 hours or perhaps longer, depending on the pace and distance.

The remainder of the week's training consists of runs of various distances, speed, or intensity. These may include hill workouts and some type of speed training (intervals, fartlek, tempo runs). For the average ultramarathoner, interval training is probably not necessary and increases the risk of injury; many runners use local 5K and 10K races as speed workouts.

Rest is also a very important part of training. This is especially true after a hard workout, such as a long run or speed work. Rest might consist of a day off or an easy run. Rest is also important if signs of overtraining or illness are present, such as excessive fatigue, elevated resting heart rate, sore throat, and persistent myalgias.

Weekly mileage varies widely for runners competing in a 100-mile race, ranging from 50 to 200 miles per week. Training is often dictated by work schedules, demands of one's family, and history of injuries. Ignoring these factors will usually have a negative impact on training.

Mental attitude is another important part of training. The concept of running 100 miles may be a bit intimidating to a new ultramarathoner. Breaking the race down into smaller segments may make it seem more manageable. Barring significant injury or illness, the runner needs to banish all thoughts of quitting. A good support crew can be a great motivator, and using a pacer late in the race (if allowed) can be invaluable. Once a runner has completed a 100-mile race the distance is no longer feared, but it still must be respected.

NUTRITION FOR ULTRAMARATHONERS

More than 10,000 calories are needed to complete a 100-mile race, therefore a runner must consume many calories during the race. Most races have aid stations set up along the course with a wide variety of foods and liquids. Foods typically include fruit, potatoes, cookies, sandwiches, and pretzels. Soup is often served at night and during races in cooler weather. Most aid stations will have salt and most runners will use this liberally. Fluids typically include one or more sports drinks, caffeinated sodas, and water, with coffee often available at night. Additionally, most runners carry a supply of fluid and food (typically compact food like sports bars and gels). A runner should practice eating and drinking during training runs. New foods or liquids should not be ingested for the first time during a race.

Nausea is a common problem during the longer ultramarathons and is probably due to a number of factors.[20] Dehydration and hyponatremia may both cause nausea. Consuming only carbohydrates during a race causes nausea in many runners. Consuming proteins and fats will help control acidity in the GI tract. The best way to avoid or mitigate this problem is to maintain hydration, consume a variety of foods and salt, and train adequately before attempting an ultramarathon.

SUMMARY

Ultramarathons are challenging for both the runner and the medical professional caring for the athlete. Understanding the demands of the event are paramount to ensure proper training and to minimize potential problems during the race. The medical professional caring for ultramarathoners must understand the problems that may occur in training for and running ultramarathons in order to provide the best possible care for these runners.

REFERENCES

1. Laslett L, Eisenbud E: Lack of detection of myocardial injury during competitive races lasting 18 to 30 hours. *Am J Cardiol* 1997:80, 379.
2. Davila-Roman V, Guest T, Tuteur P, et al.: Transient right but not left ventricular dysfunction after strenuous exercise at high altitude. *J Am Coll Cardiol* 1997:30, 468.
3. Lind R, Eisenbud E, Lang G, et al.: CPK studies in Western States 100 Mile Endurance Runners. *UltraRunning* 1996:16, 48.
4. Lind R, Shipley J: Transient renal failure in the Western States 100 Mile Run. *UltraRunning* 1999:19, 34.
5. Seiler D, Franz H, Hellstern P, et al.: Effects of long-distance running on iron metabolism and hematological parameters. *Int J Sports Med* 1989:10, 357.
6. DePaz J, Villa J, Lopez P, et al.: Effects of long-distance running on serum bilirubin. *Med Sci Sports Exerc* 1995:27, 1590.
7. Dickson D, Wilkinson R, Noakes T: Effects of ultramarathon training and racing on hematologic parameters and serum ferritin levels in well-trained athletes. *Int J Sports Med* 1982:3, 111.
8. O'Toole M, Iwane H, Douglas P, et al.: Iron status in ultraendurance triathletes. *Phys Sportsmed* 1989:17, 90.
9. Holtzhausen L, Noakes T, Kroning B, et al.: Clinical and biomechanical characteristics of collapsed ultramarathon runners. *Med Sci Sports Exerc* 1994:26, 1095.
10. Noakes T: Dehydration during exercise: What are the real dangers? *Clin J Sport Med* 1995:5, 123.
11. Holtzhausen L, Noakes T: The prevalence and significance of post-exercise (postural) hypotension in ultramarathon runners. *Med Sci Sports Exerc* 1995:27, 1595.
12. Nelson P, Robinson A, Kapoor W, et al.: Hyponatremia in a marathoner. *Phys Sportsmed* 1988:16, 78.
13. Noakes T, Norman R, Buck R, et al.: The incidence of hyponatremia during prolonged ultraendurance exercise. *Med Sci Sports Exerc* 1990:22, 165.
14. Speedy D, Campbell R, Mulligan G, et al.: Weight changes and serum sodium concentrations after an ultradistance multisport triathlon. *Clin J Sports Med* 1997:7, 100.
15. O'Toole M, Douglas P, Laird R, et al.: Fluid and electrolyte status in athletes receiving medical care at an ultradistance triathlon. *Clin J Sport Med* 1995:5, 116.
16. Speedy D, Faris J, Hamlin M, et al.: Hyponatremia and weight changes in an ultradistance triathlon. *Clin J Sport Med* 1997:7, 180.
17. Speedy D, Noakes T, Rogers I, et al.: Hyponatremia in ultradistance triathletes. *Med Sci Sports Exerc* 1999:31, 809.
18. Barr S, Costill D, Fink W: Fluid replacement during prolonged exercise: Effects of water, saline, or no fluid. *Med Sci Sports Exerc* 1991:23, 811.
19. Noakes T: Hyponatremia during endurance running: A physiological and clinical interpretation. *Med Sci Sports Exerc* 1992:24, 403.
20. King K: Fighting nausea demons in an ultra. *UltraRunning* 1998:18, 48.
21. Moses FM, Baska RS, Peura DA, et al.: Effect of cimetidine on marathon-associated gastrointestinal symptoms and bleeding. *Dig Dis Sci* 1991:36, 1390.
22. Baska RS, Moses FM, Graeber G, et al.: Gastrointestinal bleeding during an ultramarathon. *Dig Dis Sci* 1990:35, 276.
23. Baska RS, Moses FM, Deuster P: Cimetidine reduces running-associated gastrointestinal bleeding. A prospective observation. *Dig Dis Sci* 1990:35, 956.
24. Bergeron B: A guide to blister management. *Phys Sportsmed* 1995:23, 37.

25. Knapik J, Reynolds K, Duplantis K, et al.: Friction blisters: Pathophysiology, prevention and treatment. *Sports Med* 1995:20, 136.

26. Vonhof J: *Fixing Your Feet: Preventative Maintenance and Treatments for Foot Problems of Runners, Hikers, and Adventure Racers*, Mukilteo, Wash, WinePress Publishing, 1997.

27. Hutson M: Medical implications of ultra marathon running: Observations on a six day track race. *Br J Sports Med* 1984:18, 44.

28. Fallon K: Musculoskeletal injuries in the ultramarathon: The 1990 Westfield Sydney to Melbourne run. *Br J Sports Med* 1996:30, 319.

29. Bishop GW, Fallon KE: Musculoskeletal injuries in a six-day track race: Ultramarathoner's ankle. *Clin J Sport Med* 1999:9, 216.

Chapter 38

NUTRITIONAL CONSIDERATIONS

Nancy M. DiMarco
and Matthew Samuels

INTRODUCTION

Athletes with a healthy diet and lifestyle are able to perform at peak output, recover more quickly, and reach goals faster. This nutrition chapter focuses primarily on fuel metabolism during exercise, carbohydrate loading and glycogen resynthesis, dietary needs before, during, and after the event, fluid needs and recommendations, and nutritional supplements. All these factors will help the athlete understand how to consume an optimal diet that contributes to peak performance and a healthy lifestyle.

FUEL UTILIZATION

Energy expenditure for different types of exercise depends on the duration, frequency, and intensity of the exercise. The more energy you use in activity, the more calories you will require. In general, an athlete training for a specific event, or someone committed to an exercise program, will require a greater caloric intake than a sedentary individual. The reference sedentary man, weighing 154 lb, expends 2700 to 3500 kcal a day (average 3025) between ages 20 and 29 years. The reference woman, weighing 125 lb, expends 1890 to 2000 kcal (average 1957) between ages 20 and 29 years.[1] Male athletes in training will expend 3000 to 6000 calories a day; for participation in the Ironman Triathlon (consisting of a 2.4-mile open ocean swim, 112-mile bike race, and 26.2-mile marathon), approximately 9000 kcal are required.

Energy expenditure must be balanced by energy intake. If the distance is short, fuel is not a limiting factor. However, if the muscles must contract for a long time (for example, over an hour), fuels begin to deplete. It is important to understand the types of fuels available to power different types of activities. The type of activity performed determines the predominant energy pathways, three of which (two anaerobic and one primarily aerobic) are mostly used for muscular work.

The first is the *power pathway*. Exercise duration usually lasts no longer than 4 seconds and is of high intensity. Adenosine triphosphate (ATP) and creatine phosphate provide the energy. Activities include the clean and jerk in weight lifting or a fast break in basketball. The second is the *speed pathway*; exercise duration is 4 to 60 seconds. Muscle glycogen and glucose are the main substrates used. This pathway is anaerobic and is used for track events of less than 400 meters or swimming events of less than 100 meters, for example. The third is the aerobic pathway, also referred to as the *endurance pathway*; it is used for events lasting longer than 2 minutes. Muscle and liver glycogen, fat deposits found in muscle, blood, and adipose tissue, and muscle, blood, and liver amino acids all serve as substrates for events such as a 1500-meter run, marathon, half-marathon, and so forth.

TABLE 38–1. CONTRIBUTION OF AEROBIC VS. ANAEROBIC PRODUCTION OF ATP DURING MAXIMAL EXERCISE AS A FUNCTION OF THE DURATION OF THE EVENT

	Duration of Maximal Exercise								
	Sec			*Min*					
	10	*30*	*60*	*2*	*4*	*10*	*30*	*60*	*120*
% Aerobic	10	20	30	40	65	85	95	98	99
% Anaerobic	90	80	70	60	35	15	5	2	1

Source: From Powers and Howley.[2]

In general, short-term activities are supplied by energy that is readily available in the muscle performing the activity. If the activity extends beyond 2 minutes, the body begins to switch over from primarily anaerobic systems to more aerobic ones as oxygen becomes more available.

The ATP-creatine phosphate (power) system is the immediately available source found in muscles. Glucose and muscle glycogen produce ATP rapidly through the speed system, but this rapid provision of energy cannot be sustained. Only the aerobic (endurance) system, which uses fats as a primary source of energy, can produce large amounts of ATP over considerable time via the Krebs cycle and electron transport.

The conversion of energy systems over time is shown in Table 38–1. As you can see, we can depend on anaerobic systems of ATP-creatine phosphate and lactic acid for only brief periods, and then we must use the endurance system. The change from anaerobic to aerobic systems is not abrupt, and the intensity, duration, frequency, type of activity, and fitness level of the participant determines the crossover point. After

2 hours of activity, most of the energy is derived from the endurance system (approximately 99%) and only a trace from the anaerobic system (approximately 1%).[2]

The energy sources during 1 to 4 hours of continuous exercise at 70% of maximal oxygen capacity are shown in Fig. 38–1.[3] At this level of intensity, approximately 50% to 60% of energy is derived from carbohydrate and the rest from free fatty acid oxidation. As the level of intensity decreases, a greater proportion of energy comes from the oxidation of free fatty acids, primarily those derived from muscle triglycerides.[4] Figure 38–2 shows cumulative total energy utilized during prolonged exercise before and after training.[5] Although the total energy expended does not change as a result of training, the energy derived from fat increases and the energy derived from carbohydrate decreases as fats are used more efficiently as an energy source. A trained individual uses a higher percentage of fat than an untrained person at the same workload. Long-chain fatty acids derived from stored muscle triglycerides become the preferred fuel for aerobic exercise for the individual performing mild- to moderate-intensity exercise.[4,6-8].

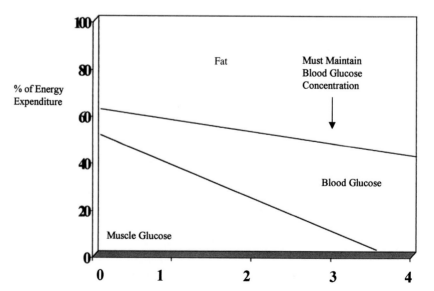

Figure 38–1. Energy sources during 1 to 4 hours of continuous exercise at 70% of V̇o₂max. Approximately 50% to 60% of energy is derived from carbohydrate, with the remaining 40% to 50% from free fatty acid oxidation. *(Source: From Coyle et al.[3])*

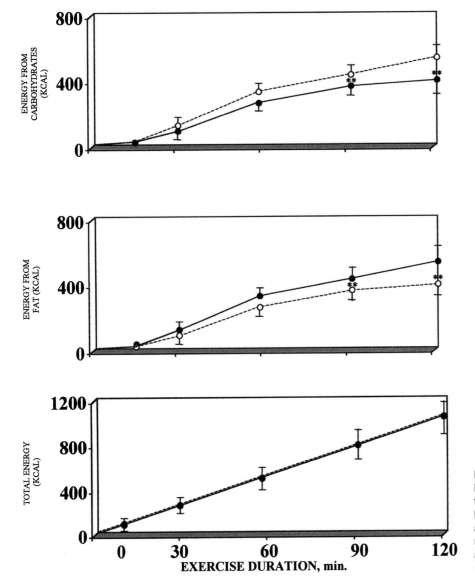

Figure 38–2. Cumulative total energy utilized, energy from fat oxidation, and energy from carbohydrate oxidation during prolonged exercise test before (open circles) and after (filled circles) training. Values are means ±SD. **Difference between before and after training significant at $P < 0.01$. (*Source: From Hurley et al.[5]*)

GENERAL DIETARY NEEDS OF THE RUNNER

The average American consumes about 46% (or about 4 g/kg body weight) of total caloric intake as carbohydrate. This amount of carbohydrate would not be sufficient to supply the needs of the endurance athlete. The general guidelines for the endurance athlete are that between 60% and 70% of total kcal, or 8 to 10 g/kg body weight, should be in the form of carbohydrates for those runners participating in training that extends beyond an hour or more.[9–12] Endurance athletes training for less than an hour a day can resynthesize glycogen adequately on dietary intakes of 6 g/kg body weight. All general dietary guidelines for endurance athletes are predicated on consumption of adequate calories to sustain daily energy expenditure. The average endurance athlete should consume approximately 55 kcal/kg body weight, so a 150-lb person (68 kg) would need about 3750 kcal a day during training, of which 1920 to 2700 kcal should be carbohydrates (480 to 675 g of carbohydrate a day).[13]

At this point, mention of the Zone Diet promulgated by Barry Sears is warranted.[14] This diet and other fad approaches to sports nutrition are very popular. The "Zone" is attained, according to the author, by consuming a diet consisting of 40% carbohydrate, 30% protein, and 30% fat. In his popular book, he asserts that this proportion of macronutrients will cause a decrease in the amount of insulin secreted, alter the production of eicosanoids, and, therefore, decrease body fat and risk for disease. He recommends three small meals not

TABLE 38–2. FOOD GUIDE FOR THE ENDURANCE ATHLETE[a]

Food Type	Serving Size	Servings/Day	Kcals	Protein (g)	CHO (g)	Fat (g)
Rice, cereal, grains, pasta, legumes	$\frac{1}{2}$ cup or 1 oz	18	80 × 18 = 1440	3 × 18 = 54	15 × 18 = 270	0
Vegetables	$\frac{1}{2}$ cup	6	25 × 6 = 150	2 × 6 = 12	5 × 6 = 30	0
Fruit/juices	1 small fruit or $\frac{1}{2}$ cup	8	60 × 8 = 480	0	15 × 8 = 120	0
2% Milk/milk products	1 cup	5	120 × 5 = 600	8 × 5 = 40	12 × 5 = 60	5 × 5 = 25
Meats (includes 1 egg, 1 T peanut butter, 1 oz low-fat cheese)	1 oz	5	75 × 5 = 375	7 × 5 = 35	0	5 × 5 = 25
Fats	1 tsp	7	45 × 7 = 315	0	0	5 × 7 = 35
Nuts and seeds	1 T	3	50 × 3 = 150	1 × 3 = 3	1 × 3 = 3	5 × 3 = 15
Sugars/sweets	1 T	4	60 × 4 = 240	0	15 × 4 = 60	0

[a]This dietary plan provides about 3750 kcals, 133 g of protein, 14% of total kcal, 1.95 g/kg body weight, 543 g of carbohydrate, 58% of total kcal, 100 g of fat, 24% of total kcal.

over 500 kcal and two snacks not over 100 kcal. Sears claims that the protein-to-carbohydrate ratio attained by following this regimen will change the balance between insulin (decreases) and glucagon (increases) and decrease the bad eicosanoids that promote heart disease, cancer, and autoimmune diseases. Unfortunately, there are few if any good research studies to back up his claims. This author contends that anyone who is active and consuming a diet of only 1700 kcal a day will lose weight but that this number of kcal will *not* support the demands of a competitive athlete's nutritional needs nor his or her needs for optimal performance.

From a dietitian's point of view, this diet is inadequate in carbohydrates, vitamins, minerals, and antioxidants. It is imbalanced in comparison with the recommendations of the American Heart Association, the American Cancer Society, the American College of Sports Medicine, the American Dietetic Association, and the U.S. Dietary Guidelines, which recommend 55% to 60% carbohydrate, 10% to 15% protein, less than 30% fat, and 20 to 35 g of fiber daily. The Zone Diet causes water loss and ketosis and may increase uric acid, blood urea nitrogen (BUN), and creatinine levels,

which in turn may increase the risk of gout and exacerbate impaired kidney function. The only sure way to lose weight effectively and permanently is a varied, balanced diet eaten in moderation in combination with a higher-activity lifestyle.

High-quality protein intake for the endurance athlete should be 1.0 to 1.5 g/kg body weight per day[15,16] or 150% to 175% of the current RDA for protein. Most endurance athletes are currently consuming large amounts of protein as part of their normal intake. A 150-lb person would therefore need about 75 to 113 g of protein a day.

Dietary fat intake should total less than 30% of the total kcal.[9,11] Endurance athletes involved in a great deal of training are advised to reduce their fat intake to 20% to 25% of the total kcal, to be able to consume the large amounts of carbohydrate necessary to prevent chronic fatigue or "staleness."[9,11] For our 150-lb athlete consuming 3750 kcal a day, fat intake at 30% of the total kcal would be 1125 kcal, or 125 g of fat. Tables 38–2 and 38–3 provide a sample menu for a 150-lb endurance athlete consuming 3750 kcal/day. This sample may easily be modified by changing the number of servings.

TABLE 38–3. SAMPLE MENU FOR 150-POUND ENDURANCE ATHLETE CONSUMING ABOUT 3750 kcal A DAY

Breakfast	*Lunch*	*Dinner*
3 cups cereal	3 oz lean ham	1$\frac{1}{2}$ cups tossed salad
2 cups 2% milk	1 oz baby Swiss cheese	2 tsp salad dressing
1 cup orange juice	lettuce	1 cup steamed broccoli
2 slices whole wheat toast	2 tsp mayonnaise	1 cup rice or couscous
2 tsp butter or margarine	4 sliced tomatoes	2 oz grilled salmon
1 T jam or jelly	2 slices sandwich bread	1 cup 2% milk
Morning snack	1 cup grapes	2 dinner rolls
1 banana	3 T almonds	*Evening snack*
1 granola bar	2 chocolate chip cookies	2 cinnamon graham crackers
$\frac{1}{2}$ cup baby carrots	*Afternoon snack*	1 cup 2% milk
	3 cups light popcorn	1 cup strawberries
	1 Granny Smith apple	

CARBOHYDRATE LOADING AND GLYCOGEN RESYNTHESIS

Carbohydrate loading is the only legal manipulation that has proven effects during long-distance events. Carbohydrate must be replaced on a regular basis for individuals training at high-intensity levels. This is true for exercising individuals as well as elite athletes. Figure 38–3 shows the effects on muscle glycogen content of a low- (40% of kcal) vs. a high-carbohydrate (70% of kcal) diet during 3 successive days of heavy training.[17] Even after 2-hour training bouts, individuals consuming a high-carbohydrate diet replenished glycogen stores almost back to baseline levels. Individuals on the low-carbohydrate diet, however, displayed continual decreases in muscle glycogen stores. It can be seen from this study that habitual high-carbohydrate intake is essential for maintenance of muscle glycogen stores for both training and endurance events. In 1966, Bergstrom and Hultman[18] performed a now classical experiment. One of them worked with his left leg and the other the right leg on bicycle ergometers. They exercised for several hours until the exercising leg was almost depleted of glycogen and the resting leg still had normal levels. They then went on a carbohydrate-rich diet for 3 days. They both saw small increases in the nonexercised leg and dramatic increases in the exercising leg until glycogen content of the exercising muscle was almost four times higher than the baseline content.

Originally, the carbohydrate loading method involved depletion of glycogen levels by exhaustive exercise 1 week prior to competition. The exhaustive exercise was followed by a low-carbohydrate diet phase (less than 100 g a day) for 3 days in addition to continued exercise and then a switch to a high-carbohydrate diet (250 to 525 g a day) for 3 days to ensure glycogen supercompensation. This method of carbohydrate loading was not without consequences. The high-fat phase was accompanied by irritability, hypoglycemia, water deposition, stiffness and heaviness of the muscles, diarrhea, and dehydration. Older marathoners often experienced chest pains.

Today, modified carbohydrate loading techniques are used quite successfully. Typically, individuals will consume diets consisting of approximately 60% of the total caloric intake as carbohydrates and manipulate the amount of exercise performed during the week prior to competition.[19] This modified regimen is shown in Table 38–4.[9] When compared with the older method, the same level of muscle glycogen is achieved without the negative consequences observed previously. A few notes of caution: glycogen loading is used for endurance-trained individuals, as the muscles loaded are those used in the event. Furthermore, training must decrease during the 3 days prior to competition to allow glycogen stores to maximize, and glycogen loading should only be used for events lasting longer than 90 minutes.

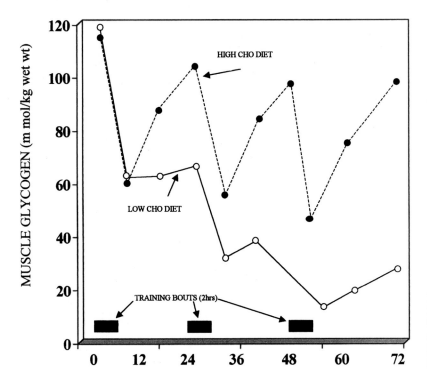

Figure 38–3. Muscle glycogen content during 3 days of heavy training and consumption of a diet whose caloric composition was 40% carbohydrate (low CHO) and 70% carbohydrate (high CHO). *(Source: From Costill and Miller.[17])*

TABLE 38–4. MODIFIED CARBOHYDRATE LOADING REGIMEN

Day	Exercise Duration	Dietary Carbohydrate (%)
1	90 min	60
2	40 min	60
3	40 min	65
4	20 min	70
5	20 min	70
6	Rest	70
7	Competition	70

Source: From Coleman.[9]

Carbohydrate intake subsequent to competition should begin immediately after fluid replacement. Costill et al.[20] have shown that the type of carbohydrate consumed during the first 24 hours after competition does not seem to matter. After 48 hours, complex carbohydrates are the preferred substrates for glycogen resynthesis. Figure 38–4 shows the results of this study, in which participants consumed a 70% carbohydrate diet consisting of either simple sugars such as pancakes, syrup, candy bars, and glucose drinks or complex carbohydrates such as pasta, potatoes, rice, and whole-wheat bread, after a 10-mile run at 80% of maximal oxygen capacity and sprints at 130% of maximal oxygen capacity to decrease gastrocnemius glycogen levels. There was no difference in glycogen resynthesis at 24 hours after exercise, but at 48 hours, significantly more glycogen was synthesized from complex carbohydrates.

The recommendation for today's active individual is that 60% of the total kcal should come predominantly from complex carbohydrates. Glycogen depletion can be prevented by consumption of a diet containing rich sources of carbohydrate (6 to 10 g/kg body weight a day) in combination with days of rest. For those individuals involved in heavy periods of training at higher intensity, the recommendation for carbohydrate is increased to 8 to 10 g/kg body weight a day to achieve glycogen replenishment while reducing fat intake to 20% to 25% of the total calories.

DIETARY NEEDS BEFORE, DURING, AND AFTER THE EVENT

The recommendations for both active individuals and athletes are based on the U.S. Department of Agriculture Food Guide Pyramid and Dietary Guidelines for Americans.[21,22]

The Meal Before the Event

Athletes often compete in early morning events; if they do not consume any food, they are at serious risk for glycogen depletion and dehydration, manifesting as poor performance.[3,23] The meal before the event should be individualized based on preferences and food digestibility, excluding high-fat and protein-containing foods for at least 3 hours prior to competition. It should

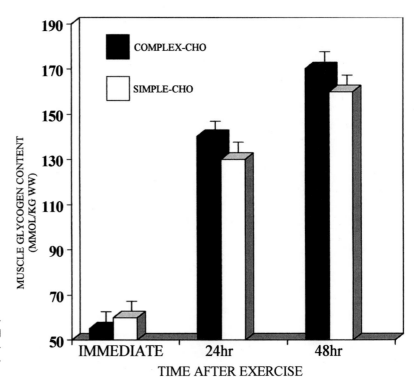

Figure 38–4. Muscle glycogen content measured immediately after, 24 hours after, and 48 hours after strenuous exercise in individuals consuming either complex or simple carbohydrates. *(Source: From Costill et al.[20])*

contain 150 to 300 g of carbohydrate (3 to 5 g/kg body weight). The form of the meal probably does not affect exercise performance. Sherman et al.[24] evaluated the effects of liquid carbohydrate 4 hours prior to 95 minutes of interval cycling followed by a performance trial. The 312 g of carbohydrate improved cycling performance by 15%.

Eating 1 Hour Prior to the Event

Although some studies have indicated positive effects of 1 g/kg body weight carbohydrate consumption 1 hour prior to competition,[25] not all studies have been conclusive. The recommendation by these authors is to encourage the athlete to experiment prior to competition to determine what works best.

Eating During the Event

Carbohydrate intake during events lasting longer than 1 hour may improve performance by helping to maintain blood glucose levels and spare muscle glycogen. Consuming approximately 60 g/hr of liquid or solid carbohydrate during events lasting longer than 1 hour has been shown to be beneficial to optimum performance.[26–30] Endurance athletes should refrain from consuming beverages containing fructose, as less fructose can be used as a source of energy in comparison with glucose during prolonged exercise.[31] Fructose is also absorbed much more slowly than glucose and can cause severe gastrointestinal distress (vomiting and diarrhea).[32] Choosing beverages that contain glucose or sucrose as the main ingredient is wise for the endurance athlete.

Eating After the Event

Once rehydration has occurred, easily digested liquid or solid foods high in carbohydrates should be consumed as quickly as possible to maximize glycogen resynthesis and provide protein for maintenance and repair of muscle tissue. The amount of food and the number of servings can be determined by using the Sports Food Swap developed by Houtkooper.[11] A range of 3.2 to 4.5 g/lb of body weight for carbohydrates and 0.5 to 0.75 g/lb of body weight for protein is recommended following heavy endurance training. Fat intake should be 30% of total kcal. Foods included represent the food groups from the Food Guide Pyramid and can be adapted to a vegetarian meal plan as well.

HYDRATION

Proper hydration is arguably the most important factor affecting performance and acute health in athletes, including runners. Although adequate hydration does not necessarily have ergogenic effects, it does allow for optimal performance. In contrast, inadequate hydration can easily lead to severe performance decrements and acute health problems.

Water is the most important nutrient for regulating hydration status in individuals. Not only does water act as a medium for cellular processes, it is also the main component of plasma and thus plays an important role in the transport of oxygen and nutrients to the tissues. Water loss during exercise occurs primarily through sweat, with the amount of loss being dependent on such factors as ambient temperature, humidity, exercise intensity, and the rate of exogenous fluid intake. This water loss occurs in both the intra- and extracellular fluid compartments of the body,[33] ultimately leading to changes in electrolyte balance (Na^{2+} and K^+) and cardiorespiratory function.

Effects of Dehydration

The average person does not consume enough fluid to offset sweat losses during exercise, often because of psychological/physiological factors and the nature of the activity.[33] In running, it can be difficult for individuals to consume adequate fluid because of the repetitive bouncing motion, especially during competition. In fact, it is not uncommon for elite runners to consume less than 200 ml of fluid during distance events in a cool environment lasting more than 2 hours.[33]

Water loss through sweat during exercise can amount to 2% to 6% of a person's body weight.[34] This state of dehydration leads to many physiological changes, including impaired heat dissipation, decreased plasma volume, and impaired skin blood flow. In severe conditions this decreased plasma volume causes decreased stroke volume, increased heart rate, and ultimately cardiac drift or heat stroke. Therefore, it is imperative that the runner be properly educated about the detriments of dehydration and various ways to maintain proper hydration during training or competition.

Maintaining Adequate Hydration

Fluid Replacement Prior to Exercise

To offset the risk of dehydration, it is recommended that individuals be adequately hydrated when they begin exercise,[35] by consuming fluid continuously throughout the day and ingesting 400 to 600 ml of fluid 2 hours before exercise or competition. The former is especially important when the individual is training on consecutive days in hot or humid weather. This 2-hour period should allow ample time for the excretion of excess water.

Fluid Replacement During Exercise

The goal for the athlete is to replace fluid at a rate equal to sweat loss. This can be monitored by changes in body weight. A 1-lb decrease in body weight signifies a loss of roughly 500 ml of water. Therefore, if a runner were to lose 2 lb during exercise, proper fluid status could be restored through the consumption of 1 L of fluid.

Since monitoring of weight loss is not always possible, a practical recommendation is to consume 150 to 300 ml of water every 15 to 20 minutes of exercise, depending on the sweat rate.[35] This is often achieved using cool fluid (between 15 and 22°C [59 to 72°F]) with a flavor enhancer.

When exercise lasts less than an hour, water is generally the recommended fluid. When exercise lasts for more than 1 hour, the addition of carbohydrate (glucose or sucrose) and/or electrolytes can be beneficial. Not only does this supply a rapid source of glucose to the working muscles (often delaying systemic fatigue), it may also promote increased fluid consumption (through increased palatability) and aid in gastric emptying. However, a few points should be made. The carbohydrate solution should not contain more than 10% carbohydrate, with 4% to 8% being optimal. This is equivalent to 10 g of carbohydrate per 100 ml of water. For example, Gatorade contains 14 g of carbohydrate per cup, or 6%, and has an osmolality of 280 mosm/kg water. This amount of carbohydrate ensures maximal stimulation of fluid absorption and improved performance. A higher carbohydrate concentration does not necessarily lead to increased glucose uptake by the cells and can also promote dehydration by pulling water into the intestinal lumen and decreasing the osmolality of the solution. Also, electrolytes are typically not necessary since any sodium and potassium loss can be replenished through a balanced diet. However, in the presence of excessive exercise duration, extreme environmental conditions, or a poor diet, electrolytes could prove to be beneficial.

Fluid Replacement After Exercise

Body weight changes are the best method of determining fluid replacement rates after exercise. As mentioned previously, 500 ml of fluid should be consumed for every 1 lb of weight loss. It is also recommended that food consumption be rich in sodium and potassium if sweat loss was particularly high. Foods particularly high in sodium and potassium include fruits and vegetables.

Summary

Proper hydration is essential for peak running performance. Dehydration can lead to such conditions as decreased heat dissipation and stroke volume, increased heart rate, and heat stroke. To ensure proper hydration it is recommended that the athlete consume 400 to 600 ml of water 2 hours prior to exercise, 150 to 300 ml every 15 to 30 minutes during exercise, and at least 500 ml/lb of body weight loss following exercise. If the activity lasts longer than 1 hour, a glucose/sucrose solution containing 4% to 8% carbohydrate is recommended.

ERGOGENIC AIDS

Creatine

Creatine is one of the most popular sports nutrition supplements on the market today. Athletes in strength and power sports consider it an effective strength and performance enhancer. It is important for the professional to explore the research data, to determine whether creatine is an effective ergogenic aid or just a hyped supplement and whether creatine may be beneficial for runners.

Overview

Creatine is synthesized from the amino acids glycine, arginine, and methionine in the kidneys, liver, and pancreas and is found primarily in skeletal muscle.[36] Creatine can be found in both free and phosphorylated forms within the tissues, with approximately 60% being in the phosphorylated form. Generally about 2 g a day is catabolized and equally consumed exogenously. Foods rich in creatine include meat and fish.

Creatine is an important source of chemical energy for muscle contraction because it can undergo rapid phosphorylation, creating phosphocreatine (CP), and also acts as a donor of a phosphate group to adenosine diphosphate (ADP) for the synthesis of ATP.[37] It is this rapid phosphorylation of ADP to ATP that makes creatine a possible ergogenic aid, especially for high-intensity, intermittent exercise lasting less than 30 seconds. Therefore, it has been hypothesized that creatine could possibly increase performance in such activities as weight training and sprinting, especially when the activity is performed repetitively.

Effect on Physical Performance

Because creatine has only been marketed to the general public within the past few years, relatively few studies have been performed specifically in runners. However, it is possible that data can still be effectively extrapolated when the mode of activity stresses the same energy systems (ATP-CP or aerobic glycolysis). Most studies have used exogenous creatine in the form of creatine phosphate, a supplemental protocol of 20 g/day for 5 to 7 days followed by a maintenance dose of 2 g a day, and various un-standardized exercise protocols. In addition, some studies have used simple carbohydrates consumed with creatine, which may enhance the transport of creatine into the intracellular compartment. In-depth reviews of many creatine studies can be found in references 36 and 37.

In general, it has been found that creatine supplementation may enhance performance in certain repetitive, high-intensity, short-term tasks that utilize the ATP-CP energy system, especially in the laboratory setting.[37] However, this has typically been found to occur using such protocols as sprints performed on a cycle ergometer and isotonic and isometric contractions. In the field setting, both Stout et al.[38] and Goldberg and Bechtel[39] found no significant effect from creatine supplementation on 40- to 100-meter sprint speed in football and track athletes. Results are also equivocal in studies that used running for 30 to 150 seconds (anaerobic glycolysis), with approximately 50% of studies showing improvements in running performance. Finally, very few studies have looked at the effects of creatine on endurance performance. Of three studies that looked at creatine and endurance performance, only one showed an improvement in 1000-meter run time performed over four trials.

Side Effects

Because creatine is degraded to creatinine in the kidney, it has been hypothesized that supplemental creatine intake may cause short-term or long-term renal problems, especially in those who have existing renal conditions. Unfortunately, to date no long-term studies have been performed to determine whether this hypothesis is valid. Short-term studies have reported no adverse effects on renal function when supplemental intake lasted up to 6 weeks.

One noticeable side effect reported in the literature and among athletes is a rapid increase in body mass after the acute loading phase, typically a weight gain of 3 to 10 lb. It is believed that this increase is due to an increase in intracellular hydration as a direct result of increased cellular creatine concentrations. Depending on the sport, this weight gain may be looked on positively or negatively.

Conclusions

Creatine may have beneficial effects on performance in activities that are intensive, less than 30 seconds in duration, and repetitive. As the length of time the activity is performed increases, the beneficial effects of creatine decrease. A typical protocol for creatine supplementation is 20 g for 5 to 7 days followed by 2 to 3 g a day during the maintenance phase. Also, creatine

uptake by the cells may be facilitated by a carbohydrate beverage or food that elicits a medium to high increase in blood sugar. Although the research is not conclusive, there is enough evidence to warrant creatine's possible use as an ergogenic aid for such athletes as sprinters.

Antioxidants

Because exercise increases oxygen consumption as much as 15-fold, there is also an increase in free radical production, which may lead to skeletal muscle damage. These free radicals include superoxides, hydroxyl radicals, and hydrogen peroxide. They induce lipid peroxidation of the membranes and an increase in macrophages and white blood cells in the damaged muscle,[40] producing even more free radicals. These free radicals may also mediate soreness and inflammation.

To decrease the damaging effects of free radicals, antioxidants donate hydrogen ions, reducing these substances and rendering them nonoxidative. These antioxidants include vitamins A, C, and E. Vitamins A and E are fat soluble and help protect the cellular membrane from oxidation, whereas vitamin C is water soluble, protects the intracellular structure, and donates hydrogen ions to vitamin E.

Antioxidants and Physical Performance

Because of their powerful properties, it has been hypothesized that antioxidants, especially vitamins C and E, may increase physical performance. However, studies to date have shown very little benefit to physical performance from antioxidant supplementation.[40] Also, very few studies have shown decreases in muscle soreness due to vitamin C or E supplementation.[41] It has been found that supplemental vitamin C may decrease upper respiratory tract infections in runners.[42] Vitamin A has not been shown to have any effect on performance.[40]

Although performance benefits have not been found from antioxidant supplementation, the decrease in lipid peroxidation from antioxidants is beneficial to athletes. Typical intakes among active individuals who use antioxidants for health purposes are approximately 500 to 1000 mg of vitamin C a day and 400 IU of vitamin E a day.

Branched Chain Amino Acids

Central fatigue is common to all athletes, manifesting by decreases in neural stimulus, concentration, and performance. It is believed that central fatigue results from the concatenation of numerous physiological changes including decreased glycogen stores, decreased branched chain amino acid (BCAA) concentrations, and increased levels of free fatty acids, free tryptophan (fTryp), and serotonin (5-HT). BCAAs have been studied to determine whether supplementation can prevent central fatigue and therefore increase athletic performance.

BCAAs include the amino acids valine, leucine, and isoleucine. These nutrients may play a role in decreasing central fatigue by preventing fTryp from crossing the blood-brain barrier in large concentrations. Because fTryp and BCAA compete for the same transporter into the brain, fTryp crosses the blood-brain barrier at a much higher rate when BCAA concentrations are low, leading to an increased production of 5-HT. As a result, the increased 5-HT causes lethargy, depresses motor neuron excitability, alters autonomic and endocrine functions, decreases muscular contraction, and may impair judgment.[43]

Research Findings

Studies using supplemental BCAA, with or without carbohydrates, have been done to determine whether they will decrease the fTryp/BCAA ratio. These studies have produced equivocal results. Some show increases in plasma ammonia[44] and no benefits on cycling times to exhaustion or perceived exertion.[45] However, it has also been reported that supplementation with BCAA (up to 10 g/hr) with or without carbohydrate minimizes the increase in the fTryp/BCAA ratio, decreases muscle protein breakdown, and improves mental performance during and/or following exercise.[43]

Recommendations

Although performance benefits of BCAA with or without a glucose solution are equivocal, the addition of BCAA (2 to 10 g/hr) to a glucose solution during prolonged exercise bouts may help to attenuate the fTryp/BCAA ratio and muscle protein breakdown, thereby reducing fatigue and increasing recovery. For adequate hydration purposes this glucose solution should contain a 4% to 8% concentration of carbohydrate.

SUMMARY

A balanced diet that provides the proper amounts of all required nutrients is essential for peak performance and a healthy lifestyle. This is especially important for the athlete who might be training intensely or competing on successive days. The three primary energy systems used during running are the power, speed, and endurance systems. The energy systems used and energy requirements will vary for each individual depending on such factors as mode of activity, intensity, duration, height, weight, and gender. To aid in peak performance, it is recommended that the athlete pay special attention to nutrient consumption before, during, and after the event. This will help ensure adequate hydration, glucose intake, and recovery. Finally, the use of such methods as glycogen loading and creatine intake may help increase performance and power output for long-distance runners and sprinters, respectively.

REFERENCES

1. Briefel RR: Total energy intake of the US population: The Third National Health and Nutrition Examination Survey, 1988–1991. *Am J Clin Nutr* 1995:62(suppl), 1072S.
2. Powers SK, Howley ET: *Exercise Physiology,* Dubuque, IA, Wm C Brown, 1990.
3. Coyle EF, Coggan AR, Hemmert MK, et al.: Muscle glycogen utilization during prolonged strenuous exercise when fed carbohydrate. *J Appl Physiol* 1986:61, 165.
4. Martin WA: Effect of endurance training on fatty acid metabolism during whole body exercise. *Med Sci Sports Exerc* 1997:29, 635.
5. Hurley BF, Nemeth PM, Martin WH, et al.: Muscle triglyceride utilization during exercise: Effect of training. *J Appl Physiol* 1986:60, 562.
6. Hargreaves M: Interactions between muscle glycogen and blood glucose during exercise. *Exerc Sport Sci Rev* 1997:25, 21.
7. Nicklas BJ: Effects of endurance exercise on adipose tissue metabolism. *Exerc Sport Sci Rev* 1997:5, 77.
8. Turcotte LP, Richter EA, Kiens B.: Increased plasma FFA uptake and oxidation during prolonged exercise in trained versus untrained humans. *Am J Physiol* 1992:262, E791.
9. Coleman EJ. Carbohydrate—the master fuel, in Berning JR, Steen SN (eds.), *Nutrition for Sport and Exercise,* Gaithersburg, MD, Aspen, 1998:21.
10. Pate RR, Branch JD: Training for endurance sport. *Med Sci Sports Exerc* 1992:24, S340.
11. Houtkooper L: Food selection for endurance sports. *Med Sci Sports Exerc* 1992:24, S349.
12. Sherman WM, Lamb DR: Nutrition and prolonged exercise,e, in Lamb DR, Murray R (eds.), *Perspectives in Exercise Science and Sports Medicine,* vol 1, *Prolonged Exercise,* Indianapolis, IN, Benchmark, 1988:213.
13. Klaas R, Saris WMH: Limits of energy turnover in relation to physical performance achievement of energy balance on a daily basis. *J Sports Sci* 1991:9, 1.
14. Sears B: *The Zone.* Harper Collins Publishers, New York, Regan Books, 1995.
15. Sherman WM, Maglischo EW: Minimizing chronic athletic fatigue among swimmers: Special emphasis on nutrition. *Sports Sci Exchange* 1991:4,1.
16. Snyder AC, Naik J: Protein requirements of athletes, in Berning JR, Steen SN (eds.), *Nutrition for Sport and Exercise,* Gaithersburg, MD, Aspen, 1998:45.
17. Costill DL, Miller JM. Nutrition for endurance sports: Carbohydrate and fluid balance. *Int J Sports Med* 1980:1, 2.

18. Bergstrom J, Hultman E. Muscle glycogen synthesis after exercise: An enhancing factor localized to the muscle cells in man. *Nature* 1996:2, 309.

19. Sherman WM, Costill DL, Fink WJ, et al.: The effect of exercise and diet manipulation on muscle glycogen and its subsequent use during performance. *Int J Sports Med* 1981:2, 114.

20. Costill DL, Sherman WM, Fink WJ, et al.: The role of dietary carbohydrates in muscle glycogen resynthesis after strenuous running. *Am J Clin Nutr* 1981:34, 1831.

21. *Food Guide Pyramid: A Guide to Daily Food Choices*, Washington, DC, U.S. Department of Agriculture and U.S. Department of Health and Human Services, 1992.

22. *Nutrition and Your Health: Dietary Guidelines for Americans*, 4th ed., Washington, DC, U.S. Department of Agriculture, U.S. Department of Health and Human Services, 1995.

23. Dohm GL. Metabolic response to exercise after fasting. *J Appl Physiol* 1986:61, 1363.

24. Sherman WM, Brodwicz G, Wright DA, et al.: Effects of 4 h preexercise carbohydrate feedings on cycling performance. *Med Sci Sports Exerc* 1989:21, 598.

25. Sherman WM, Peden, MC, Wright, DA. Carbohydrate feedings 1 h before exercise improves cycling performance. *Am J Clin Nutr* 1991:54, 866.

26. Ball TC, Headley SA, Vanderburgh PM, et al.: Periodic carbohydrate replacement during 50 min of high-intensity cycling improves subsequent sprint performance. *Int J Sport Nutr* 1995:5, 151.

27. Jeukendrup AE, Wagenmakers AJ, Stegen JH, et al.: Carbohydrate ingestion can completely suppress endogenous glucose production during exercise. *Am J Physiol* 1999:276, E672.

28. Mason WL, McConell G, Hargreaves M: Carbohydrate ingestion during exercise: Liquid vs. solid feedings. *Med Sci Sports Exerc* 1993:25, 966.

29. McConell G, Kloot K, Hargreaves M: Effect of timing of carbohydrate ingestion on endurance exercise performance. *Med Sci Sports Exerc* 1996:28, 1300.

30. McConell G, Snow RJ, Proietto J, et al.: Muscle metabolism during prolonged exercise in humans: Influence of carbohydrate availability. *J Appl Physiol* 1999:87, 1083.

31. Massicotte D, Peronnet F, Adopo E, et al.: Effect of metabolic rate on the oxidation of ingested glucose and fructose during exercise. *Int J Sports Med* 1994:15, 177.

32. Craig BW: The influence of fructose feeding on physical performance. *Am J Clin Nutr* 1993:58, 815S.

33. American College of Sports Medicine: Position Stand: Exercise and Fluid Replacement. *Med Sci Sports Exerc* 1996:28, i.

34. Noakes TD: Fluid replacement during exercise. *Exerc Sports Sci Rev* 1993:21, 297.

35. Latzka WA, Montain SJ: Water and electrolyte requirements for exercise. *Clin Sports Med* 1999:18, 513.

36. Demiant TW, Rhodes EC: Effects of creatine supplementation on exercise performance. *Sports Med* 1999:28, 49.

37. Williams MH, Branch JD: Creatine supplementation and exercise performance: An update. *J Am Coll Nutr* 1998:17, 216.

38. Stout JR, Echerson J, Noonan D, et al.: The effects of a supplement designed to augment creatine uptake on exercise performance and fat free mass in football players. (Abstract). *Med Sci Sports Exerc* 1997:29, S251.

39. Goldberg PG, Bechtel PJ: Effects of low dose creatine on strength, speed, and power events by male athletes. (Abstract). *Med Sci Sports Exerc* 1997:29, S251.

40. Clarkson P: Antioxidants and physical performance. *Crit Rev Food Sci Nutr* 1995:35, 131.

41. Kaminski M, Boal R: An effect of ascorbic acid on delayed onset muscle soreness. *Pain* 1992:50, 317.

42. Peters-Futre EM: Vitamin C, neutrophil function, and upper respiratory tract infection risk in distance runners: The missing link. *Exerc Immunol Rev* 1997:3, 32.

43. Kreider RB: Central fatigue hypothesis and overtraining, in Kreider RB, Fry AC, O-Toole ML (eds.), *Overtraining in Sport*, Champaign, IL, Human Kinetics, 1998:309.

44. Vandewalle L, Wagenmakers AJM, Smets K, et al. Effect of branched-chain amino acid supplements on exercise performance in glycogen depleted subjects. *Med Sci Sports Exerc* 1992:23, S116.

45. Galiano FJ, Davis JM, Bailey SP, et al.: Physiologic, endocrine and performance effects of adding branched-chain amino acids to a 6% carbohydrate-electrolyte beverage during prolonged cycling. *Med Sci Sports Exerc* 1991:23, S14.

Chapter 39

DISTANCE RUNNING: ORGANIZATION OF THE MEDICAL TEAM

John C. Cianca, William O. Roberts, and Deborah Horn

INTRODUCTION

In the United States, running is a popular form of exercise, and 9% of the population runs or jogs. Participation in road racing, particularly the marathon, has increased dramatically in the 1990s. It is estimated that there are 15,000 road races a year. Annual marathon finishers have increased in the United States by 1800% since 1976, with 451,000 marathon finishers in 1998 alone.[1] A large part of this increase is due to the influx of charity-based runners and the training programs developed in cities across the United States to help runners prepare for distance races like the marathon. These altruistic opportunities in distance running have created another lure for recreational runners to participate in more serious racing endeavors. As a result, the average marathon finish times at races that cater to charity runners have increased to the 4- to 5-hour range, and the finish line areas are remaining open to participants for 6 to 10 hours. The combination of increased participation and longer finishing times has increased the exposure to injury during a marathon. The likelihood of requiring medical intervention generally increases with the race distance, so the need for medical coverage, with the exception of very large mass participation races, is greater for longer distance races. Medical coverage provides a safety net for runners during distance races, especially in the mass participation races conducted in high-risk environments, and for the marathon and longer-distance races.

THE MEDICAL TEAM

A mass participation marathon requires a comprehensive medical staff and resources. Shorter races, unless held in moderate- to high-heat stress conditions or fielding a large number of participants, tend to require a less-extensive medical team, but the preparations for catastrophic medical problems are unchanged. Ultradistance races may have a significant injury rate, but they usually have fewer entrants, so the demand for medical coverage is less.

Medical Director's Position

The primary role of the medical director during the race is orchestrating the care and safety of the participants. For a mass participation distance event, this demands good "vision" and judgment. Prior to the race, the Medical Director functions as an administrator, developing an effective medical plan with adequate resources and personnel, and as a medical liaison with the race administrators. Open communication with the race administration is vital for the medical team to operate within the infrastructure of the race. The Medical Director also serves as an educator for race participants and volunteers. Prerace instructional information is useful for the runners, the medical team members, and the race volunteers. Through prerace education, injuries and illness during the race are reduced, medical team functions are coordinated, and race volunteers are prepared to interact with the medical team. During the race, the medical director coordinates the medical team in the immediate care of the runners and defines the overall medical support within the race. The Medical Director may choose to be a direct care provider, but this role is difficult in large races. Each of these roles can be fulfilled and carried out in an effective manner with good organization, adequate preparation time, and a competent staff.

Medical Team Organization

A large medical team can be divided into several groups led by Assistant Medical Directors who report to the Medical Director. Within the structure of the marathon medical team, it is common to divide the duties by area of the race into start, finish, and course operations. Nonmedical volunteers are an important part of the medical team. The nonmedical members of the medical team are assigned to central supply, inventory, medical records check-in, medical records transcription, family information, and fetching dry cloths. Logistics volunteers maintain inventory and control the dissemination of equipment and resources in the field hospital and on the course. A van is used to deliver extra supplies to aid stations or medical personnel on the course. All medical personnel should be easily identifiable with badges, shirts, jackets, vests, or caps.

The medical responsibilities at the starting area are limited. There is usually little need for medical care, but the medical team can assist with last-minute advice for runners. The primary medical function at the start is the prerace announcement, which should include medical and safety information, especially the location of medical volunteers, the current and expected weather conditions, and the medical team recommendation for competition. The location, type, and availability of fluid stations along the course, along with a caution about both under- and overhydrating, should also be given in the prerace announcement.

The primary medical care station is the medical tent/field hospital in the finish area. It should be located close to the finish line but still be accessible from other parts of the finish area. The entrances and exits should be clearly marked and monitored by a security team. The medical tent is usually divided into sections defined by anticipated type and level of care. Common designations include orthopedic and podiatric care, skin injury, medical massage, medical observation, medical intervention, and intensive medical care areas. These areas are staffed with appropriately qualified medical personnel. Medical care in the tent will necessitate interactions among physicians, nurses, physical therapists, podiatrists, paramedics, emergency medical technicians (EMTs), and athletic trainers. Nursing staff will provide much of the direct medical care; these staff members are often expert at establishing intravenous (IV) lines. Satisfactory staffing numbers for the medical tent are difficult to judge without a race injury rate and previous race experience for injury type and severity. At the Twin Cities Marathon, which has a 19-year average injury rate of <20/1000 entrants, the tent is staffed by 10 to 15 physicians, 15 to 20 registered nurses, 4 physical therapists, 10 EMTs, and 15 to 20 nonmedical volunteers. The Houston Marathon has an average injury rate of 40/1000 entrants in 1998 to 2000. The medical tent is staffed with 10 to 15 physicians, 5 podiatrists, 35 to 40 registered nurses, 5 to 7 physical therapists, 15 to 20 EMTs, and 50 nonmedical volunteers.

The finish line is an area of heavy runner and volunteer traffic, which requires close cooperation between race and medical personnel. Runners may be crossing the finish line at a rate of more than 100 a minute. The number of finish line attendants must match the peak finisher rate. A group of 20 to 30 is usually adequate for a race of 6000 to 8000 entrants, assuming a peak number of finishers between $3\frac{1}{2}$ to 5 hours into the marathon race. Finish line medical personnel should be ready to offer immediate assistance to ailing runners. Runners should be moved out of the runner flow and transported via gurney or wheelchair to the medical tent. A medical tent triage physician should quickly assess the runners and assign them to the appropriate treatment area within the medical tent. Medical emergencies may necessitate immediate resuscitation, and it is recommended that an advanced cardiac life support ambulance be stationed at the finish line.

Additionally, it is recommended that a small team of triage personnel patrol the area surrounding the finish line to aid or transport collapsed or ill runners. These teams should have a radio contact with the communications team and a medical kit.

Depending on the layout of the race, medical team members are placed at various positions along the course. Typically, this is every other mile in the early stages of a marathon. This may vary from race to race, and more frequent placement of aid stations may be necessary in very large field races to ensure access to first aid and fluids. The Houston Marathon employs medical aid stations at every other mile from mile 5 through mile 19 and then every mile thereafter. For shorter races, such as 5K and 10K distances, one or two aid stations should suffice on the course. For "out and back" courses, the aid stations can double up to provide care in both directions.[2] Ideally, aid stations should be located next to water stations, allowing medical team members access to an adequate supply of water for treatment. Water stations are common stopping points for runners and are an effective area for medical intervention. At the Twin Cities Marathon, there are medical teams at each water stop and smaller medical teams with assigned communications personnel spaced every $1/4$ to $1/2$ mile between the aid stations.

Medical aid stations can be staffed by three or more medical providers for immediate care of runners on the course. Aid station personnel are usually physicians, nurses, or athletic trainers. Additionally, teams of paramedics or EMTs traveling the course by bicycle can assist downed runners away from stationary aid stations. The mobile teams provide the initial care of runners while awaiting the arrival of ambulance services for transportation off the course. Mobile teams allow the stationary aid personnel to remain at their stations and speed the transition of care to the local emergency medical service.[3] Communication with the ambulance service on the course can be handled through the medical committee communications system or by interaction with a local emergency medical transport service. The number of participants, length of the race, race injury rate, and anticipated weather conditions dictate how many ambulances are necessary. One ambulance per 1000 entrants on the course is an adequate starting point for a marathon, but the Twin Cities Marathon, with 7500 entrants, utilizes only two dedicated ambulances with close proximity of two ambulance stations that can respond if necessary. The on-course ambulance responds and stabilizes while another ambulance is brought to the scene for transport to the emergency medical facility. This allows the dedicated ambulances to be free for emergencies while other ambulances are in the process of transport. Shorter races require fewer ambulances, with a minimum of one dedicated to the finish area.[4–6] These vehicles can directly transport runners to community hospitals or the race field hospital. The medical operations group should decide in advance of the race whether downed runners on the course will be transferred to the finish area medical station or to an emergency medical facility. It is the policy of the Twin Cities

Marathon to transport all on-course casualties to an emergency facility because access to the finish line medical area is limited during the race. The Houston Marathon, on the other hand, sends only runners in imminent danger to hospitals directly from the course. The ability to transport both well and ill runners from the course to the medical tent, the finish area, or an emergency medical facility improves runner safety, especially in cold weather.

The presence of medical aid stations or additional runner advisory stations along the race course allows runners to stop and ask questions regarding their physical condition as well as the current and predicted weather conditions for the remainder of the race. These stations should be staffed with people who can address medical and running issues. Stations may provide medical intervention and advice on continuing or dropping out of the race.

Coordination of care between the course and the medical tent is of great concern during the race. A communication system within the medical team is of vital importance before and during the race to coordinate the medical care between personnel on the course and in the medical tent. Communications among the course, the transportation vehicles, and the medical tent are best monitored by a dedicated team of communication specialists via a central radio command post in the medical area.[3–6] Fax machines and phone lines can be established within this area as well. The Medical Director, Assistant Directors, and finish line captain should each have a radio to allow them to give advice and direction to the medical team. If possible, each major area of the medical team should have its own radio channel. Specifically, separate channels are established for aid stations, cycling teams, ambulances, and finish line personnel. These channels are monitored by the communications team, which in turn has direct contact with the Medical Director and the Assistant Medical Directors. Since there are a limited number of channels available on most hand-held radios, the needs of the rest of the race operations may limit the medical team to a single channel, and a ham radio network can be used to extend the communications of the medical team. Each aid station, cycle team, ambulance, and pick-up vehicle should have its own radio or ham radio communicator. Aid station personnel, cyclists, and ambulances can identify runners who appear to be struggling and pass the information along the course to the aid stations and response teams. Additionally, the Medical Director should maintain radio contact with the Race Director for updates between the two groups regarding race operations and race injuries. A portable phone should also be available for medical tent personnel to communicate with the area emergency facilities to ensure a safe transfer of care.

Medical Planning and Organization

The organization of duties should be established well before the race. Monthly meetings beginning several months prior to the race are helpful for organizing the medical team and should include at least one meeting to check and update the race medical inventory. However, in newly established medical teams, it may be necessary to have more frequent meetings until a level of preparation has been achieved that would ensure the delivery of effective care on race day. Effective race day medical care will require the deployment of appropriate medical staff on the course to ensure adequate care for the runners. The primary goal of the medical team is always to identify and triage injured runners, and the medical committee should anticipate the medical challenges of race day. With greater numbers of participants and more stressful meteorologic conditions, the need for advanced medical care will increase. The usual weather conditions should be considered with provisions for the historical extremes of temperature and humidity. A well-coordinated medical team reduces the number of minor injuries and treatable illnesses, which could overwhelm local emergency facilities, leaving little room for the community members at large.[7]

It is important to have the philosophy of treatment defined prior to the race with accompanying protocols designed to establish consistent and effective treatment for common and expected race injuries. The treatment delivered will be based on the race size, climate, resources, and available medical staff.

Medical coverage can be as basic as first aid support with triage to local hospitals for more significant illness or as involved as on-site care of all but the most ill athletes, with transfer of only the critically ill runners. Specifically, the decision to treat most of the runners on site, including the use of IV fluids, should be decided well in advance of the race, as the decision dictates the extent of medical supplies, staffing, and ambulance coverage required to provide care for the runners. It may be more efficient, in some circumstances, to triage runners who require intensive treatment to local hospitals. First aid can involve the treatment of minor musculoskeletal injuries, resuscitation from mild to moderate exercise-associated collapse, initial cooling for exertional heat stroke, and cardiopulmonary resuscitation (CPR). All members of the medical staff should be trained in basic cardiopulmonary life support, and a cardiac arrest team trained in advanced cardiac life support (ACLS) should be designated for the medical tent and finish area.

More comprehensive on-site treatment is possible and may involve the measurement of glucose, electrolytes, and O_2 saturation with portable devices. Protocols for fluid replacement, cooling, warming, cardiac monitoring, and emergent care should be established and discussed with medical staff prior to race day. If more involved care is to be provided, decisions regarding automatic transfer criteria, the type and amount of IV fluids administered, medications, specific warming and cooling protocols, and equipment issues need to be resolved prior to race day.[7,8] All body temperature measurements should be done rectally.[9] Protocols for transport of well and ill runners must be in place, and quick interface with local emergency rooms must be readily available. Ultimately the medical care at a race should be individualized and not exceed the capabilities of the medical team.

The medical staff should be aware of road racing rules regarding the treatment of struggling runners, as medical evaluation can result in disqualification in some instances. As a general rule in the marathon, runners can be evaluated and allowed to return as long as no "invasive" treatment is rendered. Policies that address the removal of a runner from the race course for medical reasons should be considered and implemented prior to the race. Criteria for removal from the course combine both mental and physical function, including the ability to proceed in a direct path to the finish, good running posture, adequate thermoregulation and hydration status, and verbal responses to basic orientation questions regarding the runner's name and location.[10,11] Prerace education packets should include a clear statement of race rules regarding the evaluation and removal from the course due to medical impairment.

Medical Liability

The subject of medical liability is another important consideration when staffing the medical team. It is uncommon for road race insurance policies to cover medical team volunteers. The Road Race Club of America provides liability coverage for race volunteers, but this specifically excludes medical personnel.[12] Although medical liability insurance will cover many physicians in the role of a race volunteer, other health care professionals often will not have professional liability. Registered nurses, physical therapists, and other medical volunteers may not be covered by their individual or job-related medical liability insurance while acting as a volunteer for events. The race administration should pursue medical liability coverage for its health care volunteers. Some states will place medical volunteers at nonprofit road races, including physicians, under the Good Samaritan laws.

Runner Education

The running boom has attracted novice runners to the sport who may underestimate the preparation needed for racing at the marathon distance. The Medical Director can oversee the race-generated education materials for both novice and veteran racers. The entry form and prerace literature should include sections on the safety and medical aspects of the race including a description of the medical support that will be available during the race. Race entry forms, confirmation replies, race-day packets, and the race Web site serve as useful ways to disseminate pertinent race medical information. Topics for the publications can include general running issues, proper preparation for race day, medical coverage during the race, anticipated race-day weather conditions, hyperthermia, hypothermia, exercise-associated collapse, exercise exhaustion, exercise-associated muscle cramping, hyponatremia, overuse injuries, and injury prevention. Runners should be warned not to start the race with an illness and not to continue the race if they develop chest pain, chest pressure, or severe dyspnea. The race participants should be instructed to record important personal medical information on the back of their race numbers including allergies and medications.

The longer a runner is on the course the greater the risk of injury or illness.[13] As the number of runners with finish times greater than 4 hours increases, the need for education on overhydration and electrolyte replacement has become a critical issue. The incidence of hyponatremia in slow marathon runners is increasing. Overhydration with water alone or in combination with an electrolyte replacement drink seems to be the primary cause of hyponatremia in long-distance runners. This is particularly important in warm weather races, in which the tendency to drink extra fluids is greater among the slower runners. The usual sweat rate in a runner is 1 to 2 L/hr, greater than the average runner fluid replacement and gastric emptying rate. Basic fluid replacement recommendations include 500 ml at least 2 hours prior to a race and 600 to 1200 ml/hr during a race.[14–16] If the fluid loss is exceeded by the fluid intake, it is possible to dilute the normal body sodium level, resulting in fatal cerebral edema and pulmonary edema. Data from an unpublished study at the Houston Marathon show that all cases of diagnosed hyponatremia occurred in runners with finish times greater than $4\frac{1}{2}$ hours in high heat and humidity conditions. Slower runners should be cautioned to match fluid intake to estimated sweat losses and consider using the electrolyte drink while racing. The fluid losses can be estimated by taking a nude weight 30 minutes before a run. At the end of the run, the nude weight is repeated after toweling off the sweat. The weight loss in ounces is doubled and represents the fluid volume to be replaced per hour of running. The incidence of low postrace sodium was decreased in a triathlon by decreasing the number of water stations.[17]

The Medical Director or other medical team members can also deliver educational lectures to local training groups and running clubs on the same topics published in the prerace literature. Many larger races have prerace expositions that include educational programs. This is an opportune time for the Medical Director to present information to race participants regarding last-minute preparation for the race and to reiterate information included in the prerace printed materials. Injury screening clinics can also be arranged for running clubs or the race exposition and can serve as an effective means of increasing participant awareness of common running injuries.

SUPPLIES

In the months prior to race day, the medical team should develop a list of equipment and supplies required to support the medical protocols and should arrange to purchase, rent, or borrow the necessary items. The inventory should be updated, replenished, and repaired from year to year. A well-organized and documented inventory will make race-day utilization and postrace updating more efficient. At the end of each race, the remaining inventory should be cataloged, inspected for damage or wear, and replaced or appropriately cleaned and stored. Cots, blankets, and other reusable items that have come into contact with patients must be washed and disinfected. Perishable items, such as IV fluids and medications, will need to be replenished before the expiration date. Portable electrolyte and glucose monitors should be recalibrated prior to the next use, and used cartridges should be replaced. Digital rectal thermometers, blood pressure cuffs, O_2 regulators, and suction devices will need to be serviced regularly. The upkeep and resupply of an inventory is expensive, and the race budget should reflect this expense, otherwise the race will have to depend on donations to support the needs of the medical team. The medical team can solicit hospitals and medical facilities for the medical equipment and supplies. Wheelchairs, gurneys, blankets, towels, and other equipment can be rented or loaned from local medical supply houses and linen distributors.

RACE COVERAGE

Preparation for Race Day

The medical tent should be set up, stocked, and prepared to function before the finishers begin to arrive (Table 39–1). The day before the race is a good time to

TABLE 39–1. EQUIPMENT: MEDICAL TENT[a]

Item	Quantity/1000 Runners
Ambulance	1
Stat kit with oxygen	1
Electrocardiographic monitor	2
Wool or synthetic blankets	25–30
Biomedical waste bags	5–10
Sharps containers	5–10
Electrolyte monitor	1–2
Moleskin	10 sheets
Thermometers (rectal)	20–30
Blood pressure cuffs	1/staff member
Stethoscopes	1/staff member
Arm/leg splints	2–3 each
Suction unit	1–2
IV poles	1/4 beds
Band-Aids, tape, gauze (4 × 4), Ace wraps, Betadine	In abundance
Beds	10
IV solution (normal saline)	25
Mylar blankets	40
IV starter kit	25
Clean T-shirts	20
Medical records	50
Stretchers/gurneys	3–4
Wheelchairs	2–3
Petroleum jelly	2–3 jars

[a]Based on 60 medical encounters per 1000 entrants at the Houston Marathon.

set up the medical tent and, as soon as the medical area is secured, to organize the medical equipment and supplies. Often setup will be limited to the day of the race, when the area cannot be secured in advance. Pre–race-day setup allows for a more comprehensive setup and provides additional time for unexpected adjustments. A central supply area established in the medical tent will be useful in tracking equipment and disseminating inventory to the various care areas in the finish area and along the course. Portable toilets should be positioned within the medical area, as runners will frequently need to urinate during medical care and will occasionally develop diarrhea from the stress of the run.

Similarly, aid stations and course equipment can be distributed and/or signed out prior to race day to allow for early setup on the morning of the race. The equipment for the course aid stations and bicycles can be packaged and inventoried in suitable containers and portable packs (Tables 39–2 and 39–3). When the containers and packs are distributed, the aid station or cycle team personnel can recheck the prerace inventory and replace any missing equipment prior to the race. A postrace inventory can be used to estimate supply needs for the next race, based on the use per number of participants in similar race conditions. Aid stations should be staffed and ready to operate before runners pass through the area. Bicycle and ambulance crews

TABLE 39–2. EQUIPMENT: AID STATIONS[a]

Item	Quantity/1000 Runners
Sign with station no.	1
Stethoscopes	2
Blood pressure cuffs	1
Tongue depressors	10
Kling (roll), 4 x 4	1
Sterile	20
Nonsterile	20
Vaseline	16 oz
Band-Aids	10
Alcohol wipes	10
Ace wraps	6
Triangle bandage	2
Ice coolers	1
Ice	20 lb
Plastic bags	20
Topical antibiotic packet	20
Betadine swab sticks	10
Pocket mask	1
Peroxide (bottle)	1
Cots	1
Clip board	1
Tape (rolls)	4
Cups	20
Thermometer (rectal)	1
Thermometer covers	4
Medical records	25
Mylar blankets[b]	10
Radio, 900 MHz	1
Trash bag	1

[a]In a warm weather marathon.
[b]For cold weather marathons, have garbage bags with head holes to provide wind and cold protection.

should be on the course before the runners (Tables 39–4 and 39–5). If there is wheelchair competition during the race, the medical team will need to be on station earlier to accommodate the faster pace of the wheelers.

TABLE 39–3. EQUIPMENT: CYCLIST'S PACK[a]

Item	Quantity
Blood pressure cuffs, 4 × 4	1
Sterile	6
Nonsterile	10
Band-Aids	10
Alcohol wipes	6
Ace wraps	2
Triangle bandage	2
Topical antibiotic packet	10
Betadine swab sticks	2
Pocket mask	1
Tape (rolls)	2
Thermometer (rectal)	1
Thermometer covers	4
Medical records	5
Mylar blankets	4
Radio, 900 MHz	1

[a]Based on 40 medical encounters per 1000 entrants at the Houston Marathon. Also an automatic external defibrillator if available.

TABLE 39–4. PERSONNEL: COURSE[a]

Personnel	No.
Aid stations	
Physicians	1–2
Athletic trainers/nurses	2–4
Bicycle EMTs	3–4/1000 runners
Ambulances	1–2/1000 runners
Paramedics/EMTs per ambulance	2–3
Advisory station	2–3 staff/station
(includes nurses, physicians, coaches)	

[a]Based on 40 medical encounters per 1000 entrants at the Houston Marathon.

A thermal injury flag system should be employed and set up at the start of the race along the course in areas designated in the prerace literature. The American College of Sports Medicine (ACSM) advocates a system to alert runners to current weather conditions using the wet bulb globe temperature (WBGT) formula incorporating ambient temperature, radiant heat, and humidity.[18] The WBGT can be taken off a heat stress monitor or calculated from the individual factors. The temperature-based flag system developed by the ACSM corresponds to a risk scale for heat stress including extreme-, high-, moderate-, and low-risk (Table 39–6). These warning flags should be placed either at aid stations or advisory stations on the course if there will be significant changes in heat stress during the race. At the Houston Marathon, flags are placed at the starting line, mile 3, mile 7, and mile 20. These locations are at or near aid stations so that flags can be changed by medical personnel throughout the race as the heat stress changes. WBGT readings should be taken every 30 to 60 minutes and updates communicated to aid-station personnel. At the Twin Cities Marathon, where the temperatures do not vary significantly from the start temperature, the flags are displayed only at the starting line, and the prerace announcements include the anticipated change in temperature during the race. A recommendation for modification or cancellation of the race should be considered in high-risk conditions in consultation with the Race Director.

TABLE 39–5. PERSONNEL: MEDICAL TENT[a]

Personnel	No.
Triage/technical assistance	8–10
EMTs	2–4
Podiatry	2
Physicians	2
Physical therapists	
Medical	1
Massage	10–20
Nurses	5–6

[a]Based on 40 medical encounters per 1000 entrants at the Houston Marathon.

A final communication check of the radios and phones should be done before the race start. Contact with local emergency rooms should be made 2 to 3 weeks before race day and again just before the start of the race to alert emergency rooms of possible incoming injuries. A fax machine is an effective method of communicating with emergency rooms during the race to relay information for a runner in transport. Communication between the race medical staff and emergency room personnel is vital to ensure continuity of care for ill runners. In critical cases it may be necessary for a medical team member to ride in the ambulance with the runner.

Race Operations

A medical record should be devised for use during the race (Fig. 39–1) and should be initiated at first contact with an ill runner. The record should remain with the runner during all phases of evaluation and treatment. The medical record used by the Houston Marathon medical team has a perforated tag for each medical area. These tags can then be detached and sent to a central data entry area where the runner's progress and treatment can be recorded. This method of tracking provides information for the family members who may be trying to locate a missing runner. Once the runner is checked out of the medical area, the entire record is entered into the computer database for more comprehensive documentation of the medical encounter. The medical record for the Twin Cities Marathon is double-sided and tailored to the common medical and musculoskeletal problems seen in the finish area tent. Data are transcribed into the computer database after the race.

After the initial triage, a runner is sent to the appropriate area of the medical tent for definitive treatment. Podiatry/Orthopedics/Skin can be combined as one treatment unit to care for musculoskeletal and skin complaints. Simple home-care instructions are given to runners for minor injuries, and treatment is rendered when appropriate.

The minor medical area or tent serves as an observation site for runners who do not feel well but are obviously not ill or unstable. After an initial evaluation, vital signs are recorded periodically during the observation period, and fluids and food are provided. The runner may be discharged when feeling recovered, exhibiting stable vital signs, tolerating fluids, and, ideally, urinating without difficulty.[7] Nurses and other paraprofessionals can provide most of the care in the minor medical area under the supervision of a physician. The medical massage area is staffed by massage therapists and physical therapists and is utilized for runners with cramps and tight muscles. The physical therapists often rotate to other treatment areas within the medical tent to assist cramping runners utilizing neuromuscular inhibition techniques. Massage for

TABLE 39–6. ACSM COLOR-CODED FLAG SYSTEM

Flag	Temperature	Recommendation
Black	WBGT >82°F (28°C)	Extreme high risk for hyperthermia No competition recommended Cancellation should be considered
Red	WBGT 73°F–82°F (23°C–28°C)	High risk for hyperthermia Heat-sensitive participants should withdraw Consider slowing pace or intensity
Yellow	WBGT 65°F–73°F (18°C–23°C)	Moderate risk for hyperthermia Heat-sensitive participants should slow pace
Green	WBGT 50°F–65°F (10°C–18°C)	Low risk for heat injury Hyperthermia can occur Hypothermia can occur postevent
White	WBGT <50°F (10°C)	Very low-risk hyperthermia Hypothermia risk rises as WBGT decreases Wind and wet conditions increase risk of hypothermia

WBGT (wet bulb globe temperature) = (0.7 Twb) + (0.2 Tbg) + (0.1 Tdb); Twb = temperature, wet bulb thermometer; Tbg = temperature, black globe thermometer; Tdb = temperature, dry bulb thermometer.
Source: Adapted from Armstrong et al.[18]

well runners is done by physical therapists and massage therapists in a separate area adjacent to the medical area at the Houston Marathon. At the Twin Cities Marathon, massage is conducted in a separate area away from the medical tent only after rehydration and rest in well runners. Physical therapists are utilized to relieve cramping using neuromuscular inhibition techniques and acupressure.

The major medical area within the medical tent provides more intensive assessment and intervention techniques for medically ill runners, including IV rehydration and electrolyte monitoring (Fig. 39–2). A team of one or two nurses, one physician, one paramedical professional, and one nonmedical volunteer can usually staff four cots. Roving nurses and physicians can assist teams caring for too many acutely ill runners.

A critical care area can be set up adjacent to the major medical area. The critical care area serves as a location for rapid assessment and stabilization of runners prior to transport to the local emergency room. An ambulance should be stationed immediately adjacent to the critical care area for prompt transfer of unstable runners.

The medical area should be protected and secured for privacy, confidentiality, and control of hazardous waste. Security personnel are essential to enforce an "ill runner–only" policy. A family waiting area with an information service near the medical treatment area will take some of the pressure off the security team. The waiting area should be staffed by volunteers who can communicate with both the medical tent and data entry personnel to keep family members informed of an ill runner's condition. Family members should not

be routinely allowed into the medical area for confidentiality and blood-borne pathogen control reasons. Family members are often anxious, usually uninformed, and frequently tired by the end of a long race. An escorted visit by one family member into the tent for a short visit will often allay the family fears and help the image of the medical team. The staff in the family waiting area will need to be well versed in patient interaction and the art of diplomacy.

INJURY/ILLNESS

Race Characteristics

Medical encounter rates are influenced by a variety of factors, and the race distance and running environment will influence the rate and type of illness and injury seen.[7] As the race length increases, the risk of illness increases; however, the risk of exertional heat stroke is greater in faster-paced, shorter-distance races in the same running environment.[19] Weather changes can increase the incidence of thermal and hydration problems in a race of any distance. As the temperature and relative humidity rise, the medical-encounter rate will increase, as demonstrated by the contrast in environment conditions and encounter rates at the Houston (warm) and Twin Cities (cool) Marathons. Medical team encounter data over a 3-year period from the Houston Marathon show a 3.9% encounter rate, with an average start temperature of 68°F and relative humidity of 90% RH. In contrast, the Twin Cities Marathon has a 12-year average encounter rate of 1.8%, with an average start temperature of 41°F and 84% RH.[20] Race distance and starting time have been linked

Houston Marathon Medical Information Tag | Podiatry

1551

_____
Runner Number

Location: __GRB __Van (#___) __ Course (?_____)

Runner Number

Last Name_____First_____M.I.___

Address _____

City _____ State _____ Zip Code _____

Phone (___) _____   Social Security # _____

1551

Chief Complaint _____

Allergies _____ Medications _____

Past Medical Hx. _____

_____

Massage

Runner Number

Time	B/P	Pulse	Resp	Temp	Initials

1551

Patient admitted to **triage** at _____am/pm & transfered to:

( ) **Massage** ( ) **Minor** ( ) **Major** ( ) **Podiatry**
  at _____am/pm. Initials _____   Patient transfered to:
( ) **Massage** ( ) **Minor** ( ) **Major** ( ) **Podiatry**
  at _____am/pm. Initials _____   Patient transfered to:

( ) **Hospital**_____ via _____ at _____am/pm.

( ) **Released** ( ) AMA? Initials _____ at _____am/pm.

Minor Medical

Runner Number

1551

Major Medical   1551

Runner Number _____

Triage   1551

Runner Number _____

Figure 39–1. Medical record, Houston Marathon.

Podiatry	Houston Marathon Medical Information Tag
	Narrative / Treatment **Date __/__/__**

Massage	

Minor Medical	

Time	Results (Lab Values)

Patient Refusal - I am refusing further medical evaluation and / or treatment at this time. I understand that these services are being offered to me. I also understand that I may or may not require further medical attention at this time. I have also been advised to seek appropriate medical care, if necessary, or my condition changes.

_____   _____
Patient   Witness

Major Medical

Triage

Figure 39–1. Continued.

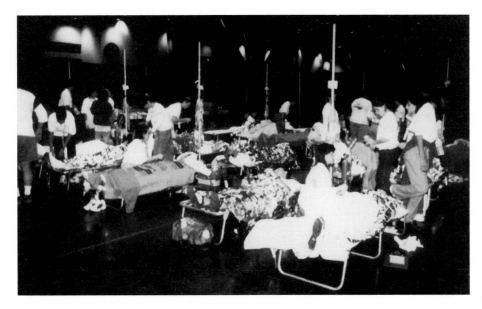

Figure 39–2. Major medical area, Houston Marathon.

to reduction of injury in a report from Grandma's Marathon in Duluth, Minnesota.[21] A half-marathon race to coincide with a marathon and a start time before 8:00 AM reduced the risk of injury. The odds ratio of requiring medical intervention doubled if the start temperature was above 55°F.[21] The incidence of musculoskeletal and skin injury may also be affected by both race distance and environmental conditions.

In addition to the calendar date, the time of day that a race starts influences the encounter rate. A preventative approach to race planning includes avoiding the hot seasons on the calendar and a start in the heat of the day. Excessive heat adversely affects medical encounters and performance.[22] The ACSM recommends that all hot weather races be scheduled with a morning start prior to 8:00 AM or, if necessary, an evening race start to avoid the heat of midday.[7,18] The International Amateur Athletic Federation suggests that all races planned for days during which the historical average high temperature is above 65°F utilize an early morning "sunrise" start. This allows most participants to finish before noon and minimizes exposure to the midday heat and solar radiation. Races with traditionally slow runners or walkers in hot climates, like the Honolulu Marathon, start at 5:00 AM to avoid the heat of the day.

Musculoskeletal/Dermatologic Injuries

Musculoskeletal injuries are largely confined to the lower extremities and include muscle cramps, sprains, and strains. The treatment of musculoskeletal injuries is usually rest, ice, compression, elevation, and occasional pain medications. Traumatic injuries are not common, with the ankle sprain occurring

most frequently, and fractures or joint dislocations occurring infrequently. Dislocations and other bony injuries should be reduced if experienced personnel are available; otherwise the runner should be stabilized and transported to an emergency room for diagnostic imaging and definitive care.

Skin injury is common in marathon races and involves the feet, inner thighs, axilla, and nipples. Blisters are the most common and account for 289 of 316 skin injuries in the Twin Cities Marathon database.[20] Blister care involves aspiration of the vesicle, without deroofing, and covering with a sterile bandage and bacitracin. On the course, blisters can be covered with high adhesive tape or moleskin to allow the runner to finish the race.[7,23] Falls can result in abrasions. Treatment consists of cleaning the abrasions with saline, removing road debris, applying antibiotic ointment, and dressing the area with clean gauze. Subungual hematomas can be decompressed with a needle or hot cautery pen. Chafing is another common minor complaint. It typically occurs in the axilla, medial thigh, and over the nipples. Chafing can be easily prevented by applying petroleum jelly to friction areas and using Band-Aids over nipples. The pain of friction sores, once they are irritated, can be reduced with the additional application of petroleum jelly or dressings.[10]

Medical Illness

Exercise-Associated Collapse

Exercise-associated collapse (EAC) is a classification system based on body temperature, vital signs, and clinical complaints.[24] Collapse casualties are divided into hyperthermic, normothermic, and hypothermic groups and are classified by clinical signs as mild, moderate, or severe. Treatment will be dictated by placement on the classification matrix. Dehydration, depleted energy stores, temperature regulation malfunction, loss of the leg muscle pump after stopping exercise, vasovagal responses, and peripheral vasodilation probably play a role in the etiology of EAC. The treatment protocol addresses the following areas: diagnosis and documentation, fluid redistribution and replacement, body temperature correction and maintenance, energy replacement, and disposition.[24]

Exercise exhaustion, also referred to as heat exhaustion, results from several factors including dehydration, unusual physical effort or prolonged exercise, loss of the leg muscle pump when exercise is discontinued, vasovagal responses, and venous pooling. It usually occurs immediately following sustained vigorous exertion in both warm and cool conditions and may be synonymous with normothermic EAC. Signs and symptoms include hypotension, lightheadedness, profuse sweating, muscle cramps, irritability, confusion, nausea, tachycardia, tachypnea, and decreased urine output.[18] Temperatures are normal or elevated to 104° F. Exercise exhaustion can be treated with passive venous return by elevating the legs and buttocks with the runner in the supine position, oral rehydration supportive care, and temperature monitoring. If nausea is severe, IV fluids may be required. Heat acclimatization prior to race day, proper hydration during the event, and continued walking or jogging immediately following cessation of exercise can help prevent the occurrence of this benign disorder. Transfer to an emergency room is indicated if signs and symptoms persist or worsen.

Dehydration

Dehydration can occur in long races like a marathon and can contribute to collapse and impaired heat dissipation.[14,24] Adequate hydration before and during a race can reduce the risk of dehydration. Failure to replace sustained sweat losses, particularly in hot weather, will result in dehydration. Symptoms of dehydration include lethargy, dizziness, weakness, muscle cramps, and irritability. Signs include low blood pressure, tachycardia, orthostatic hypotension, and irritable muscles. Treatment consists of rehydration with either oral fluids, preferably a glucose electrolyte mixture (i.e., sports drink), or IV fluids in more severe cases.[16] In most road racing situations, IV fluids should not be needed in moderate temperatures. The Twin Cities Marathon medical team has started only 125 IV drips in 66,000 finishers.[20] Electrolyte and glucose levels should be checked using a portable electrolyte or glucose measuring device (if available) that can test a small sample of blood in 2 to 3 minutes. This information allows the medical team to assess electrolyte and glucose levels accurately before initiating IV hydration treatment. Electrolyte and glucose evaluation can make a significant difference in treatment because dehydration, hyponatremia, and hypoglycemia can present with similar findings. The onset of urination allows the medical staff to assess whether a runner's hydration status is improving (Fig. 39–3).

Hyponatremia

Hyponatremia was once thought to be confined to ultramarathon races and ironman triathlons,[24] although there have been a few case reports of hyponatremia in marathon runners.[25] As more slow runners have entered marathons, the incidence of exertional hyponatremia

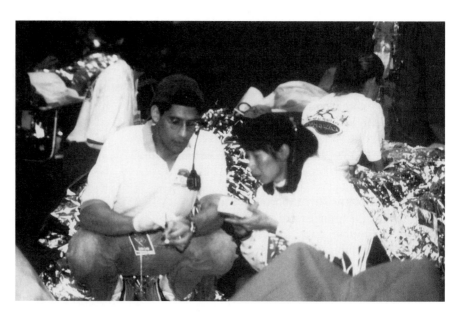

Figure 39–3. iStat device provides rapid electrolyte and glucose evaluation to assess for IV needs.

seems to be rising, particularly during hot weather races. The Houston Marathon medical team has diagnosed and managed 25 runners with of hyponatremia during the 1999 and 2000 races.

The etiology of hyponatremia is still not completely understood, but it generally results from overzealous hydration by slower runners during hot and humid conditions.[26] Salt losses may contribute to hyponatremia in some runners who sweat heavily and replace fluid losses with water. The use of fluids containing a sodium load may decrease the risk in athletes who sweat heavily (2 to 4 L/hr) or are on the race course for more than 4 hours. Speedy et al.[17] have reported prevention of hyponatremia by reducing the number of water stops in an ultramarathon. However, it should be noted that there was a corresponding increase in participants with dehydration.[17]

The presenting symptoms of exercise-associated hyponatremia are similar to other causes of collapse, with several important differences. Symptoms often include headache, nausea, dyspnea, puffiness, and/or muscle cramps. Blood pressure, pulse, and respiratory rate are usually normal in hyponatremia. Sodium levels range from 110 to 130 mEq in exertional hyponatremia. Rapid deterioration, progressing to seizure, respiratory distress, and coma due to worsening pulmonary and cerebral edema, can occur with severe hyponatremia.[27–29] The diagnosis and treatment of hyponatremia hinges on measurement of electrolyte levels. Medical teams with sufficient experience and on-site measuring devices may be able to treat runners with sodium levels below 130 mEq/L. In runners with clinical signs of dehydration and serum sodium of 125 to 130 mEq/L, rehydration with normal saline can be accomplished in the medical tent.[7] Electrolyte levels should be rechecked after each liter of IV fluid. Transfer of care to an emergency facility should be initiated for hyponatremia casualties who are unresponsive to initial therapy, who have worsening sodium levels, or who present with a sodium level below 130 mEq and are obviously fluid overloaded.[30]

Hyperthermic Illness

Exertional hyperthermia and exertional heat stroke are more severe forms of hyperthermic illness. Hyperthermic illness develops when the heat generated by exercise cannot be removed from the body and the core temperature begins to rise. When high ambient temperatures are combined with high relative humidity, the ability to dissipate metabolic body heat is markedly restricted. Dehydration impairs the cardiovascular heat transport and the sweating mechanism, further compromising the thermoregulatory system. Hyperthermic illness is progressive, and exertional heat stroke (EHS) presents with rectal temperatures greater than 104°F and central nervous system (CNS) symptoms. Once the core temperature begins to rise, organ failure can ensue, with the CNS affected early in the process. An elevated rectal temperature above 104°F associated with CNS symptoms is exertional heat stroke and should be treated emergently with on-site cooling protocols. A rectal temperature measurement is required to estimate the core temperature adequately in collapsed athletes.[31–33] CNS failure at its worst involves hypothalamic failure with inhibition of sweating and the progression of classic heat stroke. If the rectal temperature measurement is delayed, it may be <104°F and still be considered exertional heat stroke. Hyperthermic illness is worsened by poor conditioning, chronic or recent illnesses, high heat and humidity, alcohol ingestion, and prolonged sun exposure.

In exertional heat stroke, the body temperatures range from 104° to 112°F. Sweating may cease, but this is an end-stage sign in EHS.[18] The runner affected by EHS is often combative, cannot walk unassisted, has memory loss, and can deteriorate into coma and have seizures. Rapid cooling via an ice bath is the quickest way to reduce the elevated body temperatures.[34–37] In the absence of an ice bath, ice bags in the neck, axilla, and groin can be used. Electrolyte monitoring and IV rehydration with normal saline should be initiated if there are signs of severe dehydration. The core temperature should be reduced to 102°F before discontinuing cooling protocols. Seizure and muscle cramping should be treated with IV diazepam, magnesium sulfate, or dantrolene sodium. Transfer to an emergency room should be facilitated as soon as the rectal temperature has been lowered if the runner is not clinically stable.

Exercise-associated muscle cramps have long been considered a heat-related illness resulting from a combination of muscle fatigue and dehydration due to excessive sweating. A recent hypothesis for the exercise-associated muscle cramping seen in marathon and other distance runners implicates neural fatigue related to the intensity and duration of exercise affecting alpha motor neurons and Golgi tendon bodies rather than "heat" exposure, as cramping occurs in both warm and cool temperature conditions.[38] The treatment of exercise-associated muscle cramping consists of rest, rehydration, prolonged stretch with neural inhibition techniques, glucose replacement, and in some severe cases the use of IV diazepam or magnesium sulfate and/or IV rehydration with normal saline. Cramping also occurs with exertional hyponatremia from excessive water intake or salt loss, and if there are no clinical signs of dehydration a serum sodium should be checked if cramping does not respond to simple measures. Diuretic medications are also associated, implying a role for electrolyte imbalance in the etiology of muscle cramping.

Hypothermic Illness

Hypothermia is common in distance running in cool (<65°F) and cold climates. Wet and windy conditions can add to the risk of hypothermia via conductive and convective heat losses. Longer exposure time not only increases the severity of cold injury but can result in unexpected occurrences at higher temperatures.[8,24] Hypothermia tends to occur more frequently in the slower runners who do not generate as much metabolic body heat.

Initial signs of hypothermia include pale or cyanotic extremities and shivering progressing to lethargy, disorientation, clumsiness, and weakness. In its milder forms, hypothermia is difficult to distinguish from hyperthermic and normothermic collapse, so a rectal temperature measurement is the key to distinguishing the exercise-associated collapse disorders. Core temperatures below 97°F are indicative of hypothermia. Pulse and respiratory rates are depressed at very low core temperatures. Field treatment consists of removal of wet clothes, external rewarming through the use of thermal blankets, warmed water bags in the neck, axillary, and groin regions, and breathing humidified, prewarmed air. The runners should be protected from additional cold exposure. If core temperatures are below 90°F, the runner should be transferred to an emergency center for rapid rewarming. The risk of ventricular fibrillation in severe hypothermia increases if peripheral vasodilation occurs as a result of rewarming.[8]

Medical Emergencies

Other life-threatening medical conditions such as cardiac arrest can occur in road racing and the marathon, but they are rare.[39] Prerace preparation for life-threatening conditions like cardiac arrest includes recruiting a medical team trained in ACLS techniques. All first responders should be trained in CPR, and the ACLS-trained personnel need to be stationed to respond and to intervene effectively. Care protocols for asthma, hypoglycemia, and anaphylaxis should be prepared for all races. Airway maintenance and blood pressure support are vital while transport is being organized. Access to equipment including automatic external defibrillators, airway kits, suction devices, nebulizers, and drugs such as dextrose 50% in water and epinephrine is necessary to treat these medical emergencies.

Hospital Follow-up

The medical director should maintain contact with emergency rooms and hospitals that accept the more critically ill runners in transfer from the race medical team. Postrace follow-up with hospital staff and hospitalized runners establishes goodwill between the runner and the medical team. It also serves to complete the medical database for the race and allows the medical team to prepare adequately for future events.

SUMMARY

The medical administration of road races is based on prevention strategies designed to enhance the safety of the athlete. Primary prevention strategies are introduced in the prerace planning to lessen the risk of injury by scheduling the race at the safest time of the year and day, and by offering runner education to improve performance and lessen the risk of medical encounters. Secondary prevention strategies on race day are used on behalf of the runner to interrupt the progression of illness or injury on the course or in the finish area. The medical team staffing and supplies should be tailored to the event and the anticipated medical encounter rate to ensure adequate care during the peak of medical encounters. The risk of marathon racing seems to rise with increasing heat and humidity. The medical team should develop care protocols for the anticipated encounters and be prepared for the rare medical emergencies that occur on race day. The race administration in conjunction with the medical team should determine any environmental conditions that would alter or cancel the race. The safety of the runners and volunteers should be the primary concern when making these decisions. The medical team should keep records of medical encounters and environmental conditions so future participants can benefit from the past experience of the race.

REFERENCES

1. USA Track & Field Road Running Information Center: *Road Race Participation Numbers Source*, Santa Barbara, CA, 2000.
2. Cianca JC: Distance running: Organization of a medical team. *J Back Musculoskel Rehabil* 1995:6, 59.
3. Noble B, Bachman D: Medical aspects of distance race plan. *Physician Sports Med* 1979:6, 78.
4. Grollman LJ: Organization and administration of medical coverage for road races, in Fu FH (ed.), *Sports Injuries, Running: Mechanisms, Prevention and Treatment*, Baltimore, Williams & Wilkins, 1994:582.
5. Roberts WO: Medical management and administration for long distance road racing, in Brown CH, Budjonsson B (eds.), *IAAF Medical Manual for Athletics and Road*

Racing Competitions: A Practical Guide, Monaco, International Amateur Athletic Federation, 1998, 39.

6. Reid DC: *Sports Injury Assessment and Rehabilitation,* New York, Churchill Livingstone, 1992:1173.

7. Jones BH, Roberts WO: Medical management of endurance events, in Cantu RC, Micheli LJ (eds.), *ACSM: Guidelines for the Team Physician,* Philadelphis, Lea & Febiger, 1991, 266.

8. Bracker MD: Environmental and thermal injury. *Clin Sports Med* 1992:11, 419.

9. Roberts WO: Assessing core temperature in collapsed athletes. *Physician Sportsmed* 1994:22, 49.

10. Roberts WO: Medical management of athletic events, in Kibler WB (ed.), *ACSM: Handbook for the Team Physician,* Baltimore, Williams & Wilkins, 1996:17.

11. Whipkey RR, Paris PM, Stewart RD: Marathon medicine. *Emerg Med* 1985:Sept, 64.

12. Dolley JW: Professional liability coverage (medical malpractice). *Road Race Manage* 1999:Oct, 3.

13. Hughes WA, Bates Noble H, Porter M: Distance race injuries: An analysis of runner's perceptions. *Physician Sportsmed* 1985:13, 43.

14. Convertino VA, Armstrong LE, Coyle EF, et al.: ACSM position stand: Exercise and fluid replacement. *Med Sci Sports Exerc* 1996:28, I-vii.

15. Coyle EF, Montain SJ: Benefits of fluid replacement with carbohydrate during exercise. *Med Sci Sports Exerc* 1992:24, S324.

16. Shirreffs SM, Maughan RJ: Rehydration and recovery of fluid balance after exercise. *Exerc Sport Sci Rev* 2000: 28, 27.

17. Speedy DB, Rogers IR, Noakes TD, et al.: Diagnosis and prevention of hyponatremia in an ultradistance triathalon. *Clin J Sports Med* 2000:10, 52.

18. Armstrong LE, Epstein Y, Greenleaf JE, et al.: American College of Sports Medicine: Position statement on heat and cold illnesses during distance running. *Med Sci Sports Exerc* 1996:28, I-vii.

19. Noakes TD, Myburgh KH, du Pliessis J, et al.: Metabolic rate, not percent dehydration, predicts rectal temperature in marathon runners. *Med Sci Sports Exerc* 1991:23, 443.

20. Roberts WO: A twelve year profile of medical injury and illness for the Twin Cities Marathon. *Med Sci Sports Exerc* 2000:32, 1549.

21. Crouse B, Beattie K: Marathon medical services: Strategies to reduce runner morbidity. *Med Sci Sports Exerc* 1996:28, 1093.

22. McCann DJ, Adams WC: Wet bulb globe temperature index and performance in competitive distance runners. *Med Sci Sports Exerc* 1997:29, 955.

23. Cortese TA: Treatment of blisters. *Arch Dermatol* 1968:97, 717.

24. Roberts WO: Exercise-associated collapse in endurance events: A classification system. *Physician Sportsmed* 1989:17, 49.

25. Nelson PB, Robinson AG, Kapoor W: Hyponatremia in a marathoner. *Physician Sportsmed* 1988:16, 78.

26. Speedy DB, Noakes TD, Rogers IR, et al.: Hyponatremia in ultradistance triathletes. *Med Sci Sports Exerc* 1999:31, 809.

27. Mann SO, Carroll HJ: Disorders of sodium metabolism: Hypernatremia and hyponatremia. *Crit Care Med* 1992:20, 94.

28. Mulloy AL, Caruana RJ: Hyponatremic emergencies. *Endocr Emerg* 1995:79, 155.

29. Ayrus JC, Varon J, Areiff AI: Hyponatremia, cerebral edema, and noncardiogenic pulmonary edema in marathon runners. *Ann Intern Med* 2000:132, 711.

30. Sterns RH: The management of hyponatremic emergencies. *Crit Care Clin* 1991:7, 27.

31. Armstrong LE, Maresh CM, Crago AE, et al.: Interpretation of aural temperatures during exercise, hyperthermia, and cooling therapy. *Med Exerc Nutr Health* 1994:3, 9.

32. Deschamps A, Levy RD, Cosio MG, et al.: Tympanic temperature should not be used to assess exercise induced hyperthermia. *Clin J Sports Med* 1992:2, 27.

33. Roberts WO: Assessing core temperature in collapsed athletes. *Physician Sportsmed* 1994:22, 49.

34. Armstrong LE, Crago AE, Adams R, et al.: Whole-body cooling of hyperthermic runners: Comparison of two field therapies. *Am J Emerg Med* 1996:14, 355.

35. Brodeur VB, Dennett SR, Griffin LS: Exertional hyperthermia, ice baths, and emergency care at The Falmouth Road Race. *J Emerg Nurs* 1989:15, 304.

36. Costrini AM: Emergency treatment of exertional heat stroke and comparison of whole body cooling techniques. *Med Sci Sports Exerc* 1990:22, 15.

37. Roberts WO: Managing heatstroke: On-site cooling. *Physician Sportsmed* 1992:20, 17.

38. Schwellnus MP: Skeletal muscle cramps during exercise. *Physician Sportsmed* 1999:27, 109.

39. Maron BJ, Poliac LC, Roberts WO: Risk for sudden cardiac death associated with marathon running. *J Am Coll Cardiol* 1996:28, 428.

Part VI

REHABILITATION

Chapter 40

BASIC TREATMENT CONCEPTS

Francis G. O'Connor, Robert P. Wilder,
and Robert P. Nirschl

The great majority of running-related injuries are due to overuse. These injuries are often quite challenging in that runners have already sought counsel from colleagues on a variety of interventions and therapies, and thus are frequently familiar with the clinical problem by the time they present to a clinician. This chapter reviews current concepts regarding the etiology of overuse injuries, and outlines an effective strategy for diagnosing, managing, and rehabilitating overuse injuries.[1,2] In addition, we will discuss the concept of prehabilitation and its role in preventing overuse injuries that might otherwise sabotage effective running programs.

EPIDEMIOLOGY OF OVERUSE INJURIES

Overuse injuries are thought to be the most common sports-related disorders encountered by primary care physicians. A review of the literature reveals that 30% to 50% of all sports injuries are secondary to overuse.[3] Baquie and Bruckner,[4] noted Australian primary care sports medicine specialists, recently reported their center's experience over a 1-year period. They found overuse injuries to be twice as common as acute injuries, with the most common presentation being anterior knee pain.

Our experience at the Dewitt Army Community Hospital Primary Care Sports Medicine Clinic is comparable to that of similar centers. All the patients of our primary care sports medicine staff are seen by referral; they are seen initially by primary care physicians and referred only if needed. Retrospective review of our data demonstrated a predominance of overuse injuries (52%) as opposed to injuries secondary to trauma (48%). The most common injuries encountered included rotator cuff tendinitis (11.7%) and patellofemoral tracking disorders (10.6%).[5]

The epidemiology of running injuries is often difficult to ascertain because many runners do not present for professional medical attention. Postrace survey instruments have demonstrated that only a minority of runners seek care for their injuries. Koplan and colleagues[6] surveyed Peachtree Road Race competitors 1 year following completion of the event and found that while over one third of runners developed an injury requiring a change in weekly mileage, less than a third of that group consulted a physician. These data, when combined with those obtained from studies involving running and sports medicine clinics, have consistently demonstrated that the great majority of presenting clinical problems are secondary to overuse, with patellofemoral tracking disorders being most common.[7,8] One study evaluated age as a determinant for presenting injuries and found that patellofemoral dysfunction and stress fractures were more prevalent in the young, while metatarsal pain syndromes and plantar fasciitis were more prevalent in the older population.[9]

A recent review of female athletic injuries found that injuries once thought to be gender-specific (i.e., patellofemoral pain and stress fractures) are in reality more sport-specific.[10]

WHAT CAUSES OVERUSE INJURIES?

Overuse injuries result from repetitive microtrauma that leads to inflammation and/or local tissue damage in the form of cellular and extracellular degeneration. This tissue damage can be cumulative, resulting in tendinitis or tendinosis, stress fracture, joint synovitis, entrapment neuropathies, ligament strains, and muscle myositis.

In the cycle of repetitive overload, abusive tissue trauma secondary to continuous activity promotes microtraumatic tissue failure. Leadbetter describes the "principle of transition" where injury is most likely to occur, when the athlete experiences a change in mode or use of the involved extremity.[11] For the injured runner this may be an increase in mileage or a change in the phase of training. In this scenario, changing soft tissue demands, frequently accompanied by a mismatch between overload and recovery, leads to tissue breakdown. If the transition is so rapid that the tissue is unable to accommodate the ongoing demands, injury ensues. The profile of this type of injury is shown in Fig. 40–1. This unique pattern of injury seen with microtraumatic overload is underscored by the subclinical phase of failed adaptation. In theory, subclinical injury and dysfunction precede the conscious awareness of injury. The implication of this subclinical phase is that soft tissue injury has been accumulating for a long period before the first medical treatment was sought.

A condition recently described in the sports medicine literature is the *overtraining syndrome*.[12] When

TABLE 40–1. RISK FACTORS THAT CONTRIBUTE TO OVERUSE INJURIES

Intrinsic	Extrinsic
Malalignment	Training errors
Muscle Imbalance	Equipment
Inflexibility	Environment
Muscle weakness	Technique
Instability	Sports-imposed deficiencies

individuals rapidly increase their training load without adequate recovery, they may become overtrained. Overtraining is manifested by performance decrements, fatigue, poor sleep patterns, myalgias, weight loss, and neuroendocrine and immune dysfunction. Risks of unrecognized overtraining may include performance failure, premature retirement, illness, and injury, generally of the overuse type.

Both intrinsic and extrinsic factors contribute to overuse injuries (Table 40–1). Intrinsic factors are biomechanical and physiological abnormalities unique to a particular athlete. High arches in military recruits, for example, have been demonstrated to predispose to a greater risk of musculoskeletal overuse injury than low arches or flat feet.[13] A recent study involving male infantry trainees identified genu valgum, excessive Q angle, and genu recurvatum as risk factors for overuse injuries associated with vigorous training.[14] Wen and colleagues[15] studied a group of runners in a 32-week marathon-training program and found that minor variations in lower extremity alignment did not conclusively appear to contribute to overuse running injuries. Fields and coworkers[16] performed a prospective study involving 40 runners and found that type A personality features were a stronger risk factor for injury than was weekly mileage.

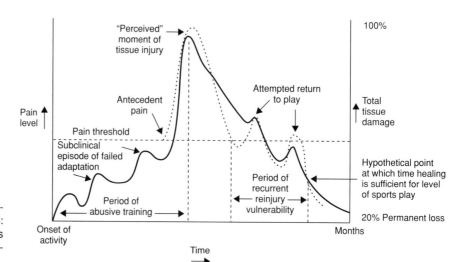

Figure 40–1. Profile of Chronic Microtraumatic Soft Tissue Injury. (Leadbetter WB: Cellmatrix response in tendon injury. Clinics in Sports Medicine 1992;11(3):533–578. Reproduced with permission.)

Poor technique, improper equipment, and changes in the duration and/or frequency of activity are common sources of extrinsic overload. Training errors are recognized as the most common cause of overuse injuries in the recreational runner.[7,17–19] Lysholm and Wilklander[17] followed 60 runners for 1 year and found that a training error alone or in combination with other factors was responsible for nearly 72% of injuries. Gardner and associates,[20] while evaluating the role of shock-absorbing insoles in preventing lower extremity stress fractures in recruits, found a slight trend toward more stress injuries with increasing age of running shoes.[20] Vulnerability to extrinsic overload varies with an individual's intrinsic characteristics, and exercise reveals these weaknesses in the form of injuries.[21]

Sports-acquired deficiencies, categorized as extrinsic risk factors, are actually the result of both biomechanical abnormalities and training errors. Sports activity can overload an athlete's musculoskeletal system in predictable patterns. Repetition without proper conditioning can propagate muscular imbalance and flexibility deficits. Throwing serves as a classic example in both baseball pitchers and water polo players.[22] Chronic overuse has been shown to create a disparity in muscular balance between the internal and external rotators of the shoulder. The external rotators, continually required to eccentrically decelerate the arm, are subject to overuse fatigue that subsequently produces strength and flexibility deficits. These maladaptive

changes are believed to play a role in the pathogenesis of rotator cuff tendinosis. While we know of no studies that clearly demonstrate predictable musculoskeletal abnormalities in runners, our experience has shown that runners acquire flexibility deficits in the hamstring, gastrocsoleus, and tensor fascia lata, with concomitant weakness in those muscle groups that are repetitively eccentrically loaded.

Kibler and associates[23] have developed a model to describe the cycle of musculoskeletal overload and injury production (Fig. 40–2). The clinical alterations produced by an injury include pain, swelling, decreased range of motion, and similar findings that produce a *clinical symptom complex*. The anatomic alterations from an injury include the actual tissue that has been damaged, the *tissue injury complex*, as well as the tissues that have been stressed or overloaded and are contributing to or exacerbating the injury, known as the *tissue overload complex*. The physiological and mechanical alterations that alter the mechanics of performance of athletic activities are known as the *functional biomechanical deficit complex*. There are motions that an athlete substitutes to compensate for the injury and associated mechanical problems. Such changes in sports motions are referred to as the *subclinical adaptation complex*. Use of this model ensures that all aspects of the primary injury and the secondary sites of injury and/or dysfunction are completely diagnosed. The complete rehabilitation program addresses the injured

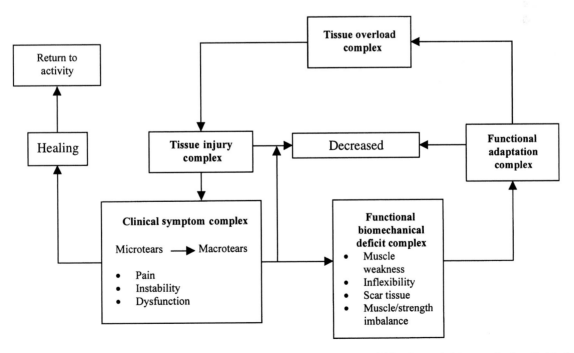

Figure 40–2. Vicious Overload Cycle. This model for the vicious overload cycle is useful for thorough injury evaluation that includes five categories: the tissue injury complex, the clinical symptom complex, functional biomechanical deficits, the functional adaptation complex, and the tissue overload complex. Reprinted with permission from Kibler.[23]

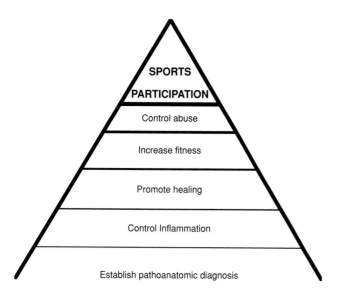

Figure 40–3. Nirschl Clinic Overuse Injury Pyramid. The five-step pyramid designed to manage overuse injuries and return runners to sports participation.

tissues, as well as the functional deficits that create abnormal biomechanics.

FIVE STEPS TO MANAGEMENT

The diagnosis and management of overuse injuries require a multidisciplinary approach. The sports medicine physician's principal responsibilities are to establish a correct pathoanatomic diagnosis and direct rehabilitation, enlisting the expertise of physical therapists, orthotists, athletic trainers, and coaches. At the Nirschl Clinic and Dewitt Army Hospital Primary Care Sports Medicine Clinic, we utilize a management pyramid with five steps that lead to a return to sports participation (Fig. 40–3).[1,2]

Step 1: Establish the Pathoanatomic Diagnosis

Successfully treating an injured athlete requires correctly identifying the injury. Vague diagnoses, such as runner's knee or shin splints, fail to clearly define the anatomic dysfunction. On the other hand, diagnoses such as patellar tendinitis and medial tibial stress syndrome assist in more clearly defining the disorder. Diagnosis of most overuse injuries requires only a thorough history, physical examination, and selected radiographs.

The history is the most important element in establishing the diagnosis; physical examination and radiographs generally confirm what is deduced from a good history. Ask the athlete questions that focus on identifying the transition that may have contributed to

the overuse. When did the injury first occur? Did the athlete recently purchase new shoes or a new racquet? Did he or she change training locations or training regimen? Questions should also focus on clarifying the quality of the pain. Does the pain occur only with sport activity, or also with activities of daily living? Perceived pain phase scales, such as the Nirschl Pain Phase Scale (Table 40–2), frequently help determine prognosis and gauge rehabilitative progress.

General health questions should identify recurrent minor illnesses, sleep patterns, nutritional habits, and overall mood states, all of which may provide clues to overtraining. Identification of the athlete's training goals and intensity may help reveal a potential endpoint for rehabilitation. Female athletes should be questioned about a history of stress fractures, menstrual abnormalities, and eating habits. These findings are manifestations of the *female athlete triad*, which if identified early, can lead to interventions that may prevent considerable morbidity.

The physical examination seeks to identify the focal problem and uncover contributing intrinsic abnormalities. This detailed examination incorporates the concept of "victims and culprits."[24] The victim represents the presenting problem and the culprit is the anatomic abnormality that created the victim. An example would be gastrocsoleus inflexibility (culprit) contributing to plantar fasciitis (victim). Accordingly, the entire extremity and/or kinetic chain needs to be thoroughly examined when evaluating a specific injury. Failure to identify muscle imbalance patterns and structural malalignment often sabotages an otherwise well-planned rehabilitation program.

The runner who presents with running-related anterior knee pain requires a detailed examination of the knee as well as an examination of the entire lower extremity including the feet. Leg length discrepancies, sacral rotations, hamstring inflexibility, gluteal weakness, and subtle forefoot pronation are only a few of the many potential culprits. The tennis player with elbow pain almost invariably demonstrates weakness of the rotator cuff. The baseball pitcher with shoulder pain needs an examination that includes the lower extremity as well as the trunk, because all are intimately involved in the throwing motion.

As described, the physical examination is biomechanical in its orientation and should include dynamic assessment, because subtle anatomic and physiologic abnormalities not evident on static examination may present during walking or running. Slow-motion video analysis may be required. Finally, the examination of the athlete with an overuse injury also requires an evaluation of equipment (e.g., running shoes, tennis racquets, etc.).

TABLE 40–2. NIRSCHL PAIN PHASE SCALE OF ATHLETE'S OVERUSE INJURIES

Phase 1. Stiffness or mild soreness after activity. Pain is usually gone within 24 hours.

Phase 2. Stiffness or mild soreness before activity that is relieved by warm-up. Symptoms are not present during activity, but return after, lasting up to 48 hours.

Phase 3. Stiffness or mild soreness before specific sport or occupational activity. Pain is partially relieved by warm-up. It is minimally present during activity, but does not cause the athlete to alter activity.

Phase 4. Pain is similar to but more intense than Phase 3 pain. Phase 4 pain causes the athlete to alter performance of the activity. Mild pain occurs with activities of daily living, but does not cause a major change in them.

Phase 5. Significant (moderate or greater) pain before, during, and after activity, causing alteration of activity. Pain occurs with activities of daily living, but does not cause a major change in them.

Phase 6. Phase 5 pain that persists even with complete rest. Phase 6 pain disrupts simple activities of daily living and prohibits doing household chores.

Phase 7. Phase 6 pain that also disrupts sleep consistently. Pain is aching in nature and intensifies with activity.

Radiographs aid diagnosis and can rule out injuries such as fractures, tumors, intraarticular abnormalities, or heterotopic calcification. Only a small minority of overuse injuries, including combined pathoanatomic presentations or those with clinical evidence of major soft-tissue disruption, require more advanced imaging techniques. Electromyographic studies and intracompartmental testing can assist when clinically warranted.

Fundamental to treating overuse injuries successfully is appropriate initial classification. Puffer and Zachazewski[25] outlined a treatment protocol based on classifying overuse injuries according to the athlete's perception of pain. Type 1 pain occurs only after activity. Type 2 pain occurs during activity, but does not impair or restrict performance. Type 3 pain occurs during activity and is severe enough to interfere with performance. Type 4 pain is classified as chronic and unremitting. Nirschl's seven-phase pain scale is somewhat more useful in gauging progress of the rehabilitative process, because activities of daily living are separated from sport performance (Table 40–2).

Step 2: Control Inflammation

Although some inflammation is required for proper healing of sports injuries, an excessive or prolonged inflammatory response can become self-perpetuating and destructive. Therefore controlling or suppressing inflammation is one of the primary goals of overuse injury treatment.

Control of inflammation has received considerable attention in the medical literature. The classic approach is RICE (rest, ice, compression, and elevation). However, at the Nirschl Clinic, we utilize PRICEMM, which adds prevention (or protection), modalities, and medications to the treatment. Nearly all protocols for managing overuse injuries begin with the athlete abstaining from or modifying exposure to injurious activity. Rest, however, should not necessarily mean a complete refrain from activity. Relative rest protects the injured area while avoiding the consequences of deconditioning and disuse atrophy. To prevent reinjury and ensure better compliance, we emphasize what athletes can do to enhance healing and maintain fitness, rather than what they cannot do. Athletes will often be able to continue some level of training if they follow a modified activity regimen (Table 40–3). Athletes with lower extremity injuries, for example, can frequently duplicate their land workouts in the pool. Pool running is an excellent supplement to a modified running schedule, and can be used to train athletes for whom running on land is contraindicated (see Chapter 45).

Modalities and medications are fundamental to controlling inflammation and are frequently incorporated into the treatment of overuse injuries. Their role in healing overuse injuries, however, has yet to be clearly established.[26,27] We incorporate the use of both agents as adjunctive therapy to assist in pain control, so the patient can sooner move on to rehabilitative exercise (see Chapters 41 to 43).

Corticosteroids are potent anti-inflammatories, and are commonly used in managing athletic injuries. However, their use in treating an athlete's overuse injuries is controversial and not well supported by scientific evidence. They can be used to treat patients who have significant (Nirschl pain phase 5 or greater) or refractory pain. However, proceed cautiously when using corticosteroids because they are thought to decrease collagen and ground substance production, weaken the tensile strength of tendons, and ultimately result in poorer healing. After injecting steroids near a weightbearing tendon, we restrict land running for 2 to 3 weeks; pool running and/or stationary bicycling may be prescribed on an individual basis. Injecting into weightbearing tendons is contraindicated. In addition, while we do not use steroid injections more than 3 times a year in an individual athlete, there are no accurate data to either support or condemn this practice.

TABLE 40–3. RELATIVE ACTIVITY MODIFICATION GUIDELINES PATIENT HANDOUT

Certain injuries (such as stress fractures, nerve trauma, or significant soft-tissue injury) necessitate complete avoidance of running. During this time you may be able to participate in certain cross-training activities to maintain your fitness while you are healing. For our runners and running athletes we recommend deep-water running as an ideal form of cross-training during the recovery period. Other lower-impact forms of cross-training such as the elliptical machine, stationary bike, and stair-climber may also be utilized to maintain fitness. Discuss cross-training options with your physician so that an optimum level of fitness can be maintained.

While rehabilitating from certain other injuries, however, the athlete is often able to continue running at some level in spite of the presence of injury, but it is important not to exceed the appropriate level of running so that proper healing is not impeded. We have devised the following relative activity modification guidelines to assist the athlete in gauging how much running they can safely do during the recovery period. However, we emphasize that the instructions given by your physician remain the ultimate guidelines to avoid worsening an injury.

1. You may be able to run with some level of discomfort, but the pain should not exceed the mild level. We define mild pain as 0 to 3 on a 10-point scale. This would correspond roughly with levels 1 through 3 on the Nirschl pain phase scale. If certain activities cause moderate level pain (4, 5, and 6 on a 10-point scale or roughly levels 4 and 5 on the Nirschl scale), you must decrease activity so that exercise produces no more than mild pain (e.g., excluding hill running). If pain is severe (7 to 10 on a 10-point scale, or 6 to 7 on the Nirschl scale) you should not run at all.

2. If you find that pain is present only at the beginning of activity and once you warm-up the pain has resolved, most often this represents mild soft-tissue injury. If, however, you find that there is a point at which pain becomes progressively worse, do not attempt to run beyond that point.

3. If you find that the pain causes you to limp or change your gait mechanics in any way, in order to prevent worsening the injury you must not run at all. Seek the advice of your physician.

Additionally, you should not run if you are experiencing active swelling, redness, fever, or nerve symptoms including numbness and weakness. You may often supplement a decreased level of running with cross-training activities such as the deep-water running mentioned above. If you are unsure of the safety of a particular activity, please discuss it with your physician before continuing it.

Source: Courtesy of Dr. Robert P. Wilder, MD, FACSM.

Step 3: Promote Healing

Ekstrand and Gillquist[28] demonstrated that failure to properly rehabilitate an athlete's initial injury can be an important risk factor for recurrent injury. All too often, efforts to control inflammation successfully relieve a patient's pain, and he or she prematurely returns to athletic activity and is reinjured. Athletes and health care professionals may fail to appreciate that rest and anti-inflammatory medications do not heal. Clinicians can ensure a successful return to sport only when inflammation control is used in concert with aggressive efforts to promote healing.

Promotion of healing involves enhancing the proliferative invasion of vascular elements and fibroblasts to create successful collagen deposition and maturation. This is best accomplished with rehabilitative exercise and cardiovascular conditioning.[29] The goal of rehabilitative exercise is to restore injured tissue to normal or near-normal function. Early exercises enhance tissue oxygenation and nutrition, minimize unnecessary atrophy, and align collagen fibers so they can withstand the sports-induced stresses that will be imposed upon them. Progression through a rehabilitative exercise program is best facilitated by a physical therapist or a certified athletic trainer, because each patient's regimen is individualized based on the nature of the injury and the athlete's specific needs (see Chapter 44).

Ultimately, successful rehabilitative exercise programs incorporate full-motion strengthening to balance antagonistic forces to allow the athlete to meet the demands of his or her sport. As previously described, overuse injuries are commonly the result of eccentric overload. Accordingly, eccentric exercise should be the cornerstone of the rehabilitative exercise program. Curwin and Stanish[30] have outlined an effective eccentric exercise program.

In addition to rehabilitative exercises, good overall conditioning is important in promoting healing. A good conditioning program combines strength training of an athlete's uninjured parts with acceptable forms of aerobic exercise. General body conditioning enhances rehabilitation of specific injuries by

- increasing regional perfusion through central and peripheral aerobics;
- providing neurologic stimuli to the injured tissue through neurophysiologic synergy and overflow;
- minimizing weakness of adjacent uninjured tissue (decreases or eliminates the destructive "domino effect");
- minimizing negative psychological effects; and
- minimizing accumulation of unwanted fat and extra weight

Exercises commonly used for general body conditioning include stationary bicycling, stair climbing, upper body ergometry, and aqua therapy.

Generally, rehabilitative exercise successfully restores an athlete's previous level of function. However, a small minority of patients fail to respond to rehabilitation and may require surgical intervention. In cases of chronic tendinosis, surgery is designed to resect pathologic soft tissue that has failed to respond to conservative therapy, and correct underlying risk factors such as pathologic instability. Surgery thereby provides a more suitable biological environment for a successful rehabilitative effort. Consider surgery for a patient when his or her rehabilitative program has failed for at least 3 to 6 months; quality of life is unacceptable; or weakness, atrophy, and dysfunc-tion persist. Patients who fail to improve with conservative therapy warrant a second opinion to ensure all possible causes have been identified and treated before considering surgical options (see Chapter 50).

Step 4: Increase Fitness

People who have tissue that has above normal (supranormal) strength, endurance, and power are optimally suited for the demands of sport. To elevate patient's rehabilitated normal tissue to above normal levels, introduce fitness exercises. These exercises involve sport-specific rehabilitative exercises and further general body conditioning.

A patient can begin sport-specific exercises once he or she achieves near pain-free range of motion, and strength and endurance tests indicate a return to the preinjury state. Sport-specific activities work the athlete's target tissues, providing neurophysiologic stimulus and redeveloping proprioceptive skills. Sport-specific agility, speed, and skill drills such as plyometrics, interactive eccentric/concentric muscle loading, anaerobic sprints, and interval training coordinate interaction of the athlete's antagonistic and supporting muscles (see Chapter 48).

Step 5: Control Abuse

The final step of overuse injury management is to control force loads to the previously injured rehabilitated tissue. Controlling abusive overload requires modifying both intrinsic and extrinsic risk factors that were identified through the patient's history and physical examination. Control of abusive force loads is best accomplished by

- improving the athlete's sport technique;
- bracing or taping the injured part;
- controlling the intensity and duration of the activity; and
- appropriately modifying equipment

Because abnormal biomechanics quickly promote reinjury, modifying an athlete's improper sport technique is critical before allowing a return to sport.

Bracing and/or taping are used to control abuse during rehabilitation and when the athlete first resumes sport activity. Counterforce bracing helps control strain an athlete's muscle balance. Groppel and Nirschl[31] have shown that elbow counterforce braces decrease elbow angular acceleration and electromyogram muscle activity, and thus are of value in treating tennis elbow. We have successfully used counterforce bracing to treat patients with tennis elbow, plantar fasciitis, and patellar tendinitis.

Modifying equipment requires paying attention to shoes, sport-specific equipment, and playing or training surfaces. Subtle abnormalities in an athlete's foot biomechanics can contribute to numerous lower extremity overuse injuries. Physicians need to attempt to correct these abnormalities through rehabilitation, proper footwear, and if necessary, custom orthotics. Lower-extremity injuries such as plantar fasciitis and stress fractures often result from poor or hard playing surfaces. Optimal running environments should enhance proper footing and provide adequate cushioning and an even surface to minimize abnormal forces.

Training errors, specifically those of excessive intensity and duration, represent the principal risk factors for overuse injury. The clinician must emphasize that more is not always better. Encourage athletes to follow basic training principles of progression and periodization. Explain that overtraining is not only a precipitator of injury, but also fosters fatigue and decreased performance.

BACK IN ACTION

Traditionally, athletes have been allowed to return to activity when they can demonstrate full range of motion and when the injured extremity showed 80% to 90% of the strength (objectively measured with functional lower extremity testing) of the uninjured extremity. These criteria, however, represent only the minimum required for return to sport. Before allowing athletes to return to activity, sports physicians should also focus on these questions: (1) Does the athlete demonstrate sports-specific function? and (2) Is the athlete psychologically ready? When the athlete, coach, trainer, and physician are satisfied that the answer to both of these questions is "Yes," the athlete can safely return to full activity (see Chapter 49).

PREHABILITATION AND THE PREPARTICIPATION EXAMINATION

Overuse injuries can be quite perplexing and frustrating to athletes, coaches, trainers, and health care professionals. Accordingly, prevention by risk-factor identification and modification has been the focus of numerous authors. Kibler and associates have coined the term "prehabilitation," implying rehabilitation before clinical injury.[32] Kibler and coworkers, among others, believe that the preparticipation examination can be utilized to identify weakness and flexibility deficits and intervene before injury occurs.[33] Hartig and Henderson recently demonstrated that improving hamstring flexibility in military basic trainees resulted in a significant reduction of lower extremity overuse injuries.[34] These concepts are currently utilized at the Nirschl Clinic with elite tennis players and runners, and at the Dewitt Army Community Hospital Primary Care Sports Medicine Center with active duty soldiers. We hope that data from well-controlled studies will continue to support what we have observed anecdotally.

CONCLUSION

The management pyramid outlined in this chapter describes a process of evaluation and management that we have found quite helpful in treating runners with overuse injuries. The basic concepts elucidated in this strategy ensure a functional approach to the patient-athlete, and optimize the opportunity for a successful return to sport activity. In addition, we are currently incorporating these concepts into our preparticipation assessments in an attempt to prevent these frustrating injuries.

REFERENCES

1. O'Connor FG, Howard TM, Fieseler CM, et al.: Managing overuse injuries: A systematic approach. *Physician Sports Med* 1997:25, 88.
2. O'Connor FG, Nirschl RP, Sobel JR: Five-step treatment of overuse injuries. *Physician Sports Med* 1992:21, 128.
3. Herring SA, Nilson KL: Introduction to overuse injuries. *Clin Sports Med* 1987:6, 225.
4. Baquie P, Bruckner P: Injuries presenting to an Australian sports medicine centre: A 12 month study. *Clin J Sports Med* 1997:7, 28.
5. Butcher JA, Zukowski CA, Bramnen SJ, et al.: Patient profile, referral sources, and consultant utilization in a primary care sports medicine clinic. *J Fam Pract* 1996:43, 556.
6. Koplan JP, Powell KE, Sikes RK, et al.: An epidemiologic study of the benefits and risks of running. *JAMA* 1982:248, 3118.
7. Brody DM: Running injuries. *Clin Symposia* 1980:32, 1.
8. MacIntyre JG, Taunton JE, Clement OR, et al.: Running injuries: A clinical study of 4173 cases. *Clin J Sports Med* 1991:1, 81.
9. Matheson GO, MacIntyre JG, Taunton JE, et al.: Musculoskeletal injuries associated with physical activity in older adults. *Med Sci Sports Exerc* 1989:21, 379.
10. Arendt EA: Common musculoskeletal injuries in women. *Physician Sportsmed* 1996:24, 39.
11. Leadbetter WB: Cell-matrix response in tendon injury. *Clin Sports Med* 1992:11, 533.
12. Fry RW, Morton AR, Keast D: Overtraining in athletes. *Sports Med* 1991:12, 32.
13. Cowan DN, Jones BH, Robinson JR: Foot morphologic characteristics and risk of exercise-related injury. *Arch Fam Med* 1993:2, 773.
14. Cowan DN, Jones BH, Frykman PN: Lower limb morphology and risk of overuse injury among male infantry trainees. *Med Sci Sports Exerc* 1996:28, 945.
15. Wen DY, Puffer JC, Schmalzreid TP: Injuries in runners: A prospective study of alignment. *Clin J Sports Med* 1998:8, 187.
16. Fields KB, Delaney M, Hinkle JS: A prospective study of type A behavior and running injuries. *J Fam Pract* 1990:30, 425.
17. Lysholm J, Wilklander J: Injuries in runners. *Am J Sports Med* 1987:15, 168.
18. Hoeberigs JH: Factors related to the incidence of running injuries. A review. *Sports Med* 1992:13, 408.
19. Shawayhat AF, Linenger JM, Hofherr LK, et al.: Profiles of exercise history and overuse injuries among United States Navy Sea, Air, and Land (SEAL) recruits. *Am J Sports Med* 1994:22, 835.
20. Gardner LI, Dziados JE, Jones BH, et al.: Prevention of lower extremity stress fractures: A controlled trial of a shock absorbent insole. *Am J Public Health* 1988:78, 1563.
21. McKeag DB: Overuse injuries: The concept in 1992. *Primary Care* 1991:18, 851.
22. McMaster WC, Long SC, Caiozzo VJ: Isokinetic torque imbalances in the rotator cuff of the elite water polo player. *Am J Sports Med* 1991:19, 72.
23. Kibler WB, Chandler TJ, Pace BK: Principles of rehabilitation after chronic tendon injuries. *Clin Sports Med* 1992: 11, 661.
24. Macintyre JG, Lloyd-Smith DR: Overuse running injuries, in Renstrom PA (ed.), *Sports Injuries—Basic Principles of Prevention and Care*, Boston, Blackwell Scientific, 1993:139.
25. Puffer JC, Zachazewski JE: Management of overuse injuries. *Am Fam Physician* 1988:38, 225.
26. Rivenburgh DW: Physical modalities in the treatment of tendon injuries. *Clin Sports Med* 1992:11, 645.
27. Weiler JM: Medical modifiers of sports injury: The use of nonsteroidal anti-inflammatory drugs in sports soft tissue injury. *Clin Sports Med* 1992:11, 625.
28. Ekstrand J, Gillquist J: Soccer injuries and their mechanisms: A prospective study. *Med Sci Sports Exerc* 1982: 15, 267.
29. Hess GP, Capiello WL, Poole RM, et al.: Prevention and treatment of overuse injuries. *Sports Med* 1989:8, 371.
30. Curwin S, Stanish WD: *Tendinitis: Its Etiology and Treatment*, Lexington, Mass, DC Health & Co, 1984.
31. Groppel JL, Nirschl RP: A mechanical and electromyographic analysis of the effects of various counterforce

braces on the tennis player. *Am J Sports Med* 1986:14, 195.

32. Kibler WB, Chandler JJ, Stracener ES: Musculoskeletal adaptations and injuries due to overtraining. *Exerc Sports Sci Rev* 1992:20, 99.

33. Fleck SJ, Falkel JE: Value of resistance training for the reduction of sports injuries. *Sports Med* 1986:3, 61.

34. Hartig DE, Henderson JM: Increasing hamstring flexibility decreases lower extremity overuse injuries in military basic trainees. *Am J Sports Med* 1999:27, 173.

Chapter 41

MEDICATIONS AND ERGOGENIC AIDS

Scott D. Flinn

INTRODUCTION

Rehabilitation of the injured runner may entail the use of medications, which are commonly used in the acute injury phase to limit pain and inflammation and presumably to speed healing. For chronic injuries, both oral medications and corticosteroid injections are used. Many runners self-medicate without medical supervision using both traditional medications and ergogenic aids. Alternative methods are used in an attempt to develop optimal performance as well as to prevent and heal injuries. This chapter discusses the current literature and evidence-based medicine with regard to the use of common medications in injury healing. Ergogenic aids used by runners are likewise examined. Current National Collegiate Athletic Association (NCAA) and International Olympic Committee (IOC) guidelines regarding banned substances are also reviewed.

MEDICATIONS

Various medications are used to aid rehabilitation of running injuries, two of the most common being nonsteroidal anti-inflammatory drugs (NSAIDs) and corticosteroids. These medicines are used in an attempt to decrease pain and inflammation, with the ultimate goal of promoting healing and a more rapid return to sport. Some athletes also use anabolic steroids, albeit illegally, in an attempt to speed healing of injuries. What does the literature show regarding these purported benefits, what are the risks, and what is the best way to enhance the risk/benefit profile of these medications?

NSAIDs

NSAIDs are commonly used to treat both acute and chronic injuries. Over 50 million people in the United States take daily prescription NSAIDs, and more than 100 million Americans use prescription NSAIDs during a year.[1] The rationale for using NSAIDs has been to decrease pain and inflammation at the injury site. Recent research on the mechanisms of action of NSAIDs and the pathophysiology of acute and chronic injuries have led both to advances in treating these injuries and to questions regarding their routine use in treatment.

Mechanism of Action

NSAIDs are a broad class of drugs that have anti-inflammatory, antipyretic, and analgesic properties. Common NSAIDs are listed in Table 41–1. The major pharmacologic effect of NSAIDs is to inhibit the enzyme cyclooxygenase (COX), thus decreasing prostaglandin production, which decreases inflammation and promotes analgesia in the injured tissue.

TABLE 41–1. NONSTEROIDAL ANTI-INFLAMMATORY DRUGS

Regular
Aspirin
Diclofenac
Etodolac
Indomethacin
Ibuprofen
Ketorolac
Ketoprofen
Mefenamic acid
Naproxen
Oxaprozin
Piroxicam
Sulindac
Tolmetin
Combination
Diclofenac/misoprostol
COX2-selective
Celebrex
Vioxx

COX-1 AND COX-2. There are at least two forms of the COX enzyme, COX-1 and COX-2.[2] COX-1 is important in the production of prostaglandins involved in the homeostasis of various tissues including renal parenchyma, gastric mucosa, and platelets.[3] COX-2 produces prostaglandins involved in pain and inflammation. Most NSAIDs inhibit both COX-1 and COX-2 at various levels; newer agents (e.g., celecoxib) have been developed to be more COX-2 selective. Theoretically, this enhances the desired effects while limiting the side effects.[2]

OTHER MECHANISMS. Inhibition of prostaglandin synthesis may not be the only method by which NSAIDs work. Articular cartilage synthesis of glycosaminoglycans may be inhibited by NSAIDs.[4] Neutrophil adherence to endothelial cells is also affected,[5] although neutrophil metabolic activity does not seem to be affected.[6] NSAIDs also affect a number of cellular processes, all of which may influence the inflammatory process.[4] What does all this mean in terms of controlling pain, inflammation, and promoting healing?

Rationale for Use

Decreasing pain may be of benefit in the rehabilitation and healing of injuries. Controlling pain will not only allow progression of rehabilitation but may also help avoid disuse atrophy. Decreasing inflammation may be beneficial if the inflammation is causing destruction of normal tissues. However, the inflammation and repair process is necessary for ideal long-term healing of an injury. To what extent do NSAIDs preserve normal tissue, and do they inhibit repair of an injury?

ACUTE INJURIES. Over the years, many studies have been conducted on the efficacy of NSAIDs in treating acute injuries, with some earlier studies showing no clinical benefit.[3] Two of the most common acute injuries investigated are ankle sprains and muscle strains. In 1995, a metaanalysis reviewing 84 articles on ankle soft-tissue injuries concluded that early use of NSAIDs relieved pain and shortened the time to recovery.[7] In a 1997 randomized study on Australian Regular Army recruits, subjects treated with piroxicam had less pain, were able to return to training more rapidly, and had better exercise endurance compared with subjects treated with placebo.[8] Two recent studies evaluating the effect of naproxen on exercise-induced, delayed-onset muscle soreness showed a decrease in the perception of soreness and improved muscular performance after injury.[9,10] However, a study using moderately trained men who had exercise-induced quadriceps injury showed no decrease in pain.[11] There was a more rapid return to voluntary knee extension at 48 hours after injury.[11] Another study looking at acute hamstring injuries showed no difference in healing or pain at 1, 3, and 7 days after the injury, and the subgroup that had more severe injuries actually had better pain control.[12] One study looking at healing in an animal model suggested that the proliferative phase of healing in an injured muscle was delayed with NSAIDs,[13] and another suggested overall histologic delay in muscle repair.[14] The conclusion to be drawn from reviewing the studies appears to be that judicious use of NSAIDs for pain control in the acute phase of an injury probably speeds return to sport while not delaying healing.

CHRONIC INJURIES. It has traditionally been thought that chronic overuse tendinopathies are caused by repetitive overload, resulting in tissue injury and inflammation. NSAIDs are commonly used in these injuries to treat the chronic inflammation. However, this concept has recently been challenged. Histopathologic studies of Achilles', patellar, extensor carpi radialis brevis, and rotator cuff tendons involved in chronic overuse injuries have shown an absence of inflammatory cells.[15] It appears that there are disorganized fibroblastic or myofibroblastic cells and prominent capillary cell proliferation, often with discontinuity of these cells. What has been correlated with these injuries is increasing age and tendon vascularity.[16] This has led to a suggestion to change the name of chronic tendon injuries to tendonosis, which refers to a degenerative process, instead of tendinitis since inflammation is not a major factor.[15] Thus, treatment for chronic tendon injuries should be directed at correcting the underlying biomechanical cause and properly rehabilitating the injury. Judicious short-term use of NSAIDs to control pain may still be warranted.[17]

Common Side Effects and Complications

Side effects due to NSAID toxicity have a significant impact, with more than 100,000 estimated hospitalizations occurring each year.[18] The most common side effect is dyspepsia, occurring in about 15%.[19] The most common serious side effect is gastrointestinal (GI) ulceration, which occurs in 2% to 4% of patients taking the medicine for a year. In elderly patients with history of ulcers, there is a four to sixfold relative risk of a fatal GI bleed.[19] Most serious side effects are not seen in young, otherwise healthy athletes.

Chronic NSAID use has also been associated with the development of chronic renal disease[20] and (rarely) with acute renal failure.[21] Rarely, severe liver injury may occur.[22] NSAIDs have also been associated with asthma in non–IgE-mediated responses, a reaction that has been termed aspirin-induced asthma (AIA)[23] and that is seen in 10% to 15% of all asthmatics.[24] Sometimes platelet function may be impaired, resulting in prolonged bleeding times.[2]

Strategies to Limit Side Effects

Various strategies exist to combat NSAID complications (Table 41–2). Most of the bad side effects of NSAIDs are related to long-term use. Therefore, the most obvious way to limit NSAID toxicity is to limit prescription use for sports injury to short-term use or not prescribe them at all. Physical therapy modalities and other medicines may be useful in controlling pain. If NSAIDs are given, limit the amount and duration to that necessary to achieve analgesia and inflammation control.

Since GI ulceration is the most common serious side effect, most strategies have focused on reducing this complication. Drug therapy to prevent this in the form of H2 blockers is largely ineffective except for perhaps duodenal ulcers.[25,26] The role of omeprazole and sucralfate is not well defined.[25] Misoprostol, a prostaglandin E_1 (PGE_1) analog, has been shown to decrease ulcers and serious GI complication rates up to 40%.[27,28] It is cost-effective in high-risk groups, those over 75 with previous ulcer disease, but is not very cost-effective in the typically younger otherwise healthy athlete.[25,27] A combination drug of misoprostol with diclofenac shows similar efficacy in pain control compared with plain NSAIDs, with significantly fewer GI ulcers and bleeds, but it should probably also be used in the high-risk patient.[29] Furthermore, misoprostol cannot be used in women who might become pregnant.

Because GI protection seems to be dependent on the prostaglandins produced by COX-1, the COX-2-selective agents were developed to provide pain and inflammation relief without increasing GI ulceration rates. The first drug of this class, which has been released (celecoxib), has been shown to do exactly that.[2] Until postmarketing reporting and long-term follow-up studies are performed, it will not be known how other NSAID effects, such as those on kidneys, brain, and platelets, will be modified and what new toxicities will be experienced.[30]

Another attempt to limit side effects is to use topical preparations of NSAIDs. Topical NSAIDs have serum drug levels of only about 10% of oral medication while showing equivalent tissue concentrations.[31,32] Many different formulations have been used with some success. For example, one study on osteoarthritis patients compared eltenac gel with oral diclofenac and found that both reduced pain significantly more than placebo.[33] However, the topical product had one-third fewer GI side effects. A study on rheumatoid arthritis patients compared a 2-week treatment of flurbiprofen patch with oral diclofenac and found the flurbiprofen patch more efficacious, with reduced side effects.[34] A metaanalysis of 86 trials using up to 2 weeks of treatment concluded that topical nonsteroidals are effective in relieving pain in both acute and chronic conditions and have a low incidence of local side effects with systemic side effects no different from those of placebo.[35]

Corticosteroids

Mechanism of Action

Corticosteroids are a class of medications that act on a number of body systems including inflammation. They can inhibit inflammation in a number of ways. Glucocorticoids down-regulate the expression of inflammatory genes in cells, thus decreasing inflammatory cytokines, enzymes, and adhesion molecules.[36] They also up-regulate anti-inflammatory genes that produce anti-inflammatory proteins such as interleukin-1 receptor antagonist and interleukin-10.[36]

Rationale for Use

Steroids can be given orally, by injection, or transdermally through the use of cremes, iontophoresis or

TABLE 41–2. STRATEGIES TO COMBAT NSAID COMPLICATIONS

Limit amount
Limit duration
Use alternative medication (e.g., acetaminophen)
Use alternative modality for pain control (e.g., ice, electrical stimulation)
Use with GI-protective medication, e.g., misoprostol
Use combination medication, diclofenac/misoprostol
Use COX2-selective medication
Use topical NSAID

NSAID = nonsteroidal anti-inflammatory drugs; COX2 = cyclooxygenase 2.

phonophoresis. They are commonly used for a variety of acute and chronic injuries.[17] Unfortunately, most of the literature evaluating steroids for treating sports medicine injuries is retrospective in nature, involves case series, or is anecdotal.

ACUTE INJURIES. The literature has no prospective studies that evaluate the effectiveness of steroids in treating acute injuries. Anecdotally, some clinicians use short courses of oral steroids from 3 to 5 days on acute injuries including radicular back pain, but this has not been evaluated prospectively. Because of the potential side effects from steroid use, treatment with corticosteroids for acute injuries in the sports setting should be of short duration, and the individual clinician should develop any treatment protocol until better information becomes available.

CHRONIC INJURIES. As previously discussed, many chronic tendon injuries seem to be tendonoses of a degenerative nature and do not involve classic chronic inflammatory cells.[15,16] Even so, clinicians frequently use corticosteroids for these conditions, which often provides the patient with temporary pain control. However, the effectiveness of steroids in chronic injuries has not been well investigated by prospective trials. An uncontrolled retrospective trial of steroid injection in acromioclavicular joint arthropathy suggested that corticosteroid injection provided short-term pain relief but did not affect the long-term outcome.[37] A case series reported that corticosteroid injection for treating recalcitrant osteitis pubis was mostly helpful in a case series of 12 intercollegiate athletes.[38] A review of the literature on the use of epidural corticosteroid injections for treating low back pain suggested it may help in some patients with radicular pain for 2 to 12 weeks but stated that more good research was needed.[39] Two rigorous studies evaluating steroid injection for Achilles' tendinitis found no benefit over placebo.[40]

Phonophoresis uses ultrasound waves to propel steroid-containing gel through the skin into the subcutaneous tissue.[32] There appears to be little systemic absorption with this technique and few prospective data evaluating its efficacy in treatment.[32] Iontophoresis uses electrical current to drive the charged particles through the skin. One of the few prospective double-blind trials available showed that iontophoresis using 0.4% dexamethasone provided superior pain relief over 2 weeks of treatment in patients with plantar fasciitis, but 1 month later both groups had improved equally.[41] Overall, the literature suggests that if steroids are used to treat chronic sports injuries, they should be considered a pain-control method.

Common Side Effects and Complications

Steroid injection has a low complication rate of 1% to 2%, with hypopigmentation and fat pad atrophy being the most common long-term ill effects.[40] Steroids may also produce ill effects on tendons. In a review on the use of steroid injection for Achilles' tendinitis, the authors found that steroid injection directly into a tendon weakens it, whereas injection into the paratenon does not have that effect.[40] The effect of systemic steroids on healing muscle tissue has been studied in some animal models. One study showed that in acute muscle injury, corticosteroid-treated muscle had greater strength at day 2 but developed complete muscle degeneration at day 14.[42]

Long-term therapy or extremely high dosages of steroids causes well-known complications. Avascular necrosis has been associated with long-term use, with cases due to short-term use perhaps being underreported. Other side effects such as adrenal suppression, GI ulcer, diabetes, cataracts, hypertension, and increased risk of infection generally occur with use for 2 to 3 weeks or much longer.[43]

Strategies to Limit Side Effects

As with NSAIDS, use of corticosteroids should be done judiciously. Short-term treatment may help with pain control, but long-term therapy often raises the specter of worsening an injury or creating serious complications. Corticosteroids should be considered an adjunct and the underlying cause identified so that proper rehabilitation and healing may occur. Direct injection into the tendon should probably be avoided, although injection into the paratenon appears to be safe.

Anabolic Steroids

Anabolic steroids are synthetic derivatives of testosterone. They have both anabolic properties of increasing lean muscle mass and androgenic qualities.[44] Because of their muscle growth-enhancing properties, some athletes have used them in an attempt to speed healing of injuries.

Mechanism of Action

Anabolic steroids increase protein synthesis in skeletal muscle and inhibit breakdown through unknown mechanisms.[44] To produce increases in muscle mass and strength, supraphysiologic doses are taken while performing strength training.[45]

Rationale for Use

No studies have looked at healing of injuries in humans. Studies performed on rat tendons in 1992 showed that anabolic steroid rats had tendons that were stiffer and failed with less elongation than controls.[42,46] Changes in tendon crimp morphology were also reported.[47] The rat Achilles' tendon and soleus muscle also showed collagen changes when treated with testosterone.[48] However, two studies showed that anabolic steroids aided muscle recovery from injury in rats.[49,50] Obviously, one should be cautious when extrapolating animal data to humans.

Complications

The many complications of anabolic steroids are reviewed in the section on ergogenic aids. One of the greatest complications at the present is the possibility of incarceration. The Anabolic Steroids Control Act of 1990 made anabolic steroids a controlled substance that may be legally obtained only through prescription.[44] Until much more research is done on the potential healing effects of anabolic steroids, their use is not indicated in treating injuries.

ERGOGENIC AIDS

Definition

Throughout history, athletes have used various ergogenic aids in an attempt to gain a competitive edge or to promote healing. Ergogenic aids are defined as items designed to increase work or improve performance above that of regular training and diet and are usually classified as mechanical, psychological, physiologic, pharmacologic, and nutritional aids (Table 41–3). Mechanical aids may be as simple as running flats for racing. Physiologic aids are substances that naturally occur in the body, such as fluids and blood. The differentiation between nutritional and pharmacologic aids can be difficult but pharmacologic aids may be considered drugs, with no nutritional value, requiring Food and Drug Administration (FDA) approval in the United States. Some ergogenic aids, like racing flats, are allowed in competition, whereas others, such as blood doping or anabolic steroids, are not.

History

Ergogenic aids have been used at least as early as the ancient Greek Olympics, for which athletes used certain herbs and mushrooms in attempts to win.[51,52] Warriors would use products such as deer's liver to gain speed or lion's heart for courage.[51] Aztecs would likewise consume human hearts.[52] In the late 1800s and early 1900s, runners, including 1904 Olympic marathon champion Tom Hicks, would use alcohol and a popular stimulant of the time, strychnine.[52,53]

Since the early 1900s, science has vastly improved our understanding of how muscles work and metabolize fuel. Previously, protein had been thought to be the major energy source for muscles.[51] The basics of fuel metabolism and the function of protein, carbohydrates, fats, as well as the discovery of vitamins spurred further interest in the search for ergogenic substances. The 1950s and 1960s saw the development and widespread use of synthetic anabolic steroids. In 1994, Congress passed the Dietary Health and Supplement Education Act (DHSEA), which substantially changed the regulation and marketing of dietary supplements.[54] Essentially, many of the regulatory controls were lifted, and the multibillion dollar industry blossomed. These substances can be sold without USFDA approval as long as the products are labeled and sold as dietary supplements and the labels make no claims for drug activity. They are not held to the same quality control standards as FDA-approved drugs; the content and purity of these products is not regulated, and they may contain too much of the product or none at all.[45] Furthermore, these substances do not require evaluation for safety nor efficacy.

Even so, ergogenic aids are commonly used, sometimes with dire consequences. For example, cyclist Knut Jensen died in the 1960 Olympic bicycle road race, and Tommy Simpson died in the 1967 Tour de France from taking amphetamines.[52] Recent deaths of European cyclists have been attributed to the use of blood doping with recombinant erythropoietin.[53] Before an ergogenic aid is used, it should be evaluated with respect to three parameters: (1) Does it work? (2) Is it safe? (3) Is it ethical, legal, or banned by the sports governing body? (Table 41–4).

Evaluation

Evaluation of ergogenic aids can be a difficult proposition. The scientific literature can differ significantly from the lay press and advertising propaganda for many products.[55] Studies looking at dietary substances can be

TABLE 41–3. ERGOGENIC AIDS

Type of Aid	Example
Mechanical	Running flats
Psychological	Hypnosis
Pharmacologic	Caffeine
Physiologic	Blood doping
Nutritional	Carbohydrate loading

TABLE 41–4. CONSIDERATIONS IN USING ERGOGENIC AIDS

1. Does scientific research show that it is effective?
2. Is it safe?
3. Is it legal and ethical to use it?

hard to perform. With the deregulation following DHSEA, there is no burden of proof on the manufacturer to prove efficacy or product content like as is for drugs.[54] Products may contain lower amounts of the product than that listed on the label, with some products having zero amount of the supposedly ergogenic substance.[56] Furthermore, the placebo effect can have a huge impact on the perceived benefits derived by the user.[57]

Efficacy

Ergogenic aids can affect various aspects of physical fitness to improve performance. Six components of fitness that may be affected include aerobic fitness, anaerobic fitness, strength, body composition, psychological factors, and healing of injuries (Table 41–5). Aerobic metabolism uses oxygen whereas anaerobic metabolism does not. During running, both the aerobic and anaerobic systems are used to varying degrees throughout a run. Aerobic fitness is of importance, especially to distance runners. Aerobic fitness is the ability to produce work using aerobic metabolism, generally lasting longer than 1 minute and often lasting for hours.[58] It is composed of two parts, maximal aerobic power and aerobic capacity. The maximum rate at which muscles can uptake and utilize oxygen is measured by $\dot{V}o_2$max.[58] Aerobic capacity, also called aerobic endurance, is the maximum amount of work that can be done using aerobic metabolism.

Anaerobic fitness is more important to short- and middle-distance runners. Brief activities generally lasting less than a minute are fueled primarily through anaerobic metabolism.[58] Anaerobic capacity refers to the amount of work that can be done anaerobically and is often thought of as muscular endurance.[58] Maximum strength, usually measured by the one repetition maximum, refers to the amount of power that can be generated in a brief burst fueled by anaerobic metabolism.[58] Strength is important, especially to sprinters and jumpers.

Body composition is an important fitness component for all athletes. It can affect performance in two ways. Increasing lean muscle mass produces more muscles to do the work. Decreasing body fat decreases the weight that has to be carried through space to the finish line.

Psychological factors may affect performance through various mind-body mechanisms. The placebo effect alone may cause an enhancement of performance. Decreasing the mind's perception of fatigue and pain may also improve performance or allow additional training. Enhancing the healing of injuries promotes a more rapid return to training and maintenance of fitness.

Safety Considerations

Ergogenic aids can have side effects like any other substance. Many of these may be insignificant, and others may be catastrophic. Heart attacks, seizures, coma, and death have been attributed to the use of ergogenic products.[52] Also, injectable products carry the risk of disease transmission if needles are shared.[53]

Ethical and Legal Considerations

Athletes are constantly caught in the dilemma of wondering what the other guy is up to. If another competitor is using a product that may make him or her stronger or faster and then beats the athlete, was it due to that product, better athletic ability, better training, or some other factor? Many athletes will try these products even though the product has not been shown to work, has serious side effects, or is banned by the particular sport's governing body. Winning simply through training and ability should be the athletic ideal; it is often not the reality.

In an attempt to keep the playing field level, various amateur and professional organizations have instituted drug policies. These policies are targeted toward substances that may be dangerous or illegal and/or give an unfair competitive advantage. For example, the use of anabolic steroids had become so widespread by the 1964 Olympics that drug testing began at the 1968 Olympic Games in Mexico City.[53] Athletes have been disqualified and have had medals revoked, probably most notably Ben Johnson in the 1988 Olympics.[53] The NCAA began testing for steroids in 1986.[59] The American College of Sports Medicine (ACSM) has taken a position stand on anabolic steroids,

TABLE 41–5. FITNESS COMPONENTS OF ATHLETIC PERFORMANCE

Component	Definition
Aerobic fitness	Performance of work using aerobic metabolism
	May last from 1–2 min to hours
	Comprised of maximum aerobic power ($\dot{V}o_2$max) and aerobic capacity
Anaerobic fitness	Performance of work using anaerobic metabolism
	Usually lasting less than 1–2 min
	Composed of maximum anaerobic power (muscular endurance) and anaerobic capacity
Strength	Maximum force that can be generated in a brief burst
	Also an anaerobic function
	Lasts less than 5 sec
	Often measured by 1 rep maximum
Body habitus	Body composition
	Lean muscle mass to perform work
	Body fat percentage
Psychological	Involves aspects of performance such as pain tolerance, aggressiveness
Healing	Speed of recovery from training and injuries

stating that they are unethical and have dangerous side effects and that their use should be deplored.[60]

The government also has regulations regarding some substances used as ergogenic aids. Anabolic steroids were made a schedule III controlled substance by the Anabolic Steroids Control Act of 1990.[45] This puts anabolic steroids on the same legal footing as other controlled medicines such as narcotics and amphetamines, with athletes and physicians subject to applicable laws. Anabolic steroids may be prescribed for certain medical indications and have certain contraindications to their use (Table 41–6). As with other substances that may be obtained through illegal methods, the products obtained through the black market may contain little or none of the sought-after steroid.[45]

Anabolic steroids are not the only substances banned by sports governing bodies such as the IOC and NCAA. The IOC developed their list in 1967.[61] As research and development continued, various substances were added to or deleted from the lists. The list of banned substances for the IOC can be viewed on their website at http://www.nodoping.org/medch2_e.html.[62] The NCAA likewise has a list on their website at http://www.ncaa.org/sports_sciences/drugtesting/

banned_list.html.[63] The U.S. Olympic Committee (USOC) has a program that mirrors the IOC program. The USOC has a telephone hotline to answer any questions, 800-233-0393. Table 41–7 lists some of the more common banned substances. Because the lists are continually changing, physicians caring for athletes in these or other organizations should always consult them before writing a prescription or suggesting

TABLE 41–6. INDICATIONS AND CONTRAINDICATIONS FOR ANABOLIC STEROIDS

Indications
  Primary hypogonadism
  Hypogonadotropic hypogonadism
  Hereditary angioedema
  Antithrombin III deficiency
  Anemia from renal disease
  Catabolic disease such as AIDS
  Delayed onset puberty
Contraindications
  Known or suspected prostate cancer
  Breast cancer in females with high Ca^{2+}
  Breast cancer in males
  Nephritis
  Pregnancy or nursing

TABLE 41–7. COMMON ERGOGENICS BANNED BY THE IOC AND NCAA

Ergogenic Aid	Banned by IOC	Banned by NCAA
Stimulants		
Amphetamines	Yes	Yes
Caffeine	Dose limited	Dose limited
Ephedrine	Yes	Yes
Beta 2 agonists		
Clenbuterol	Yes	Yes
Salbutamol	May use inhaler for asthma	May use inhaler for asthma
Albuterol	May use inhaler for asthma	May use inhaler for asthma
Salmeterol	May use inhaler for asthma	May use inhaler for asthma
Anabolic/androgenic		
Testosterone	Yes	Yes
Nandrolone	Yes	Yes
Androstenedione	Yes	Yes
DHEA	Yes	Yes
Diuretics	Yes	Yes
Hormones		
Growth hormone	Yes	Yes
Erythropoietin	Yes	Yes
Insulin	Yes	Yes
Processes		
Blood doping	Yes	Yes
Narcotics		
Morphine	Yes	No
Corticosteroids		
Oral/systemic	Yes	Yes
Topical	No	No
Local injection	No	No
Intraarticular	No	No

IOC = International Olympic Committee; NCAA = National Collegiate Athletic Association; DHEA = dehydroepiandrosterone.

over-the-counter remedies. For example, commonly used cold medicines containing pseudoephedrine or phenylpropanolamine are banned and would disqualify an athlete found to have these drugs in the urine test sample. Another important point to remember is that at the bottom of each list is the statement " and related substances." When in doubt, contact the organization.

For testing, urine samples are analyzed by a number of methods; most confirmatory tests are performed using gas chromatography/mass spectometry.[53] In the future, blood or hair samples may be used to detect banned substances.[53,61,64–67]

As testing has become more widespread, athletes have become more sophisticated in their methods of avoiding detection. In addition to potential health risks, using diuretics to mask urine results became so common that diuretics had to be banned. An effective drug testing program is difficult to plan and implement and requires availability of random year-round testing. An effective program can make athletes feel that the program works and that they can compete in a drug-free environment. A recent survey of NCAA athletes suggests that the drug control program is working at their level.[61] This type of environment may help athletes successfully wrestle with the ethical problems associated with drug use in sports.

Specific Ergogenic Aids

Specific ergogenic aids are reviewed here in terms of their efficacy, safety, and legality. Table 41–8 gives an overview of many ergogenic aids, their effects on the six fitness components, and their safety. Carbohydrates, fluids, branched chain amino acids (BCAA), and creatine are reviewed in Chapter 38.

Amphetamines

EFFICACY. Amphetamine and dextroamphetamine are stimulants sometimes used to treat obesity and attention deficit/hyperactivity disorder. Despite their widespread use, few studies have been performed to examine their effect on athletes. One study reported a mild improvement in swimming and throwing events.[68] Another study on six runners showed increased strength, muscular power (endurance), and time to exhaustion, possibly due to the masking of fatigue.[69] However, there was no improvement in aerobic power ($\dot{V}O_2$max) or running speed. Amphetamines also act as appetite suppressants.

SAFETY. As previously noted, amphetamines can be fatal. Fatalities can be caused by cardiovascular complications including myocardial infarctions and arrhythmias, cerebrovascular accidents, and heat stroke.[64] Other problems include hypertension, restlessness, and seizures.

LEGALITY. Amphetamines are banned by both the IOC and the NCAA.[62,63] Amphetamine and dextroamphetamine are class CII medications and are considered potentially addicting.

Anabolic/Androgenic Steroids and Androstenedione

EFFICACY. Anabolic steroids have both anabolic (tissue-building) and androgenic effects. Androstenedione is

---

TABLE 41–8. ERGOGENIC AIDS: EFFECTS ON FITNESS COMPONENTS AND DANGEROUS SIDE EFFECTS

Product	Aerobic	Anaerobic	Strength	Body Comp.	Psych.	Healing	Danger
Amphetamines	+	+	+	+	+		+
Anabolic steroids			+	+	+	?	+
Antioxidants						?	
Bicarbonate		+			+		
Blood doping	+						+
Caffeine	+	+			?		
Caffeine + ephedrine	+			+	?		
Carbohydrate	+					?	
Clenbuterol			?	?	?		
CoQ10						?	
DHEA			?	?			
Ephedrine	+			+	?		+
Ginseng					?		
Glycerol							rare
Hydration	+						
Vitamins							

CoQ10 = coenzyme Q10; DHEA = dehydroepiandrosterone; Body Comp.= body composition; Psych. = psychological factors.

one of the few ergogenic aids that are converted into testosterone when ingested.[45] Anabolic steroids have been shown to increase lean muscle mass and strength when used with an adequate diet and with progressive weight training.[60] The effects seem even more pronounced in athletes who use supraphysiologic doses.[45] There appears to be no effect on aerobic power, aerobic capacity, or athleticism.[60] Enhancement of aggression may also occur.[45] Anabolic steroids have been found to increase strength and lean muscle mass in men infected with HIV when used with progressive resistance training.[70] Athletes have long thought that steroids speed healing from injuries, and a recent study on muscle injury in rats suggested that they do indeed help in healing from muscle contusion injury.[71] However, other studies have shown that they affect rat tendon morphology adversely.[46]

SAFETY. Contraindications to steroids are listed in Table 41–6. Anabolic steroids have a long list of reported side effects, some of which may have been exaggerated in the literature. Probably the most harmful side effect is the impact on cardiac risk factors, with elevated blood pressure and alteration in blood cholesterol levels. An increase in low-density lipoprotein (LDL) and a decrease in high-density lipoprotein (HDL) of 50% on average in both male and female users have been widely reported.[44] No direct link with increased cardiovascular mortality has been established to date.[44] Adverse effects have been noted in the liver including jaundice, benign tumors, and (rarely) peliosis hepatis (blood-filled cysts in the liver), which has caused a few fatalities when the cysts ruptured.[60] Causation of malignant liver tumors has not been proved.[44] Other side effects include acne, female masculinization (alopecia, hirsutism, clitoromegaly, deepening of the voice), and enhancement of aggression.[44] Side effects of androstenedione are likely to be similar to those of anabolic steroids.

Long-term side effects have been harder to establish. The biggest problem seems to be that when the anabolic steroids are stopped, the lean muscle and strength gains resolve. A study of 16 chronic users showed that their blood pressure, cholesterol levels, and liver enzymes returned to normal after 3 months of steroid cessation.[72] However, a study compared rats given comparable supraphysiologic doses of steroids for 6 months with those given low doses and those given none. At age 20 months, 1 year after stopping the steroids, 52% of the high-dose steroid rats had died compared with 35% of the low-dose rats and only 12% of steroid-free rats.[73]

LEGALITY. Steroids are a class III controlled substance. Most organizing bodies including the IOC and NCAA have banned them.[62,63] Users could avoid detection by tapering in advance of announced tests, staying within the 6:1 testosterone-to-epitestosterone level, or using masking agents like diuretics.[61] Recent development of a hair test may change the way testing is done in the future.[65] Androstenedione, although banned, is not often specifically tested for the moment.[44]

Bicarbonate

EFFICACY. Sodium bicarbonate is found naturally in the body. It is thought to act ergogenically by helping to buffer lactic acid during high-intensity exercise or through some action of the sodium ion on intravascular volume.[74,75] Bicarbonate appears to be effective in reducing acidosis of the muscle cell and blood, decreasing the perception of fatigue, and improving performance and delaying time to exhaustion in high-intensity events.[74,75] Studies have shown improved performance in 400-, 800-, and 1500-meter runs in highly trained runners.[74,76]

SAFETY. Bicarbonate appears safe at doses needed to produce ergogenic effects.[74,75] Excessive doses could lead to alkalosis. The major side effect at ergogenic doses is GI distress and diarrhea, which may prevent the ergogenic effect.[76]

LEGALITY. Bicarbonate is currently not a banned substance.[62,63]

Blood Doping and Recombinant Erythropoietin

EFFICACY. Blood doping refers to the process of artificially increasing red blood cell (RBC) mass to improve exercise performance. RBC mass can be increased by infusion of RBCs or by use of the recombinant human hormone erythropoietin (rEPO), which stimulates RBC production.[77] By increasing the RBC mass, oxygen-carrying capacity is increased, with a resultant increase in both maximal aerobic power and aerobic capacity. The increased $\dot{V}O_2$max and time to exhaustion cause improvements in race performance, especially in distance runners.[77,78] Blood doping also seems to help performance in the heat, especially in acclimatized individuals.[77]

SAFETY. The major risk from blood transfusions is transfusion reactions. Although rare, transfusion reactions from both autologous and homologous blood reactions can occur due to clerical errors or mishandling of blood. Infections may occur if the blood is improperly handled. Transfusion of homologous blood also carries the risk of transmitting communicable diseases.[77]

Hyperviscosity can occur with hemoglobin levels over 55%. This may increase the risk of thrombosis, causing strokes or myocardial infarction in athletes using rEPO or blood transfusions. Although it has not been proved, numerous deaths among cyclists have been attributed to the ability of rEPO to cause vascular sludging and myocardial artery occlusion.[53,77,79] Blood pressure may also be increased by rEPO and is contraindicated in uncontrolled hypertension.[78]

LEGALITY. Blood doping through transfusion or rEPO is banned by most governing bodies including the IOC and NCAA.[62,63] Blood transfusions can be detected if homologous blood is used, but autologous blood use is harder to detect.[77] rEPO is likewise hard to detect. Indirect findings of doping using rEPO include a higher transferrin level and younger RBC population.[53,66] Direct measurement of erythropoietin isoforms can be done on blood samples.[66] However, since rEPO currently can only be detected for a few days after administration but has effects that last for weeks, reliable testing is difficult.[64,77]

Caffeine

EFFICACY. Although there are some conflicting studies, caffeine seems to enhance performance during both prolonged activity and shorter intense activity.[74,75,80–84] The effectiveness of caffeine may not be as great in habitual users or in hot humid environments.[83,85] Caffeine is a central nervous system stimulant that may cause ergogenic effects through numerous mechanisms. It has been hypothesized to work for runners by increasing free fatty acid production, which would spare muscle glycogen, elevating cyclic adenosine monophosphate (AMP) levels in cells, altering the movement of calcium by the sarcoplasmic reticulum, increasing levels of catecholamines, increasing neuromuscular transmissions, and decreasing perceived effort and fatigue.[53,75,83,86,87]

SAFETY. In normal doses (5 to 8 mg/kg) caffeine appears to be safe and produces only a few side effects such as diarrhea, insomnia, restlessness, and anxiety.[64] Caffeine does not appear to increase risk for heat stroke or to compromise cardiovascular activity in endurance performance.[88] High doses, over 10 mg/kg, may cause seizures, and overdosing may lead to death.[89]

LEGALITY. Caffeine, although ergogenic at 5 to 10 mg/kg, is not completely banned by the IOC and NCAA. Habitual users may consume their usual caffeine in small amounts. Ingestion of around 7 mg/kg, roughly 2 cups of coffee, produces urinary levels close to the limit of 12 μm/ml for the IOC.[75,62] The NCAA levels are slightly more liberal, at 15 μm/ml.[63]

Caffeine Plus Ephedrine

EFFICACY. Caffeine plus ephedrine has been shown to improve exercise time to exhaustion.[90] Caffeine, when combined with ephedrine, may also be beneficial in weight loss.[91]

SAFETY. Caffeine and ephedrine side effects are listed under those single items. Because caffeine potentiates ephedrine, it may also potentiate its side effects.

LEGALITY. Both substances are on the banned substance list.[62,63]

Clenbuterol and Beta Agonists

EFFICACY. Clenbuterol and other beta$_2$ agonists like salmeterol and albuterol are widely used as bronchodilators for the treatment of many types of asthma including exercise-induced asthma.[92] Nonasthmatic athletes use them, especially clenbuterol, for their potential anabolic effects, either as an anabolic steroid substitute or to prevent some of the muscle loss after cessation of anabolic steroids.[52,53,64] Animal studies have shown that clenbuterol in high doses increases lean body mass and decreases adipose tissue.[64,93] However, human studies are not available that show these effects. Prolonged administration of oral beta$_2$ agonists have been shown to have a mild ergogenic effect on strength in nonasthmatic athletes.[94] One study showed that a sustained-release oral dose of salbutamol taken for 3 weeks increased quadriceps and hamstring strength.[95] Another showed that 6 weeks of oral albuterol may augment strength gains in isokinetic strength training of the knee.[96] In contrast, studies looking at short-term inhalant therapy of salmeterol and albuterol showed no effect on anaerobic power output or strength in nonasthmatics.[96–98] One study on inhaled salmeterol and salbutamol actually showed a decrease in running time to exhaustion.[99] Taken together, these studies imply that there may be an ergogenic effect of prolonged oral beta$_2$ agonists on strength, but no ergogenic effect of short-term administration of inhaled medicines. Confirmatory studies on humans remain to be done regarding their potential anabolic effects.

SAFETY. Side effects of beta$_2$ agonists are common and include tachycardia, tremor, palpitations, anxiety, headache, anorexia, and insomnia. Serious side effects include dysrhythmias, cardiac muscle hypertrophy, myocardial infarction, or stroke.[53,64,93]

LEGALITY. Because of its potential ergogenic effect, clenbuterol in all its forms and all oral beta$_2$ agonists are banned by the IOC and NCAA.[62,63] Advances in testing may eventually allow detection of these drugs through hair analysis.[67] Clenbuterol is not FDA approved. It is interesting to note there was an increase in the percentage of U.S. Olympic athletes with exercise-induced asthma from 10% in the 1984 Summer Olympics to over 20% in the 1996 Summer Olympics, thus greatly increasing the number of athletes who can "legally" use these products.[52,100]

Coenzyme Q10

EFFICACY. Coenzyme Q10 (CoQ10), also called ubiquinone, is part of the electron transport system and functions as an antioxidant.[74] In cardiac patients with congestive heart failure, cardiac function is improved, including increased stroke volume, ejection fraction, cardiac output, and cardiac index, although total work output does not appear to be increased.[101] The data on athletes are generally negative for an ergogenic effect of CoQ10. A double-blind Finnish study did show an increase in anaerobic and aerobic indices in 25 top-level cross country skiers.[102] However, four other studies examining CoQ10 either alone or in combination with other antioxidants did not show any effect on anaerobic or aerobic performance.[103–106] It may serve some role in injury healing/prevention due to its antioxidant properties, especially in heart attack patients.[107] More research is required.

SAFETY. CoQ10 seems safe, although there are no long-term studies.

LEGALITY. CoQ10 is not on the list of banned substances.[62,63]

Dehydroepiandrosterone

EFFICACY. DHEA is a hormone secreted by the adrenal gland that is a precursor to both androgens and estrogens.[45,108,109] The FDA banned the manufacture of DHEA as a drug due to insufficient evidence of efficacy and safety, but it continues to be available as a nutritional supplement.[109] DHEA levels peak in at puberty and young adulthood and gradually fade as aging progresses.[108] Studies showed that physiologic doses (50 mg/day) and supraphysiologic doses (1600 mg/day) of DHEA increased circulating androgen levels in older women but not in older men.[109,110] DHEA increased androstenedione levels but not testosterone levels and nonstatistically increased lean body mass when given at supraphysiologic doses to five young males.[111] DHEA did not appear to affect energy or protein metabolism in young males.[112] In summary, DHEA does not appear to increase testosterone in young healthy males, and its ergogenic properties in the young athletic population are largely unknown.

SAFETY. Short-term use of DHEA has been associated with few side effects.[108] If DHEA does work to increase serum androgens and estrogens in an unopposed manner, there is a theoretical risk of prostate and endometrial cancer.[45,108] DHEA may also produce a favorable cholesterol profile.[108] However, these are hypothetical risks and benefits, and there is no information on long-term use, especially at supraphysiologic doses.

LEGALITY. DHEA is currently banned by both the NCAA and IOC and is available only as a nutritional supplement in the United States.[62,63,109]

Ephedrine (Ma Huang) and Related Sympathomimetics

EFFICACY. Ephedrine is a sympathomimetic drug that is the active ingredient in the Chinese herb Ma huang.[113] Ephedrine, and other sympathomimetics like pseudoephedrine and phenylpropanolamine, are commonly found in over-the-counter cold medicines. Ephedrine acts physiologically to increase heart rate and blood pressure.[114] When used with caffeine, ephedrine has been shown to improve time to exhaustion during exercise tests.[90] When used with caffeine, it also seems to be effective in producing weight loss.[91] However, ephedrine by itself when given at a low dose (24 mg) did not favorably affect performance.[115] Likewise, pseudoephedrine and phenylpropanolamine have not been shown to improve aerobic performance in controlled trials.[116,117] More research at therapeutic nontoxic doses of ephedrine would need to be done to determine its ergogenic potential for anaerobic and aerobic performance.

SAFETY. Ephedrine has caused fatalities even at recommended over-the-counter doses, prompting the FDA to issue a warning against its consumption in 1996.[118–121] Other serious side effects have been reported including nephrolithiasis and (rarely) hepatitis.[122,123] Common side effects include tachycardia, hypertension, anxiety, and arrhythmias.[124]

LEGALITY. Ephedrine and related compounds are banned by the NCAA and IOC.[62,63] The IOC allows a small amount of ephedrine in the urine, 5 mg/ml.[62]

Ginseng

EFFICACY. Ginseng is a shrub whose root is often used as an ergogenic aid. At least four varieties of the plant are used in the preparation of products including *Panax ginseng C.A. Meyer,* known as Chinese ginseng, and *Eleutherococcus senticosus,* known as Siberian ginseng.[74,125] The saponin extracts or glycosides from the root are considered to provide most of the biologic activity. There have been conflicting reports on effi-cacy, with a few placebo-controlled studies showing improvement in maximum aerobic capacity whereas others did not.[74] However, recent well-designed placebo-controlled, double-blind studies have failed to demonstrate any improvement in aerobic exercise.[126–129] The largest problem with this nutritional supplement, as with most supplements, is the lack of quality control and standardization in the amount of saponins available in the products.[130]

SAFETY. There are few reported side effects with ginseng. Hypertension, anxiety, acne, edema, and diarrhea have been reported with long-term high-dose use.[74]

LEGALITY. Ginseng is not banned by the NCAA or the IOC.[62,63]

Glycerol and Hyperhydration

EFFICACY. Glycerol can be used to induce a state of hyperhydration, which may theoretically aid in distance running in warm environments.[74,131] In a thermoneutral environment, glycerol hyperhydration did not improve performance in prolonged exercise.[131] Another study was performed in which subjects were placed in an experimental setting of exercise in uncompensable heat stress.[132] Hyperhydration with water alone and with glycerol was compared with euhydration with water. Both hyperhydration states significantly prolonged time to heat exhaustion to 34 minutes compared with water at 29 minutes. However, all physiologic parameters were equal, and heat exhaustion occurred at similar body core temperatures. The authors concluded that hyperhydration with glycerol provided no advantage over hyperhydration with water. Furthermore, the only advantage to hyperhydration over euhydration was to delay hypohydration during uncompensable heat stress.[132] More research needs to be done to delineate under which circumstances, if any, hyperhydration with glycerol or water alone is indicated.

SAFETY. Glycerol may increase the risk of intraocular and intracerebral dehydration and should not be used in persons with renal disease.

LEGALITY. Glycerol is not banned by the NCAA or IOC.[62,63]

Vitamins and Antioxidants

EFFICACY. Vitamin and mineral supplementation has been used by athletes for years, even though there is no evidence of effectiveness. If an athlete consumes a well-balanced diet, vitamin supplementation for 3 months does not seem to affect blood concentrations of the vitamins.[133] After 3 to 9 nine months of multivitamin and mineral supplementation no effect on exercise performance was seen.[134,135] Unless a nutritional deficiency exists, routine supplementation of vitamins and minerals is not recommended.

Antioxidants include vitamin E, vitamin C, beta-carotene (a vitamin A precursor), and CoQ10, among others. Animal studies and some human studies have suggested that muscle injury places oxidative stress on muscles.[136] However, almost all studies on humans to date have not reported a beneficial effect of antioxidant supplementation on performance.[136–139] The lone study that did show an effect used N-acetyl-cysteine as the antioxidant and showed an improvement on tibialis anterior contraction force following stimulation to fatigue.[140] Until more studies show an ergogenic effect, routine supplementation with antioxidants does not appear to be warranted.

SAFETY. Supplementation with a multivitamin or antioxidant appears to be safe. However, in large doses they may become toxic. At high doses, vitamin C and beta-carotene may actually become prooxidant.[136]

LEGALITY. Vitamins and antioxidants are not banned by the NCAA or IOC.[62,63]

Glucosamine and Chondroitin Sulfate

EFFICACY. Glucosamine and chondroitin sulfate are used in the synthesis of glycosaminoglycans, a significant part of the extracellular matrix of articular cartilage.[141] Many studies have been performed evaluating the efficacy of these substances in treating osteoarthritis compared with placebo and with NSAIDs. For example, one study comparing chondroitin sulfate with diclofenac sodium in a 6-month randomized double-blind double-dummy study found chondroitin to be equal to diclofenac with respect to function as measured by the Lequesne Index and in treatment of pain.[142] The reduction of symptoms took longer but lasted after treatment was stopped. A randomized placebo-controlled double-blind study on U.S. Navy Seals showed that supplementation with chondroitin sulfate, glucosamine HCl, and manganese ascorbate significantly decreased pain, although run times did not improve.[143] Over the years, numerous other studies have shown that supplementation with chondroitin sulfate and glucosamine reduces pain in osteoarthritis patients equal to that of NSAIDs and may also have some intrinsic anti-inflammatory properties.[141] Some of the studies may show differences in efficacy due to the differences in the amount of glucosamine and chondroitin sulfate in the product.[141] Glucosamine HCl is usually given as 1500 mg/day; glucosamine sulfate requires around 2600 mg to be an equivalent bioactive dose.[141] Chondroitin sulfate is usually given as 1200 mg/day. Combination products are probably better than using one product alone.[141]

SAFETY. Short-term studies have not shown any adverse side effects, but there are no long-term studies evaluating safety.[141]

LEGALITY. Glucosamine and chondroitin sulfate are not banned by the IOC or NCAA.[62,63]

Growth Hormone

EFFICACY. Growth hormone (GH) is secreted by the hypothalamus and is important in the growth and development of normal bones and muscle. GH seems to be intricately related to insulin-like growth factor-I (IGF-I) and the regulation of insulin.[144] GH appears to provide an anabolic effect and increases bone mass and lean body mass while decreasing adipose tissue.[144–146] GH supplementation is anabolic in HIV-positive adolescents.[147] Administration of GH in GH-deficient individuals such as those with Prader-Willi syndrome has been shown to increase height, decrease body fat, and improve respiratory muscle function, strength, and agility.[148] However, in normal individuals, supplementation with GH has never been shown to improve athletic performance. Although there are myocardial receptors for GH, administration of recombinant human growth hormone (rhGH) did not affect cardiovascular performance as measured by left ventricular ejection fraction, heart rate, or blood pressure in seven normal male volunteers.[149]

Previously supplementation with GH was accomplished by using extract from primates; now the recombinant human form (rhGH) is used. In addition to supplementation, GH levels can be increased by exercise, and the level of release is directly related to exercise intensity.[150] The duration of GH release after exercise and the effects of long-term training on this release are not well known.[151] It has been reported that more fit individuals have higher levels of GH and IGF-I.[152] However, the decline of GH and IGF-I during aging was not reported to be offset by exercise.[153,154]

SAFETY. The safety of long-term administration of GH in nondeficient individuals has not been established. High GH levels cause acromegaly and gigantism.

LEGALITY. GH supplementation is banned by the IOC and NCAA.[62,63]

SUMMARY

Many medicines and ergogenic aids are used in an attempt to speed healing and gain a competitive edge. NSAIDs should be used acutely for pain and inflammation; their chronic use should be relegated to truly inflammatory conditions. Likewise, corticosteroids should be used judiciously. Anabolic steroids are not only banned from sport but carry further legal consequences if an individual is caught using or distributing them. Their use is appropriate in certain medical situations, and it will be interesting to see what the research shows regarding their ability to help heal injury.

Ergogenic aids are used widely. However, since they are deregulated, quality control is not the same as it is for drugs. What is on the label is not necessarily what is in the bottle. Some products have proven efficacy whereas others have only advertising claims or hype to validate their use. All products should be used with the three basic principles in mind: (1) Do they work? (2) Are they safe? (3) What are the legal and ethical consequences of using the product? In the end, the race is always against yourself.

REFERENCES

1. Simon LS, Smith TJ: NSAID mechanism of action, efficacy, and relative safety, in *Managing Arthritis: A Postgraduate Medicine Special Report*, 1998:March, 17.
2. Lefkowith JB: Cyclooxygenase-2 specificity and its clinical implications. *Am J Med* 1999:106, 43S.

3. Stanley KL, Weaver JE: Pharmacologic management of pain and inflammation in athletes. *Clin Sports Med* 1998:17, 375.

4. Abraham SB, Weissman G: The mechanics of action of nonsteroidal anti-inflammatory drugs. *Arthritis Rheum* 1989:32, 1.

5. Diaz-Gonzalez F, Gonzalez-Alvero I, Companero MR, et al.: Prevention of in-vitro neutrophil-endothelial attachment through shedding of L-selectin by NSAIDs. *J Clin Invest* 1995:95, 1756.

6. Pizza FX, Cavender D, Stockard A, et al.: Anti-inflammatory doses of ibuprofen: Effect on neutrophils and exercise-induced muscle injury. *Int J Sports Med* 1999:20, 98.

7. Ogilvie-Harris DJ, Gilbart M: Treatment modalities for soft tissue injuries of the ankle: A critical review. *Clin J Sports Med* 1995:5, 175.

8. Slatyer MA, Hensley MJ, Lopert R: A randomized controlled trial of piroxicam in the management of acute ankle sprain in Australian Army Regular Army recruits. The Kapooka Ankle Sprain Study. *Am J Sports Med* 1997:25, 544.

9. Dudley GA, Czerkawski J, Meinrod A, et al.: Efficacy of naproxen sodium for exercise-induced dysfunction muscle injury and soreness. *Clin J Sports Med* 1997: 7, 3.

10. Lecomte JM, Lacroix VJ, Montgomery DL: A randomized controlled trial of the effect of naprosyn on delayed onset muscle soreness and muscle strength. *Clin J Sports Med* 1998:8, 82.

11. Bourgeois J, MacDougall D, MacDonald J, et al.: Naproxen does not alter indices of muscle damage in resistance-exercise trained men. *Med Sci Sports Exerc* 1999:31, 4.

12. Reynolds JF, Noakes TD, Schwellnus MP, et al.: Nonsteroidal anti-inflammatory drugs fail to enhance healing of acute hamstring injuries treated with physiotherapy. *South Afr Med J* 1995:85, 517.

13. Almekinders LC, Baynes AJ, Bracey LW: An in vitro investigation into the effects of repetitive motion and nonsteroidal antiinflammatory medication on human tendon fibroblasts. *Am J Sports Med* 1995:23, 119.

14. Obremsky WT, Seaber AV, Ribbeck BM, et al.: Biomechanical and histological assessment of a controlled muscle strain injury treated with piroxicam. *Am J Sports Med* 1994:22, 558.

15. Khan KM, Cook JL, Bonar F, et al.: Histopathology of common tendinopathies. Update and implications for clinical management. *Sports Med* 1999:27, 393.

16. Almekinders LC, Temple JD: Etiology, diagnosis, and treatment of tenodonitis: An analysis of the literature. *Med Sci Sports Exerc* 1998:30, 1183.

17. Leadbetter WB: Anti-inflammatory therapy in sports injury. The role of nonsteroidal drugs and corticosteroid injection. *Clin Sports Med* 1995:14, 355.

18. Schieman JM: Gastrointestinal effects of NSAIDs: Therapeutic implications of Cox-2-selective agents, in *Managing Arthritis: A Postgraduate Medicine Special Report*, 1998:March, 17.

19. Smalley WE, Griffin MR: NSAIDs, eicosanoids, and the gastroenteric tract. *Gastroenterol Clin* 1996:25, 373.

20. Delzell E, Shapiro S: A review of epidemiologic studies of nonnarcotic analgesics and chronic renal disease. *Medicine (Baltimore)* 1998:77, 102.

21. Feldman HI, Kinman JL, Berlin JA, et al.: Parenteral ketorolac: The risk for acute renal failure. *Ann Intern Med* 1997:126, 193.

22. Walker AM: Quantitative studies of the risk of serious hepatic injury in persons using nonsteroidal antiinflammatory drugs. *Arthritis Rheum* 1997:40, 201.

23. Szczeklik A, Stevenson DD: Aspirin-induced asthma: Advances in pathogenesis and management. *J Allergy Clin Immunol* 1999:104, 5.

24. Joint Task Force on Practice Parameters: Practice parameters for the diagnosis and treatment of asthma. *J Allergy Clin Immunol* 1995:96, 707.

25. Hollander D: Gastrointestinal complications of nonsteroidal anti-inflammatory drugs: Prophylactic and therapeutic strategies. *Am J Med* 1994:96, 274.

26. Raskin JB, White RH, Jaszewski R, et al.: Misoprostol and ranitidine in the prevention of NSAID-induced ulcers: A prospective, double blind, multicenter study. *Am J Gastroenterol* 1996:91, 223.

27. Maetzel A, Ferraz MB, Bombadier C: The cost-effectiveness of misoprostol in preventing serious gastrointestinal events associated with the use of nonsteroidal antiinflammatory drugs. *Arthritis Rheum* 1998:41, 16.

28. Silverstein FE, Graham DY, Senior JR, et al.: Misoprostol reduces serious gastrointestinal complications in patients with rheumatoid arthritis receiving nonsteroidal anti-inflammatory drugs. A randomized, double-blind, placebo controlled trial. *Ann Intern Med* 1995:123, 24.

29. McKenna F: Diclofenac/misoprostol: The European clinical experience. *J Rheumatol Suppl* 1998:51, 21.

30. Golden BD, Abramson SB: Selective cyclooxygenase-2 inhibitors. *Rheum Dis Clin North Am* 1999:25, 359.

31. Dominkus M, Nicolakis M, Kotz R, et al.: Comparison of tissue and plasma levels of ibuprofen after oral and topical administration. *Arzneimittelforschung* 1996:46, 1138.

32. Rosenstein ED: Topical agents in the treatment of rheumatic disorders. *Rheum Dis Clin North Am* 1999:25, 899.

33. Sandelin J, Harilainen A, Crone H, et al.: Local NSAID gel (eltenac) in the treatment of osteoarthritis of the knee. A double blind study comparing eltenac with oral diclofenac and placebo gel. *Scand J Rheumatol* 1997:26, 287.

34. Martens M: Efficacy and tolerability of a topical NSAID patch (local action transcutaneous flurbiprofen) and oral diclofenac in the treatment of soft-tissue rheumatism. *Clin J Rheumatol* 1997:16, 25.

35. Moore RA, Tramer MR, Caroll D, et al.: Quantitative systematic review of topically applied non-steroidal anti-inflammatory drugs. *BMJ* 1998:316, 333.

36. Barnes PJ: Anti-inflammatory actions of glucocorticoids: molecular mechanisms. *Clin Sci* 1998:94, 557.

37. Jacob AK, Sallay PI: Therapeutic efficacy of corticosteroid injections in the acromioclavicular joint. *Biomed Sci Instrum* 1997:34, 380.

38. Holt MA, Keene JS, Graf BK, et al.: Treatment of osteitis pubis in athletes. Results of corticosteroid injections. *Am J Sports Med* 1995:23, 601.

39. Spaccarelli KC: Lumbar and caudal epidural corticosteroid injections. *Mayo Clin Proc* 1996:71, 169.

40. Shrier I, Matheson GO, Kohl HW 3rd: Achilles tendonitis: Are corticosteroid injections useful or harmful? *Clin J Sports Med* 1996:6, 245.

41. Gudeman SD, Eisele SA, Heidt RS, et al.: Treatment of plantar fascitis by iontophoresis of 0.4% dexamethasone. A randomized, double blind, placebo controlled study. *Am J Sports Med* 1997:25, 312.

42. Beiner JM, Jokl P, Cholewicki J, et al.: The effect of anabolic steroids and corticosteroids on healing of muscular contusion injury. *Am J Sports Med* 1999:27, 2.

43. Gabriel SE, Sunku J, Salvarani C, et al.: Adverse outcomes of antiinflammatory therapy among patients with polymyalgia rheumatica. *Arthritis Rheum* 1997:40, 1873.

44. Blue JG, Lombardo JA: Nutritional aspects of exercise. Steroids and steroid-like compounds. *Clin Sports Med* 1999:18, 667.

45. Bhasin S, Storer TW, Berman N, et al.: The effects of supraphysiologic doses of testosterone on muscle size and strength in normal men. *N Engl J Med* 1996:335, 1–7.

46. Miles JW, Grana WA, Egle D, et al.: The effect of anabolic steroids on the biomechanical and histological properties of rat tendon. *J Bone Joint Surg* 1992:74, 411.

47. Inhofe PD, Grana WA, Egle D, et al.: The effects of anabolic steroids on rat tendon. An ultrastructural, biomechanical, and biochemical analysis. *Am J Sports Med* 1995:23, 227.

48. Laseter JT, Russell JA: Anabolic steroid-induced tendon pathology: A review of the literature. *Med Sci Sports Exerc* 1991:23, 1.

49. Karpakka JA, Pesola MK, Takala TE: The effects of anabolic steroids on collagen synthesis in rat skeletal muscle and tendon. A preliminary report. *Am J Sports Med* 1992:20, 262.

50. Ferry A, Noirez P, Page CL, et al.: Effects of anabolic/androgenic steroids on regenerating skeletal muscles in the rat. *Acta Physiol Scand* 1999:166, 105.

51. Applegate EA, Grivetti LE: Search for the competitive edge: A history of dietary fads and supplements. *J Nutr* 1997:127, 869S.

52. Eichner ER: Ergogenic aids. *Physician Sportsmed* 1997:25, 70.

53. Thein LA, Thein JM, Landry GL: Ergogenic aids. *Phys Ther* 1995:75, 426.

54. Glade MJ: The dietary supplement health and education act of 1994—focus on labeling issues. *Nutrition* 1997:13, 999.

55. Butterfield G: Ergogenic aids: Evaluating sport nutrition products. *Int J Sport Nutr* 1996:6, 191.

56. Schardt D: Relieving arthritis, can supplements help? *Nutr Action* 1998:Jan/Feb, 3.

57. Brown WA: The placebo effect. *Sci Am* 1998:Jan, 90.

58. Cahill BR, Misner JE, Boileau RA: The clinical importance of the anaerobic energy system and its assessment in human performance. *Am J Sports Med* 1997:25, 863.

59. Woolley AH: The latest fads to increase muscle mass and energy. *Postgrad Med* 1991:89, 195.

60. American College of Sports Medicine: The use of anabolic-androgenic steroids in sports. *Med Sci Sports Exerc* 1987:19, 453.

61. Bowers LD: Sports pharmacology. Athletic drug testing. *Clin Sports Med* 1998:17, 299.

62. International Olympic Committee Medical Code, Lausanne, Switzerland, 1999.

63. National Collegiate Athletic Association, Sports Sciences, Indianapolis, IN, 1999.

64. Knopp WD, Wang TW, Bach BR: Ergogenic drugs in sports. *Clin Sports Med* 1997:16, 375.

65. Klintz P, Cirimele V, Sachs H, et al.: Testing for anabolic steroids in hair from two bodybuilders. *Forens Sci Int* 1999:101, 209.

66. Birkeland KI, Hemmersbach P: The future of doping control in athletes. *Sports Med* 1999:28, 25.

67. Polettini A, Montagna M, Segura J, et al.: Determination of beta 2-agonists in hair by gas chromatography/mass spectrometry. *J Mass Spectrom* 1996:31, 47.

68. Smith GM, Beecher HK: Amphetamine sulfate and athletic performance. *JAMA* 1959:170, 524.

69. Chandler JV, Blair SN: The effect of amphetamines on selected physiological components related to athletic success. *Med Sci Sports Exerc* 1980:12, 65.

70. Sattler FR, Jaque SV, Schroeder ET, et al.: Effects of pharmacological doses of nandrolone decanoate and progressive resistance training in immunodeficient patients infected with human immunodeficiency virus. *J Clin Endocrinol Metab* 1999:84, 1268.

71. Beiner JM, Jokl P, Cholewicki J, et al.: The effect of anabolic steroids and corticosteroids on healing of muscle contusion injury. *Am J Sports Med* 1999:2791, 2.

72. Hartgens F, Kuipers H, Wijnen JA, et al.: Body composition, cardiovascular risk factors and liver function in long-term androgenic-anabolic steroids using body builders three months after drug withdrawal. *Int J Sports Med* 1996:17, 429.

73. Bronson FH, Matherne CM: Exposure to anabolic-androgenic steroids shortens life span of male mice. *Med Sci Sports Exerc* 1997:29, 615.

74. Williams MH: Nutritional ergogenics in athletics. *J Sports Sci* 1995:13, S63.

75. Clarkson PM: Nutrition for improved sports performance. *Sports Med* 1996:21, 393.

76. Bird SR, Wiles J, Robbins J: The effect of sodium bicarbonate ingestion on 1500-m racing time. *J Sports Sci* 1995:13, 399.

77. Sawka MN, Joyner MJ, Miles DS, et al.: The use of blood doping as an ergogenic aid, ACSM position stand. *Med Sci Sports Exerc* 1996:28, i.

78. Ekblom B: Blood doping and erythropoietin. *Am J Sports Med* 1996:24, S40.

79. Eichner ER: Sports anemia, iron supplementation, and blood doping. *Med Sci Sports Exerc* 1992:24(9 suppl), S315.

80. Spriet LL: Caffeine and performance. *Int J Sport Nutr* 1995:5(suppl), S84.

81. Doherty M: The effects of caffeine on the maximal accumulated oxygen deficit and short-term running performance. *Int J Sport Nutr* 1998:8, 95.

82. Applegate E: Effective nutritional ergogenic aids. *Int J Sports Nutr* 1999:9, 229.

83. Tarnopolsky MA, Atkinson SA, MacDougall JD, et al.: Physiological responses to caffeine during endurance running in habitual caffeine users. *Med Sci Sports Exerc* 1989:21, 418.

84. Pasman WJ, van Baak MA, Jeukendrup AE, et al.: The effect of different dosages of caffeine on endurance performance time. *Int J Sports Med* 1995:16, 225.

85. Cohen BS, Nelson AG, Prevost MC, et al.: Effects of caffeine ingestion on endurance racing in heat and humidity. *Eur J Appl Physiol* 1996:73, 358.

86. Cole KJ, Costill DL, Starling RD, et al.: Effect of caffeine ingestion on perception of effort and subsequent work production. *Int J Sport Nutr* 1996:6, 14.

87. Hogervorst E, Reidel WJ, Kovacs E, et al.: Caffeine improves cognitive performance after strenuous physical exercise. *Int J Sports Med* 1999:20, 354.

88. Gordon NF, Myburgh JL, Kruger PE, et al.: Effects of caffeine ingestion on thermoregulatory and myocardial function during endurance performance. *South Afr Med J* 1982:62, 644.

89. FitzSimmons CR, Kidner N: Caffeine toxicity in a bodybuilder. *J Accid Emerg Med* 1998:15, 196.

90. Bell D, Jacobs I: The effects of ingesting caffeine, ephedrine and their combination on exercise time to exhaustion at 85% $\dot{V}o_2$max. *Can J Appl Physiol* 1995: 20, 5.

91. Carek PJ, Dickerson LM: Current concepts in the pharmacological management of obesity. *Drugs* 1999:57, 883.

92. Smith BW, LaBotz M: pharmacologic treatment of exercise-induced asthma. *Clin Sports Med* 1998:17, 343.

93. Prather ID, Brown DE, North P, et al.: Clenbuterol: a substitute for anabolic steroids? *Med Sci Sports Exerc* 1995:27, 1118.

94. Martineau L, Horan MA, Rothwell NJ, et al.: Salbutamol, a beta 2 adrenoceptor agonist, increases skeletal muscle strength in young men. *Clin Sci* 1992:83, 615.

95. Caruso JF, Signorile JF, Perry AC, et al.: The effects of albuterol and isokinetic exercise on the quadriceps muscle group. *Med Sci Sports Exerc* 1995:279, 1471.

96. Lemmer JT, Fleck SJ, Wallach JM, et al.: The effects of albuterol on power output in non-asthmatic athletes. *Int J Sports Med* 1995:16, 243.

97. Morton AR, Joyce K, Papalia SM: Is salmeterol ergogenic? *Clin J Sports Med* 1996:6, 220.

98. McDowell SL, Fleck SJ, Storms WW: The effects of salmeterol on power output in nonasthmatic athletes. *J Allergy Clin Immunol* 1997:99, 443.

99. Carlsen KH, Ingjer F, Kirkgaard H, et al.: The effect of inhaled salbutamol and salmeterol on lung function and endurance performance in healthy well-trained athletes. *Scand J Med Sci Sports* 1997:7, 160.

100. Weiler JM, Layton T, Hunt M: Asthma in United States Olympic athletes who participated in the 1996 Summer Games. *J Allergy Clin Immunol* 1998:102, 722.

101. Soja AM, Mortensen SA: Treatment of congestive heart failure with coenzyme Q10 illuminated by meta-analysis of clinical trials. *Mol Aspects Med* 1997:18(suppl), S519.

102. Ylikoski T, Piiraninen J, Hanninen O, et al.: The effect of coenzyme Q10 on the exercise performance of cross-country skiers. *Mol Aspects Med* 1997:18(suppl), S283.

103. Snider IP, Bazzarre TL, Murdoch SD, et al.: Effects of coenzyme athletic performance system as an ergogenic aid on endurance performance to exhaustion. *Int J Sports Nutr* 1992:2, 272.

104. Porter DA, Costill DL, Zachwieja JJ, et al.: The effect of oral coenzyme Q10 on the exercise tolerance of middle aged, untrained men. *Int J Sports Med* 1995:16, 421.

105. Weston SB, Zhou S, Weatherby RP, et al.: Does exogenous coenzyme Q10 affect aerobic capacity in endurance athletes? *Int J Sport Nutr* 1997:7, 197.

106. Nielsen AN, Mizuno M, Ratkevicius A, et al.: No effect of antioxidant supplementation in triathletes on maximal oxygen uptake, ^{31}P-NMRS detected muscle energy metabolism and muscle fatigue. *Int J Sports Med* 1999:20, 154.

107. Singh RB, Wander GS, Rastogi A, et al.: Randomized, double blind placebo controlled trial of coenzyme Q10 in patients with acute myocardial infarction. *Cardiovasc Drug Ther* 1998:12, 347.

108. Sturmi JE, Diorio DJ: Sports pharmacology. Anabolic agents. *Clin Sports Med* 1998:17, 261.

109. Stricker PR: Sports pharmacology. Other ergogenic aids. *Clin Sports Med* 1998:17, 283.

110. Mortola JF, Yen SS: The effects of oral dehydroepiandrosterone on endocrine-metabolic parameters in postmenopausal women. *J Clin Endocrinol Metab* 1990:71, 696.

111. Nestler JE, Barlascini CO, Clore JN, et al.: Dehydroepiandrosterone reduces serum low density lipoprotein levels and body fat but does not alter insulin sensitivity in normal men. *J Clin Endocrinol Metab* 1988:66, 57.

112. Welle S, Jozefowicz R, Statt M: Failure of dehydroepiandrosterone to influence energy and protein metabolism in humans. *J Clin Endocrinol Metab* 1990:71, 1259.

113. Mack RB: All but death can be adjusted. *N C Med J* 1997:58, 68.

114. White LM, Gardner SF, Gurley BJ, et al.: Pharmacokinetics and cardiovascular effects of ma-huang in normotensive adults. *J Clin Pharmacol* 1997:37, 116.

115. Sidney KH, Lefcoe NM: The effects of ephedrine on the physiological and psychological responses to submaximal and maximal exercise in man. *Med Sci Sports* 1977:9, 95.

116. Gillies H, Derman WE, Noakes TD, et al.: Pseudoephedrine is without ergogenic effect during prolonged exercise. *J Appl Physiol* 1996:81, 2611.

117. Swain RA, Harsha DM, Baenziger J, et al.: Do pseudoephedrine or phenylpropanolamine improve maximum oxygen uptake and time to exhaustion? *Clin J Sports Med* 1997:7, 168.

118. Litovitz TL, Klein-Schwartz W, Caravati EM, et al.: 1998 annual report of the American Association of Poison Control Centers toxic exposure surveillance system. *Am J Emerg Med* 1999:17, 435.

119. Backer R, Tautman D, Lowry S, et al.: Fatal ephedrine intoxication. *J Forens Sci* 1997:42, 157.
120. US Department of Health and Human Services: Adverse effects associated with ephedrine containing products. *MMWR* 1996:45, 689.
121. US Department of Health and Human Services: FDA statement on street drugs containing the botanical ephedrine. April 10, 1996.
122. Nadir A, Agrawal S, King PD, et al.: Acute hepatitis associated with the use of a Chinese herbal product, ma-huang. *Am J Gastroenterol* 1996:91, 1436.
123. Powell T, Hsu FF, Turk J, et al.: Ma-huang strikes again: Ephedrine nephrolithiasis. *Am J Kidney Dis* 1998:32, 153.
124. Fugh-Berman A: Clinical trials of herbs. *Primary Care Clin Office Pract* 1997:24, 889.
125. Sprecher E. Ginseng—miracle drug or phytopharmacon? *Apotheker J* 1997:9, 52.
126. Morris AC, Jacobs I, McLellan TM, et al.: No ergogenic effect of ginseng ingestion. *Int J Sport Nutr* 1996:6, 263.
127. Dowling EA, Redondo DR, Branch JD, et al.: Effect of *Eleutherococcus senticosus* on submaximal and maximal exercise. *Med Sci Sports Exerc* 1996:28, 482.
128. Engels HJ, Wirth JC: No ergogenic effect of ginseng during graded maximal aerobic exercise. *J Am Diet Assoc* 1997:97, 1110.
129. Allen JD, McLung J, Nelson AG, et al.: Ginseng supplementation does not enhance healthy young adult's peak aerobic exercise performance. *J Am Coll Nutr* 1998:17, 462.
130. Cui J, Garle M, Eneroth P, et al.: What do commercial ginseng preparations contain? *Lancet* 1994:334, 134.
131. Inder WJ, Swanney MP, Donald RA, et al.: The effect of glycerol and desmopressin on exercise performance and hydration in triathletes. *Med Sci Sports Exerc* 1998:30, 1263.
132. Latzka WA, Sawka MN, Montain SJ, et al.: Hyperhydration: Tolerance and cardiovascular effects during uncompensable exercise-heat stress. *J Appl Physiol* 1998:84, 1858.
133. Weight LM, Noakes TD, Labadarios D, et al.: Vitamin and mineral status of trained athletes including the effects of supplementation. *Am J Clin Nutr* 1988:47, 186.
134. Weight LM, Myburgh KH, Noakes TD: Vitamin and mineral supplementation: Effect on running performance of trained athletes. *Am J Clin Nutr* 1988:47, 192.
135. Singh A, Moses F, Deuster PA: Chronic multivitamin-mineral supplementation does not enhance physical performance. *Med Sci Sports Exerc* 1992:24, 726.
136. Powers SK, Hamilton K: Nutritional aspects of exercise. Antioxidants and exercise. *Clin Sports Med* 1999:18, 525.
137. Ji LL: Exercise, oxidative stress, and antioxidants. *Am J Sports Med* 1996:24(6 suppl), S20.
138. Kanter MM, Williams MH: Antioxidants, carnitine, and choline as putative ergogenic aids. *Int J Sport Nutr* 1995:5(suppl), S120.
139. Clarkson PM: Antioxidants and physical performance. *Crit Rev Food Sci Nutr* 1995:35, 131.
140. Reid MB, Stokic DS, Koch SM, et al.: N-acetylcysteine inhibits muscle fatigue in humans. *J Clin Invest* 1994:94, 2468.
141. Deal CL, Moskowitz RW: Nutraceuticals as therapeutic agents in osteoarthritis. *Rheum Dis Clin North Am* 1999:25, 379.
142. Morreale P, Manopulo R, Galati M, et al.: Comparison of the anti-inflamatory efficacy of chondroitin sulfate and diclofenac sodium in patients with knee osteoarthritis. *J Rheumatol* 1996:23, 1385.
143. Leffler CT, Philippi AF, Leffler SG, et al.: Glucosamine, chondroitin, and manganese ascorbate for degenerative joint disease of the knee or low back: A randomized, double-blind, placebo-controlled pilot study. *Military Med* 1999:164, 85.
144. Berneis K, Keller U: Metabolic actions of growth hormone: Direct and indirect. *Baillieres Clin Endocrinol Metab* 1996:10, 337.
145. Casanueva FF, Dieguez C: Interaction between body composition, leptin and growth hormone status. *Baillieres Clin Endocrinol Metab* 1998:12, 297.
146. Scacchi M, Pincelli AI, Cavagnini F: Growth hormone in obesity. *Int J Obesity Rel Metab Disord* 1999:23(3), 260.
147. Dreimane D, Gllagher K, Nielsen K, et al.: Growth hormone exerts potent anabolic effects in an adolescent with human immunodeficiency virus wasting. *Pediatr Infect Dis J* 1999:18, 167.
148. Carrel AL, Myers SE, Whitman BY, et al.: Growth hormone improves body composition, fat utilization, physical strength and agility, and growth in Prader-Willi syndrome. *J Pediatr* 1999:134, 215.
149. Bisi G, Podio V, Valetto MR, et al.: Acute cardiovascular and hormonal effects of GH and hexarelin, a synthetic GH releasing peptide, in humans. *J Endocrinol Invest* 1999:22, 266.
150. Pritzalff CJ, Wideman L, Weltman JY, et al.: Impact of acute exercise intensity on pulsatile growth hormone release in men. *J Appl Physiol* 1999:87, 498.
151. Roemmich JN, Rogol AD: Session V: National cooperative growth study experience and reason: Anabolic effects of growth hormone. *Journal of Pediatrics* 1997:131, S75.
152. Eliakim A, Brasel JA, Mohan S, et al.: Physical fitness, endurance training, and growth hormone insulin like growth factor I system in adolescent females. *J Clin Endocrinol Metab* 1996:81, 3986.
153. Deuschle M, Blum WF, Frystyk J, et al.: Endurance training and its effect upon the activity of the GHIGFs system in the elderly. *Int J Sports Med* 1998:19, 250.
154. Taafe DR, Jin IH, Vu TH et al.: Lack of effect of recombinant human growth factor on muscle morphology and GH insulin like growth factor on expression in resistance trained elderly men. *J Clin Endocrinol Metab* 1996:81, 421.

Chapter 42

PHYSICAL AGENTS

Jeffrey R. Basford

INTRODUCTION

Running places unique demands on the musculoskeletal system. With these demands come health, satisfaction, and occasionally injury. This chapter reviews the role of physical agents in the treatment and rehabilitation of musculoskeletal injuries relevant to running.

The physical agents use physical forces to speed healing, avoid complications, and return an athlete to as full a level of function possible. These agents are not used in isolation: they can do much to improve recovery but are ineffective alone and are used as a complement to conventional medicine and surgery and a therapy program that typically includes exercise and education.

These agents can seem complex. Nevertheless, they are, at heart, quite simple. Moreover, they all rely on a restricted number of natural phenomena (e.g., heat, cold, and electromagnetic waves) to produce a limited number of effects: heating, cooling, analgesia, muscle movement, and tissue healing. This chapter examines these modalities with an emphasis on their clinical use and scientific basis. We begin with the superficial and deep heating agents, progress to cooling, and conclude with treatments that use electrical currents and electromagnetic forces to achieve effects directly. The emphasis is on established agents, but unconventional and poorly established treatments pertinent to runners and athletes will also be addressed.

HEAT AND COLD

Biophysics

Heat and cold have profound effects on the body; performance in a sport degrades rapidly with relatively small changes in core temperature. Elevation of a few more degrees centigrade may lead to heat exhaustion, heat stroke, and even death. Localized temperatures of 45°C may injure tissue and even denature protein.[1] Temperature decreases may also be important. Core temperatures below 28°C may be fatal,[1] and ambient temperatures lower than 13°C are uncomfortable. Small and localized temperature changes may also have important implications. A 3°C elevation in joint temperature increases collagenase activity significantly.[2] Changes of 13°C to 15°C in the finger joint may change joint viscosity by about 20%.[3] Nerve function is also temperature dependent; conduction velocities slow about 1 meter a second per degree of cooling, and changes in temperature of 5°C to 7°C produce clinically meaningful changes in blood flow, pain perception, sudomotor response, and collagen extensibility.[4–8]

Tissue is warmed by the addition of energy. The laws of physics restrict the ways that this can occur to three processes: conduction, convection, and conversion. Cooling, on the other hand, involves the removal of energy from tissue. As this cannot be done by conversion (i.e., cold, the absence of energy, cannot be

TABLE 42–1. THERAPEUTIC HEAT

General indications
    Pain
    Muscle spasm
    Contracture
    Tension myalgia
    Hematoma resolution
    Bursitis
    Tenosynoitis
    Fibromyalgia
    Superficial thrombophlebitis
    Vasodilation
    Acceleration of metabolic process
General contraindications and precautions
    Acute inflammation, trauma, or hemorrhage
    Bleeding dyscrasia
    Ischemia
    Insensitivity
    Atrophic skin
    Scar tissue
    Inability to communicate
    Poor thermal regulation (systemic applications)
    Malignancy
    Edema

radiated or converted to another form), cooling therapies are restricted to conductive and convective means.

The heating agents produce analgesia, increase soft-tissue extensibility, promote hyperemia, and reduce muscle tone. As a result, they share many of the same indications and contraindications (Table 42–1). The cooling agents are often used for their analgesic, metabolic, and perfusion-limiting effects. Thus these agents also share many common indications and contraindications (Table 42–2).

Superficial Heat

We review the common superficial heating agents below. Each has unique attributes, but all are limited by tissue tolerance to localized effects that may or may not be augmented by distal and local reflexes.

TABLE 42–2. THERAPEUTIC COLD

General indications
    Acute musculoskeletal trauma
    Pain
    Muscle spasm
    Spasticity
    Reduction of metabolic activity
General contraindications and precautions
    Ischemia
    Insensitivity
    Cold intolerance
    Raynaud's phenomenon and disease
    Severe cold pressor responses
    Cold allergy

Hot Packs

Hot packs maintain their place in the clinic due to their low cost, easy use, long life, and patient acceptance (Fig. 42–1). The most common type of pack consists of a canvas envelope filled with a hygroscopic silicon dioxide that absorbs many times its own weight of water.[2] Packs are typically rectangular and segmented but are available in various shapes and sizes to conform to specific parts of the body.

When not in use these packs are kept in thermostatically controlled water baths at 70°C to 80°C. During treatment, they are removed from the bath, and excess water is allowed to drip off. They are then placed in terry cloth insulating covers or wrapped in towels and placed on the patient for periods of 20 to 30 minutes.

Hot water can produce burns and scalds. However, except for the need to avoid direct exposure to hot water (i.e., by careful draining before use and placing the packs on, not under, the patient), they are safe agents and subject to the restrictions of Table 42–1. Alternative agents such as electric heating pads, circulating water heaters, and various moist heat home-heating products are available. Most of these are no more dangerous to use than hot packs, the one exception perhaps being pads that do not cool spontaneously or are particularly hot.

Heat Lamps

In theory hot packs and heat lamps should be equally effective superficial heating agents. In practice, however, hot packs (perhaps due to their "moistness") are far more popular. Nevertheless, infrared heat sources (as well as occasionally simply incandescent light bulbs) are used at times and deserve a few brief comments.

Heat lamps are simple to use but require some attention to avoid injuries or burn. Skin temperatures are controlled either by adjusting the power applied to the heating elements or by changing the separation between the heat source and the patient. In practice, therapeutic temperatures are usually obtained when the heat sources are about 50 cm from the skin. Nevertheless, differences exist. It is important to remember that the intensity of heating of point heat sources, such as incandescent bulbs, drops off in accordance with the inverse squared ($1/r^2$) law, whereas the heating effectiveness of linear sources, such as some quartz lamps, may follow a more slowly decreasing $1/r$ relationship.

SAFETY. The general precautions of Table 42–1 apply to all the superficial heating agents. In addition, these agents produce erythema (known as *erythema ab igne* and *erythema calor*), and chronic use may produce a permanent brownish skin discoloration.

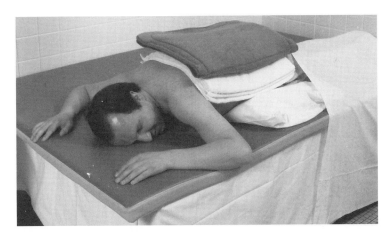

Figure 42–1. Low-back hot-pack therapy. Note that the pack is covered with an insulated wrapper and separated from the patient with several layers of toweling. *(Source: From Basford.[147])*

Hydrotherapy

Hydrotherapy uses a fluid medium to apply heat, cold, physical forces, or pharmaceutical agents to the body. The medium is usually water, but a variety of fluids or fluid-like materials may be used.

Temperature choice depends on the amount of the body immersed, treatment goals, medium motion (an agitated medium conducts heat to or from the body far more rapidly than a stationary one), and the patient's tolerance. Immersion of large portions of the body in water at "neutral temperatures" (33°C to 36°C) is usually well tolerated, and higher temperatures extending up to 43°C to 45°C are possible on restricted portions of the body. Systemic temperatures can be altered by hydrotherapy, and even for the healthy athlete, water temperatures are limited to about 39°C if a significant fraction of the body is immersed.

Regardless of its composition, the hydrotherapy medium may be stationary (with temperature changes occurring primarily by conduction) or in motion (with changes occurring by convection). Whirlpool baths, for example, use water as the medium to provide heat and agitation, whereas other, less common, agents may use fine particles suspended ("fluidized") in a turbulent air stream (Fluidotherapy[R]). Contrast, paraffin, and sitz baths, on the other hand, require no turbulence and utilize a stationary medium.

Hydrotherapy is an effective sports medicine modality, and this section discusses the more common approaches. As water is the most frequent medium, its properties are emphasized.

Whirlpool Baths and Hubbard Tanks

Baths and tanks range in size and construction from small portable units intended to treat a portion of a limb to fixed Hubbard tanks in which the entire body is immersed. Hydrotherapy is expensive in terms of labor and resources. As a result, therapists try to use the smallest tanks possible (Fig. 42–2).

WOUNDS AND BURNS. Although research has typically been done on surgical wounds or debilitated patients with decubitus ulcers, there is support for the idea that hydrotherapy may lessen the pain and speed the healing of open wounds in general.[9,10] Whirlpools and Hubbard tanks (and sometimes also water jets and showerheads) are often used for wounds and treatments when gentle mechanical debridment, heat, and solvent action are desired. Although truly aseptic treatment is not possible, a "sterile" tank should be filled with tap water, which is amazingly sterile; in combination with careful cleansing between treatments and the diluting effects of the water, disease transmission is unlikely.[11]

Treatment is surprisingly comfortable. Neutral to somewhat warmer temperatures are chosen, and, after the patient or body part is submerged, agitation is begun, to provide gentle debridement and aid in dressing removal. If wounds are large, or if there is significant exposure of internal tissue, sodium chloride may be added to the water to produce a 0.9% NaCl solution, which improves comfort and lessens the risks of hemolysis and electrolyte imbalance. Additional agents such as potassium permanganate and gentle detergents may also be used in some circumstances.

MUSCULOSKELETAL APPLICATIONS. Hydrotherapy is often used as an adjunct to joint mobilization after cast removal or prolonged mobilization. Sitz baths (a small warm water bath) are well established in the treatment of perineal and anal pain. It is interesting that their benefits, despite their simple nature, are well supported by research.[12] Hydrotherapy is widely used to treat musculoskeletal pain, "muscle spasms," and diffuse tension myalgia. These uses are well supported by clinical observations, but they have a surprisingly meager scientific basis.[13]

SAFETY. Hydrotherapy is a safe modality. Drowning is theoretically possible in the larger baths, and

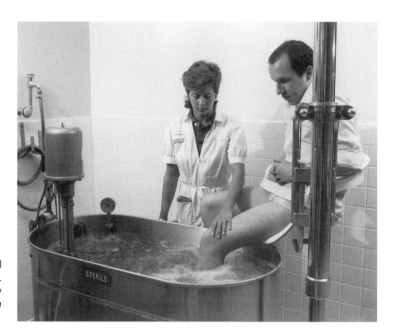

Figure 42–2. Lower-extremity whirlpool therapy. Many different pools are available. This pool uses a hydraulic chair to simplify entering and exiting the water. *(Source: From Basford.[147])*

temperatures must be monitored, with allowances made for the enhanced heat-exchanging abilities of agitated mediums. Disease transmission is a concern and does occur in public baths.[14,15] However, in clinical institutions where disinfecting procedures are followed and areas of stagnant water are avoided, infection appears to be rare. As an example, in a study in which the investigators specifically sought to isolate pathogenic bacteria (i.e., *Staphylococcus aureus*, *Pseudomonas aeruginosa*, and *Escherichia coli*) from hydrotherapy tanks, only 2 of 96 cultures were positive at locations that the investigators felt might lead to transmission.[11]

Contrast Baths

Contrast baths consist of two baths: a warm bath at about 43°C and a cool reservoir at about 16°C. Treatment begins by soaking the involved limb in the warm reservoir for about 10 minutes and then progressing to about four cycles of 1- to 4-minute cold and 4- to 6-minute warm soaks.[16] Patients may initially find the conventional temperatures of the hot and cold baths too extreme. In this case treatment can begin with the warm bath somewhat cooler and the cold bath somewhat warmer, with progression to the normal range as treatment progresses. These baths are not a common sports therapy modality but are useful in producing reflex hyperemia and desensitization in patients with complex regional pain syndrome I (CRPS I or RSD).

Water-Based Exercise

The benefits of the water environment for cross-training purposes are discussed in Chapter 45. Additional advantages of the reduced weightbearing aspects of water-based exercise also seem obvious for situations such as postoperative knee rehabilitation. Nevertheless, the intuitive benefits of this approach have been more difficult to establish than we might expect. For example, a comparison of postsurgical anterior cruciate rehabilitation programs found that a water-based program resulted in less pain but produced slower gains in knee strength than a land-based program.[17] Degenerative arthritis of the hip is not a common running injury, but it has also been suggested that the addition of twice-a-week pool exercises to a home hip osteoarthritis program did not improve outcome.[18]

Spa Therapy (Balneotherapy)

The potential effects on recovery from musculoskeletal injury of gases (e.g., CO_2, methane), elements (magnesium, cobalt, etc.), and substances such as hydrogen sulfide dissolved in water often intrigue athletes interested in alternative/complementary medicine.[19,20] Little research has addressed these issues for athletes, but some relevant information is available. First of all, we know that penetration of these solutes though intact skin is minimal and that in most cases measurable concentrations after a spa bath are found only in patients with impaired skin integrity.[21] Although patients with rheumatoid arthritis may benefit from treatment with mineral-rich hot packs,[22] information on athletes is limited. In addition, a comparison of the effects of spa therapy, underwater traction, and water jets on low-back pain found no specific benefits attributable to balneotherapy.[23] Thus, although a number of less rigorously controlled studies find benefits from balneotherapy for musculoskeletal back pain,[24,25] it is difficult to isolate spa therapy effects from those of hydrotherapy with "normal" water and a physical therapy program.

Fluidotherapy

As noted above, fine particles "fluidized" by turbulent, high-velocity hot air may also be used as a treatment medium. These treatments are frequently used in hand rehabilitation after injury and surgery. Despite widespread use (and undeniable comfort) the benefits of this high-temperature, low-heat–capacity approach remain poorly established.[26,27]

Hyperthermia

Runners are typically healthy people. However, not all runners are young and healthy, and even in younger athletes there are legitimate concerns about the sequela of systemic hyperthermia following immersion in a Hubbard tank or time in a sauna. Fortunately, research offers reassuring information for both the healthy and the impaired athlete.

CARDIAC DISEASE. There is no question that sauna baths and hot tubs elevate heart rates, increase sweating, raise body temperatures, and produce orthostatism. More specifically, 20 minutes in a hot bath at 40°C results in a 37.8°C core temperature and a pulse rate of 108 beats/min. Immersion at 41.5°C, on the other hand, raises core temperature to 38.3°C and heart rate to 123 beats/min.[28] Nevertheless, this degree of hyperthermia may not be contraindicated even for athletes with heart disease. For example, contrary to intuition, sauna bathing can reduce the symptoms of congestive heart failure.[29] In addition, 15 minutes in a 40°C hot tub results in electrocardiographic and blood pressure alterations similar to those that occur during stationary bicycle exercise in cardiac rehabilitation.[29] Epidemiology studies corroborate these findings. Finnish researchers found that sauna bathing after a myocardial infarction does not lead to increased cardiovascular risk.[30,31]

FERTILITY. Systemic hyperthermia does have some effects on the reproductive system. Single or repeated episodes of sauna bathing may lower sperm counts in men,[32] and neural tube defects may be more common in women who sauna bathe during the early portion of their pregnancies.[33]

Paraffin Baths

Paraffin baths are occasionally helpful in the treatment of scars and hand contractures following injury. Treatment temperatures (52°C to 54°C) are higher than those of water-based hydrotherapy (<40°C to 45°C) but are well tolerated due to the low heat capacity of the 7:1 paraffin-mineral oil mixture and a lack of convection.

TREATMENT. There are three approaches to paraffin treatment. The first of these, dipping, is the most frequent and involves repeatedly dipping the treated region in the paraffin with a pause between each dip to allow the wax to harden. After about 10 dips the paraffin-coated region is wrapped with a layer of plastic and placed in an insulating mitt.

Dipping initially increases skin temperatures by about 15°C. Cooling is rapid, however, and within 20 to 30 minutes skin temperature will return to within a few degrees of its predipped value. Temperature changes decrease with depth. A 15°C skin temperature elevation is mirrored by only a 3°C subcutaneous and a <1°C intramuscular temperature increase.[34]

Immersion is another common technique. With this method, the treated area is dipped once and then kept submerged for remainder of the session. Although this approach produces the same initial 15°C skin temperature elevation as dipping, temperatures decline more slowly. By the end of a session, skin temperatures may be still elevated by 8°C to 9°C and subcutaneous and intramuscular temperatures are about 5°C and 3°C higher than would occur from dipping.[34]

Paraffin is occasionally brushed onto the area of treatment. This approach is relatively rare, but it is used when circulation may be poor or on portions of the body that can not be dipped or immersed.[35]

SAFETY. Burns are the main safety concern with paraffin treatment. Bath temperatures should be monitored carefully with a thermometer. Visual inspection is also important: an open paraffin bath should have a thin film of white paraffin on its surface or an edging around the edges of the reservoir.

Diathermy

Ultrasound (US) and electromagnetic diathermy each heat deep tissue vigorously. US diathermy (USD) is the most widely used and is discussed in detail. Electromagnetic (EM) diathermy, on the other hand, is gradually losing favor: microwave diathermy (MWD) is no longer used in the physical therapy clinic. Short-wave diathermy (SWD), although less common than it once was, is still widely used and is reviewed here. It should be remembered that the popularity of agents tends to wax and wane. Thus, MWD, although now rare in physical therapy, still has a place in the treatment of prostatic cancer and hypertrophy as well as in potentiating the cytotoxic effects of chemotherapy and radiation.[36]

Ultrasound

USD uses sound waves to heat tissues. A wide range of frequencies are potentially useful, but in the United

States most machines operate between 0.8 and 1 MHz. US machines use piezoelectric transducers to convert electrical energy into sound. Output frequencies are relatively stable with time, but powers are more variable and may change with time or during a session by 20% or more.[37–39] US at frequencies as low as 30 and 45 kHz has potential benefits for superficial applications such as wound healing and ankle sprains.[40] However, these devices are still relatively rare and are not reviewed here in detail.

BIOPHYSICS. US is merely sound at frequencies above the 17-kHz limit of human hearing. As a result, it can be focused, bent (refracted), and reflected. The velocity of sound depends on the medium and the frequency. The velocity of sound in soft tissue in the 1-MHz range is about 1500 m/sec, and its wavelength (λ = velocity/frequency) is about 1.5 mm. As this wavelength is small relative to the several centimeters diameters of the applicators, US beams are very focused and limited in extent.

US is the most vigorous and deeply penetrating heating agent and can elevate the intramuscular temperatures of large muscles such as the gastrocsoleus by about 3.5°C to 4.0°C.[41] (The application of superficial heat before treatment may accelerate this process.) Penetration, however, is not uniform and depends markedly on tissue properties, frequency, and direction of travel. Tissue composition is remarkably important: a US beam that travels several centimeters in muscle and 7 to 8 cm in fat may penetrate less than 1 mm.[42,43] In addition, US penetration depth decreases by about 85% as frequency increases from 0.3 to 3.3 MHz.[42] Penetration also depends on direction: US may penetrate 7 cm in a direction parallel to a muscle's fibers, but less than half that perpendicular to them.[42] Tissue discontinuities are also important, as large amounts of energy are converted to heat at these sites: 5°C temperature increases are easily possible at a bony–soft-tissue interface.[43,44]

The ability of US to heat tissue by the conversion of sound energy into heat is its best understood capability. Nonthermal processes such as cavitation, shock waves, streaming, and mechanical deformation also occur and are briefly outlined due to their implications for safety and alternative treatments.

The first of these, cavitation, occurs when small gaseous bubbles are formed in the presence of a high-intensity US beam and either oscillate stably or grow rapidly in size and collapse.[45] This bubble oscillation and collapse can disrupt and damage tissue but can be easily avoided by restricting US intensities to those of common clinical use and keeping the soundhead in constant motion during treatment. US may also produce "streaming" movements in water-rich tissues and standing waves. Streaming may damage tissue or possibly speed healing. Standing waves can produce quite intense forces and, at least in the laboratory, can produce alternating bands of red blood cell aggregation in small vessels that resolve when treatment is stopped.[42,46,47]

Most US therapy relies on thermal effects. However, nonthermal mechanisms have potential benefits. The stimulatory effects of specific US regimens on bone healing are well known. What is less well known is that low-intensity US (15 to 400 mW/cm^2) may also stimulate cell proliferation, protein synthesis, and cytokine production.[48] Although these findings are limited to the laboratory, they furnish some support for the clinical interest in low-intensity US in wound healing.

TECHNIQUE. US treatment begins with cleaning the skin at the site of treatment and applying a coupling gel to the applicator to reduce skin-applicator interface heating. Commercial agents are usually used, but substances such as mineral oil are also effective.[49–51] The applicator head is placed in firm contact with the skin and moved in slow (a few centimeters a second) overlapping strokes for about 5 to 7 minutes. US therapy is labor intensive and is restricted to small areas of 50 to 100 cm^2.

US intensity is determined by the goal of treatment. Thermal treatments require the most energy: in these situations continuous-wave US is used at intensities between 0.5 and 2 W/cm^2 depending on tissue geometry and patient comfort. The effects of nonthermal treatment are less established. However, if the nonthermal aspects of US are to be emphasized, the US machine is either set at a low intensity or adjusted to deliver a low average power by delivering brief pulses of high-intensity US separated by longer pauses of no power.

"Indirect" US is an alternative, less-common, technique that is used to treat uneven surfaces such as the ankle, where it is difficult to maintain good applicator-skin contact. In this approach, the extremity to be treated is placed in a container of "degassed" tap water (tap water allowed to sit for several hours to allow dissolved gases to escape, thus avoiding the formation of energy-attenuating bubbles on the applicator head). The applicator is then moved, at a short separation, over the treatment area. Higher power intensities may be necessary than with direct contact treatment due to energy losses caused by the separation and poorer applicator-skin coupling.

INDICATIONS. US has been extensively studied. Even so, except in the case of contracture treatment, conclusive evidence of benefit is elusive. In fact, a recent systematic review of therapeutic US concluded that there was little overall evidence for effectiveness in musculoskeletal treatment.[52]

TENDINITIS AND BURSITIS.   Even though US is frequently used for tendinitis and bursitis, the research supporting this application is limited. Some does exist, however. For example, one controlled study of 50 patients treated with 1 MHz US at 1.2 to 1.8 W/cm^2 found that >85% had fair or better improvement in terms of pain and range of motion.[53] Although some studies suggest that US may be more effective than corticosteroids in the treatment of shoulder pain, its benefits may[54] or may not[55–59] be supported by other work.

MUSCLE PAIN AND OVERUSE.   US is frequently used in sports medicine to treat exercise-induced muscle pain and trauma (Fig. 42–3). Here again, conditions vary and representative studies are difficult to do. Controlled studies on delayed-onset muscle soreness following exercise offer limited support for an effect on the onset of pain or recovery of strength.[60–62] Thus, despite its widespread acceptance, US treatment of muscle pain may be more problematic than we would like.

CONTRACTURES.   Contractures occur after prolonged immobilization such as may occur after a fracture or a painful shoulder injury. Here the evidence supporting US use is stronger and probably reflects the ability of US to heat deeper joints such as the hip and the proven effects of heat on collagen extensibility. Technique is important, as collagen and tendon extensibility increase as temperatures increase and fall as they fall. As a result, heating should be vigorous and prolonged, and stretching should be maintained well into the cooling phase to allow the tissue a chance to "set" at its elongated length.[7]

US, in conjunction with stretching, is effective in increasing the range of motion of periarthritic shoulders and contracted hips.[44,63–65] Effects in healthy tissue appear more limited. For example, in healthy subjects US combined with stretching is more effective than stretching alone in increasing ankle dorsiflexion. Effects, however, are transient.[66]

US is frequently used to treat superficial contractures. Benefits here are arguable. Thus, although some feel that burns and finger contractures may be too superficial to benefit from US treatment,[67,68] some research shows that 4 minutes of 3-MHz, 1-W/cm^2 US increases temperatures of relatively superficial tissues by 4°C to 8°C.[69]

INFLAMMATION AND TRAUMA.   US is typically avoided in the acute stages of an injury due to concerns that it may aggravate bleeding, tissue damage, and swelling. The subacute situation may be different, as many feel that US may speed healing and the resolution of symptoms in the later stages of injury.

There is mixed evidence for this latter view. Delayed-onset muscle soreness may be a good example of subacute muscle injury: unfortunately, studies in healthy volunteers find that pulsed US of about 1 W/cm^2 has no effect on the onset of pain or recovery of strength.[61,62] Myofascial trigger points are markers for chronic musculoskeletal pain: studies in the neck and shoulder regions may not find clinically significant benefits. Ankle and heel pain may also be resistant to treatment.[70,71] On the other hand, there is some support for the idea in that injection indurations[72] and subacute hematomas[73] may improve more rapidly following US treatment. Despite widespread use, calcific shoulder tendinitis also seems to be resistant to 0.8-W/cm^2 US treatment in combination with acetic acid iontophoresis. Carpal tunnel syndrome is another chronic condition thought to be associated with inflammation and swelling, but clinical studies

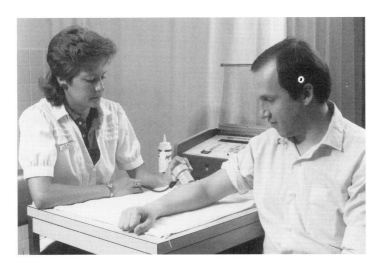

Figure 42–3. US treatment of the elbow. Note the use of a folded towel to provide comfortable support for the arm. *(Source: From Basford.[147])*

may[74] or may not[75] find treatment beneficial. US is used as a treatment for scars and keloids. Here there is evidence showing that 3 MHz of US produces significant superficial tissue temperature elevations,[69] but clinical support is limited, and one small study found treatment with 0.5 to 0.8 W/cm^2 US ineffective.[76] Postpartum perineal pain is more acute, and it is interesting that there is evidence both supporting[77] and against[78] US benefits in this situation. Thus, the evidence is mixed. In most cases, US comparisons have been done against placebo controls; the relative effectiveness of this agent over that of other conventional approaches is unknown.

Whether US can accelerate the healing of injured but otherwise healthy tissue is arguable, and convincing evidence in healthy individuals with an isolated injury, such as an ankle sprain, is limited. However, research in older and sicker populations may be relevant. Unfortunately, even here in relatively frequently studied conditions such as decubitus[79-82] and stasis ulcers,[83-86] results are inconclusive and limited by the variable research design and quality. An attempt at systemic analysis echoes this impression but suggests that US might be most effective when done at low intensities and around the margins of the wounds.[87] Subacute inflammation and swelling are also arguable US indications, as some feel that the heating and increased membrane-permeability effects of US preclude this approach, whereas others feel it is beneficial. Research involving humans (the jaw and perineum)[88,89] and rats[90] is not persuasive.

FRACTURES. Low-intensity US (e.g., 30 mW/cm^2) accelerates bone healing and is approved by the Food and Drug Administration (FDA) for the treatment of some fractures.[91] However, as electromagnetic stimulation is also effective and can be incorporated into the patient's cast, it is unclear how useful a labor-intensive approach like US will be.

PHONOPHORESIS. US may be used to deliver medication into tissues. In this case the active substance is mixed into the coupling medium, and US is used to "drive" (phonophores) the material through the skin. In concept, the idea is intriguing, and phonophoresis with corticosteroids is frequently used in sports medicine. However, quantitative research is limited, and penetration into deeper tissues is arguable. Some things are known, however. Although some studies find increased concentrations of substances such as lidocaine and hydrocortisone at depths of several centimeters after treatment, our own research as well as that of others finds penetration depth limited.[92-94]

Clinical studies are equally conflicting. Thus, a study that compared US phonophoresis of 0.05% fluocinonide with US alone at the same 1.5-W/cm^2 intensity found both treatments beneficial but indistinguishable in their effects on a variety of superficial musculoskeletal conditions.[95] Another study did not find lidocaine and corticosteroid phonophoresis more effective than the same treatment with an inert coupling agent.[96] Other studies, however, find phonophoresis with substances such as carbocaine, phenylbutazone, and chymotrypsin beneficial.[97,98]

PRECAUTIONS AND CONTRAINDICATIONS. US can produce intense heating, and the precautions of Table 42–1 are particularly important. In addition, shock waves, cavitation, beam hot spots, and other mechanical tissue effects are possible. These dangers of these effects range from theoretical to real, but all can be avoided using clinically appropriate intensities and constantly moving the applicator. Fluid-filled areas such as the eyes and pregnant uterus should not be treated. Growth plates, immature or inflamed joints,[99-101] and acute hemorrhages are avoided, as are ischemic tissue, tumors, laminectomy sites, infections, and implanted devices such as pacemakers and pumps. Many do not use US near metal plates or cemented artificial joints, as the effects of localized heating[102-104] or mechanical forces on prosthetic-cement interfaces is not well known.

Electromagnetic Diathermy

EM diathermy uses EM energy to interact with tissue. Both thermal and nonthermal effects are possible. Tissue warming is produced by two processes. One is resistive heating, which occurs when electrical eddy currents induced by EM waves pass through the body. The other is produced by the degradation of molecular oscillatory motions that EM waves induce when they interact with tissue. Nonthermal effects, which are complex and variable, are less-well understood and are discussed in the appropriate sections below.

SWD is the dominant EM diathermy sports medicine. As a result our discussion focuses on short-wave devices, most of which operate at 27.12 MHz. Frequencies of 13.56 and 40.68 MHz are also approved for use by the U.S. Federal Communications Commission.

BIOPHYSICS. An SWD machine is essentially a signal generator that uses either inductive or capacitive electrodes to deliver energy to the body (Fig. 42–4). Inductive electrodes act as an antenna, and the body absorbs energy from an EM field produced by the short-wave machine. With capacitive electrodes, on the

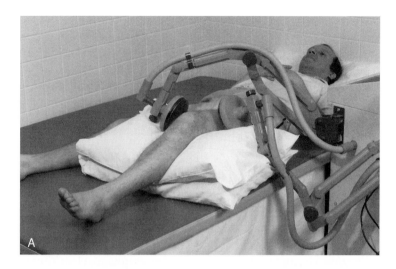

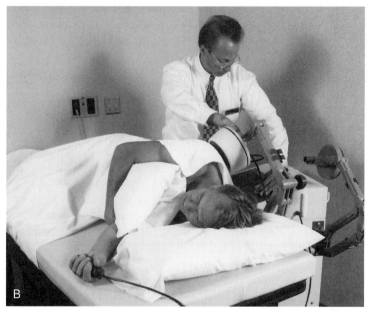

Figure 42–4. (*A*) Short-wave diathermy treatment with a capacitive plate applicator. Careful positioning is necessary. (*B*) SWD with an inductive applicator. The patient should wear no jewelry and lie on a non-conductive table. Note the emergency cutoff switch in the patient's hand. *(Source: From Basford.[147])*

other hand, the portion of the body being treated is placed in series between the electrodes and serves as the dielectric (resistance) between two plates of a capacitor.

The differences between these applicators are not merely academic. Inductive applicators induce currents that preferentially flow in water-rich tissues such as muscle that are highly conductive. Capacitive applicators, on the other hand, heat poorly conductive substances such as fat the most.[105] Significant heating is possible. For example, SWD can increase subcutaneous fat temperatures by 15°C and intramuscular temperatures at depths of 4 to 5 cm by 4°C to 6°C.[106,107]

As is true for US, nonthermal effects exist and can be emphasized by using low-output powers or a pulsing field. Nonthermal phenomena such as "pearl chains" have been known since the 1950s, and the ben-

efits of low-intensity EM fields on fracture healing are well known.[108] Nevertheless, it remains difficult to generalize this approach to musculoskeletal therapy.

TECHNIQUE. There are two common inductive applicators. Pad applicators are moderately flexible mats that contain a coil. They may have dimensions of 0.5 × 0.75 meters and are used to treat large areas such as the low back. Drum applicators consist of fixed coils connected by hinges. These devices are smaller and permit treatment to more limited areas such as the knee and shoulder. Capacitive electrodes are also typically used over limited areas such as the shoulder and knee.

INDICATIONS. EM diathermies are used to produce heating in tissues that are either too deep or too extensive to be treated by other modalities. Subacute musculoskeletal dysfunction involving the low back, the knee, and the shoulder are particularly common today, whereas in the past pelvic diathermy with vaginal and rectal electrodes was common.

Some might consider using the diathermies for more acute conditions. However, at least for the higher-power applications, these indications seem limited since damage might be augmented. This concern is particularly true for joints, due to the increase in enzyme activity that occurs with temperatures. However, temperatures >42°C may denature these enzymes, and patients may find treatment improves comfort.[100,101] Overall, the risk seems high, and most practitioners do not heat acute injuries aggressively.

PRECAUTIONS AND CONTRAINDICATIONS. EM diathermy is primarily a heating modality and the contraindications of Table 42–1 should be noted. In addition, conductive materials may result in localized heating. As a result, jewelry is removed, treatment is performed on nonconductive tables, and towels are used to absorb moisture and perspiration. Metal implants or electrical devices (e.g., joints, pacemakers, pumps, and metallic intrauterine devices), contact lenses, and the menstruating or pregnant uterus are contraindications. The risk of localized heating by metallic surgical clips in an EM field is unclear, but 3°C to 4°C temperature elevations are possible during diathermy at 90 MHz.[36] Although the risk may be small, the effects of EM diathermy on the immature skeleton are not well established.[109,110]

EM field leakage varies depending on the applicators involved and the intensity of the field. However, field intensities drop rapidly and are usually <10 mW/cm² 0.5 m from the treatment site.[105,111] American National Standards Institute (ANSI) guidelines for SWD at 27.12 MHz are about 1 mW/cm² on a time-averaged basis.[105,112,113] As therapists work only intermittently with these agents, their exposures seem to be minimal.[114–116]

Low-Power and Pulsed EMF

The nonthermal benefits of EM field waves are highly debatable. Nevertheless, many people want to harness their effects either in isolation or to augment tissue warming during musculoskeletal treatments. Pulsing offers an opportunity to do this, since with this approach, heating capability can be preserved by alternating pulses of high-intensity SWD with periods of no power.

Nonthermal effects can be obtained and tissue heating avoided altogether by using low-power fields delivered in either continuous or pulsed modes. These lower-intensity fields can be optimized to emphasize either electric or magnetic field characteristics and are often chosen in musculoskeletal dysfunction and wound-healing situations. Research offers little to support the specificity or certainty of benefits. For example, one wound-healing study found no difference in effects of pulsed electric or magnetic fields at either 20 or 110 Hz in small groups of patients with trochanteric or sacral pressure sores.[117]

Cryotherapy

Chilling has potent physiologic effects. Superficial cold produces analgesia[6]; reduces metabolic activity; slows and may block nerve conduction[4]; decreases muscle tone and spasticity[118–120]; and increases gastrointestinal motility.[121] Ice is the most common cryotherapy agent, and its effects are emphasized in this section.

Skin temperatures initially fall rapidly following the application of ice and then decrease more slowly toward an equilibrium value of 12°C to 13°C 10 minutes later. Subcutaneous and intramuscular temperatures follow a less marked but similar pattern: temperatures just under the skin decrease by 3°C to 5°C and intramuscular temperatures by a degree or less over the same period.[122] Longer periods of cooling have a more pronounced effect. For example, ice cooling for 20 to 180 minutes can lower relatively superficial intramuscular temperatures by 6 to 16°C.[4,99,118,123] Other tissues behave similarly: knee intraarticular temperatures decrease by 6°C after being packed in ice for 3 hours, and its bone and soft tissue blood flow decrease by 20% and 30%, respectively, after 25 minutes.[123]

TECHNIQUE. Ice packs, compression wraps, and slushes cool tissue rapidly. Sessions typically last 20 to 30 minutes before additional treatment is begun. If ice packs are used, a towel is usually placed around them, and the skin may be coated with mineral oil.

Ice massage is a very vigorous approach suitable for limited portions of the body. Treatment is simple and consists of rubbing a piece of ice (e.g., water frozen in a small cup) over the painful area for 7 to 10 minutes. Most patients find treatment effective and report a sequence of cold, burning, and aching that persists until analgesia is reached.

Iced whirlpools cool large areas vigorously. Although a motivated athlete may accept this approach, many people find temperatures below 13°C uncomfortable and tolerate sessions poorly. Neoprene boots or gloves may increase tolerance if it is not necessary to expose the feet or hands to the cold.

Other cooling agents have a place in sports medicine. One, for example, circulates chilled water through compression sleeves to deliver both pressure

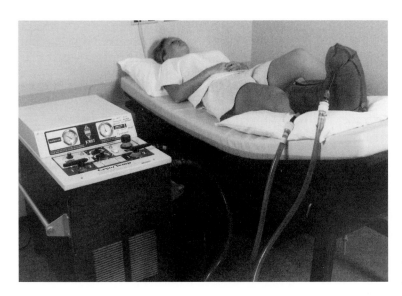

Figure 42–5. Cryotherapy. This machine circulates chilled water through an inflated cuff to apply pressure and cooling to an ankle injury. (*Source: From Basford.[147]*)

and cold analgesia (Fig. 42–5). This device has obvious benefits, but whether it is more effective than less complex treatment with Ace wraps and an ice pack is unclear. Vapocoolant and liquid nitrogen sprays produce large (as much as 20°C), rapid drops in skin temperature and are used at times to produce superficial analgesia as well as in "spray and stretch" treatments.[123,124]

Chemical ice packs are also common. These packs have the benefit of convenience but tend to be expensive and may not cool particularly well. It is useful to remember that plastic bags of frozen vegetables such as peas conform well to the body (after being hit on a flat surface) and that 12-oz cans of frozen orange juice, when wrapped in a towel, remain cold for extraordinary lengths of time.

TRAUMA. Research tends to support the central role of ice in the treatment of acute musculoskeletal injury. Although some argument exists, cooling has a long list of apparent benefits.[125–127] In particular, cooling applied soon after trauma may decrease edema, lessen metabolic activity, reduce blood flow, lower compartmental pressures, diminish tissue damage, and accelerate healing.[128–133]

In any event, rest, ice, compression, and elevation (RICE) are the mainstay of treatment. A variety of approaches are recommended, but most involve variations of immediate compression, elevation, and cyclic ice application (e.g., 20 minutes on, 10 minutes off, or 30 minutes on, 2 hours off) for 6 to 24 hours.[6,134–136] Acute sprains and fractures are often splinted or placed in padded Robert Jones dressings. While splints and cushioning slow the rate of tissue cooling (progressively moreso as one goes from plaster to synthetic casts and then to compressive wraps), therapeutic

temperatures are obtainable with all but the bulky Robert Jones dressings.[137]

Opinions begin to diverge 24 to 48 hours following an injury. Emphasis is on mobilization and strengthening as rapidly as possible in view of injury severity. Some, however, use ice for prolonged periods, whereas others switch to warming agents. Taste, experience, and patient motivation all play a role in the ultimate treatment plan.

CHRONIC PAIN. Although most patients with chronic musculoskeletal pain seem to prefer heating agents, cryotherapy may also have a role. For example, ice massage may be as effective as transcutaneous electrical nerve stimulation (TENS) for those with chronic low-back pain,[138] and ice massage or hot packs appear to be equally effective as an adjunct to exercise in patients hospitalized with low-back pain.[139]

PRECAUTIONS AND CONTRAINDICATIONS. The precautions of Table 42–2 apply. Nevertheless, healthy, well-perfused tissue tolerates 20- to 30-minute ice therapy sessions without difficulty.[118,134] Cooling is more dangerous when sensation is compromised, circulation is impaired, or tissues are compressed.[140] Rare but possible problems include pressor responses aggravating cardiovascular disease, Raynaud's phenomenon, cold hypersensitivity, urticaria, and cold allergy/cryoprecipitation.

ELECTROTHERAPY

The ability of electric eels, rays, and catfish to produce analgesia has been known for thousands of years.[141]

However, the role of electricity in this process did not begin to be understood until an amazing burst of knowledge in the 18th and 19th centuries resulted in the invention of the electrostatic generator; the work of Ampere, Faraday, and Ohm; and, ultimately, Maxwell's electromagnetic field equations.

The general population was entranced as well. Tricks such as the "electrostatic boy" were popular, in which a young boy was suspended by ropes and electrically charged with a generator; the public was then allowed to draw sparks from him and watch bits of paper be attracted. Road shows, quacks, and charlatans proliferated and contributed to an enthusiastic reception of electrostatic baths and galvanically induced limb movement.[141,142] Unfortunately, benefits did not meet expectations, and therapeutic electricity fell into a disrepute that persists today.

Today, high-intensity electrical stimulation is used to strengthen muscles and to move paralyzed limbs. Less-intense stimulation produces analgesia and delivers medications percutaneously. Stimulation at still lower intensities has gained FDA approval for fracture healing. Soft-tissue wounds, osteoporosis, and musculoskeletal pain represent additional potentially important, but still investigational, applications. This section discusses these agents.

Electrical Analgesia

Electrical analgesia is thought to produce its effects by one of two mechanisms. The first of these, the gate theory, postulates that cells in the spinal cord substantia gelatinosa inhibit the passage of nociceptive information to the brain if nonpainful sensory afferent signals are present.[143] The second, the opioid hypothesis, is based on the concept that the production of analgesia at stimulation intensities higher (e.g., moderately uncomfortable) than those involved in the gate theory can reduce pain by stimulating central nervous system opioid production. TENS, percutaneous electrical nerve stimulation (PENS), and H-wave therapy (HWT) are all used.[144,145] This chapter emphasizes TENS, as PENS requires percutaneous needle placement, HWT is relatively rare, and surgically implanted units are not germane to sports medicine.

TENS

It is difficult to design adequate controlled studies of electrical analgesia. Nevertheless, it is clear that TENS stimulation produces localized analgesia, and research suggests that stimulation at 110 Hz (as well as HWT at 2 and 60 Hz) results in a hypoalgesia that persists for up to 5 minutes after stimulation is stopped.[145] Research finds that dorsal horn cell activity is reduced following stimulation.[146] As noted above, conventional ("high-frequency") TENS (barely or not perceptible, 10 to 100+ Hz) may work more according to the gate theory than higher intensity ("low-frequency") (1 to 4 Hz) stimulation, which may be more dependent on endorphins.

TENS units are typically about the size of a large pager and consist of a rechargeable battery, an adjustable signal generator, and usually two sets of electrodes. Units generate a variety of stimuli, with currents of ≤100 mA, pulse rates between 1 and 200 Hz, and pulse widths ranging from 10 to a few hundred microseconds. A variety of ramping, burst-mode, and wave-train modulation options are available to improve comfort and effectiveness, but their utility has not been established. Asymmetric, biphasic waveforms are favored as they seem to be more comfortable and seem to reduce the possibility of electrolytic and iontophoretic effects.

Electrodes are usually placed over the painful region, but other locations are common. Alternative placements (in roughly decreasing order of use) include spinal nerve origins, afferent nerves, acupuncture and trigger points, sites contralateral to the pain, and auricular locations.

Parameter choice is somewhat standardized, but still personalized. Many begin a TENS evaluation with a conventional setting (barely perceptible stimulus; 40 to 100 Hz; <100 μs duration pulse). If benefits are limited, a higher intensity trial (uncomfortable stimulus; 1 to 4 Hz, >100 μs pulse duration) will be evaluated. A number of sessions may be necessary to establish effectiveness. As TENS units are expensive (often as much as $800) and annoying to put on and as benefits often wane with time, purchase is not warranted unless its improvements persist for several months.

INDICATIONS. Research dating from the 1970s and extending up to the present often finds that TENS use reduces pain in a variety of situations. For example, treatment lessens the severity of dysmenorrhea, reduces postoperative and first-stage labor pain and narcotic use by as much as two-thirds, shortens intensive care needs, and improves mobility.[147–150] Unfortunately, evaluation is difficult due to the subjective nature of pain, differences in parameter choice, and outcome measures. In addition, success seems to drop off with the length of follow-up, and study quality ranges from well-designed randomized controlled trials to uncontrolled retrospective series.

Musculoskeletal low-back pain provides a good example of this uncertainty. In four studies of TENS, one found it no more effective than manipulation, corsets, and massage[151]; two found it no more effective than exercise[152,153]; and a fourth found (high-intensity) TENS more effective than a control treatment.[154] Studies of knee osteoarthritis and temporomandibular joint pain have found TENS beneficial but no more effective than nonsteroidal medication or mouth splints.[152,155,156]

Benefits of chronic use are also difficult to establish. Some patients will find TENS helpful in suppressing pain for prolonged periods, but overall use decreases with time and of those who buy a unit less than a third may be using it 3 years later.[157–159]

Although TENS appears to have physiologic effects in addition to analgesia, support for the clinical benefit of such effects is limited. Vasodilation provides an interesting example. Here, although clinical proof of benefits is limited, stimulation may increase cutaneous perfusion and distal skin temperatures in patients with scleroderma and diabetic neuropathy.[160,161] Spasticity is another refractory problem that may benefit from stimulation. Unfortunately, research may[162] or may not[163] find benefits. There is no evidence it has any musculoskeletal curative effects.

In summary, TENS seems to be helpful in a limited number of patients. Acute conditions may be more susceptible to treatment than more chronic ones, and psychogenic pain seems particularly resistant.[159] A rough rule of thumb may be that about a third of patients will find significant benefit from TENS during an initial trial of a few sessions. Of this group roughly a third will find that benefits persist (or that continued treatment is necessary) after a month. Thus at the end of a month, only about one ninth of patients evaluated with TENS may be still using it regularly. However, a significant proportion of these may continue to use it, despite its inconvenience, for prolonged periods.

PRECAUTIONS AND CONTRAINDICATIONS. TENS is a relatively safe modality, and safety issues are mostly minor. Skin irritation and contact dermatitis can occur and usually respond to changes in electrode placement or composition. Pain may be caused by too high a current density as the result of an inadvertently high stimulating current or an incompletely adherent electrode, but this is easily corrected. Cardiac pacemakers may be relatively resistant to TENS signals, but there is at least one report that an intracardiac defibrillator was triggered by a TENS unit.[164] Caution suggests that patients with pacemakers, electrical implants, and dysrhythmias avoid TENS[148,165] and that areas near the carotid sinus, the epiglottis, and the pregnant uterus should not be treated. These precautions are probably too restrictive, but as TENS is not curative, and results are often problematic, it seems wise to err on the side of caution.

Muscle Stimulation

Electrical currents have been used for almost 40 years to improve or maintain muscle strength and function. The first, at least the first well-known report, appeared in 1961 when Liberson et al.[166] showed that electrical stimulation could help compensate for tibialis anterior weakness and improve the gait in patients with hemiparesis. Over the years investigators have extended and improved the applications of electrical stimulation to both healthy and impaired muscle.

The use of electrical stimulation to restore function (FES), rather than improve the strength of muscle, is the most developed of these applications. Electrical stimulation is most refined for patients with spinal cord injury: it is used to improve upper as well as lower extremity function and has been shown to reduce spasticity and edema and facilitate cardiovascular exercise. In particular, FES, in conjunction with bracing, can improve functional activities such as walking and transfers,[167] strengthen paretic muscle, increase lean body mass,[168] improve cardiovascular fitness, and perhaps enhance proprioception and muscle reeducation.[169] Practicality is limited, however. The FES apparatus is difficult to don, stimulates a limited number of muscles, may require surgically placed electrodes, and often necessitates concomitant bracing. FES may be suitable to less-extensive applications also. For example, a palatal appliance delivering 3 mA to the soft palate can reduce snoring and might be a potential treatment for sleep apnea.[170]

MUSCLE STRENGTHENING. Electrical stimulation can retard the atrophy of injured or immobilized muscle.[168] Unfortunately, although the concept of improved athletic performance as the result of electrically based strengthening is enticing, there are physiologic limitations to this approach. In particular, although electrical stimulation does induce muscle contractions, the contractions are limited in power by comfort and a limited region of recruitment. In addition, electrically stimulated contractions do not mimic normal recruitment patterns, and rapid muscle fatigue limits functional benefits.[171]

In summary, electrical muscle stimulation is more effective in maintaining muscle mass after an injury than it is in reversing atrophy once it is established.[172] Whether it will have a useful role in the strengthening of healthy muscle (much less muscle involved in highly coordinated activity) remains to be established.

Iontophoresis

Electric fields exert forces on charged particles that are proportional to their charge (i.e., $F = qE$). Iontophoresis takes advantage of this fact and uses electrical fields to force charged or polarized substances into tissue. Basic rules of physics apply to this process. The force on a substance and hence the speed that it moves into the skin is dependent on its charge-to-mass ratio and the applied voltage. The quantity of material driven into the tissue, on the other hand, is a function of the current. Skin resistance is also important, and permeability is increased if superficial wounds, abrasions, rashes, and sweat glands are present.[173–175]

Iontophoretic devices consist basically of a direct-current (possibly pulsed) power source and two electrodes. A dilute solution of the active substance (which must exist in an ionized or polar form) is placed under the electrode of the same polarity, and the device is turned on. The currents involved vary with the situation but are adjusted so that they produce current intensities at the active electrode that are <0.5 mA/cm^2.

Medication is not always required as the electric current alone may have therapeutic benefits. Thus, iontophoresis with tap water alone can inhibit hyperhydrosis for prolonged periods[176] and increase skin blood flow under the cathode by more than 800%.[177] The mechanism for these actions may be the concentration of current flow in low-resistance sweat ducts.

WOUND HEALING. Many studies find that iontophoresis increases the concentration of antibiotics such as gentamicin, penicillin, and (some) cephalosporins in poorly vascularized tissue such as burns and cartilage.[178–180] The utility of these findings for healthy wounds is doubtful. However, it is interesting that other studies support such findings for poorly perfused tissue. For example, iontophoresis three times a week with vasoactive intestinal protein and calcitonin gene-related peptide produced a healing rate in patients with venous stasis ulcers 30% greater than that in a control group.[181] Less-rigorous studies found that iontophoresis with iodine or zinc may reduce scar tissue formation and accelerate the healing of ischemic ulcers.[182,183]

It has been known for more than a century that iontophoresis is effective in reducing pain from localized superficial trauma such as injections and minor surgery.[177] Nevertheless, despite generalization to materials other than analgesics and rather widespread use, including use in tendinitis, bursitis, and sprains, research support is limited. Nonsteroidal anti-inflammatory iontophoresis of lateral epicondylitis may be helpful.[178] However, acetic acid iontophoresis combined with US for calcific tendinitis does not appear to be beneficial, and corticosteroid iontophoresis has limited support from randomized clinical trails.[184] Direct comparison of iontophoresis with oral medication, transdermal patches, or alternative physical therapy approaches is rare.

SAFETY. With reasonable care and safe equipment, iontophoresis should be safe. Allergies to the materials (pads, electrodes, medication) used are always possible, and the passage of electrical current into the skin can cause erythema, rashes, and, if the current intensity is high, pain.[177]

Low-Intensity Electric and Electromagnetic Fields

WOUND HEALING. The use of electrical stimulation to heal wounds has a long history. Systematic investigation began 30 to more than 40 years ago with reports that low-intensity direct current (LIDC) promoted the healing of ischemic wounds.[185–189] LIDC, however, did not gain general use, perhaps because the studies were poorly controlled and emphasized arcane rules for electrode polarity choice.

Despite the lack of success of LIDC, it is important to remember that electricity and wound healing are physiologically intertwined. For example, bony and soft-tissue trauma results in small (1 V/m) electric fields that may gain their effects through changes in cell-wall permeability that alter a variety of cellular functions such as growth, proliferation, movement, and orientation.[190,191] High-intensity fields also have effects that may influence healing, and fields $>10^5$ V/m can increase cell-wall permeability, perhaps due to electroporation.[192,193]

Interest in electrically stimulated soft-tissue healing continues and has benefited from improvements in electronics. Low-frequency microcurrent (e.g., 10 to 200 Hz, <10 mA/cm^2) electric currents and fields designed to accelerate wound healing by neutralizing injury currents or reducing free radical concentrations have gained some currency.[194] Success remains elusive, but there is some support for these approaches. For example, tap water iontophoresis increases perfusion in healthy tissue,[177] and TENS may improve healing and elevate the skin temperatures of people with neuropathies or scleroderma.[195,196] Unfortunately, study size tends to be small, design and blinding arguable, and comparison with alternative treatment minimal. Acceptance of electrical and EM field stimulation as a mainstream treatment option depends on clearer evidence of effectiveness.

Interferential and Kilohertz Frequency Currents

Skin impedance falls as frequency increases. As a result, stimuli that are painful at the low <70-Hz frequencies of TENS and many muscle simulators are well tolerated at a few thousand hertz. There are at least two ways to take advantage of this fact. One of these arranges two sets of electrodes so that two sine waves in the low-kilohertz range differing by 20 to

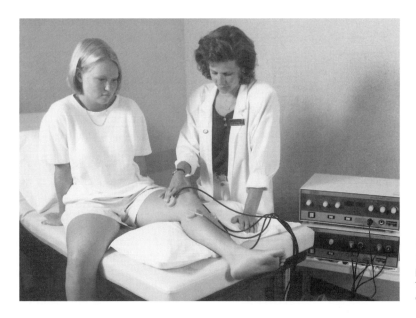

Figure 42–6. Interferential current treatment. This approach uses the interference pattern of two higher-frequency sine waves to apply electrical stimulation at physiological frequencies. *(Source: From Basford.[147])*

100 Hz cross. The waves thus interfere with each other and produce beneath the skin barrier a "difference" frequency comparable to that of TENS units and muscle stimulators (Fig. 42–6). Another approach that permits painless penetration of the skin consists of pulsing high-frequency carrier waves at frequencies comparable to those of TENS and muscle stimulators. These devices have theoretical advantages for many situations in which analgesia or muscle stimulation is desired. The extent of their clinical advantages remains to be fully determined.

Safety

There are two issues of concern. The electrical devices used in these applications operate at low powers, and the safety issues are similar to those outlined above in conjunction with TENS. The second issue is that of the safety of low-intensity EM fields. Again, risk seems minimal. Thus, although early epidemiologic studies suggested an association between low-intensity EM fields and increased rates of cancer, more recent, and better designed, studies tend to echo the findings of a 1996 National Research Council review panel concluding that there is "no conclusive and consistent evidence" that EM field exposure causes a significant increase in the risk of cancer, neurobehavioral, or reproductive dysfunction.[197,198]

Complementary and Alternative Therapies

Athletes as well as the general population are intrigued by the potentials of complementary and alternative medicine. A wide variety of these approaches are pertinent to sports medicine. We have dealt with a number of them already in our discussion of electrotherapeutic and EM devices. There are many other possible approaches with potential benefits, a few of which are discussed below.

Static Magnetic Fields

Magnetic discs, pads, bandages, and blankets are promoted in sports, veterinary, and general circulation magazines as a cure for a variety of musculoskeletal injuries. Unfortunately, although an occasional study finds treatment beneficial (Vallbona), support from well-controlled clinical trials is limited, and the mechanism of action remains obscure. We do know that there are limitations on potential mechanisms, however. For example, the mechanism cannot be based on either magnetically induced currents or direct blockage of nerve transmission: a static magnetic field cannot induce a current, and the 24-T fields required to produce a 10% reduction in nerve conductivity are orders of magnitude larger than those produced by these devices.[199] Other possibilities such as electronic spin state alterations,[200,201] changes in the physical state of water,[202] and Hall effect charge separation do not seem plausible under reasonable physiologic conditions.[203,204] Further research and clinical experience will help to identify possible mechanisms and indications for magnet therapy.

Low-Intensity Laser Therapy

Low-power lasers are widely used to treat musculoskeletal injuries, speed healing, and lessen pain. Over the years a variety of devices have been used, but now most treatments involve 30 to 100+ mW devices, wavelengths between 630 and 1000 μm (i.e., visible red to infrared), and treatments of 1 to 4 J/cm^2. Laboratory studies offer some support for the approach: radiation stimulates cellular function and collagen production and may improve the recovery of damaged nerve tissue. Unfortunately, demonstration of clinical benefits has been difficult, and these devices have yet to gain FDA approval for clinical use.[205]

Shock-Wave Therapy

Many therapeutic approaches such as injections and cross-fiber massage can be viewed as controlled applications of forces designed to stimulate healing or break up scars. Lithotripsy was developed initially for renal stone treatments but is now being generalized to other areas such as the gallbladder. Attempts to extend this approach to musculoskeletal conditions such as calcific tendinitis of the shoulder, lateral epicondylitis, and plantar fasciitis are intriguing, but benefits are still in the investigational stage.[206–208]

Vibration

Vibration is a potential analgesic agent that is already in use for neuromuscular rehabilitation to facilitate muscle function. An assortment of vibrators is used, but many feel that amplitude and frequency choices of 1.5 mm and 150 Hz may be particularly effective.[209–211] Research is intriguing, but limited. Vibration may be as effective as TENS or aspirin for musculoskeletal pain,[212,213] and studies in mice suggest that it may lessen edema and improve lymphatic and venous repair.[214]

CONCLUSIONS

Most of what we know about the physical agents is based on poorly controlled or conflicting clinical trials, extrapolations from basic science, habit, and prejudice. Treatment is thus far more subjective than we would like to admit. However, there are some general rules. For example, cooling is emphasized for acute musculoskeletal injuries. Heat and hydrotherapy tend to be used for larger areas, whereas more vigorous agents such as ice massage and US are restricted to smaller sites. SWD is losing currency, but new modalities such as lasers and low-intensity EM fields are intriguing but remain unproved. In the end, it is essential to remember that physical agents are not used alone: a well-designed treatment plan involves consideration of the place a physical agent should have in a program that may include exercise, massage, and education.

REFERENCES

1. Franchimont P, Juchmes J, Lecomte J: Hydrotherapy—mechanisms and indications. *Pharmacol Ther* 1983:20, 79.
2. Harris ED Jr, McCroskery PA: The influence of temperature and fibril stability on degradation of cartilage collagen by rheumatoid synovial collagenase. *N Engl J Med* 1974:290, 1.
3. Wright V: Quantitative and qualitative analysis of joint stiffness in normal subjects and in patients with connective tissue diseases. *Ann Rheum Dis* 1961:20, 36.
4. Denys EH: AAEM minimonograph :14: The influence of temperature in clinical neurophysiology. *Muscle Nerve* 1991:14, 795.
5. Guyton A: *Textbook of Medical Physiology,* 7th ed., Philadelphia, WB Saunders, 1986:336.
6. Knight K: *Cryotherapy: Theory, Technique and Physiology,* 1st ed., Chattanooga, TN, Chattanooga Corporation, 1985:83.
7. Lehmann JF, Masock AJ, Warren CG, et al.: Effect of therapeutic temperatures on tendon extensibility. *Arch Phys Med Rehabil* 1970:51, 481.
8. On AY, Colakoglu Z, Hepguler S, et al.: Local heat effect on sympathetic skin responses after pain of electrical stimulus. *Arch Phys Med Rehabil* 1997:78, 1196.
9. Burke DT, Ho CH, Saucier MA, et al.: Effects of hydrotherapy on pressure ulcer healing. *Am J Phys Med Rehabil* 1998:77, 394.
10. Juve Meeker B: Whirlpool therapy on postoperative pain and surgical wound healing: An exploration. *Patient Educ Counseling* 1998:33, 39.
11. Stanwood W, Pinzur MS: Risk of contamination of the wound in a hydrotherapeutic tank. *Foot Ankle Int* 1998:19, 173.
12. Jiang JK, Chiu JH, Lin JK: Local thermal stimulation relaxes hypertonic anal sphincter: Evidence of somatoanal reflex. *Dis Colon Rectum* 1999:42, 1152.
13. Sjogren T, Long N, Storay I, et al.: Group hydrotherapy versus group land-based treatment for chronic low back pain. *Physiother Res Int* 1997:2, 212.
14. Luttichau HR, Vinther C, Uldum SA, et al.: An outbreak of Pontiac fever among children following use of a whirlpool. *Clin Infect Dis* 1998:26, 1374.
15. Kuroki T, Sata S, Yamai S, et al.: [Occurrence of free-living amoebae and Legionella in whirlpool baths]. *Kansenshogaku Zasshi J Jpn Assoc Infect Dis* 1998:72, 1056.
16. Woodmansey A, Collins DH, Ernst MM: Vascular reactions to the contrast bath in health and in rheumatoid arthritis. *Lancet* 1938:2, 1350.
17. Tovin BJ, Wolf SL, Greenfield BH, et al.: Comparison of the effects of exercise in water and on land on the rehabilitation of patients with intra-articular anterior cruciate ligament reconstructions [published erratum appears in *Phys Ther* 1994:74, 1165]. *Phys Ther* 1994:74, 710.
18. Green J, McKenna F, Redfern EJ, et al.: Home exercises are as effective as outpatient hydrotherapy for osteoarthritis of the hip [see comments]. *Br J Rheumatol* 1993:32, 812.
19. Forster MM: Mineral springs and miracles. *Can Fam Physician* 1994:40, 729.
20. Tishler M, Brostovski Y, Yaron M: Effect of spa therapy in Tiberias on patients with ankylosing spondylitis. *Clin Rheumatol* 1995:14, 21.

21. Sukenik S, Giryes H, Halevy S, et al.: Treatment of psoriatic arthritis at the Dead Sea. *J Rheumatol* 1994:21, 1305.
22. Sukenik S, Buskila D, Neumann L, et al.: Mud pack therapy in rheumatoid arthritis. *Clin Rheumatol* 1992:11, 243.
23. Konrad K, Tatrai T, Hunka A, et al.: Controlled trial of balneotherapy in treatment of low back pain. *Ann Rheum Dis* 1992:51, 820.
24. Constant F, Collin JF, Guillemin F, et al.: Effectiveness of spa therapy in chronic low back pain: A randomized clinical trial. *J Rheumatol* 1995:22, 1315.
25. Guillemin F, Constant F, Collin JF, et al.: Short and long-term effect of spa therapy in chronic low back pain [see comments]. *Br J Rheumatol* 1994:33, 148.
26. Alcorn R, Bowser B, Henley EJ, et al.: Fluidotherapy and exercise in the management of sickle cell anemia. A clinical report. *Phys Ther* 1984:64, 1520.
27. Borrell RM, Parker R, Henley EJ, et al.: Comparison of in vivo temperatures produced by hydrotherapy, paraffin wax treatment, and fluidotherapy. *Phys Ther* 1980:60, 1273.
28. Allison TG, Reger WE: Comparison of responses of men to immersion in circulating water at 40.0 and 41.5 degrees C. *Aviat Space Environ Med* 1998:69, 845.
29. Tei C, Horikiri Y, Park JC, et al.: Acute hemodynamic improvement by thermal vasodilation in congestive heart failure. *Circulation* 1995:91, 2582.
30. Luurila OJ: Cardiac arrhythmias, sudden death and the Finnish sauna bath. *Adv Cardiol* 1978:25, 73.
31. Romo J: Factors related to sudden death in acute ischemic heart disease: A community study in Helsinki. *Acta Med Scand (Suppl)* 1972:547, 1.
32. Kauppinen K, Vuori I: Man in the sauna. *Ann Clin Res* 1986:18, 173.
33. Pleet H, Graham JM Jr, Smith DW: Central nervous system and facial defects associated with maternal hyperthermia at four to 14 weeks' gestation. *Pediatrics* 1981:67, 785.
34. Abramson DI, Tuck S, Chu LSW, et al.: Effect of paraffin bath and hot fomentations on local tissue temperatures. *Arch Phys Med Rehabil* 1964:45, 87.
35. Helfand AE, Bruno J: Therapeutic modalities and procedures. Part I: Cold and heat. *Clin Podiatr* 1984:1, 301.
36. Lee ER, Sullivan DM, Kapp DS: Potential hazards of radiative electromagnetic hyperthermia in the presence of multiple metallic surgical clips. *Int J Hyperthermia* 1992:8, 809.
37. Stewart HF, Harris GR, Herman BA, et al.: Survey of use and performance of ultrasonic therapy equipment in Pinellas County, Florida. *Phys Ther* 1974:54, 707.
38. Coakley WT: Biophysical effects of ultrasound at therapeutic intensities. *Physiotherapy* 1978:64, 166.
39. Allen KG, Battye CK: Performance of ultrasonic therapy instruments. *Physiotherapy* 1978:64, 174.
40. Ward AR, Robertson VJ: Comparison of heating of nonliving soft tissue produced by 45 kHz and 1 MHz frequency ultrasound machines. *J Orthop Sports Phys Ther* 1996:23, 258.
41. Draper DO, Harris ST, Schulthies S, et al.: Hot-pack and 1-MHz ultrasound treatments have an additive effect on muscle temperature increase. *J Athletic Training* 1998:33, 2.
42. Goldman DE, Heuter TF: Tabular data of the velocity and absorption of high-frequency sound in mammalian tissues. *J Acoust Soc Am* 1956:28, 35.
43. Lehmann JF, Delateur BJ, Stonebridge JB, et al.: Therapeutic temperature distribution produced by ultrasound as modified by dosage and volume of tissue exposed. *Arch Phys Med Rehabil* 1967:48, 662.
44. Lehmann JF, DeLateur BJ, Warren CG, et al.: Heating of joint structures by ultrasound. *Arch Phys Med Rehabil* 1968:49, 28.
45. Flint EB, Suslick KS: The temperature of cavitation. *Science* 1991:253, 1397.
46. Dyson M: Non-thermal cellular effects of ultrasound. *Br J Cancer (Suppl)* 1982:45, 165.
47. Dyson M, Pond JB, Woodward B, et al.: The production of blood cell stasis and endothelial damage in the blood vessels of chick embryos treated with ultrasound in a stationary wave field. *Ultrasound Med Biol* 1974:1, 133.
48. Doan N, Reher P, Meghji S, et al.: In vitro effects of therapeutic ultrasound on cell proliferation, protein synthesis, and cytokine production by human fibroblasts, osteoblasts, and monocytes. *J Oral Maxillofac Surg* 1999:57, 409.
49. Balmaseda MT, Fatehi MT, Koozekanani SH, et al.: Ultrasound therapy: A comparative study of different coupling media. *Arch Phys Med Rehabil* 1986:67, 149.
50. Reid DC, Cummings GE: Efficiency of ultrasound coupling agents. *Physiotherapy* 1977:63, 255.
51. Warren CG, Koblanski JN, Sigelmann RA: Ultrasound coupling media: Their relative transmissivity. *Arch Phys Med Rehabil* 1976:57, 218.
52. van der Windt DA, van der Heijden GJ, van den Berg SG, et al.: Ultrasound therapy for musculoskeletal disorders: A systematic review. *Pain* 1999:81, 257.
53. Echternach JL: Ultrasound: An adjunct treatment for shoulder disabilities. *Phys Ther* 1965:45, 865.
54. Ebenbichler GR, Erdogmus CB, Resch KL, et al.: Ultrasound therapy for calcific tendinitis of the shoulder [see comments]. *N Engl J Med* 1999:40, 1533.
55. Downing DS, Weinstein A: Ultrasound therapy of subacromial bursitis. A double blind trial. *Phys Ther* 1986:66, 194.
56. Dijs H, Mortier G, Driessens M, et al.: A retrospective study of the conservative treatment of tennis-elbow. *Acta Belg Med Phys* 1990:13, 73.
57. Lundeberg T, Abrahamsson P, Haker E: A comparative study of continuous ultrasound, placebo ultrasound and rest in epicondylalgia. *Scand J Rehabil Med* 1988: 20, 99.
58. Taube S, Ylipaavalniemi P, Kononen M, et al.: The effect of pulsed ultrasound on myofascial pain. A placebo controlled study. *Proc Finn Dent Soc* 1988:84, 241.
59. van Der Heijden GJ, Leffers P, Wolters PJ, et al.: No effect of bipolar interferential electrotherapy and pulsed ultrasound for soft tissue shoulder disorders: A randomised controlled trial. *Ann Rheum Dis* 1999:58, 530.

60. Tiidus PM: Massage and ultrasound as therapeutic modalities in exercise-induced muscle damage. *Can J Appl Physiol* 1999:24, 267.

61. Craig JA, Bradley J, Walsh DM, et al.: Delayed onset muscle soreness: Lack of effect of therapeutic ultrasound in humans. *Arch Phys Med Rehabil* 1999:80, 318.

62. Plaskett C, Tiidus PM, Livingston L: Ultrasound treatment does not affect postexercise muscle strength recovery or soreness. *J Sport Rehabil* 1999:8, 1.

63. Lehmann JF, Erickson DJ, Martin GM: Comparison of ultrasonic and microwave diathermy in the physical treatment of periarthritis of the shoulder. *Arch Phys Med Rehabil* 1954:35, 627.

64. Lehmann JF, Fordyce WE, Rathbun LA, et al.: Clinical evaluation of a new approach in the treatment of contracture associated with hip fracture after internal fixation. *Arch Phys Med Rehabil* 1961:42, 95.

65. Lehmann JF, McMillan JA, Brunner GD, et al.: Comparative study of the efficiency of short-wave, microwave and ultrasonic diathermy in heating the hip joint. *Arch Phys Med Rehabil* 1959:40, 510.

66. Draper DO, Anderson C, Schulthies SS, et al.: Immediate and residual changes in dorsiflexion range of motion using an ultrasound heat and stretch routine. *J Athletic Training* 1998:33, 141.

67. Markham DE, Wood MR: Ultrasound for Dupuytren's contracture. *Physiotherapy* 1980:66, 55.

68. Ward RS, Hayes-Lundy C, Reddy R, et al.: Evaluation of topical therapeutic ultrasound to improve response to physical therapy and lessen scar contracture after burn injury. *J Burn Care Rehabil* 1994:15, 74.

69. Chan AK, Myrer JW, Measom GJ, et al.: Temperature changes in human patellar tendon in response to therapeutic ultrasound. *J Athletic Training* 1998:33, 130.

70. Williamson JB, George TK, Simpson DC, et al.: Ultrasound in the treatment of ankle sprains. *Injury* 1986:17, 176.

71. Crawford F, Snaith M: How effective is therapeutic ultrasound in the treatment of heel pain? *Ann Rheum Dis* 1996:55, 265.

72. Mune O, Thoseth K: Ultrasonic treatment of subcutaneous infiltrations after injections. *Acta Orthop Scand* 1963:33, 347.

73. Oakley EM: Evidence for effectiveness of ultrasound treatment in physical medicine. *Br J Cancer (Suppl)* 1982:45, 233.

74. Ebenbichler GR, Resch KL, Nicolakis P, et al.: Ultrasound treatment for treating the carpal tunnel syndrome: Randomised "sham" controlled trial. *BMJ* 1998:316, 731.

75. Oztas O, Turan B, Bora I, et al.: Ultrasound therapy effect in carpal tunnel syndrome. *Arch Phys Med Rehabil* 1998:79, 1540.

76. Wright ET, Haase KH: Keloids and ultrasound. *Arch Phys Med Rehabil* 1971:52, 280.

77. Foulkes J: The application of therapeutic pulsed ultrasound to the traumatised perineum. *Br J Clin Pract* 1980:34, 114.

78. Hay-Smith EJ, Reed MA: Physical agents for perineal pain following childbirth: A systematic review. *Phys Ther Rev* 1997:2, 115.

79. ter Riet G, Kessels AG, Knipschild P: Randomised clinical trial of ultrasound treatment for pressure ulcers [published erratum appears in *BMJ* 1995:310, 1300] [see comments]. *BMJ* 1995:310, 1040.

80. Nussbaum EL, Biemann I, Mustard B: Comparison of ultrasound/ultraviolet-C and laser for treatment of pressure ulcers in patients with spinal cord injury. *Phys Ther* 1994:74, 812.

81. Paul BJ, Lafratta CW, Dawson AR, et al.: Use of ultrasound in the treatment of pressure sores in patients with spinal cord injury. *Arch Phys Med Rehabil* 1960:41, 438.

82. ter Riet G, Kessels AG, Knipschild P: A randomized clinical trial of ultrasound in the treatment of pressure ulcers. *Phys Ther* 1996:76, 1301.

83. Rozsivalova V, Nozickova M, Jelinkova R, et al.: Management of painful leg ulcers by ultrasound therapy. *Sbornik Vedeckych Praci Lekarske Fakulty Karlovy Univerzity V Hradci Kralove* 1987:30, 325.

84. Dyson M, Franks C, Suckling J: Stimulation of healing of varicose ulcers by ultrasound. *Ultrasonics* 1976:14, 232.

85. Callam M, Harper D, Dale J, et al.: A controlled trial of weekly ultrasound therapy in chronic leg ulceration. *Lancet* 1987:25, 204.

86. Peschen M, Weichenthal M, Schopf E, et al.: Low-frequency ultrasound treatment of chronic venous leg ulcers in an outpatient therapy. *Acta Derm Venereol* 1997:77, 311.

87. Johannsen F, Gam AN, Karlsmark T: Ultrasound therapy in chronic leg ulceration: A meta-analysis. *Wound Repair Regeneration* 1998:6, 121.

88. Hashish I, Hai HK, Harvey W, et al.: Reduction of postoperative pain and swelling by ultrasound treatment: A placebo effect. *Pain* 1988:33, 303.

89. Grant A, Sleep J, McIntosh J, et al.: Ultrasound and pulsed electromagnetic energy treatment for perineal trauma. A randomized placebo-controlled trial. *Br J Obstet Gynecol* 1989:96, 434.

90. Goddard DH, Revell PA, Cason J, et al.: Ultrasound has no anti-inflammatory effect. *Ann Rheum Dis* 1983:42, 582.

91. Hadjiargyrou M, McLeod K, Ryaby JP, et al.: Enhancement of fracture healing by low intensity ultrasound. *Clin Orthop* 1998:S216, 29.

92. Novak EJ: Experimental transmission of lidocaine through intact skin by ultrasound. *Arch Phys Med Rehabil* 1964:45, 231.

93. Griffin JE, Touchstone JC, Liu A: Ultrasonic movement of cortisol into pig tissue: II. Movement into paravertebral nerve. *Am J Phys Med* 1965:44, 20.

94. Bare AC, McAnaw MB, Pritchard AE, et al.: Phonophoretic delivery of 10% hydrocortisone through the epidermis of humans as determined by serum cortisol concentrations [see comments]. *Phys Ther* 1996:76, 738.

95. Klaiman MD, Shrader JA, Danoff JV, et al.: Phonophoresis versus ultrasound in the treatment of common mus-

culoskeletal conditions. *Med Sci Sports Exerc* 1998:30, 1349.

96. Moll MJ: A new approach to pain: Lidocaine and decadron with ultrasound. *USAF Med Service Dig* 1977:30, 8.

97. Cameroy BM: Ultrasound enhanced local anesthesia. *Am J Orthop* 1966:8, 47.

98. Wanet G, Dehon N: [Clinical study of ultrasonophoresis with a topical preparation combining phenylbutazone and alpha-chymotrypsin]. *J Belge Rhumatol Med Phys* 1976:31, 49.

99. Dussick CT, Fritch DJ, Kyraizidan M, et al.: Measurement of articular tissues with ultrasound. *Am J Phys Med* 1958:37, 160.

100. Weinberger A, Fadilah R, Lev A, et al.: Deep heat in the treatment of inflammatory joint disease. *Med Hypotheses* 1988:25, 231.

101. Weinberger A, Fadilah R, Lev A, et al.: Treatment of articular effusions with local deep microwave hyperthermia. *Clin Rheumatol* 1989:8, 461.

102. Brunner GD, Lehmann JF, McMillan JA, et al.: Can ultrasound be used in the presence of surgical metal implants: An experimental approach. *Phys Ther* 1958:38, 823.

103. Gersten JW: Effect of metallic objects on temperature rises produced in tissue by ultrasound. *Am J Phys Med* 1958:37, 75.

104. Skoubo-Kristensen E, Sommer J: Ultrasound influence on internal fixation with a rigid plate in dogs. *Arch Phys Med Rehabil* 1982:63, 371.

105. Kantor G: Evaluation and survey of microwave and radiofrequency applicators. *J Microw Power* 1981:16, 135.

106. Lehmann JF, DeLateur BJ, Stonebridge JB: Selective muscle heating by shortwave diathermy with a helical coil. *Arch Phys Med Rehabil* 1969:50, 117.

107. Draper DO, Knight K, Fujiwara T, et al.: Temperature change in human muscle during and after pulsed shortwave diathermy. *J Orthop Sports Phys Ther* 1999:29, 13.

108. Wildervanck A, Wakim KG, Herrick JF, et al.: Certain experimental observations on a pulsed diathermy machine. *Arch Phys Med Rehabil* 1959:40, 45.

109. Rubin A, Erdman WJ: Microwave exposure of the human female pelvis during early pregnancy and prior to conception. *Am J Phys Med* 1959:38, 219.

110. Worden RE, Herrick JF, Wakim KG, et al.: The heating effects of microwaves with and without ischemia. *Arch Phys Med Rehabil* 1948:29, 751.

111. Stuchly MA, Repacholi MH, Lecuyer DW, et al.: Exposure to the operator and patient during short wave diathermy treatments. *Health Phys* 1982:42, 341.

112. American National Standards Institute: *I. Safety Levels With Respect to Human Exposure to Radio Frequency Electromagnetic Fields, 300 kHz to 100 GHz*, Washington, DC, American National Standards Institute, 1982.

113. Moseley H, Davison M: Exposure of physiotherapists to microwave radiation during microwave diathermy treatment. *Clin Phys Physiol Measure* 1981:2, 217.

114. Ouellet-Hellstrom R, Stewart WF: Miscarriages among female physical therapists who report using radio- and microwave-frequency electromagnetic radiation [see comments]. *Am J Epidemiol* 1993:138, 775.

115. Larsen AI: Congenital malformations and exposure to high-frequency electromagnetic radiation among Danish physiotherapists. *Scand J Work Environ Health* 1991:17, 318.

116. Guberan E, Campana A, Faval P, et al.: Gender ratio of offspring and exposure to shortwave radiation among female physiotherapists. *Scand J Work Environ Health* 1994:20, 345.

117. Seaborne D, Quirion-DeGirardi C, Rousseau M, et al.: The treatment of pressure sores using pulsed electromagnetic energy (PEME). *Physiother Can* 1996:48, 13.

118. Hartviksen K: Ice therapy in spasticity. *Acta Neurol Scand* 1962:38, 79.

119. Knutsson E, Mattsson E: Effects of local cooling on monosynaptic reflexes in man. *Scand J Rehabil Med* 1969: 1, 126.

120. Miglietta O: Action of cold on spasticity. *Am J Phys Med* 1973:52, 198.

121. Bisgard JD, Nye D: The influence of hot and cold application upon gastric and intestinal motor activity. *Surg Gynecol Obstet* 1940: 71, 172.

122. Lehmann JF, de Lateur BJ: Diathermy and superficial heat and cold therapy, in Kottke FJ, Stillwell GK, Lehmann JF (eds.), *Krusen's Handbook of Physical Medicine and Rehabilitation*, 3rd ed., Philadelphia, WB Saunders, 1982:275.

123. Oosterveld FG, Rasker JJ: Effects of local heat and cold treatment on surface and articular temperature of arthritic knees. *Arthritis Rheum* 1994:37, 1578.

124. Travell J: Ethyl chloride spray for painful muscle spasm. *Arch Phys Med Rehabil* 1952:33, 291.

125. Whitelaw GP, DeMuth KA, Demos HA, et al.: The use of the Cryo/Cuff versus ice and elastic wrap in the postoperative care of knee arthroscopy patients. *Am J Knee Surg* 1995:8, 28.

126. Daniel DM, Stone ML, Arendt DL: The effect of cold therapy on pain, swelling, and range of motion after anterior cruciate ligament reconstructive surgery [see comments]. *Arthroscopy* 1994:10, 530.

127. Matsen FA, Questad K, Matsen AL: The effect of local cooling on postfracture swelling: A controlled study. *Clin Orthop* 1975:109, 201.

128. Ho SS, Illgen RL, Meyer RW, et al.: Comparison of various icing times in decreasing bone metabolism and blood flow in the knee. *Am J Sports Med* 1995:23, 74.

129. Basur RL, Shephard E, Mouzas GL: A cooling method in the treatment of ankle sprains. *Practitioner* 1976:216, 708.

130. Moore CD, Cardea JA: Vascular changes in leg trauma. *South Med J* 1977:70, 1285.

131. Schaubel HJ: The local use of ice after orthopedic procedures. *Am J Surg* 1946:72, 711.

132. Bert JM, Stark JG, Maschka K, et al.: The effect of cold therapy on morbidity subsequent to arthroscopic lateral retinacular release. *Orthop Rev* 1991:20, 755.

133. Hirase Y: Postoperative cooling enhances composite graft survival in nasal-alar and fingertip reconstruction. *Br J Plast Surg* 1993:46, 707.

134. Knight KL: *Cryotherapy: Theory, Technique and Physiology,* 1st ed., Chattanooga, TN, Chattanooga Corporation, 1985:15.

135. Sloan JP, Hain R, Pownall R: Clinical benefits of early cold therapy in accident and emergency following ankle sprain. *Arch Emerg Med* 1989:6, 1.

136. Hocutt JE Jr, Jaffe R, Rylander CR, et al.: Cryotherapy in ankle sprains. *Am J Sports Med* 1982:10, 316.

137. Weresh MJ, Bennett GL, Njus G: Analysis of cryotherapy penetration: A comparison of the plaster cast, synthetic cast, Ace wrap dressing, and Robert-Jones dressing. *Foot Ankle Int* 1996:17, 37.

138. Melzack R, Jeans ME, Stratford JG, et al.: Ice massage and transcutaneous electrical stimulation: Comparison of treatment for low-back pain. *Pain* 1980:9, 209.

139. Landon BR: Heat or cold for the relief of low back pain. *Phys Ther* 1967:47, 1126.

140. Barlas D, Homan CS, Thode HC Jr: In vivo tissue temperature comparison of cryotherapy with and without external compression. *Ann Emerg Med* 1996:28, 436.

141. Kane K, Taub A: A history of local electrical analgesia. *Pain* 1975:1, 125.

142. Geddes LA: A short history of the electrical stimulation of excitable tissue. Including electrotherapeutic applications. *Physiologist* 1984:27, S1.

143. Melzack R, Stillwell DM, Fox EJ: Trigger points and acupuncture points for pain: Correlations and implications. *Pain* 1977:3, 3.

144. Ghoname EA, Craig WF, White PF, et al.: Percutaneous electrical nerve stimulation for low back pain: A randomized crossover study [published erratum appears in *JAMA* 1999:281, 1795]. *JAMA* 1999:281, 818.

145. McDowell BC, McCormack K, Walsh DM, et al.: Comparative analgesic effects of H-wave therapy and transcutaneous electrical nerve stimulation on pain threshold in humans. *Arch Phys Med Rehabil* 1999:80, 1001.

146. Garrison DW, Foreman RD: Effects of transcutaneous electrical nerve stimulation (TENS) on spontaneous and noxiously evoked dorsal horn cell activity in cats with transected spinal cords. *Neurosci Lett* 1996:216, 125.

147. Basford JR: Physical agents, in DeLisa JA, Gans BM, Currie DM, et al. (eds.), *Rehabilitation Medicine: Principles and Practice,* 2nd ed., Philadelphia, JB Lippincott, 1993:404.

148. Chen D, Philip M, Philip PA, et al.: Cardiac pacemaker inhibition by transcutaneous electrical nerve stimulation [published erratum appears in *Arch Phys Med Rehabil* 1990:71, 388]. *Arch Phys Med Rehabil* 1990:71, 27.

149. Chen L, Tang J, White PF, et al.: The effect of location of transcutaneous electrical nerve stimulation on postoperative opioid analgesic requirement: Acupoint versus nonacupoint stimulation. *Anesth Analg* 1998:87, 1129.

150. Kaplan B, Rabinerson D, Pardo J, et al.: Transcutaneous electrical nerve stimulation (TENS) as a pain-relief device in obstetrics and gynecology. *Clin Exp Obstet Gynecol* 1997:24, 123.

151. Pope MH, Phillips RB, Haugh LD, et al.: A prospective randomized three-week trial of spinal manipulation, transcutaneous muscle stimulation, massage and corset in the treatment of subacute low back pain. *Spine* 1994:19, 2571.

152. Deyo RA, Walsh NE, Martin DC, et al.: A controlled trial of transcutaneous electrical nerve stimulation (TENS) and exercise for chronic low back pain [see comments]. *N Engl J Med* 1990:322, 1627.

153. Herman E, Williams R, Stratford P, et al.: A randomized controlled trial of transcutaneous electrical nerve stimulation (CODETRON) to determine its benefits in a rehabilitation program for acute occupational low back pain. *Spine* 1994:19, 561.

154. Marchand S, Charest J, Li J, et al.: Is TENS purely a placebo effect? A controlled study on chronic low back pain [see comments]. *Pain* 1993:54, 99.

155. Lewis B, Lewis D, Cumming G: The comparative analgesic efficacy of transcutaneous electrical nerve stimulation and a non-steroidal anti-inflammatory drug for painful osteoarthritis. *Br J Rheumatol* 1994:33, 455.

156. Linde C, Isacsson G, Jonsson BG: Outcome of 6-week treatment with transcutaneous electric nerve stimulation compared with splint on symptomatic temporomandibular joint disk displacement without reduction. *Acta Odontol Scand* 1995:53, 92.

157. Fishbain DA, Chabal C, Abbott A, et al.: Transcutaneous electrical nerve stimulation (TENS) treatment outcome in long-term users. *Clin J Pain* 1996:12, 201.

158. Verdouw BC, Zuurmond WWA, DeLange JJ, et al.: Long-term use and effectiveness of transcutaneous electrical nerve stimulation in treatment of chronic pain patients. *Pain Clin* 1995:8, 341.

159. Meyler WJ, de Jongste MJ, Rolf CA: Clinical evaluation of pain treatment with electrostimulation: A study on TENS in patients with different pain syndromes. *Clin J Pain* 1994:10, 22.

160. Nolan MF, Hartsfield JK Jr, Witters DM, et al.: Failure of transcutaneous electrical nerve stimulation in the conventional and burst modes to alter digital skin temperature. *Arch Phys Med Rehabil* 1993:74, 182.

161. Kaada B, Helle KB: In search of mediators of skin vasodilation induced by transcutaneous nerve stimulation: IV. In vitro bioassay of the vasoinhibitory activity of sera from patients suffering from peripheral ischemia. *Gen Pharmacol* 1984:15, 115.

162. Goulet C, Arsenault AB, Bourbonnais D, et al.: Effects of transcutaneous electrical nerve stimulation on H-reflex and spinal spasticity. *Scand J Rehabil Med* 1996:28, 169.

163. Levin MF, Hui-Chan CW: Relief of hemiparetic spasticity by TENS is associated with improvement in reflex and voluntary motor functions. *Electroencephalogr Clin Neurophysiol* 1992:85, 131.

164. Curwin JH, Coyne RF, Winters SL: Inappropriate defibrillator (ICD) shocks caused by transcutaneous electronic nerve stimulation (TENS) units [letter, comment]. *Pacing Clin Electrophysiol* 1999:22, 692.

165. Eriksson M, Schuller H, Sjolund B: Hazard from transcutaneous nerve stimulation in patients with pacemakers [letter]. *Lancet* 1978:1, 1319.

166. Liberson WT, Holmquest HJ, Scot D, et al.: Functional electrotherapy: Stimulation of the peroneal nerve synchronized with the swing phase of the gait of hemiplegic patients. *Arch Phys Med Rehabil* 1961:42, 101.

167. Bonaroti D, Akers JM, Smith BT, et al.: Comparison of functional electrical stimulation to long leg braces for upright mobility for children with complete thoracic level spinal injuries. *Arch Phys Med Rehabil* 1999:80, 1047.

168. Hjeltnes N, Aksnes AK, Birkeland KI, et al.: Improved body composition after 8 wk of electrically stimulated leg cycling in tetraplegic patients. *Am J Physiol* 1997:273, R1072.

169. Rakos M, Freudenschuss B, Girsch W, et al.: Electromyogram-controlled functional electrical stimulation for treatment of the paralyzed upper extremity. *Artif Organs* 1999:23, 466.

170. Schwartz RS, Salome NN, Ingmundon PT, et al.: Effects of electrical stimulation to the soft palate on snoring and obstructive sleep apnea. *J Prosthet Dent* 1996:76, 273.

171. Mourselas N, Granat MH: Evaluation of patterned stimulation for use in surface functional electrical stimulation systems. *Med Eng Phys* 1998:20, 319.

172. Baldi JC, Jackson RD, Moraille R, et al.: Muscle atrophy is prevented in patients with acute spinal cord injury using functional electrical stimulation. *Spinal Cord* 1998:36, 463.

173. Chantraine A, Ludy JP, Berger D: Is cortisone iontophoresis possible? *Arch Phys Med Rehabil* 1986:67, 38.

174. O'Malley EP, Oester YT: Influence of some physical chemical factors on iontophoresis using radio isotopes. *Arch Phys Med Rehabil* 1955:36, 310.

175. Hill AC, Baker GF, Jansen GT: Mechanism of action of iontophoresis in the treatment of palmar hyperhidrosis. *Cutis* 1981:28, 69.

176. Peterson JL, Read SI, Rodman OG: A new device in the treatment of hyperhidrosis by iontophoresis. *Cutis* 1982:29, 82.

177. Berliner MN: Reduced skin hyperemia during tap water iontophoresis after intake of acetylsalicylic acid. *Am J Phys Med Rehabil* 1997:76, 482.

178. Demirtas RN, Oner C: The treatment of lateral epicondylitis by iontophoresis of sodium salicylate and sodium diclofenac. *Clin Rehabil* 1998:12, 23.

179. Greminger RF, Elliott RA Jr, Rapperport A: Antibiotic iontophoresis for the management of burned ear chondritis. *Plast Reconstruct Surg* 1980:66, 356.

180. LaForest NT, Cofrancesco C: Antibiotic iontophoresis in the treatment of ear chondritis. *Phys Ther* 1978:58, 32.

181. Gherardini G, Gurlek A, Evans GR, et al.: Venous ulcers, improved healing by iontophoretic administration of calcitonin gene-related peptide and vasoactive intestinal polypeptide. *Plast Reconstruct Surg* 1998:101, 90.

182. Tannebaum M: Iodine iontophoresis in reducing scar tissue. *Phys Ther* 1980:60, 792.

183. Cornwall MW: Zinc iontophoresis to treat ischemic skin ulcers. *Phys Ther* 1981:61, 359.

184. Perron M, Malouin F: Acetic acid iontophoresis and ultrasound for the treatment of calcifying tendinitis of the shoulder: A randomized control trial. *Arch Phys Med Rehabil* 1997:78, 379.

185. Wolcott LE, Wheeler PC, Hardwicke HM, et al.: Accelerated healing of skin ulcer by electrotherapy: Preliminary clinical results. *South Med J* 1969:62, 795.

186. Gault WR, Gatens PF Jr: Use of low intensity direct current in management of ischemic skin ulcers. *Phys Ther.* 1976:56, 265.

187. Hewitt GK: Chronic leg ulcers. *Physiotherapy* 1956: 42, 43.

188. Burr HS, Taffel M, Harvey SC: An electrometric study of the healing wound in man. *Yale J Biol Med* 1940:12, 483.

189. Weiss DS, Kirsner R, Eaglstein WH: Electrical stimulation and wound healing. *Arch Dermatol* 1990:126, 222.

190. Cheng N, Van Hoof H, Bockx E, et al.: The effects of electric currents on ATP generation, protein synthesis, and membrane transport of rat skin. *Clin Orthop* 1982, 264.

191. Robinson KR: The responses of cells to electrical fields: A review. *J Cell Biol* 1985:101, 2023.

192. Marcer M, Musatti G, Bassett CA: Results of pulsed electromagnetic fields (PEMFs) in ununited fractures after external skeletal fixation. *Clin Orthop* 1984, 260.

193. Albanese R, Blaschak J, Medina R, et al.: Ultrashort electromagnetic signals: Biophysical questions, safety issues, and medical opportunities. *Aviat Space Environ Med* 1994:65, A116.

194. Barron JJ, Jacobson WE, Tidd G: Treatment of decubitus ulcers. A new approach. *Minn Med* 1985:68, 103.

195. Vodovnik L, Karba R: Treatment of chronic wounds by means of electric and electromagnetic fields. Part 1. Literature review. *Med Biol Eng Comput* 1992:30, 257.

196. Kaada B: Vasodilation induced by transcutaneous nerve stimulation in peripheral ischemia (Raynaud's phenomenon and diabetic polyneuropathy). *Eur Heart J* 1982:3, 303.

197. Kaiser J: Panel finds EMFs pose no threat [news] [see comments] [published erratum appears in *Science* 1997:275, 741]. *Science* 1996:274, 910.

198. Kaiser J: NIH panel revives EMF-cancer link [news]. *Science* 1998:281, 21.

199. Wikswo JP, Barach JP: An estimate of the steady magnetic field strength required to influence nerve conduction. *IEEE Trans Biomed Eng* 1980:27, 722.

200. Schulten K: Magnetic field effects in chemistry and biology. *Adv Solid State Phys* 1982:22, 61.

201. Steiner UE, Ulrich T: Magnetic field effects in chemical kinetics and related phenomena. *Chem Rev* 1989:89, 51.

202. Beall PT, Hazlewood CF, Rao PN: Nuclear magnetic resonance patterns of intracellular water as a function of HeLa cell cycle. *Science* 1976:192, 904.

203. Frankel RB, Liburdy RP: Biological effects of static magnetic fields, in Polk C, Postow E (eds.), *Handbook of Biological Effects of Electromagnetic Fields*, 2nd ed., Boca Raton, FL, CRC Press, 1996:149.

204. Porter M: Magnetic therapy. *Equine Vet Data* 1997:17, 371.

205. Basford JR: Low intensity laser therapy: Still not an established clinical tool. *Lasers Surg Med* 1995:16, 331.

206. Loew M, Jurgowski W, Mau HC, et al.: Treatment of calcifying tendinitis of rotator cuff by extracorporeal shock waves: A preliminary report. *J Shoulder Elbow Surg* 1995:4, 101.

207. Rompe JD, Hopf C, Nafe B, et al.: Low-energy extracorporeal shock wave therapy for painful heel: a prospective controlled single-blind study. *Arch Orthop Trauma Surg* 1996:115, 75.

208. Rompe JD, Hope C, Kullmer K, et al.: Analgesic effect of extracorporeal shock-wave therapy on chronic tennis elbow. *J Bone Joint Surg Br* 1996:78, 233.

209. Bishop B: Vibratory stimulation: Part I. Neurophysiology of motor responses evoked by vibratory stimulation. *Phys Ther* 1974:54, 1273.

210. Bishop B: Vibratory stimulation. Part II. Vibratory stimulation as an evaluation tool. *Phys Ther* 1975:55, 28.

211. Bishop B: Vibratory stimulation. Part III. Possible applications of vibration in treatment of motor dysfunctions. *Phys Ther* 1975:55, 139.

212. Lundeberg T, Nordemar R, Ottoson D: Pain alleviation by vibratory stimulation. *Pain* 1984:20, 25.

213. Lundeberg T: The pain suppressive effect of vibratory stimulation and transcutaneous electrical nerve stimulation (TENS) as compared to aspirin. *Brain Res* 1984:294, 201.

214. Leduc A, Lievens P, Dewald J: The influence of multidirectional vibrations on wound healing and on regeneration of blood and lymph vessels. *Lymphology* 1981:14, 179.

Chapter 43

MASSAGE AND MANUAL MEDICINE

Marcy Schlinger and Michael Andary

INTRODUCTION

As therapeutic techniques, both massage and manipulation (or manual medicine) have been used extensively for many kinds of injuries. For the active runner, there are specific applications and indications for both massage and manual medicine. These techniques are used for treatment of injury, to promote recovery, to enhance well-being, and to optimize performance. This chapter contains a description of both modalities, a review of the literature that addresses their use in sports-related injury, and a description of practical and technical approaches for diagnosis and treatment.

Before initiating treatment with massage or manual medicine, it is prudent and clinically imperative to diagnose or rule out orthopedic, neurological, or other systemic etiologies for a given injury. While both modalities can be used in the adjunctive treatment of an athlete with fractures, tendon or ligament disruption, or neurologic impairment, they should not be used in lieu of comprehensive medical care. For purposes of the discussion that follows, it is assumed that appropriate screening and treatment measures have been implemented.

THERAPEUTIC PRINCIPLES

While manipulation and massage are considered distinctly different healing modalities, they have many overlapping characteristics. These include the following:

- Many techniques and some technical aspects are similar because both are hands-on manual treatments.
- They have therapeutic principles in common—they are both restorative approaches directed at improving tissue integrity, and in a general sense at re-establishing homeostasis.
- The end points of treatment are similar because both approaches are used to relieve pain, improve mobility, and restore symmetry of function.

MASSAGE

History

Massage has been used as a therapeutic modality for centuries, and the medical literature is replete with references to massage. It is mentioned in what is thought to be the oldest existing medical text, *The Yellow Emperor's Classic of Internal Medicine* (1000 B.C.). The use of massage is addressed in the writings of Hippocrates, Asclepiades, and Galen.[1] In particular, sports-specific massage was valued by the ancient Greeks and subsequently by the Romans. It was used in preparation for exercise by athletes in the gymnasia of Sparta and Athens.[2]

The fall of the Roman Empire was followed by many centuries of stilted development in the occidental world. The time of the Renaissance ushered in sequential eras of scientific development and inquiry. In the ensuing centuries (the 16th through 19th) many European physicians of historical renown described the beneficial use of massage in their writings (Pare, Hoffman, Ling, Mezger, Estradere, and others).[1] In the United States, massage has not been widely recognized by the medical establishment, nor was it well publicized until the latter part of this century.

Applications of Massage

As a hands-on restorative approach, massage encompasses various techniques affecting multiple physical systems and psychological states. Proponents of massage report many positive therapeutic effects. In a general sense, pain relief, tissue healing, restoration of normal function, and enhancement of optimum performance are the major areas of perceived benefit.[3]

More specifically, these benefits include control of soft-tissue swelling and edema, increased arterial flow and venous exchange, relief of pain and muscle spasm, resolution of inflammatory processes, and the enhancement of relaxation and improvement in one's sense of well being. In addition, the blood clotting cascade, lymphatic drainage, and general functions of the somatic and autonomic nervous systems are all thought to be influenced by massage.[3]

Massage Technique

Central to the approach of Western massage therapy are several basic techniques directed at soft tissues of the body. These are described below and may be used in various combinations.[3–5]

EFFLEURAGE. Effleurage consists of long strokes which may be delivered slowly or rapidly. The strokes are applied in a peripheral to central direction, facilitating the return of blood to the heart. The strokes may be applied with either firm or light pressure. This technique is one of the most commonly used. It is used to enhance relaxation, as well as to maintain continuity of operator contact while moving from one area of the body to another.

PETRISSAGE. Petrissage is a technique used on discrete areas of skin and underlying subcutaneous tissue. Compared with effleurage, it is applied more deeply and involves the compression of tissue that is lifted from the underlying somatic structures.

KNEADING. Kneading utilizes both light and firm compression of soft tissues in relatively confined areas. Kneading is similar to petrissage; however, more tissue is lifted and compressed in each area.

FRICTION. This technique uses deep, penetrating, directed pressure. With enough pressure to stabilize the loose surface tissue, attention can be directed to a deeper level. The action is one of shearing in small, confined areas. The pressure, directed at underlying structures, is applied in a circular or transverse manner.

PERCUSSION. Percussion (or tapotement) consists of a variety of soft blows (striking, hacking, slapping, beating, and tapping) applied to the skin and underlying musculature. These are delivered rhythmically from a short distance away from the body. While specifically directed, they are not forceful. They are considered to be vibratory techniques.

In addition, there are other approaches that may be categorized as types of massage. These include, among others, rolfing (deep tissue work that is reported to affect somatic structures and posture), reflexology, and acupressure (directed at affecting Chi, the energy that travels along the twelve meridians of the body as defined in the Chinese system of medicine).

Sport-Specific Massage

Sport-specific massage has applications that are different from those associated with massage delivered for purposes of therapeutic relaxation. While massage therapists may utilize the techniques above for sport-specific treatment, they also employ trigger point pressure, cross fiber techniques (strokes applied in a direction that is perpendicular to the longitudinal muscle fibers), and jostling (oscillating maneuvers).[6] In addition, they may use contract relax techniques to loosen tight muscles, as well as to facilitate reciprocal inhibition and relaxation. Massage therapists in these settings may use a more diagnostic approach to clinical presentations and work in a more focused manner on particular areas of injury.

Pre-event massage is utilized by athletes to loosen muscles and for invigoration. It is also used to aid, but not substitute for, warm-up exercise. Massage of this type may be applied with long, gliding strokes. Pre-event massages are not long (30 minutes or less) and do not involve deep tissue work; they are not intended to facilitate deep relaxation.

Postevent massage is utilized to loosen tight muscles, provide relaxation, decrease muscle spasm, and alleviate pain. Runners commonly injure hamstrings, quadriceps and gastrocnemius muscles, hip musculature, and the low back muscles, and postevent massage is helpful with these kinds of injuries. Ice massage is also utilized in these circumstances.

Research

Investigators have evaluated the effects of massage on blood flow, lymphatic drainage, serum levels of beta-endorphin and beta-lipotrophin, and general muscle tone. The results of the these investigations have been somewhat difficult to compare.[7]

The efficacy of sport-specific massage has been investigated as it relates to both performance and recovery. Drews and colleagues[8] reported in 1990 that pre- and postexercise massage as compared with placebo (microwave) was found to have no significant effect on the performance times of six elite cyclists in a 4-day stage race. Rest periods between daily sequential trials may have countered the effects of massage in this commentary study.[8,9] There have been contradictory results in studies conducted by Drews and associates (no significant effect)[10,7] and Weinberg and co-workers (positive effect)[11,7] that evaluated the effect of postrace massage on mood. Massage was reported to have an effect on perception of recovery, but not on actual performance parameters or lactate or glucose levels in a controlled trial with eight amateur boxers treated with either rest or massage between two sequential bouts.[9]

In assessing the effects of pre-event massage, warm-up, and stretching, on joint range of motion, and quadriceps and hamstring strength in eight male volunteers, Wiktorsson-Moller and Oberg[12] found that warm-up and stretching had a superior effect overall on increasing flexibility (as measured with goniometry) than warm-up alone, massage alone, or massage combined with warm-up.

Investigating the efficacy of massage in alleviating DOMS (delayed-onset muscle soreness), Weber and colleagues[13] did not find that massage, as compared with upper body ergometry or microcurrent electrical stimulation, had any effect on the course of DOMS. This was a randomized study with 40 female volunteers assigned to one of the three treatment groups or a control group. Smith and associates,[14] in a controlled trial with seven treatment and control subjects, evaluated the effects of massage versus rest on DOMS following upper extremity isokinetic eccentric exercise. In a trend analysis, serial evaluations revealed significantly decreased levels of creatinine kinase, decreased diurnal reduction of cortisol, prolonged elevation of neutrophils, and decreased DOMS in the treatment subjects. Yackzan and co-workers[15] reported that ice massage after eccentric exercise was not helpful in relieving DOMS in 30 subjects. In a controlled study on 25 treated subjects, Rodenburg and associates[16] also did not find massage to be helpful in reducing DOMS after eccentric exercise. Ernst,[17] in a review of studies on DOMS, found seven controlled studies that, although methodologically flawed, suggest that massage may have some therapeutic effect on DOMS.

Augmented soft-tissue mobilization (ASTM; friction massage) has been used with clinical effect to treat tendinitis. Studies in a rat model by Gehlsen and colleagues[18] revealed a statistically significant difference in the number of fibroblasts in rat Achilles' tendons following deep pressure massage. Fibroblast proliferation is associated with tendon healing.

Blackman and associates[19] investigated the effect of massage on chronic anterior compartment exertional syndrome in seven symptomatic athletes. Massage was found to significantly delay the onset of pain from work performed in dorsiflexion. Postexercise anterior intracompartment pressures did not change. Studies by Balke and colleagues[20] of seven subjects and by Rinder and Sutherland[21] of 20 subjects (in a randomized, crossover trial) found that massage was effective in reducing muscular fatigue. In 1995, Tiidus and Shoemaker[22] reported that massage was not helpful in enhancing long-term restoration of postexercise muscle strength over a 96-hour period. Gupta and associates[23] reported that short-term massage was not more effective than rest followed by activity for lactate removal in 10 male subjects. In 1990, Cafarelli and coworkers[24] reported that there was no significant effect on rate of recovery from fatigue when vibratory massage was compared with rest in 12 subjects. Shoemaker and colleagues[25] reported that manual massage had no effect on muscle blood flow as evaluated with Doppler ultrasound in 10 healthy subjects. Investigation of the effect of massage on the expenditure of energy or oxygen consumption at rest was not shown to have any significant effect in 10 healthy adult males.[26] Conclusions reached in a review by Tiidus in 1997 indicate that light exercise is more effective than massage for recovery of function.[27]

Morelli and colleagues[28] and Sullivan and associates,[29] in separate studies evaluating the effect of massage on muscle tone, found a decrease in (Hoffman) H-reflex amplitudes during massage in healthy subjects. The H-reflex or spinal reflex arc includes sensory afferent and motor efferent nerves from the first sacral vertebral spinal cord structures. In Morelli and colleagues' controlled study of 20 subjects, the researchers observed statistically significantly decreased H-reflex amplitudes while massage was being administered.[28] Sullivan and coworkers, in their controlled study of 16 subjects, evaluated the effect of massage on H-reflex amplitudes and also found a significant reduction in amplitude in the trials in which subjects received massage.[29] There is no known clinical significance to these H-reflex changes.

As noted previously, the long-term efficacy of massage therapy has not been validated with research.[4] There is little consistency in research design among the studies, making it difficult to compare results. Most of the studies have had relatively small sample sizes. In addition, studies published in languages other than English are not readily available.[30] Other caveats to consider in the critical review of the literature include the varying individual styles of treatment methods used by therapists, as well as the potential placebo effect.

Comments and Guidelines

The use of massage in traditional Western medicine has been limited by many factors, including lack of cultural context, lack of belief in its efficacy, and lack of insurance reimbursement for massage services. Physicians and other health care providers may not perceive or appreciate the benefits of massage. The variety of social connotations of massage outside of a medical context (e.g., massage parlors) detract from the perception that massage is valuable.

Health care providers may voice skepticism about this hands-on modality that is directed at what is presumed to be a passive recipient. Athletes (professional and nonprofessional) may carry less of a stigma of passivity and thus may be thought of as more deserving of treatment modalities such as massage. In contrast to massage, many physicians prescribe treatment with analgesic medications, many of which have similar costs but more side effects. Comparisons of side effects, costs, and efficacy of medications versus massage demonstrate advantages to massage in many cases. One should keep in mind the current medical cultural milieu when considering massage as a therapeutic modality.

When seeking a massage therapist, one needs to find out, either from professional referrals or by word of mouth, which therapists in the community are effective and reputable practitioners. The training, certification, licensing, and skill level of massage therapists are not uniform. There may be a significant variance of levels of medical, anatomic, and physiological expertise of massage practitioners. Licensing requirements for massage therapists vary from state to state (25 states and the District of Columbia require licensure).

The American Massage Therapy Association (AMTA), founded in 1943, is the largest professional organization of massage therapists. The AMTA is well recognized and has developed educational criteria for membership, as well as practice standards for massage therapists. Write the AMTA at 820 Davis Street, Suite 100, Evanston, IL 60201-4444. The AMTA maintains a comprehensive, informative web site at www.amta-massage.org.

The AMTA requires a minimum of 500 hours of classroom instruction or passage of a certifying exam-

ination for membership. The National Certification Board for Therapeutic Massage and Bodywork (NCBTMB) administers a certifying examination that is recognized by the National Commission of Certifying Agencies. COMTA (Commission on Massage Therapy Accreditation) is the AMTA affiliate that accredits national training programs. AMTA also has within its membership the National Sports Massage Team, composed of massage therapists who have expertise and experience in sports massage.

In summary, massage does have empirically recognized benefits. Massage is useful for relief of pain, induction of relaxation, and promotion of rest. It is also helpful in inducing warmth and enhancing joint and connective tissue mobility.[2] Massage is a modality that is highly valued by athletes and perceived to provide benefit. The specific reasons for its efficacy, as well as measures of its efficacy, have yet to be well delineated.

MANIPULATION (MANUAL MEDICINE)

You can't trim the sails if the anchor is down.[31]
—*Kurt Heinking*

Introduction

A 44-year-old marathon runner with low back pain, a 23-year-old athlete with shin splints, and a 38-year-old runner with hip pain may appear to have isolated musculoskeletal injuries. From an osteopathic or chiropractic manipulative approach, however, musculoskeletal pain, injury, or dysfunction are considered systemically within the context of surrounding somatic structures and their relative functions.

The most common types of manual medicine used in the United States are osteopathic and chiropractic forms of manipulation. While they have common endpoints, they have different philosophical bases. Historically, osteopathic practice is predicated on the intent to optimize circulatory (vascular) integrity, while chiropractic practice is based on the intent to restore neurological function. This distillation is probably an oversimplification of a complex and poorly understood intervention. In fact, in a physiological sense, they are not mutually exclusive concepts, and this distinction is somewhat artificial. The discussion below primarily describes the care provided by osteopathic physicians. Most osteopathic physicians who utilize manual medicine do so within the larger, holistic context of osteopathic philosophy and science. Manual medicine techniques, to varying degrees, may also be used by physical therapists, massage therapists, and athletic trainers.

There are many techniques and approaches that fall within the rubric of the practices of both osteopathic manual medicine and chiropractic manipulation. The common goals of these approaches are the restoration of motion, the reduction of tissue/texture tension, relief of pain, and restoration of function. For the athlete, facilitating return to training or competition and improving motor control and coordination are additional goals of treatment.

Research

The efficacy of manipulation for low back pain has been addressed in prior studies and reviews.[4,32–36] Spinal manipulation is one of the recommended treatments for acute low back pain in the 1994 Agency for Health Care Policy and Research (now the Agency for Healthcare Research and Quality) guidelines.[37]

There are very few controlled interventional trials analyzing the efficacy of manipulation for sports injuries. Cibulka and Delitto[38] reported a statistically significant difference between hip mobilization versus sacroiliac manipulation in 20 runners with hip pain and sacroiliac dysfunction. There are several studies that have attempted to clarify the relationship between lower extremity function, lumbopelvic mobility, and sacroiliac and low back pain. These studies are primarily descriptive; however they have clinical relevance. Many of them have been reviewed comprehensively elsewhere.[39,40]

Cibulka and associates[39] reported unilateral asymmetry of hip range of motion in 100 patients with sacroiliac dysfunction. LaBan and colleagues[41] identified pubic symphysis instability in 50 subjects with lumbosacral pain; 20 had decreased hip mobility on the symptomatic side. Bachrach has described the biomechanical relationship of maladaptive patterns of movement and lower extremity joint injury to lumbopelvic dysfunction and psoas restriction in dancers.[42] Ellison and coworkers[43] reported statistically significant differences in hip rotational patterns (reduced range of motion) in 50 subjects with low back pain as compared with 100 asymptomatic patients.[43] In contrast, Brier and Nyfield did not find a correlation between hip and low back inflexibility in 108 runners and cyclists.[40]

Piriformis syndrome and short leg syndrome are both controversial diagnoses. While they may be clinically apparent problems, the efficacy of treatment with manual medicine has not been prospectively addressed.

Muscle imbalances, with their resultant pain and dysfunction, have been described by Janda and others.[44,45] The collaborative efforts of Greenman, Janda, and Bookhout have provided a working clinical paradigm which, when utilized diagnostically and as a basis for exercise prescription, enhances osteopathic treatment.[46] The exact physiological reasons for the efficacy of manual treatments are not understood. There are theoretical constructs that address bone alignment, muscle length, muscle and spindle tone, neurological and nociceptive input, central nervous system processing, and psychological factors, as well as many others. The intimacy of the human touch undoubtedly contributes to the patient's positive experience. This is an extremely complicated phenomenon, incorporating nearly all aspects of the human experience, including pain, function, behavior, philosophy, psychology, and socialization. As these issues are more rigorously researched, it is likely that the efficacy of manual manipulation (as in other aspects of medicine) will be found to be a multifactorial phenomenon.

Referral

Athletes with either acute or chronic problems may benefit from manual medicine evaluation and treatment. Acute injuries not requiring surgical intervention and/or neurological evaluation include sprains, strains, and ligamentous injuries. These injuries, in addition to causing pain, may affect mechanical function and movement. Initial treatment with manual medicine is contraindicated for acute fractures and neurologic injury. However, once the primary etiology and treatment for serious injuries has been determined, osteopathic treatment may be implemented to facilitate recovery and address compensatory biomechanical changes.

Chronic problems in the runner that warrant treatment with manual medicine include persistent pain or dysfunction exacerbated by running or exercising. Activity may exacerbate pain in a variety of different areas of the musculoskeletal system, from the cervical spine to the feet. The comprehensive osteopathic structural evaluation that addresses posture, gait, symmetry, efficiency of movement, and pelvic and lower extremity function, including foot and ankle mechanics, will help the athlete to address and resolve chronic compensatory patterns that exacerbate pain and affect performance.

In osteopathic terminology, *somatic dysfunction* is defined as impaired or altered function of related components of the somatic (body framework) system: the skeletal, arthrodial, and myofascial structures and their related vascular, lymphatic, and neural elements.[46,47] Somatic dysfunction may occur in almost anyone and does not necessarily cause pain. The structural findings that one identifies on physical examination in a patient with pain, discomfort, or restricted function are evaluated in light of their particular presentation. There are specific physical examination findings that, as a constellation, formulate the diagnosis of somatic dysfunction (see below).

History of Symptoms

Prior to the structural examination or initiation of treatment, the history of injury or dysfunction must be elicited. The clarity of understanding the mechanism of injury helps direct and modify treatment. The history includes particular attention to

1. Circumstances of injury or dysfunction: position, impact, direction of impact, gravitational forces at time of injury, patterns of movement, and compensatory strategies
2. Timing and progression of injury (sudden or insidious)
3. Pain: location, quality, duration, localization, radiation, and provocative and palliative factors
4. Associated symptomatology
5. Patterns of restricted movement; problems with training
6. Specific activities the athlete is unable to do
7. Current treatment measures
8. History of previous trauma or dysfunction
9. History of previous treatment and response to previous treatment
10. Previous hospitalizations/emergency department evaluations
11. Past medical history, menstrual history, and comorbidities
12. Past surgical history
13. Psychosocial and psychological stressors
14. Drug and medication use, including efficacy of medications
15. Red flag review of systems: Neurological: symptoms including weakness, numbness, tingling, gait abnormalities, upper extremity functional changes, atrophic changes, bowel or bladder symptoms, and cognitive deficits; General: weight changes, malaise, fatigue, fevers, and chills; Rheumatological: joint abnormalities (swelling, pain, and erythema).

This is a basic working framework for gathering pertinent historical details; it is not an exhaustive list.

Structural Examination and Diagnosis

The osteopathic manual medicine evaluation starts with a structural examination that may appear deceptively simple. What follows is a brief outline of the components of the osteopathic structural examination. These are much more comprehensively described elsewhere and the reader is encouraged to use references listed at the end of this chapter.[46–51] The focus of the structural examination is to detect areas of tissue tension and to determine patterns of restriction of movement.

The hallmark of osteopathic structural diagnosis is summarized by the mnemonic *TART*[47]: *Tissue texture abnormality, Asymmetry of bony landmarks, Restriction of motion, and Tenderness or soreness to examiner pressure*. The purpose of the physical examination is to identify areas with these characteristics that will be addressed with treatment.

Osteopathic Structural Examination for the Runner (Utilizing Visual Inspection, Palpation, and Motion Testing)

Standing:
- Posture (sagittal and frontal views)
- Shoulder, hip crest, and trochanteric heights
- Static pelvic position/rotational tendency
- Pelvic shift (side to side)
- Standing flexion tests
- Schober's and stork tests
- Active range of motion of the lumbar spine (side bending, rotation, flexion, and extension)
- Balance

Seated:
- Seated flexion test
- Lumbar and thoracic range of motion (side bending, rotation, flexion, and extension)
- Lumbar vertebral segmental abnormalities
- Tissue texture abnormalities in the paravertebral structures
- Passive range of motion of the thoracic and lumbar spines
- Cervical active and passive range of motion
- Passive range of motion of the fibular head; assessment of joint mobility of the ankle and foot

Supine:
- Malleolar levels (assessed by comparing the inferior aspects of the malleoli—side to side)
- Anterior superior iliac spine and pubic symphysis positions
- Hip, knee, and ankle range of motion
- Qualitative motion testing of lumbar-sacral and thoracolumbar side bending and rotational tendencies
- Hamstring length and tightness
- Hip external and internal rotator restriction (hip and knee flexed to 90 degrees)
- Adductor tightness/asymmetry

- Patellar tracking
- Anterior tender points (Jones' anterior lumbar tender points)
- Psoas tender points
- Inspiratory and expiratory ranges of the upper and lower thoracic cage
- Shoulder range of motion (range of internal and external rotation with arm abducted to 90 degrees, elbow flexed to 90 degrees)

Prone:

- Malleolar levels (assessed by comparing the inferior aspects of the malleoli—side to side)
- Ischial tuberosity levels; sacral tuberous ligament asymmetry and laxity
- Iliac crest levels
- Posterior superior iliac spine levels
- Sacral position and mobility
- Lumbar vertebral segmental abnormalities
- Gluteal tender points
- Psoas and quadriceps tightness
- Firing patterns of the hip extensors

Sidelying:

- Firing patterns of the hip abductors
- Quadratus lumborum tender points
- Tensor fascia lata tightness

Gait analysis:

- Gait patterns, walking and running: Patterns and tendencies of symmetrical or asymmetrical movement in the pelvis and lower extremities, trunk movement and position, head posture and movement

As information is gathered from the structural examination, restrictions may be named for their particular positional tendencies (i.e., posteriorly rotated innominate, flexed and side bent vertebral segment, superior ischial tuberosity). Once the examination is completed, the specific areas of somatic dysfunction are identified, yielding the osteopathic structural diagnosis. Throughout the process, one attempts to identify those areas of restriction that are primary and those that are secondary and compensatory.

There are specific areas of injury and patterns of restriction that runners may encounter, as follows:

1. Persistent patterns of innominate rotations
2. Sacral motion restrictions
3. Upslips or downslips in the sacroiliac joint
4. Sacral tuberous ligament abnormality
5. Pubic symphysis asymmetry (inferior/superior shear)
6. Lumbar vertebral rotational restrictions

7. Leg length abnormality (either structural/skeletal or muscular)
8. Restrictive, tight muscles (hamstrings, quadriceps, psoas, adductors)
9. Paraspinal hypertonicity
10. Impaired gluteus maximus and medius firing patterns
11. Hip, knee, ankle, and foot joint mobility restrictions
12. Impaired unilateral balance

The above are structural problems amenable to treatment that optimally will facilitate recovery of function.

Treatment

After osteopathic structural diagnostic findings are clarified, treatment may be initiated and directed toward

1. Restoring range of motion
2. Reducing pain and muscle spasm
3. Enhancing optimal mobility and efficiency of movement
4. Restoring confidence and decreasing psychological stress related to injury

Osteopathic practitioners use a variety of approaches to treatment. Their individual armamentarium of treatment techniques depends on their training, their study with mentors, and the integration of and comfort level with particular techniques. Choice of technique is also dependent on the population served. There are many different treatment orientations. The reader is encouraged to refer to selected references for further study.[46,47,52–54]

At the heart of individual treatment paradigms is the concept of a barrier, which is in fact the end point of motion. Barriers may be anatomic, elastic, physiologic, or restrictive.[46]

Osteopathic manual medicine techniques are distributed along a spectrum of direct and indirect techniques, the maneuvers of which, respectively, move restricted segments to points of restriction (toward the barrier) or into positions of ease (away from the barrier). Seemingly diametrically opposed, these approaches may be utilized in complementary ways. A brief, general discussion of several primary osteopathic manipulative techniques follows.

Muscle Energy Technique[52]

The muscle energy technique was initially developed by Fred Mitchell, Sr., and further elucidated by Fred Mitchell, Jr., among others. Muscle energy uses isometric muscle contraction followed by passive stretch to restore motion. This direct technique requires active patient participation; pain may limit cooperation.

As a muscle is held in sequential isometric contraction, relaxation and lengthening are progressively enhanced. This technique can be applied in all regions of the somatic musculature where a muscle crosses a joint. Following each sequential release, motion is facilitated to a higher degree and progressively restored. For example, restrictively tight quadriceps muscles can be progressively lengthened with sequential isometric contraction resisted (by the operator) at increasing degrees of knee flexion. Muscle energy technique is very useful for treating rotational restrictions in the spine, asymmetrical restriction of motion in the sacrum, asymmetry and restriction of the ilia, and restrictions of the pubic symphysis, among others.

High-Velocity Low-Amplitude Thrust[46]

This is one of the most commonly used osteopathic and chiropractic techniques. It is primarily a direct technique, also known as mobilization with impulse. A restricted segment is brought directly to its final point of restriction of movement. A high-velocity low-amplitude thrust (controlled maneuver) moves the restricted segment through the barrier in order to restore motion. In the best of circumstances, it is a finely localized treatment. Although one can apply high-velocity low-amplitude thrust maneuvers incidentally throughout many areas of the bony skeleton, a high level of diagnostic acumen is helpful for the identification of specific areas causing restriction.

Myofascial Release[47]

Fascial restrictions, as they occur with injury, restrict motion. By using direct and indirect myofascial approaches to the fascia, restricted tissues can be released and mobilized, restoring motion.

Counterstrain[53]

Counterstrain, developed by Dr. Lawrence Jones, incorporates theoretical principles of afferent reduction (reduction of afferent aberrant stimulation to the peripheral nervous system). A series of tender points have been identified that correlate with regions of musculoskeletal discomfort and pain. The body is positioned in a way that reduces tenderness at a particular point, providing relief. Counterstrain is a very effective treatment for presentations of acute pain. It requires little active participation except relaxation on the part of the patient.

Functional Technique[54]

Functional technique is an indirect method, utilizing principles of afferent reduction, that facilitates movement in the direction of ease. Operator-induced movement in the direction of ease helps to restore movement in the direction of restricted motion. This is a very useful technique, especially for patients with pain or muscle spasm that limits their participation and active engagement with treatment.

Craniosacral Therapy[55]

Craniosacral therapy is an osteopathic treatment developed by Dr. William Sutherland. It is a treatment modality that has at its core several key principles. They include a) re-establishment of the craniosacral rhythm (an inherent homeostatic mechanism); b) restoration of cranial suture mobility, and c) restoration of internal homeostasis.

Other techniques include, among others, soft-tissue mobilization, articulatory/oscillation, joint play/mobilization, and facilitated positional release.

The use of osteopathic manual medicine to treat running injuries is a natural extension of the use of manual medicine in the general population. The pain, injury, and dysfunction that an athlete experiences are viewed contextually. As a constellation of symptoms, they may be a red herring, masking the underlying structural limitations on movement.

COMMENTARY

Treatment Goals

For athletes, the primary treatment goal is usually a return to sports or training. Other goals that can be achieved are pain relief, an increase in function (including return to work), improved sleep, and improved quality of life. More focused goals of intervention are improvement in somatic dysfunction, improvement in range of motion, decreased tenderness, and alleviation of soft-tissue palpatory abnormalities. We strongly support the concept of linking the focused goals of treatment with functional activities (i.e., return to running or work). If the manipulation or massage is helping, this should be reflected by an increase in activity. If the manipulation/massage is making the patient feel better, but he or she is not doing more or has not regained his or her previous functional status, this is a red flag that treatment is not truly helping the patient.

Duration and Frequency of Therapy

This topic can be controversial, and is often dependent on the desired goals of the clinician and patient. If there is little or no progress toward achieving the treatment goals within 3 to 6 visits, the treatment should be re-evaluated both from a diagnostic and therapeutic point of view. One would expect at least a slight improvement in symptoms in 2 to 4 weeks or 3 to 6 visits.

Most clinicians support a time-limited course, but there are examples of abuses of the system, in which patients are seen two to five times per week for many months. It appears that many of these treatments are focused on psychological gratification, temporary relief, or financial gain.

Long-term follow-up needs to be determined on an individual basis. Some patients can benefit from one or two interventions per month. Others are best managed at the time of acute occurrence of their problem. Exercises to maintain mobility, strength, and coordination are frequently prescribed. These give patients a way of controlling their symptoms. In contrast to treatment with manipulation or massage, active exercise is needed more often, usually three to five times or more per week.

When and Where to Refer

This is an extremely individualized decision based on numerous factors, including expectations and attitudes of both patients and physicians, geographic location, economic incentives, ethical issues, and availability of skilled clinicians. Identifying a clinician whose treatment will benefit a particular athlete is important and not always easy to accomplish. The differences in skill level and philosophical orientations of osteopathic physicians, chiropractors, physical therapists, massage therapists, and athletic trainers are considerable. For example, there are many osteopathic physicians who do no manipulation, while some athletic trainers and physical therapists are well trained in the use of manipulation techniques. This makes it impossible to accurately predict what treatment a patient will receive based only on a practitioner's educational degree. This requires referring doctors, health care providers and patients to screen carefully to determine if the practitioner is able to meet their individual needs.

CONCLUSIONS

Although there is limited research definitively proving the efficacy of massage or manipulation in athletes, there is considerable anecdotal evidence to support its use. Most commonly, a short course of these treatments along with other medical care can help improve function enough to justify their use. More rigorous research will help identify the roles of manipulation and massage in patient care.

ACKNOWLEDGMENTS

The authors would like to thank Lynn Brumm, D.O.; Professor of Family Medicine and Athletic Department Consultant, Michigan State University College of Osteopathic Medicine; Stanley Daniels, D.C., Lansing, Michigan; Kurt Heinking, D.O., Chicago College of Osteopathic Medicine; Whitney Lowe, Licensed Massage Therapist, Orthopedic Massage Education and Research Institute; Chris Reay, Licensed Massage Therapist, Creative Wellness Holistic Health Center; and Gail Shafer, OTR, Assessment Rehabilitation Management, for their time and valuable input.

REFERENCES

1. Kamenetz HL: History of massage, in Basmajian JV (ed.), *Manipulation, Traction and Massage*, 3rd ed., Baltimore, Williams & Wilkins, 1985:214, 228.

2. Braverman DL, Schulman RA: Massage techniques in rehabilitation medicine. *Phys Med Rehabil Clin North Am* 1999:10, 631.

3. Goats GC: Massage—the scientific basis of an ancient art: Part 2. Physiological and therapeutic effects. *Br J Sports Med* 1994:28, 153.

4. Rechtien JJ, Andary M, Holmes TG, et al.: Manipulation, massage and traction, in Delisa JA, Gans BM (eds.), *Rehabilitation Medicine: Principles and Practice*, Philadelphia, Lippincott, 1998:521.

5. Goats GC: Massage—the scientific basis of an ancient art: Part 1. The techniques. *Br J Sports Med* 1994:28, 149.

6. Phaigh R, Perry P: *Athletic Massage*, New York, Simon and Schuster, 1984:22.

7. Callaghan MJ: The role of massage in the management of the athlete: A review. *Br J Sports Med* 1993:27, 28.

8. Drews T, Krieder B, Drinkard B, et al.: Effects of post event massage therapy on repeated endurance cycling. *Int J Sports Med* 1990:11, 407.

9. Hemmings B, Smith M, Graydon J, et al.: Effects of massage on physiological restoration, perceived recovery, and repeated sports performance. *Br J Sports Med* 2000:34, 109.

10. Drews T, Krieder RB, Drinkard B, et al.: Effects of post event massage therapy on psychological profiles of exertion, feeling and mood during a four day ultraendurance cycling event. *Med Sci Sports Exerc* 1991:23, 91.

11. Weinberg RE, Jackson A, Kolodny K: The relationship of massage and exercise to mood enhancement. *Sports Psychol* 1988:2, 202.

12. Wiktorsson-Moller M, Oberg B, Eksrand J, et al.: Effects of warming up, massage and stretching on range of motion and muscle strength in the lower extremity. *Am J Sports Med* 1983:11, 249.

13. Weber MD, Servedio FJ, Woodall WR: The effects of three modalities on delayed onset muscle soreness. *J Orthoped Sports Phys Therapy* 1994:20, 236.

14. Smith LL, Keating MN, Holber D, et al.: The effects of athletic massage on delayed onset muscle soreness, creatinine kinase, and neutrophil count: A preliminary report. *J Orthoped Sports Phys Ther* 1994:19, 93.

15. Yackzan L, Adams C, Francis KT: The effects of ice massage on delayed muscle soreness. *Am J Sports Med* 1984:12, 159.

16. Rodenburg J, Steenbeek D, Schiereck P, et al.: Warm-up, stretching and massage diminish harmful effects of eccentric exercise. *Int J Sports Med* 1994:15, 414.

17. Ernst E: Does post-exercise massage treatment reduce delayed onset muscle soreness? A systematic review. *Br J Sports Med* 1998:32, 212.

18. Gehlsen GM, Ganion LR, Helfst R: Fibroblast responses to variation in soft tissue mobilization pressure. *Med Sci Sports Exerc* 1999:31, 531.

19. Blackman PG, Simmons LR, Crossley KM: Treatment of chronic exertional anterior compartment syndrome with massage: A pilot study. *Clin J Sports Med* 1998:8, 14.

20. Balke B, Anthony J, Wyatt F: The effects of massage treatment on exercise fatigue. *Clin Sports Med* 1989:1, 189.

21. Rinder A, Sutherland C: An investigation of the effects of massage on quadriceps performance after exercise fatigue. *Complementary Ther Nursing Midwifery* 1995:1, 99.

22. Tiidus PM, Shoemaker JK: Effleurage massage, muscle blood flow and long-term post-exercise strength recovery. *Int J Sports Med* 1995:16, 478.

23. Gupta S, Goswami A, Sadhukhan AK, et al.: Comparative study of lactate removal in short term massage of extremities, active recovery and a passive recovery period after supramaximal exercise sessions. *Int J Sports Med* 1996:17, 106.

24. Cafarelli E, Sim J, Carolan B, et al.: Vibratory massage and short-term recovery from muscular fatigue. *Int J Sports Med* 1990:11, 474.

25. Shoemaker JK, Tiidus PM, Mader R: Failure of manual massage to alter limb blood flow: Measures by doppler ultrasound. *Med Sci Sports Exerc* 1997:29, 610.

26. Boone T, Cooper R: The effect of massage on oxygen consumption at rest. *Am J Chinese Med* 1995:23, 37.

27. Tiidus P: Manual massage and recovery of muscle function following exercise: A literature review. *J Orthopaed Sports Phys Ther* 1997:25, 107.

28. Morelli M, Seaborne DE, Sullivan J: H-reflex modulation during manual massage of human triceps surae. *Arch Phys Med Rehabil* 1991:72, 915.

29. Sullivan SJ, Williams LRT, Seaborne DE, et al.: Effects of massage on alpha motoneuron excitability. *Phys Ther* 1991:71, 555.

30. Personal communication, Whitney Lowe, massage therapist.

31. Personal communication, Kurt Heinking, D.O.

32. Brunarski DJ: Clinical trials of spinal manipulation: A critical appraisal and review of the literature. *J Manipulative Physiol Ther* 1984:7, 243.

33. Koes BW, Assendelft WJJ, Heijden GJMG, et al.: Spinal manipulation and mobilization for back and neck pain—a blinded review. *Br Med J* 1991:303, 1298.

34. Shekelle PG, Adams AH, Chassin MR, et al.: Spinal manipulation for low back pain. *Ann Intern Med* 1992:117, 590.

35. Di Fabio RP: Efficacy of manual therapy. *Phys Ther* 1992:72, 853.

36. Twomey L, Taylor J: Exercise and spinal manipulation in the treatment of low back pain. *Spine* 1995:5, 615.

37. U.S. Department of Health and Human Services: Acute low back problems in adults. AHCPR Publication No. 95-0642, Washington, U.S. Government Printing Office, 1994.

38. Cibulka MT, Delitto A: A comparison of two different methods to treat hip pain in runners. *J Orthopaed Sports Phys Ther* 1993:17, 172.

39. Cibulka MR, Sinacore DR, Cromer GS, et al.: Unilateral hip rotation range of motion asymmetry in patients with sacroiliac joint regional pain. *Spine* 1998:23, 1009.

40. Brier SR, Nyfield B: A comparison of hip and lumbopelvic inflexibility and low back pain in runners and cyclists. *J Manipulative Physiol Ther* 1995:18, 25.

41. LaBan MM, Meerschaert JR, Taylor RS, et al.: Symphyseal and sacroiliac joint pain associated with pubic symphysis instability. *Arch Phys Med Rehabil* 1978:59, 470.

42. Bachrach RM: Team physician #3. The relationship of low back/pelvic somatic dysfunctions to dance injuries. *Orthopaed Rev* 1988:17, 1037.

43. Ellison JB, Rose SJ, Sahrmann SA: Patterns of hip rotation range of motion: A comparison between healthy subjects and patients with low back pain. *Phys Ther* 1990:70, 537.

44. Janda V: *Muscle Function Testing*, Butterworths, London, 1983.

45. Geraci MC: Rehabilitation of pelvis, hip and thigh injuries in sports. *Phys Med Rehabil Clin North Am* 1994:5, 157.

46. Greenman P: *Principles of Manual Medicine*, Baltimore, Williams & Wilkins, 1996.

47. Ward R (ed.): *Foundations of Osteopathic Medicine*, Baltimore, Williams & Wilkins, 1997.

48. Kuchera ML, Goodridge JP: Lower extremities, in Ward R (ed.), *Foundations of Osteopathic Medicine*, Baltimore, Williams & Wilkins, 1997.

49. Bourdillon JF, Day EA, Bookhout MR: *Spinal Manipulation*, Oxford, Butterworth-Heinemann, 1992.

50. English WR: Manual medicine techniques used in the management of musculoskeletal (somatic) dysfunction of the lower extremities. *Phys Med Rehabil Clin North Am* 1996:7, 811.

51. Prokop LL, Wieting MJ: The use of manipulation in sports medicine practice. *Phys Med Clin North Am* 1996:7, 915.

52. Mitchell FL Jr, Moran PS, Pruzzo NA: *An Evaluation and Treatment Manual of Osteopathic Muscle Energy Procedures*, Valley Park, Mo, Mitchell, Moran and Pruzzo Associates, 1979.

53. Jones LH: *Strain and Counterstrain*, Colorado Springs, Colo, American Academy of Osteopathy, 1981.

54. Johnston WL, Friedman HD: *Functional Methods*, Indianapolis, American Academy of Osteopathy, 1994.

55. Magoun HI: *Osteopathy in the Cranial Field*, Kirksville, Mo, Journal Printing Company, 1976.

Chapter 44

THERAPEUTIC EXERCISE

Josef H. Moore and
Gregory P. Ernst

INTRODUCTION

To address the basic principles of therapeutic exercise, providers should remember that athletes in general and runners in particular react differently to injury, from both a physiological and psychological perspective. This, however, should not affect the overall goals of therapeutic exercise in returning patients to asymptomatic movement and function, permitting them to resume a safe and normal running schedule. Ideally, providers should implement an evidenced-based approach when establishing criteria to administer an effective therapeutic exercise program. In principle, rehabilitation through exercise prescription should be based on randomized clinical trials. Unfortunately, whereas the scientific methods of exercise are ideal, they are not always available. Therefore clinicians must also rely on theoretical and anecdotal applications of therapeutic exercise, in a sense the art of sports medicine. The fundamental premise of incorporating one's knowledge regarding the physiological effects of therapeutic exercise on the neuromusculoskeletal, cardiovascular, and respiratory systems, combined with current clinical and scientific research, provides an excellent foundation on which to rehabilitate all runners, from elite athletes to recreational joggers.

This chapter is designed to give clinicians a useable criterion-based approach for treating both surgical and nonsurgical running-related pathologies. This approach is presented as an established model with an overview of the physiological principles for therapeutic exercise, based on available and current scientific evidence. The University of Virginia (UVA)-Baylor Model (Fig. 44–1) for intervention and progression, first conceptualized by Dr. Joe Gieck at the University of Virginia, provided clinicians with a guide for using accepted criteria for implementation and progression of therapeutic exercise in injured athletes. The authors and faculty of the U.S. Army-Baylor University Physical Therapy Program have maintained Dr. Gieck's original concepts of the model but have modified it to incorporate the respective responsibilities for both providers and patients. The model assumes that the provider is competent in performing a diagnostic and functional evaluation for neuromusculoskeletal injury, in understanding the physiology of healing tissues, and in implementing the basic concepts of exercise physiology for musculoskeletal injuries.

FOUNDATION FOR THERAPEUTIC EXERCISE

The foundational concepts for proper implementation of therapeutic exercise encompass not only the role and responsibilities of the provider in formulating an accurate diagnosis and effective intervention, but also the patient's inherent responsibilities for recovery and well-being. Clinicians have long understood the

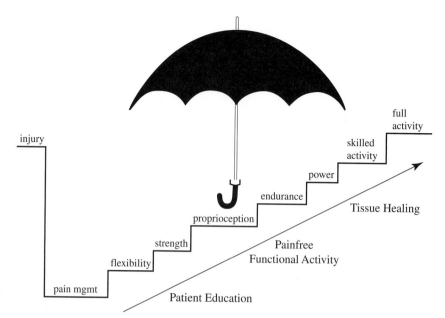

Figure 44–1. The UVA-Baylor Model for intervention and progression.

necessity of educating and encouraging patients to be more self-reliant. Unfortunately, it is an area in which we sometimes put too little emphasis both clinically and in research. Ultimately the goal is to return the patient to preinjury running status in the most effective and efficient manner, with the hope of educating the patient on the safe return to running and on preventative measures for potential future injuries.

Role of the Provider

Providers play a unique role in attempting to manage patients with running-related injuries. It is probably not enough simply to perform a comprehensive examination and prescribe an intervention limited to the injury itself. Runners, whether they are recreational or elite athletes, typically do not have the patience to allow for proper tissue healing, or for the time necessary to capitalize on the benefits of therapeutic exercise for a variety of impairments. Therefore, providers should also assume the role of a counselor. It helps to counsel a patient on the physical nature of the injury, and on the psychological component as well, which sometimes is just as perplexing. Runners as patients typically respond better when they are educated about their injury and *why* the intervention is being prescribed.

Provider's Responsibilities

Each of us in our own way has developed a methodology by which we implement a patient care plan. The plan usually involves a problem-solving process whereby clinical decisions are made based on the patient's signs and symptoms, functional limitations, and personal goals for returning to running. To implement

an effective plan, which may or may not incorporate therapeutic exercise, providers have inherent responsibilities to their clients. Although responsibilities vary based on location and level of practice, the following seven are identified as fairly generic for most providers.

First, providers should remain current through scientific literature on all aspects of running-related pathology and proposed interventions. Second, providers must comprehend the interrelationships among the anatomy, biomechanics, and pathomechanics of the injured segment. They must have a thorough understanding of tissue healing and its relationship to exercise prescription. Next, providers must be able not only to perform a competent and comprehensive examination of the patient, but also to interpret the findings properly in order to prescribe an effective intervention. Providers must have an understanding of the potential adverse effects and contraindications to exercise based on the nature of the injury, the stages of tissue healing, and the overall health of the patient. In establishing therapeutic goals, providers must take into consideration the needs of the patient. Finally, but certainly not last in terms of importance, providers must educate the patient regarding management of the condition, injury prevention, and overall wellness. The patient as a consumer needs to buy into the plan, which means he or she must also assume responsibilities.

Patient's Responsibilities

Although not all patients seek magical cures, expecting to be healed instantly, our society seems more inclined to be passive when it comes to health care, passive in the sense that patients expect (and sometimes demand) that health care providers assume full responsibility for recovery and, in a sense, cure. It probably goes without saying that patients deserve competent providers who will effectively diagnose and prescribe an appropriate intervention. However, patients must assume responsibilities for recovery and well-being. This is certainly true when therapeutic exercise is a part of the intervention. The umbrella in the UVA-Baylor Model is symbolic of the patient's responsibility to comply with the prescribed intervention and guidance from the provider.

BASIC CONCEPTS

When describing the basic concepts of therapeutic exercise, authors may vary their content based on area of specialization or experience. This section incorporates those concepts, which provide a basis on which to understand and implement the basic principles of therapeutic exercise, regardless of specialty.

Skeletal Muscle Anatomy and Physiology

It is beyond the scope of this chapter to provide an in-depth discussion on skeletal muscle anatomy and physiology. However, a quick review of skeletal muscle structure and function as it relates to therapeutic exercise should be useful. Running requires the functional use of several skeletal muscles, which not only produce moments about joints but also assist with joint stabilization.[1] It is seldom difficult to discuss with patients the mobility function of skeletal muscle in that most people understand that movement is linked to muscular contraction. However, the physiology and potential for injury and recovery involved with different types of muscular contractions are less-well appreciated by patients and providers alike. An equally important function of skeletal muscle, which is even less appreciated by most individuals, is the contribution of muscle to joint stability.[2] Muscular contraction not only generates rotational forces at the joints being moved but also assists in joint stability through compressive forces at the joint.[2] This is certainly true in closed-chain exercise or weightbearing of the lower extremities during running. The following sections briefly review the structural components of skeletal muscle and its relationship to neural mechanisms and function. Readers are encouraged to consult anatomy texts for more detail, which would include muscle fiber composition.

Structure

Skeletal muscles are microscopically striated and considered to be voluntary in nature.[3] They are enclosed within connective tissues and grouped into bundles of fibers, which are referred to as fascicules. The arrangement of fascicules in terms of length and diameter varies throughout the body. The fascicules may present either parallel to the long axis (strap or fusiform), at an angle to the long axis (unipennate, bipennate, or multipennate), or spiraling around the long axis.[2,3] The arrangement of muscle fibers is functionally important in that it affects the length-shortening relationship of skeletal muscle. Therefore one must remember that there is not always a direct relationship between the length of a muscle fiber and the distance it is able to move a bony lever.[2]

There are three primary types of muscle fibers in skeletal muscles.[4] For purposes of discussion in this section the fiber types will be referred to as type I or slow-twitch oxidative (SO), type IIB or fast-twitch glycolytic (FG), and type IIA or fast-twitch oxidative glycolytic (FOG). Fiber types may be differentiated based on their oxidative metabolic capabilities, fiber diameters, and other properties. A fourth fiber type has been identified histologically by McDonagh et al.[5] as fast intermediate (FI), which is intermediate in fatigability. Table 44–1 provides a summary of the three primary fiber types and nomenclature in general use. Muscle

TABLE 44–1. BASIC CLASSIFICATION OF SKELETAL MUSCLE FIBER TYPES

	Type		
	I (SO)	*IIB (FG)*	*IIA (FOG)*
Muscle color	Red	White	Red
Oxidative capacity	High	Low	Very high
Glycolytic capacity	Moderate	High	High
Diameter	Small	Large	Intermediate
Motor unit size	Small	Large	Intermediate to large
Rate of fatigue	Slow	Fast	Intermediate
Contraction rate	Slow	Fast	Fast
Nerve conduction	Slow	Fast	Fast

SO = slow-twitch oxidative; FG = fast-twitch glycolytic; FOG = fast-twitch glycolytic.

fiber type and arrangement vary throughout the body. These structural variations have an affect on the function of various muscles.

The anatomical relationship of skeletal muscle fibers as a part of the motor unit is also important for normal function. The motor unit consists of the cell body of an alpha motor neuron, the motor nerve itself, and all the muscle fibers innervated by that nerve.[3] The number of motor units allocated to each fiber type varies considerably. This variation in terms of the number, size, and rate of motor units firing has an impact on muscle function.[6] Strength and speed of contraction, as well as fatigability, are related to the motor unit. Theoretically, these variations are believed to be genetically determined.

Body movement in general and running in particular are intimately related and controlled by neural mechanisms. Although the contractile process is initiated by a stimulus transmitted through an alpha motor neuron, various peripheral receptors are responsible for modifying or influencing the quality of movement. The stretch reflex provides an important contribution to the maintenance of upright posture. The primary receptor responsible for affecting this reflex appears to be the muscle spindle.[3,7] The muscle spindle, located within the muscle, is parallel to the skeletal muscle fibers.[3,7] Its primary function is to perceive length or change in length of the muscle fibers.[3,7]

Physiology

Skeletal muscle's functional role in movement is related to its ability to develop tension and exert force on a bony segment, thereby generating torque about a joint axis.[2,8] Understanding the normal mechanical principles that produce this function are essential when considering tissue dynamics of injured muscle. This section focuses on the length-tension relationship of skeletal muscle as it relates to types of muscular contraction used while running.

There is a direct relationship between tension generated within the muscle and the length of the muscle.[2,9] This relationship exemplifies that tension generated in skeletal muscle is a direct function of the magnitude of overlap between the actin and myosin filaments.[10,11] The optimal length at which a muscle is most efficient at developing tension is approximately 1.2 times longer than resting length.[2] Muscle tension and efficiency are therefore reduced when the muscle is lengthened or shortened beyond optimal length. The amount of tension generated and the length of muscle are essential in producing torque about a joint, in conjunction with biomechanical variables such as angle of pull, the moment arm, and lever arm length.[8,11] These factors are important considerations when prescribing

therapeutic exercises for runners with limited range of motion or decreased strength.

Skeletal muscle contraction is typically discussed as it relates to muscle length and angular velocity of a given joint, such as isometric, isotonic, or isokinetic contraction.[2,11,12] When considering skeletal muscle action during running, primarily in the lower extremities, it seems more useful to look at concentric and eccentric contractions. Certainly the latter of the two is very important when discussing injury prevention and rehabilitation in that eccentric contractions are theorized to be associated more with muscle injury and soreness.[11,12] Eccentric action of muscle produces more work, generating more muscle force for the same velocity of movement that is activated concentrically (Fig. 44–2). Concentric contraction or positive work results when the internal force produced by the muscle exceeds the external resistance placed on the muscle.[13,14] In this situation the muscle shortens, producing angular motion at a particular joint, whereas eccentric muscle contraction or negative work results from an already shortened muscle in which the external force applied to the muscle exceeds the internal force of the muscle.[14] During this type of contraction the muscle lengthens while continuing to maintain tension. This lengthening contraction primarily works to decelerate a limb, essentially producing a braking function by the muscle.[2,11,12] For example, during running the quadriceps are eccentrically loaded during heel strike to absorb the momentum of the body. Likewise, the hamstring muscles eccentrically contract during the swing phase of running to control and decelerate the lower leg. Therapeutic

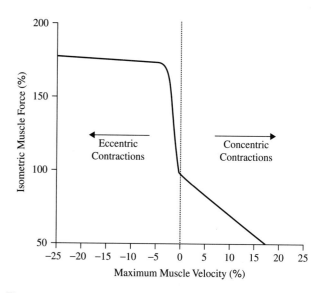

Figure 44–2. Relationship between velocity of movement and torque development capability.

exercises should take into account both concentric and eccentric work.

Physiology of Tissue Repair

A variety of cellular and tissue responses usually take place postoperatively or following a musculoskeletal injury. Appropriate examination of the injury, with a thorough understanding of wound healing and tissue repair, forms the basis for therapeutic intervention. Providers must recognize the vast number of variables that may confound wound healing, which then negate any "cookbook" intervention for every runner. The goal of managing running injuries should be to promote tissue repair and safe functional return to work/play while minimizing the potentially harmful effects of a traumatic inflammatory response. Providers are increasingly challenged to understand cellular responses to injury in order to justify the value of any therapeutic intervention.

Musculoskeletal trauma, regardless of the tissue(s) involved and mechanism of injury, responds similarly throughout the stages of healing, although the times may vary somewhat.[15,16] When considering repair of skeletal muscle, remember to differentiate between contractile and noncontractile (connective tissue) components since both have respective cells responsible for tissue regeneration. The bottom line is that providers should be able to recognize the physiological processes associated with injuries in order to establish a basis for initiating or changing a treatment program to ensure proper healing and the earliest safe return to activity. The inflammatory response denotes the earliest stage of wound healing, followed by the proliferative and maturation and remodeling stages.[15-17] The following description of the stages of tissue healing is only a brief review of the physiological responses involved.

Inflammatory Stage

The inflammatory or acute stage of tissue healing occurs within the first 0 to 6 days.[15-18] Inflammation is a vascular, cellular, and humoral response to trauma. The classic description of the inflammatory response includes the cardinal signs of inflammation: redness (rubor), swelling (tumor), pain (dolor), warmth (calor), and loss of function (functio laesa).[15-18] This response is important for tissue healing to begin and to prepare the injured site for the repair process. It partially accomplishes this through the clotting mechanism, which is precipitated by fibrin production, and through phagocytosis of debris within and around the wound.[15-18] During this stage new capillary beds are formed, and early fibroblastic activity is initiated. The inflammatory process is normal and *cannot* be prevented. Although as providers we cannot speed up the healing process, we can intervene to reduce the deleterious effects of prolonged tissue inflammation and provide for optimal healing of the injured tissues.

Typically during this stage, intervention according to the UVA-Baylor Model is limited to the first step of pain management and sometimes includes the second step of gentle pain-free motion to restore flexibility. There are several means by which pain is managed, ranging from oral and injectable medications, modalities such as transcutaneous nerve stimulation (TENS) and ice, and temporary rest or immobilization. The goal of intervening at this point is to protect the injured tissues, control the inflammatory response, and provide an optimal environment within the tissues for healing.

The use of ice with rest, ice, compression, and elevation (RICE) is effective in managing inflammation early in the healing process. The concept of cryokinetics, motion with ice, also formulated by Dr. Gieck, works very well when beginning early motion. Pain-free nonweightbearing motion may also help during this stage by reducing adhesions and promoting early healing. However, caution must be used not to exacerbate the patient's symptoms and prolong the inflammatory response. Temporary rest or immobilization may be necessary but should be used judiciously due to its deleterious effects, particularly for mild soft tissue injuries. For many runners this is a difficult period in which they frequently attempt to ignore their symptoms and run through the pain, frequently prolonging their recovery.

Proliferative Stage

The proliferative or subacute stage of tissue healing marks the beginning of the repair process. This stage may begin as early as the second day after trauma and coincides with the resolution of tissue inflammation.[15-18] Depending on the extent of tissue damage and early management, this stage usually lasts 1 to 2 weeks after injury, but it may last up to 6 or 8 weeks. During this stage collagen formation and granulation tissue within the wound provide the early framework for repair and tissue regeneration.[15-18] The general method of healing for soft tissues is fibrous repair.

Several factors affecting tissue healing during this stage should be taken into consideration before implementing an effective intervention. If healing tissue is kept absolutely immobile, the resultant fibrous repair may be weakened. When there are no natural forces on healing tissue, collagen is laid down haphazardly. Fibrous healing is stronger if natural movements are encouraged. In applying Wolff's law, gentle normal movements provide natural tensions in healing tissue, resulting in a stronger fibrous healing.

Wound closure takes approximately 5 to 8 days in muscle and skin, and 3 to 5 weeks in tendon and ligament. Fibrous healing will be poor in the presence of continued inflammation, a finding that is unfortunately not uncommon as a result of improper intervention or overzealous runners who don't listen to their bodies.

During this stage, pain-free controlled motion is important, which now includes the steps through endurance in the UVA-Baylor Model. Gentle natural tension should be transmitted to the new collagen bundles as they are laid down, to ensure correct architectural lineup. These movements are usually appropriate as early as the fourth day postinjury. It is important to remember that patients shouldn't progress with exercise if they're experiencing pain at rest. As Dr. Gieck often stresses, "sometimes less is more." The types of therapeutic exercise are discussed in more detail later in this chapter, but they could consist of a variety of open and closed-chain exercises for strengthening, proprioception, and muscular endurance.

Maturation and Remodeling Stage

Wound maturation and remodeling, associated with the chronic stage of tissue repair, occur late in the healing process. This stage may overlap with the proliferative stage as early as the second week postinjury.[15–18] There should be no signs of inflammation present; the patient typically feels asymptomatic with normal activities of daily living and low-intensity exercise. Some runners may be able to resume running at a pace and distance less than normal for their level. Again, care is in order to prevent reinjury to the healing tissues. During this stage connective tissue maturation results from collagen fiber production.[15–18] There is a continued increase in wound strength while the scar tissue begins to contract and remodel. Wound strength is related to the tensile and shear forces placed on the connective tissue, which aligns the collagen fibers to the applied stress.[15–18] This level of therapeutic exercise corresponds to the upper steps on the UVA-Baylor Model and positions the patient to resume full activity.

Effects of Immobilization and Deconditioning

Just as an athlete's body responds to training, it also responds to lack of training. These changes can occur both locally within the affected joints or muscles and also centrally involving the cardiovascular system and motor control areas of the central nervous system. These changes are most pronounced when an athlete suffers a significant injury that requires immobilization of a joint. When this occurs, significant changes occur in the bone, cartilage, ligaments, tendons, and muscle surrounding the immobilized joint. Bone surrounding an immobilized joint undergoes regional

osteoporosis.[19] Ligaments weaken at insertion sites as Sharpey's fibers are affected.[20] Water content of the cartilage is decreased, and the proteoglycan content decreases.[20] This may lead to cartilage softening and thinning, which makes the cartilage more susceptible to injury. Tendons and ligaments become weaker and less stiff.[21] It has been demonstrated in animal studies that tendons can decrease in strength up to 50% with only 8 weeks of immobilization.[22] Finally, muscles will obviously atrophy and weaken with immobilization, fast twitch fibers more so than slow twitch fibers.[23] There will also be an increase in the connective tissue component in muscle with immobilization, reducing the extensibility of muscle.[2] Aerobic capacity can also decrease with immobility. One study showed that maximum oxygen consumption decreased 25% with 20 days of bed rest.[24]

The clinician needs to consider all these significant changes that occur with immobilization when working with a runner who is recovering from surgery or other significant injury. Obviously, most running injuries do not require such immobilization. However, when a runner's activity decreases from his or her intense training regimen, the tissues of the musculoskeletal system can certainly suffer. In a strength training study, strength decreased to pretraining levels within 8 weeks of discontinuing training.[25] The clinician needs to come up with an alternative activity that will minimize this degradation and to return the runner gradually to full activity, which will allow the musculoskeletal system to rebuild and adapt to the new stresses.

Weaklink

The weaklink concept refers to the fact that when a runner has an injury, he or she can only fully rehabilitate to a level that is tolerated by the injured tissue. This concept has an implication that clinicians often neglect. If a runner has an acute tendinitis, for example, most clinicians recognize that this tendon is a weaklink and are careful about not overloading the tendon. However, often the entire lower extremity is rested, which results in deconditioning of joints and muscles throughout the rest of the lower extremity. The clinician must provide a rehabilitation program that will continue to apply loads to other muscles and joints of the extremity while appropriately resting the injured tissue.

Transfer of Training

The transfer of training concept allows for training effects to occur in a limb not capable of exercise. As stated above, it is desirable to exercise the affected lower extremity in alternate ways to prevent weakening in surrounding joints and muscles. This is sometimes not possible for various reasons such as immobilization of an extremity. In these cases, the athlete can exercise the opposite limb. Although this does not provide as strong a benefit as actually exercising the involved limb, studies have shown that training effects occur in a resting limb while the opposite limb trains.[25] Transfer of training may also refer to the mode or type or exercise. Strength training may have some effect on endurance, and training at a fast speed can also increase strength at slower speeds.[18] However, because of one additional concept to be discussed below, the best effect of training is accomplished by training in a manner that is specific to the athlete's event.

Proximal Stability

Proximal stability before distal mobility is a concept clinicians cannot neglect. This concept is often mentioned in regard to rehabilitation of upper extremity injuries. Although the proximal lower extremity is highly stable due to its body configuration, the concept of proximal muscle strength, even when rehabilitating distal lower extremity injuries, is vitally important. Foot and ankle injuries make up the majority of running injuries. Many of these injuries are due to the repetitive pounding of the body weight on the joints. This force can be as much as three times body weight.[26] The proximal muscle groups, particularly the hip and knee extensors, play a vital role in absorbing this impact through eccentric contractions. Weakness of these proximal muscles may place more demand on distal musculotendinous units to absorb the shock or may place additional stress on bones and joints. Therefore, strengthening proximal lower extremity muscle groups may improve the shock absorption capability of the lower extremity. This is a key component of a rehabilitation program for a runner with a distal lower extremity injury.

Overload

The overload principle means that by exercising at a level above normal for that individual, adaptations will occur. These adaptations can mean greater muscle strength or endurance, aerobic capacity, and even greater bone, ligament, or tendon strength. Overload does not necessarily imply increasing the amount of resistance during a strength training exercise, but refers to changing any combination of intensity, frequency, mode of exercise, or duration. The overload principle is highly individualized and is applicable to the most elite runner and the geriatric population. The amount of overload sufficient to result in a physiologic change is usually expressed in a percent of maximum capacity. In regard to strength training, the amount of resistance needs to be at least 60% to 80% of the

athlete's maximum to result in strength gains. To increase aerobic capacity, intensity should be at least 70% of the athlete's maximal heart rate (220 − age).[27]

Specificity of Training

Specificity of training is probably the most important concept to consider when designing a rehabilitation program. This concept basically means that athletes need to train in a manner consistent with their activity. If one desires to improve jump height, he or she should train by jumping. A distance runner needs to train by running. This concept has also been termed the SAID principle, which stands for specific adaptations to imposed demands. In regard to running injuries, if a distance runner cannot run due to a foot or knee injury, the clinician needs to include an activity that will closely simulate the running action and has a cardiovascular component. Not only must the runner perform isolated, specific therapeutic exercises for his or her specific injury, but also should perform an activity like pool running, work on a stepping machine, or cross-country ski machine. Also, when planning the runner's rehabilitation program, the clinician should keep the mechanism of injury in mind. For example, if the runner has an overuse injury related to deceleration, the athlete should train the musculotendinous unit in this manner. In the case of a posterior tibialis tendinitis resulting from trying to control excessive pronation, the athlete should train the posterior tibialis with eccentric exercise, preferably with a strong endurance component. Since most musculotendinous injuries are the result of strong, repetitive eccentric exercise, the athlete must train and prepare the musculotendinous unit for this demanding role. This is the basis for specificity of training: train the athlete in a manner similar to the demands of the sport.

PRINCIPLES OF THERAPEUTIC EXERCISE: INTERVENTION PROGRESSION

Up to this point the UVA-Baylor Model has been addressed in terms of the overall concept as it relates to the provider's responsibility to prescribe an effective intervention and the inherent responsibilities, which must be assumed by patients. The earlier discussion on tissue healing mentioned the progressive steps of the model, which are now addressed more fully.

Pain Management

In 1979 the International Association for the Study of Pain defined pain as an "an unpleasant sensory and emotional experience associated with actual or potential tissue damage." Pain is certainly subjective in nature and varies in description in terms of sensation and intensity. Managing pain is an important aspect of working with patients. Although some studies have attempted to provide us with insights into pain mechanisms and modulation through the use of certain modalities, unfortunately few good randomized clinical trials have been performed. We are still looking at the tip of the iceberg, and more research is needed to address this complex issue. However, until the time comes that we have scientific evidence to support our anecdotal claims, we will continue to use certain modalities in treating patients, with the caveat that our rationale for using them is grounded in theory. One effective modality for reducing pain that has been used for decades is ice. Ice packs or ice massage should be administered throughout the inflammatory stage and after exercise or running as the patient progresses.

Pain management theories such as the gate control theory proposed by Melzak and Wall[27a] in 1965, central biasing, or noxious pain modulation, and the theory of pain modulation through neurochemical inhibitory mechanisms exceed the scope of this chapter. It is important to remember that pain serves a purpose in identifying that a problem exists; patients should pay attention to these signals during the recovery process and when returning to full activity. To have a patient progress up the steps of the UVA-Baylor Model when pain is still present at rest or with limited activity may predispose the patient to increased risk of further injury while prolonging the healing process. The problem is that pain can also be used by less-motivated individuals to maximize their disability. Once again, herein lies the art and science of providers in determining an appropriate intervention and patient goals.

Flexibility

Numerous contributing factors have been proposed for various overuse injuries in runners, the most common ones often associated with flexibility. Thus, most treatment programs include some form of stretching, generally static, ballistic, or proprioceptive neuromuscular facilitation (PNF) techniques. Static stretching involves placing the musculotendinous unit in a comfortable stretch position and holding the position for at least 15 to 30 seconds. Research has shown that holding a stretch longer than 30 seconds does not provide any additional benefit.[28] The emphasis when doing a static stretch is on the duration of the stretch. If the athlete cannot hold the stretch for at least 15 seconds, he or she should decrease the intensity so that the stretch can be held for the minimum time period. Static stretching is very safe due to the low intensity of the force applied.

Ballistic stretching involves small oscillations at the end of the range of motion of a joint. This form of stretching can improve flexibility; however, it is generally discouraged because of the greater risk of injury due to the quick stretch. The quick stretch may also cause a reflex muscle contraction due to stimulation of the muscle spindles.

The final stretching method uses PNF techniques commonly called hold-relax or contract-relax. In hold-relax stretching, the musculotendinous unit is usually put on a stretch by an assistant, another athlete, or a therapist. The athlete then contracts the muscle group being stretched while the assistant resists the motion so an isometric contraction occurs. The muscle contraction theoretically stimulates the Golgi tendon organs, resulting in relaxation of the muscle. The athlete holds this contraction for approximately 5 seconds; upon relaxing, the assistant usually notes a decrease in tension in the musculotendinous unit and takes up the slack by applying a greater stretch to that unit. This process is repeated until a maximal length change occurs. The contract-relax procedure is exactly the same, but instead of an isometric contraction, a concentric contraction is allowed before the stretch.

Several research studies have compared these stretching methods. Wallin et al.[29] showed that the contract-relax method was more effective than the ballistic method. Studies comparing PNF techniques with static stretching have been contradictory, although both have been shown to increase flexibility.[30,31]

A prerequisite for all types of stretching is proper preparation of the joint or musculotendinous unit to be stretched. It is very important that the area to be stretched be warmed up first. Active warm-up through low-intensity exercise is thought to warm tissue more thoroughly than passive heating, as in applying a heating pad. It has been shown that heating collagenous tissue while stretching and maintaining the stretch while the tissue cools results in the most elongation of tissue.[32] Stretching while the extremity is warm not only helps one get the most out of the stretch, but also helps prevent injury.

Strength Training

Some form of strength training is often indicated during rehabilitation of a running injury. Muscular weakness may develop during the rest period of relative inactivity, or muscular weakness may have been a contributing factor to the injury. There are numerous factors to consider when designing a resistive training program for a runner with an injury.

One concern is whether the resistance should be isometric, isotonic, or isokinetic. Most rehabilitation programs will include a combination of these types depending on the patient's needs and the time course in the rehabilitation program. In isometric resistance, the athlete applies resistance against an immovable object or performs a cocontraction (contracting the agonist and antagonist simultaneously). Because the amount of resistance applied is under the control of the athlete and no joint motion occurs, isometric resistance is considered a very safe and effective mode of exercise and is often used early in the rehabilitation of an injury. The disadvantage of isometric exercise is that it is nonfunctional. A runner rarely performs an isometric contraction of a muscle during his or her sport. This is the advantage of isotonic exercise.

Isotonic exercise is the traditional "weight-lifting" exercise. This type of resistance is more functional since the joint is moving. Isotonic resistance training is conducive to progression, as the athlete can gradually increase the amount of weight lifted. Another advantage is that isotonic resistance allows acceleration and deceleration of the weight through the range of motion, which simulates functional activity better than isometric and isokinetic resistance. Another advantage is that isotonic exercise has demonstrated a positive carryover effect for joint position sense, which improves balance.[33] There are a few disadvantages. The first is that isotonic exercise is not as safe as isometric or isokinetic resistance. While lifting a weight in the midrange, an athlete may discover that it is too heavy; the athlete may try to control it, and injury may result. Therefore, heavy isotonic resistance is not appropriate in the early phases of rehabilitation. Another disadvantage is that resistance is only maximal at a small part of the complete range of motion; therefore, strength increases may not occur throughout the range of motion.

The final type is isokinetic resistance, in which the speed of the exercise is adjustable and constant throughout the range of motion. Thus, an amount of resistance is not set. As the athlete moves through the range of motion at a set speed, the isokinetic machine will match the resistance of the athlete. This is termed accommodative resistance and is considered very safe. Another advantage is that the resistance will be maximal throughout the range of motion. The main disadvantage of isokinetic resistance is that although it does allow movement throughout the range of motion, it does not allow acceleration of the joint through the range.

When using isotonic or isokinetic resistance, the clinician must also consider whether concentric, eccentric, or both types of contractions should be used. An eccentric, or lengthening, contraction is more stressful to the musculotendinous unit than a concentric, or shortening, contraction. Eccentric exercise is, however, a very important part of the rehabilitation program. Many running injuries involving musculotendinous units are the result of strong and fast eccentric contractions. A runner with excessive or prolonged pronation may get a posterior tibialis tendinitis from the overuse of this muscle in an attempt to control the pronation through eccentric contraction. Foot orthotics are often used to control this pronation, but any muscle groups that decelerate pronation should also be strengthened in a manner specific to the demands that will be placed on them (principle of specificity). Therefore, those musculotendinous units must be strengthened in an eccentric manner. Since eccentric contractions with heavy resistance are stressful to a musculotendinous unit, athletes should start with light concentric exercise. Once the athlete achieves near normal strength, emphasis should be placed on eccentric exercise. Both increasing resistance and/or increasing the speed of the exercise can increase the intensity of eccentric exercise.

Finally, the provider should determine whether strength training should be performed in a weightbearing or nonweightbearing position (also referred to as closed and open kinetic chain exercise, respectively). There are several advantages and disadvantages to each type of exercise. In the nonweightbearing position, the ankle is free to move, which is more conducive to work on mobility. The nonweightbearing position also allows isolation of specific muscle groups. For example, if the athlete wanted to work on strengthening the posterior tibialis, he or she could easily perform a combination of plantarflexion-inversion to strengthen this muscle specifically. In a weightbearing position, isolation of muscle groups is very difficult. For example, one may perform a partial squat to strengthen the quadriceps muscle group. If, however, the quadriceps are inhibited due to pain or swelling, the hip extensors and/or soleus can compensate and perform much of the knee extension.[34] This would leave very little strengthening stimulus for the quadriceps.

Nonweightbearing exercise is often best in the early stages of rehabilitation. Mobility is encouraged, isolated strengthening of weak muscles can occur, and the stress of weightbearing is removed. Strengthening in the weightbearing position does have many advantages, however. The weightbearing position simulates the athlete's activity much better than nonweightbearing activity. The muscle groups being used can be trained together to work in optimal synchrony. During running, the synchronous action of all lower extremity muscle groups is important to control motion, especially during deceleration. When a runner's heel strikes the ground, many muscle groups (including the ankle dorsiflexors, invertors, soleus, quadriceps, hip extensors, and external rotators) all contract at quite specific times to decelerate the lower extremity and control lower extremity internal rotation and pronation. If these muscle groups are trained together in a manner specific to the athlete's activity, not only does strengthening result, but also improved neuromotor skills for optimal recruitment of muscle groups.

Proprioception

Joint proprioception is often a concern for any athlete with a joint injury. Proprioception refers to the afferent and efferent volley between joint or muscle receptors and skeletal muscle. Proprioception is important for joint stability and injury prevention. When a joint is stressed to near its end range, the joint or muscle receptors are stimulated. This information is sent to the appropriate motor neurons, resulting in contraction of muscles that will stabilize the joint. Proprioception is most important in sports like soccer or basketball: quick stops or cutting activities are routine. Because running is a straight-ahead activity, proprioception is typically not a problem. However, when the athlete is running on trails or uneven surfaces, proprioception is important to stabilize the foot/ankle complex. This may be especially important for long-distance runners, as it has been shown that joint proprioception can decrease with muscle fatigue.[35] Cross-country runners or other runners who will return to running on uneven surfaces following their rehabilitation should include activities that will train their proprioceptive system. Exercises such as balancing on one leg on the floor or a balance board are helpful. The trainer or therapist can also challenge the patient further by playing catch with the athlete while he or she is balancing on one leg or gently pushing the athlete off balance and allowing him or her to regain balance. The provider can find many types of proprioceptive rehabilitation activities for the athlete in the literature on ankle instability.

Endurance

Endurance is a component of the runner's rehabilitation program that can usually be progressed at the earliest stages of injury. Cardiovascular endurance can be performed in many ways without using the affected joint or extremity. The athlete can perform stationary bicycling with the unaffected extremity or can swim with minimal or no use of the affected extremity. Endurance activities with the upper extremities such as those using an upper-body ergometer can also be performed. Muscular endurance with the affected extremity can be more difficult in the early stages of rehabilitation. As shown in the UVA-Baylor Model, once pain, flexibility, strength, and proprioception have been developed, the athlete can easily be progressed to exercises that will improve specific muscular endurance.

Muscular endurance exercise should emphasize high repetition (25 to 50) and low resistance (about 60% of maximum).

Power

The final component of rehabilitation before skilled activity is the development of power. Power is defined as work per amount of time. Power can be increased either by increased amount of work or by speed. With the high rate of joint velocity during most athletic activities, it is more functional to work on power by emphasizing speed rather than work or amount of resistance. Although power is more important for sprinters and middle-distance runners, it is also important for long-distance runners. Power workouts can initially be performed on a stationary bike, pool, stair-step machine, or similar activity. To develop power using these machines, resistance should be light, with emphasis on speed. Power workouts should also be quickly progressed to activity-specific exercise, namely, running on flat surfaces. However, the provider should keep in mind that higher-ground reaction forces are associated with increases in running speed.[36] If hills are an important component of the athlete's event, power work on hills can be gradually added to the training regime.

THERAPEUTIC EXERCISE WITH FUNCTIONAL INTEGRATION

Skilled Activity

There are almost as many protocols for the early phase of return to running as there are providers who design and implement these protocols. A single model that has been validated through a randomized clinical trial is yet to be published. Since it is so difficult to design a study addressing specific therapeutic exercises and functional activities for every possible scenario of running-related pathology, it is perhaps best for providers to prescribe an intervention based on the individual needs of the patient. This concept (not a new one) allows providers the flexibility of adapting an appropriate therapeutic exercise plan to the needs of the patient. Having said this, we still need to pursue evidence-based criteria to give all providers an effective guide in returning runners to their roads and tracks. To accompany the UVA-Baylor Model, we have provided criteria (Table 44–2) that may assist providers in advancing runners up the steps to full activity.

Full Activity: Return to Running

The fundamental idea that patients can resume their normal running routine when they are asymptomatic is seriously flawed. Findings on physical examination

TABLE 44–2. CRITERIA NECESSARY TO ADVANCE TO THE LISTED STEP IN THE UVA-BAYLOR MODEL[a]

Step	Criterion
Flexibility	Pain-free passive range of motion
Strength	Pain-free active range of motion
Proprioception	75% strength
Endurance	75% strength
Power	90% strength
Skilled activity	90% strength with normal proprioception and endurance
Full activity	90% strength with normal proprioception and endurance; successfully performs skilled activity without symptoms

[a]Criteria may vary depending on the athlete's injury and sport.

such as normal range of motion, strength, no pain, and complete willingness on the patient's part to resume running should serve as the beginning of a progressed running program. In fact some patients may have to begin with a walk-and-run program by which they are only walking for part of the time on the track or road (Table 44–3). As the late Col. Douglas A. Kersey, PT, use to emphasize frequently to all his patients, "your body will adapt to any stresses if you give it time and

TABLE 44–3. PHASES IN WALK-TO-RUN PROGRESSION AFTER AN INJURY

General Guidelines
1. Use running shoes and not court or cross-trainers.
2. Begin at an easy pace on level surfaces; no hills until at least 3–5 weeks after phase VIII.
3. Stop if increased pain, swelling, or stiffness are noted, especially while running and if symptoms are present by the next morning. Do not resume running until cleared by provider.
4. Do not run more than 3 times a week and do not run daily until 3 to 5 weeks after phase VIII.
5. Try each phase at least twice. Progress to the next phase if no increase in pain, swelling, or stiffness.
6. After phase VIII: gradually begin to increase running without walking.
7. All increments for walk-to-run progression are based on miles.

Phase	Instruction
I	Walk 2 miles at your own pace
II	Progress to walking 2 miles in 35 minutes
III	Walk ¼ Run ¼ Walk ¼ Run ¼
IV	Walk ¼ Run ¼ Walk ¼ Run ¼ Walk ¼ Run ¼ Walk ¼ Run ¼
V	Walk ¼ Run ½ Walk ¼ Run ½ Walk ¼ Run ½
VI	Walk ¼ Run ¾ Walk ¼ Run ¾
VII	Walk ¼ Run 1 Walk ¼ Run 1
VIII	Walk ¼ Run 1 Walk ¼ Run 1 Walk ¼ Run 1

gradually increase your training." In other words, moderation is the key in prescribing a safe and effective running program. One physical stress most runners should avoid in the early phase of returning to running is to run up and down hills, particularly down hills. A safe clinical prescription has been to have patients not run hills until they have resumed pain-free running for at least 3 weeks.

REFERENCES

1. Farley CT, Ferris DP: Biomechanics of walking and running: Center of mass movements to muscle action, in *Exercise and Sports Sciences Reviews*, vol 26, Philadelphia, Lippincott Williams & Wilkins, 1998:253.
2. Norkin CC, Levangie PK: *Joint Structure and Function: A Comprehensive Analysis*, 2nd ed., Philadelphia, FA Davis, 1992:1.
3. Berne RM, Levy MN: *Physiology*, 3rd ed., St. Louis, Mosby, 1993.
4. Clamann HP: Motor unit recruitment and the gradation of muscle force. *Phys Ther* 1993:73, 830.
5. McDonagh JC, Binder MD, Reinking RM, et al.: Tetrapartite classification of motor units of cat tibialis posterior. *J Neurophysiol* 1970:44, 696.
6. Sanders B: Exercise and rehabilitation concepts, in Malone TR, McPoil T, Nitz AJ (eds.), *Orthopedic and Sports Physical Therapy*, 3rd ed., St. Louis, Mosby, 1997:211.
7. Rowinski MJ: Neurobiology for orthopedic and sports physical therapy, in Malone TR, McPoil T, Nitz AJ (eds.), *Orthopedic and Sports Physical Therapy*, 3rd ed., St. Louis, Mosby, 1997:47.
8. Cornwall MW: Biomechanics of orthopedic and sports therapy, in Malone TR, McPoil T, Nitz AJ (eds.), *Orthopedic and Sports Physical Therapy*, 3rd ed., St. Louis, Mosby, 1997:65.
9. Fredericks CM: Skeletal muscle: the somatic effector, in Fredericks CM, Saladin LK (eds.), *Pathophysiology of Motor Systems: Principles and Clinical Presentations*, Philadelphia, FA Davis, 1996:30.
10. Lutz GJ, Lieber RL: Skeletal muscle myosin II structure and function, in *Exercise and Sports Sciences Reviews*, vol 27, Philadelphia, Lippincott Williams & Wilkins, 1999:63.
11. Lieber RL, Bowdin-Fowler SC: Skeletal muscle mechanics: implications for rehabilitation. *Phys Ther* 1993:73, 844.
12. Faulkner JA, Brooks SV, Opiteck JA: Injury to skeletal muscle fibers during contractions: Conditions of occurrence and prevention. *Phys Ther* 1993:73, 911.
13. O'Connel AL, Gowitzke B: *Understanding the Scientific Basis of Human Movement*, Baltimore, Williams & Wilkins, 1972.
14. Bouisset S: EMG and muscle force in normal motor activities, in Desmedt JE (ed.), *New Developments in Electromyography and Clinical Neurophysiology*, vol 1, Basle, Karger, 1973.
15. English T, Wheeler ME, Hettinga DL: Inflammatory responses of synovial joint structures, in Malone TR,

McPoil T, Nitz AJ (eds.), *Orthopedic and Sports Physical Therapy*, 3rd ed., St. Louis, Mosby, 1997:81.

16. Kloth LC, McCulloch JM: The inflammatory response to wounding, in McCulloch JM, Kloth LC, Feedar JA (eds.), *Wound Healing: Alternatives in Management*, Philadelphia, FA Davis, 1995:3.

17. Boissonnault WG: Introduction to pathology of the musculoskeletal system, in Goodman CC, Boissonnault WG (eds.), *Pathology: Implications for the Physical Therapist*. Philadelphia, WB Saunders, 1998:571.

18. Kisner C, Colby LA: *Therapeutic Exercise: Foundations and Techniques*, Philadelphia, FA Davis, 1996.

19. Enneking WF, Horowitz M: The intra-articular effects of immobilization of the human knee. *J Bone Joint Surg Am* 1972:54A, 973.

20. Akeson WH, Amiel D, Dip I, et al.: Effects of immobilization on joints. *Clin Orthop* 1987:219, 28.

21. Woo S, Gomez MA, Seguchi Y, et al.: Measurement of mechanical properties of ligament substance from a bone-ligament-bone preparation. *J Orthop Res* 1983:1, 22.

22. Enwemeka CS: Conective tissue plasticity: Ultrastructural, biomechanical and morphometric effects of physical factors on intact and regenerating tendons. *J Orthop Sports Phys Ther* 1991:14, 198.

23. Booth F: Physiologic and biomechanical effects of immobilization on muscle. *Clin Orthop* 1986:219, 15.

24. Saltin B, et al.: Response to exercise after bed rest and after training. *Circulation* 1968:38(suppl).

25. Weir JP, Houch DJ, Housh TJ, et al.: The effect of unilateral concentric weight training and detraining on joint angle specificity, cross-training, and the bilateral deficit. *J Orthop Sports Phys Ther* 1997:25, 264.

26. Ounpuu S: The biomechanics of walking and running. *Clin Sports Med* 1994:13, 843.

27. McArdle WD, Katch FI, Katch VL: *Exercise Physiology*. Philadelphia, Lea & Febiger, 1991.

28. Melzack R, Wall PD. Pain mechanisms: a new theory. Science, 150:971–979, 1965.

29. Wallin D, Ekblom B, Grahn R, et al.: Improvement of muscle flexibility: A comparison between two techniques. *Am J Sports Med* 1985:13, 263.

30. Sullivan MK, Dejulia JJ, Worrell: Effect of pelvic position ans stretching method on hamstring muscle flexibility. *Med Sci Sports Exerc* 1992:24, 1383.

31. Tanigawa MC: Comparison of the hold-relax procedure and passive mobilization on incresing muscle length. *Phys Ther* 1972:52, 725.

32. Warren CJ, Lehmann JF, Koblanski JN: Elongation of rat tail tendon: Effect of load and temperature. *Arch Phys Med Rehabil* 1971:52, 465.

33. Docherty CL, Moore JH, Arnold BL: Effects of strength training on strength development and joint position sense in functionally unstable ankles. *J Athletic Training* 1998:33, 310.

34. Ernst GP, Saliba E, Diduch D, et al.: Lower extremity compensations following anterior cruciate ligament reconstruction. *Phys Ther*, 2000:80, 251.

35. Voight ML, Hardin JA, Blackburn TA, et al.: The effects of muscle fatigue on the relationship of arm dominance to shoulder proprioception. *J Orthop Sports Phys Ther* 1996:23, 348.

36. Munro CI, Miller DI, Fuglerand AJ: Ground reaction forces in running: A reexamination. *J Biomech* 1987:20, 147.

37. Barber SD, Noyes FR, Mangine RE, et al.: Quantitative assessment of functional limitations in normal and anterior cruciate ligament-deficient kness. *Clin Orthop* 1990:225, 204.

38. Noyes F, Barber SD, Mangine RE: Abnormal lower limb symmetry determined by function hop tests after anterior cruciate ligament rupture. *Am J Sports Med* 1991:19, 513.

Chapter 45

AQUA RUNNING

Robert P. Wilder and
David K. Brennan

INTRODUCTION

Aqua running is an effective form of cardiovascular conditioning for both injured athletes and those who desire a low-impact aerobic workout. Sufficient cardiovascular responses have been demonstrated to result in a training effect. Deep-water exercise is thus being used in treatment and conditioning programs for a number of rehabilitation populations. This is especially true in the field of sports medicine, in which aqua running is used as an effective form of cardiovascular conditioning for injured athletes as well as for others who desire a low-impact aerobic workout.

Aqua running, or deep-water running, consists of simulated running in the deep end of a pool aided by a flotation device (vest or belt) that maintains the head above water. The participant may be held in one location by a tether cord, essentially running in place, or may actually run through the water across the width of the pool. The tether serves to increase resistance, to assist in maintaining a nearly vertical posture, and to facilitate monitoring of exercise by a physician, therapist, or coach. No contact is made with the bottom of the pool, thus eliminating impact. The elimination of weight load on joints makes this an ideal method for rehabilitating or conditioning injured athletes, particularly those with foot, ankle, or knee injuries for whom running on land is contraindicated.

Several positive effects of incorporating aqua running into a training program are summarized below:

1. Improvement or maintenance of fitness without associated risk of impact loading
2. Improvement of biomechanics for running (especially upper-body mechanics)
3. Decrease in thermal stress
4. Active recovery on days following hard workouts or races
5. Avoidance of training boredom through creative workouts
6. Increase in social component by allowing runners of all abilities to train together

An understanding of the bioengineering principles of the aquatic environment, proper technique, physiologic response, and methods of exercise prescription help practitioners incorporate aqua running into rehabilitation and training programs.

PRINCIPLES OF HYDROTHERAPY

Several properties of water make it an ideal environment for exercise.[1]

Buoyancy
Buoyancy supports a body submerged in water from the downward pull of gravity. The submerged body

seems to lose weight equal to the weight of the water displaced, resulting in less stress and pressure on bone, muscle, and connective tissue.

Drag Force

The viscosity and drag force of water provides a resistance that is proportional to the effort exerted, much like running into a stiff wind. This adds to the cardiovascular challenge of aquatic exercise without having impact stress on joints and soft tissue.

Hydrostatic Pressure

Hydrostatic pressure (i.e., pressure exerted by water on a submerged body) is proportional to depth and equal in all directions. It is thought to aid cardiovascular function by promoting venous return.

Specific Heat

Specific heat is the amount of heat needed to raise the temperature of a substance by 1°C. The specific heat of water is several times that of air; therefore, the rate of heat loss in water is much greater than the rate of heat loss to air at the same temperature. This is an especially important consideration in warmer climates, where heat illness is a significant source of morbidity. It is also helpful in training injured athletes who are deconditioned and not acclimated to exercise in warm environments.

Temperature

The aquatic environment allows regulation of the temperature during exercise. An ideal range appears to be 82°C to 86°F (28°C to 30°C), where little heat is stored and performance is not impaired. In our experience, competitive athletes typically prefer a slightly cooler environment.

BIOMECHANICS OF AQUA RUNNING

The form of running in water is patterned as closely as possible after that used on land (Fig. 45–1). For the runner (or any athlete whose sport requires running), aqua running therefore represents a biomechanically specific means of conditioning during a rehabilitation program or when supplementing regular training. This has special importance, as the effects of training include not only improvement in cardiac and pulmonary performance but also improvement in those muscle groups that undergo enzyme, capillary density, and other adaptations to exercise. Compared with land-based running, the elimination of weightbearing and the addition of resistance in aqua running change the relative contribution of each muscle group. Every effort is made, therefore, to reproduce the running

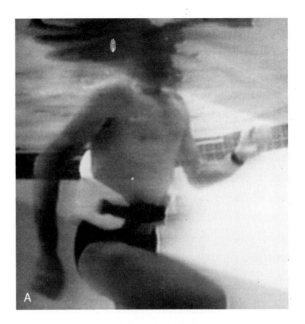

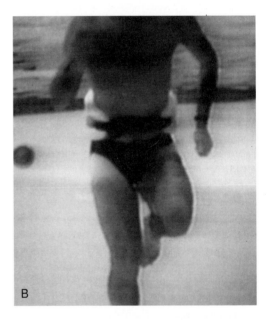

Figure 45–1. The form of running in water closely mimics the form used on land. Notice that the arm carriage is identical to that used with land-based running. (*a*) Lateral view (closeup). (*b*) Frontal view. (*Courtesy of Houston International Running Center, Houston TX; used with permission.*)

form used on land and to ensure the use of the same muscle groups.

The following guidelines will assist the patient in maintaining proper form during aqua running[2]:

1. The water line should be at the shoulder level. The mouth should be comfortably out of the water without cervical spine extension. The head should be looking straight ahead, with the neck unflexed.

2. The body should assume a position slightly forward of the vertical, with the spine maintained in a neutral position.

3. Arm motion is identical to that used on land, with primary motion at the shoulder. Hands are held lightly clenched.

4. Hip flexion should reach 60 to 80 degrees. As the hip is being flexed, the leg is extended at the knee (from the flexed position). When end hip flexion is reached, the lower leg should be perpendicular to the horizontal. The hip and knee are then extended together, the knee reaching full extension when the hip is in a neutral position (0 degrees flexion). As the hip is extended, the leg is flexed at the knee. These movements are repeated, and throughout the cycle the foot undergoes dorsiflexion and plantarflexion at the ankle. The ankle is in a position of dorsiflexion when the hip is in a neutral position and the leg extended at the knee. Plantarflexion is assumed as the hip is extended and the leg flexed. Dorsiflexion is reassumed as the hip is flexed and the leg extended. Underwater viewing demonstrates that inversion and eversion accompanies dorsiflexion and plantarflexion, similar to land-based running.

EXERCISE RESPONSE TO AQUA RUNNING

The metabolic responses to aqua running and land-based running differ significantly.[3,4] Nonetheless, aqua running elicits sufficient cardiovascular response to result in a training effect, thus supporting anecdotal evidence of its usefulness in the rehabilitation of the athlete. The American College of Sports Medicine Guidelines for Exercise Prescription state that to obtain a training effect, one must exercise three to five times a week at an intensity level between 40% and 85% of maximum oxygen uptake ($\dot{V}O_2max$) or 55% to 90% of maximum heart rate. This level should be maintained for 15 to 60 minutes.[5] Studies have demonstrated that aqua running elicits responses well within these suggested ranges.

Maximal Physiologic Responses
Several studies have compared the maximal physiologic responses with aqua running and land-based running.[6–16] Important measures of response to exercise of maximal intensity include $\dot{V}O_2max$ and maximal heart rate. $\dot{V}O_2max$ values during supported deep-water running (with a flotation device) are 73% to 92% of those values obtained during land-based running. Heart rates during deep-water running range from 86% to 95% of those values obtained during land-based running.

Similar rating of perceived exertion (RPE) values have been reported for both deep-water running and treadmill running consistent with maximal effort. Cardiorespiratory efficiency as evidenced by O_2 pulse can be calculated as $\dot{V}O_2/HR$. Maximal O_2 pulse during deep-water running has been reported to be lower than during treadmill running.[8,15] Reports have varied regarding lactate and ventilation. Blood lactate concentrations following deep-water running have been reported as higher,[8] lower,[9,14,15] and similar[12] to those following maximal treadmill running. Ventilation during deep-water running has been reported as both similar[4,12] and lower[4,6,13,14] than during treadmill running.

Submaximal Physiologic Responses
Important relationships have also been noted during deep-water running at submaximal intensities. For a given level of perceived exertion, heart rates and oxygen uptake levels tend to be lower during deep-water running than during treadmill running. During graded exercise testing, Svedenhag and Seger[8] noted higher central and peripheral RPEs during deep-water running at any given $\dot{V}O_2$ or heart rate compared with treadmill running at the same intensity. Navia[11] reported a similar relationship between RPE and physiologic responses during graded exercise. Higher RPE values were expressed during deep-water running at any given heart rate than during treadmill running. A similar relationship was noted for RPE and $\dot{V}O_2$. These differences should be noted if perceived exertion is used as the sole measure of exercise intensity.

During submaximal deep-water running for 45 minutes, Bishop et al.[17] recorded lower mean $\dot{V}O_2$ and ventilation and respiratory exchange rate (RER) values than those recorded during a 45-minute treadmill run at a comparable perceived exertion ($\dot{V}O_2$: 29.8 ml/kg/min vs. 40.6 ml/kg/min; ventilation 58.1 L/min vs. 79.1 L/min). Heart rates were also lower during deep-water running (122 vs. 157 beats/min); however, this was not deemed statistically significant with the small sample involved ($n = 7$). Two participants, who were described as the most accomplished and enthusiastic deep-water runners, achieved similar responses during deep-water running and treadmill running, suggesting that motivation or familiarity may play a role in attaining levels of physiologic response.

Ritchie and Hopkins[18] noted that perceived exertion and perceived pain during a 30-minute deep-water run at a "hard" pace were comparable to those ratings obtained during "hard" treadmill running. These ratings were significantly greater than perceived exertions during treadmill running or road running at a "normal" training pace.

Examining the relationship between heart rate and $\dot{V}O_2$ during submaximal graded exercise, Svedenhag and Seger[8] reported lower heart rates during deep-water running than treadmill running at any given level of oxygen uptake. Oxygen pulse was higher during submaximal exercise in the water. A similar relationship between heart rate and $\dot{V}O_2$ was noted by Navia[11] at higher workloads. These results suggest that an aerobic training effect may occur at lower heart rates during deep-water running than during treadmill running at submaximal levels. Svedenhag and Seger[8] also reported higher RER and similar ventilation during deep-water running at submaximal intensity compared with land running.

Yamaji et al.[19] noted significant interindividual variability in heart rate responses as a function of $\dot{V}O_2$ during unsupported deep-water running. Although group data revealed a similar heart rate-$\dot{V}O_2$ relationship for both deep-water running and treadmill running, two of the more skilled participants did have lower heart rate values during deep-water running than during treadmill running at a comparative $\dot{V}O_2$. Ritchie and Hopkins[18] obtained heart rate values during a 30-minute session of hard deep-water running that were lower than those during hard treadmill running (159 vs. 176 beats/min). Oxygen uptake values, however, were similar (49 ml/kg/min vs. 53 ml/kg/min). The heart rate values obtained during hard deep-water running were similar to those obtained during treadmill running at a normal training pace; however, corresponding oxygen uptake was greater during hard deep-water running. This study also supports the contention that deep-water running at submaximal levels may result in greater overall aerobic response if heart rate is used as the measure of exercise intensity.

Frangolias and Rhodes demonstrated lower heart rate and $\dot{V}O_2$ values during aqua running than during treadmill running at the ventilatory threshold. RPE, RER, and ventilation were similar during both aqua running and treadmill running at the ventilatory threshold.[12]

Michaud et al.[20] examined eight trained runners completing three separate 15-minute tests as follows: (1) treadmill run at 75% treadmill $\dot{V}O_2$max; (2) water run at 75% water run $\dot{V}O_2$max; and (3) water run at 75% treadmill $\dot{V}O_2$max. HR and $\dot{V}O_2$ were similar during both deep-water running and treadmill running. Blood lactate, RER, and RPE were greater during deep-water running.[20] This study suggests that heart rate may be more reflective of the aerobic demands of deep-water running as opposed to RPE.[20,21]

Gerhing et al.[22] demonstrated that competitive runners were able to maintain similar $\dot{V}O_2$ values during 20-minute submaximal treadmill and water running sessions, whereas noncompetitive runners had lower $\dot{V}O_2$ values in the water compared with the land. This study suggests that more accomplished runners may be able to utilize aqua running with greater efficiency than noncompetitive runners.

During submaximal running at heart rates equivalent to 60% and 80% of treadmill $\dot{V}O_2$max, DeMaere and Ruby[21] demonstrated higher RER and carbohydrate metabolism and lower fat oxidation during deep-water running than during land-based running. Ventilation was higher during deep-water running compared with treadmill running at 80% $\dot{V}O_2$max. $\dot{V}O_2$, RPE, and energy expenditure did not differ significantly between trials.[21]

Long-Term Training Effects

Several studies have reported on the long-term effects of a deep-water exercise program. Michaud et al.[10] reported that 10 subjects who underwent an 8-week training program of aqua running showed improvements in $\dot{V}O_2$ during both water-based and land-based graded exercise testing (19.6% and 10.7%, respectively), thus demonstrating training as well as crossover effects to land-based exercise. Eyestone et al.[23] demonstrated that deep-water running was comparable to land-based running and cycling for preserving levels of fitness during a 6-week training period at maintenance duration (20 to 30 minutes) and frequency (three to five times/week). Although a small decrease in $\dot{V}O_2$max was noted for each group, this was much less than the 16% to 17% loss previously reported during a 6-week rest period.

Wilber et al.[24] demonstrated no significant differences in treadmill $\dot{V}O_2$max, ventilatory threshold, running economy, and blood lactate at $\dot{V}O_2$max following 6 weeks of training in two groups, one training on land, the other training exclusively in water. Additionally, glucose and norepinephrine levels were similar between the two groups. Notably, both groups improved treadmill $\dot{V}O_2$max levels, the land-based training group improving 13.8% and the water training group improving 9.2%. Bushman et al.[25] found no significant differences in simulated 5-km run time, submaximal and maximal oxygen consumption, or lactate threshold following 4 weeks of deep-water training in recreationally competitive distance runners.

Quinn et al. reported a 7% decrease in $\dot{V}O_2$max following a 4-week deep-water training program. Their subjects, however, were previously unfamiliar with deep-water running and exercised at minimum maintenance levels of intensity, duration, and frequency only. Furthermore, the technique described as a "high knee bicycle motion" suggests that the less than full range of running motion during aqua running may have influenced results.[26]

These training studies suggest that when performed with proper technique and intensity, deep-water running can provide a stimulus great enough to maintain and even improve running fitness.

Discussion

There are several possible explanations for the differences in metabolic response to deep-water and land-based running. Differences in muscle use and activation patterns contribute to these differences in exercise response. Furthermore, because weightbearing is eliminated and resistance is increased, the larger muscle groups of the lower extremities do less work, and a comparatively greater proportion of work is done by the upper extremities. This may contribute to the lower maximal oxygen uptakes recorded during deep-water running. It has also been suggested that lower perfusion pressures in the legs during immersion, with resultant decreases in total muscle blood flow, influence the higher anaerobic metabolism during deep-water running.[8]

Hydrostatic pressure is thought to assist in cardiac performance by promoting venous return; thus, the heart does not have to beat as fast to maintain cardiac output. This may contribute to the lower heart rates observed during both submaximal and maximal deep-water running. Temperature also has been demonstrated to have an effect on heart rate during exercise, with higher temperatures correlating with higher heart rates.

Town and Bradley[9] have suggested that decreased blood flow to the lower extremities during deep-water running may be responsible in those cases in which lower blood lactate was measured. Frangolias and Rhodes,[4] however, have suggested that the level of familiarity with deep-water running may play the most important role in the variability in blood lactate response. It has also been suggested that in those cases in which ventilation is reduced during deep-water running, an increase in intrathoracic blood volume and hydrostatic chest compression results in an increase in the force required for inspiration by reducing total lung compliance and vital capacity. However, it has also been suggested that a proportionally greater increase in central blood flow during water immersion may accommodate for the reduced lung compliance in those cases in which ventilation is similar.[12]

Familiarity with this form of exercise appears to be an important factor in maximizing physiologic response to deep-water running when measured at a particular level of perceived exertion. In our experience at The Runner's Clinic at UVa and the Houston International Running Center, strict adherence to proper form and technique ensures a higher physiologic response as measured by $\dot{V}O_2$ and heart rate.

EXERCISE PRESCRIPTION FOR AQUA RUNNING

Three measures are used for grading aqua running exercise intensity: (1) heart rate, (2) rating of perceived exertion, and (3) cadence. Workout programs are typically designed to reproduce the work the athlete would do on land and to incorporate both long runs and interval/speed training.

Heart Rate

There is a high correlation between heart rate and oxygen uptake. The American College of Sports Medicine guidelines recommend that for a training effect, one should exercise at a level between 55% and 90% of the maximum heart rate (the target heart rate range).[5] The maximum heart rate can be estimated (220 minus age) or can be based on heart rate levels attained during exercise of maximum effort. Although heart rate levels in the water tend to be lower than those on land, it is possible to approach land-based values by adherence to proper technique. Heart rate can be monitored by a waterproof heart rate monitor or periodically by palpation.

Rating of Perceived Exertion

The RPE refers to the patient's subjective grading of level of exertion.[27,28] Perceived exertion for jogging is rated as low, whereas that for sprinting is rated as high. A high correlation has been identified between perceived exertion and physiologic variables during deep-water running.[2,29] The most commonly used scale of perceived exertion is the Borg Scale, a 15-point scale with verbal descriptors ranging from very, very light to very, very hard (Table 45–1). For distance

TABLE 45–1. BORG SCALE OF PERCEIVED EXERTION

Level	RPE
6	
7	Very, very light
8	
9	Very light
10	
11	Light
12	
13	Somewhat hard
14	
15	Hard
16	
17	Very hard
18	
19	Very, very hard
20	

RPE = rating of perceived exertion.
Source: From Borg.[27] For correct use of the Borg RPE scale it is necessary to follow instructions given by Borg. Borg G: Borg's perceived exertion and pain scales. Human Kinetics, 1998.

TABLE 45–2. BRENNAN SCALE OF PERCEIVED EXERTION FOR DISTANCE RUNNERS

Level	Description	RPE	CPM[a]	Land Equivalent
1	Very light	1.0	<55	Recovery jog
		1.5	55–59	
2	Light	2.0	60–64	Easy run
		2.5	65–69	
3	Somewhat hard	3.0	70–74	Brisk run
		3.5	75–79	
4	Hard	4.0	80–84	5–10K pace
		4.5	85–89	Long track intervals
5	Very hard	5.0	>90	Short track intervals

[a]CPM = cycles per minute, measured as the number of times each limb moves through a complete gait cycle per minute.
Source: From Brennan and Wilder.[2]

TABLE 45–3. MODIFIED BRENNAN SCALE FOR SPRINTERS

Description	RPE	CPM	Land Equivalent (m)
Very light	1.0	<74	>800
	1.5	75–79	
Light	2.0	80–84	600–800
	2.5	85–90	
Somewhat hard	3.0	90–94	400–600
	3.5	95–99	
Hard	4.0	100–104	200–400
	4.5	105–109	
Very hard	5.0	>110	50–200

RPE = rating of perceived exertion.

runners, we use the Brennan Scale, a 5-point scale designed exclusively for aqua running; verbal descriptors for this scale range from very light to very hard (Table 45–2).[2] We further instruct our athletes that level 1 (very light) corresponds to a recovery jog, level 2 (light) to a long easy run, level 3 (somewhat hard) to a brisk run, level 4 (hard) to speeds of 5 to 10 km, and level 4.5 to 5 (very hard) to track intervals. The Brennan Scale facilitates the incorporation of both speed and distance work into workouts in a manner easily understood by both coach and athlete. A sample workout protocol is presented in Fig. 45–2. A separate perceived exertion scale is utilized for sprinters (Table 45–3).

Cadence

Wilder et al.[30] demonstrated a very high correlation between cadence and heart rate, with intraindividual correlations averaging 0.98. Competitive athletes undergo a graded exercise test of aqua running following our standard protocol (Fig. 45–3). Cadence is controlled by an auditory metronome. By recording heart rate responses to various levels of cadence, we can anticipate an expected physiologic response to a particular cadence level. Workouts can then be

designed that use timed intervals at particular cadence levels.

Studies that have measured leg speed (cadence) as a measured variable of deep-water running intensity reported lower cadences than during land running at submaximal levels (60% to 70% of peak $\dot{V}O_2$ and heart rate).[2] As subjects in the water approach peak workloads, cadences begin to match those on land more closely. For the elite athlete this may suggest a higher degree of biomechanical specificity for deep-water running at intensities that approach 80% to 90% of peak workloads. Additional studies are needed to evaluate and standardize sport-specific biomechanical models for deep-water running.

Measurement of heart rate is used primarily during long runs: prolonged periods of exercise at a specified rate (the target heart rate). RPE and cadence ratings are most often used for interval sessions. RPE is most helpful in group settings, whereas cadence is most appropriate for individual sessions.

PRACTICAL GUIDELINES FOR CLINICIANS

Our athletes typically undergo one or two individual sessions for familiarization and to ensure proper

Total workout time and workout no.	No. of Repetitions	x	Duration of repetitions (mins)	@	Exertion	Level	(Recovery periods)
(37:00) 1	5	x	2:00	@	RPE	SH	(:30)
	8	x	1:00	@	RPE	H	(:30)
	5	x	2:00	@	RPE	SH	(:30)

Figure 45–2. Sample workout protocol. (*Source: From Brennan and Wilder.*[2])

Name: _____   Date: _____

Predicted 90% Max Heart Rate: _____

Stage	End Point	Cadence	Heart Rate	RPE	Comments
1	3:00	66			
2	6:00	72			
3	9:00	78			
4	12:00	84			
5	15:00	90			
6	18:00	96			
7	21:00	102			
Post	1:00				
	2:00				
	5:00				

Figure 45–3. Houston International Running Center Data Collection Sheet: Modified Wilder Graded Exercise Test for Aqua Running. Post (values), postexercise values during cool-down. (*Courtesy of Houston International Running Center, Houston, TX, copyright 1990; used with permission.*)

technique. A flotation device is used because it is difficult to adhere to proper technique without support. The athletes then undergo our graded exercise test (GXT), allowing us to correlate cadence and perceived exertion to heart rate responses. Workouts are then designed using perceived exertion and cadence to effect a particular level of physiologic response. Training schedules are designed to follow closely the work that the athlete would do on land. Thus, for example, if an athlete was scheduled to run 6 × 600 meters at a pace of 2 minutes each on the track, the athlete would perform six 2-minute intervals in the water at a Brennan Perceived Exertion level of 4. Longer runs may call for aqua running up to 1 to 2 hours at a Brennan Perceived Exertion level of 2.

For nonrunners and athletes seeking general conditioning and fitness maintenance only, three to four sessions a week are performed at maintenance duration (15 to 60 minutes) and intensity (55% to 90% maximum heart rate). Aqua running is also effectively incorporated into cross-training programs involving other forms of exercise such as biking and stair climbing.

As the athlete gradually returns to land-based running, sessions are tapered; however, many athletes choose to incorporate one or two sessions of aqua running a week into their regular training programs. Sample training programs for both distance runners and sprinters are illustrated below.

Distance Programs

Long Continuous Running

This type of running simulates long slow distance runs up to tempo runs. One should be able to hold a conversation while performing this workout. The RPE level will range from 2.0 to 3.0. Running economy can be practiced during this "steady-state," low-intensity workout. The athlete should try to focus on the correct running mechanics. Music can enhance the workout if it is done alone. Five sample workouts are listed below:

- Workout #1: 40 min @ RPE 2.0–3.0
- Workout #2: 50 min @ RPE 2.0–3.0
- Workout #3: 60 min @ RPE 2.0–3.0
- Workout #4: 70 min @ RPE 2.0–3.0
- Workout #5: 80 min @ RPE 2.0–3.0

Long Intervals

Long intervals improve the runner's ability to sustain a faster pace without acquiring excessively high blood-lactate levels. A single session each week can familiarize the runner with the muscular as well as cardiovascular demands of both short and long distances (5K through marathon). Long-interval training should be at 80% to 90% of maximum. Several intervals of greater than 3:00 to 15:00 minutes' duration are usually performed with 1 to 2 minutes of recovery. Total run time should be 30 to 60 minutes. This training would stimulate intervals of 800 meters up to 5 km on the track.

SAMPLE WORKOUTS
- Workout #1 (31 minutes)
  8:00 @ RPE 3.0 (1:00 @ RPE2)
  6:00 @ RPE 3.5 (1.00 @ RPE2)
  5:00 @ RPE 3.5 (1.00 @ RPE2)
  4:00 @ RPE 4.0 (1:00 @ RPE2)
  3:00 @ RPE 4.0 (1.00 @ RPE2)
- Workout #2 (36 minutes)
  4 × 8:00 @ RPE 3.0–3.5 (1:00 @ RPE2)
- Workout #3 (40 minutes)
  9:00 @ RPE 3.5 (1:00 @ RPE2)
  8:00 @ RPE 3.5 (1:00 @ RPE2)
  7:00 @ RPE 3.5 (1:00 @ RPE2)
  6:00 @ RPE 4.0 (1:00 @ RPE2)
  5:00 @ RPE 4.0 (1:00 @ RPE2)
- Workout #4 (44 minutes)
  2 × 6:00 @ RPE 3.5 (1:00 @ RPE2)
  2 × 5:00 @ RPE 4.0 (1:00 @ RPE2)
  2 × 4:00 @ RPE 4.0 (1:00 @ RPE2)
  2 × 3:00 @ RPE 4.5 (1:00 @ RPE2)
- Workout #5 (48 minutes)
  8 × 5:00 @ RPE 4.0 (1:00 @ RPE2)

Short Intervals

Short-interval training usually involves running at 90% to 99% of the maximum at an interval of 30 seconds up to 2 minutes, with recovery periods that may range from 30 seconds up to 5:00 minutes depending on the intensity and length of the intervals and whether the training interval calls for "incomplete" recovery. This type of training allows the runner to feel comfortable at high leg speeds and helps the muscular and circulatory system "tolerate" very high workloads for short periods of time. Short intervals in the pool simulate 200- to 800-meter track intervals and should be preformed once or twice every 7 to 10 days depending on the training objectives at the time.

SAMPLE WORKOUTS
- Workout #1 (30 minutes)
  10 × 2:00 @ RPE 4.0–4.5 (1.00 @ RPE2)
- Workout #2 (46 minutes)
  4 × 3:00 @ RPE 4.0 (1:00 @ RPE2)
  6 × 2:00 @ RPE 4.0–4.5 (1:00 @ RPE2)
  8 × 1:00 @ RPE 4.5 (0:30 @ RPE2)
- Workout #3 (36 minutes)
  4 × 2:00 @ RPE 4.0 (1:00 @ RPE2)
  4 × 1:30 @ RPE 4.5 (1:00 @ RPE2)
  4 × 1:00 @ RPE 4.5 (1:00 @ RPE2)
  4 × 0:30 @ RPE 4.0–4.5 (1:00 @ RPE2)

- Workout #4 (38 minutes)
  4 × 2:00 @ RPE 4.0 (1:00 @ RPE2)
  6 × 1:00 @ RPE 4.5 (0:30 @ RPE2)
  5:00 @ RPE 2.0
  8 × 0:30 @ RPE 4.5–5.0 (1:00 @ RPE3)
- Workout #5 (45 minutes)
  10 × 1:00 @ RPE 4.0 (1:00 @ RPE2)
  5:00 @ RPE 2.0
  10 × 1:00 @ RPE 4.5–5.0 (1:00 @ RPE2)

SPRINT WORKOUTS. Water-based training can be used effectively for sprint training whether for track or other sports that require explosive-type running. We have used a three-phase approach to sprint training in the pool.

1. *Transitional phase (1 to 2 weeks).* This phase allows progressive loading of the musculoskeletal system and provides biomechanical familiarization with specific moving patterns required for deep-water running. Even if the athlete is very fit, we recommend spending at least two to three sessions over the course of a week or two before moving to the next phase.
   - *Sample program:*
     Warm-up: 5:00 @ 1.0–1.5/stretch 5–10 min
     Intervals: 2 × 3:00 @ RPE 2.0 (1:00 @ RPE 1.0)
              2 × 2:00 @ RPE 2.5 (1:00 @ RPE 1.0)
              4 × 1:30 @ RPE 3.0 (1:00 @ RPE 1.0)
              6 × 1:00 @ RPE 3.5 (1:00 @ RPE 1.0)
     Cool-down: 5:00 @ 1.0–1.5/stretch 5–10 min

2. *Base phase (4 to 6 weeks).* Sprinters can benefit from a base phase in precompetition preparation. These base phase workouts simulate a 400- to 800-meter type of training, ensuring the development of an efficient cardiovascular system and specific muscular endurance. Base workouts also enhance the circulatory system, thus possibly aiding an athlete's recovery from strenuous longer track intervals, which often are a major component of early season sprint training and a source of potential injury.
   - *Sample program:*
     Warm-up: 5:00 @ 1.0–1.5/stretch 5–10 min
     Intervals: 2 × 2:00 @ RPE 3.0 (0:30 @ RPE 1.0)
              2 × 1:30 @ RPE 3.5 (0:30 @ RPE 1.0)
              4 × 1:00 @ RPE 4.0 (1:00 @ RPE 1.0)
              4 × 0:45 @ RPE 4.5 (1:00 @ RPE 1.0)
     Cool-down: 5:00 @ 1.0–1.5/stretch 5–10 min

3. *Speed phase (4 to 6 weeks).* Specific training enhances leg turnover, limb range of motion, and coordination between the upper and lower extremities while maintaining high speeds.

- *Sample program:*
  Warm-up: 5:00 @ 1.0–1.5/stretch 5–10 min
  Intervals: 3:00 @ RPE 3.0 (1:00 @ RPE 1.0)
                2:00 @ RPE 3.5 (1:00 @ RPE 1.0)
                4 × 1:30 @ RPE 4.0 (2:00 @ RPE 1.0)
                6 × 0:30 @ RPE 5.0 (2:00 @ RPE 1.0)
  Cool-down: 5:00 @ 1.0–1.5/stretch 5–10 min

AQUA RUNNING FOR SPECIAL POPULATIONS

We have also incorporated aqua running into fitness and rehabilitation programs for nonathletes. These include patients with lumbar spine disorders, arthritis and degenerative joint disease (DJD), postoperative orthopedic patients, lower-extremity amputees, and women with uncomplicated pregnancies. We emphasize neutral spine mechanics for patients with lumbar spine disease. These mechanics are then incorporated into land-based exercises. The technique is generally modified in patients with arthritis and DJD as well as in postoperative orthopedic patients in order to exercise within pain-free ranges. In pregnant women who do not have contraindications to exercise during pregnancy, mild to moderate exercise may be performed consistent with fitness level; however, women are counseled not to exercise to exhaustion and to stop exercising if they experience any signs of overexertion, hyperthermia, dehydration, or fetal distress[31] (see Chapter 34).

CONCLUSIONS

Despite the differences between deep-water and land-based running, deep-water running does elicit the physiologic responses necessary to promote a training effect as defined by the American College of Sports Medicine (40% to 85% $\dot{V}O_2$max or 55% to 90% maximum heart rate). These responses can be maximized by adherence to proper technique and by the use of environment-specific means of exercise prescription (established specifically for deep-water exercise). Deep-water running also offers additional benefits, most notably the maintenance of quick turnover (rapid gait cycling) as well as coordinated movements between the arms and legs. These aspects facilitate return to land-based training.

Maintaining conditioning is a challenge for the injured athlete. Aqua running is an effective way to continue training during rehabilitation and can later be incorporated into a regular training program, providing a low-stress form of additional cardiovascular exercise.

Further research will help define the effect of aqua running on physiologic parameters other than oxygen uptake and heart rate as well as responses in special populations. Questions have also been raised regarding differences between shallow-water and deep-water exercise. The increasing interest in aquatic exercise and research will help us answer these questions and expand the use of aquatic exercise in rehabilitation and fitness.

REFERENCES

1. Edlich RF, Towler MA, Goitz RJ, et al.: Bioengineering principles of hydrotherapy. *J Burn Care Rehabil* 1987:8, 580.
2. Brennan DK, Wilder RP: *Aqua Running: An Instructor's Manual,* Houston, TX, Houston International Running Center, 1999.
3. Wilder RP, Brennan DK: Physiologic responses to deep water running in athletes. *Sports Med* 1993:16, 374.
4. Frangolias DD, Rhodes EC: Metabolic responses to mechanisms during water immersion running and exercise. *J Sports Med* 1996:22, 38.
5. American College of Sports Medicine: *Guidelines for Graded Exercise Testing and Prescription,* 4th ed. Philadelphia, Lea & Febiger, 1991.
6. Butts NK, Tucker M, Smith R: Maximal responses to treadmill and and deep water running in high school female cross country runners. *Res Q Exerc Sports* 1991:62, 236.
7. Butts NK, Tucker M, Greening C: Physiologic responses to maximal treadmill and deep water running in men and women. *Am J Sports Med* 1991:19, 612.
8. Svedenhag J, Seger J: Running on land and in water: Comparative exercise physiology. *Med Sci Sports Exerc* 1992:24, 1155.
9. Town GP, Bradley SS: Maximal metabolic responses of deep and shallow water running in trained runners. *Med Sci Sports Exerc* 1991:23, 238.
10. Michaud TJ, Brennan DK, Wilder RP, et al.: Aqua running and gains in cardiorespiratory fitness. *J Strength Conditioning Res* 1995:9, 78.
11. Navia AM: Comparison of energy expenditure between treadmill running and water running. Thesis, University of Alabama at Birmingham, 1986.
12. Frangolias DD, Rhodes EC: Maximal and ventilatory threshold responses to treadmill and water immersion running. *Med Sci Sports Exerc* 1995:27, 1007.
13. Dowzer CN, Reilly T, Cable NT, et al.: Maximal physiological responses to deep water and shallow water running. *Ergonomics* 1999:42, 275.
14. Nakanishi Y: Maximal physiologic responses to deep water running at thermonuclear temperature. *Appl Human Sci* 1999:18, 3.
15. Nakanishi Y: Physiologic responses to maximal treadmill and deep water running in young and middle age males. *Appl Human Sci* 1999:18, 81.

16. Melton-Rogers S: Cardiorespiratory responses of patients with rheumatoid arthritis during bicycle riding and running in water. *Phys Ther* 1996:76, 1058.

17. Bishop PA, Frazier S, Smith J, et al.: Physiologic responses to treadmill and water running. *Physician Sportsmed* 1989:17, 87.

18. Ritchie SE, Hopkins WG: The intensity of exercise in deep water running. *In J Sports Med* 1991:12, 27.

19. Yamaji K, Greenly M, Northey DR, et al.: Oxygen uptake and heart rate responses to treadmill and deep water running. *Can J Sports Sci* 1990:15, 96.

20. Michaud TJ, Rodriguez-Zayas J, Andres FF, et al.: Comparative exercise responses of deep water running and treadmill running. *J Strength Cond Res* 1995:9, 104.

21. DeMaere JM, Ruby BC: Effects of deep water running and treadmill running on oxygen uptake and energy expenditure in seasonally trained cross-country runners. *J Sports Med Phys Fitness* 1997:37, 175.

22. Gehring MM, Keller BA, Brehm BA: Water running with and without a flotation vest in competitive and recreational runners. *Med Sci Sports Exerc* 1997:29, 1374.

23. Eyestone ED, Fellingham G, George J, et al.: Effect of water running and cycling on maximum oxygen consumption and 2-mile run performance. *Am J Sports Med* 1993:21, 41.

24. Wilber RL, Moffat RJ, Scott BE, et al.: Influence of water run training on the maintenance of physiological determinants of aerobic performance. *Med Sci Sports Exerc* 1996:28, 1056.

25. Bushman BA, Flynn MG, Andres FF, et al.: Effect of four weeks of deep water run training on running performance. *Med Sci Sports Exerc* 1997:29, 694.

26. Quinn TJ, Sedory DR, Fisher BS: Physiological effects of deep water running following a land-based training program. *Res Q Exerc Sport* 1994:65, 386.

27. Borg GV: Psychophysical basis of perceived exertion. *Med Sci Sports Exerc* 1982:14, 377.

28. Carlton RL, Rhodes EC: Critical review of the literature on rating scales for perceived exertion. *Sports Med* 1985:2, 198.

29. Brown SP, Chitwood LF, Beason KR, et al.: Physiological correlates with perceived exertion during deep water running. *Percept Mot Skills* 1996:83, 155.

30. Wilder RP, Brennan DK, Schotte DE: A standard measure for exercise prescription for aqua running. *Am J Sports Med* 1993:21, 45.

31. American College of Obstetricians and Gynecologists: Exercise during pregnancy and the postpartum period. Technical Bulletin 189. Washington, DC, ACOG, 1994.

Chapter 46

THE RUNNING SHOE

John A. Johnson

INTRODUCTION

The number of people who participate in both recreational and/or competitive running has increased dramatically over the last several years. This increase has led to a concomitant increase in running injuries,[1,2] which are caused by intrinsic or extrinsic factors or the interaction between the two.[3,4] Intrinsic factors are those conditions unique to each athlete and include instability, malalignment, inflexibility, and muscle weakness and/or imbalance.[5] Extrinsic factors include weather conditions, training errors, surface conditions, and running shoes.[6] The athlete's vulnerability to extrinsic conditions varies with their intrinsic characteristics.

This chapter deals exclusively with the importance of the running shoe. Proper running shoe selection is important for both prevention and treatment of running injuries. The proper shoe can compensate for intrinsic abnormalities of an athlete, thus decreasing susceptibility to injury.[7–10]

RUNNING SHOE ANATOMY

Shoes are divided into uppers and bottoms. The upper is the part of the shoe that is above the sole and is designed to cover and secure the foot to the bottom. The bottom provides cushioning, stability, and protection from the running surface (Fig. 46–1).

Uppers

Most uppers are made from a lightweight nylon mesh that allows the foot to breathe. The main components of the uppers are the vamp in the front, the quarters, which form the majority of the midsection of the upper, and the heel counter, which is the reinforced area in the back of the shoe.

The vamp forms the front part of the shoe and is sewn to the eyestays and the quarters. The front portion of the vamp forms the toe box. The toe box needs to be deep enough to protect the toes from chafing. Some athletic shoes have stiffeners or reinforcements in the toe box to prevent it from collapsing. These are usually not found in running shoes because they add unnecessary weight. Some manufacturers add material called foxing to the front of the shoe, forming the toe cap. The toe cap protects the toes and increases the durability of the toe box.

The top of the vamp just in front of the instep is referred to as the throat. This is usually the narrowest part of the shoe and must be checked carefully during shoe fitting to avoid excessive pressure on the instep.

The quarters form the midportion of the uppers. They form the majority of the sides of the shoes. They are sewn to the vamp anteriorly and conform to the arch area and midfoot. The quarters may have stabilizing bars or arch braces added for increased side-to-side stability.

The tongue extends under the laces of the shoe. It is sewn to the vamp anteriorly and in some shoes has

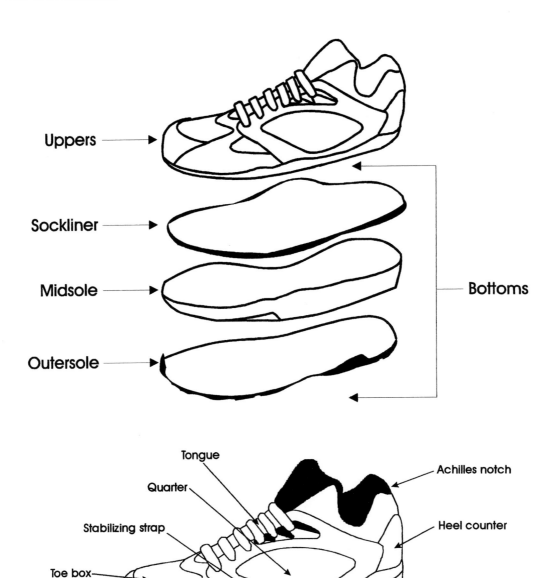

Figure 46–1. Running shoe anatomy.

an elastic material that connects it to the bottoms. The tongue is padded to reduce irritation to the dorsum of the foot from the laces.

The heel counter is a reinforced area in the back of the shoe. It is usually made of stiffened fiberboard or plastic and is molded to the heel. This allows the heel counter to withstand the torsional forces during running. Stiffer heel counters increase rearfoot stability and can reduce the speed of pronation and rotation.

Bottoms

The bottom of the shoe consists of the outersole, the midsole, and the sockliner or insole. The outersole is designed to provide traction and protection from the running surface. Outersoles are primarily made of carbon rubber, blown rubber, or hard rubber. Carbon rubber is very dense and durable. It is the same material used in the construction of Indy racecar tires. Carbon rubber wears very well but is not very flexible. Blown rubber is less dense than carbon rubber. It has small air bubbles blown into the rubber. It is lighter and more flexible than carbon rubber but not as durable. Hard rubber outersoles are made from a mixture of carbon and blown rubber.

The midsole is the heart of the running shoe. Most of the recent changes in the running shoe industry have been in the design and materials of the midsole. Midsoles provide the main cushioning and stability. Midsoles are manufactured from a combination of materials, the most common being ethyl vinyl acetate (EVA) and polyurethane. Most state-of-the art running shoes have some amount of EVA in the midsole. EVA is light and resilient and has good cushioning properties. EVA is first heated and then compressed into the shape of the midsole. EVA can also be manufactured in varying densities. Denser EVA is firmer but provides less cushioning. Dual- and triple-density midsoles alter the density of EVA in different areas of the midsole to provide either more motion control or more shock absorption. For example, denser EVA is used in the rearfoot for durability and firmness, and less dense material is used in the forefoot for cushioning and flexibility. Polyurethane is heavier, denser, and more durable than EVA. Other less-used midsole materials include newer foam polymers including Elvalite, Phylon, and Hytrel.

Shoewear is not determined by the wear on the outersole but by the wear of the midsole. Midsoles break down under the repetitive stresses of running, for example, EVA midsoles lose about 40% of their initial shock absorption at 250 to 500 miles.[11] Midsoles also lose compressibility with age. This dual mechanism of midsole breakdown means that runners should change their running shoes every 6 months or 500 miles.[12]

Advances in attenuating heel-load dispersion were made with Nike's introduction of the "airsole."[13,14] Airsoles use freon or other gases encapsulated in pockets in the midsole. These provide greater cushioning and break down slower than foam polymers. These encapsulated units may be in the heel, the forefoot, or both. These systems have superior shock absorption and are not as susceptible to compression as polyurethane or EVA, making them more durable. The tradeoff is that these systems provide less stability.[15] Other manufacturers use gel or mechanical plastics to achieve the same effect (Table 46–1).

The insole or sock liner provides cushioning and reduces friction. Most insoles are removable for cleaning or for replacement. Insoles should also be removed when a runner is using an orthotic. Insole materials include neoprene foam, viscoelastic materials, or polyethylene foams. Examples are shown in Table 46–2.

TABLE 46–1. ENCAPSULATED MATERIALS

Manufacturer	Material
Asics	Gel
Brooks	Silicone
New Balance	Ethyl vinyl acetate (EVA)
Nike	Air bags
Puma	Honeycomb pads
Reebok	Honeycomb pads

TABLE 46–2. SAMPLE INSOLE MATERIALS

Insole Material	Brand Name
Polyethylene foam	Plastizote
Viscoelastic	Sorbothane
Neoprene foam	Spenco

Data are conflicting as to the effectiveness of different insoles. Viscoelastic insoles have been shown to reduce the force of impact at heel strike,[16] but other studies have shown that this has no effect on the musculoskeletal system and, when compared with conventional running shoes, does not significantly reduce the vertical impact forces.[17] One study showed that using neoprene foam insoles for shock absorption in the standard military footwear of new recruits reduced the incidence of overuse injuries including a significant reduction in the number of tibial stress fractures.[18] In another study comparing viscoelastic to neoprene insoles, it was found that the neoprene insoles were less rigid, reduced transmitted forces better, and were more resistant to shear forces.

Construction

Shoes are manufactured on a wood, metal, or plastic form known as a last, which is made to approximate an average foot. The last gives the shoe its basic shape, size, and proportions. This basic shape affects the shoe's support characteristics and fit. Shapes vary from straight to slightly curved, semicurved, and curve-lasted.

The other "lasting" referred to in shoes describes how the uppers are attached to the bottoms. In board-lasted shoes, the periphery of the upper is glued to a fiberboard sole. These shoes are usually also straight lasted, i.e., have no forefoot adduction, and are fairly stiff. Slip or curve-lasted shoes have a "moccasin" upper sewn to the midsole material. They have a forefoot adduction of approximately 25 degrees and are very flexible and mobile. Combination lasted shoes are usually semicurved and have a board-lasted rear with a slip-last in the forefoot. They are constructed with approximately 7 to 10 degrees of forefoot adduction.

The differing shape and construction give the shoes predictable characteristics. Straight or board-lasted shoes have the most medial stability and rigidity. These shoes provide the greatest amount of motion control but are heavier and less flexible than other shoes. Curve or slip-lasted shoes provide the greatest amount of flexibility and shock absorption. They are lighter but less stable than the straight-lasted shoes. Combination or semicurve-lasted shoes are designed to be more flexible and lighter than straight-lasted shoes, but they provide more stability than curve- or slip-lasted shoes. They provide good rearfoot control

**TABLE 46–3. RELATIONSHIPS AMONG LASTS
AND FUNCTIONS**

Last	Flexibility	Stability	Weight	Comfort
Board (straight)	Least	Most	Most	Least
Combination	↓	↓	↓	↓
Slip (curved)	Most	Least	Least	Most

and allow for forefoot flexibility and cushioning. The relationships among last, flexibility, stability, weight, and comfort are summarized in Table 46–3.

BIOMECHANICS

To understand the function of the running shoe, we need to review briefly the biomechanics of the foot in running. During running, the foot contacts the ground at heel strike. At heel strike, the vertical forces on the heel are three times the runner's weight, for example, a 150-lb runner has an impact force of 450 lb. At heel strike the foot is in supination and the tibia is externally rotated. The subtalar joint of the foot acts as an oblique hinge joint that converts the subsequent internal rotation of the tibia into pronation, which consists of rearfoot eversion, forefoot abduction, and slight ankle dorsiflexion. This pronation brings the axis of the subtalar joint parallel to the axis of the midtarsal joint and "unlocks" it, allowing the forefoot to become more flexible. This flexibility is what allows the foot to adapt to the ground and to absorb some of the vertical and horizontal forces generated at heel strike and subsequent loading on the foot. As the foot progresses through the stance phase to toe-off, the tibia rotates externally, resupinating the subtalar joint, and locks the midtarsal, which again makes the foot a more rigid structure. This allows the foot to become a rigid lever for toe-off and propulsion.

The ability of the subtalar joint to pronate and supinate allows the foot to go from a rigid landing platform at heel strike, to a more flexible shock-absorbing and adaptive mechanism during midstance, and then return to a rigid lever at toe-off. This allows the foot to perform five distinct and necessary functions during locomotion: adaptation, shock absorption, torque conversion, stability, and rigidity. A runner's intrinsic characteristics can limit the foot's ability to perform these functions properly. The choice of an appropriate shoe can help minimize the effects of an intrinsic abnormality.

FOOT TYPE AND INJURY PATTERNS

Runners with a high fixed arch, or pes cavus, are underpronators. In underpronators the foot is unable to reach or spends too little time in pronation. Underpronators have a stable and rigid foot that lacks flexibility and adaptability. Underpronation has been associated with tibial and femoral stress fractures,[19] Achilles' tendinitis,[20] and plantar fasciitis.[21] Achilles' tendinitis and plantar fasciitis result from the relative tightness and inflexibility of these tendons in a cavus foot. The tibial and femoral stress fractures result from poor shock absorption in the foot, allowing greater forces to be transmitted up the kinetic chain. Normal feet with lower arches act as better shock absorbers than normal feet with a higher arch.[22]

Overpronators spend too much time in pronation, leaving the foot in a flexible but unstable position. Weightbearing is shifted to the medial side of the foot, leading to excessive internal rotation of the tibia and increasing stress on the medial portions of the foot, leg, and knee. Overpronation has been associated with patellofemoral pain, popliteal tendinitis,[23] posterior tibial tendinitis,[24] Achilles' tendinitis,[25] plantar fasciitis,[26] and metatarsal stress fractures.[27–29]

Determination of a runner's foot type can be made after a thorough examination, as detailed in earlier chapters. Additional information can be gathered by examining the runner's shoes. In runners with a neutral gait the shoe should wear on the lateral aspect of the heel and have uniform wear under the toes. An overpronator's shoe will show excessive wear on the medial portion of the heel and forefoot due to the increased weightbearing on the medial portion of the foot. The shoe of an underpronator will have more wear on the lateral heel and the entire lateral portion of the outsole.

SHOE SELECTION BY FOOT TYPE

By matching the characteristics of different shoes to the foot type, practitioners and runners are able to select shoes that will compensate for the functions that the foot can not intrinsically accomplish.

In overpronators, those with a hypermobile and unstable foot, the shoes need to provide motion control or decrease the speed at which pronation occurs. Motion control shoes need more medial support. They should have a multidensity, firm midsole with a medial heel stabilizer. A medial forefoot wedge may be incorporated to provide greater forefoot control. The shape should be fairly straight to slightly curved and have board-last construction. The heel flare should be wide on the medial side and can be shaved down on the lateral side to decrease the moment arm that can force the foot into pronation faster. If only rearfoot control is needed, a combination last shoe is appropriate.

For underpronators, those with a rigid foot that is a poor shock absorber and inflexible, shoes should be chosen to maximize cushioning and flexibility. They should have soft midsoles with a lateral heel stabilizer. They should be slip lasted and have a semicurved to curved shape (forefoot adduction). This will give the shoe a soft, torsional flex. Replacement of a stock sockliner or insole with a neoprene or viscoelastic insole should also be considered to provide more shock absorption.

Some features should be looked for in all running shoes. The uppers should be lightweight and breathable. Besides the traditional nylon, some manufacturers have begun to incorporate materials such as Lycra, Gore-Tex, and spandex, which may be more snug, secure, and comfortable. The insole should be comfortable and reduce friction. It should also be removable if the runner needs orthotics. The heel and tongue should be well padded.

Since some shoe manufacturers change models on an annual basis, practitioners should prescribe shoes by specifying the components that a runner needs rather than by specifying a model. An example of a preprinted prescription form is shown in Figure 46–2.

A knowledgable running store representative can then recommend specific shoes. Running magazines are an excellent source of information about shoes and their components. *Runner's World*, for example, publishes a list of new shoes and their features in the spring and fall. The shoes are listed by type, i.e., if you have this foot type, buy this shoe. Runners should be advised to shop for shoes in a reliable athletic footwear store that specializes in running shoes. The staffs in

PATIENT FOOTWEAR RECOMMENDATION

Type Of Shoe (Activity):

Foot Structure: _____

Foot Function:

    O Over Pronation   O Neutral   O Under Pronation

SHOE FEATURES:

LAST (Shape):
O Straight   O Semi Curved   O Curved

CONSTRUCTION:
O Board   O Combination   O Slip

MIDSOLE:
O Firm Medial Midsole (Dual Density)   O Compression Molded EVA

FOOT FRAME:
O Rearfoot Cushioning   O Forefoot Cushioning

UPPERS:
O 3/4 height   O High Top

O Medial/Lateral Stability Straps O Reinforced/Extended Heel Counter

O Deep Toe Box   O Wide Toe Box

OUTSOLE:
O High Density Carbon Heel   O Lightweight Blown Rubber

O Rubber   O Polyurethane

INSOLE:
O Removable Insole for Orthotics

SPECIAL NEEDS: _____

Figure 46–2. Example of a preprinted footwear prescription form.

these stores are more knowledgable about shoe construction and choosing the proper shoe for the runner's particular foot type and running style.

FITTING

Foot size should be measured in a standing position. Sizing should be done later in the day since the feet will be larger than in the morning due to swelling. Runners should try shoes on with the socks that they wear when they run. Both shoes should be tried on since the runner's feet may be different sizes or the shoes may not be the same size. The toe box should be wide and deep enough for the toes to move around. There should be $1/4$ inch from the end of the longest toe to the front of the toe box to allow for swelling during runs. Heel counters should fit snugly so the heel will not slip or rub. Runners should pay close attention to the construction of the shoe during the fitting, avoiding shoes with bad seams or improper gluing, since the quality of production is not always the same for shoes even in the same product line. The runner should look for a shoe that fits and has the right features rather than buying by price, brand name, or cosmetics. One study showed no difference in the incidence of injury with shoes costing over \$40 versus those costing less than \$25.[30] Above all, the shoe should fit comfortably.

REFERENCES

1. Jacobs SJ, Berson BL: Injuries to runners: A study of entrants to a 10,000 meter race. *Am J Sports Med* 1986:14, 151.
2. James SL, Bates BT, Osternig LR: Injuries to runners. *Am J Sports Med* 1978:6, 40.
3. Stanish WD: Overuse injuries in athletes: A perspective. *Med Sci Sports Exerc* 1987:16, 1.
4. Herring SA, Nilson KL: Introduction to overuse injuries. *Clin Sports Med* 1987:6, 225.
5. Brody D: Running injuries, in Nicholas JA, Hershman EB (eds.), *The Lower Extremity and Spine in Sports Medicine,* St. Louis, CV Mosby, 1986:1534.
6. Hess GP, Cappiello WL, Poole RM, et al.: Prevention and treatment of overuse tendon injuries. *Sports Med* 1989:8, 371.
7. Brody D: Techniques in the evaluation and treatment of the injured runner. *Orthop Clin North Am* 1982:13, 541.
8. Lutter LD: Shoes and orthoses in the runner. *Techn Orthop* 1990:5, 57.
9. Cavanagh P: *The Running Shoe Book,* Mountain View, CA, World Publications, 1987.
10. Clarke TC: The effect of shoe design on rearfoot control in running. *Med Sci Sport Exerc* 1983:15, 376.
11. Cook SD, Kester MA, Brunet, ME: Shock absorption characteristics of running shoes. *Am J Sports Med* 1985:13, 248.
12. McKeag D: Overuse injuries. *Prim Care* 1991:18, 851.
13. Cavanagh PR, Lafortune MA: *Biomechanics* 1980:143, 397.
14. Schwellnus MP, Jordan G, Noakes TD: Prevention of common overuse injuries by the use of shock absorbing insoles. *Am J Sports Med* 1990:18, 636.
15. Sharkey NA, Ferris L, Smih TS, et al.: Strain and loading of the second metatarsal during heel lift. *J Bone Joint Surg Am* 1995:77A, 1050.
16. Jorgensen U: Body lad in the heel strike running: The effect of a firm heel counter. *Am J Sports Med* 1990:18, 177.
17. Nigg BM, Nurse MA, Stefanyshyn DJ: Shoe inserts and orthotics for sport and physical activities. *Med Sci Sports Exerc* 1999:31(7, suppl), S421.
18. Lutter LD: Cavus foot in runners. *Foot Ankle* 1981:1, 225.
19. Torg JS, Pavlov H, Torg E: Overuse injuries in sport: The foot. *Clin Sports Med* 1987:6, 291.
20. Lutter LD: Shoes and orthoses in the runner. *Techn Orthop* 1990:5, 57.
21. Roy S: How I manage plantar fasciitis. *Phys Sports Med* 1983:11, 127.
22. Frey C, Stress fractures: Footwear and stress fractures. *Clin Sports Med* 1997:16, 249.
23. Andrews JR: Overuse syndromes of the lower extremity. *Clin Sports Med* 1983:2, 137.
24. Krisoff WB, Ferris WB: Runner's injuries. *Phys Sports Med* 1979:7, 53.
25. Smart GW, Taunton JE, Clement DB: Achilles tendon disorders in runners: A review. *Med Sci Sport Exerc* 1980:12, 231.
26. Campbell JW, Inman VT: Treatment of plantar fasciitis and calcaneal spurs with the UC-BL shoe insert. *Clin Orthop* 1974:103, 57.
27. Hulkko A, Orava S: Stress fractures in athletes. *Int J Sports Med* 1987:8, 221.
28. Milgrom C, Giladi M, Stien M, et al.: Stress fractures in military recruits: A prospective study showing an unusually high incidence. *J Bone Joint Surg Br* 1985:65B, 732.
29. Simkin A, Leichter I, Giladi M, et al.: Combined effect of foot arch structure and an orthotic device on stress fractures. *Foot Ankle* 1989:10, 25.
30. Gardner L, Dziados JE, Jones BH, et al.: Prevention of lower extremity stress fractures: A controlled trial of a shock absorbent insole. *Am J Public Health* 1988:78, 1563.

Chapter 47

FOOT ORTHOTICS

Steven I. Subotnick

INTRODUCTION

At some point in their career, most runners will develop lower extremity problems that interfere with running. As runners age, many find that although few problems arose in the initial years of participation in distance running, they suddenly have nagging injuries, even though the mileage and intensity of running may have actually decreased.

Often the injury is short-lived, a minor nuisance that can be readily linked to training errors or inappropriate gear with premature weardown of running shoes. Simply replacing worn-out shoes or changing brands or style along with some modest training intensity changes will take care of the problem.

In other cases, however, minor discomfort may steadily progress to a chronically painful sports-related injury that does not readily respond to changes in training or foot gear. These more chronic problems are often associated with abnormal biomechanics. Modest biomechanical imbalances, which when the runner was younger caused few problems, are now causing major problems as the athlete ages and has been engaged in running for over 3 to 5 years. Even more notable is the athlete who has run pain free for 10 to 15 years and now needs to find solutions for chronic repetitive running injuries that are not responsive to new shoes or training schedule changes.

Sooner or later, all injured runners consider new shoes, shoe modification, inner soles, or foot orthotics. A visit to the family doctor often leads to a referral to a sports podiatrist or sports medicine physician. It is widely believed that a foot orthotic will alter foot function and allow runners to return to running. Even though the exact effect of orthotics on running biomechanics and/or the prevention or rehabilitation of running injuries is unknown, runners and doctors nonetheless feel that orthotics will be beneficial.

ORTHOTICS AND INJURY REDUCTION

Although orthotics have been used for years, little scientific or clinical evidence has been published in the literature to support their use. Orthotics have been commonly used for the following reasons:

- To reduce the frequency of movement-related injuries
- To align the skeleton properly
- To provide improved cushioning
- To improve sensory feedback
- To improve comfort.

Several studies have noted our limited knowledge of the specific function of orthotic devices but have provided patient-oriented evidence suggesting that orthotics improve the injury condition of runners.

Gross and associates[1] found that foot orthoses may be very effective in providing symptomatic relief of lower extremity complaints including knee, foot, ankle, and hip problems. Of the 347 runners who answered their questionnaire, 30.8% reported complete relief of symptoms, 44.7% great improvement, 15.8% slight improvement, 7.5% no improvement, and 1.2% a worsening. Ninety percent of these runners given a foot orthotic still wore it after their symptoms had subsided. Unfortunately, the type of orthotic was not clearly indicated, and the details on the presenting indications for orthotic usage were reported by the study participants. Even so, because 90% of the runners continued to use the orthotic devices after symptom resolution, the authors found a high degree of overall satisfaction. The results of treatment were independent of diagnosis or the runner's level of participation. Orthotic shoe inserts were most effective in the treatment of symptoms arising from biomechanical abnormalities such as excessive pronation or leg-length discrepancy.[1]

In general, a satisfactory level of symptom relief from the use of orthoses has been reported in overuse injuries.[1–3] After wearing orthoses for 3 months, 81% of 43 patients with painful heels treated with a customized rigid plastic foot orthosis reported complete symptom relief.[4] Blake and Denton[5] reported that a functional foot orthosis effectively reduced pain by 80% in patients with plantar fasciitis. Orthotic devices have also been reported to hasten return to full function of injured runners.[6]

In contrast to these positive findings, other studies have shown little symptom relief. In fact, in the study of Gross et al.,[1] 24.5% of the participants had slight or no improvement, and 13.5% experienced increased severity of symptoms or developed new complaints during the period of orthotic usage. D'Ambrosia[3] has noted that when orthotics are unsatisfactory, a poorly fitted orthosis or poor diagnosis is the cause in more than half of the cases.

GENERAL PRINCIPLES

Orthotic intervention is believed to influence the pattern of lower extremity movement through a combination of mechanical control and biofeedback.[7] It has been speculated that orthoses placed under the mid- and forefoot may increase the afferent feedback from cutaneous receptors, which may lead to reduced eversion due to muscle contraction of the inverting muscles.[8] More recently, the new concept of "minimizing muscle activity" has been proposed to explain the

effect of applying shoe inserts and orthoses in sporting activities.[9] The present author has explored the biomechanics of running in relation to the prevention of foot injuries and has also discussed flatfoot in relation to foot injury.[10,11]

In their review article on the biomechanical effects of orthotic shoe inserts, Razeghi and Batt[12] concluded that little agreement exists on the specific effect of orthoses on kinematic foot variables. Variations and findings may be attributed to differences in the type of orthosis, the material used, the speed and cadence of running, and the method of measuring. Furthermore, the interaction between foot and orthosis may be more subtle than expected; individual variations may not be quantifiable with the present techniques.[12]

In general, orthotics may serve the following clinical purposes:

1. Motion control (by controlling excessive pronation, force transmission up the kinetic chain is limited)
2. Shock absorption
3. Pressure relief in a specific area (such as the plantar heel or great toe metatarsophalangeal/sesamoid region)
4. Redistribution of forces away from a specific area (i.e., use of a metatarsal pad to redistribute forces associated with metarsalgia or a Morton's neuroma; Figs. 47–1 and 47–2).

ORTHOTIC FABRICATION

Most long-distance runners as well as physicians treating long-distance runners are not aware of the most

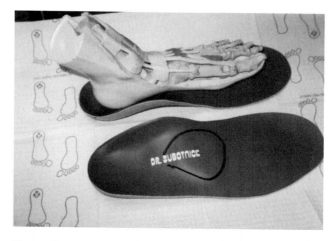

Figure 47–1. Full-length running orthotic with skeleton showing the 17-mm-deep heel seat, extended medial longitudinal arch, and metatarsal pad under cover to elevate the second, third, and fourth metatarsals. The metatarsal pad is outlined in black.

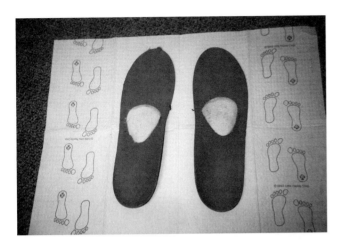

Figure 47–2. Full-length ready-made soft runners' orthotics with bilateral felt metatarsal pads.

recent research studies exploring the various effects of orthotics. They simply know empirically that some type of foot insert (be it an over-the-counter device or a more sophisticated custom-designed biodynamic running foot orthosis) will often help to ameliorate the current running-related injury and sometimes prevent further injuries by decreasing abnormal forces, excessive shock, or excessive abnormal motion.

The author agrees that this empirical type of reasoning is often useful and justified. In the face of increasing overuse running injuries, running shoe therapy and foot orthoses can be an important adjunct to physical rehabilitation and training modification that will help in returning an athlete to full function and preventing further injury (Figs. 47–3 and 47–4).

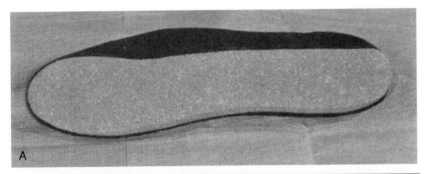

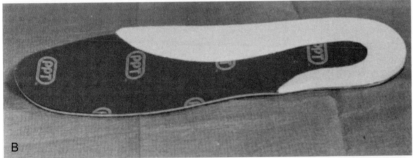

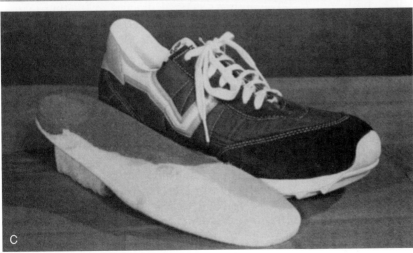

Figure 47–3. Modification of inner soles in running shoes and soft temporary running orthoses. (*A*) Full-length foot support system from a running shoe with additional medial wedging. Medial wedging is with rubber-cork mixture. (*B*) Full-length soft temporary orthotics with a Cobra pad. Note how this pad provides for an increased medial arch and a heel-cup effect. The Cobra pad is formed of a medium durometer foam material. (*C*) Bottom of soft temporary full-length orthoses showing increased medial arch and medial heel extending to the lateral heel using rubber-cork material. (*Source: From Subotnick.*[14])

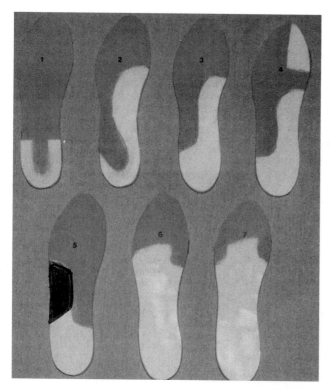

Figure 47–4. Bottom of soft temporary orthotics showing variations of medium durometer foam accommodations and postings. (*1*) Horseshoe padding to accommodate for heel spur and provide for heel stability. (*2*) Cobra pad for medial longitudinal arch and heel stability. Excellent for pronation, plantar fasciitis, or heel spur syndrome. (*3*) Full heel posting with increased medial wedging and medial longitudinal arch. Excellent for heel stability, increased heel lift, and medial longitudinal arch. (*4*) Addition of kinetic wedge to the heel posting with medial longitudinal arch. This allows for accomodation of first metatarsal head and plantarflexion of the first metatarsal head during propulsion; it also accommodate sesamoids. (*5*) Heel posting with lateral extension and cuboid pad. This is utilized for lateral column instability. The cuboid pad is outlined in black and stabilizes the calcaneal cuboid fourth and fifth metatarsal articulation. Increased heel height and lateral wedging increases pronation and lateral column stability. This is good for a moderate cavus foot deformity. (*6*) Heel posting with increased medial longitudinal arch and runner's wedge extending under metatarsal heads two, three, four, and five. This allows for stability of the lesser metatarsal heads while accommodating the first metatarsal head. With increased lateral wedging, this accommodation is good for forefoot valgus and cavus-type feet. (*7*) Full plantar extension under metatarsal heads two, three, and four. This allows for accommodation of plantarflexed first and fifth metatarsals. It can also be fitted with a metatarsal pad to increase the transverse metatarsal arch and allow for treatment of neuromas of the second or third interspace. These types of soft temporary orthotics are also excellent when more durable materials are used in orthotic foot devices for track or short-distance cross-country running when most of the running is done on the ball of the foot. Note that these orthotics are all full length so that accommodation and/or posting can control propulsion. The author finds that full-length orthoses are preferable for treating runners. (*Source: From Subotnick.*[14])

The term *foot orthoses* covers a wide spectrum of externally applied devices ranging from simple arch supports to custom-made dynamic ankle-foot drop splints. The goal of the orthotic prescription varies depending on the specific need. However, functional orthoses are usually prescribed in an attempt to alter foot function with the expectation that they will guide the foot through the weightbearing stance phase of gait to promote overall biomechanical efficiency.[13]

A useful guide to the subject is *Sports Medicine of the Lower Extremity*,[14] which outlines the use of orthotics, the clinical and sagittal plane biomechanics, and the normal patterns of walking and running, as well as the forces acting on the lower extremity; this book also discusses sports-specific biomechanics, with a multidisciplinary presentation of treatment of lower-extremity injuries related to running and other sports. In Chapter 24 of this text, Valmassy and Subotnick[13] discuss various casting techniques, as well as the indications for and use of orthotics in treating the injured runner (Fig. 47–5).

The present author feels that a soft, temporary orthotic is a sensible measure before the use of a more expensive custom-made biodynamic running device. Over-the-counter prefabricated devices, which can often be modified in the dispensing physician's office, have become available; these make the practicality and use of softer, noncustom orthotics more desirable and practical. Most runners will report improvement in comfort and decrease in symptoms with the use of these devices. If the problems go away completely and reinjury is reduced, these devices may suffice.

However, if some but not complete improvement occurs, and the treating sports clinician is aware of the probability of incomplete control of abnormal (or unwanted) pronation with the temporary devices, then more permanent custom biodynamic devices are understandably desirable and indicated (Fig. 47–6).

The author's general practice in treating injured runners is to use the soft temporary orthotics first, either prefabricated or fabricated in the office. These devices are altered with increase or decrease in rearfoot control depending on foot type. Additional indications for specific modifications include the following:

1. A medial longitudinal arch is added for hyperpronators.
2. Additional forefoot varus is added for hypermobile first ray with excessive pronation.
3. The higher arch cavus foot or foot with plantarflexed first ray is treated with additional lateral forefoot wedging and accommodation of the first metatarsal head.

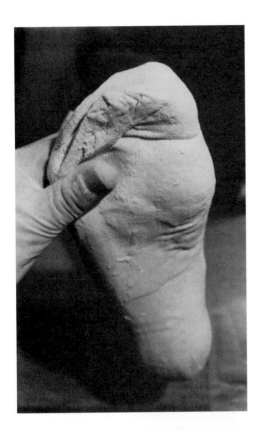

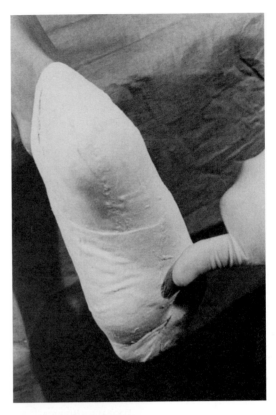

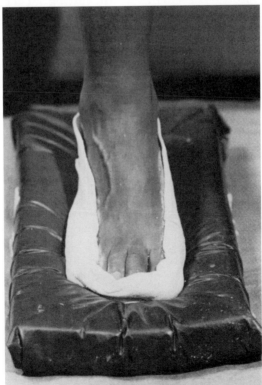

Figure 47–5. Casting technique for custom-made runners, orthotic foot devices. (*1*) Supine. (*2*) Prone casting technique (preferred by author). (*3*) Semipronated casting technique. This is a weightbearing technique that allows an orthosis to be made for a semi-rigid pronated foot that will not accommodate full control. This type of device is excellent for an osteoarthritic or rheumatoid arthritic foot or that of a senior runner. These devices range in their degree of control and allow for increased comfort and accommodation as well as increased shock absorbance (with the appropriate material). (*Source: From Subotnick.*[14])

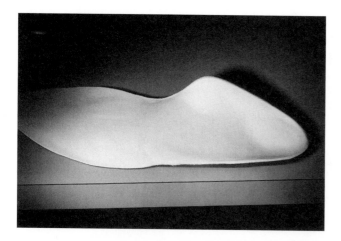

Figure 47–6. Full-length running orthotic with extended medial flange. This type of device is used for the moderate to severe pronator. The extended medial flange helps to provide for midtarsal joint stability. The high heel cup helps to keep the calcaneal fat pad in place, improving the shock-absorbing capability of the heel fat-pad complex.

4. Runners complaining of lateral arch pain, the so-called peroneal cuboid syndrome, are treated with a cuboid pad or increased lateral arch support on the soft temporary devices.[15]

After the use of soft devices with various modifications, the patient is then casted, neutrally, for a more permanent biodynamic device. These devices are as soft as possible to provide biomechanical control and likewise dampen excessive contact forces. In general, the older the athlete, the softer the device. Although firmer devices are tolerated in younger athletes, as the athlete ages, softer devices are generally preferred for comfort and tolerance. Furthermore, it has been observed over many years of treating athletes that the foot often becomes longer and flatter over the years. Therefore various modifications and orthotic devices as well as a change in shoe size are often indicated.

ORTHOTIC MODIFICATION

The author prefers the use of a treadmill with a video playback device to help in determing the effectiveness of changing shoes, the use of soft temporary devices, over-the-counter devices, and more permanent biodynamic devices in actually providing some form of rearfoot and forefoot stability during running. Often an alteration in the angle of gait will be noted as the sophistication of biomechanical control and effectiveness increases. For example, athletes who pronate often toe out, and with the use of biodynamic-

specific devices to control abnormal pronation, the angle of gait often changes, with increased toeing in and more biomechanical efficiency. Examination of the athlete running with and without orthotics therefore allows the clinician to assess orthotic efficacy better, as well as the possible need for further modification.

High Arched Cavus Foot

Treatment of the high arched cavus foot is difficult. The goal in treating this foot is to provide for increased heel height, especially when the foot has anterior equinus, a dropped forefoot. In addition, most cavus feet have plantarflexed first metatarsal and forefoot valgus, either localized or in general. This requires lateral wedging on the orthotic.

The orthotic devices for the higher arch cavus foot, which is usually also more rigid with decreased subtalar joint range of motion, are intended to increase shock absorbance and decrease lateral instability. Accommodation of the plantarflexed first ray is almost always necessary. In addition, an increased lateral arch is necessary to stabilize the cuboid. In the higher arch cavus foot or the foot with a peroneal cuboid syndrome, an extended lateral flange is often helpful in allowing for increased lateral rearfoot stability as well as midfoot stability.

Pronated Foot

In the pronated foot, an extended medial arch is desirable. In addition, a high rearfoot cup is helpful in preventing excessive motion of the plantar calcaneal fat pad and in stabilizing the rearfoot (Figs. 47–7 to 47–11). In most runners, orthotic accommodation of the first

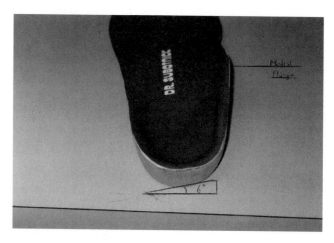

Figure 47–7. Custom-made orthotics with a deep heel cup (18 mm) and extended medial flange. Rearfoot varus posting is 6 degrees medial. There is accommodation of the first metatarsal head with a kinetic wedge.

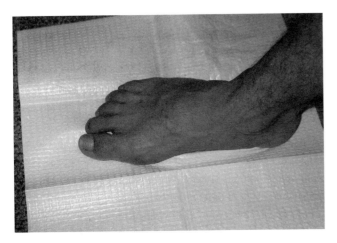

Figure 47–8. Foot with moderate pronation.

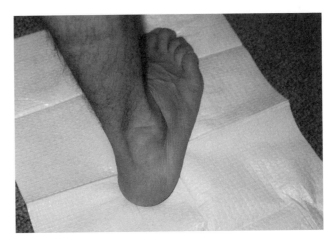

Figure 47–10. Rear view of moderate pronation foot in a runner.

ray, to allow for a kinetic wedge as described by Dannanberg,[16] is desirable (Figs. 47–12 to 47–15).

Even though an injured runner has an orthotic from another health care specialist (even a sports podiatrist), failure of this device in helping to treat a running-related injury or prevent subsequent injury does not mean orthotics will be ineffective. The author has seen countless patients with ineffective orthotics from various health care providers, some of them quite well made. The reasons for failure are often subtle and require much trial and error, knowledge of the various

types and materials, and sometimes shoe modification. A persistent sports podiatrist will usually find a device that will improve the comfort of the runner while decreasing symptoms.

The treatment of a runner with foot orthotic devices requires an on-site biomechanical foot orthotic lab to allow the individual practitioner to modify devices, check their effectiveness immediately by having the athlete run on a treadmill, and (if needed) video the results. Lack of the ability to modify devices on site is one of the major reasons for failure of orthoses in the treatment of runners. Another cause of failure is the shoe-orthotic interface.

Furthermore, failure to evaluate fully the various needs of different runners and to use a soft temporary device initially while assessing these needs is another reason for failure. Also, a running orthosis may not be appropriate for everyday use or dress shoes. Different

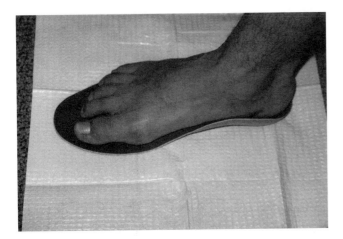

Figure 47–9. Same foot with orthotic foot control. A full-length runner's orthosis has been used with a deep 18-mm heel, increased rearfoot posting of 6 degrees medial, medial longitudinal arch filler with extended medial arch, and kinetic wedge with accommodation of the first metatarsal head. In addition, a runner's platform that is 6 degrees varus extends from behind the first metatarsal head to beyond the second, third, fourth, and fifth metatarsal heads. Six degrees is medial, decreasing gradually to 0 degrees at the lateral aspect of the foot. This type of runner's wedge under the forefoot provides for control of propulsive pronation.

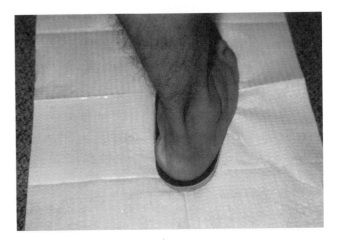

Figure 47–11. Same foot from the rear view showing control of moderate pronation with a full-length runner's orthotic. Note that the heel valgus and midfoot pronation have been controlled.

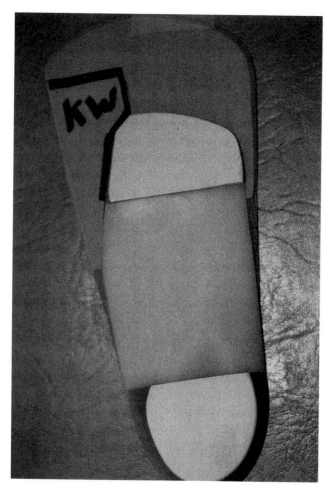

Figure 47–12. Running orthotic with rearfoot and forefoot posting and kinetic wedge after the method of Dannenberg. (*Source: From Subotnick.[14]*)

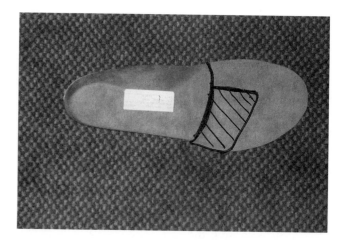

Figure 47–14. Kinetic wedge and accommodation of the first metatarsal head. Combination polypropylene and rubber-cork filler to provide for biomechanical control and increased shock absorbance. This type of device is preferable in that it allows for the best properties of the molded polypropylene orthotic and the softer, more accommodative leather cork rubber devices. The amount of softness, biomechanical control, and shock absorbance can be modified by changing the various materials. For instance, for a very large 220-lb runner with excessive pronation, 3.5-mm polypropylene may be necessary with a leather-cork filler. A lighter runner might do well with 2- to 2.5-mm polypropylene and a lighter poron-type rubber filler. Since these devices are full length and have soft material under the metatarsal heads and toes, accommodation of lesions is easily carried out.

orthotic devices are necessary for different functions, and thus the runner may require two sets of orthoses, as it is important to control biomechanics during everyday activity as well as during running.

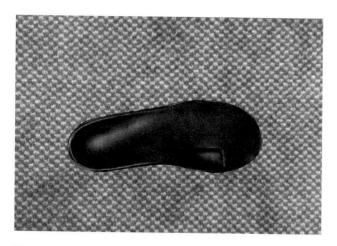

Figure 47–13. Full-length running orthotic with kinetic wedge and suspension of the first metatarsal head. This allows for plantarflexion of the first metatarsal head during running and provides for increase in the "windlass" effect of plantarflexion of the first metatarsal head with tightening of the medial plantar fascia.

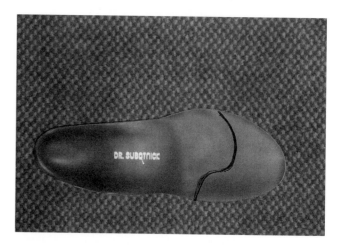

Figure 47–15. Full-length running orthotic with forefoot runner's platform. Note that the bottom material, as outlined on the top, extends well beyond the metatarsals into the base of the toes. It likewise provides for accommodation of the first metatarsal head. This type of device is optimal in that it allows for accommodation of propulsive biomechanical abnormalities. It also improves shock absorbance under the metatarsal heads.

CONCLUSIONS

The fabrication of orthotic foot devices for runners requires both skill and experience and still remains an art as well as a science. Although there is scientific evidence of the effectiveness of orthotics, there also are papers describing failure. Such failure may be due to imprecise orthotic prescriptions. Although various health care providers can become proficient in the basics of orthotic devices for runners, a sports medicine specialist such as a sports podiatrist or orthotist with experience in treating runners (as well as training in running biomechanics and the utilization of foot orthotics) will have the most success; such a practitioner is thus a valuable member of the treatment team.

Treatment of runners is often best performed by health care providers who are or have been runners. Since they have usually suffered through various injuries themselves, these providers have an understanding of runners' needs and specific problems. They also understand the importance of the sport in the life of the runner. When this personal connection to running is absent, it becomes more difficult to identify with the runner and to summon the fortitude to stick with it until the appropriate orthotic foot control can be found for optimal treatment.

REFERENCES

1. Gross ML, Davlin LB, Evanski PM: Effectiveness of orthotic shoe inserts in the long-distance runner. *Am J Sports Med* 1991:19, 409.
2. James SL, Bates BT, Ostering LR: Injuries to the runners. *Am J Sports Med* 1987:6, 40.
3. D'Ambrosia RD: Orthotic device in running injuries. *Clin Sports Med* 1985:4, 611.
4. Schere PR: Heel spur syndrome; pathomechanics and non-surgical treatment. Biomechanics Graduate Research Group for 1988. *J Am Podiatr Med Assoc* 1991:81, 68.
5. Blake RL, Denton JA: Functional foot orthoses for athletic injuries, a retrospective study. *J Am Podiatr Med Assoc* 1985:75, 359.
6. Bates BT, Ostering LR, Masson B, et al.: Foot orthotic devices to modify selected aspects of lower extremity mechanics. *Am J Sports Med* 1979:7, 338.
7. Nawockzenski DA, Saltezman CL, Cook TM: Effect of foot structure on the dimensional kinematic coupling behavior of the leg and rear foot. *Phys Ther* 1998:78, 404.
8. Stacoff A, Reinschmidt C, Nigg BM, et al.: Effects of foot orthoses on skeletal motion during running. *Clin Biomech* 2000:15, 54.
9. Nigg BM, Nurse MA, Stefanyshyn DJ: Shoe inserts and orthotics for sports and physical activities. *Med Sci Sports Exerc* 1999:31(suppl), S421.
10. Subotnick SI: The biomechanics of running: Implications for prevention of foot injuries. *Sports Med* 1985:2, 144.
11. Subotnick SI: The flat foot. *Physician Sports Med* 1981:9, 85.
12. Razeghi M, Batt ME: Biomechanical analysis of the effect of orthotic shoe inserts. *Sports Med* 2000:29, 425.
13. Valmassy R, Subotnick SI: Orthoses, in Subotnick SI (ed.), *Sports Medicine of the Lower Extremity*, 2nd ed., Philadelphia, Churchill Livingstone, 1999:465.
14. Subotnick SI (ed.): *Sports Medicine of the Lower Extremity*, 2nd ed., Philadelphia, Churchill Livingstone, 1999.
15. Subotnick SI: Peroneal cuboid syndrome: An often overlooked cause of lateral column foot pain. *Chiro Tech* 1998:10, 1556.
16. Dannanberg HJ: Sagittal Plans Biomechanics, in Subotnick SI (ed.), *Sports Medicine of the Lower Extremity*, 2nd ed., Philadelphia, Churchill Livingstone, 1999:137.

Chapter 48

PRINCIPLES OF STRENGTH TRAINING

Eric M. Chumbley

INTRODUCTION

For some time a gulf has separated strength and endurance training, in both theory and practice. Some authors[1] have held that training in one mode could not contribute to gains in the other and may even diminish those gains. Endurance athletes have sometimes resisted the idea of performing serious strength training. Current thought, however, reverses that position and indicates that strength training can actually improve endurance performance.[2] This chapter outlines the health benefits of strength training, examines the evidence supporting strength training as an adjunct to running, and gives current strength training recommendations for runners.

HEALTH BENEFITS

Overall Function

The ability of strength training to influence strength, functionality, and bone mineral density (BMD) favorably, especially in the elderly, is well documented.[3–5] Considering the aging population of the United States, this is emerging as an important area in health care. As adults grow older, they tend to lose muscle mass, strength,[3] and BMD, with subsequent loss of mobility and increased risks of falls and fractures. Resistance training has been proposed to help reduce the risk of

falls and the injury rate through increased muscle strength, gait velocity, and stair climbing power.[5] Although most weightbearing exercises seem capable of improving BMD, the increase is site specific.[4] Accordingly, aerobic exercises such as running can improve lower extremity BMD, but activities such as strength training are necessary to improve the BMD of upper extremities.[6] Taken as a whole, these data indicate that an increased emphasis on strength training could potentially result in fewer fractures, less morbidity, and more independence as individuals live farther into their ninth and tenth decades.

Cardiovascular Function

Aerobic exercise has long been recognized as an effective means of positively influencing the cardiovascular system, but many clinicians may fail to appreciate the cardiovascular benefits of strength training. Indeed, some myths persist that strength training may actually adversely affect resting blood pressure. However, the literature supports strength training as a means of reducing cardiac stress and improving cardiovascular risk factors.

In a study that has implications for daily living, McCartney et al.[7] examined the effects of strength training on two common cardiovascular parameters. They showed that strength training decreases the heart rate and blood pressure responses to the performance of submaximal leg presses after 12 weeks, suggesting that improved strength lessens the load on the heart during routine lifting tasks. The increased tolerance to strenuous work implied by these data may have wide-ranging applications, from carrying groceries to shoveling snow or even completing a cardiac rehabilitation program.

The potential to modify cardiac risk factors with strength training appears to center on an increase in muscle mass. Body composition improves in strength-trained individuals, as muscle mass increases relative to fat.[7–9] Higher muscle mass places a greater energy demand on the body, raising the caloric expenditure required to maintain body weight (increasing the resting metabolic rate).[9] This can be especially important in the mature population, as the resting metabolic rate usually declines with age when fat-free mass decreases. Strength training therefore plays an important role in preventing and treating obesity, a risk factor for diabetes mellitus and coronary artery disease.[10] It has also been shown to have a more direct role in preventing diabetes by improving glucose tolerance and the insulin response to an oral glucose tolerance test just as effectively as aerobic training. The decrease in insulin is directly correlated with an increase in lean body mass.[11]

Finally, strength training has not been proved to cause resting hypertension.[12] Studies of training with Olympic lifts have even shown modest reductions in resting systolic and diastolic blood pressures.[13]

RUNNING ADVANTAGES

Improved Performance

Although the health benefits are worthwhile, the serious runner may already feel healthy and may question why he or she should divert time from running to another form of training. The answer is simple: a competitive edge. Evidence indicates that when aerobic conditioning is equal, the anaerobic energy system contributes to improved race performance in college cross-country runners.[14] The reason for this advantage is probably the ability to perform extended high-intensity exercise.

When exercising at a high percentage of $\dot{V}O_2max$, endurance seems to be related more to lactate metabolism and glycogen use than to $\dot{V}O_2max$ itself.[15] This has been demonstrated by an increase in short-term endurance with strength training, without any significant change in $\dot{V}O_2max$.[16,17] Both the lactate threshold and the onset of blood lactate accumulation are extended by high-volume weight training,[18,19] allowing high-intensity exercise to be sustained longer. These changes provide the runner who has better anaerobic conditioning with the "kick" essential for climbing hills, accelerating, and sprinting.[2,14]

Injury Prevention

Athletes seem to be at higher risk for injuries when muscle imbalances exist, either side to side, or agonist group to antagonist group.[20] Some authors note that strength training may indeed help prevent medial tibial stress syndrome, plantar fasciitis, and patellofemoral dysfunction.[21] Strength training also has the potential to decrease injuries by its effect on other connective tissues. Tendons and ligaments are known to become thicker, heavier, and stronger through strength training.[22,23] Articular cartilage function improves as well.[23] Interestingly, strength training may be of even more benefit to runners than power athletes with regard to injury prevention, given the higher volume and frequency of endurance training.[24]

STRENGTH TRAINING DEFINITIONS

To be able to speak with authority to athletes and coaches, the clinician must be familiar with the language of strength training.

Strength is the ability to produce maximal force in a one-time, all-out effort, whereas power is maximum strength in relation to time (power = work/time). Muscular endurance is the ability to continue muscular contractions over prolonged periods.

A concentric contraction of the muscle occurs as the muscle body shortens and the athlete overcomes resistance. It is sometimes called the *positive*. The eccentric contraction is the muscle contraction that occurs as the muscle body lengthens. This occurs as the athlete lowers the weight and is often termed the *negative*. Together, the concentric and eccentric contractions make up one repetition.

A set is a number of repetitions performed consecutively without rest, usually in a predetermined amount. Doing two sets of 10 repetitions of the squat means that the athlete will perform 10 squats, stop for a period of time (to spot his or her partner on the same exercise, perform another set with a different exercise, or simply rest), and then perform another 10 squats.

The repetition maximum (RM or rep max) is the highest amount of resistance that can be correctly performed for a given number of repetitions. For instance, if an athlete can perform 10 correct repetitions of leg presses with 200 lb, but not 11, his or her 10 repetition maximum (10 RM) for the leg press is 200 lb. If he or she can perform one correct repetition of the bench press with 150 lb, but not two, his or her 1 RM for the bench press is 150 lb. The RM is frequently used as a guide to training intensity.

The volume of training is the total amount of repetitions done with a specific load for a given exercise.

It is usually expressed as sets × repetitions × load (resistance in pounds).

Overload is the basic principle of exercise by which the body is stressed beyond its normal requirements. It is required for improvement in any type of exercise. In strength training, overload is achieved by adding volume (sets, repetitions, or load).

Intensity is the power output of an exercise. The highest intensity exercises rely almost solely on the phosphagen energy system (adenosine triphosphate and creatine phosphate interacting via a biochemical loop to produce energy at a very high rate) and can only be sustained for brief periods of about 6 seconds or less.[15] Heavy intensity relies on the phosphagen system as well, but more on the anaerobic glycolytic pathways (carbohydrate breakdown with lactate formation, also known as fast glycolysis) and can be sustained up to 2 minutes. Light-intensity exercise is mostly oxidative, lasting over 3 minutes. In general, strength training is much more intense exercise than distance running, relying much more heavily on the phosphagen and anaerobic glycolytic pathways than the oxidative, but the intensity can be varied depending on the desired results.

Muscles are composed of two main categories of fibers, type I and type II.[12,25] Type I fibers are red in color because of their high density of myoglobin and mitochondria; they rely primarily on oxidative metabolism. They are adapted to prolonged exercise at low intensity and are sometimes called *slow twitch* fibers. Type II fibers are white in color and are dependent on glycolytic metabolism to provide short, intense bursts of powerful contractions. They contract at two to three times the speed of type I fibers and are often referred to as *fast twitch.* Type II fibers are subdivided into type IIa (intermediate between aerobic and anaerobic), type IIb (primarily anaerobic; the largest and most powerful fibers), and type IIc (undifferentiated). Type I fibers are recruited early in a muscle contraction, whereas type II fibers are recruited later, when more strength is required.

Strength training causes predictable changes in skeletal muscle, according to the SAID principle—specific adaptation to imposed demand.[12,25] Muscles grow in response to training by hypertrophy, with increased number and size of myofibrils (components of muscle fibers). Increased strength results. Type I fibers respond well to prolonged, lower-intensity training, whereas type II fibers are better stimulated by brief, high-intensity bouts of exercise.

TRAINING RECOMMENDATIONS

To promote muscular fitness for all adults, the American College of Sports Medicine (ACSM) recommends one set of 8 to 12 repetitions of 8 to 10 resistance exercises, two or three times a week, to include all major muscle groups.[26] The guidelines of this chapter are in agreement with those of the ACSM and are intended to help the clinician put the ACSM position stand into practice.

As with any exercise prescription, the first consideration must be the mode of training. If the athlete will not stay with the program, the most carefully planned routine will fail to produce results. The clinician making recommendations to the runner, then, must be responsive to the runner's desires. Indeed, flexibility should be viewed as a great asset, since the large range of exercises and regimens in strength training can yield tremendous variety and therefore increased compliance.

Machines vs. Free Weights

In creating a strength training regimen, one of the first choices faced is whether to work with machines or free weights. Both options offer advantages and drawbacks. Machines are typically easier to use and do not require a partner, or spotter, for safe use (Fig. 48–1). The time needed to master them is therefore shorter, making them more attractive to novice lifters. Using machines may allow a quicker workout, since resistance is quickly and easily changed. However, each

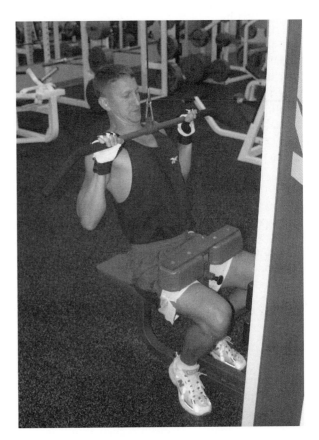

Figure 48–1. Lateral pulldown, a common machine.

machine often exercises only one muscle group or joint. In addition, many machines link both left and right extremities in their design, so that asymmetric strength may never be detected and could actually be magnified. Free weight exercises, on the other hand, are often multijoint, which may more closely replicate athletic activity than isolated, single-joint exercises. Balance, so key in symmetric development, is emphasized with free weights, as both the right and left sides of the body must work equally to perform exercises with barbells. Free weights demand more practice and coordination, though, and a spotter is mandatory for many types of exercises. Finally, sessions with free weights may take longer to complete, as bars must be loaded and unloaded with plates before and after each exercise. Of course, availability of each mode plays a role, as all gyms are equipped differently. In the end, the specific workout to be performed will be the product of the runner's interest in and experience with strength training, as well as the equipment available.

Exercise Selection

Two primary principles must be recognized when choosing the exercises to be performed. Modifications can then be made depending on individual preferences, such as his or her specific goals (overall health only, improved running performance and injury prevention, developing his or her physique) and the amount of time to be dedicated to lifting. Again, interest and equipment will play the pivotal roles in deciding which exercises to include.

First, any program intended to increase overall strength must address all major muscle groups. For the runner, it could be tempting to cut the workout short by only exercising the lower extremities, using the simple reasoning that the legs do all the work. However, the body is held erect during the running gait by the abdominal and back muscles, and the arms are in constant motion. It may be true that most exertion occurs below the waist, but the rest of the body must also be addressed to avoid undue fatigue and potential secondary overuse problems.

Second, opposing muscle groups should always be worked. For instance, runners depend on hip extensors (gluteals, hamstrings) to move the leg backward and thus generate forward motion during the propulsion phase of running, whereas the hip flexors (iliopsoas, rectus femorus) are needed to recover the leg to a forward position during the swing phase. Both groups must be exercised to avoid muscle imbalance that could potentially lead to overuse injuries.

Table 48–1 gives a brief list of common exercises to work the basic muscle groups. Although it is by no

TABLE 48–1. EXERCISES

Muscle Group	Machine	Free Weights/ Body Weight
Quadriceps	Leg press Leg extension	Squat Lunge
Hamstrings	Leg press Leg curl	Squat Lunge
Calves	Seated calf	Calf raises
Chest	Chest press Butterfly Decline press	Bench press Incline press Decline press Dumbbell flies Dips
Shoulders	Overhead press Lateral raise	Shoulder press Shrugs Dumbbell lateral raises
Upper back	Compound row Lat pulldown Seated row	Bent over row Pull-ups
Triceps	Chest press Overhead press Triceps pushdown	Lying triceps extension Shoulder press Dips
Biceps	Compound row Preacher curl	Biceps curl Preacher curl (with bar)
Lower back	Low back extension	Straight leg dead lift Hyperextension
Abdominals	Abdominal Rotary torso	Bent-leg sit-ups
Neck	Four-way neck	Resistance with partner

means exhaustive, it gives a good idea of available options. A review of these exercises should reveal that several are effective at working more than one muscle group. This information becomes important when designing a program that will make the most efficient use of the runner's time. It should also be noted that some exercises involve neither weights nor machines but effectively rely on body weight alone. Changing the specific exercises used in the routine every 4 to 8 weeks is encouraged to prevent boredom and provide different muscle stimulation. Table 48–2 shows samples of programs that exercise all major muscle groups.

Order

Many authorities recommend placing exercises that work the largest muscle groups earliest in the workout.[12,25,27] These exercises are more often multijoint and require both more energy to complete and the input of smaller muscle groups for control. Working smaller muscle groups first would both deplete the energy reserves necessary for large movements and fatigue the smaller groups, making the multijoint,

TABLE 48–2. SAMPLE ROUTINES

Machines Only	Free Weights Only	Combination
Leg extension	Squat	Squat
Leg curl	Lunge	Leg extension
Seated calf	Calf raises	Calf raises
Chest press	Inclined bench press	Chest press
Overhead press	Shoulder press	Overhead press
Lat pulldown	Bent over row	Lat pulldown
Triceps pushdown	Lying triceps extension	Triceps pushdown
Preacher curl	Biceps curl	Biceps curl
Low back extension	Hyperextension	Low back extension
Abdominal	Crunches	Bent leg sit-ups
Four-way neck	Neck with partner	Four way neck

large-muscle exercises less productive. The exercises in Table 48–2 are placed in appropriate order.

Another strategy is to alternate lower body and upper body exercises.[27] This regimen has been used during circuit weight training to allow for rest of one group of muscles while another is working. Circuit weight training is discussed in more detail later in the chapter.

Frequency

Muscle groups tend to respond to training differently. The muscles supporting the extremities may require training 3 days a week or more for maximum development, whereas those supporting the spine seem to do as well with fewer sessions.[28] In the interest of time and compliance, though, recommendations for the runner should be streamlined. Forty-eight hours of rest between training sessions is recommended as a general guideline for most muscle groups and most athletes.[28] This usually translates into three sessions per week, with 1 or 2 days off between sessions, such as Monday-Wednesday-Friday. The runner who wants to devote less time to strength training can still gain over 80% of the strength benefits by training only twice a week.[29] Runners who choose this course should allow either 2 or 3 days off between sessions, such as Monday-Thursday. When possible, strength training sessions should be performed on days of light running or no running at all.

Volume

To remain competitive, runners perform high-volume aerobic training regularly. The addition of resistance training should be at a relatively low volume, especially when beginning, to keep the risk of overtraining low. In addition, high-volume strength training is known to result in a large degree of muscle hypertrophy,[12] which could conceivably slow the runner. Like many forms of exercise, response to strength training

is highly individualized, and each runner must experiment to some extent in order to reach optimal results.

Sets

In 1962, Berger[30] demonstrated significantly increased strength gains when multiple bench press sets vs. one set were performed; all other studies have failed to show such an advantage. However, these studies have been mainly conducted on previously untrained individuals and over relatively short periods of 4 to 20 weeks.[28] Experienced athletes and coaches involved in traditionally power- and strength-oriented sports (field events, wrestling, football, etc.) tend to recommend multiple sets, based more on experience than scientific data. Even in this setting, though, initial recommended exercise volumes are held low, typically using one to three sets.[31] For overall health benefits, the President's Council on Physical Fitness and Sports recommends one set of 8 to 15 repetitions, two or three times a week.[32] Because of the concerns of overtraining in runners, one set of each chosen exercise should be adequate initially. Later in training, after the athlete has become confident with strength training techniques and accustomed to the new addition to his or her routine, extra sets may be added if desired.

Repetitions

The best number of repetitions to perform with each set depends on the goal of strength training. There is an inverse relationship between the number of repetitions that can be performed and the load that can be lifted. Because the number of repetitions determines the duration of the exercise, it also determines the intensity and therefore the energy system required. Assuming that sets are performed to momentary muscle failure, the fewer the repetitions that can be performed, the higher the relative contribution from the phosphagen system (higher intensity), and the more strength is developed. With higher repetitions, the oxidative system is taxed more, and endurance is emphasized. Distance runners are not power athletes, so very intense training in the under 30-second range would be of little value, and possibly dangerous since high loads are used. At the other extreme, runners already engage in large volumes of endurance training, so little is to be gained by prolonged workouts of moderate to light intensity lasting 2 minutes or more per set. The best duration of sets for runners is probably 30 to 120 seconds, which primarily utilizes the anaerobic (fast) glycolytic pathway. This translates into sets of 5 to 20 repetitions when standard 6-second repetitions (2 seconds concentric contraction, 4 seconds eccentric) are performed. Again, flexibility in design and variety are key.

The lower end of this range represents greater gains in strength, and the upper end increases muscle endurance. To standardize a workout and keep it brief, a repetition range of 8 to 12 a set should be adopted. At an average of 1 minute a set (6 seconds × 10 repetitions), and allowing roughly a minute between exercises, a 12-exercise session can be completed in under 25 minutes. This scheme should be effective to build strength over the initial 3 to 4 months of training[28] and may easily be manipulated later as the runner progresses in strength training.

Load

Although sets and repetitions may be predetermined for large groups of people, the actual load lifted must be highly individualized. To gain the greatest benefit from each set of every exercise, overload must be achieved. The resistance selected must fatigue the muscle group exercised within the predetermined range of repetitions, meaning that sets are performed to momentary muscular failure. When performing sets of 8 to 12 repetitions, the correct load is determined by how many repetitions the runner is capable of doing with a given weight. If the runner cannot perform eight repetitions, he or she should decrease the weight. If the runner can perform 12 or more repetitions, he or she should increase the weight.

Circuit Weight Training

Circuit weight training is a method of strength training that combines benefits of both anaerobic and aerobic exercise, although not to the fullest extent of either. In this form of strength training, exercises are performed with minimal rest (15 to 30 seconds) in between, progressing in a specific sequence. Gains in V̇o₂max are modest, and the brief rest periods do not allow repletion of the phosphagen system, preventing maximum strength benefits. This is potentially the quickest method of strength training, though, and is well suited to individuals who have little time.

Form and Safety

Runners embarking on a new strength training program should spend the first 2 to 3 weeks becoming acquainted with the regimen. This includes keeping initial volume and intensity low, to help prevent excessive muscle soreness, which could lead to poor compliance.[12] Strict form should be emphasized, both to become familiar with the equipment and to ingrain good training habits. During this period, the runner should concentrate on working through the full range of motion of each exercise.

Proper breathing and repetition speed are also essential. Inhalation should coincide with the eccentric contraction, and exhalation should accompany the concentric contraction. Although for years, many authorities have held that breath holding should be avoided because of acute, extraordinarily high blood pressure, recent evidence suggests that in some cases it may be appropriate if the breath is held briefly in the initial concentric contraction.[33] This may serve to decrease cardiac afterload and reduce transmural cerebral artery pressure. Repetitions should be performed slowly, taking 4 seconds for the eccentric and 2 seconds for the concentric contractions. This practice emphasizes the stronger eccentric contraction rather than ignoring it by simply rapidly lifting and then dropping the weight (Fig. 48–2).

Adequate warm-up includes 5 to 10 minutes of easy aerobic activity, followed by stretching specific to the exercises to be performed. Stretching should also be included in cool-down[34] (see Chapter 44, on therapeutic exercise).

Finally, as noted earlier, having a spotter is mandatory for free weight use and some forms of

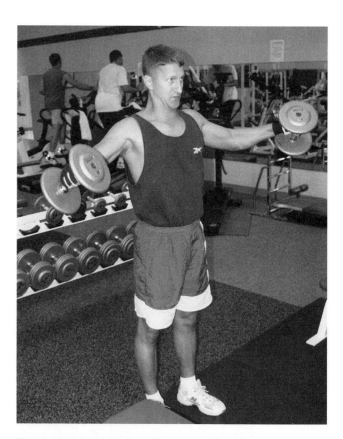

Figure 48–2. Lateral raises. Emphasizing the slow, eccentric contractions during the lowering phase increases the difficulty of the exercise and may help prevent injury.

high-intensity training. There are also other, less-tangible benefits to having a training partner. Knowing that someone else will be waiting for you at the gym is incentive to show up regularly. In addition, training partners can be great motivators for improvement.

Advanced Training Techniques

For the runner interested in more advanced means for muscle building by altering the order of exercise, several techniques are available.[27,35] Some require performance of multiple sets of exercises. Supersetting involves alternating agonist and antagonist groups at the same joint with little rest between sets (Figs. 48–3 and 48–4). Compound setting alternates two different exercises with the same muscle group with little rest and is a more intense form of training. Preexhaustion is used to make multijoint exercises more difficult by first performing a single-joint exercise (Fig. 48–5) with the same muscle group. It is most useful when the multijoint exercise is not achieving desired results. These techniques are advanced and should not be used until the athlete has become comfortable with the basic strength training techniques and is willing to devote more energy to strength training.

Other techniques can be done with only one set of each exercise. Breakdown training, for example,

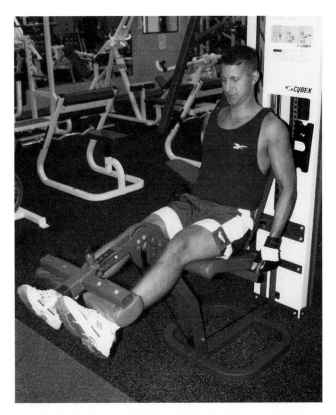

Figure 48–3. Leg extension. All exercises should always be balanced by their antagonist movements.

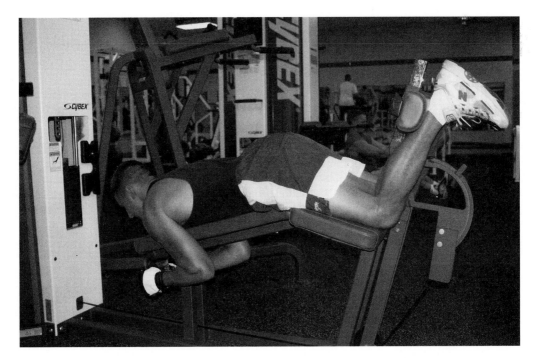

Figure 48–4. Leg curl, the antagonist movement to the leg extension.

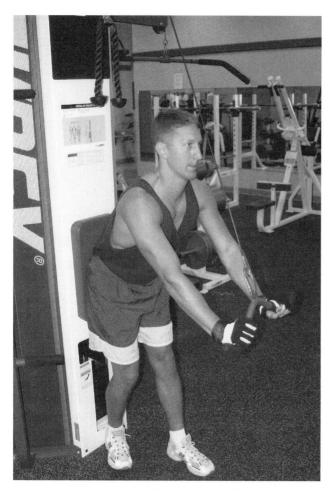

Figure 48–5. Triceps extension, a machine exercise that fatigues the triceps and can be used in the preexhaustion technique with the bench press.

increases the difficulty of training without significantly increasing the length of the workout. At the end of a set (when no more repetitions can be completed), the resistance is decreased by 10% to 20%, and two to four additional repetitions are performed to exhaustion. This method has been shown to increase strength development by 30% over standard training[36] and is most quickly and easily accomplished while using machines. Assisted training can achieve similar results, with the training partner giving enough assistance to perform two to four extra concentric repetitions at the end of a set. The eccentric repetitions are unassisted.

SUMMARY

Strength training can be an effective adjunct for serious runners in both improved performance and decreased injuries. The very nature of strength training allows tremendous variety in exercise choice and flexibility in workout schedule. When beginning, runners should perform strength training sessions two or three times a week and do a single set of 8 to 12 repetitions using exercises that will work each major muscle group. As they see improvements in strength, decreases in injuries, or faster times, they may wish to add extra exercises, more sets of the same exercises, or an additional training session during the week, allowing a day of rest from strength training in between sessions. In short, strength training for runners can be a relatively small investment in time for potential gains in health and performance.

REFERENCES

1. Kraemer WJ, Patton JF, Gordon SE, et al.: Compatibility of high-intensity strength and endurance training on hormonal and skeletal muscle adaptations. *J Appl Physiol* 1995:78, 976.
2. Tanaka H, Swensen T: Impact of resistance training on endurance performance: A new form of cross-training? *Sports Med* 1998:25, 191.
3. Evans WJ: Exercise training guidelines for the elderly. *Med Sci Sports Exerc* 1999:31, 12.
4. Layne JE, Nelson ME: The effects of progressive resistance training on bone density: A review. *Med Sci Sports Exerc* 1999:31, 25.
5. Fiatarone MA, O'Neill EF, Ryan ND, et al.: Exercise training and nutritional supplementation for physical frailty in very elderly people. *N Engl J Med* 1994:330, 1769.
6. Hamdy RC, Anderson JS, Whalen KE, et al.: Regional differences in bone density of young men involved in different exercises. *Med Sci Sports Exerc* 1994:26, 884.
7. McCartney N, McKelvie RS, Martin J, et al.: Weight-training-induced attenuation of the circulatory response of older males to weightlifting. *J Appl Physiol* 1993:74, 1056.
8. Dolezal BA, Potteiger JA: Concurrent resistance and endurance training influence basal metabolic rate in nondieting individuals, *J Appl Physiol* 1998:85, 695.
9. Pratley R, Nicklas B, Rubin M, et al.: Strength training increases resting metabolic rate and norepinephrine levels in healthy 50- to 65-yr-old men. *J Appl Physiol* 1994:76, 133.
10. Smutok MA, Reece C, Kokkinos PF, et al.: Aerobic versus strength training for risk factor intervention in middle-aged men at high risk for coronary heart disease. *Metabolism* 1993:42, 177.
11. Miller WJ, Sherman WM, Ivy JL: Effect of strength training on glucose tolerance and post-glucose insulin response. *Med Sci Sports Exerc* 1984:16, 539.
12. Lillegard WA, Terrio JD: Appropriate strength training. *Clin Sports Med* 1994:78, 457.
13. Stone MH, Wilson GD, Blessing D, et al.: Cardiovascular responses to short-term Olympic style weight-training in young men. *Can J Appl Sports Sci* 1983:8, 134.

14. Bulbulian R, Wilcox AR, Darabos BL: Anaerobic contribution to distance running performance of trained cross-country athletes. *Med Sci Sports Exerc* 1986:18, 107.

15. Stone MH, Conley MS: Bioenergetics, in Baechle TR (ed.), *Essentials of Strength Training and Conditioning,* Champaign, IL, Human Kinetics, 1994:67.

16. Hickson RC, Rosenkoetter MA, Brown MM: Strength training effects on aerobic power and short-term endurance. *Med Sci Sports Exerc* 1980:12, 336.

17. Hickson RC, Dvorak BA, Gorostiaga M, et al.: Potential for strength and endurance training to amplify endurance performance. *J Appl Physiol* 1988:65, 2285.

18. Marcinik EJ, Potts G, Schlabach G, et al.: Effects of strength training on lactate threshold and endurance performance. *Med Sci Sports Exerc* 1991:23, 739.

19. Stone MH, O'Bryant HS: *Weight Training: A Scientific Approach,* Minneapolis, MN, Burgess International, 1987.

20. Knapik JJ, Bauman CL, Jones BH, et al.: Preseason strength and flexibility imbalances associated with athletic injuries in female collegiate athletes. *Am J Sports Med* 1991:19, 76.

21. Putukian M: Track and field, in Mellion MB, Walsch WM, Shelton GL (eds.), *The Team Physician's Handbook,* 2nd ed., Philadelphia, Hanley and Belfus, 1997:754.

22. Astrand PO: Exercise physiology and its role in disease prevention and in rehabilitation. *Arch Phys Med Rehabil* 1987:68, 305.

23. Fleck SJ, Falkel JE: Value of resistance training for the reduction of sport injuries. *Sports Med* 1986:3, 61.

24. Wathan D: Load assignment, in Baechle TR (ed.), *Essentials of Strength Training and Conditioning,* Champaign, IL, Human Kinetics, 1994:435.

25. DiNubile NA: Strength training. *Clin Sports Med* 1991: 10, 33.

26. American College of Sports Medicine Position Stand on The Recommended Quantity and Quality of Exercise for Developing and Maintaining Cardiorespiratory and Muscular Fitness, and Flexibility in Healthy Adults. *Med Sci Sports Exerc* 1998:30, 975.

27. Wathen D: Exercise order, in Baechle TR (ed.), *Essentials of Strength Training and Conditioning,* Champaign, IL, Human Kinetics, 1994:431.

28. Feigenbaum MS, Pollock ML: Prescription of resistance training for health and disease. *Med Sci Sports Exerc* 1999:31, 38.

29. Braith R, Graves J, Pollock M, et al.: Comparison of two versus three days per week of variable resistance training during 10 and 18 week programs. *Int J Sports Med* 1989:10, 450.

30. Berger RA: Effect of varied weight training programs on strength. *Res Q* 1962:33, 168.

31. Wathen D: Training volume, in Baechle TR (ed.), *Essentials of Strength Training and Conditioning,* Champaign, IL, Human Kinetics, 1994:447.

32. Pollock ML, Vincent KR: Resistance training for health. *The President's Council on Physical Fitness and Sports Research Digest* 1996:2, 1.

33. McCartney N: Acute responses to resistance training and safety. *Med Sci Sports Exerc* 1999:31, 31.

34. Allerheiligen WB: Stretching and warm-up, in Baechle TR (ed.), *Essentials of Strength Training and Conditioning,* Champaign, IL, Human Kinetics, 1994:290.

35. Westcott WL: *Building Strength and Stamina: New Nautilus Training for Total Fitness,* Champaign, IL, Human Kinetics, 1996.

36. Westcott W: High intensity strength training. *Nautilus* 1994:4, 5.

Chapter 49

PSYCHOLOGY AND THE INJURED RUNNER: RECOVERY-ENHANCING STRATEGIES

Christopher S. Robinson

As you ought not to attempt to cure the eyes without the head, or the head without the body, then neither ought you attempt to cure the body without the soul . . . for the part will never be well unless the whole is well.

Plato

INTRODUCTION

Running and other healthy behaviors have dramatically increased. Unfortunately, the incidence rates of running injuries have also increased and are estimated to be between 35% and 85% for the nations' regular runners.[1-3] As a result, there have been increased attempts to further the awareness of both preventive and early intervention efforts. Surprisingly, however, injuries still increase. Since more and more people are participating in running, there are quite simply going to be more and more overuse injuries.[4] The injured runner can present to the sports medicine provider with a variety of complaints and concerns. There is, of course, the ever-present focus on the injured area. Concerns about the injury quickly become the center of attention for both the runner and the sports medicine provider. There are very real concerns regarding the return to previous running levels and the impact the injury may have on future performance. There are additional concerns about pain and coping with the stress of the injury. Finally, there are often concerns about both the rigors of a rehabilitation program and the loss of running as part of a daily routine. These concerns are paramount with the injured runner and can influence many subsequent rehabilitation behaviors.

These concerns need to be addressed in a comprehensive rehabilitation program. What does a comprehensive rehabilitation program entail? Pointing to the extent of psychological factors in the recovery from an injury, Thompson et al.[5] argue, "Rehabilitation is 75% psychological and 25% physical" (p. 265). Steadman[6] maintains that complete rehabilitation from an injury involves three distinct areas also designed to address these concerns. The first area is the *physical recovery* from the injury and involves aerobic, strength, and flexibility training. Second, *specific rehabilitation* to the injured area is critical and may involve prescribed physical therapy. Finally, *psychological rehabilitation* is critical and will shape the outcome of the rehabilitation program in many ways. A growing consensus is emerging in the literature regarding the importance of these psychological factors in the rehabilitation process.[7-13]

What are these psychological factors and how do they manifest in the rehabilitation of the injured runner? The runner's particular actions, emotions, and cognitions can work either for or against rehabilitation behaviors.[14,15] A psychological rehabilitation program using mental training focusing on development of sports-related images, for example, will address both the physical aspects of the injury and speed up the recovery process.[9] This approach has been demonstrated to provide both a quicker and less stressful recovery and a better understanding of the rehabilitation process.[16,17] Although a particular "injured athlete personality style" has not been identified, there are particular behaviors that certainly can and do contribute to rehabilitation problems.[18] For example, many researchers and practitioners advocate the use of certain behaviors such as goal setting, utilizing social support, implementing relaxation training, educating about specific medical actions, and other psychological treatment measures.[19,20] These are the behaviors that become the targets for a psychological intervention designed to facilitate recovery. Ievleva and Orlick[21] have concluded that the athlete's personal response to the injury ultimately separates the recovery rates between any two runners with similar injuries. Even with the best intentions to reassure the injured runner, difficulties can be plentiful. Therefore, just as the physical aspects of the runner's injury are important to address, so too are the emotional, cognitive, social, and behavioral components.[22-26]

Communicating this approach to the injured runner is critical and may involve a variety of strategies. Ahern and Lohr[18] argue that the "mental game" is a key element during rehabilitation. Taylor and Taylor[11] make use of a similar metaphor in their discussion of "rehabilitation as athletic performance." This notion of a game, or contest, can easily resonate with the runner as an appropriate metaphor for psychological rehabilitation. The provider can then introduce and emphasize these psychological techniques, allowing the athlete to focus on and/or be aware of them. Undeniably a multidisciplinary treatment approach, including the use of a trained psychologist, can be critical to returning the injured runner to previous functioning.

In this chapter I attempt to highlight the current literature regarding the psychological rehabilitation of the injured runner. The appropriate application of education and self-management training, goal setting,

the use of imagery and other mental devices, stress management, relaxation training, social support, pain management, and the ruling out of more relevant psychological problems are addressed. Initially, however, an introduction to functional analysis and case conceptualization will be presented.

FUNCTIONAL ANALYSIS AND CASE CONCEPTUALIZATION

As mentioned, neglect of the emotional, cognitive, social, and behavioral reactions to an injury can result in a slower and less effective recovery process. How can the psychologist aid the multidisciplinary team in the conceptualization and treatment of the runner with a musculoskeletal injury? A useful and well-known psychological tool is the functional analysis. This is simply an assessment outline designed to teach the multidisciplinary team to conceptualize the injured runner using the biopsychosocial model. Important influences on the injury and rehabilitation are assessed focusing on those factors preceding the injury (e.g. medical and psychological history, life stress), factors associated with the injury (e.g. emotional reaction, pain, injury), and factors following the injury (e.g. compliance with treatment, pain, medication use, social support, psychological state).[27] The biopsychosocial conceptual model goes on to assess the emotional, cognitive, physical, behavioral, and social aspects of the runner's athletic life and then uses these factors to guide rehabilitation. This model offers a different and more comprehensive view of the individual with an injury, which promotes adherence and effective rehabilitation.[28] These five biopsychosocial factors are explained more fully below.

Physical Factors

Where is the injury? How frequently does it hurt? How long does the pain last? How much does it hurt? Do you have any other significant medical problems? Is there muscle tension and bracing evident? How is your energy level? Are there any persistent illnesses present? Is your sleep restful?

Behavioral Factors

What do you *do* as a result of your injury? For example, have you ever skipped important responsibilities because of your injury? Do you have any unhealthy habits (substance abuse, abnormal eating behavior, too much or too little exercise, etc.) that may be negatively influencing your rehabilitation? How much were you running prior to your injury and how much do you run now? Are you adhering to the prescribed rehabilitation? Do you give your best effort at every rehabilitation session?

Cognitive Factors (Beliefs, Thoughts, Attitudes)

What do you *believe* needs to be done about your injury? Do you *think* "hurt" is the same as "harm?" (In other words, are you limiting your rehabilitation because you *think* the normal pain associated with rehabilitation is harmful?) Do you know the difference between benign pain (to be expected during exercise and rehabilitation) and harmful pain (as a result of overuse and possible reinjury)? Does it make sense to approach your rehabilitation with an *attitude* that can work better for you? Do you *believe* you will fully recover? Do you always *think* and talk positively about your rehabilitation? Are you excited about returning to running?

Emotional Factors

Have you recently gotten yourself more anxious, sad, or upset than you would like as a result of your injury? Do you have any fears about returning to running? Are you grieving your running loss as an activity outlet?

Relationship Factors (Social Support)

Are you having any relationship problems due to your injury? Do your significant others respond differently to you as a result of your injury? Have you been withdrawing from your family and friends as a result of your injury? Do you have a constructive social support system?

Once these domains have been thoroughly assessed, target areas for treatment can be better identified. A comprehensive treatment plan can then be developed to target these areas in order to supplement the runner's physical rehabilitation program.

EDUCATION AND SELF-MANAGEMENT TRAINING

Following the functional analysis, the injured runner must develop a solid understanding of the general nature of the injury, the rehabilitation program itself, and the prognosis for recovery.[13,28] Taylor and Taylor[11] point out that the elements of a successful rehabilitation program include education about the following three elements: *understanding + organization + progress*. In order for the program to be successful, the individuals must *understand* the recovery process, *organize* themselves to increase rehabilitation adherence, and monitor their rehabilitation *progress*. These steps involve education. It

has been argued that the injured athlete cannot give the required effort unless he or she understands what is wrong and why the prescribed rehabilitation program makes sense.[19] Although it is useful to make the most of a multidisciplinary team approach, this approach can bewilder the athlete. There may be times when the athlete has an incomplete understanding of his or her injury and as a result remains unclear about rehabilitation. Working closely with the treatment team, the psychologist can help elucidate the often bewildering array of new requests and information. Here is an area where the psychologist can facilitate the development of a treatment plan and ensure that the injured runner is made aware of both the total package and how to negotiate the different treatment requests.

Taylor and Taylor's[11] second step concerns organization. Combining the necessary use of medical care with self-management training best accomplishes this step. Self-management has been established as a useful tool designed to help individuals increase a sense of control both in their lives and in the management of health concerns, injury, and rehabilitation.[23,29,30] Self-management involves teaching specific skills to the athlete in terms they can understand and can then implement on their own. It often involves collaborating closely with the athletes and the multidisciplinary treatment team on the treatment goals and then devising a specific rehabilitation plan. The use of goal setting is a central component of self-management training.

GOAL SETTING

A goal has been defined as the attainment of a specific standard of proficiency in a task within a specified time limit.[31] Goal setting links motivation to action[19] and is the most advocated technique to increase athlete motivation in order to enhance recovery.[11] It gives injured athletes the sense that the rehabilitation program is simply another competition in which they prepare to be successful. Goal setting provides the runner with clear direction and aids short- and long-term goal attainment. Examples include physical rehabilitation goals, psychological rehabilitation goals, and particular performance goals. It is important to note that outcome goals focused on winning a competition ("I will be in the top 10 in next month's 5K race") can work against successful rehabilitation and are not recommended. Such a goal involves too many variables that are outside the runner's control and therefore much more difficult to direct. Performance goals, on the other hand, are much easier to control and to keep within attainable reach of the runner ("Today I will run four laps at 2½ minutes a lap"). Performance goals involve improvements on the individual's *own* past performance.

Treatment goals may also include helping reduce the use of ineffective or problematic coping responses such as poor compliance to rehabilitation or frequent requests for pain medication. An additional goal may be to help increase the use of positive coping skills. For example, the injured runner can set such goals as increasing physical and social activity, increasing the use of distraction and relaxation techniques to cope with intense pain episodes, and/or increasing the ability to manage increased emotional reactions. The overall purpose of goal setting is to increase the use of effective coping strategies as the runner negotiates rehabilitation. Empirical evidence supports this notion of goal setting to increase motivation, to ensure quicker and more effective injury recovery, and to facilitate performance clearly and consistently.[21,32–35] Goal setting is a critical part of the injured runner's rehabilitation program.

Figure 49–1 provides an example of the following important goal guidelines:

Goal #1 Complete the Spring 5 Kilometer Race 6 Months from Now

Running
My 6-Month Running Goal:
Running Frequency: In 6-Months I will run 3-4 times per week
Running Duration: In 6-Months I will run 4 miles each time I run
Running Intensity: In 6-Months I will run an 8 ½ min mile pace for each of my runs

Goal for this Week	Goal for Next Week	Goal for 2 Weeks from Now
Running Frequency: 3 times per week	**Running Frequency:** 3 times per week	**Running Frequency:** 3 times per week
Duration: 10 min	**Duration**: 13 min	**Duration**: 16 min
Intensity: *10 ½ min/mile	**Intensity:** *10 min/mile	**Intensity:** *9 ¾ min/mile

*Run at a pace where you can still talk (Not too fast!)

Strength Training
My 6-Month Strength Goal:
In 6-Months I will Perform 3 Sets of 10 Leg Extensions using 75 pounds
In 6-Months I will Perform 3 Sets of 10 Squats Using 100 pounds

This Week	Next Week	2 Weeks
3 Sets of 5 Leg Extensions using 35 pounds	**3 Sets of 7 Leg Extensions using 35 pounds**	**3 Sets of 5 Leg Extensions using 40 pounds**
3 Sets of 5 Squats using 60 pounds	**3 Sets of 7 Squats using 60 pounds**	**3 Sets of 5 Squats using 65 pounds**

Goal #2 Relaxation\Imagery Performance Enhancement

Relaxation/Performance Enhancement Training
My 6-Month Relaxation/Performance Enhancement Goal:
In 6 Months I will Use Relaxation and Imagery Effectively During Training and Races

This Week	Next Week	2 Weeks
Relaxation 5 Minutes Prior to Home Work-Out	**Relaxation 5-10 Minutes Prior to Home Work-Out**	**Relaxation 10 Minutes Prior to Home Work-Out**

Figure 49–1. Goal guidelines example.

- Goals should be challenging but realistic.
- Goals should be specific, measurable, and set in behavioral terms.
- Goals should be set in a positive rather than a negative framework.
- Goals should be related to the individual's own performance areas and not competitive outcome areas.
- Focus should be more on *degree* of attainment of the goal rather than the *absolute* attainment of all goals.
- Goal setting should be a dynamic process. Goals can and will change during the course of rehabilitation.
- A target date for goal attainment should be set.
- A written copy of the goals should be given directly to the runner.
- Regular feedback should be provided.

UTILIZING IMAGERY AND OTHER MENTAL DEVICES

Taylor and Taylor[11] argue that "rehabilitation imagery has perhaps the greatest ability to address the diverse concerns and challenges that injured athletes experience during rehabilitation" (p. 197). Imagery is a mental technique designed to program the mind to respond to certain events in a certain way.[36] Many professionals in the field of injury rehabilitation are now advocating the central role of imagery during rehabilitation.[37–40] Psychoneuromuscular theory reasons that sustained mental activity can result in muscle innervations similar to those produced by actual physical execution of the movement.[36] Mental imagery involves the use of one's imagination to replay and rehearse athletic maneuvers.[41] For example, the runner may imagine running fluidly and effortlessly at a healthy pace, rehearsing all the different movements in the mind. This can occur in one's living room to the sounds of soft music accompanied by relaxed breathing. This is an ideal task both for the runner rehabilitating from injury and for the runner interested in performance enhancement.

The use of imagery is clearly underused, generally due to misunderstanding on the best implementation strategies. In fact, it is a simple technique to put into practice. For example, the injured runner can be taught the use of healing imagery, soothing imagery, and/or performance imagery. Healing imagery involves imagining that the specific injured area is mending and healing. Soothing imagery can be used as a distracter for pain and/or as a supplement to relaxation training.[42] The runner is taught to imagine a peaceful or soothing scene while practicing slow, deep breathing. Finally, performance imagery uses imagery to enhance performance and can be quite effective.[25,36,38] It can enhance techniques, mental preparation, and competitive performance, even when the runner is unable to actually run. This is clearly a useful skill that can be taught and developed with practice in both the injured and noninjured runner.

COGNITIVE-BEHAVIORAL TRAINING

One of the consistent findings in the literature is that successful performance in any activity, including rehabilitation, is correlated with self-confidence.[43] Self-assured runners will convince themselves they can master the rehabilitation program and that they will ultimately be successful. Can self-assurance be taught, or is it something with which we are simply born? These specific cognitive activities can indeed be taught to the runner and are critical to successful rehabilitation.[44] Since thoughts precede a feeling, which precedes behavior, it makes sense to learn to control thoughts as a central element to improve performance. The key to cognitive control is self-talk.[25,43,45] Self-talk involves the use of specific self-statements designed to increase concentration and focus and to improve one's mood.[41] Taylor and Taylor[11] present four cognitive levels of self-talk to improve the injured runner's confidence in the rehabilitation program (program confidence, adherence confidence, physical confidence, and return to sport confidence). A treatment program must assess these important variables and include them in the psychological rehabilitation program. Confidence is emphasized by learning to challenge alarming thoughts and change them to reassuring thoughts.

Motivation is another important cognitive factor involving self-talk. Motivation is one of the psychological factors likely to have the greatest impact on adherence to the rehabilitation process.[46] If the runner is not motivated to stick to the rehabilitation program and hopeful of a positive outcome, adherence becomes unlikely. Taylor and Taylor[11] describe motivation as the ability to offer sustained effort in the face of compelling and competing obstacles. Obvious signs of low motivation are failure to attend scheduled exercise sessions and related appointments. The rehabilitating runner with this particular problem could benefit from self-talk training designed to increase motivation.

Another important cognitive area includes the assessment and monitoring of grief reactions. If the runner believes a terrible and awful loss has occurred due to the injury, a grief reaction could occur that may ultimately work against rehabilitation. Therefore, effective treatment programs will assess this area and provide cognitive treatment interventions as needed.[13,47]

The interface of the mind and the body is thought of as the stress response, and self-talk is a central component of this as well. The stress response is where the psychological and physical factors interact, and it can influence the likelihood of successful rehabilitation or of reinjury.[48] The concept of psychological influence on injury and rehabilitation is a synthesis of the stress-illness, stress-injury, and stress-accident literature.[49] During the stress response, very real physiological and psychological changes can work against the injured and the noninjured runner. A stress management intervention, including recognition of stress early warning signs, relaxation training, and reassuring self-talk, is a critical part of the successful rehabilitation program.

IMPLEMENTING A RELAXATION PROGRAM TO ENHANCE REHABILITATION OF THE RUNNER

A typical response during stress that reduces performance is to hold one's breath and/or to begin shallow, rapid breathing.[50] This stress response can result in muscle tension and consequent reinjury.[51] In addition, the injury itself can actually become a stressor, further impeding rehabilitation.[4,52] Anxiety and worry can also have a deleterious effect on the injured athlete in two ways. During times of anxiety and worry it is difficult for muscles to relax completely, and thus excessive muscle tension is maintained. In addition, oxygen deprivation, caused by vascular constriction, can slow the healing of the injured area.[11] The fluctuation of mental control and arousal greatly impacts performance during competition and rehabilitation.[50] The ability to control arousal, to concentrate, and to focus on reassuring self-talk is critical. Each of these areas involves the effective use of relaxation. When the runner learns to communicate with the body through relaxation, many helpful and healing mechanisms can occur. As a result, it makes sense for the injured runner to keep stress and anxiety at a minimum during rehabilitation. The effectiveness of relaxation training has been demonstrated for postsurgical anxiety, pain, and physical rehabilitation.[17] Relaxation training can increase body awareness, deepen muscular relaxation at rest, and increase muscular performance during competition and rehabilitation.[41]

A quick and simple way to decrease muscle tension and improve injury rehabilitation is diaphragmatic breathing (Fig. 49–2). This simply involves a slow, deep inhalation, holding the inhaled breath for a few moments, and then a somewhat quicker exhalation. Sitting still with one's eyes lightly closed, trying not to make any excessive movement, and practicing rhythmic breathing can contribute to this process. This should be practiced for 5 to 10 minutes a day in order to gain and maintain proficiency.

SOCIAL SUPPORT

An injured runner's social support network is critical in the rehabilitation process. Social support has been defined as "an exchange of resources between at least two individuals perceived by the provider or the recipient to be intended to enhance the well-being of the recipient."[53] The runner's social network often includes running partners, teammates, coaches, parents, spouses, and/or friends.[8,22] A runner with an injury may quickly require extra positive support during recovery; criticism and social isolation may be very difficult for some runners. It is critical for the multi-disciplinary treatment team to assess for and develop awareness of this important piece of the runner's rehabilitation.

PAIN MANAGEMENT

Pain at the injury site can have significant impact on the runner. An injured runner can easily become frustrated or depressed when the injury is compounded by unremitting and recalcitrant pain,[9] for several reasons. The runner may continue to seek medical care for the same injury, feeling either that little benefit is seen or that recovery is taking longer than anticipated. The injured runner with pain may request increased levels of pain medication and/or more frequent contact with the doctor, again with only minimal relief. The runner with pain may also become overly upset about the pain and abandon rehabilitation altogether. These runners can benefit from psychological interventions designed to alter their reaction to the pain.[54] The athlete who is responding to the pain and the injury with depression, hopelessness, and withdrawal is less likely to follow through with the rehabilitation program. This piece of the rehabilitation program will target both the depression and activity levels by helping individuals to change their reaction to the pain and to become more actively involved with the rehabilitation program. Again, a combination of medical care and self-management training is the best approach.

Treatment goals for pain management include helping the injured runner reduce ineffective or problematic coping responses (e.g., heavy pain-medication

DIAPHRAGMATIC BREATHING EXERCISE

1. Sit in a comfortable position.

2. Take 3 deep cleansing breaths.

3. Place one hand on your stomach and the other on your chest.

4. Try to breathe so that only your stomach rises and falls.

    a. As you inhale, concentrate on your chest remaining relatively still while your stomach rises. It may be helpful to imagine that your pants are too big and you need to push your stomach out to hold them up.

    b. When exhaling, allow your stomach to fall in and the air to fully escape.

5. Take some deep breaths, concentrating on only moving your stomach. Hold each breath for 2 seconds.

6. Return to regular breathing, continuing to breathe so that only your stomach moves.

The CALM Reminder

Chest: Breathing slower and deeper

Arms: Shoulders sag

Legs: Loose and flexible

Mouth: Jaw drop

Figure 49–2. Diaphragmatic breathing.

use, depression, poor rehabilitation adherence). An additional goal may be to help increase the use of positive coping skills. This could include increasing physical and social activity, distraction and relaxation techniques to cope with intense pain episodes, and the ability to manage emotional reactions associated with a pain episode.

The two general categories of nonpharmacologic pain management are pain reduction and pain distraction strategies.[9] Pain reduction strategies may include deep breathing, relaxation training, biofeedback, imagery, and massage. Pain distraction techniques can be equally fruitful in teaching the injured runner techniques designed to modify the reaction to the aversive stimuli of pain.[42] This can include changing one's focus from the pain to external events, the use of pleasant and soothing imagery, relaxation training, pain acknowledgment, and reassuring self-talk. The overall goal of this treatment approach is to increase general activity levels and to teach the runner to react to a pain episode with effective (vs. ineffective) responses.

RULING OUT MORE SERIOUS PSYCHOLOGICAL PROBLEMS

A referral to the psychologist is not appropriate for every person with an injury. Many injured runners' lives are only minimally disrupted, and they manage to enjoy a good, healthy recovery. Other runners, however, tend to have difficulty with rehabilitation and could benefit from psychological treatment. The psychologist is trained to detect and treat psychological problems associated with the injury. Brewer et al.[46] reported a 19% prevalence rate of self-reported clinically elevated levels of distress in a clinical sample of orthopedic patients of which 58% considered themselves athletes. Thirty-one percent of this sample evidenced anxiety, and 20% evidenced depression. In addition, 33% of the sample of injured football players were regarded as depressed. Therefore, the sports medicine provider should be constantly aware of elevated symptoms of distress that may warrant referral for more extensive psychological treatment. Again, successful use of functional analysis can discern this level of distress in the runner.

Substance abuse problems (including alcohol and drug use and abuse) can occur with this population. Three behavior categories are used in the *Diagnostic and Statistical Manual of Mental Disorders* to determine the extent of a substance abuse problem.[55] These are continued use of the substance despite recurrent problems, impaired control, and tolerance and withdrawal. The stage of problem development is important and should drive the type of intervention posed for the athlete.[22] The individual in the at-risk or hazardous use stage can generally benefit either from abstinence or from moderate use. Individuals in the problem-use or dependent-use groups often need to be referred for specialized treatment. A helpful screening tool is the CAGE acronym for substance use, defined by the following questions[56]:

1. Have you ever felt you should *Cut down* on your substance use?
2. Have people ever *Annoyed* you by criticizing your substance use?
3. Have you ever felt bad or *Guilty* about your substance use?
4. Have you ever used the substance first thing in the morning to steady your nerves or to get rid of a hangover *(Eye-opener)*?

A score of one or more yes answers is positive for hazardous substance use. Two or more yes answers constitutes positive screening for substance abuse and perhaps dependence. These individuals should be referred for additional assessment and treatment.

Eating disorders are another potential psychiatric problem worth mentioning. Eating disorders can be quite disruptive and even deadly if not noted and treated. Two types of eating disorders are described in the *Diagnostic and Statistical Manual of Mental Disorders.*[55] Anorexia nervosa is characterized by a refusal to maintain a normal body weight, an intense fear of gaining weight or becoming fat, a disturbance in the way one's body weight or shape is experienced, and amenorrhea in females. Bulimia nervosa is characterized by recurrent binge eating, recurrent inappropriate purging attempts to prevent weight gain following a binge episode, binging and purging occurring at least twice a week for 3 months, the undue influence on self-esteem by body shape and weight, and the absence of

anorexia nervosa. If the injured runner manifests these signs or symptoms, referral for a more extensive psychological evaluation and treatment is in order.

CONCLUSIONS

In conclusion, it is clear that the psychologist has much to offer the injured runner in negotiating the difficult path from injury to recovery. A careful functional analysis focusing on the biopsychosocial influences on rehabilitation and recovery can highlight areas where treatment may prove beneficial. After the collaborative selection of specific treatment goals, the treatment team can choose from the different techniques described here and tailor the rehabilitation program to the unique needs and concerns of each runner. This will enhance the rehabilitation process, providing more efficient and more effective recovery, a faster return to running, and a runner who is more content.

REFERENCES

1. Wexler RK: Lower extremity injuries in runners. *Postgrad Med Running Injuries* 1995:98, 185.
2. O'Toole ML: Prevention and treatment of injuries to runners. *Med Sci Sports Exerc* 1992:24, S360.
3. Booth W: Arthritis institute tackles sport. *Science* 1987:237, 846.
4. Crossman J: Psychological rehabilitation from sports injuries. *Sports Med* 1997:23, 333.
5. Thompson TL, Hershman EB, Nicholas JA: Rehabilitation of the injured athlete. *Pediatrician* 1990:17, 262.
6. Steadman JR: A physician's approach to the psychology of injury, in Heil J (ed.), *Psychology of Sport Injury,* Champaign, IL, Human Kinetics Publishers, 1993:25.
7. Doyle J, Gleeson NP, Rees D: Psychobiology and the athlete with anterior cruciate ligament (ACL) injury. *Sports Med* 1998:26, 379.
8. Weinberg RS, Gould D: *Foundations of Sport and Exercise Psychology,* Champaign, IL, Human Kinetics Publishers, 1995:529.
9. Heil J: *Psychology of Sport Injury,* Champaign, IL, Human Kinetics Publishers, 1993.
10. Williams JM, Roepke N: Psychology of injury and injury rehabilitation, in Singer RN, Tennant LK, Murphey M (eds.), *Handbook of Research in Sports Medicine,* New York, Macmillan, 1993:815.
11. Taylor J, Taylor S: *Psychological Approaches to Sports Injury Rehabilitation,* Gaithersburg, MD, Aspen Publishers, 1997.
12. Ford IW, Gordon S: Perspectives of sport physiotherapists on the frequency and significance of psychological factors in professional practice: Implications for curriculum design in professional training. *Aust J Sci Med Sport* 1997:29, 34.

13. Gordon S, Potter M, Ford IW: Toward a psychoeducational curriculum for training sport-injury rehabilitation personnel. *J Appl Sports Psychol* 1998:10, 140.

14. Morrey M: *Predicting Injury Recovery Is a Function of Affect and Pain Perception in Athletes Who Have Undergone Anterior Cruciate Ligament Reconstruction Surgery: An Exploratory Study,* Williamsburg, VA, Association for the Advancement of Applied Sport Psychology (AAASP), 1996.

15. Smith A, Scott S, Wiese D: Emotional responses of athletes to injury. *Mayo Clin Proc* 1990:65, 38.

16. Larson GA, Starkey C, Zaichkowsky LD: Psychological aspects of athletic injuries as perceived by athletic trainers. *Sports Psychologist* 1996:10, 37.

17. Ross MJ, Scott BR: Effects of stress inoculation training on athletes' postsurgical pain and rehabilitation after orthopedic injury. *J Consult Clin Psychol* 1996:64, 406.

18. Ahern DK, Lohr BA: Psychosocial factors in sports injury rehabilitation. *Clin Sports Med* 1997:16, 755.

19. Heil J: A comprehensive approach to injury management, in Heil J (ed.), *Psychology of Sport Injury,* Champaign, IL, Human Kinetics Publishers, 1993:137.

20. Heil J, Bowman JJ, Bean B: Patient management and the sports medicine team, in Heil J (ed.), *Psychology of Sport Injury,* Champaign, IL, Human Kinetics Publishers, 1993:237.

21. Ievleva L, Orlick T: Mental links to enhanced healing: An exploratory study. *Sports Psychologist* 1991:5, 25.

22. Ray R, Wiese-Bjornstal DM: *Counseling in Sports Medicine,* Champaign, IL, Human Kinetics Publishers, 1999:361.

23. Wiese D, Weiss M, Yukelson D: Sport psychology in the training room: A survey of athletic trainers. *Sports Psychologist* 1991:5, 15.

24. Nideffer R: The injured athlete: Psychological factors in treatment. *Orthop Clin North Am* 1993, 373.

25. Weiss M, Troxell R: Psychology of the injured athlete. *Athletic Training* 1986:21, 104.

26. Lampton CC, Lambert ME, Yost R: The effects of psychological factors in sports medicine adherence. *J Sports Med Phys Fitness* 1993:33, 292.

27. Heil J: A framework for psychological assessment, in Heil J (ed.), *Psychology of Sport Injury,* Champaign, IL, Human Kinetics Publishers, 1993:73.

28. Fisher CA: Adherence to sports injury rehabilitation. *Sports Med* 1990:9, 151.

29. Bender BG: Establishing a role for psychology in respiratory medicine, in Resnick RJ, Rozensky RH (eds.), *Health Psychology Through the Life Span: Practice and Research Opportunities,* Washington, DC, American Psychological Association, 1996:232.

30. Rehm LP: Self-management therapy for depression. *Adv Behav Ther Res* 1984:6, 83.

31. Locke E, Shaw K, Saari L, et al.: Goal setting and task performance. *Psychol Bull* 1981:90, 125.

32. Gould D: Goal setting for peak performance, in Williams JM (ed.), *Applied Sport Psychology: Personal Growth to Peak Performance,* Mountain View, CA, Mayfield Publishing Company, 1993:158.

33. Weinberg R: Goal-setting and motor performance: A review and critique, in Roberts GC (ed.), *Motivation in Sports and Exercise* Champaign, IL, Human Kinetics Books, 1993:177.

34. Burton D, Weinberg R, Yukelson D, et al.: The goal effectiveness paradox in sport: Examining the goal practices in collegiate athletes. *Sports Psychologist* 1998:12, 404.

35. Brewer BW: Psychological applications in clinical sports medicine: Current status and future directions. *J Clin Psychol Med Settings* 1998:5, 91.

36. Vealey RS, Walter SM: Imagery training for performance enhancement and personal development, in Williams JM (ed.), *Applied Sport Psychology: Personal Growth to Peak Performance,* Mountain View, CA, Mayfield Publishing Company, 1993:200.

37. Lynch GP: Athletic injuries and the practicing sport psychologist: Practical guidelines for assisting athletes. *Sports Psychologist* 1988:2, 161.

38. Rotella RJ, Heyman SR: Stress, injury, and the psychological rehabilitation of athletes, in Williams JM (ed.), *Applied Sport Psychology: Personal Growth to Peak Performance,* Mountain View, CA, Mayfield Publishing Company, 1993:338.

39. Hall C, Rodgers W: Enhancing coaching effectiveness in figure skating through a mental skills training program. *Sports Psychologist* 1989:2, 142.

40. Gould D, Tammen V, Murphy S, et al.: An examination of US Olympic sport psychology consultants and services they provide. *Sports Psychologist* 1989:3, 300.

41. Heil J: Mental training in injury management, in Heil J (ed.), *Psychology of Sport Injury,* Champaign, IL, Human Kinetics Publishers, 1993:151.

42. Turk DC, Meichenbaum D, Genest M: *Pain and Behavioral Medicine: A Cognitive-Behavioral Perspective.* New York, Guilford Press, 1983:452.

43. Bunker L, Williams JM, Zinsser N: Cognitive techniques for improving performance and building confidence, in Williams JM (ed.), *Applied Sport Psychology: Personal Growth to Peak Performance,* Mountain View, CA, Mayfield Publishing Company, 1993:225.

44. Taylor AH, May S: Threat and coping appraisal as determinants of compliance with sports injury rehabilitation: An application of protection motivation theory. *J Sports Sci* 1996:14, 471.

45. Wiese DM, Weiss MR: Psychological rehabilitation and physical injury: Implications for the sports medicine team. *Sports Psychologist* 1987:1, 318.

46. Brewer B, Jeffers K, Petitpas A: Perceptions of psychological interventions in the context of sport injury rehabilitation. *Sports Psychologist* 1994:8, 176.

47. Evans L, Hardy L: Sport injury and grief responses: A review. *J Sport Exerc Psychol* 1995:17, 227.

48. Anderson M, Williams J: Psychological risk factors and injury prevention, in Heil J (ed.), *Psychology of Sport Injury,* Champaign, IL, Human Kinetics Publishers, 1993:49.

49. Durso-Cupal D: Psychological interventions in sport injury prevention and rehabilitation. *J Appl Sport Psychol* 1998:10, 103.

50. Harris DV, Williams JM: Relaxation and energizing techniques for relaxation of arousal, in Williams JM (ed.), *Applied Sport Psychology: Personal Growth to Peak*

Performance, Mountain View, CA, Mayfield Publishing Company, 1993:185.

51. Hardy L: Psychologic stress, performance, and injury in sport. *Br Med Bull* 1992:48, 615.

52. Kulund D: *The Injured Athlete.* Philadelphia, Lippincott, 1982.

53. Shumaker SA, Brownell A: Toward a theory of social support: Closing conceptual gaps. *J Soc Issues* 1984:40, 11.

54. Taylor J, Taylor S: Pain education and management in the rehabilitation from sports injury. *Sports Psychologist* 1998:12, 68.

55. APA: *Diagnostic and Statistical Manual of Mental Disorders,* 4th ed., Washington, DC, American Psychiatric Association, 1994:886.

56. Fleming MF, Barry KL: *Addictive Disorders,* St. Louis, Mosby, 1992.

Part VII

SURGICAL CONSIDERATIONS IN THE RUNNER

Chapter 50

OVERVIEW: SURGICAL CONSIDERATIONS IN THE RUNNER

Robert P. Nirschl

The basics of nonoperative treatment are well chronicled in preceding chapters. This care is described in the sequential treatment algorithm depicted in Table 50–1. If nonoperative treatment proves unsuccessful, certain possibilities must be assessed. These include adequacy of the treatment plan as prescribed by the medical professionals and due diligence to the plan by the patient.

If the prescription as outlined in Table 50–1 was implemented properly, treatment failure indicates that the problem exceeds the capacity of nonoperative care.

At this point, indications for surgery must be considered, including the definition of treatment success, the timeliness of maximum treatment benefit, and the possible outcome of treatment measured in function (both short- and long-term) and durability (Table 50–2).

In the event that nonoperative treatment fails, the athlete has several choices: consider surgical intervention or modify and/or eliminate sport participation. Surgical intervention might also be considered when nonsurgical options might offer some treatment success but with some compromise of function, durability, or timeliness of sports return.

TABLE 50–1. NONOPERATIVE TREATMENT ALGORITHM

1. Accurate pathoanatomic diagnosis
2. Appropriate pain and inflammation control
3. Functional counterforce and protective bracing
4. Rehabilitation of injured part dedicated to cure
   a. Neovascularization
   b. Fibroblastic infiltration
   c. Collagen production and maturation
   d. Restoration of strength, endurance, flexibility, and proprioception
5. Maintenance of general fitness (aerobic, anaerobic, strength, endurance, and flexibility)
6. Transitional exercise for return to sport
7. Modification of sport activity to eliminate abuse
   a. Technique of activity
   b. Intensity and frequency of activity
   c. Proper equipment
   d. Functional counterforce bracing

TABLE 50–2. INDICATIONS FOR SURGICAL INTERVENTION

1. Failure of adequate nonsurgical approach
2. Obvious problem beyond the capacity of nonsurgical care
   Example: Displaced fracture
3. Compromised unacceptable functional level by nonsurgical approach
   Example: Ruptured Achilles' tendon
4. Compromised durability by nonsurgical approach
   Example: Increased Achilles' tendon rerupture rate with nonsurgical treatment
5. Delayed return to sport by nonsurgical approach
   Example: Jones' fracture at base of fifth metatarsal
6. Inability to comply with nonoperative approach
   Example: Need for prolonged immobilization with nonoperative approach

In most instances, with the above factors in mind, the ultimate decision for surgical intervention is made by the athlete on the basis of individual goals, wants, and needs. The role of the physician is to define the problem, outline the options, including risks, and, as best as possible, prognosticate the outcome, including satisfactory return to high-level sport participation.

Since running sports are extremely demanding, full function is not always achieved, depending on the severity of the problem. Conversely, in many instances, the current level of surgical technology in association with dedicated postoperative rehabilitation offers an opportunity to return to the level of sport activity enjoyed before the injury.

Chapter 51

HIP/PELVIS

**Bradley J. Nelson
and Dean C. Taylor**

INTRODUCTION

Hip pain affects as many as one fourth of competitive and recreational runners.[1] MacIntyre and coauthors[2] reported a 6% incidence of hip injury in a group of over 4000 runners. Most of these hip injuries can be managed nonoperatively with training modifications, stretching, physiotherapy, and nonsteroidal anti inflammatory medications (NSAIDs). Occasionally, patients have recalcitrant injuries that require operative management. This chapter discusses the operative management of some of the more common hip injuries that affect the runner.

STRESS FRACTURES OF THE FEMUR

Stress fractures are relatively common overuse injuries in runners. Incidence rates in runners ranging from 8% to 37% have been reported in the literature.[1,3–5] Bennell and coworkers[4] demonstrated a 21% incidence of stress fractures in a recent prospective study of track and field athletes.

Femoral stress fractures can involve the femoral neck, the subtrochanteric area, the midfemoral shaft, and the distal femur. Matheson et al.[6] demonstrated that the femur was involved in 7.2% of collegiate athletes with stress fractures. In their study, the femur was the fourth most commonly involved location, after the

tibia, tarsals, and metatarsals. Johnson and coworkers[7] have shown a surprisingly high incidence of femoral shaft stress fractures in a series of collegiate athletes. These authors reported involvement of the femoral shaft in 20.6% of athletes who presented with stress fractures.

Making the diagnosis of a femoral stress fracture can be difficult. Symptoms may be vague and usually develop over a prolonged period. Runners may present with groin pain, anterior thigh pain, or pain referred to the knee. The pain is usually exacerbated by activity, and the history may reveal a recent change in the training regimen. The physical examination usually reveals an antalgic gait, and tenderness on palpation may be present. Patients with femoral neck stress fractures may have pain with hip range of motion, particularly maximum internal rotation. Johnson et al.[7] have described the fulcrum test to aid in the clinical diagnosis of femoral shaft stress fractures. To perform the fulcrum test the examiner places the patient's thigh across his or her knee and applies pressure to the proximal and distal thigh. Pain in the thigh suggests a femoral shaft stress fracture.

Plain radiography is the first imaging modality obtained in the evaluation of femoral stress fractures. However, plain films are not sensitive in the initial time period. Technetium-99 diphosphonate bone scintiography has been commonly used for the early diagnosis of femoral stress fractures.[8] Recently,

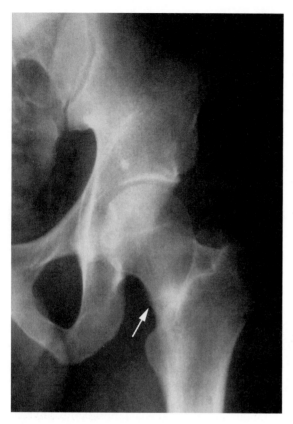

Figure 51–1. Typical appearance of a compression femoral neck stress fracture with the fracture line at the inferior (compressive side) aspect of the femoral neck.

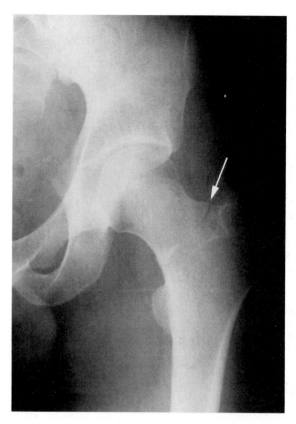

Figure 51–2. Typical appearance of a distraction/tension femoral neck stress fracture with the fracture line at the superior (tension side) aspect of the femoral neck and resulting distraction.

magnetic resonance imaging has been shown to be superior to bone scintiography in the diagnosis of femoral neck stress fractures because of its improved specificity.[9]

The treatment of femoral stress fractures depends on the location and the presence of displacement. Femoral neck stress fractures can be classified as compression femoral neck fractures, distraction/tension femoral neck fractures, or displaced fractures[10,11] (Figs. 51–1 to 51–3). Most compression-type fractures can be treated nonoperatively with rest and protected weightbearing followed by a gradual return to full activity.[11,12] However, patients with compression-type stress fractures demonstrating radiographic findings of a fracture involving a significant portion of the femoral neck or radiographic worsening of the fracture may be candidates for operative intervention. Additionally, patients who are unable to comply with the protected weightbearing regimen should be offered operative stabilization. Surgical fixation involves placement of cannulated screws across the femoral neck. (Fig. 51–4). Postoperatively, patients are placed on crutches and allowed protected weightbearing until the fracture is healed.

The treatment of tension or distraction stress fractures is more controversial. Some authors recommend immediate operative stabilization with cannulated screws for any femoral stress fracture on the tension side of the femoral neck.[8] However, two separate studies have demonstrated the efficacy of nonoperative treatment of this type of fracture.[11,13] Nonoperative treatment involves strict bed rest until the patient is asymptomatic. Radiographs are obtained daily during this time period. Surgical stabilization with cannulated screws is undertaken if there is any evidence of fracture progression or if bed rest is not feasible. We believe that operative stabilization should be considered for all stress fractures on the tension side of the femoral neck. The operative morbidity is minimal, and the complications from a displaced femoral neck fracture can be disastrous.

Displaced fractures of the femoral neck are managed with emergent operative intervention. Avascular necrosis and nonunion are common after displaced femoral neck fractures.[14,15] Anatomic reduction and surgical stabilization should be performed within 8 to 12 hours of fracture displacement to reduce the chance of avascular necrosis and nonunion.[16] Closed reduction

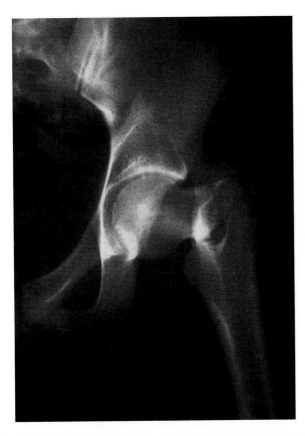

Figure 51–3. Displaced femoral neck fracture following an untreated stress fracture.

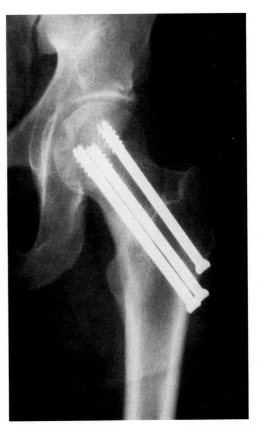

Figure 51–4. Postoperative radiograph of surgical fixation of femoral neck stress fracture with three cannulated screws.

is attempted initially, followed by open reduction if anatomic alignment cannot be obtained. The fracture is stabilized using cannulated screws or a compression hip screw and side plate. Supplemental bone grafting has been recommended by some authors.[17]

The prognosis is not uniformly good following operative management of a femoral neck stress fracture in an athlete, especially following displaced fractures. Johansson and coworkers[18] reported on 16 athletes who required surgical stabilization for femoral neck stress fractures. Most of them were runners. There were seven nondisplaced fractures and nine displaced fractures. Three patients developed avascular necrosis, two patients had a refracture, and one patient had a nonunion. No elite level athlete returned to his or her preinjury level of activity. In addition, 70% of patients rated their ability to perform sports as poor. Thus, the goal of operative treatment should be limited to restoring or maintaining the anatomy of the femoral neck to minimize the probability of avascular necrosis and nonunion.

Femoral shaft stress fractures can be classified as either nondisplaced or displaced. Nondisplaced fractures are managed nonoperatively. Butler et al.[19] reported on seven collegiate track athletes with subtrochanteric

femoral stress fractures. All fractures were nondisplaced and healed with a period of rest. Similar success of nonoperative therapy for nondisplaced femoral shaft fractures has been demonstrated in separate studies by Hershman et al.[20] and Lombardo and Benson.[21]

Displaced femoral shaft stress fractures are rare. These injuries are best managed with surgical stabilization. The surgical techniques are the same as those used to manage traumatic fractures of the femoral shaft. Nearly all displaced fractures of the femoral shaft are best treated with closed intramedullary nailing.[22] More proximal fractures in the subtrochanteric region may require a reconstruction-type nail or a compression hip screw and side plate.

Few reports of displaced femoral shaft fractures in athletes are available for review in the literature. Luchini and coauthors[23] reported on two long-distance runners with displaced fractures of the femoral shaft. The patients were treated with intramedullary nails, and one was able to return to running. Leinberry et al.[24] reported on a displaced subtrochanteric stress fracture in an amenorrheic runner. The authors stabilized the fracture with an intramedullary nail. The fracture healed, but the patient was instructed not to return to her preinjury level of running.

In conclusion, femoral stress fractures can usually be managed nonoperatively if they are diagnosed early. Operative management of femoral neck stress fractures is occasionally required to minimize serious complications and fracture displacement; however, following operative treatment it is uncommon for runners to return to their previous level of activity.

BURSITIS

Inflammation of the bursae around the hip is a common source of pain in runners. The bursae overlying the greater trochanter, the iliopectineal eminence, and the ischium are the most commonly involved. In the vast majority of cases, symptomatic treatment is all that is required. Occasionally, chronic bursitis can be accompanied by an audible snap. This so-called snapping hip is discussed separately in a later section.

Trochanteric Bursitis

Trochanteric bursitis is a common cause of lateral hip pain. Tenderness localized over the greater trochanter and increased pain with hip adduction are frequently present. Patients usually respond to a program that includes correction of training errors, rest, ice, stretching, and NSAIDs. Occasionally corticosteroid injections are required. This condition rarely requires surgical treatment.

In the rare instance in which nonoperative treatment is unsuccessful, incision of the iliotibial band and resection of the underlying bursal sac may be required for symptomatic relief.[25,26] Slawski and Howard[26] reported good results with this technique in an athletic population.

Bradley and Dillingham[27] have published a recent case report utilizing bursoscopy to resect symptomatic trochanteric bursae with good results. The procedure is performed in the lateral decubitus position with a 4.0-mm arthroscope. A motorized resector and laser are used to perform the bursectomy. This is the only report in the literature discussing this technique.

Iliopectineal Bursitis

Inflammation of the iliopectineal bursa results in groin and anterior hip pain. Patients may present with an antalgic gait and hold the lower extremity in a position of hip flexion and external rotation.[28] Snapping of the iliopsoas over the iliopectineal eminence is often present. Nonoperative treatment is nearly always successful. The surgical management of iliopectineal bursitis involves lengthening of the iliopsoas tendon and is discussed further in the section on snapping hip.

Ischial Bursitis

Patients with ischial bursitis present with buttock and proximal hamstring pain. Localized ischial tenderness is present, and patients may have difficulty sitting. Nonoperative therapy is the mainstay of treatment, and corticosteroid injections may be useful in refractory cases. Debridement of the ischial bursal tissue has been described[28] but is rarely necessary for treatment.

Puranen and Orava[29] have coined the term *hamstring syndrome* to describe buttock pain in the area of the ischial tuberosity. The pain radiates down the posterior thigh and is exacerbated with sitting and hamstring stretching. Most patients in the authors' series had sustained multiple hamstring strains, and sprinters are most commonly affected. Compression of the sciatic nerve by tight bands of the biceps femoris tendon is thought to result in this syndrome. The authors surgically divided the tight bands in 59 patients with good results.

SNAPPING HIP

Coxa saltans or snapping hip can be a source of pain in the runner. Patients complain of an audible snap with hip range of motion, and this snapping is often associated with pain. Snapping hip can be classified as external, internal, and intraarticular.[30]

External Snapping Hip

The external type of coxa saltans is usually due to the iliotibial band or the anterior portion of the gluteus maximus snapping over the greater trochanter. Lateral hip pain associated with the snapping is due to inflammation of the trochanteric bursa. Clinical examination reveals tenderness over the greater trochanter. The examiner can palpate the iliotibial band snapping over the trochanter with flexion and extension of the hip. The snapping can also be palpated with the patient standing on the normal limb and mimicking the running motion with the involved extremity.[31]

Most patients with the external type of coxa saltans will respond to nonoperative therapy. Stretching, rest, NSAIDs, and avoiding those activities that result in snapping are usually helpful in relieving patients' symptoms. Injection with a local anesthetic and a corticosteroid is usually effective in those patients who have persistent symptoms.

Surgical treatment may be considered for the external snapping hip only after all nonoperative means have failed, including activity restriction for at least 6 months. Operative treatment includes debridement of the thickened, inflamed bursal tissue over the greater trochanter. In addition, several techniques to eliminate the snapping have been proposed. Brignall

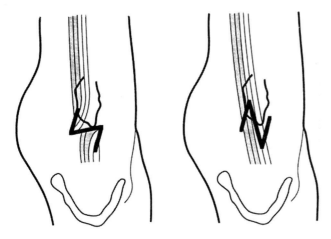

Figure 51–5. Diagram of surgical technique for Z-plasty lengthening of the iliotibial band. (*Source: From Brignall and Stainsby.*[32])

and Stainsby[32] described a Z-plasty lengthening of the iliotibial band (Fig. 51–5). The authors reported excellent results in six patients; however, no mention was made of activity level or athletic participation.

Zoltan and coauthors[31] reported on a surgical technique that involved resection of an elliptically shaped portion of the iliotibial band overlying the greater trochanter (Fig. 51–6). The procedure is performed in the lateral decubitus under local anesthetic. The patient actively flexes and extends the hip, allowing intraoperative assessment of the snapping. The elliptical resection is enlarged until no further snapping is observed. The authors reported excellent results in six of seven athletes who underwent this procedure.

One patient required a second, more extensive resection that resulted in symptomatic relief.

In summary, surgical management of the external type of snapping hip is rarely required. If required, both Z-plasty lengthening and elliptical resection techniques have shown good results in small series.

Internal Snapping Hip

The internal type of coxa sultans is usually due to the iliopsoas tendon snapping over the femoral head, the iliopectineal eminence, or an exostosis of the lesser trochanter (Fig. 51–7).[30] This results in painful inflammation of the underlying iliopectineal bursa. Patients typically complain of groin pain associated with an audible snap that occurs with extension of the flexed, abducted, and externally rotated hip.[33] This snapping can be palpated on physical examination. Iliopsoas bursography is a useful radiographic procedure that can aid in the diagnosis of internal snapping hip.[34]

Nonoperative, symptomatic treatment emphasizing stretching with the hip in extension is routinely successful.[35] Corticosteroid injections can also be useful in patients with persistent symptoms. Only rarely is operative intervention required.

Operative management of the internal type of coxa saltans involves lengthening or release of the iliopsoas tendon.[35,36] Jacobson and Allen[35] have described a technique that lengthens the iliopsoas tendon by partial transection of the posteromedial tendinous portion of the iliopsoas. In 6 of 18 patients who had the procedure, snapping recurred but to a lesser

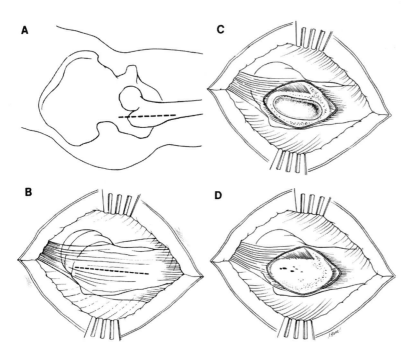

Figure 51–6. Diagram of surgical technique for resection of the iliotibial band in the treatment of external snapping hip. (*A*) Incision. (*B*) Exposure of iliotibial band. (*C*) Partial excision of iliotibial band. (*D*) Trochanteric bursa excised. (*Source: From Zoltan et al.*[31])

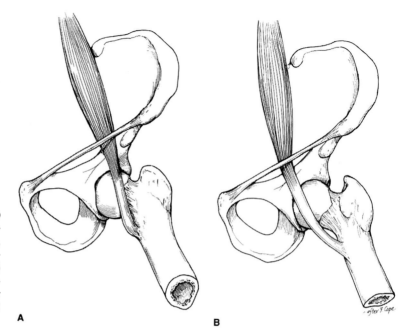

Figure 51–7. Diagram showing lateral to medial shift of the iliopsoas tendon with flexion and extension. (*A*) With flexion of the hip, the iliopsoas tendon shifts laterally in relation to the center of the femoral head. (*B*) With extension of the hip, the iliopsoas tendon shifts medially in relation to the center of the femoral head. (*Source: From Allen and Cope.*[30])

degree. All but two patients improved and were able to return to full activity. Three patients reported weakness of hip flexion, and two patients had injury to the lateral femoral cutaneous nerve.

Taylor and Clarke[36] published their results with iliopsoas tendon transection. The iliopsoas tendon was approached between the pectineus and adductor brevis, and the tendinous portion of the iliopsoas was divided. This procedure was performed on 22 patients with good results in all. However, six patients had persistent snapping, albeit to a lesser degree. Two patients had subjective weakness of hip flexion, but no other complications were reported.

Like the external type, the internal form of snapping hip nearly always responds to nonoperative treatment. Lengthening or transection of the iliopsoas tendon results in improvement in most patients. However, some degree of residual snapping is not uncommon.

Intraarticular Snapping Hip

Acetabular labral tears or loose bodies can cause snapping hip. These intraarticular etiologies present with intermittent clicking and pain.[30] Frequently, labral tears and loose bodies cause pain without snapping and are discussed in the next section.

INTRAARTICULAR CONDITIONS

Loose bodies and acetabular labral tears are intraarticular lesions that can cause hip pain in the runner. Patients usually present with pain and intermittent mechanical symptoms. Many patients will have a his-

tory of trauma. A loss of hip motion and pain with resisted straight-leg raising is frequently seen on physical examination.[37] Imaging modalities that can aid in the diagnosis include plain radiographs, computed tomography, and magnetic resonance imaging. However, the diagnosis may remain in doubt despite an extensive workup in over 50% of cases.[38] Pain relief following an injection of local anesthetic into the hip joint is helpful in predicting whether an intraarticular condition exists as a source of hip or groin pain. Hip arthroscopy has been shown to be useful in diagnosing intraarticular lesions.[37,38]

Hip arthroscopy can be performed in the supine or lateral position. A fracture table or specialized hip distractor is used to distract the hip joint. Distention of the joint with normal saline can aid in distraction. Fluoroscopic imaging confirms proper placement of arthroscopic instrumentation. Careful portal placement is necessary due to the close proximity of large neurovascular structures. In most instances, peritrochanteric portals and an anterior portal are used[39] (Fig. 51–8). Visualization of most of the hip joint can be accomplished by alternating the arthroscope between portals and using both the 30- and the 70-degree arthroscope. Longer, specialized instruments allow debridement of acetabular labral tears and removal of loose bodies. Patients are usually allowed to go home the day of surgery and can bear weight as tolerated with crutches.

Loose bodies in the hip can result from posttraumatic fragments, osteochondritis dissecans, or synovial chondromatosis.[37] Arthroscopic removal of loose bodies avoids the morbidity of a hip arthrotomy and allows earlier return to activity.

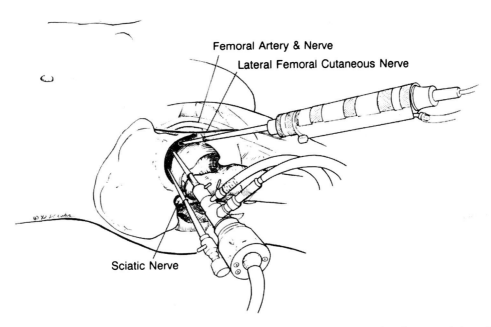

Figure 51–8. Diagram demonstrating a shaver in the anterior portal and an arthroscope and outflow cannula in peritrochanteric portals. The lateral femoral cutaneous nerve traverses close to the anterior portal. (*Source: From Byrd.[39]*)

Acetabular labral tears have become an increasingly recognized cause of hip pain. Much of this new awareness is due to hip arthroscopy. The clinical diagnosis of an acetabular labral tear can be difficult, and imaging studies are often nonspecific. An arthroscopic evaluation of the hip joint can visualize the labrum, and debridement of labral tears can be accomplished with arthroscopic techniques (Fig. 51–9). Farjo and

coauthors[40] reported their results of hip arthroscopy on 28 patients with acetabular labral tears. Most of them were located anteriorly and were radial flap tears. Debridement of the labral tear resulted in good pain relief in 71% of patients who had no evidence of arthritis. Patients who had arthroscopic evidence of arthritis did not benefit significantly from tear debridement. These results are consistent with our hip arthroscopy experience at West Point.

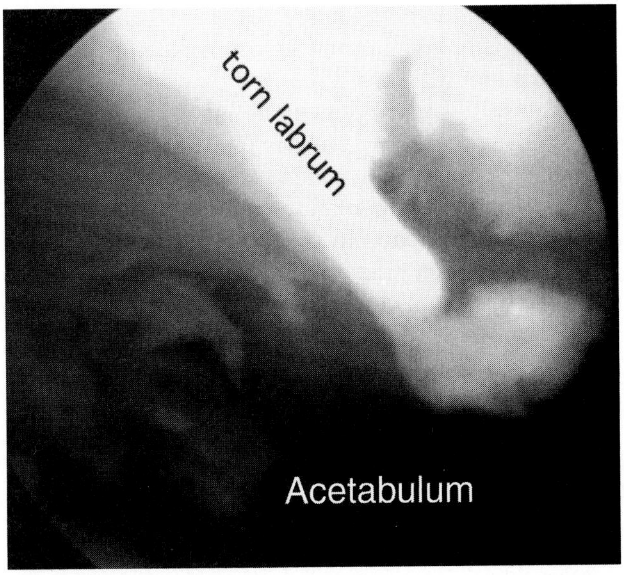

CHRONIC GROIN PAIN

Chronic groin pain in the runner can result from incomplete treatment of the conditions discussed above. Other causes of chronic groin pain include ilioinguinal neuralgia, genitourinary afflictions (prostatitis, epididymitis, urethritis, hydrocele, etc.), and osteitis pubis. These problems can almost always be treated nonoperatively. Muscle injuries, including chronic adductor muscle strains and abdominal muscle wall injuries, can also cause groin pain and may require operative treatment. Obturator nerve entrapment is another painful condition that has been treated surgically.

Adductor Longus Injury

Adductor longus tendinopathy is a common cause of groin pain.[41] Patients complain of an insidious onset of groin pain that gradually worsens. There is usually localized tenderness and pain with resisted adduction of the hip. Nonoperative treatment consists of rest,

Figure 51–9. Arthroscopic photograph of an anterolateral labral tear in the right hip of a college soccer player. The arthroscope is in the anterior portal. A 4.5-mm shaver is entering the joint through the lateral peritrochanteric portal.

physiotherapy, correction of training errors, NSAIDs, and corticosteroid injections.

Surgical management of adductor longus injury is rarely required. In fact, only one recent publication is available for review.[42] Akermark and Johansson[42] reported their results of adductor longus tenotomy in 16 competitive athletes. Three of these were runners. The procedure is performed through an incision distal and parallel to the groin crease. The adductor longus tendon is incised 1 cm from the muscle origin. All patients in this series were improved or symptom free, and all but one patient were able to return to athletic activity. Adductor weakness was noted on isokinetic testing. The authors recommended this procedure for chronic groin pain due to adductor longus injury but cautioned that other etiologies of groin pain must be excluded.

Abdominal Musculature Abnormalities

Groin pain due to abnormalities in the abdominal wall has been termed "pubalgia,"[43] "sportsmen's hernia,"[44] and "Gilmore's groin."[45] The exact nature of the injury is controversial, as is the surgical management. Most authors feel that the pathology is attributable to an indirect hernia or hernia precursor due to disruption of the conjoined tendon.[43,44,46]

The diagnosis of pubalgia can be difficult. Patients usually complain of groin pain that worsens with activity. Coughing or sit-ups may exacerbate the symptoms. Palpation of the inguinal ring and pubic tubercle results in tenderness. In many patients a palpable hernia is not present. Resistance of the hip adductors and Valsalva's maneuver may elicit discomfort.[48] Adductor tendinosis is excluded because adductor tendon tenderness is absent. Herniography can aid in the diagnosis.[47]

Herniorrhaphy has been recommended in patients with chronic groin pain if no other diagnosis can be made.[43,44,46] Malycha and Lovell[44] have published a large series of 50 athletes who underwent herniorrhaphy for chronic groin pain. Seventy-five percent of patients reported their result as good, and an additional 23% felt they were improved. Ninety-three percent of patients were able to return to normal activities.

Two recent reports have demonstrated good results with laparoscopic herniorrhaphy.[48,49] Ingoldby[49] has published a report comparing laparoscopic and conventional herniorrhaphy in athletes with chronic groin pain. The results of the procedures were similar, but laparoscopic repair resulted in less pain and earlier return to sport.

Obturator Nerve Entrapment

Bradshaw and McCrory[50] have recently published their experience with obturator nerve entrapment in athletes. Patients in their series complained of groin pain that radiated down the medial side of the thigh and was worse after exercise. Patients complained of weakness after exercise, and physical examination revealed adductor muscle weakness and paresthesias over the medial thigh. Electrophysiology studies revealed denervation in the short and long adductor muscles. The diagnosis was confirmed with a local anesthetic block. Nonoperative measures for obturator nerve entrapment were not successful.

The authors performed neurolysis of the obturator nerve in 32 athletes. Postoperatively, all 32 patients were improved and returned to athletic activities. In addition, the electrophysiology studies returned to normal in all patients.

In summary, the management of chronic groin pain in the runner can be difficult. Adductor tendinosis is a common problem and usually responds to nonoperative measures. However, other less well-known entities like pubalgia and obturator nerve entrapment need to be included in the differential diagnosis. Surgical management of these problems that fail to respond to nonoperative measures can often allow the runner to return to full activity.

OSTEOARTHROSIS

The risk of hip osteoarthrosis in runners is controversial. A review of the literature by Boyd et al.[51] concluded that most studies demonstrated no increased incidence of osteoarthrosis in runners. However, a more recent study has shown an increased risk of osteoarthrosis in female distance runners compared with a control group.[52]

The initial management of hip osteoarthrosis is nonoperative. Activity modification and oral medications may improve the patient's symptoms. Most runners will need to diminish or cease their running significantly. Nonimpact exercises such as swimming and bicycling are recommended in place of running. Total hip replacement is very successful in relieving pain in older patients with hip osteoarthrosis. Running is discouraged after total hip replacement due to the risk of component wear and prosthetic failure.

SUMMARY

Hip problems in the runner consist of a wide spectrum of soft tissue and osseous injury. The vast majority of these problems will improve without surgical intervention. Correction of training errors, rest, physiotherapy, and NSAIDs will frequently allow the athlete to return to running. Occasionally surgical management is indicated in athletes who fail to improve with these measures. In many instances, operative management can improve patients' symptoms and allow runners to return to sport. However, the surgical management of femoral neck fractures and hip osteoarthrosis usually results in the cessation of running.

REFERENCES

1. Brunet ME, Cook SD, Brinker MR, et al.: A survey of running injuries in 1505 competitive and recreational runners. *J Sports Med Phy Fit* 1990:30, 307.
2. MacIntyre JG, Taunton JE, Clement DB, et al.: Running injuries: A clinical study of 4173 cases. *Clin J Sports Med* 1991:1, 81.
3. Barrow GW, Saha S: Menstrual irregularity and stress fractures in collegiate female distance runners. *Am J Sports Med* 1988:16, 209.
4. Bennell KL, Malcolm SA, Thomas SA, et al.: The incidence and distribution of stress fractures in competitive track and field athletes. A twelve-month prospective study. *Am J Sports Med* 1996:24, 211.
5. Bennell KL, Brukner PD: Epidemiology and site specificity of stress fractures. *Clin Sports Med* 1997:16, 179.
6. Matheson GO, Clement DB, McKenzie DC, et al.: Stress fractures in athletes. A study of 320 cases. *Am J Sports Med* 1987:15, 46.
7. Johnson AW, Weiss CB, Wheeler DL: Stress fractures of the femoral shaft in athletes—more common than expected. A new clinical test. *Am J Sports Med* 1994:22, 248.
8. Boden BP, Speer KP: Femoral stress fractures. *Clin Sports Med* 1997:16, 307.
9. Shin AY, Morin WD, Gorman JD, et al.: The superiority of magnetic resonance imaging in differentiating the cause of hip pain in endurance athletes. *Am J Sports Med* 1996:24, 168.
10. Devas MB: Stress fractures of the femoral neck. *J Bone Joint Surg* 1965:47B, 728.
11. Fullerton LR, Snowdy HA: Femoral neck stress fractures. *Am J Sports Med* 1988:16, 365.
12. Hajek MR, Noble HB: Stress fractures of the femoral neck in joggers. Case reports and review of the literature. *Am J Sports Med* 1982:10, 112.
13. Aro H, Dahlstrom S: Conservative management of distraction-type stress fractures of the femoral neck. *J Bone Joint Surg Br* 1986:68B, 65.
14. Kuslich SD, Gustilo RB: Fractures of the femoral neck in young adults. *J Bone Joint Surg Am* 1976:58A, 724.
15. Protzman RR, Burkhalter WE: Femoral neck fractures in young adults. *J Bone Joint Surg Am* 1976:58A, 689.
16. Swiontkowski MF, Winquist RA, Hansen ST: Fractures of the femoral neck in patients between the ages of twelve and forty-nine years. *J Bone Joint Surg Am* 1984:66A, 837.
17. DeLee JC: Fractures and dislocations of the hip, in Rockwood CA, Green DP, Bucholz RW, et al. (eds.), *Rockwood and Green's Fractures in Adults,* 4th ed, Philadelphia, Lippincott-Raven, 1996:1659.
18. Johansson C, Ekenman I, Tornkvist H, et al.: Stress fractures of the femoral neck in athletes. The consequence of a delay in diagnosis. *Am J Sports Med* 1990:18, 524.
19. Butler JE, Brown SL, McConnell BG: Subtrochanteric stress fractures in runners. *Am J Sports Med* 1982:10, 228.
20. Hershman EB, Lombardo J, Bergfeld JA: Femoral shaft stress fractures in athletes. *Clin Sports Med* 1990:9, 111.
21. Lombardo SJ, Benson DW: Stress fractures of the femur in runners. *Am J Sports Med* 1982:10, 219.
22. Bucholz RW, Brumback RJ: Fractures of the shaft of the femur, in Rockwood CA, Green DP, Bucholz RW, et al. (eds.), *Rockwood and Green's Fractures in Adults,* 4th ed, Philadelphia, Lippincott-Raven, 1996:1827.
23. Luchini MA, Sarokhan AJ, Micheli LJ: Acute displaced femoral-shaft fractures in long-distance runners. *J Bone Joint Surg Am* 1983:65A, 689.
24. Leinberry CF, McShane RB, Stewart WG, et al.: A displaced subtrochanteric stress fracture in a young amenorrheic athlete. *Am J Sports Med* 1992:20, 485.
25. Brooker AF: The surgical approach to refractory trochanteric bursitis. *Johns Hopkins Med J* 1979:145, 98.
26. Slawski DP, Howard RF: Surgical management of refractory trochanteric bursitis. *Am J Sports Med* 1997:25, 86.
27. Bradley DM, Dillingham MF: Bursoscopy of the trochanteric bursa. *Arthroscopy* 1998:14, 884.
28. Gross ML, Nasser S, Finerman GA: Hip and pelvis, in DeLee JS, Drez D (eds.), *Orthopaedic Sports Medicine,* 1st ed. Philadelphia, WB Saunders, 1994:1063.
29. Puranen J, Orava S: The hamstring syndrome. A new diagnosis of gluteal sciatic pain. *Am J Sports Med* 1988:16, 517.
30. Allen WC, Cope R: Coxa saltans: The snapping hip revisited. *J Am Acad Orthop Surg* 1995:3, 303.
31. Zoltan DJ, Clancy WG, Keene JS: A new operative approach to snapping hip and refractory trochanteric bursitis in athletes. *Am J Sports Med* 1986:14, 201.
32. Brignall CG, Stainsby GD: The snapping hip: Treatment by z-plasty. *J Bone Joint Surg Br* 1991:73B, 253.
33. Schaberg JE, Harper MC, Allen WC: The snapping hip syndrome. *Am J Sports Med* 1984:12, 361.
34. Harper MC, Schaberg JE, Allen WC: Primary iliopsoas bursography in the diagnosis of disorders of the hip. *Clin Orthop* 1987:221, 238.
35. Jacobson T, Allen WC: Surgical correction of the snapping iliopsoas tendon. *Am J Sports Med* 1990:18, 470.
36. Taylor GR, Clarke NM: Surgical release of the 'snapping iliopsoas tendon'. *J Bone Joint Surg Br* 1995:77B, 881.
37. McCarthy JC, Day B, Busconi B: Hip arthroscopy: Applications and technique. *J Am Acad Orthop Surg* 1995:3, 115.
38. Baber YF, Robinson AN, Villar RN: Is diagnostic arthroscopy of the hip worthwhile? A prospective review of 328 adults investigated for hip pain. *J Bone Joint Surg Br* 1999:81B, 600.
39. Byrd JWT: Hip arthroscopy utilizing the supine position. *Arthroscopy* 1994:10, 275.
40. Farjo LA, Glick JM, Sampson TG: Hip arthroscopy for acetabular labral tears. *Arthroscopy* 1999:15, 132.

41. Renstrom P, Peterson L: Groin injuries in athletes. *Br J Sports Med* 1980:14, 30.
42. Akermark C, Johansson C: Tenotomy of the adductor longus tendon in the treatment of chronic groin pain in athletes. *Am J Sports Med* 1992:20, 640.
43. Taylor DC, Meyers WC, Moylan JA, et al.: Abdominal musculature abnormalities as a cause of groin pain in athletes. Inguinal hernias and pubalgia. *Am J Sports Med* 1991:19, 239.
44. Malycha P, Lovell G: Inguinal surgery in athletes with chronic groin pain: The 'sportsman's' hernia. *Aust N Z J Surg* 1992:62, 123.
45. Gilmore J: Groin pain in the soccer athlete: Fact, fiction, and treatment. *Clin Sports Med* 1998:17, 787.
46. Hackney RG: The sports hernia: A cause of chronic groin pain. *Br J Sports Med* 1993:27, 58.
47. Smedberg SG, Broome AE, Gullmo A, et al.: Herniography in athletes with groin pain. *Am J Surg* 1985:149, 378.
48. Azurin DJ, Go LS, Schuricht A, et al.: Endoscopic preperitoneal herniorrhaphy in professional athletes with groin pain. *J Laparoendosc Adv Surg Tech* 1997:7, 7.
49. Ingoldby CH: Laparoscopic and conventional repair of groin disruption in sportsmen. *Br J Surg* 1997:84, 213.
50. Bradshaw C, McCrory P: Obturator nerve entrapment. A cause of groin pain in athletes. *Am J Sports Med* 1997:25, 402.
51. Boyd KT, Peirce NS, Batt ME: Common hip injuries in sport. *Sports Med* 1997:24, 273.
52. Spector TD, Harris PA, Hart DJ, et al.: Risk of osteoarthritis associated with long-term weight-bearing sports: A radiologic survey of the hips and knees in female ex-athletes and population controls. *Arthritis Rheum* 1996:39, 988.

Chapter 52

SURGICAL TREATMENT OF KNEE DISORDERS IN RUNNERS

Barry P. Boden

INTRODUCTION

Running is one of the oldest forms of exercise, dating back to preclassical Greek times. Over the last 30 years, there has been a tremendous resurgence in the popularity of running, because of its low cost, minimal time requirement, and advantageous health effects. Unfortunately, running is also associated with a risk of injury to the lower extremity, usually the knee.[1] For athletes who run more than 25 miles a week, the annual injury rate may approach 30%, with one third of these injuries involving the knee.[2] This chapter reviews the most common disorders of the knee in runners, with the focus on surgical treatment.

Epidemiologic studies on distance runners have found that most running injuries occur in the knee.[1] During running, the knee (especially the patellofemoral joint) is subjected to tremendous forces. Training errors such as a sudden increase in the duration or intensity of exercise are responsible for most injuries. Improvement in running shoes has reduced the number of leg and foot injuries but has had little effect in protecting the knee. Knee injuries in runners may be classified as disorders of the patellofemoral joint, soft-tissue injuries, and osteoarthritis (Table 52–1). Although most knee conditions resolve with conservative treatment, surgery is often necessary in refractory cases.

PATELLAR TILT

Patellar tilt, a common disorder, has been referred to as lateral patellar compression syndrome (LPCS) or excessive lateral pressure syndrome (ELPS). This disorder is characterized by a tight lateral retinaculum, resulting in abnormally high forces between the lateral facet of the patella and the lateral trochlea. The onset of symptoms is often insidious and may be associated with minor antecedent trauma. Patients typically present with diffuse anterior knee pain that is greatest over the lateral retinaculum during knee flexion. Chronic lateral patella tilt can lead to degeneration of the articular cartilage on the lateral facet of the patella.

Patellar tilt is assessed by attempting to raise the patient's lateral patellar facet away from the lateral femoral trochlea. An inability to raise the lateral facet to the horizontal is suggestive of lateral retinacular tightness and tethering of the lateral patella. Frequently, patients with patellar tilt demonstrate tenderness along the lateral patellar facet secondary to wear of the articular cartilage. The axial radiograph is the most helpful plain radiograph to diagnose patellar tilt and demonstrates a diminished joint space between the lateral facet of the patella and the lateral trochlea (Fig. 52–1).[3]

TABLE 52–1. CLASSIFICATION OF KNEE INJURIES IN RUNNERS

Anterior knee pain (patellofemoral disorders)
    Patellar tilt
    Patellar instability
        Dislocation
        Subluxation
    Chondral injuries
Soft-tissue injuries
    Patellar tendinopathy
    Quadriceps tendinopathy
    Iliotibial band friction syndrome
    Plica
    Meniscal injuries
Osteoarthritis

In patients with patellar tilt, the treatment of choice after an unsuccessful trial of nonoperative therapy is an arthroscopic lateral release. This procedure has been shown to be more effective in the management of patellar tilt than patellar subluxation.[4] The lateral release does not significantly reduce the active lateral vector of the quadriceps and therefore less satisfactory results are seen in patients with subluxation. The entire lateral retinaculum, vastus lateralis obliquus, and distal patellotibial band should be released.[5,6] The release is performed 5 mm lateral to the lateral patellar border covering the distance from 1 cm superior to the patella to the anterolateral portal. The author's preferred technique employs electrocautery or bipolar electroablation.

Although a lateral release is a routine technical operation, the procedure may be associated with several potential complications. Hemarthrosis is the most common postoperative complication. A hemarthrosis inhibits the quadriceps and delays rehabilitation. The incidence of postoperative hemarthroses from injury to the superior lateral geniculate artery can be diminished by performing the release with electrocautery. If a tourniquet is used, it should be deflated prior to closure in order to cauterize any bleeding vessels. Incising the vastus lateralis tendon or performing a lateral release on patients with pathology other than patellar tilt may lead to medial patellar subluxation. Release of

the main vastus lateralis tendon should not be performed; otherwise, the muscle may retract and atrophy, leading to an imbalance of the patellar stabilizers. This is avoided by angling the release 45 degrees in a lateral direction proximal to the superior margin of the patella.

PATELLAR INSTABILITY

Patellar Subluxation

Instability disorders of the patella may be classified as patellar dislocation or subluxation.[7] In runners subluxation is the more prevalent condition. Lateral translation of the patella is the most common direction of patellar subluxation and is usually associated with malalignment of the lower extremity. Patients present with a history of "giving way" as the patella jumps from a centralized position in the trochlear groove to a lateral position with full extension. Lateral subluxation is a condition that predominantly affects individuals with preexisting malalignment, such as genu valgum or hyperlaxity. Medial subluxation is uncommon and usually iatrogenic.

Patients with patellar subluxation should be assessed for any physical signs that may serve as prognosticators for patellar instability (Table 52–2). The presence of femoral anteversion, genu valgum, external tibial torsion, and foot pronation can be documented by observing the patient in a standing position and during the gait cycle. Hip muscular strength and

---

TABLE 52–2. PREDISPOSING RISK FACTORS FOR PATELLOFEMORAL SUBLUXATION

Generalized hyperlaxity
Femoral anteversion
Femoral dysplasia
Genu valgum
Patellar dysplasia
Patella alta
VMO atrophy
High Q-angle
Pes planus

VMO = vastus medialis obliquus muscle.

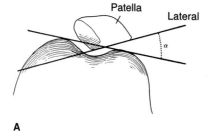
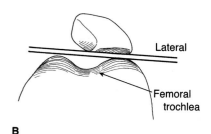

Figure 52–1. Illustration of the axial view of the patellofemoral joint demonstrating normal patellofemoral congruity (*A*) and lateral patellar tilt (*B*) with diminished joint space between the lateral facet of the patella and the lateral trochlea. (*Source: From Fulkerson.*[27])

A   B

joint range of motion are evaluated with the patient in the supine position to exclude referred knee pain originating from hip pathology. The Q-angle, the angle between the quadriceps tendon and the patellar tendon, should be measured with the knee in flexion, as measurements of the Q-angle in full extension may result in falsely low values.

Patellar tracking is assessed as the patient sits on the edge of the examining table and flexes and extends his or her knee. Normally, the patella is centered within the femoral trochlea with slight knee flexion and traces a straight line as the knee is brought into extension. In patients with patellar subluxation, however, the patella travels from a central position within the femoral trochlea at 30 degrees of flexion to a laterally subluxated position in full extension. Excessive lateral excursion during terminal knee extension is referred to as a positive J-sign and is indicative of lateral patellar subluxation. In equivocal cases, computed tomography may aid in the determination of malalignment of the tibial tubercle or the patella at knee flexion angles less than 20 degrees.[8]

Surgery may be indicated in patients with subluxation only if symptoms persist after a quality nonoperative rehabilitation program. Determination of the optimal surgical procedure is based on the type of subluxation. For most patients with subluxation secondary to skeletal malalignment, a distal realignment procedure produces a good outcome. The primary goal of surgery is to transfer the tibial tubercle medially to correct the Q-angle. The Hauser procedure is performed by transferring the tibial tubercle medially onto the tibia and is cited only for historical reasons. Results with this procedure have been disappointing due to posteriorization of the tubercle, which increases the patellofemoral contact forces and predisposes the joint to degenerative changes.

For isolated subluxation without significant degenerative changes, the Elmslie-Trillat procedure provides good results. A transverse osteotomy is employed to shift the tibial tubercle onto the medial aspect of the tubercle eminence. In contrast to the Hauser procedure, the tibial tubercle is left attached distally by an intact hinge of bone to avoid any posteriorization. In extreme cases with both subluxation and chondromalacia, the author recommends the Fulkerson procedure or an anteromedial transfer of the tibial tubercle (AMTT).[9,10] This procedure corrects the Q-angle via an oblique osteotomy, which medializes the tibial tubercle and unloads the patellofemoral articulation with anteriorization of the tibial tubercle (Fig. 52–2). The results of the procedure have been reported to be good and excellent in 90% of cases.[10] Meticulous attention to detail is critical since the potential complications

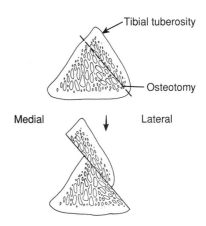

Figure 52–2. Diagrammatic representation of AMTT osteotomy. Cross section of tibia illustrating how the oblique cut allows anterior and medial displacement of tibial tuberosity. (*Source: From Fulkerson.*[27])

include skin slough, infection, peroneal nerve injury, and compartment syndrome.

Before the open procedure is performed, an arthroscopic evaluation of the entire knee joint should be completed. The superomedial portal is particularly helpful for evaluating patellar tracking.[11] The lateral facet should align with the trochlea by 20 to 25 degrees of knee flexion followed by the midpatellar ridge by 35 to 40 degrees of knee flexion. Any lateral overhang of the patella should be documented while the patella is engaging the femoral trochlea. After observing passive patellar tracking, a muscle stimulator can be applied to the quadriceps to evaluate active patellar tracking. Prior to fixation of the osteotomized tibial tubercle, the arthroscope may be inserted into the joint to reassess patellar tracking.

In skeletally immature patients with subluxation, an AMTT procedure should be avoided until closure of the proximal tibial growth plates. Nonoperative therapy prior to skeletal maturity should include vastus medialis obliquus (VMO) strengthening exercises, a patellar stabilizing brace, and restriction of provocative activities. For the subgroup of patients with normal patellar alignment who have subluxation secondary to trauma, a proximal repair or reconstruction of the medial structures may be more appropriate.

Patellar Dislocation

Patellar dislocation is an uncommon malady in runners. Osteochondral lesions, which may be detected by the presence of fat droplets in the knee aspirate, are often found after an acute patellar dislocation. In patients treated nonoperatively for an initial episode of patellar dislocation, the chance of recurrent dislocation ranges from approximately 15% to 44%.[12–14] The medial patellofemoral ligament (MPFL) is the major medial

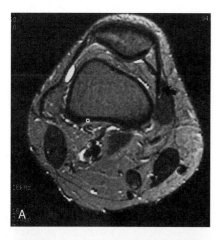

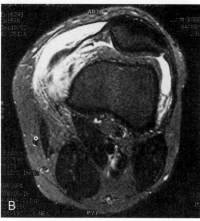

Figure 52–3. Axial MRI of normal MPFL in the right knee (*A*) and MPFL avulsion of the medial femoral epicondyle in the left knee (*B*). (*Source: From Boden et al.[7]*)

stabilizer of the patella (Fig. 52–3).[15] Management of patellar instability due to an acute patellar dislocation is controversial. Advances in the understanding of the pathoanatomy associated with an acute patellar dislocation, combined with the high incidence of recurrent patellar redislocation, have led to a renewed interest in acute surgical repair. Candidates for surgical repair of the MPFL include young, athletic patients who sustained the dislocation by an indirect mechanism.

Prior to operative repair of the MPFL, arthroscopy should be performed to evaluate the knee for any osteochondral lesions. Large articular lesions are optimally fixed in the acute setting, while small fragments are removed. The surgical procedure for MPFL repair is performed through a 4-cm incision just anterior to the medial epicondyle at the distal edge of the VMO muscle belly. The MPFL is identified deep to the VMO fascial layer. Most injuries to the MPFL are avulsions off the femur and may be repaired directly to the bone with suture anchors. A lateral release or AMTT is not routinely performed with this procedure. In patients

with patellar tilt symptoms prior to their acute dislocation, as well as intraoperatively confirmed patellar tilt after MPFL repair, a lateral release may be required. Similarly, for patients with significant anatomic malalignment, and a history of patellofemoral subluxation before their acute dislocation, a realignment procedure may be necessary in addition to the MPFL repair.

Short-term results of surgical repair of the MPFL reveal redislocation rates of less than 10%.[16,17] Although the incidence of instability is markedly reduced with operative repair, many patients continue to report pain and swelling. Chronic symptoms are most likely secondary to osteochondral lesions from the original injury.[18] Surgery is accepted as the treatment of choice for recurrent patellar dislocations. Although no prospective studies exist documenting the optimal procedure, arthroscopy combined with repair of the essential lesion, the MPFL, may provide the best outcome.

ARTICULAR CARTILAGE LESIONS (CHONDROMALACIA)

The articular cartilage of the patellofemoral joint is a frequent site of traumatic and degenerative lesions in runners. Several etiologic factors are involved: trauma, malalignment, and aging. In athletes competing in sports that require frequent pivoting and decelerating motions, delamination lesions are common (Fig. 52–4). These injuries occur as a result of shear stresses and involve a separation of the uncalcified articular cartilage from the calcified cartilage. In runners, patellofemoral lesions are usually a result of chronic, abrasive wear, which damages the cartilage in a superficial to deep direction, and are classified as partial or full thickness. Abrasive, degenerative changes secondary to malalignment primarily involve the lateral facet. Presenting symptoms of articular surface lesions include anterior knee pain, swelling, and a grinding sensation. The pain may be reported as diffuse and nonspecific, or as a sharp, stabbing sensation during a specific angle of knee flexion.

The patient's patella should be palpated for any crepitus that may suggest an articular cartilage injury. Compression of the patella during full range of motion of the knee may reproduce the pain. Based on the knee flexion angle in which symptoms are experienced, the location of the chondral injury may be estimated. Articular lesions on the distal patella are painful during early knee flexion, whereas proximal patella lesions manifest with further flexion. Radiographs may be helpful in diagnosing advanced chondral lesions.

Management of patellofemoral arthritis refractory to conservative measures is based on the patient's age, activity level, extent and location of cartilage damage,

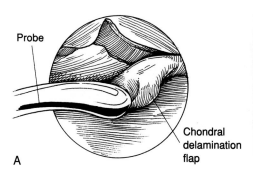

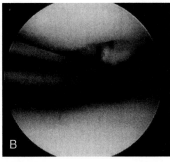

Figure 52–4. Delamination of an articular cartilage lesion on the patella as visualized through the arthroscope. (*Source: From Boden et al.*[7])

and patellofemoral mechanics. Traumatic delamination lesions may be arthroscopically debrided to a stable margin. Lesions smaller than 1.5 cm have a more favorable prognosis. Subchondral drilling is controversial and is left to the discretion of the surgeon. Return to sports may be allowed as early as 2 to 3 months postoperatively, although complete resolution of symptoms often is not achieved for 6 months.

In patients with degenerative, abrasive changes of the articular cartilage, the underlying cause of the abnormal forces on the patella should be identified and corrected. Lateral facet arthrosis is common in patients with long-standing patellar tilt or subluxation. A lateral release may help relieve symptoms in patients with patellar tilt and secondary arthrosis. In patients with subluxation resulting in lateral facet arthrosis, an AMTT may improve both maladies. Anterior displacement of the tibial tubercle unloads the distal and lateral facets of the patella and shifts the forces to the proximal and medial facet of the patella. Optimal results are obtained in patients with some preservation of the proximal and medial patellar articular cartilage.

QUADRICEPS AND PATELLAR TENDINOSIS

Overuse or traction injuries to the extensor mechanism can produce lesions in the quadriceps or patellar tendons. Complete quadriceps ruptures typically occur in older individuals with preexisting degenerative changes in the tendon, whereas patellar tendon ruptures usually result from trauma in younger athletes. In skeletally mature runners, repetitive submaximal overload forces may result in quadriceps tendinosis or patellar tendinosis. The pathology in partial thickness tears of the patellar tendon is located in the posterior half of the tendon at its insertion site into the patella. In adolescents, the same forces may produce a traction injury of the tibial tubercle known as Osgood-Schlatter disease.

Pain on palpation of the superior pole of the patella is often diagnostic of quadriceps tendinosis, whereas pain at the inferior pole is indicative of patellar tendi-

nosis. Runners with partial thickness lesions experience weakness of the extensor mechanism, whereas complete ruptures lead to an inability to extend the knee from a flexed position on extreme extension weakness. Diagnosis of most patella and quadriceps lesions can be made by a thorough history and physical. When in doubt, a magnetic resonance image may be helpful in identifying degenerative or partial thickness tendon lesions.

Most overuse injuries to the patella and quadriceps tendons can be successfully treated by nonoperative treatment consisting of avoidance of the inciting activity followed by a rehabilitation program. In refractory partial thickness injuries, debridement of degenerative tissue and plication of the tendon may be necessary. For complete tendon ruptures, surgical repair is performed through a longitudinal incision over the affected tendon. The site of reattachment on the patella is prepared by removing overlying periosteum and abrading the bone to create a bleeding surface. The tendon may be repaired with suture anchors or multiple holes drilled through the patella. The author prefers to drill three longitudinal holes through the patella and repair the tendon with nonabsorbable suture.

ILIOTIBIAL BAND FRICTION SYNDROME

Iliotibial band (ITB) friction syndrome is an overuse injury caused by excessive friction between the ITB and the lateral femoral condyle. The ITB lies anterior to the lateral femoral condyle with the knee in extension and posterior in flexion. At 20 to 30 degrees of knee flexion, the ITB may impinge on the lateral femoral condyle or the overlying bursa. Predisposing factors include overuse running, a tight ITB, excessive foot pronation, and/or genu varum.

Clinically, athletes present with lateral knee pain 3 cm proximal to the joint line. Activities such as running downhill in which the knee repetitively flexes from 20 to 40 degrees may aggravate the symptoms. Physical examination reveals pain with the compression test and ITB tightness with the Ober test. The differential diagnosis includes lateral meniscal pathology, biceps femoris or popliteus tendinosis, stress fracture, and lumbar disc pathology.

Most patients respond to nonoperative therapy consisting of anti-inflammatory medications, ITB stretching, activity modification, and an orthotic for athletes with excessive foot pronation. Only rarely is surgical intervention required.[19,20] The procedure is performed through a longitudinal incision at the level of the lateral femoral condyle with the knee placed in 30 degrees of flexion. The lateral condyle should be palpated for any bony spurs or osteochondromas that may need to be excised. Next a triangular piece of the posterior half of the ITB is resected. The leg is moved through a range of motion to ascertain that there is no further impingement. Postoperatively, running is gradually resumed, with full return to competition by 3 to 4 weeks. The surgical technique results in a high success rate.[19]

PATHOLOGIC PLICA

A plica is a residual embryologic synovial septum that persists into adult life. Although most synovial plicae are asymptomatic and are noted as incidental findings during arthroscopy, occasionally a plica may become inflamed and painful in a runner. In chronic cases the fibrotic plica may produce articular cartilage damage as it rubs against the medial femoral condyle. Of the four types of plica described, the medial parapatellar plica or medial plica is most often symptomatic.

In distance runners symptoms usually are insidious and aggravated by activity. On examination tenderness is present over the inflamed plica. A snapping sensation may be experienced as the pathologic plica rubs against the medial femoral condyle between 45 and 60 degrees of flexion. Relief of symptoms after an injection of local anesthetic into the pathologic plica is diagnostic.

The goal of treatment is to decrease inflammation through anti-inflammatory medications and restriction of running. Resistive knee exercises in the symptomatic range of motion should be avoided. Surgical intervention is indicated only after a failed trial of conservative therapy and exclusion of all other pathology. Meticulous arthroscopic inspection of the entire joint, especially the meniscus and articular cartilage, should be performed prior to plica resection. Often plica are overdiagnosed clinically only to find other intraarticular pathology during arthroscopy. The medial plica is best visualized with the arthroscope in the superolateral portal.[21] The plica is resected only if it appears thickened, avascular, and greater than 12 mm in

width.[22] An anterolateral portal is recommended for resection of a pathologic medial plica. The entire plica should be removed to prevent recurrence. Satisfactory to excellent results have been reported in 75% to 90% of cases.[23,24]

MENISCAL INJURIES

Meniscal injuries typically affect middle-aged and older runners. The onset of symptoms may be insidious in a degenerative tear or acute after a misstep causing a traumatic tear. There may be a history of mechanical symptoms such as "locking" or "catching." Physical signs include a small effusion, joint line tenderness, and occasionally a positive McMurray's test.

Symptomatic full-thickness mensical tears usually require arthroscopic treatment. For meniscal lesions in the avascular, central zone, partial meniscectomy is performed, preserving healthy meniscal tissue (Fig. 52–5). Meniscal repair is the preferred procedure

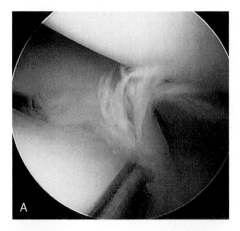

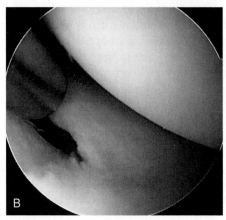

Figure 52–5. Arthroscopic photograph of radial tear of the lateral meniscus before (*A*) and after (*B*) partial meniscectomy.

for tears in the peripheral, vascular zone. The traditional inside-outside technique involves making a small incision close to the meniscal tear in order to tie the vertical mattress stitches. Advances in arthroscopic equipment allow the surgeon to repair the meniscus with an all-inside technique using biodegradable fixation devices. The long-term efficacy of this procedure has yet to be determined. Rehabilitation typically requires 4 to 6 weeks after partial meniscectomy, and 4 to 6 months after meniscal repair. For athletes with complete absence of the meniscus, meniscal transplantation offers restoration of the shock-absorbing function of the meniscus.

OSTEOARTHRITIS

There is no evidence in the literature that a lifetime of long-distance running is associated with the development of premature tibiofemoral osteoarthritis.[25,26] However, there is a risk of accelerating degenerative changes in a preexisting arthritic knee. With the increased participation in running in older patients, this condition is being seen more frequently in the office. Unless it is possible to limit running to a tolerable level, alternative low-impact activities such as swimming, biking, and cross-country skiing are recommended.

In patients with no mechanical symptoms, the results of arthroscopic debridement for osteoarthritis are poor. Newer techniques to treat localized full-thickness articular cartilage lesions hold promise. Osteochondral autogenous transplantation (OATS) is performed by transferring a plug of articular cartilage from a minimally weightbearing area into the weightbearing defect. Another more experimental salvage technique that involves two surgical procedures is autologous chondrocyte implantation. The first operation involves debridement of the lesion and biopsy of normal cartilage from the intercondylar notch. After the tissue is cultured and properly prepared, the cells are reimplanted into a contained articular cartilage defect and covered with a sleeve of periosteum.

SUMMARY

Disorders of the knee constitute a common source of pain in distance runners. The spectrum of pathologic conditions includes patellofemoral disorders, soft-tissue abnormalities, and osteoarthritis. A trial of nonoperative treatment that includes rehabilitation and activity modification often provides good results for most disorders. When indicated, surgical treatment can yield significant improvement in symptoms and patient satisfaction.

REFERENCES

1. van Mechelen W: Running injuries: A review of the epidemiological literature. *Sports Med* 1992:14, 320.
2. Jacobs SJ, Berson BL: Injuries to runners: A study of entrants to a 10,000 meter race. *Am J Sports Med* 1986:14, 151.
3. Laurin CA, Dussault R, Levesque HP: The tangential x-ray investigation of the patellofemoral joint: X-ray technique, diagnostic criteria, and their interpretation. *Clin Orthop* 1979:144, 16.
4. Kolowich PA, Paulos LE, Rosenberg TD, et al.: Lateral release of the patella: Indications and contraindications. *Am J Sports Med* 1990:18, 359.
5. Fulkerson JP, Hungerford DS: *Disorders of the Patellofemoral Joint*, 2nd ed., Baltimore, Williams & Wilkins, 1990.
6. Hallisey MJ, Doherty N, Bennett WF, et al.: Anatomy of the junction of the vastus lateralis tendon and the patella. *J Bone Joint Surg* 1987:69, 545.
7. Boden BP, Pearsall AW, Feagin JA, et al.: Patellofemoral instability: Evaluation and management. *J Am Acad Orthop Surg* 1997:5, 47.
8. Inoue M, Shino K, Hirose H, et al.: Subluxation of the patella. *J Bone Joint Surg Am* 1988:70, 1331.
9. Fulkerson JP: Anteromedialization of the tibial tuberosity for patellofemoral malalignment. *Clin Orthop* 1983:177, 176.
10. Fulkerson JP, Becker GJ, Meaney JA, et al.: Anteromedial tibial tubercle transfer without bone graft. *Am J Sports Med* 1990:18, 490.
11. Schreiber SN: Technical note: Proximal superomedial portal in arthroscopy of the knee. *Arthroscopy* 1991:7, 246.
12. Hawkins RJ, Bell RH, Anisette G: Acute patella dislocations: The natural history. *Am J Sports Med* 1986:14, 117.
13. Cofield R, Bryan R: Acute dislocation of the patella: Results of conservative treatment. *J Trauma* 1977:17, 526.
14. Hughston JC, Deese M: Medial subluxation of the patella as a complication of lateral retinacular release. *Am J Sports Med* 1988:16, 383.
15. Conlan T, Garth WP, Lemons JE: Evaluation of the medial soft-tissue restraints of the extensor mechanism of the knee. *J Bone Joint Surg Am* 1993:75, 682.
16. Salley PI, Poggi J, Speer KP, et al.: Acute dislocation of the patella: A correlative pathoanatomic study. *Am J Sports Med* 1996:24, 52.
17. Vainionpaa S, Laasonen E, Silvennoinen T, et al.: Acute dislocation of the patella: A prospective review of operative treatment. *J Bone Joint Surg Br* 1990:72, 366.
18. Gomes JLE: Medial patellofemoral ligament reconstruction for recurrent dislocation of the patella: A preliminary report. *J Arthrosc* 1992:8, 335.

19. Martens M, Lebbrecht P, Burssens A: Surgical treatment of the iliotibial band friction syndrome. *Am J Sports Med* 1989:17, 651.

20. Noble C: Iliotibial band friction syndrome in runners. *Am J Sports Med* 1980:8, 232.

21. Brief LP, Laico JP: The superolateral approach: A better view of the medial patellar plica. *Arthroscopy* 1987:3, 170.

22. Ewing JW: Plica: Pathologic or not? *J Am Acad Orthop Surg* 1993:1, 117.

23. Dorchak JD, Barrack RL, Kneisl JS, et al.: Arthroscopic treatment of symptomatic synovial plica of the knee: Long-term follow-up. *Am J Sports Med* 199:19, 503.

24. Richmond JC, McGinty JB: Segmental arthroscopic resection of the hypertrophic mediopatellar plica. *Clin Orthop* 1983:178, 185.

25. Kondradsen L, Hansen EB, Sondergaard L: Long distance running and osteoarthrosis. *Am J Sports Med* 1990:18, 379.

26. Newton PM, Mow VC, Gardner TR: The effect of life-long exercise on articular cartilage. *Am J Sports Med* 1997:25, 282.

27. Fulkerson JP: Patellofemoral pain disorders: Evaluation and management. *J Am Acad Orthop Surg* 1994:2, 124.

Chapter 53

THE LEG

Keith S. Albertson and
Gregory G. Dammann

INTRODUCTION

As the number of recreational athletes involved in running and jumping sports has increased, so has the number of patients presenting with lower leg pain. Three diagnoses that need to be considered are compartment syndrome, tibial stress fracture, and posterior tibial tendinitis. This chapter reviews the workup, surgical evaluation and management, and return to running criteria.

COMPARTMENT SYNDROME

Chronic compartment syndrome is activity-related pain caused by increased intermuscular pressure within an anatomic compartment. The exact nature of the pain is uncertain, but it probably results from ischemia, during which the blood flow in muscle arterioles is compromised. A muscle may expand approximately 20% during contraction. In patients with tight or thickened fascia, the compartment cannot expand to accommodate this increased muscle size so tissue pressure increases instead. When this pressure increases above the arteriolar blood pressure, blood flow is compromised. Repetitive contractions continue to elevate the tissue pressure and disrupt blood flow. Eventually the muscle becomes ischemic and pain is felt.[1]

A confusing plethora of terms is used to describe this condition. Exertional compartment syndrome, exercise-induced compartment syndrome, and chronic compartment syndrome are certainly synonymous. Vaguer terms such as shin splints or medial tibial stress syndrome should be avoided. The etiology of these terms is varied and may not be related to compartment pressure changes and ischemia.

Anatomy

There are four major compartments in the leg. Each is bound by bone and fascia, and each contains a major nerve. The anterior compartment contains the extensor hallucis longus, extensor digitorum longus, peroneus tertius, and anterior tibialis muscles, as well as the deep peroneal nerve. The lateral compartment contains the peroneus longus and brevis as well as the superficial peroneal nerve. Posteriorly there are two compartments, the superficial posterior and the deep posterior compartments. The superficial compartment contains the gastrocnemius and soleus muscles and the sural nerve. The deep posterior compartment contains the flexor hallucis longus, flexor digitorum longus, and posterior tibialis muscles, as well as the posterior tibial nerve. Some authors believe that the posterior tibialis should be considered a separate compartment, since it is surrounded by its own fascia.

Surgical Evaluation

History

Patients will complain of diffuse pain within one or more compartments that begins during exercise. The patient is asymptomatic initially, but pain will begin at a predictable time during the workout. The pain worsens with continued exercise and persists for a variable time after exercise stops. This pain is described as dull, aching, or cramping in nature. It frequently radiates down into the foot or ankle and may be associated with dysesthesias along the nerve within the affected compartment. There is frequently a sensation of swelling, fullness, or tightness within the compartment. Patients cannot "run through" their pain. Their pain usually has gotten progressively worse despite nonsteroidal anti-inflammatory drugs (NSAIDs), shoe modification, and stretching, and the onset begins earlier and earlier during their workout.

Physical Examination

Examination at rest is usually normal. There may be some tenderness along the compartment with deep palpation. There may be a palpable fascial defect within the affected extremity. Such defects have been found in up to 60% of patients with chronic compartment syndrome.[2,3] Examination immediately after exercise usually reveals a firm, tender compartment with some increased pain on passive stretch. Fascial defects and resultant small muscle herniations are more identifiable. There may be some transient altered sensation in the distribution of the nerve that traverses the affected compartment (Table 53–1).

Imaging

Plain radiographs are required to rule out tibial stress fracture. Ultrasound can be useful to rule out deep venous thrombosis (DVT), although this is unlikely to be confused with chronic compartment syndrome. Nuclear medicine studies have been advocated by some to confirm the diagnosis of chronic compartment syndrome, but these are costly and unnecessary in most patients.[4,5]

Compartment Pressure Testing

This is the most useful diagnostic test in the evaluation of a patient with chronic compartment syndrome.

We prefer to use the Stryker Compartment Pressured Monitor since it is easy to use, portable, and requires minimal materials. Pressures are taken before exercise, 1 minute after exercise, and, if necessary, 5 minutes after exercise. If the history clearly suggests that only the anterior compartment is involved, then only that compartment is measured. If the pain is posterior, we measure both the superficial and deep posterior compartments. If the symptoms are extremely vague it may be necessary to measure all four compartments. Compartment pressure testing is uncomfortable, and the relatively large-bore needle can damage neurovascular structures.

Nonoperative Care

Nonoperative care is usually ineffective. Although rest, NSAIDs, orthotics, stretching, and altered activities may improve symptoms, pain invariably returns with exercise. Patients must either give up the aggravating activity entirely or undergo surgery.

Indications for Surgery

Surgical indications include the following factors: (1) an appropriate history for chronic compartment syndrome; (2) a 1-minute postexercise compartment pressure greater than 30 mmHg; and (3) the presence of a fascial defect. Stress fractures must be ruled out before surgery. The most important indication is an appropriate history for compartment syndrome. A postexercise compartment pressure greater than 30 mmHg is helpful. However, patients with a classic history for compartment syndrome should not be shunned just because their compartment pressure measurements are not confirmatory. Any symptomatic patient with a palpable fascial hernia should be offered surgical release.

Surgical Procedures

Surgery entails a fasciotomy that divides the fascia longitudinally over the entire length of the involved compartment. A one- or two-incision technique may be used. The benefit of the single-incision technique is that there is a smaller skin wound. The disadvantage is that it is more difficult to ensure that the compartment is completely released. The benefit of the two-incision approach is that it allows good visualization of the most proximal and distal portions of the

TABLE 53–1. SENSORY DISTRIBUTION OF THE MAIN NERVE IN EACH COMPARTMENT

Compartment	Nerve	Sensory Distribution
Anterior	Deep peroneal	First web space
Lateral	Superficial peroneal	Dorsum of foot
Superficial posterior	Sural	Lateral surface of foot
Deep posterior	Tibial	Plantar surface of foot

compartment and ensures that the compartment will be fully released. Its disadvantage is that there is more scarring for the patient. Regardless of the technique, any fascial hernias must be included in the fascial incision.

Anterior and Lateral Compartment Fasciotomy

TWO-INCISION TECHNIQUE. The two-incision technique exposes the most proximal and distal portions of the compartments and allows the fascia to be divided subcutaneously under the skin bridge between them. The proximal incision begins at the level of the fibular neck, whereas the distal incision terminates about 5 cm above the lateral malleolus. Each incision is about 4 cm long, oriented longitudinally, and centered between the anterior tibial crest and the fibula. The fascia is exposed and the anterior intermuscular septum is palpated. To release the anterior compartment, the fascia in each wound is incised longitudinally 1 cm anterior to the intermuscular septum. The fascial incisions are then connected using long Metzenbaum scissors. Care must be taken to avoid the terminal branch of the deep peroneal nerve where it comes through the intermuscular septum, about two thirds of the way down the leg. The lateral compartment may be released through

the same incisions. The fascia is incised 1 cm posterior to the intermuscular septum in both incisions. Scissors connect these fascial incisions in the same manner as for the anterior compartment.

ONE-INCISION TECHNIQUE. The one-incision, or Mubarak, technique,[6] which is the author's preferred method, uses a single 5-cm longitudinal skin incision centered over the leg, midway between the anterior tibial crest and the fibula. The fascia is exposed and incised longitudinally 1 cm anterior to the intermuscular septum. Scissors extend the fasciotomy proximally to the level of the fibular head and distally to the extensor retinaculum just above the ankle. Long retractors lift the skin and subcutaneous tissue to allow direct vision of the scissors tips. The fasciotomy must release the entire compartment, especially distally. Otherwise, the muscle can be irritated where it herniates against the V in the fascial incision.[7] The lateral compartment is released in similar fashion through a fascial incision 1 cm posterior to the intermuscular septum. Extend the fasciotomy proximally to just below the level of the fibula head to avoid the peroneal nerve, and distally to about 5 cm above the ankle. Stay lateral distally to avoid the superficial peroneal nerve (Fig. 53–1).

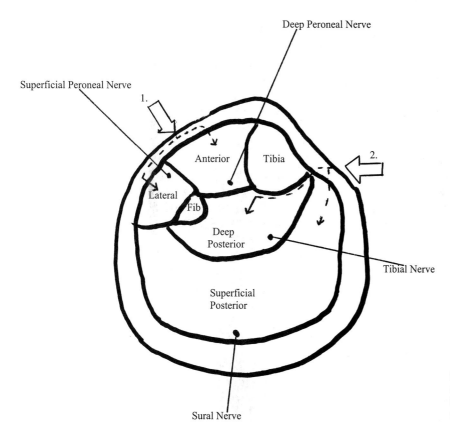

Figure 53–1. One-incision technique for 1. Anterior and lateral compartment fasciotomy 2. Superficial and deep posterior compartment fasciotomy.

Superficial and Deep Posterior Compartment Fasciotomy

TWO-INCISION TECHNIQUE. Two longitudinal incisions, one proximal and one distal, and each about 4 cm long, are made 1 cm posterior to the medial border of the tibia. The fascia overlying the superficial compartment is incised at this level. Scissors connect these fascial incisions underneath the skin bridge. To release the deep posterior compartment, the soleus bridge must be detached from the distal one third of the tibia. Then the fascia over the flexor digitorum longus is incised. Neurovascular structures are immediately deep to this fascial incision, so stay up against the tibia. Expose the posterior tibialis and incise the fascia over this muscle as well. Although the posterior tibialis is not classically in its own compartment, the fascia over this muscle must be released independently to decompress it.

SINGLE-INCISION TECHNIQUE. The single-incision technique is the author's preferred method. A single incision 5 to 6 cm long is made medially 1 cm posterior to the medial border of the tibia. The underlying saphenous nerve and vein are protected. The fascia overlying the superficial compartment is released proximally and distally. The soleus bridge is incised where it attaches to the distal tibia, and the deep posterior compartment is identified. The fascia is incised longitudinally, staying right on the tibia. Retractors are used to expose the posterior tibialis, and the fascia over this deep muscle is incised along its length.

Postoperative Care

A compressive dressing is applied. Drains are not normally necessary. Crutches are used for comfort for a few days, but the patient begins active and passive motion immediately. Once the wound is healed, walking and bicycling are encouraged. Patients may begin a light jog in 2 weeks, but no actual running for 6 weeks. It usually takes 3 months for full rehabilitation, but patients with deep posterior compartment fasciotomies may need longer.[8]

Complications

Most surgical complications are due to neurovascular injury. A transected sensory nerve is likely to result in permanent numbness and possibly a painful neuroma. Symptoms may return if the compartment is not fully released or is allowed to scar because of immobilization. There have been reports of persistent nerve irritation because a sensory nerve is rubbing against the fasciotomy. Proper placement of the fascial incision will mitigate this. Reoperation with removal of a fascial window may be required. Some patients complain of a feeling of fullness or puffiness in the leg. Patients may also experience some mild weakness.

STRESS FRACTURE

Stress fractures may occur on either the compression or tension side of the cortex. Fractures of the proximal and distal third of the tibia are more likely to occur in compression. These fractures are frequently seen in undertrained or "forced" athletes, such as new military recruits. On the other hand, midshaft tibial stress fractures occur on the tension side of the bone and usually affect the well-conditioned athlete involved in running and jumping sports. As these sports have become more popular, tibial stress fractures have become more common.[9] Although the vast majority of stress fractures will heal with nonoperative treatment, surgery can be considered for selected individuals.

Surgical Evaluation

History

Patients with stress fractures report dull, achy pain over the shin that began after strenuous exercise. The pain gradually worsened and now occurs with nonathletic activities or during rest. Symptoms usually improve with rest, ice, and NSAIDs, but the pain returns as soon as activity resumes. On questioning, many patients will admit to a rapid increase in the intensity or duration of their workouts 1 or 2 months prior to the onset of symptoms.

Physical Examination

The hallmark of a stress fracture is localized point tenderness directly over bone. There may be some slight edema, warmth, and even erythema over the area. Occasionally there is a palpable bony bump or fullness representing periosteal new bone formation. A tuning fork placed on the bone distant from the suspected fracture site will elicit pain at the fracture site. Most patients will have antalgic gait.

Imaging

Plain radiographs should be included as part of the initial evaluation of leg pain in athletes. These can be used to evaluate the width of the tibia, since a narrow tibia has been found to be a risk factor for developing a subsequent stress fracture.[10] Although a complete fracture line may be visualized, this is usually not the case. Instead, there may be cortical thickening, narrowing of the intermedularry canal, or evidence of periostitis. A linear, unicortical radiolucency in the anterior tibia represents the "dreaded black line" of a tension side stress fracture with its prolonged and unpredictable healing.[11]

Although a bone scan is the most sensitive test for stress fracture, it has poor specificity. A triple-phase bone scan will improve specificity. Medial tibial stress syndrome, periostitis, and contusion can all cause increased uptake, but the uptake in these conditions is more diffuse whereas that of stress fractures is more focal. Magnetic resonance imaging (MRI) is both specific and sensitive for stress fractures. It is very costly and rarely required.

Nonoperative Treatment

Rest is the mainstay of treatment. For compression fractures of the fibula and tibia, simply limiting impact loading is usually sufficient. Crutches are used until the limp resolves. The patient must abstain from running for 8 to 12 weeks. Nonimpact conditioning activities such as water running, cycling, and selected exercise machines are permissible if they do not cause pain. A splint or pneumatic brace may be worn for comfort. A cast may provide the most comfort but should be used for the shortest duration possible to avoid stiffness and atrophy. The midshaft anterior fracture of the tibia is prone to nonunion and requires more aggressive treatment. These fractures should be treated with immobilization in a nonweightbearing cast for a minimum of 3 to 6 months. Electrical stimulation devices may be beneficial, but their efficacy is far from certain. These devices are bulky and expensive. They are best reserved for fractures that show no evidence of healing after 3 to 6 months.

Patients may return to athletic activity when they have no pain with unprotected daily activity, there is no bony tenderness, and the radiographs show evidence of healing. This return must be gradual. When patients can walk without pain, they may jog. When they can jog without pain, they may run. When they can run without pain, they may compete. A thorough evaluation of equipment and training techniques is mandatory to prevent further stress fractures.

Indications for Surgery

Surgery should be reserved for patients with anterior tibial stress fractures who fail to heal after at least 6 months on nonoperative treatment. Surgical consideration can also be given to the high-performance athlete who is unwilling or unable to comply with a prolonged period of inactivity. Surgery is not indicated in compression side stress fractures since they will heal without difficulty.

Surgical Procedures

Cortical Drilling

The anterior cortex of the tibia is poorly vascularized. As a result, it has a weak inflammatory response to injury. Cortical drilling attempts to stimulate the reparative process. Multiple transverse 2- to 3-mm drill holes are made a few centimeters proximal and distal to the fracture gap. This may be done either percutaneously or via small skin incisions over the anterior compartment. Cortical drilling is frequently combined with bone grafting at the fracture site.

Bone Grafting

Bone grafting may improve healing in anterior tibial stress fractures.[12] Autogenous cancellous bone is harvested from the ipsilateral iliac crest. The fracture site is exposed through a small incision over the anterior compartment about 2 cm from the tibial border. A curette removes any fibrous tissue from the fracture site. The cancellous bone graft is then packed into the fracture gap and around the sides of the fracture site. Healing time is usually 5 months from surgery.

Author's Preferred Method

We prefer intermedullary nailing of tibial stress fractures if surgery is indicated. The actual surgical procedure depends on the nail used, but there are some important general principles. Use of a reamed nail is recommended. Reaming provides a larger contact area between the bone and the implant. Reamed nails are also stiffer than their unreamed counterparts. The larger contact area and the increased stiffness should resist tension forces across the fracture area better than an unreamed nail. When exposing the proximal tibia, care should be taken to preserve the integrity of the knee joint. Preserve as much of the fat pad as possible, and be sure to bury the proximal rod below the level of the cortex. These measures will help eliminate the anterior knee pain sometimes associated with tibial nailing. Interlocking is not necessary since anterior tibial stress fractures are stable fractures under tension. This eliminates the possibility of irritation from the interlocking screws.

Postoperative Care

A soft dressing is applied about the knee. This dressing is removed after 3 days, and a smaller dressing is applied. Sutures are removed within 10 days. A short leg splint may provide some initial postoperative comfort, but this splint is exchanged for a hinged "walking boot" orthosis as soon as possible. Knee and ankle motion exercises are begun immediately. Crutches are used for comfort only and are discontinued when weightbearing is well tolerated. Conditioning with bicycling, swimming, or water walking can begin within a few weeks. Impact loading and running may begin as early as 6 weeks with full fracture healing usually taking 6 months.

Complications

Nailing should not be undertaken lightly. Patients face the standard operative and anesthetic risks associated with any surgical procedure. There is a potential to shatter the tibial cortex, turning a nondisplaced stable fracture into a displaced, unstable fracture. Most patients will complain of some vague anterior knee pain with strenuous activity. This usually improves over time and rarely prohibits return to full activity. Patellar tendinitis may occur if the nail rides "proud" at the proximal tibia. A few patients have complained that their nailed leg was not as good at "absorbing shock" as their unnailed leg. Some patients complain of vague leg discomfort, which they associate with the nail. If the patients insist, we will remove the nail after 1 year provided there is radiographic evidence of complete healing. However, we generally discourage nail removal because of the operative risks, recovery time, and potential for refracture. The only exception to this is patients engaged in sports that present a risk of high-energy lower extremity trauma such as parachuting or motor racing.

POSTERIOR TIBIAL TENDON INJURY

The posterior tibial tendon needs to be considered when a patient presents with medial ankle pain. Injury to the posterior tibial tendon can be from an acute traumatic event, which may signify tendon disruption, or as part of a chronic overuse syndrome, which could signify posterior tibial tendinitis. A number of surgical options are available for those who fail nonsurgical management of posterior tibial tendon injuries.

Surgical Evaluation

History

Patients report pain along the medial aspect of the leg posterior to the medial malleolus. The onset of the pain is typically gradual. Pain increases with activities that require push-off with the affected extremity such as walking, running, or jumping.

Physical Examination

There may be loss in height of the medial longitudinal arch and a planovalgus deformity, as evidenced by the "too many toes sign." When observing the patient from behind, the affected side will reveal more toes lateral to the heel than the unaffected side. There is usually tenderness and swelling over the course of the tendon. Pain and weakness are present with resisted inversion or with the heel raise test. In this test, foot supination and heel inversion are diminished during heel raise.

Imaging

The x-ray evaluation should include standing anteroposterior and lateral views. On the anteroposterior view, look for medial talar displacement in relation to the navicular bone. On the lateral view, look for decreased height of the longitudinal arch. Further evaluation can include computed tomography (CT) or MRI. MRI is the method of choice for evaluation of soft tissues. Ultrasound can be sensitive and specific in diagnosing posterior tibial tenosynovitis, which appears as a hypoechoic and swollen tendon.[13]

Nonoperative Care

Initial management of posterior tibial tendinitis should be nonsurgical. Options vary from activity modification to casting. Rest and NSAIDs are indicated as first-line therapy. Orthotics should be used to support the arch and relieve stress on the tendon. Immobilization with the use of a boot brace or short-leg walking cast for 3 weeks may relieve symptoms.[14] Local steroid injections may improve symptoms but have been implicated in tendon rupture and are not recommended.

Patients may return to running gradually once symptoms resolve. Orthotics should be used.

Indications for Surgery

Surgery should be considered in those who do not respond to nonsurgical management after 6 to 12 weeks or those with loss of an arch.

Surgical Procedures

A skin incision is made over the posterior tibial tendon beginning at the posterior portion of the medial malleolus and extending distally about 4 cm. The underlying tendon sheath is opened longitudinally with scissors, and all the inflamed synovium is removed. If the synovitis extends more proximally, it must be removed. Extend the skin incision in a proximal direction over the tendon. The underlying flexor retinaculum is divided except for a small 1-cm band at the posterior border of the malleolus, which will keep the tendon from subluxing. Alternatively, the entire retinaculum can be divided, but this requires repair prior to closure. The tendon is then inspected, and any synovitis or degenerative tissue is removed from the tendon. Any longitudinal fissures or splits must be repaired using 5-0 nonabsorbable sutures.

In cases of posterior tibial dysfunction with loss of longitudinal arch, reconstruction of the posterior tibial tendon using the flexor digitorum longus tendon may be needed. A skin incision is made over the posterior tibial tendon beginning at the posterior portion of the medial malleolus and extending to the navicular. The tendon sheath is opened, and the tendon is inspected for abnormalities. The flexor digitorum longus tendon is identified proximal to the medial malleolus and followed distally into the midfoot area. The master knot of Henry is dissected to expose the flexor digitorum longus in its entirety.[15] The flexor digitorum longus and flexor hallucis longus are sutured together where they cross. The flexor digitorum is then cut proximal to the suture and is ideally passed into the posterior tibial tendon sheath; however, the flexor digitorum tendon is kept in its own sheath if the posterior tibial tendon is scarred down. A drill hole is made in the navicular large enough to accommodate the flexor digitorum longus tendon. The tendon is brought through the drill hole with the foot in a plantarflexed and inverted position. Tenodesis of the proximal portion of the posterior tibial tendon to the flexor digitorum longus is performed if the posterior tibial tendon has good elasticity.[16]

Postoperative Course

Postoperative care for synovectomy involves immobilization for 10 days to allow wound healing, followed by 3 weeks in a short-leg walking cast. After the walking cast is removed, range of motion exercises and weightbearing are begun as tolerated.

Postoperative care for the flexor digitorum longus tendon transfer involves a plantar splint applied to the foot in full inversion and 20 degrees of plantar flexion for about 10 days. The patient is then placed in a short-leg nonwalking cast for 4 weeks. A short-leg walking cast in a plantigrade position is used for another 4 weeks. Physical therapy is begun initially with range of motion exercises and followed by strengthening exercises for 3 to 4 months. Some patients require an orthotic to support the medial arch after surgery.[16]

Complications

Complications of the surgical procedure include infection, DVT, pain, edema, ecchymosis, and wound dehiscence. Adhesions may restrict range of motion. Large suture knots may cause irritation of tendon sheaths. Subluxation of the posterior tibial tendon may occur if the tendon sheath or retinaculum is not reconstructed. Patients also need to be counseled that the

longitudinal arch may not be corrected in up to one-third of patients undergoing flexor digitorum longus tendon transfer.[16]

REFERENCES

1. Rorabeck CH: The diagnosis and management of chronic compartment syndromes. *Instructor Course Lecture* 1989: 38, 466.
2. Davey JR, Fowler PJ, Rorabeck CH: The tibialis posterior muscle compartment: An unrecognized cause of exertional compartment syndrome. *Am J Sports Med* 1984:12, 391.
3. Jones DC, James SL: Overuse injuries of the lower extremity: Shin splints, iliotibial band friction syndrome, and exertional compartment syndromes. *Clin Sports Med* 1987:6, 273.
4. Takebayashi S, Takazawa H, Sasaki R, et al.: Chronic exertional compartment syndrome in lower legs: Localization and follow-up with thallium-201 SPECT imaging. *J Nucl Med* 1997:38, 972.
5. Ota Y, Senda M, Hashizume H, et al.: Chronic compartment syndrome of the lower leg: A new diagnostic method using near-infrared spectroscopy and a new technique of endoscopic fasciotomy. *Arthroscopy* 1999:15, 439.
6. Mubarak SJ, Owne CA: Double incision fasciotomy of the leg for decompression in compartment syndromes. *J Bone Joint Surg Am* 1977:59A, 184.
7. Detmer DE, Sharpe K, Sufit RL, et al.: Chronic compartment syndrome: Diagnosis, management and outcomes. *Am J Sports Med* 1985:13, 162–70.
8. Rorabeck CH: The diagnosis and management of chronic compartment syndromes. *Instructor Course Lecture* 1989: 38, 466.
9. Chang PS, Harris RM: Intramedullary nailing for chronic tibial stress fractures. *Am J Sports Med* 1996:24, 688.
10. Giladi M, Milgrom C, Simkin A, et al.: Stress fractures: Identifiable risk factors. *Am J Sports Med* 1991:19, 647.
11. Andrish JT: The leg, in DeLee JC, Drez D (eds.), *Orthopaedic Sports Medicine—Principles and Practice*, Philadelphia, WB Saunders, 1994:1603.
12. Green NE, Rogers RA, Lipscomb AB: Nonunion of stress fractures of the tibia. *Am J Sports Med* 1985:13, 171.
13. Wang CL, Wang TG, Hsu TC, et al.: Ultrasonographic examination of the posterior tibial tendon. *Foot Ankle Int* 1997:18, 34.
14. Trevino S, Baumhauer JF: Tendon injuries of the foot and ankle. *Clin Sports Med* 1992:11, 727.
15. Quinn MR, Mendicino SS: Surgical treatment of posterior tibial tendon dysfunction. *Clin Podiatr Med Surg* 1991:8, 543.
16. Mann RA: Flatfoot in adults, in Mann RA, Coughlin MJ (eds.), *Surgery of the Foot and Ankle*, 6th ed., St. Louis, Mosby, 1993:757.

Chapter 54

SURGICAL CONSIDERATIONS OF ANKLE INJURIES

Robert P. Nirschl

INTRODUCTION

The etiology of running injuries to the ankle region ranges from repetitive overuse to single-event trauma. The traumatic pathology of this anatomic area includes skeletal, intraarticular, and soft-tissue elements. The goal of this chapter is not to discuss every possible malady but to focus on the common and statistically significant problems that confront runners, including (in decreasing order), tendon overuse, ligament sprain, intraarticular problems, stress fractures, and tarsal tunnel syndrome. Table 54–1 outlines the more common pathoanatomic problems.

DISORDERS OF TENDONS

By far the most common tendon problems involve the Achilles' tendon. In addition, the posterior tibial and peroneal tendons are more problematic than the remaining tendons. Overall, 11 tendons cross or insert at or about the ankle. These include the Achilles', plantaris, tibialis anterior, extensor hallucis longus, extensor digitorum longus, posterior tibialis, flexor digitorum longus, flexor hallucis longus, peroneus brevis, peroneus tertius, and peroneus longus. With the exception of the Achilles' and plantaris tendons, all have

true synovial sheaths and pass through retinacular or retinacular-osseous canals. The Achilles' and plantaris tendons do not pass through a canal but are surrounded by paratenon as they proceed to insertion, with some bursal separation from the posterior proximal os calcis.

It is important to appreciate the anatomic distinctions between the tendons themselves and their surrounding tissue, namely, the paratenon, synovial sheaths, fibroosseous retinaculum, and bursa, as each tissue may have pathoanatomic distortions that contribute to symptoms. In the case of the Achilles' tendon, combinations of peritendinitis may occur in association with tendinosis. In this circumstance, for best surgical success, treatment must be directed to both tissues. The same concept is also applicable in the distinction between tenosynovitis and tendinosis. From an etiologic point of view, pathologic change can occur through overuse, single-event trauma, subluxation, or dislocation. Partial pathoanatomic tendon alteration is the usual situation, but complete rupture can and does occur.

Pathoanatomy
In runners the most common etiology of tendon pathoanatomic change is repetitive microoveruse, with single-event macroinsult a very distant second.

TABLE 54–1. COMMON ANKLE INJURIES

Soft tissue
  Tendon
    Achilles'
      Tendinosis
      Peritendonitis
      Calcific tendinosis at os calcis
      Rupture
      Haglund deformity (or retrocalcaneal bursitis or advential bursitis)
    Peroneus brevis and longus
      Tendinosis
      Subluxation
      Synovitis
    Posterior tibial
      Tendinosis
      Synovitis
      Rupture
    Extensor tendons (tibialis anterior and digitorum longus)
      Tendinosis
      Synovitis
    Flexor hallucis longus
      Tendinosis
      Synovitis
  Neural
    Tarsal tunnel
  Ligament
    Lateral sprains
    Medial sprains
    Tibial fibular syndesmosis sprains
Intraarticular
  Synovitis
  Soft-tissue impingement
  Osteochondritis dissecans talus
  Chip fracture talus
  Traumatic osteoarthritis
  Exostosis
Skeletal
  Malleolar fracture
  Stress fracture talus (lateral malleolus)

Stress fractures: Talus, lateral malleolus

Although the sequence from normal to progressive pathologic tendon alteration is not completely understood, the hypotheses advanced by Paddu et al.,[1] Kraushaar and Nirschl,[2] Plattner et al.,[3] and Clancy[4] are helpful for a basic understanding of this sequence (see Chapter 4). Overuse probably results in an initial external inflammatory cascade. Indeed, healing seems to be dependent on an orderly inflammatory sequence. Failure of the sequence results in pathoanatomic change causing persistent and chronic symptoms. In overuse injury the bursa, paratenon, retinaculum, and synovial tissues retain an unproductive inflammatory mode, whereas the body of the tendon displays a quite different histopathologic response, namely, noninflammatory degenerative angiofibroblastic tendinosis. A subset of pathologic Achilles' tendons may have additional calcific presentation at the insertion to the os calcis.

Achilles' Tendon Overuse Tendinosis/ Peritendinitis

The typical Achilles' tendon overuse location is at the apex of the Achilles' tendon curve some 4 to 5 cm proximal to the os calcis insertion. It is my hypothesis that force loads are greatest in this location, although Lagergren and Lindholm[5] and others[6] have suggested that diminished vascular supply to the area may play a role. The tendon is tender and characteristically thickened in this area. The diagnosis of abnormality is clinically evident but not specific as to whether the pathoanatomy is peritendinitis, tendinosis, or both. Clarification of the diagnosis is aided by ultrasonography; magnetic resonance imaging (MRI) is even better, since it gives clearer images.

A subset of calcific Achilles' tendinosis cases differs from the classical in that the symptoms and pathology are at the Achilles' tendon insertion to the os calcis. The pathology invariably includes calcification extending from the os calcis into the tendon. It should be noted that this calcification is intratendinous and is clearly different from the traction spur presentations of plantar fasciitis/fasciosis. Clinical location of tenderness, os calcis calcific prominence, and routine x-ray easily differentiate this subset form of calcific Achilles' tendinosis from the more typical noninsertional tendinosis presentation.

The indications for surgical intervention are outlined in Chapter 50. As noted, the patient must make the ultimate decision based on quality of life for issues. In general, surgery is chosen when pain alters the activities of daily living and an MRI reveals a quantity of tendinosis damage equivalent to 50% of the diameter of the tendon. Concern for the potential of progression to full rupture also contributes to the decision-making process. In the situation of peritendinitis, fluid between the peritendon and the body of the tendon indicates significant histopathology.

The specifics of surgical technique are determined by the pathoanatomy. In comparison with a straight incision a curvilinear incision is better, as healing is enhanced and keloid-type skin scarring is minimized (Fig. 54–1). If the issue is peritendinitis, excision of the inflammatory peritendon is undertaken (Fig. 54–2). The degenerative changes of angiofibroblastic tendinosis requires resection of the tendinosis and suture repair of remaining healthy tendon (Fig. 54–3). In the case of insertional calcific tendinosis, resection includes the calcification that characteristically infiltrates the areas of tendinosis in the region of the os calcis.

Postoperative care depends on the volume of tendinosis resection. In the typical situation of 50% of normal tendon remaining, a cam walker brace with crutch ambulation is used for approximately 2 to 3 weeks.

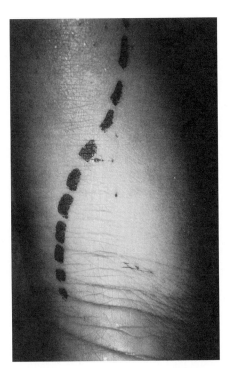

Figure 54–1. Clinical photograph. Recommended gentle curved incision. (*Courtesy of Nirschl Orthopedic Sportsmedicine Clinic.*)

Thereafter functional counterforce bracing is used. Gradual rehabilitative and water exercises may start at 10 to 14 days. When toe raises are accomplished (approximately 10 weeks), jogging may be contemplated.

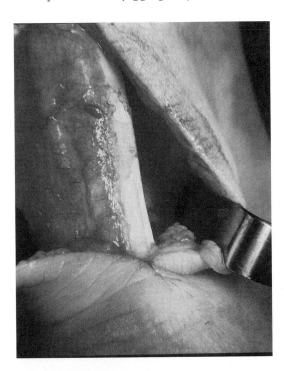

Figure 54–2. Surgical photograph. Peritendinitis. Note the inflammatory red adhesion on the parent white-appearing body of the Achilles' tendon. (*Courtesy of Nirschl Orthopedic Sportsmedicine Clinic.*)

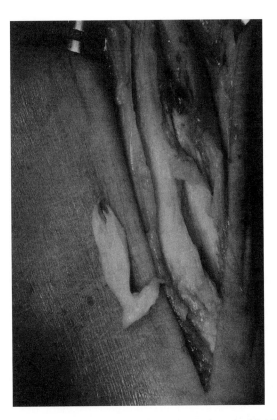

Figure 54–3. Surgical photograph. Resection and repair of Achilles' tendinosis. The tendinosis tissue depicted on skin has been resected from the central body of the Achilles' tendon. Normal tendon is not disturbed. (*Courtesy of Nirschl Orthopedic Sportsmedicine Clinic.*)

Progression to full competitive function occurs on average at 6 months.

The result of resection and repair of Achilles' peritendinitis and tendinosis surgery are quite positive for return to running provided all the pathologic tissue is identified and adequately resected.[7,8] If the resection is inadequate, however, residual symptoms can be expected. The most common complication in my experience is a sensitive skin scar if a straight incision is utilized. As noted, to avoid this complication a curvilinear incision is recommended.

Achilles' Tendon Rupture

Orthopedic community consensus opinion has tended to accept the premise that the presence of tendinosis precedes a full rupture of the Achilles' tendon. My experience deviates somewhat from this concept, however, as close questioning of patients presenting with a full rupture does not always elicit a history of prodromal tendinosis signs or symptoms. A full rupture usually occurs as a sudden event. The offending macroforce invariably occurs through one of two scenarios: a sudden and forceful push-off at the start of jumping or running or a sudden ankle dorsiflexion from a plantarflexed position (e.g., stepping in an unanticipated pothole). I once saw a 35-year-old patient who recounted the story of attempting to overtake and beat the legendary and then 70-year-old Dr. George Sheehan to the finish line in a 10-mile race. As the patient's competitive and macho juices flowed, his Achilles' tendon popped when he was just a few paces behind George and some 20 yards from the finish. Dr. Sheehan finished the race and then kindly returned to assist the patient across the finish line.

As noted in the above anecdote, Achilles' tendon rupture is usually a dramatic event. A pop or snap is often heard, not only by the patient but also by bystanders. Sudden loss of push-off function is clearly noted as well. The only (uncommon) deviation from this scenario occurs in a chronically infirm individual who suffers gradual attritional dysfunction, hardly the presentation of an active runner. Usual clinical signs include a palpable tendon defect, weakness of plantarflexion, and a positive Thompson sign (e.g., absence of passive plantarflexion with squeezing of the calf in a relaxed prone-positioned patient).

Although the history and clinical signs are usually clear-cut (Figs. 54–4 and 54–5), delayed diagnosis does occur. This is noted especially with medical personnel of less experience in musculoskeletal diagnosis when swelling obscures the palpable defect and some plantarflexion is observed secondary to toe flexor function. In a difficult presentation, any diagnostic confusion is resolvable by MRI or ultrasonography.

Accurate and prompt diagnoses are important determinants of treatment selection, as delayed diagnosis may compromise surgical success. Some treatment options are controversial. There are proponents of the nonsurgical approach of immobilization: placing the ankle in an initial extreme plantarflexed position with gradual progression to neutral dorsiflexion immobilization over a period of 3 to 4 months. The presumption is

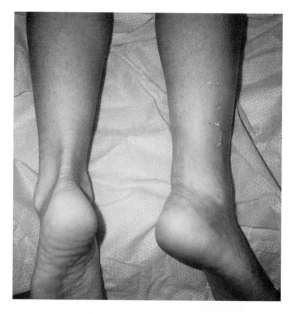

Figure 54–4. Clinical photograph. Achilles' tendon rupture. Without edema, the diagnosis is usually evident by visual inspection. A normal Achilles' tendon profile is noted on the left; the abnormal Achilles' tendon profile on right indicates a complete rupture. (*Courtesy of Nirschl Orthopedic Sportsmedicine Clinic.*)

that this form of immobilization consistently results in healing apposition of the tendon ends. Evidence exists, however, that this is not always the case, as suggested by published reports of the rerupture rate and also commonly noted long-term power and flexibility functional deficiencies.[9–12] My personal observation is that casting in plantarflexion is inferior in terms of rerupture and long-term function. The casting approach also delays rehabilitation and return to function for inordinate periods, in comparison with surgical repair.

Overall, more than 400 articles have been published concerning the treatment of Achilles' tendon

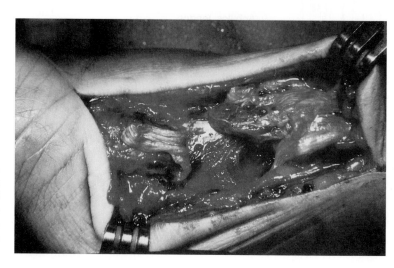

Figure 54–5. Surgical photograph. Full rupture Achilles' tendon. Complete dissociation in center of tendon. Note that a total lack of tendon continuity plus significant hemorrhage is noted in the ruptured tendon ends. (*Courtesy of Nirschl Orthopedic Sportsmedicine Clinic.*)

rupture.[13,14] Proponents of the surgical approach are many, including this author. More recently a modified percutaneous surgical approach has been advanced,[15,16] with the suggestion that results are equal to direct open suturing. In my opinion this claim needs further proof and consistent reduplication by other authors.

Haglund's Deformity and Retrocalcaneal and Adventital Bursitis

Haglund's deformity, retrocalcaneal bursitis, adventital bursitis, and insertional Achilles' tendinosis can be interrelated and can produce symptoms individually or collectively. Haglund's deformity (an underlying excessive bony prominence of the posterior superior os calcis) is often an underlying factor since osseous prominence in this area can stress the Achilles' tendon insertion, impinge on the adjacent retrocalcaneal, bursa or subject the subcutaneous tissue to extreme pressure, resulting in an adventital bursa (Fig. 54–6).

The retrocalcaneal bursa is an anatomically consistent normal synovium-lined structure situated between the posterior-superior os calcis and the under side of the Achilles' tendon just proximal to the tendon insertion. This bursa can become inflamed by overuse trauma, but evidence of more systemic inflammatory disease such as a prodrome to rheumatoid disease or Reiter's syndrome should be ruled out.[17–19] The signs of retrocalcaneal bursitis include thickening and palpable tenderness anterior to the insertion of the Achilles' tendon.

Adventital bursitis is distinct and quite different from retrocalcaneal bursitis. Adventital bursitis is not normally occurring and is not a synovium-lined bursa. The pathoanatomy is an inflammatory and fibrotic response of the superficial subcutaneous and peritendinous tissue overlying the Achilles' tendon at its insertion. The skin

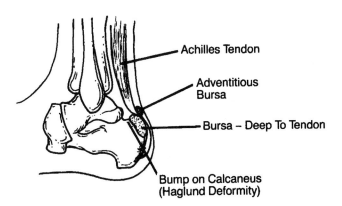

Figure 54–6. Illustration of Haglund's deformity with (1) a retrocalcaneal bursa between the Achilles' tendon and the superior bursal prominence and (2) an adventitious bursa between the Achilles' tendon and the skin. (*Source: From Bordelon RL: Heel pain, in Mann R, Coughlin M (eds.), Surgery of the Foot and Ankle, 6th ed., St. Louis, CV Mosby, 1993, 848.*)

itself may also thicken. The malady is invariably caused by impingement and friction from ill-fitting shoes. It is more common in women than men.[4]

The treatment for these posterior-superior os calcis maladies is usually nonoperative, with surgical intervention reserved for recalcitrant cases. Conservative care options include proper and well-fitting shoewear, orthotics or heel lifts, heel pads, anti-inflammatory drugs and modalities, alteration of running modes, and rehabilitation (strength and flexibility exercises). In recalcitrant cases, surgery may be considered. This might include resection and repair of underlying Achilles' tendinosis, ostectomy of a prominent Haglund's prominence, removal of a fibrotic or inflamed retrocalcaneal bursitis, trimming of an adventital bursa, or all of the above.

Peroneal Tendons

Peroneal tendon abnormalities are probably more common than is appreciated, since they can go unrecognized in association with ankle sprain. Any lingering lateral ankle symptoms should raise the potential of peroneal tendon abnormalities. The differential diagnosis should also include subtalar joint arthritis or sinus tarsi impingement.

The pathoanatomic issues include overuse attritional tendinosis, synovitis, fibroosseous retinacular fibrostenosis, and subluxation-dislocation. The usual nonpathologic anatomic presentations of the two peroneal tendons (longus and brevis) include containment in a fibroosseous canal starting with a proximal superior retinaculum, lateral malleolar fibrocartilaginous sulcus, and separate sheaths for each tendon distal to the lateral malleolus. It should be noted that additional peroneal muscle tendon units can occur, as described by Sobel et al.[20] The importance of additional tendons or distorted tendon geography is an increased potential for tenosynovitis.

The repetitive overuse of running can cause peroneal tenosynovitis, the most common type including stenosis in the fibroosseous canal, either in the peroneal sulcus posterior to the lateral malleolus or at the level of the peroneal tubercle of the calcaneous sulcus. The signs and symptoms include pain, tenderness, and swelling about the fibroosseous canal. Pain is usually aggravated by plantarflexion and inversion.

Along with stenosing tenosynovitis, the peroneus brevis may undergo attritional tendinosis and ultimately either partial or complete rupture, usually at the fibular groove.[20,21] Interestingly, many of these are longitudinal and partial rather than complete transverse ruptures. The signs of partial or complete rupture include substantial eversion weakness. Diagnosis of either tenosynovitis or rupture can be aided by MRI.

Treatment of peroneal tendon abnormalities includes the conservative efforts of anti-inflammatory medications, physical therapy modalities, control of overuse by running modification, foot posture control via orthotics, and enhancement of strength, endurance, and flexibility through rehabilitation. If conservative treatment proves unsuccessful, surgical intervention may be indicated: debridement of tenosynovitis, release of canal stenosis, and debridement with resection of the tendinosis and repair of the affected tendons, usually the brevis. If a complete rupture occurs, tenodesis of the proximal brevis tendon to the peroneus longus is indicated. It should be noted that major tendinosis problems may be associated with chronic lateral ankle instability. In these instances, surgical repair of the lateral ankle ligaments is indicated as an adjunctive treatment.

A final consideration concerning the peroneal tendons is subluxation dislocation. These maladies are more commonly associated with single-event trauma rather than overuse by running. There are, however, some patients who have the anatomic variant of a very shallow lateral malleolar sulcus,[22] making subluxation a possibility without single-event macrotrauma. Persistent peroneal subluxation or dislocation requires surgical repair or reconstruction of the fibroosseous retinaculum. The success of such surgery has been improved and simplified by technical advances in surgery including the use of bone suture anchors.

Posterior Tibial Tendon

Posterior tibial dysfunction is not uncommon and is probably the most common cause of acquired flat feet in adults. The main function of the tibialis posterior is inversion of the subtalar joint and adduction of the forefoot. It also acts as a normal antagonist of the peroneus brevis.

The pathoanatomy of the posterior tibial tendon is similar to that of other tendons traveling through fibroosseous tunnels. This includes synovitis of the peritendinous sheath, fibrous distortion of the retinacular tunnel tissues, and degenerative tendinosis of the body of the tendon, progressing to rupture or (rarely) avulsion of the tendon from the navicular.[23] The usual etiology of the most common pathology (e.g., tendinosis and perisynovitis) is repetitive overuse.

The typical clinical presentation is one of gradual onset, although occasionally some single traumatic event can be an inciting factor. Pain and swelling with local tenderness occurs over the track of the tendon starting proximally posterior to the medial malleolus and exiting distally toward the medial midfoot. Gradual collapse of the foot arch may be noted over time.

Progressive symptoms result in diminution of participation in running sports.

Physical findings include flattening of the foot arch with significant medial sag of the hindfoot. Toe raises are difficult to do and, if they are accomplished, the heel does not invert. Ankle motion is usually normal, but subtalar motion varies from normal to absent secondary to valgus ankylosis in chronic cases. Inversion muscle strength is typically weak on manual or the more sophisticated isokinetic testing. A key aspect of the evaluation is the amount and character of swelling along the posterior tendon sheath. A thickened tender sheath is pathognomonic of tenosynovitis and possibly tendinosis. Full rupture of the tendon is more likely determined by functional evaluation rather than a palpable defect. Imaging evaluation includes weightbearing foot and ankle x-rays to assess skeletal element relationships and evidence of traumatic osteoarthritis. MRI evaluation may aid in determining the magnitude of soft-tissue distortion including full rupture.

Treatment includes inflammation control, diminution of abuse by bracing and orthotics, and gradual strengthening. If synovitis persists, surgical intervention in the form of synovectomy and debridement of tendinosis is strongly recommended, as expansion of the problem to full rupture is a major problem, for which tendon transfer or subtalar fusion may be needed.[24]

Extensor Tendons (Tibialis Anterior and Digitorum Longus)

The extensor tendons are anatomically similar to the peroneal and posterior tibial tendons in that they travel through a synovial retinacular sheath. The pathoanatomic diagnoses therefore include tenosynovitis and tendinosis. Overall, tenosynovitis and retinacular stenosis are much more common than tendinosis. As a rule, these tendons are more likely affected by the compressive activities of footwear such as ice skates and ski boots rather than repetitive overuse activities. Of the two, the tibialis anterior tendon is more likely to be involved in running injuries than the extensor longus.[25]

Treatment follows the same conservative and surgical algorithms as the other tendons. Appropriate shoe design and fit are a must. The surgical concepts are dedicated primarily to decompression of any retinacular stenosis and debridement of synovitis. It is highly unusual, however, that surgery would be indicated.

Flexor Hallucis Longus

Abnormality of the flexor hallucis longus is uncommon in runners. This author has never seen a case in runners, although complete rupture has been reported in the literature in a pronated midfoot of a long-distance runner with prodromal tenosynovitis.[26]

The most common problem is stenosing tenosynovitis in ballet dancers. The most usual ankle sites are at the beginning of the fibroosseous canal on the posterior aspect of the talus and within the tendon sheath behind the medial malleolus. Symptoms of stenosis include triggering of the great toe in flexion. Surgical treatment focuses on decompression of the tendon in the area of fibroosseous canal entrapment.

TARSAL TUNNEL SYNDROME

Tarsal tunnel syndrome is a posterior tibial nerve entrapment neuropathy in or just distal to the tarsal tunnel just behind the medial malleolus. The syndrome is somewhat analogous to wrist carpal tunnel syndrome but much less common. The symptoms are medial area ankle pain and diffuse vague neurologic symptoms such as burning, tingling, and numbness in the posterior tibial nerve distributions of the lateral and medial plantar and medial calcaneal nerves. The pain and symptoms are most often aggravated with weight-bearing activities in association with flat feet.

Specific causes of tarsal tunnel syndrome may include such space-occupying lesions as ganglia, lipomas, bone fragments, and enlarged venous varicosities.[27] In runners major hindfoot pronation and repetitive overuse may stretch the posterior tibial nerve in a compromised fibroosseous tunnel. In a review of the literature, Climino[28] noted that 20% of cases had no identifiable cause.

The diagnosis can be somewhat subtle and may require supplemental diagnostic help with electrodiagnostic studies. These studies include plantar nerve conduction, motor-evoked potential amplitude, and duration and sensory conduction velocities. The tests are not always confirmatory and must be correlated with history and physical examination.

Treatment includes conservative approaches for mechanical problems, e.g., hindfoot pronation control by bracing and orthotics and strength training. If space-occupying lesions are present, surgical removal is indicated. Decompression of a tight fibroosseous tunnel may also be indicated followed by pronation control.

ANKLE SPRAIN

Classification

Classifications of ankle sprains have traditionally used grading systems such as I, II, and III (mild, moderate, and severe).[29,30] This system usually reflects a minor

stretch without laxity, a stretch with partial tear and some inversion laxity, or a complete rupture with major inversion laxity (>15 degrees) and associated anterior drawer laxity. Ordinarily inversion and anterior drawer laxity indicate a complete rupture of the anterior fibular talar and fibulocalcaneal ligaments.

Treatment is usually nonsurgical in the initial acute phase or first-time injury: protective functional bracing, inflammation, and pain control, followed by rehabilitative strength and endurance training for the entire leg. Chronic pain and repetitive instability may indicate the need for a more permanent solution with surgical intervention. This eventuality is more likely to be needed when clinical signs include a positive anterior drawer test and x-rays reveal a talar tilt exceeding 15 degrees.

Lateral Ankle Sprain

Lateral ankle sprains are the most common specific injury in sports.[31,32] In comparison with twisting and landing sports such as basketball, soccer, and dance, running may be less likely to cause sprains, but they are still possible, especially on cross-country runs over uneven ground.

The lateral ligamentous complex of the ankle consists of three ligaments: the anterior talofibular, the calcaneal-fibular, and the posterior talofibular. It is also important to consider the subtalar joint, which has five supporting ligaments. The most common ligament disruption involves the anterior fibulotalar ligament and the second most common a combination of the fibulotalar and calcaneal-fibular ligaments. Additional injuries such as tears or subluxation of the peroneal tendons, talar chip fractures, medial or syndesmotic ligament disruption, and fracture of the base of the fifth metatarsal may occur in combination.

The controversy concerning surgical intervention for acute lateral injury has been put to rest in the literature. Even with complete grade III tears, the results of functional rehabilitation are as effective as primary surgical repair, with the exception of lateral rupture combined with medial ligament or tibial fibular syndesmosis ruptures.[33]

Lateral Ankle Surgical Options

The surgical options for unacceptable lateral ligament instability are basically two: either reconstruction with an autogenous peroneus brevis tendon graft or direct repair as popularized by Brostrom.[34] For most cases the small-incision modified Brostrom direct ligament repair works well (Figs. 54–7 and 54–8).[35,36] Reconstruction techniques are successful but require an extensive incision with harvesting of the peroneus brevis tendon as the usual donor.[31] The postoperative

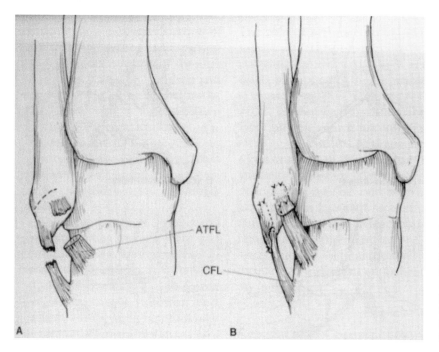

Figure 54–7. Karlsson modification of Brostrom's technique of direct late repair. (*A*) The ATF and CF ligament scar are incised to healthy tissue. (*B*) Attachment to the roughened fibula through drill holes. The proximal flaps are oversewn to reinforce the repair. (*Source: From Colville MR: Surgical treatment of the unstable ankle.* J Am Acad Orthop Surg *1998:6, 373.*)

morbidity of reconstruction is considerable in comparison with the Brostrom direct repair; therefore reconstruction should be reserved for extreme cases or failed direct repair.

It should be noted that combination pathoanatomic abnormalities might occur in addition to ligament deficiency. The most common additional comorbidity involves intraarticular abnormalities including intraarticular synovitis and talar chip fractures. Under these circumstances intraarticular arthroscopic debridement in association with direct ligament repair is indicated.

Medial Ankle Sprain

Medial collateral ligament sprains usually occur in combination with lateral ligament sprains. The medial ligament is a strong, fan-shaped structure and is rarely injured in an isolated manner or subject to chronic

functional insufficiency. The function of the medial ligament is to control ankle and foot abduction and to act as a restraint against lateral talar translation, especially if lateral malleolar fracture is an associated injury. The usual presentation of patients with medial ligament injuries includes the copathologies of lateral ligament sprain or fibular fracture, usually caused by activities more violent than running.

Treatment of medial ligament sprains is largely dependent on companion injuries. Lateral talar displacement is usually associated with fibular fracture or talofibular syndesmosis instability. Surgical fixation of these deficiencies generally avoids the necessity to repair the deltoid ligament. For the rare isolated deltoid injury or injury in association with lateral ligament sprain, the functional rehabilitation approach discussed for lateral ligament treatment is recommended. Return

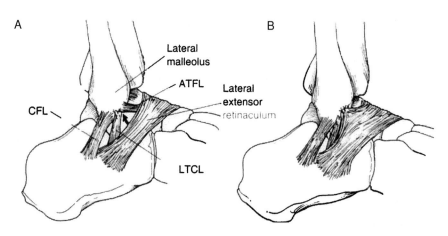

Figure 54–8. Gould modification of Brostrom's technique. (*A*) Anatomy after ATF and CF ligament repair. (*B*) The ligament repair is reinforced by suturing the lateral extensor retinaculum and the LTCL to the distal fibula. (The LTCL is variable and may not be reparable.) (*Source: From Colville MR: Surgical treatment of the unstable ankle.* J Am Acad Orthop Surg *1998:6, 373.*)

to sports is somewhat delayed if lateral and medial ligament injuries occur in combination.

In the rare instance that a complete deltoid ligament rupture has occurred, direct repair and/or imbrication are recommended. This author has never needed to repair an isolated deltoid ligament rupture surgically.[33]

Syndesmosis Sprains

Sprains of the syndesmosis (high ankle sprain) usually occur in association with fractures about the ankle but not always. A wide variation in the clinical spectrum can occur from simple sprains to rupture if the syndesmosis injury is of major magnitude. Diastasis can occur with separation of the distal ends of the tibia and fibula.

Syndesmosis sprains occurring in association with severe but more typical lateral ankle inversion sprains can be overlooked. Often the diagnosis is made later when the normal healing pattern of a typical lateral sprain does not occur. It is therefore important to be highly cognizant of the potential of injury to the syndesmosis. Clinical examination will localize tenderness over the anterior syndesmosis at and just proximal to the anterolateral ankle. It is important as well to palpate the malleoli and the entire fibula to rule out fracture. In the absence of fracture, pain in the syndesmosis area while squeezing the middistal fibula is quite suggestive of syndesmosis injury. A better clinical test for syndesmosis injury is external rotation of the foot with the knee at 90 degrees and the leg stabilized. Pain at the syndesmosis site is indicative of injury.

The diagnosis of syndesmosis sprain with diastasis is confirmed by x-ray. There is some controversy in x-ray interpretation, however. Harper and Keller,[37] on the basis of cadaver dissection, have suggested that a tibiofibular clear space of less than 6 mm on the anteroposterior and mortise x-rays is the best criterion. If routine x-rays are normal and the diagnosis is still suspected, stress radiographs with application of external rotation and abduction force are recommended. Additional diagnostic tools include arthrography, scintigraphy, computed tomography (CT), and MRI.

Treatment of syndesmosis disorders depends on the magnitude of the injury. The basic classification of acute injury by Edwards and Delee[38] is sprain without diastasis, latent diastasis, and frank diastasis. Injuries without diastasis or reducible diastasis can be treated nonoperatively.[39] If unreducible diastasis is present, surgical intervention is recommended.[38] The basic concepts of surgery include clearance of soft-tissue impingement or blockage, repair of soft-tissue elements if possible, and stabilization of the fibula in an anatomic position by screw fixation. Any other bony abnormalities such as fracture of adjacent tissues should be corrected as well.

INTRAARTICULAR ANKLE CONDITIONS

Intraarticular problems of the ankle generally fall into two categories: synovial soft tissue and talar osteochondral. Soft-tissue problems account for as much as 50% of ankle joint pathology. Many of these problems are synovial and clinically elusive and may require arthroscopic investigation for definitive diagnosis. The causes of synovial abnormality are varied and may be congenital, traumatic, rheumatic, infectious, degenerative, and neuropathic. In runners the etiologic synovial issues are traumatic overuse or trauma superimposed on congenital plica.

Ankle Arthroscopy Overview

Many of the pathoanatomic ankle maladies amenable to surgical intervention are well served by current arthroscopic approaches. These maladies include the intraarticular lesions of synovitis, soft-tissue impingement, osteochondral abnormalities, loose bodies, osteophytes including bony impingement, arthrofibrosis, and osteoarthritis. The advantages of arthroscopy are small incisional portals, limited postoperative morbidity, and rapid rehabilitation.

Modern arthroscopic surgical techniques can generally use two portals. Current technology includes improved visualization with digital optics and fluid pumps, easily applied traction, and improved operating instrumentation, all enhancing the surgical corrective opportunities. These advantages make the decision for surgery much more attractive as arthroscopic treatment, for the maladies outlined can be quite successful. Depending on the underlying pathoanatomy, a week or less of nonweightbearing protection is usually required in the immediate postoperative period. Return to running on a graduated basis is therefore quite rapid in many instances.

The risks of ankle arthroscopy are the risks of any surgery. The most likely local complications are infection and disruption of digital nerves adjacent to arthroscopy portals. The latter complication can be minimized by care in portal placement. The only absolute contraindications to ankle arthroscopy are the presence of underlying sepsis or peripheral vascular disease, which threatens healing or invites postoperative infection.

Generalized Synovitis

Generalized synovitis may occur following repetitive trauma as well as ankle sprains and fracture. The signs and symptoms are nonspecific and include generalized pain, swelling, and tenderness. Lack of response to functional rehabilitation may indicate the need for ankle arthroscopy. Arthroscopic evaluation invariably

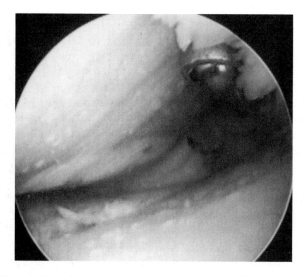

Figure 54–9. Surgical photograph. Arthroscopic debridement of intraarticular ankle pathology (synovitis). Note the remaining synovitis in the lower left corner adjacent to the shaving instrument. The underside of the tibial articular surface is above. The articular surfaces of both the tibia and talus are totally devoid of articular cartilage in this ankle. (*Courtesy of Nirschl Orthopedic Sportsmedicine Clinic.*)

reveals reddened and thickened synovium and fibrous adhesions. Chondromalacia and loose bodies may also be present and may be debrided and removed (Fig. 54–9).

Anterolateral Soft-Tissue Impingement

The intraarticular synovial tissue is vulnerable to impingement in the anterolateral corner made by the talus, fibula, and tibia. Instability following ankle sprain, especially in association with a pronated hindfoot, is a common etiologic contributor. Repetitive entrapment of the synovium may result in thickened cord-like lesions as well as a hyalinized meniscoid band between the fibula and talus, as described by Wolin et al.[40] Variations of synovial adhesions, fibrosis, inflammatory synovium, and even osteocartilaginous loose bodies may occur in combinations.[41]

The treatment for these synovial lesions is arthroscopic debridement of the tibial joint and the anterolateral gutter between the talus and fibula.[42] Postoperative strengthening of the peroneus brevis and orthotic control of hindfoot pronation is critical to long-range cure. In cases of major lateral ligament instability, surgical correction of the lateral ankle ligaments should be added to the arthroscopic debridement.

Osteochrondral Lesions of the Talus

Several lesions may be termed osteochondral. Osteochondritis dissecans is reflective of subchondral ischemia and instability followed by articular cartilage

softening and instability, with progression to fragmentation and detachment to a loose body. The other common problem is a single-event traumatic chip-type fracture. Chondromalacia and synovitis may accompany both lesions. The most common location is the anterolateral talar dome, although other locations are seen.

Diagnosis may be challenging, as the signs and symptoms may mimic synovitis. An x-ray may define the lesions, but CT scan or MRI may be needed as well.

Treatment is invariably arthroscopic debridement to a healthy subchondral base with removal of any loose osteocartilaginous fragments. As with the surgical treatment of synovitis, postoperative care includes pronation control and aggressive lower-extremity strengthening.

Osteophytes

The typical symptomatic osteophytic spurs are usually anterior tibial talar and may be associated with a progressing osteoarthritis (Fig. 54–10). In running and/or jumping sports, however, traumatic issues tend to predominate. This author's experience with runners, especially competitive sprinters and soccer and basketball players, parallels the literature on football players[43] and dancers.[44] The traumatic etiologic factor appears to be impingement by forced dorsiflexion of the bare area of the distal upper talus against the anterior lip of the distal tibia, with resulting kissing lesions on the talus and anterior tibia. An alternative etiology of a single tibial osteophyte could result from forced plantarflexion with an anterior capsular traction spur. Repetitive injury would probably be the mechanism in

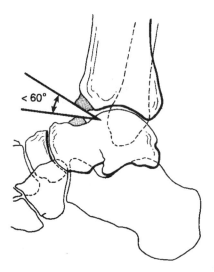

Figure 54–10. Tibial-talar osteophytes. Illustration of tibial talar osteophytes with bony impingement osteophytic formation of the distal tibia and talar neck and angle diminished to under 60 degrees. (*Source: From Ferkel.[42]*)

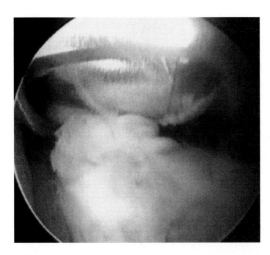

Figure 54–11. Arthroscopic debridement ankle osteophyte. Surgical photograph illustrates shaving instrument on a tibial osteophyte just prior to removal. (*Courtesy of Nirschl Orthopedic Sportsmedicine Clinic.*)

an activity such as ballet. Overall, the most common symptom-producing pathoanatomic osteophyte is that of the anterior lip of the tibia.

The presence of osteophytic spurs is problematic from several points of view. Associated impingement of osteophytes with accompanying synovitis is pain producing. In addition, osteophytes are space occupying, with resultant dorsiflexion bony blockade. The normal dorsiflexion clearance between the talus and the anterior tibia is 60 degrees or greater.[42] Compromise of this range of motion is potentially pain producing and also functionally distorting.

Other osteophytes at the tips of both the medial and lateral malleoli are also commonly noted, usually in association with chronic ankle sprain. In the author's experience these osteophytes tend not to be problematic and ordinarily do not require surgical treatment unless they are associated with the surgical correction of ankle instability.

The signs and symptoms of intraarticular tibial talar osteophytes are similar to those of synovitis, which is also an accompanying comorbidity. The additional signs of decreased and painful dorsiflexion with associated anterior tibial talar joint tenderness clearly indicate an osteophytic presence. The diagnosis is usually confirmed by x-ray, although on occasion CT scan can be helpful. A lateral x-ray with the ankle in forced dorsiflexion may demonstrate the impingement of kissing tibial talar osteophytes.

The treatment of symptomatic tibial talar osteophytes depends on functional needs and magnitude of pain. In general, patients who have aspirations to participate in athletic activities or running will opt for surgical intervention, as nonsurgical approaches cannot

resolve bony blockade or impingement. The surgical options include open arthrotomy or arthroscopic debridement of the ankle with removal of the osteophytes and loose body removal as needed (Fig. 54–11). The advantages of arthroscopy are many, and it is the author's recommended approach.

The success of arthroscopic osteophytic removal is quite satisfying provided major tibial talar articular arthritic erosion is not present. Postoperative rehabilitation is often quite rapid, with motion exercises initiated in 48 hours and weightbearing to tolerance within 3 to 4 days.

ANKLE FRACTURES AND DISLOCATIONS

Any running sport is subject to single-event trauma of the ankle. As noted, sprain is more common, but fracture and dislocation can occur in running. Fracture itself can take the form of stress fracture from overuse or complete fracture from single-event macrotrauma. The purpose of this section is not to present a comprehensive discussion but to review basic principles of more common problems.

In general, fractures or dislocations in running occur through an untoward event such as stepping unexpectedly in a hidden pothole or twisting on uneven ground. Stress fractures usually occur in the fibula (lateral malleolus) when an increase in pace or distance has been instituted. Surgery is ordinarily not needed with stress fractures.

The differential diagnosis of fracture or dislocation and ankle sprain can be obvious or subtle. Dislocation and displaced fractures have obvious anatomic distortions. Minimally displaced or nondisplaced fractures do not have such distortions. The clinical distinction from sprain resides in significant palpable tenderness over bone rather than soft tissue. Crepitus and the inability to bear weight are also indicators of fracture. In either sprain or fracture, significant swelling may be present. The x-ray examination, including anteroposterior, lateral, and oblique views, is the gold standard for ultimate skeletal diagnosis, and CT scan may be indicated in more complex situations. If clinical signs of foot injury are present, additional foot x-rays should be taken.

In runners the most likely fracture pattern would be a bimalleolar fracture of the lateral and medial malleolus with lateral talar displacement or an isolated fracture of the lateral malleolus. In the x-ray presentation of an isolated lateral malleolar fracture, the examiner should always be suspicious of companion ligamentous injuries of the deltoid and tibial fibular syndesmosis.

The indications for surgery depend on the anatomic position and stability of the fracture. Dislocations of course should be reduced promptly. The more typical fracture pattern of lateral malleolar fracture with lateral talar displacement indicates deltoid ligament rupture. Bimalleolar fracture may leave the ligament intact.

The treatment of nondisplaced fractures is usually cast immobilization for 4 to 6 weeks followed by functional bracing and rehabilitation. Nondisplaced fractures need careful x-ray monitoring, however, as displacement can occur even under casting. The treatment goal is restoration of an anatomic relationship between the tibia and talus. Any lateral talar displacement should be reduced either by closed manipulation and casting or by open reduction and internal fixation. In the typical bimalleolar fracture, this usually requires a lateral fibular plate and screws and a medial malleolar screw. In an isolated lateral malleolar fracture with lateral talar displacement, which is nonreducible, the deltoid ligament is usually ruptured and entrapped between the medial malleolus and talus. Surgical intervention in this instance would require open reduction and fixation of the lateral malleolus plus surgical repair of the deltoid ligament.

Overall anatomic reduction of ankle fractures generally results in a favorable outcome allowing return to running. The exception would be associated intraarticular damage with subsequent traumatic osteoarthritic changes.

SUMMARY

Ankle injuries in runners cover a wide pathoanatomic spectrum from the soft-tissue issues of nerve, ligament, and tendon to intraarticular damage to skeletal element distortion. In most cases, nonsurgical approaches suffice. When an injury does not respond to conservative efforts, surgical intervention has proved successful for return to running in most cases. (For detailed surgical techniques, see Mann and Coughlin.[45])

REFERENCES

1. Puddu G, Ippolito E, Postacchini F: A classification of Achilles' tendon disease. *Am J Sports Med* 1976:4, 145.
2. Kraushaar B, Nirschl R: Current concepts review. Tendinosis of the elbow (tennis elbow). Clinical features and findings of histological, immunohistochemical, and electron microscopy studies. *J Bone Joint Surg Am* 1999:81-A, 259.
3. Plattner PF, Johnson KA: Tendons and bursa, in Helal B, Wilson D (eds.), *The Foot*, London, Churchill Livingstone, 1988:581.
4. Clancy WG: Runners injuries. Part two. Evaluation and treatment of specific injuries. *Am J Sports Med* 1980:8, 287.
5. Lagergren C, Lindholm A: Vascular distribution in the Achilles' tendon: An angiographic and microangiographic study. *Acta Chir Scand* 1958:116, 491.
6. Schatzicer J, Branemark P: Intravital observation on the microvascular anatomy and microcirculation of the tendon. *Acta Orthop Scand Suppl* 1969:126, 1.
7. Leach R: Achilles' tendon ruptures, in Mack RP (ed.), *Symposium on the Foot and Leg in Running Sports*, St. Louis, Mosby Year Book, 1982:99.
8. Schepsis A, Leach R: Surgical management of Achilles' tendinitis. *Am J Sports Med* 1987:15, 308.
9. Haggmark T, Eriksson E: Hypotrophy of the soleus muscle in man after Achilles' tendon rupture: Discussion of findings obtained by computer tomography and morphologic studies, *Am J Sports Med* 1979:7, 121.
10. Lea R: Achilles' tendon rupture: Results of closed management, in Moore M (ed.), *Symposium on Trauma to the Leg and Its Sequelae*, St. Louis, Mosby Year Book, 1981: 353.
11. Lea R, Smith L: Non-surgical treatment of Achilles' tendon rupture. *J Bone Joint Surg Am* 1972:54, 1398.
12. Nistor L: Conservative treatment of fresh subcutaneous rupture of the Achilles' tendon. *Acta Orthop Scand* 1976:47, 459.
13. Barfred T: Achilles' tendon rupture: Aetiology and pathogenesis of subcutaneous rupture assessed on the basis of the literature and rupture experiments on rats. *Acta Orthop Scand Suppl* 1973:152, 1.
14. Editorial: Achilles' tendon rupture. *Lancet* 1973:1, 189.
15. Ma G, Griffith T: Percutaneous repair of acute closed ruptured Achilles' tendon: A new technique. *Clin Orthop* 1997:128, 247.
16. Hubbell J, Brogle P, Seyla L: Experience With A New Technique for Percutaneous Achilles Tendon Repair. Presented as a poster at the American Academy of Orthopaedic Surgeons Annual Meeting. Orlando, Florida, March 2000.
17. Brahms MA: Common foot problems. *J Bone Joint Surg* 1967:49, 1659.
18. Bywaters EG: Heel lesions of rheumatoid arthritis. *Ann Rheum Dis* 1954:13, 42.
19. Canoso JJ, Wohlgetidm JR, Newberg AH: Aspiration of the retrocalcaneal bursa. *Ann Rheum Dis* 1984:43, 308.
20. Sobel M, Bohne WH, Leviche R: Longitudinal attrition of the peroneus brevis tendon in the fibular groove: An anatomic study. *Foot Ankle* 1990:11, 124.
21. Larsen E: Longitudinal rupture of the peroneus brevis tendon. *J Bone Joint Surg* 1987:69, 340.
22. Marti R: Dislocation of the peroneal tendons. *Am J Sports Med* 1977:5, 19.
23. Frey C, Shereff M, Greenigie N: Vascularity of the posterior tibial tendon. *J Bone Joint Surg* 1990:72, 884.
24. Mann RA, Thompson FM: Rupture of the posterior tibial tendon causing flatfoot: Surgical treatment. *J Bone Joint Surg* 1985:67, 556.

25. Burman M: Subcutaneous strain or tear of the dorsiflexor tendons of the foot. *Bull Hosp Joint Dis Orthop Inst* 1943:4, 44.

26. Holt KW, Cross MJ: Isolated rupture of the flexor hallucis longus tendon: A case report. *Am J Sports Med* 1990:18, 645.

27. Mann RA: Tarsal tunnel syndrome, Proceedings of the American Orthopedic Foot Society. *Orthop Clin North Am* 1974:5, 109.

28. Cimino WR: Tarsal tunnel syndrome: Review of the literature. *Foot Ankle* 1990:11, 47.

29. Leach RE, Schepsis AA: Acute injuries to ligaments of the ankle, in Evarts CM (ed.), *Surgery of the Musculoskeletal System*, vol. 4, New York, Churchill Livingstone, 1990:3887.

30. Jackson DW, Ashley RL, Powell JW: Ankle sprains in young athletes. Relation of severity and disability. *Clin Orthop* 1974:101, 201.

31. Brand RL, Collins MD: Operative management of ligamentous injuries to the ankle. *Clin Sports Med* 1982:1, 117.

32. Garrick JG: The frequency of injury, mechanism of injury, and epidemiology of ankle sprains. *Am J Sports Med* 1977:5, 241.

33. Kannus P, Renstrom P: Current concepts review. Treatment for acute tears of lateral ligaments of the ankle. Operation, cast, or early controlled mobilization. *J Bone Joint Surg* 1991:73, 305.

34. Brostrom L: Sprained ankles. VI. Surgical treatment of chronic ligament ruptures, *Acta Chir Scand* 1966:132, 551.

35. Gronmark T, Johnsen D, Kogstado: Rupture of the lateral ligaments of the ankle: A controlled clinical trial. *Injury* 1980:11, 215.

36. Gould N, Seligson D, Gassman J: Early and late repair of the lateral ligament of the ankle. *Foot Ankle* 1980:1, 84.

37. Harper MC, Keller TS: A radiographic evaluation of the tibiofibular syndesmosis. *Foot Ankle* 1989:10, 156.

38. Edwards GS, Delee JC: Ankle diastasis without fracture. *Foot Ankle* 1984:4, 305.

39. Hopkinson WJ, St Pierre P, Ryan JB: Syndesmosis sprains of the ankle. *Foot Ankle* 1990:10, 325.

40. Wolin I, Glassman F, Sideman F, et al.: Internal derangement of the talofibular component of the ankle. *Surg Gynecol Obstet* 1950:91, 193.

41. Bassett F, Gates H, Billys J: Talar impingement by anteroinferior tibio-fibular ligament. *J Bone Joint Surg Am* 1990:72A, 55.

42. Ferkel R: Arthroscopy of the ankle and foot, in Mann R, Coughlin M (eds.), *Surgery of the Foot and Ankle*, 6th ed., St Louis, Mosby, 1993:1289.

43. O'Donoghue D: Chondral and osteochondral fractures. *J Trauma* 1966:6, 469.

44. Stoller S: A comparative study of the frequency of anterior impingement exostosis of the ankle in the dancer and non-dancer. *Foot Ankle* 1984:4, 201.

45. Mann R, Coughlin M: *Surgery of the Foot and Ankle*, 6th ed., St. Louis, Mosby, 1993.

Chapter 55

THE FOOT

Frederick G. Lippert III

INTRODUCTION

The foot is a weightbearing structure that provides support, shock absorption, adaptation to the contour of the weightbearing surface, and push-off. It is highly sensitive to rotational and angulatory alignment as well as the weightbearing presentation of the metatarsal heads. Abnormalities in any of these parameters may be tolerated in nonrunners, but can be incapacitating in the runner. One must take into account the type of foot involved (pes planus-normal-cavovarus) when confronted by the conditions described below.

PLANTAR FASCIITIS

Plantar fasciitis has historically been known as an inflammation of the plantar fascia at its origin on the medial calcaneal tubercle. More recently, further pathological analysis supports the concept of a degenerative process rather than an inflammatory one.

The plantar fascia inserts on the bases of the proximal phalanges and acts to support the forefoot during push-off. It also acts to neutralize the bending moments on the second metatarsal, which is at risk for stress fracture. The heel spur seen on the lateral x-ray is usually located in the flexor hallucis brevis and does not contribute to the problem. This is a myth that is hard to dispel.

Risk Factors

Some risk factors for plantar fasciitis are tight heel cords that force the foot into a pronated abducted position during stance phase, thereby abnormally stretching the plantar fascia; pes planus foot; and obesity.

Conservative Treatment

Conservative treatment begins by making the diagnosis and ruling out other causes of heel pain, such as one of the inflammatory arthritides, calcaneal stress fracture, calcaneal cysts, or degenerative joint disease of the subtalar joint. The main approach is to reduce the stretch of the plantar fascia by decreasing pronation with orthoses, providing firm hindfoot control with well-fitted footwear, and avoiding excessive dorsiflexion of the toes during push-off with a rocker sole and rigid shank in the shoe. Toe dorsiflexion during push-off tightens the plantar fascia due to the windlass effect. Wearing a night splint prevents the foot from falling into plantar flexion that may allow the fascia to contract during sleep. This phenomenon contributes to the intense heel pain experienced during the first steps in the morning. Lo-dye taping is a common sports medicine technique for supporting the arch during athletic activities.

For acute cases the quickest approach to relieving pain and restoring some ambulatory function is to put the patient in a well-molded walking cast for several weeks. The patient can then be transitioned to a fracture boot with a medial arch orthotic and subsequently to a supportive running shoe.

Physiological goals are to revitalize the fascial tissue by encouraging neovascularization, fibroplastic infiltration, and collagen production, and increasing strength, endurance, and flexibility.

Surgical Indications and Treatment

Plantar fascia release is not advised until at least 6 months of carefully supervised conservative treatment has been undertaken. Some authors favor waiting for a full year. The problem can be particularly bothersome to the runner who is often desperate for relief from pain. Patients who have tried activity modification, orthoses, footwear modifications such as a rigid shank with rocker bottom sole to decrease the windlass effect, anti-inflammatory regimens, and night splints, all to no avail are candidates for release.

Surgery for plantar fasciitis consists of releasing the medial third of the tendinous tissue at the medial calcaneal tubercle. Some authors advocate releasing the first branch of the lateral plantar nerve to the abductor digiti quinti (Baxter's nerve). Excising the bone spur is part of the release.

Current Techniques

Surgical release can be accomplished through a medial approach that provides exposure to remove the heel spur and release Baxter's nerve at the same time. A direct plantar approach gives good visibility of the plantar fascia, but leaves a scar that can be troublesome if it is on the weightbearing surface. The author prefers a percutaneous approach through the bottom of the heel. The advantage of the latter is that there is almost no morbidity from the surgery.

Complications

Complications arise when the extent of the release eliminates the function of the plantar fascia. The plantar fascia acts like a bowstring and has a major role in supporting the medial arch. Without it the foot elongates and requires medial arch support. Scarring about the calcaneal nerves with intractable heel pain can result from extensive dissection to remove the heel spur.

Criteria for Return to Running

The criteria for returning to running must be tailored to fit the individual patient. Some heal faster than others, but in general the plantar fascia release takes 6 to 8 weeks to heal. Patients progress from walking, to fast walking, to light jogging, and finally to running. I require them to demonstrate no pain or limp for a week before advancing to the next level of activity. If pain returns, they drop down to a lower level of activity.

Some patients continue to have pain despite an adequate surgical release. This is probably due to the effects of any residual degenerative tissue. Those patients may need to avoid running for a protracted period (i.e., up to a year) before trying again.

ACHILLES' TENDON

The Achilles' tendon is made up of the gastrocnemius and the soleus. They come together in the calf to form a conjoined tendon that provides the main force for plantarflexion of the foot. The runner causes a series of microtears of the tendon with overuse that result in cumulative damage over time. The pathology may be located in the tendon itself or at its insertion on the os calcis. The process tends to shift from an acute inflammatory phase to a degenerative phase. The terminology can be confusing. Generally Achilles' tendon problems can be classified into damage to the tendon itself above the calcaneus and damage at the tendon's insertion. When acute, it is called tendinitis and insertional calcific tendinitis. When chronic, it is called tendinosis and insertional tendinosis. Peritendinitis, subperitenon edema, and tendinosis in the body of the tendon are other terms used to describe these disorders.

Risk Factors

Some risk factors for Achilles' tendon disorders are cavovarus foot configuration, Haglund's deformity, tight heel cord syndrome, a training program that progresses too rapidly, and poor healing capacity in older runners.

Conservative Treatment

Conservative measures consist of heel cord stretching, ensuring that the counter of the running shoe does not have a seam pressing against the back of the heel, and rest to allow the inflamed and damaged tissues to heal. This may take as long as 4 to 6 months. During that period, the patient may need to wear a fracture boot for all ambulatory activities. Deficits in strength of the anterior tibialis or posterior tibialis also may require rehabilitation.

Surgical Indications and Treatment

Patients with degenerative Achilles' tendinosis who have tried activity modifications and the protective measures described above for at least 3 months under careful supervision are candidates for surgical debridement of the tendon.

Surgery is directed at stimulating healing by inciting a reparative response; eliminating all abnormal tissue that perpetuates the degenerative process; and removing spurs, ridges, and bony prominences, such as a Haglund's deformity. These bony irregularities are thought to cause frictional attrition of the tendon that leads to further degenerative changes. Failure of surgical treatment is often due to inadequate excision of abnormal bone and tissue.

Technique

At surgery the tendon is inspected and the areas that are swollen and discolored are addressed. These are incised longitudinally and peeled open and all degenerated tendon is removed. Up to 50% of the tendon may be removed without jeopardizing its tensile strength. When more than 50% needs to be removed, augmentation with the flexor hallucis longus tendon is considered. Sometimes just making a series of longitudinal incisions in the tendon is enough to stimulate a healing response.[2]

For insertional Achilles' tendinosis, the back of the calcaneus is widely exposed by incising the tendon longitudinally and then teeing the distal end to create two flaps that can be peeled back. The medial and lateral attachments of the tendon are not disturbed. The Haglund's deformity (an enlarged posterior tuberosity) is removed along with intratendinous calcifications and all bony ridges, and the remaining surfaces are filed smooth. All degenerated tendon tissue is removed and the distal tendon ends are reattached to the periosteal cuff. When gapping prevents reattachment, the ends are attached to bone with suture passed through holes drilled in the os calcis or bone anchors.[3] This surgery is a much more radical approach than used in the past and has been found to be highly successful.

Complications

The main complication is inadequate pain relief usually resulting from incomplete resection of tendon tissue or bone. Harvesting the flexor hallucis longus is difficult and may result in posterior tibial nerve traction symptoms, but these usually subside over time. Incisions that curve across the back of the heel create a tenuous healing situation at the apex of the curve if the surgeon does not preserve adequate thickness of the flap. Sometimes these incisions take weeks to heal. The scars usually don't cause a problem even if a keloid develops.

Criteria for Return to Running

Patients need to understand that healing may take up to 6 months before unrestricted running can be done safely. Augmentations with the long toe flexor and reattachment to bone with sutures through drill holes or anchor sutures take longer to heal. Calf muscle atrophy can be profound, causing a calcaneous gait for 6 months or longer. Returning to running must be done with a graduated program, starting with slow walking, and progressing to fast walking and then to jogging and running.

The criteria for return to unrestricted running are full calf muscle and leg strength restored as evidenced by the ability to do single stance heel rises; no calcaneus gait or limp; absence of pain or inflammatory signs in the morning following after exercise; and well-healed incisions.

MORTON'S NEUROMA

Morton's neuroma is a painful lesion of the conjoined nerve to the third web space. This includes the junction of the plantar digital nerves and the communicating branch from the lateral planar nerve. The exact etiology is unknown, but Morton's neuroma is thought to be a form of entrapment neuropathy associated with perineural fibrosis. While it is possible to have a neuroma in other interspaces, 97% are in the third space. One needs to think twice before making this diagnosis in the other interspaces.[4]

Conservative Treatment

Conservative treatment is directed at eliminating tension and pressure against the conjoined nerve described above. This includes wearing shoes with a wider toebox, placing a pad behind the third and fourth metatarsal heads to spread them apart during weightbearing, and avoiding high heels. Steroid injections into the area of the nerve through the dorsum of the foot at the third interspace are common, but this author is cautious about using steroids due to the risk of producing fat necrosis.

Surgical Treatment

Surgical treatment either removes the neuroma or provides more room for it. The main problem is identifying all the branches of the conjoined nerve and resecting them back behind the metatarsal heads. Even though the severed nerve endings sprout new nerve fibrils, these will not be symptomatic unless they are subject to weightbearing forces. The traditional approach to the nerve is through the dorsum of the foot. This requires sectioning the transverse metatarsal ligament and contending with sometimes difficult exposure. The main risk is failing to resect the nerve far enough posteriorly.

The plantar approach has gained increasing popularity due to its ease of exposure. The myth about painful scarring of the plantar surface is unfounded as long as the closure is not placed over a metatarsal head. The downside of this approach is a longer period before the patient can put full weight on the ball of the foot, but this author favors the plantar approach nonetheless. Some surgeons advocate only doing a division of the intermetatarsal ligament, thinking that the metatarsal heads will spread and make more room for the neuroma. In the author's experience this approach is highly unpredictable and unreliable.

Current Technique

While most types of anesthesia are satisfactory, the author prefers a posterior tibial nerve block behind the medial malleolus. The morbidity of this nerve block is minimal compared with other types of anesthesia.

Plantar Approach

A longitudinal incision is made between the third and fourth metatarsal heads and the nerve is exposed along with all of its branches. It is followed up into the third and fourth toes and divided. All branches are then mobilized and retracted posteriorly until they are posterior to the metatarsal heads. With traction applied the nerve is divided as far proximally as possible.

Dorsal Approach

An incision is made dorsally in the third web space, extending part way down the fourth toe. Dissection is carried down to the intermetatarsal ligament which is divided. The conjoined nerve can be seen by pushing in on the skin of the plantar web space. The branches are mobilized and resected as far posteriorly as possible.

The criteria for a return to running are a healed pain-free incision, no swelling or edema of the wound, and the ability to walk and jump up and down on the ball of the foot without pain.

Complications

Recurrence of symptoms about 3 months postsurgery is the most common complication, and it is caused by remaining residual nerve branches and failure to resect the neuroma far enough proximal to the metatarsal heads. Dehiscence of the plantar incision is possible if weightbearing is allowed too early.

ACCESSORY NAVICULAR

An accessory navicular is an ossicle within the posterior tibial tendon just posterior to the medial pole of the navicular that varies from being part of an enlarged medial pole to a separate "pebble" attached to the medial pole by a synchondrosis. Sometimes it is an isolated ossicle located more posteriorly in the tendon. The type attached by a synchondrosis is the one that is prone to injury. Three problems arise with accessory naviculars. The first is chronic pain following a hyperpronation injury affecting the synchondrosis. These rarely heal. The second type is insidious and is related to the more medial than plantar position of the tendon at the navicular. This positioning results in weaker support of the medial arch. Patients with this anatomic variation are more susceptible to medial arch problems, especially if they are involved in running activities. Vague medial arch symptoms are the usual complaint. The third problem is pain due to the medial prominence when wearing certain types of footwear such as ski boots. Other risk factors for accessory navicular problems are obesity and a pronated foot.

Conservative Treatment

Temporary immobilization in a cast or fracture boot protects the injured synchondrosis and gives it the best chance to heal. Pressure from footwear on a prominent accessory navicular can be relieved by modifying the footwear to accommodate the medial prominence using a ball-and-ring tool. When the patient presents with medial arch pain, arch supports and a firm heel counter along with avoidance of high-impact activities usually help.

Surgical Indications and Technique

Persistent pain in the region of the accessory navicular despite the measures described above, especially when there is accompanying posterior tibial tendon insufficiency, requires surgical intervention. Removal of the ossicle is often enough, unless it is associated with posterior tibial tendon insufficiency. In that case augmentation with the flexor digitorum longus will help re-establish support of the medial arch.

Complications

The tendon may be catastrophically weakened if removal of the ossicle leaves a large defect in the tendon. If the tendon lengthens as a result of ossicle removal it will not be as effective in supporting the arch. The surgeon must be careful to repair the defect and restore normal tendon length. Attempts at reattaching the ossicle may fracture the ossicle or it may pull off.

The criteria for a return to running activity are no tenderness on palpation of the accessory navicular, the ability to walk without a limp and do a single stance heel rise on the affected side, correction or support of medial arch deficiency, and the ability to fast walk without pain.

NAVICULAR STRESS FRACTURES

Navicular stress fractures can be difficult to diagnose. These fractures usually occur in athletes and military recruits, and they usually present with vague pain in the dorsum of the foot. The diagnosis is often missed, resulting in considerable delay before treatment. One must always consider this diagnosis and look for sclerosis in the navicular on plain x-rays. Tomograms or a CT scan are often needed to see the fracture

Conservative Treatment and Surgical Indications

These fractures will usually heal on their own with protected weightbearing in a cast, but if the fracture displaces or does not heal after a minimum of 3 months' protection in a cast, surgical intervention is required.

Current Surgical Technique

The approach is through a dorsal-medial incision. Holes are drilled on both sides of the fracture to establish communication with cancellous bone. Then a strain-relieving bone graft is applied by burring a small cylindrical hole across the fracture and filling it with cancellous bone taken from the lateral side of the calcaneus. One or more screws placed from medial to lateral or dorsal to plantar are used to achieve a stable repair. The fracture is protected in a nonweightbearing cast until it has healed.[5]

Complications

The main complication is degenerative joint disease of the talonavicular joint. This complication occurs when a step-off occurs and a good reduction is not obtained.

Criteria for a return to running are no pain on percussion of the fracture site or with weightbearing; no swelling, erythema, or increased warmth over the area; and healing of the fracture seen on an x-ray as a loss of definition of the fracture lines and no movement of the screws if internally fixed.

METATARSAL STRESS FRACTURES

Stress fractures of the lesser toe metatarsals occur most often in the neck region of the second and third and the base of the fifth metatarsal. The cause is repetitive overload in association with foot deformity, altered gait, or loss of the normal protective biomechanics of the plantar structures. Fatigue, trauma, and surgery can compromise the function of these structures.

A stress fractures of the base of the fifth metatarsal is often confused with a Jones fracture. The condition can be an enigma, and failure to make the diagnosis of a stress fracture will result in inadequate treatment and

chronicity. Once the diagnosis is made, the usual pitfall is assuming an overuse syndrome is responsible, and trying to heal it with rest and protection. To the clinician's surprise the patient returns 6 months later with the same problem and no clear history of trauma or overuse. An unrecognized contributing factor is a varus hindfoot that rolls outward during gait. This alignment overloads the lateral border of the foot during running. It should be corrected with a valgus calcaneal osteotomy to decrease the lateral column loading.[6]

Some risk factors for metatarsal stress fractures are planovalgus and cavovarus foot configurations, obesity, asymmetrical weightbearing parabola of the metatarsal heads, long second or short hypermobile first ray, tight gastrocnemius, loss of toe flexors or plantar fascia, and sustained strenuous loading of the foot without a period of gradual stress adaptation.

Conservative Treatment

Conservative treatment consists of protecting the stress fracture from overloading. This is accomplished by activity modification, casting, a fracture boot, or footwear with a rigid sole. Wedging the heel can help shift weight away from the affected side of the foot. Attention should also be directed at eliminating any of the risk factors listed above to prevent recurrence.

Surgical Treatment

Most stress fractures will heal if properly protected, but will tend to recur if the foot alignment or gait dynamics are abnormal. For instance, stress fractures will persist at the base of the fifth metatarsal in cavovarus feet that overload the fifth ray. An incompetent first ray will transfer weight to the second and third metatarsals. The surgeon reduces and internally fixes displaced fractures and bone grafts nonunions. Alignment problems can be corrected at the same time. Shifting the heel laterally with a valgus calcaneal osteotomy will reduce stress on the fifth metatarsal. Adjusting the length of the lesser metatarsals or their presentation to the weightbearing surface, along with making the first ray accept more load, are also necessary to ensure a successful outcome, in addition to treatment of the fracture itself.

COMPLICATIONS

Failure to treat a stress fracture can cause a chronic condition with sclerotic fracture margins that impede healing. The fracture can also displace, making treatment more difficult. Patients will often be incapacitated for months because they do not receive or refuse to follow a definitive treatment plan. Surgery on the fifth metatarsal is always risky because of sural nerve injury, entrapment by scar tissue, and irritation of the incision by the shoe.

The criteria for return to running are clinical and radiographic evidence of healing, compensation for or correction of weightbearing asymmetry, and patient awareness of the warning signs of recurrence.

REFERENCES

1. Sammarco J, Helfrey RB: Surgical treatment of recalcitrant plantar fasciitis. *Foot Ankle Int* 1996:17, 520.

2. Clancy WG, Heiden EA: Achilles' tendinitis treatment in the athlete. *Foot Ankle Clin* 1997:3, 429.

3. Gerken AP, McGarvey WC, Baxter DE: Insertional Achilles' tendonitis. *Foot Ankle Clin* 1996:1, 237.

4. Bendetti RS, Baxter DE, Davis PF: Clinical results of simultaneous adjacent interdigital neurectomy. *Foot Ankle Int* 1996:17, 264.

5. Herscovici D, Sanders R: Fractures of the tarsal navicular. *Foot Ankle Clin* 1999:4, 587.

6. Lawrence SJ, Botte MJ: Jones' fractures and related fractures of the proximal fifth metatarsal. *Foot Ankle* 1993: 14, 358.

Appendix

The American College of Sports Medicine (ACSM) has developed a number of Position Stands and Current Comments, several of which have direct application in the medical care of runners. Position Stands are referenced as they appear in the ACSM Journal Medicine and Science in Sports and Exercise. Current Comments are available from the American College of Sports Medicine (ACSM) or in writing:

ACSM Public Information Department
P.O. Box 1440
Indianapolis, IN 46206-1440

Position Stands:

Albright A, Franz M, Hornsby G, et al: American College of Sports Medicine position stand. Exercise and type 2 diabetes. Med Sci Sports Exerc. 2000:32,1345.

Cardinal BJ: ACSM/AHA Joint Position Statement. American College of Sports Medicine. American Heart Association. Med Sci Sports Exerc. 1999:31,353.

Balady GJ, Chaitman B, Driscoll D, et al: American College of Sports Medicine Position Stand and American Heart Association. Recommendations for cardiovascular screening, staffing, and emergency policies at health/fitness facilities. Med Sci Sports Exerc. 1998:30,1009.

Mazzeo RJ, Cavanagh P, Evans WJ, et al: American College of Sports Medicine position stand. Exercise and physical activity for older adults. Med Sci Sports Exerc. 1998:30,992.

Pollock ML, Gaesser GA, Butcher JD, et al: American College of Sports Medicine Position Stand. The recommended quantity and quality of exercise for developing and maintaining cardiorespiratory and muscular fitness and flexibility in healthy adults. Med Sci Sports Exerc. 1998:30,975.

Convertino VA, Armstrong LE, Coyle EF, et al: American College of Sports Medicine position stand. Exercise and fluid replacement. Med Sci Sports Exerc. 1996:28,i.

Otis CL, Drinkwater B, Johnson M, et al: American College of Sports Medicine Position Stand. The Female Athlete Triad. Med Sci Sports Exerc. 1997:29,i.

Armstrong LE, Epstein Y, Greenleaf JE, et al: American College of Sports Medicine position stand. Heat and cold illnesses during distance running. Med Sci Sports Exerc. 1996:28,i.

Oppliger RA, Case HS, Horswill CA, et al: American College of Sports Medicine position stand. Weight loss in wrestlers. Med Sci Sports Exerc. 1996:28,ix.

Sawka MN, Joyner MJ, Miles DS, et al: American College of Sports Medicine position stand. The use of blood doping as an ergogenic aid. Med Sci Sports Exerc. 1996:28,i.

Drinkwater BL, Grimston SK, Raab-Collen DM, et al: American College of Sports Medicine position stand. Osteoporosis and exercise. Med Sci Sports Exerc. 1995:27,i.

Van Camp SP, Cantwell JD, Fletcher GF, et al: American College of Sports Medicine position stand. Exercise for patients with coronary artery disease. Med Sci Sports Exerc. 1994:26,i.

Hagberg JM, Blair SN, Ehasani AA, et al: American College of Sports Medicine position stand. Physical activity, physical fitness, and hypertension. Med Sci Sports Exerc. 1993:25,i.

American College of Sports Medicine position stand on the use of anabolic-androgenic steroids in sports. Med Sci Sports Exerc. 1987:19,534.

Current Comments:

- Anabolic Steroids
- Athletes and Pesticides
- Caffeine
- Chromium Supplements
- Cocaine Abuse in Sports
- Corporate Wellness
- Creatine Supplementation
- Dehydration and Aging
- Dehydration Estrogen
- Eating Disorders
- Exercise and Age-Related Weight Gain
- Exercise and the Common Cold

- Exercise and the Older Adult
- Exercise during Pregnancy
- Exercise for Persons with Cardiovascular Disease
- Exercise in Health Clubs
- Exercise-Induced Asthma
- Explosive Exercise
- Health-Related Fitness for Children and Adults with Cerebral Palsy
- Menstrual Dysfunction
- Preparticipation Physical Examinations
- Preseason Conditioning for Young Athletes
- Safety of the Squat Exercise
- Sickle Cell Trait
- Skiing Injuries
- Stress Fractures
- Vitamin and Mineral Supplements and Exercise
- Weight Loss in Wrestlers
- Women's Heart Health and a Physically Active Lifestyle
- Youth Strength Training

Index